Oncoplastic Flap Surgery

Zan Li • Dajiang Song
Editors

Oncoplastic Flap Surgery

Breast Reconstruction

SSTP
Springer

Editors
Zan Li
Department of Oncology Plastic Surgery
Hunan Cancer Hospital
Changsha, Hunan, China

Dajiang Song
Department of Oncology Plastic Surgery
Hunan Cancer Hospital
Changsha, Hunan, China

ISBN 978-981-19-8925-4 ISBN 978-981-19-8926-1 (eBook)
https://doi.org/10.1007/978-981-19-8926-1

This Springer imprint is published by the registered company Springer Nature Singapore Pte Ltd.
The registered company address is: 152 Beach Road, #21-01/04 Gateway East, Singapore 189721, Singapore

Foreword 1

Thriving in the 1960s, microsurgery has pushed forward the developed traditional pedicled skin flap that has been used in plastic surgery for more than 100 years to the free flap transplantation with vascular anastomosis and the flap transplantation with vascular pedicle revolutionizing the traditional concept of tissue transplantation in plastic surgery.

In oncological treatment, Professor Zhou Xiao perfectly combines "surgical oncology" with "plastic surgery" where the tumor is completely removed and the defect is repaired using flap transfer. In 2001, he took the lead in putting forward the concept of "oncoplastic surgery" at home and abroad, and devoted himself to completing the theoretical construction and clinical practice of this discipline. He edited and published the monograph of "Oncoplastic Surgery" in Chinese and English. He also founded the specialty of oncoplastic surgery which has trained a large number of oncoplastic surgery professionals and promoted the development of oncoplastic surgery in China.

Professor Zan Li and his team are committed to applying the concept of oncoplastic surgery to breast reconstruction and chest reconstruction. They have completed hundreds of breast reconstruction and chest wall reconstruction by using free tissue flap transplantation technique and accumulated abundant experience in the operation of advanced breast cancer and the repair and reconstruction of huge chest wall defects.

The book *Breast Reconstruction—Oncoplastic Flap Surgery Series* is compiled based on years of surgical data, records, and drawings. It introduces the application of six commonly used tissue flaps in the field of breast reconstruction. Through the introduction of typical and difficult cases, it describes the operation process and precautions in detail. The whole book is highlighted, illustrated, and easy to understand. It is worth reading!

Department of Repair and Reconstruction
Shanghai Changzheng Hospital
Shanghai, China
March 2018

Chunlin Hou

Foreword 2

Dr. Dajiang Song is a postdoctoral fellow of Professor Hou Chunlin of the Second Military Medical University. We once worked together when I was a senior postdoctoral fellow of Professor Hou Chunlin. Therefore, I am also his senior.

I know that during his postdoctoral career in the Second Military Medical University, Dajiang mastered a medical painting skill through his hard work, which is an important skill for surgeons. He recorded the operation process in the form of pictures before and after the daily clinical operation. Over time, he has accumulated a lot of precious materials and is currently influential in the professional field.

Since Dajiang joined the oncoplastic surgery department of Hunan Cancer Hospital, he has closely combined his personal expertise in skin flap with oncoplastic surgery.

Director Li Zan has been engaged in the oncoplastic repair and reconstruction for a long time and has devoted himself to clinical academic work. He has accumulated a large number of systematic and complex clinical cases and data. Together with director Zan Li, Dajiang Song sorted out these cases and compiled them into the first monograph of oncoplastic flap specialty through the collection of clinical operation and anatomical operation data and drawings.

Browsing the whole manuscript, I think the book is featured by the following:

The collection of the literature is very complete and detailed. Taking the chapter of the perforator flap of the deep inferior epigastric artery as an example, the author has read hundreds of papers and strives to have a basis and argument for each issue, thus ensuring the academic rigor of the monograph.

In order to help readers accurately understand the anatomy of the flap, the author describes the approach, anatomical characteristics, and elements of the flap in detail through the simulated surgical anatomy of fresh cadavers, so that readers can understand and master the operation and skills of the operation more easily.

The monograph focuses on the oncoplastic repair and reconstruction. The book collects the reconstruction experience and data of more than 10 years and systematically shows the theoretical technique and experience in oncological surgery and reconstruction.

Dajiang Song is a newcomer in the field of microsurgery. He has only been engaged in the field for a short time. He is also experienced in terms of acquiring good professional quality and theory and surgical technique. In particular, his spirit of being meticulous and pursuing perfection will be reflected in this book.

Director Li Zan deserves the honorary title of "Surgical Craftsman." Moreover, he spared no effort to support the young generation. I believe that director Li Zan's team will have more achievements displayed in the international medical community.

I hope this book can benefit patients suffering from diseases!

Sixth People's Hospital of Shanghai — Zhang Changqing
August 27, 2018

Preface

One of the most important techniques in oncoplastic surgery is skin flap transplantation. Oncoplastic surgeons are not only good at microsurgical techniques for repair and reconstruction using skin flap, but are also knowledgeable in the theories and clinical diagnosis and treatment of surgical oncology.

Hunan cancer hospital is the first unit in China to establish oncoplastic surgery specialty and research laboratory. Nearly 1000 skin flap operations are carried out annually, including head and neck surgery, breast surgery, ENT surgery, cardiothoracic surgery, bone and soft tissue surgery, gynecological oncology, and urological surgery. Here, plenty of clinical data and experience in oncoplastic surgery has been accumulated for many years.

This book is based on the 27-year clinical accumulation of the chief editor. After careful planning and arrangement, it focuses on the theory and clinical application of oncoplastic flap surgery from the perspective of case studies and clinical discussion.

At present, there are many theoretical monographs on plastic repair and skin flap surgery at home and abroad, but the number of monographs describing surgical procedures based on case studies is small. Apart from the basic techniques and anatomical theories of raising skin flaps, clinical surgeons are also desired to learn surgical skills and strategies in preventing and treating complications.

The skin flap technique used for oncoplastic surgery is different from that of other fields. The defect after tumor resection is often large, deep, and complex, requiring tissue flaps from diverse donors, in various patterns and in great amount. This is different from repairing the superficial wounds caused by limb trauma. The anatomy of the skin flap varies greatly, complicating the formulation of a reasonable flap cutting strategy.

Therefore, in order to help readers truly master the flap technique in terms of theory and practice, the common and uncommon anatomical conditions and corresponding management will be presented vividly in the book.

This book contains more than 100 representative cases, more than 1500 photos of the surgical details, more than 200 photos of autopsy studies, and more than 500 color surgical schematic diagrams. It elaborates the design of surgical cases, detail handling and risk management, filling the gap in surgical monographs regarding oncoplastic surgery in China.

"Sharing what we know without reserve." There are hundreds of tissue flaps that can be raised from the human body. However, this book is not a "large and all-encompassing" encyclopedia; it focuses on the breast reconstruction cases accumulated by the editor, highlighting the experience of breast reconstruction with the inferior epigastric artery perforator flap, the deep femoral artery perforator flap, and the greater omentum flap. In addition, it is planned to further publish more books in the field of oncoplastic skin flap surgery. The specific topics covers chest wall reconstruction, head and neck repair, trunk and perineal repair and limb repair. These books will cover all branches of oncoplastic surgery, systematically and profoundly introducing the surgical techniques and concepts of oncoplastic skin flap, further promoting the progress of the specialty and benefiting patients.

Changsha, Hunan, China — Zan Li
Changsha, Hunan, China — Dajiang Song
March 2019

Contents

Contributors

Jun Chai, MD Department of Plastic and Reconstructive Surgery, The Affiliated Suzhou Hospital of Nanjing Medical University, Suzhou Municipal Hospital, Gusu School, Nanjing Medical University, Suzhou, Jiangsu Province, China

Peixian Chen, PhD Department of Breast Surgery, First People's Hospital of Foshan, Foshan, Guangdong, China

Tor Woo Chiu, MD, PhD, FACS Division of Plastic Reconstructive and Aesthetic Surgery, The Chinese University of Hong Kong, Ma Liu Shui, Hong Kong

Yanni Ding Department of Breast Surgery, The Tumor Hospital of Shaanxi Province, Xi'an City, Shaanxi Province, China

Peizhi Fan Department of Breast and Thyroid Gland Surgery, Hunan Provincial People's Hospital, The First Affiliated Hospital of Hunan Normal University, Changsha, Hunan, China

Haiyan Gao, MD Department of Breast Surgery, Changzhou Tumor Hospital, Changzhou, P. R. China

Rene D. Largo, MD Department of Plastic Surgery, The University of Texas MD Anderson Cancer Center, Houston, TX, USA

Juanjuan Li, MD Department of Breast and Thyroid Surgery, Renmin Hospital of Wuhan University, Wuhan, Hubei Province, China

Dequan Liu, MD Department of Breast Surgery, Yunnan Cancer Hospital, Kunming, Yunnan, China

Shu Liu, MD Department of Breast Surgery, Affiliated Hospital of Guizhou Medical University, Guiyang, Guizhou, China

Zan Li, MD Department of Oncology Plastic Surgery, Hunan Cancer Hospital, Changsha, Hunan, China

Xiaoqing Lu, MD Center for Breast Cancer, Shanxi Provincial Cancer Hospital, Taiyuan, Shanxi Province, China

Jie Ma, MM Department of Breast Surgery, Tangshan People's Hospital, Tangshan, HeBei, China

Shihong Ma, MD Department of Thyroid and Breast Surgery, Center Hospital of Xuhui District, Shanghai, China

Narushima Mitsunaga, MD, PhD, FACS Mie University Graduate School of Medicine Plastic and Reconstructive Surgery, Tsu, Mie, Japan

Jianyun Nie, MD, PhD Breast Cancer Center, Yunnan Cancer Hospital, Kunming, Yunnan, China

Jianghua Ou, MD, PhD Department of Breast Surgery, Plastic and Reconstructive Surgery, The Affiliated Tumor Hospital of Xinjiang Medical University, Urumqi, Xinjiang, China

Georgios Pafitanis, MD, PhD, FACS Trauma, Orthoplastic, Lower Extremity and Head and Neck Reconstruction Center, London, UK

Huaihua Qi, MD Department of Breast Surgery, Tangshan People's Hospital, Tangshan, Hebei, China

Dajiang Song, MD Department of Oncology Plastic Surgery, Hunan Cancer Hospital, Changsha, Hunan, China

Pengcheng Su, MD Department of Breast and Thyroid Surgery, People's Hospital of XinJiang Uygur Autonomous Region, Urumqi, Xinjiang, P. R. China

Yiyin Tang Department of Breast Surgery, Yunnan Cancer Hospital, Kunming, Yunnan, China

Kun Wang, MD, PhD Breast-Conserving and Reconstructive Surgery, Multidisciplinary Cancer Treatment, Department of Breast Cancer, Cancer Center, Guangdong Provincial People's Hospital, Guangdong Academy of Medical Sciences, Guangzhou, Guangdong, China

Lei Wang, MD Department of Breast and Thyroid Surgery, Affiliated Hospital of Shandong University of Traditional Chinese Medicine, Jinan, China

Nengbing Wan, MD Department of Oncoplastic Surgery, Hunan Province Cancer Hospital, Changsha, Hunan, China

Huawei Yang Department of Breast Surgery, Affiliated Cancer Hospital of Guangxi Medical University, Nanning, China

Xiaomin Yang Department of Breast Surgery, Tumor Hospital of Shaanxi Province, Xi'an, Shaanxi, China

Zhuangqing Yang, MD Department of Mammary Surgery, The Third Affiliated Hospital of Kunming Medical University (Yunnan Cancer Hospital, Yunnan Cancer Center), Kunming, Yunnan, China

Tomoyuki Yano, MD, PhD, FACS Department of Plastic and Reconstructive Surgery, Cancer Institute Hospital, Tokyo, Japan

JingHua Zhang, MD Plastic, Reconstructive Surgery, Breast Health Care Specialty and General Specialty, TangShan Maternal and Child Health Care Hospital, TangShan, Hebei, China

Rui Zhang, MD Department of Oncoplastic Surgery, Hunan Province Cancer Hospital, Changsha, Hunan, China

Yixin Zhang, MD, PhD Department of Plastic and Reconstructive Surgery, Shanghai Ninth People's Hospital, Shanghai JiaoTong University School of Medicine, Shanghai, China

Department of Laser and Aesthetic Medicine, Shanghai Ninth People's Hospital, Shanghai JiaoTong University School of Medicine, Shanghai, China

Wuping Zheng, MD, PhD Department of Breast and Thyroid Surgery at the Second Affiliated Hospital of Hainan Medical College, Haikou, Hainan Province, China

Youmao Zheng Hand and Foot Surgery, Taizhou Hospital, Taizhou, Zhejiang, China

Breast Reconstruction with Autologous Tissue Transplantation

1

Yixin Zhang, Tor Woo Chiu, Peixian Chen, Rui Zhang, Jun Chai, Peizhi Fan, Jianyun Nie, JingHua Zhang, and Lei Wang

As early as 2000 BC, the breast shape that people wanted was firm, "curved," and aesthetic.

Although plastic surgeons have improved breast shape through surgery for centuries, breast reconstruction after mastectomy was not widely accepted until the middle of the twentieth century.

Nowadays breast reconstruction is an important part of the overall treatment and rehabilitation of breast cancer (BC) patients. Breast reconstruction can improve the overall satisfaction, body image, self-esteem, and quality of life, and reduce the incidence of postoperative anxiety and depression among BC patients [1, 2].

Therefore, breast reconstruction after breast cancer is popular among the diseased people.

In the past decades, technical advance and wide use of breast reconstruction after mastectomy have greatly enhanced the cosmetic effect, which further increased the popularity of autologous tissue transfer in this field.

Breast reconstruction surgery is principled and not limited to specific operation details. It requires innovation and flexible forms to solve some complex problems in order to achieve an appropriate reconstruction method.

The evolution of breast reconstruction is a turning point to promote the transformation of traditional surgery into plastic surgery. It has a long and rich history. With its continuous development, patient satisfaction, problem analysis, technical challenges, and successful cases have promoted breast reconstruction to become a legal field in plastic surgery.

Different from other monographs, here we provide an almost complete historical description to promote our reflection and improvement, and stimulate everyone's enthusiasm for the study of past history, so as to help everyone make more new discoveries in the future.

We strive to find the close relationship between art and science in oncoplastic surgery to help us better explain the evolution of breast reconstruction.

Y. Zhang (✉)
Department of Plastic and Reconstructive Surgery, Shanghai Ninth People's Hospital, Shanghai JiaoTong University School of Medicine, Shanghai, China

Department of Laser and Aesthetic Medicine, Shanghai Ninth People's Hospital, Shanghai JiaoTong University School of Medicine, Shanghai, China

T. W. Chiu
Division of Plastic Reconstructive and Aesthetic Surgery, The Chinese University of Hong Kong, Ma Liu Shui, Hong Kong
e-mail: torchiu@surgery.cuhk.edu.hk

P. Chen
Department of Breast Surgery, First People's Hospital of Foshan, Foshan, Guangdong, China
e-mail: cpxian16@fsyyy.com

R. Zhang
Department of Oncoplastic Surgery, Hunan Province Cancer Hospital, Changsha, Hunan, China

J. Chai
Department of Plastic and Reconstructive Surgery, The Affiliated Suzhou Hospital of Nanjing Medical University, Suzhou Municipal Hospital, Gusu School, Nanjing Medical University, Suzhou, Jiangsu Province, China

P. Fan
Department of Breast and Thyroid Gland Surgery, Hunan Provincial People's Hospital, The First Affiliated Hospital of Hunan Normal University, Changsha, Hunan, China

J. Nie
Breast Cancer Center, Yunnan Cancer Hospital, Kunming, Yunnan, China

J. Zhang
Plastic, Reconstructive Surgery, Breast Health Care Specialty and General Specialty, TangShan Maternal and Child Health Care Hospital, TangShan, Hebei, China

L. Wang
Department of Breast and Thyroid Surgery, Affiliated Hospital of Shandong University of Traditional Chinese Medicine, Jinan, China

Z. Li, D. Song (eds.), *Oncoplastic Flap Surgery*, https://doi.org/10.1007/978-981-19-8926-1_1

1.1 Breast Cancer and Mastectomy

The earliest evidence of breast cancer surgery was found in "Edwin Smith Surgical Principle," which was written between 3000 BC and 2500 BC. This book recorded a series of medical cases [3, 4].

During this period, ancient Egyptian doctors completed tumor resection of the breast. In other important medical literature, such as the "theaters Papyrus" in 1550 BC, where breast cancer was described as a "protuberant breast tumor... no granulation, no liquid, no liquid secretions, and... developing toward the arm" [5].

At that time, there was no cure but only to burn the breast, hoping to burn off the disease.

Such breast surgery brought great pain and trauma to patients. In addition, women completely ignored their breast diseases, which resulted in tumor growth and breast deformity, and even premature death as well as increased disease-specific mortality.

Since ancient times, there has been a great deal of controversy over the surgical treatment of breast cancer.

Hippocrates proposed non-surgical treatment for breast cancer.

Around 400 BC, he argued, "it's better to leave it alone. Do not remove occult cancer, because those who received breast removed will soon die while those who did not lived longer" [6].

Ariel also suggested that breast cancer was a systemic disease. In his humoral theory, black bile collected in breast tissue was the pathogen [7].

Black bile clot was considered to be associated with menstrual cycle in women, which increased the incidence of BC in postmenopausal women.

In contrast to Hippocrates, Ariel supported surgical treatment for BC. Moreover, his followers took other therapies to further eliminate the tumor, such as special diet, dissection, venous bleeding, and dialysis, which were methods of treating breast cancer at that time [7].

During the eighteenth and nineteenth centuries, more thorough operation was carried out for BC patients based on better understanding of the human anatomy.

Jean Louis Petit, Dean of the French Academy of surgery, firstly cleared lymph nodes, breast parenchyma, and chest muscles to cure breast cancer because he felt that the dilated lymphatic glands were the ground for cancer.

He is considered to be the first medical scientist to create a comprehensive surgical approach to breast cancer.

Le Dran from France also advocated lymph node dissection. He thought breast cancer spread through lymphatic vessels. British surgeon Martensen recommended to remove the enlarged lymph nodes caused by breast cancer.

Until the middle of the nineteenth century, modern surgical treatment of breast cancer has been well known.

Germany pathologist Virchow studied the abnormal anatomy of the breast and hypothesized that breast cancer originated from epithelial cells and spread along the fascial surface and lymphatic vessels.

In addition, Tan's theory of unregulated cell growth and the introduction of anesthesia technology paved the way for the modern breast cancer operation in the late twentieth century.

These findings constantly turned the surgical modalities of breast cancer toward being appropriate and laid the foundation for future breast surgery.

Virchow's theory had a great impact on surgery for breast cancer in the United States.

After learning from Dr. Virchow in Europe, Halsted returned to Johns Hopkins University in 1889 and developed an innovative mastectomy, which completely revolutionized the surgical treatment of breast cancer and became the standard of surgery in the 1970s.

Based on Virchow's hypothesis that "the tumor diffuses through the lymphatic tract and fascia plane," "Halsted radical mastectomy" advocates that the breast containing the tumor along with the pectoral muscle and ipsilateral axillary contents should be removed.

Halsted mastectomy was very effective in local disease control and widely accepted by surgeons in the late nineteenth and twentieth centuries.

Compared with other contemporary methods, radical mastectomy was more successful in statistics and oncology [8].

Halsted was widely known for his radical mastectomy. He believed that closed chest "may mask tumor recurrence and increase the chance of tumor dissemination."

Therefore, he usually left the incision open and closed it later or only closed the wound at single layer under high tension.

However, such operation caused significant complications, including chest wall deformity and restrictive shoulder dyskinesia. It was this wrong understanding that greatly reduced the postoperative cosmetic effect and brought devastating psychological blow to patients [1].

Since more than a century ago, surgeons have begun to reconstruct the breast with autologous tissue, but breast reconstruction after mastectomy was not popularized until the middle of the twentieth century. To some extent, it was due to the extensive negative publicity from the famous American surgeon William Stewart Halsted.

At that time, breast reconstruction after mastectomy was not accepted because Halsted thought that reconstruction "may hide the tumor and increase the probability of tumor diffusion" [9] based on his philosophical perspective of plastic surgery.

The large incision after mastectomy was either sutured under high tension or at a delayed stage. Both methods may cause some serious complications, such as chest wall deformity, upper limb edema, and limited shoulder movement [10].

Although Halsted was worried about the healing of the defect rather than the beauty of the wound, in order to reduce the degree of postoperative injury, he designed to place a huge Thiersch implant to wrap the wound and roll up the skin edge to cover the blood vessels in the armpit [11, 12].

This technology was continuously modified and popularized later, and it was widely used when the skin could not be closed [8, 13].

With the advent of the women's rights movement in the twentieth century, radical mastectomy was questioned, leading to the development of breast conserving therapy [14].

In 1948, Patey and Dyson introduced modified radical mastectomy for breast cancer, which gradually replaced the radical mastectomy as the standard treatment [15].

In the past 30 years, breast cancer surgery gradually became minimally invasive [16].

Skin and nipple preserved in breast tumor resection has been proved to be a safe, reliable, and effective scheme in prospective randomized controlled trials [17, 18].

Some breast conserving surgeries can effectively treat breast cancer and retain the skin, which improved the overall aesthetic effect of breast reconstruction.

At the same time, skin conserving mastectomy combined with immediate breast reconstruction can reduce the operation cost, preserve the breast shape, reduce the risk of anesthesia, and improve the overall aesthetic effect [19–21].

In 1917, Bartlett introduced a method of subcutaneous mastectomy and breast reconstruction using fat from the abdominal wall, lateral thigh, and hip at the University of Washington [22].

A landmark event happened in 1948 that Patey and Dyson of Middlesex Hospital in London published an article on "modified radical mastectomy," which preserved the chest muscles and minimized trauma [15].

This operation was accepted in Europe and the United States and is still used in the treatment of early breast cancer.

In the second half of the twentieth century, non-radical mastectomy developed and achieved a better cosmetic effect [23].

Breast conserving therapy became a common practice due to a new era of adjuvant therapy based on the breakthrough (+achievement?) in the biological study of breast cancer [13].

In the past 30 years, prospective controlled trials have been conducted to study the outcomes of various breast cancer surgical treatments (breast conserving surgery or total mastectomy) [18, 24–27].

These studies showed that the extent of breast tissue removal was not associated with patient survival, which laid the ground for breast conserving treatment and completely overturned the stubborn theory of Halsted radical mastectomy.

With the emergence of mastectomy, sentinel lymph node biopsy and radiotherapy, the quality of life of breast cancer patients was being increasingly valued.

As an integral part of the overall breast cancer management, breast reconstruction can reduce the psychological trauma associated with mastectomy.

Breast reconstruction after mastectomy began to develop in the past century. The purpose is to reduce the complications after mastectomy and correct the deformities of chest wall, such as sensory deficiency, axillary vacancy, and subclavicular depression [17, 28].

The current breast reconstruction techniques have gone above and beyond the aforementioned applications and now include the correction of anatomical defects and the restoration of breast shape and symmetry.

As early as the early nineteenth century, surgeons repaired wound defects by modifying skin incision and applying local flap using contralateral breast tissue, regional flap, or autologous tissue transplantation.

The ultimate goal was to make the reconstructed breast as similar to a normal one.

Over time, local flap and autologous tissue were gradually favored by surgeons because of their natural feeling and durability versus prosthesis.

The appearance of flap was several centuries earlier than anesthesia.

The word "flap" originated in the sixteenth century and derived from the Dutch word "flappe," which referred to something wide and loose hanging only on one side.

As early as 600 BC, Indian surgeon Sushruta described the forehead flap for nasal reconstruction, which was a great breakthrough in medicine at that time, especially in the era of removing the nose as a criminal punishment [29].

Breast reconstruction includes repairing insufficient skin, replacing lost breast volume, reconstructing the missing nipple areola complex, and reconstructing symmetrical and beautiful nipples. Surgeons now tend to reconstruct with simple and minimal delayed techniques to make rehabilitation possible.

The former US President William Clinton signed a 1998 budget bill which specified that insurance companies of the education department should pay for the cost of delayed adjustments in addition to that of breast reconstruction in mastectomized patients [30].

Since Halsted radical mastectomy was carried out, breast reconstruction technique has been favored by surgeons. Most patients in China still do not choose post-mastectomy reconstruction, but the technique is already mature and commonly practiced with the goal of improving appearance, imitating the function and feeling of natural breast, and minimizing donor site injury.

Plastic surgeons currently have a variety of methods for allogeneic and autologous breast reconstruction [31].

Prosthesis implantation and autologous breast reconstruction have their own advantages and disadvantages, while autologous breast reconstruction has been more widely recognized by doctors and patients.

1.2 Breast Reconstruction with Autologous Tissue Flap

With better understanding of flap physiology and anatomy, the choice of flap is more and more diverse. (The diversity of flap becomes greater as the understanding of flap physiology and anatomy deepens.)

With the continuous progress of microsurgical techniques, surgeons can use autologous tissue flap transplantation to reconstruct a breast with exactly the same appearance and self-feeling as the one before operation.

The steady improvement of cosmetic effect after breast reconstruction increases the demand for breast reconstruction of patients after mastectomy and breast mass resection [6], and balancing patients' expectation and the technical challenges ensuring the skills required to obtain satisfactory cosmetic effect also makes breast reconstruction play an important role in plastic surgery.

The conflict between sufficient blood supply of the flap and the beauty of the reconstructed breast has never stopped [32].

Over the centuries, there have been some advances in the design and use of skin flaps, including widely used facial skin flaps, cross leg skin flaps, and various breast reconstruction skin flaps.

The first myocutaneous flap for breast reconstruction was reported in 1896. Tansini, a surgeon from Italy, introduced the latissimus dorsi myocutaneous flap (LDMF) for breast reconstruction after breast cancer surgery, which is the first documented myocutaneous flap breast reconstruction [33, 34].

1.3 Free-Styled Flap

Ten years later, in 1906, Ombredanne from Paris introduced the method of using chest muscles to reconstruct the breast immediately after mastectomy [8].

In Ombredane's operation, after removing the breast, axillary lymph nodes and pectoralis major muscle, the pectoralis minor muscle was further coronally transected and flipped over downward to create a circular muscle mass at the level of the fourth rib.

He then covered the reconstructed site by rotating a thoracoabdominal flap.

In the same year, ErwinPayr, chief surgeon at Greifswald University, reported a procedure to repair a small skin defect in people with sufficient subcutaneous fat after mastectomy.

He used a large upper medial sickle flap to construct a breast on the inner side of the defect.

The flap could be rotated to the defect from the lateral side and close the donor area at the same time, but it will lead to the atrophy of the nipple center.

The medial basis of this flap limited its use while the following flaps mainly depended on lateral blood supply.

Local tissue transfer exemplified by tubular pedicle flap was one of the most successful attempts for breast reconstruction.

The lateral thoracic flap which was introduced by Louis Ombredanne in 1924 and later modified by Kleinsch Schmidt provided with an excellent result.

Webster extended the flap to the lower abdomen in 1937 to build a skin flap pedicled on the abdomen, which has been widely used in reconstructive surgery.

1.3.1 Skin Tube

In the first half of the twentieth century, randomly designed tubular flap became the mainstream of various reconstructive surgeries including breast reconstruction.

In the next half century, the exploration of using a variety of tubular flaps obtained from the contralateral breast, abdomen, or extended thoracoabdominal area for breast reconstruction never ended.

In 1924, Ombredanne introduced the axilla-abdominal flap.

A pedicled tubular flap became well known when Sir Harold Gillies improved the thoracoabdominal flap again to re-establish a breast in 1942. The vascular pedicle (from the lower half of the contralateral breast, abdomen, and chest) of this flap was fixed and transferred in several stages along the trunk [35–38].

It was first published by Sauerbruch in 1925 that he dissected the normal breast without pectoral fascia to cover the contralateral breast defect through a wide pedicle rotation.

This methodological change resulted in an acceptable clinical outcome [39, 40].

In 1950, Yannilos successfully applied the contralateral breast composite skin tube to reconstruct the breast [40].

In 1956, Holdsworth introduced his four-step skin tube technique for breast reconstruction, which resulted in satisfactory aesthetic effect as good as other contemporary methods [41].

In his method, Holdsworth established a pedicled tubular flap in the normal breast with the pedicle still attached to the armpit and sternum. He later separated the junction of armpit and sternum and placed the flap through a crescent incision into the reconstructed breast. The nipple areola complex was made in the fourth operation.

Like the contralateral breast flap, thoracoabdominal flap was transferred to the chest, and some even used umbilical valgus for nipple reconstruction [42–44].

Tubular pedicle was favored in previous years, however, the skin tube technique has been finally abandoned due to the lack of accurate design and many complications in the donor area. The pedicled axial flap appeared and gained popularity with enhanced results.

1.4 Latissimus Dorsi Flap

LDMF is one of the most widely used and reliable flaps in breast reconstruction, chest wall covering, head and neck reconstruction, and so on.

LDMF was invented by Professor Tansini from Pavia, Italy, in 1896. However, it was not widely used for most of the twentieth century until Tansini recommended it in his report "A New Method of Mastectomy for Breast Cancer." In this report, Tansini described the principles of BC treatment and breast reconstruction.

He suggested removing all the "mammary glands, muscles and lymph glands" outside the skin to further reduce the risk of breast cancer recurrence.

Tansini advocated implanting distant tissue for wound closure so as to reduce the possibility of tumor recurrence; this flap should be wide enough to cover the axillary wound.

Tansini described that persistent necrosis was present on the distal one-third of the flaps he harvested, and hence he spent several years in the anatomical laboratory studying the axial circulation of the flap and the perforating branch of the composite flap.

In "My Mastectomy Techniques" published in 1906, Tansini elaborated on LDMF and its advantages in breast reconstruction including steady viability, considerable thickness, defect filling, and substitute for pectoralis major muscle.

Radical mastectomy combined with latissimus dorsi flap (LDF) repair was popularized in Europe between 1910 and 1920.

In 1912, Stefano d'Este reported that myocutaneous flaps including latissimus dorsi, teres major, teres minor, and infraspinatus were used to repair post-mastectomy defects.

However, breast reconstruction was not widely accepted at that time, especially in the United States where Halsted's method and philosophy prevailed.

The slow transmission of medical information, the solidification of professional hierarchy, and Halsted's condemnation of plastic surgery after mastectomy had hampered the development and progress of surgical techniques and delayed the use of post-mastectomy breast reconstruction for decades [9, 45].

In 1936, Hutchins resumed the use of latissimus dorsi (LD) flap and reported the application of LD flap in the prevention of lymphedema after mastectomy.

He speculated that the LDF reconstructed axillary lymphatic vessels. In a series of case reports, he described the utility of LD flap in preventing upper limb edema in 12 patients. Interestingly, LD provided with a good foundation for skin transplantation and abdominal fat transplantation.

In 1949, Davis et al. used LDMF to repair anterior chest wall defect.

After resection of the chondrosarcoma of the rib, a size of about 30 cm X 14 cm defect extending horizontally from the axillary line to the sternum and vertically from the fourth to seventh ribs was produced and covered with fascia lata and LDF [46].

In 1950, Darrell Campbell described a case of using latissimus dorsi muscle to cover chest wall lesions after resection of giant invasive cancer [47].

Like Davis, he combined fascia transplantation with latissimus dorsi muscle, and then transplanted a layer of medium thickness skin on the tissue flap.

Davis and Campbell's discovery brought the LDF into a new era, which confirmed Hutchins's view on the anatomical reliability of perforators. LD flap not only protected the chest wall and made it elastic, but also provided the adjacent tissue with sufficient blood supply.

After understanding the relationship of blood supply between skin and muscle, the concept of myocutaneous flap was put forward, and the latissimus dorsi used was expanded into LDF with skin island [48].

In 1976, Nevin Olivari performed breast reconstruction after mastectomy using LD flap again. As Tansini previously described, the use of this flap can reduce the damage of skin and chest wall caused by radiotherapy [49].

In 1977, Olbrisch and Schneider confirmed Olivari's work in their study.

Schneider et al. performed LDF combined with prosthesis for repair in a patient receiving neoadjuvant chemotherapy [50].

In the same year, through further exploration of LDF, Olbrisch found that it had a completely separable skin island and a completely separable vascular pedicle [51] (Fig. 1.1).

John Bostwick of Emory University elaborated on the indications and strategies of breast reconstruction after mastectomy. Among 52 patients who used LDMF, three types of tissue flaps were utilized including muscle flap, muscle flap and LDMF combined with prosthesis were used [42].

His strategies offered adequate skin coverage and breast contour replacement, ensuring the symmetry and beauty of the breast.

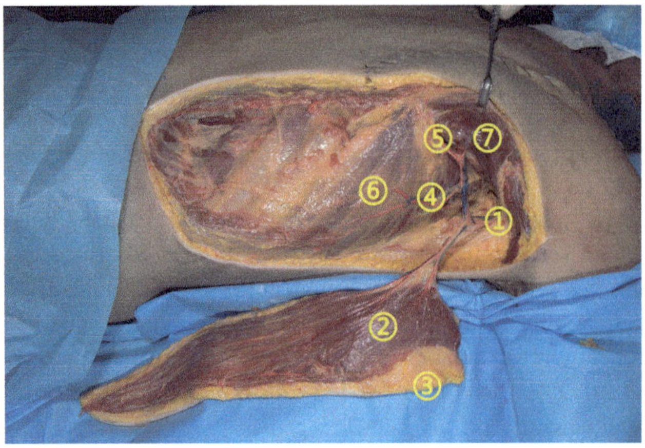

Fig. 1.1 The LDF contains a long vascular pedicle that enables transfer or free transplantation. (1) Thoracodorsal vessels; (2) Latissimus dorsi; (3) PI island; (4) Ramus serratus anterior; (5) thoracodorsal artery, scapular branch; (6) Anterior serratus muscle; (7) Teres major

Like Bostwick, Maxwell also reported other applications of LDF [52, 53].

Maxwell et al. invented free LDF which was easily dissected with a long vascular pedicle and able to cover large wounds [54, 55].

Bostwick and Maxwell were influential surgeons who played a great role in introducing latissimus dorsi muscle into breast reconstruction and other wound repair.

In the 1980s, LDF reconstruction after mastectomy achieved effective and individualized utilization [53, 56].

In 1995, Angrigiani et al. found that the skin and subcutaneous components of traditional LDF could be reliably obtained without damaging muscles [57]. Also in 1995, Hollos used LDF in breast augmentation [58].

Hammond invented a larger LDF including a layer of deep fat attached to the flap [59].

Other technical application of LDF include: (1) separation of thoracodorsal nerve to ensure breast sensation, (2) partial removal of muscle, and (3) combination of partial tissue expander and skin flap.

LDMF has been widely used in reconstructing the breast and other parts of our body ever since it was firstly reported by Tansini.

Recent research progress involved variations in flap designs and improvement of function and aesthetic results.

Although LDF may not be as popular as before, it is still an effective reconstruction method in suitable patients (Fig. 1.2).

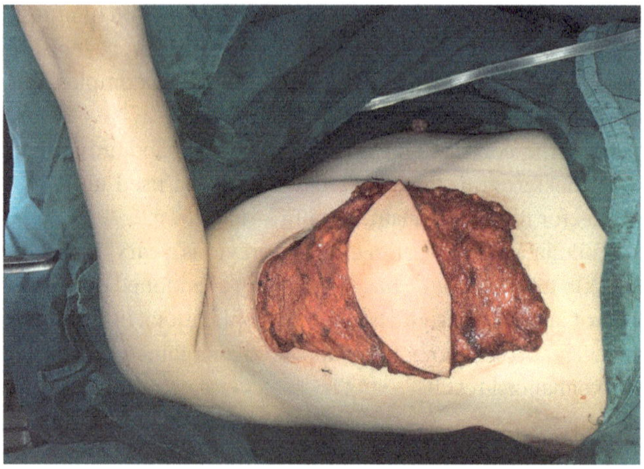

Fig. 1.2 Extended LDF for breast reconstruction

1.5 Abdominal Flap

The landmark progress of breast reconstruction with autologous tissue transplantation in the second half of the twentieth century is the development of abdominal flap in breast reconstruction.

As early as the early twentieth century, the application of the lateral thoracic and abdominal flaps were attempted in breast reconstruction; however, these flaps were finally abandoned due to poor design, large donor site damage, and low cancer-specific survival rate.

The abdomen, as the anatomical donor area for breast reconstruction, was also ignored. It was not re-examined until the abdominal wall physiology and abdominal plastic surgery techniques gained progress in the 1950s.

Further research on the physiological anatomy of abdominal flaps led surgeons to start cutting difficult abdominal flaps with more complex patterns [60, 61].

In 1957, Gillies et al. transferred a racket-like abdominal flap to the chest defect following mastectomy, and used the lateral abdomen as the pedicle and replaced the nipple with the everted navel.

Although this method was very successful, it took a very long time along with multiple delayed flap adjustments to complete the whole procedure.

Ten years later, Fernandez improved the abdominal flap design. She adjusted the flap using the perforator of the superior abdominal artery and rotated it 150° to the mastectomy site.

This flap may be one of the earliest successful attempts to use perforator vessels in breast reconstruction.

Drever [62] later changed the shape of the flap into a "spear-head" shape, expanding the pedicle of the flap to improve the blood supply, delaying the flap transfer for 10 days, and further using Z-shaped plasty to reconstruct a new navel [63].

In 1974, Tai and Hasegawa further improved an abdominal flap based on the abdomen, prepared a transverse abdominal flap pedicled with the medial rectus muscle, and retained the perforators in the upper abdominal vessels [43].

The anatomical basis of the flap was confirmed by the cadaveric study of the specimens of fatty skin or fat flap derived from the inferior superficial artery of the abdominal wall [64].

Other unique flaps such as the stage 2 thoracoabdominal flap added many options for breast reconstruction using the abdomen as a donor area [65, 66].

In the late 1970s, with the increasingly complex design of rectus abdominis myocutaneous flap and the innovation of plastic surgery, rectus abdominis myocutaneous flap became a new force among autologous tissue transplantation for breast reconstruction.

Stephen Mathes and John Bostwick firstly described the application of rectus abdominis myocutaneous flap to reconstruct abdominal wall defects and for breast reconstruction later [67].

The function of this flap was extensive and the blood supply of this flap was based on the superior or inferior vessels of the abdominal wall.

However, this bulky flap would result in weakness of abdominal wall and even abdominal hernia [68, 69].

In 1979, Robbins firstly reported breast reconstruction using rectus abdominis flap [70, 71].

In 1977, Drever firstly described a case of vertical abdominal island flap commonly known as vertical rectus abdominis flap (VRAM) for breast reconstruction.

By the late 1970s, rectus abdominis myocutaneous flap had become the main transplantation flap for breast reconstruction in multiple transplantation centers [72].

In 1982, Carl Hartrampf [73] first described and implemented the pedicled transverse rectus abdominis muscle (TRAM) flap, that is, the abdominal island flap pedicled with the blood vessels on the abdominal wall is was composed of transverse oval skin and subcutaneous tissue (Fig. 1.3).

The pedicled TRAM flap is in good blood supply and able to revolve greatly as well as contains adequate tissue amount. It can be used to reconstruct a beautiful breast without microsurgical anastomosis.

In addition, the scar on donor site can be hidden on the lower abdomen by cosmetic suture.

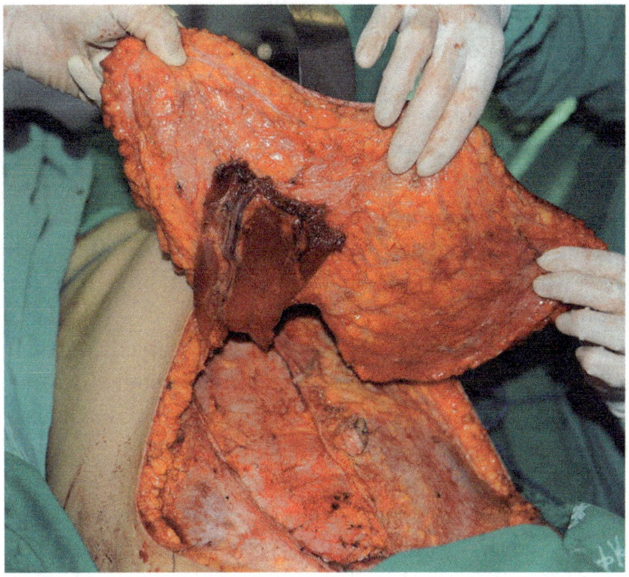

Fig. 1.3 Preparation of transverse pedicled rectus abdominis flap

Nonetheless, obvious donor site complications caused by pedicled TRAM, such as abdominal wall hernia formation and abdominal weakness, were soon recognized.

Intraoperative abdominal fascia defect is usually repaired with a synthetic mesh, if repairing fails, the long-term complications will be significant [62].

Therefore, attention was gradually focused on the development of muscle preserving flap raising technique.

In 1989, Grotting [74, 75] began to use free transverse rectus abdominis flap transplantation (free TRAM) to complete breast reconstruction, resulting with good postoperative effect.

The advantages of free TRAM over pedicled TRAM are as follows: (1) Superior inferior abdominal vascular pedicles of larger diameter were used; (2) Upper abdominal bulge was avoided; (3) Focal flap necrosis was alleviated; (4) Donor site complication rate was reduced.

Nowadays, despite the risk of donor site complications, both free and pedicled TRAM flaps are still widely used in breast reconstruction.

In conclusion, the concept of no muscle sparing in TRAM flap has been continuously developed as sparing partial rectus abdominis and fascia when obtaining the flap, so as to reduce the abdominal wall injury and retain important periumbilical vessels.

The advantages of abdominoplasty make it attractive to patients.

It was memorable in 1979 that the first rotating rectus abdominis flap was used for immediate breast reconstruction, though ugly scars were left [69, 70].

In the same year, Holmstrom reported the application of vascularized free myocutaneous flap which was first used in breast reconstruction [75, 76].

Other attempts on rectus abdominis flap also achieved great success.

In 1980, Drever made a cone in the rectus abdominis myocutaneous flap and reconstructed the areola with the patient's labia minora, creating a natural breast, and then used with a synthetic reticular structure to strengthen the abdominal wall [77].

To use the tissue that would have been discarded, Marshall et al. [69] used the excised tissue after abdominal lipoma resection to create a direct flipped flap for delayed breast reconstruction.

With the exploration of the technique of preserving muscle with rectus abdominis flap, Carl Hartrampf [73] of Emory University created a transverse elliptical abdominal island flap that was based on rectus abdominis and separated from the skin and subcutaneous tissue on the vascular pedicle.

The design of transverse rectus abdominis myocutaneous flap marks the formation of the international standard of breast reconstruction technique.

TRAM flap has rich blood perfusion, large rotation arc, and abundant abdominal fat, which can reconstruct beautiful breasts.

The natural appearance and durability of the flap (especially in patients after radiotherapy) further promote this method.

During the controversial period of transplantation, TRAM flap has always been the main way of autologous tissue transplantation.

Over the years, many technical improvements have been made to increase the blood supply of the flap and increase the survival rate of the flap, such as free TRAM, double pedicled TRAM [78], turbocharged TRAM [79], supercharged TRAM [80], and staged II surgery [81, 82].

In addition to TRAM, Hartrampf and Bennett [83] developed a risk factor algorithm to evaluate patients with TRAM flap breast reconstruction by describing the transverse rectus abdominis flap, thus making a further contribution to this field.

Firstly described by Taylor in 1976, Ruben's flap (excessive adipose tissue from the iliac crest, modeled on Paul Ruben's sixteenth century painting "the three Graces") or deep iliac circumflex artery flap is another way to shape a new breast [84, 85].

This flap provides with longer vascular pedicle and the lowest incidence rate in donor site, but it is a more challenging operation than TRAM flap in shaping a new and acceptable breast.

Traditional rectus abdominis flap is still widely used because of its simple preparation, constant anatomy, flexible transfer, and diverse cutting forms.

1.6 Free Tissue Flap Transplantation

In 1973, Taylor and Daniel [86, 87] reported a successful microvascular free flap transplantation, and the prospect of breast reconstruction was forever rewritten.

In 1975, Toyomi Fujino [88, 89] successfully applied the hip dermal fat muscle free flap anastomosed with the thoracic acromial vessels to repair congenital breast hypoplasia for the first time.

In recent years, other commonly used free flaps for breast reconstruction include deep iliac circumflex artery (groin) flap (Rubens flap) [84, 85], lateral thigh (fascia lata) flap [90], anterolateral thigh flap [91], gluteus maximus flap [92–94], gracilis myocutaneous flap [95], deltoid myocutaneous flap [96], etc. (Fig. 1.4).

The limitation and deficiency of ipsilateral LDF is one of the reasons for the development of free flap breast reconstruction technique.

In the last three decades of the twentieth century, free tissue transplantation has been greatly developed and improved in breast reconstruction.

Many scholars have described the successful conditions of free flap transplantation and the simplification of the procedure of cutting free flap.

In 1975, Fujinoet et al. [89] firstly used the free tissue flap of the upper gluteus maximus muscle for breast reconstruction after mastectomy.

He previously reported the application of a similar flap for breast hypoplasia and found that the vascular pedicle was too short to perform reliable anastomosis [88] (Fig. 1.5).

Until 1978, only several free myocutaneous flaps have been reported, including Schenck's free rectus femoris and Harri's free rectus femoris flap [97] (Fig. 1.6).

Meanwhile, Serfin and Georgiade [98, 99] firstly reported 12 micro breast reconstruction operations using ilio-groin flap (Fig. 1.7).

The first abdominal free flap was performed by Holmstrom in 1979 [100].

The abdominal free flap is designed in the umbilical area between the abdomen, the common area, and the area between the anterior superior iliac spine. It is based on one side of the inferior abdominal artery.

Of the two firstly reported cases of breast reconstruction, one failed due to venous thrombosis and the other survived due to sufficient venous anastomotic reflux.

The free rectus abdominis flap was popularized by Grotting in the 1980s [74, 75].

He firstly described the application of free inferior abdominal artery flap in breast reconstruction.

Rizzuto and Allen improved and popularized this flap for mastectomy with small defects and low damage rate at the donor site [101].

Compared with pedicled skin flap, especially for refractory wounds, free, autologous, and tissue transplantation

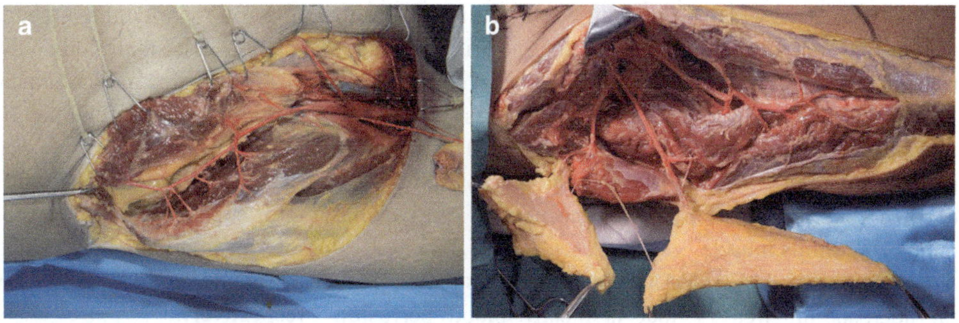

Fig. 1.4 (**a**) Preparation of tissue flap pedicled with deep iliac circumflex artery; (**b**) Tensor fascia lata flap and anterolateral femoral flap

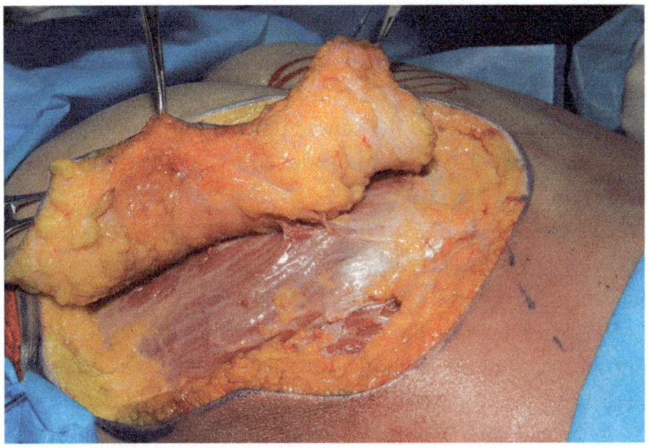

Fig. 1.5 Gluteus maximus myocutaneous flap

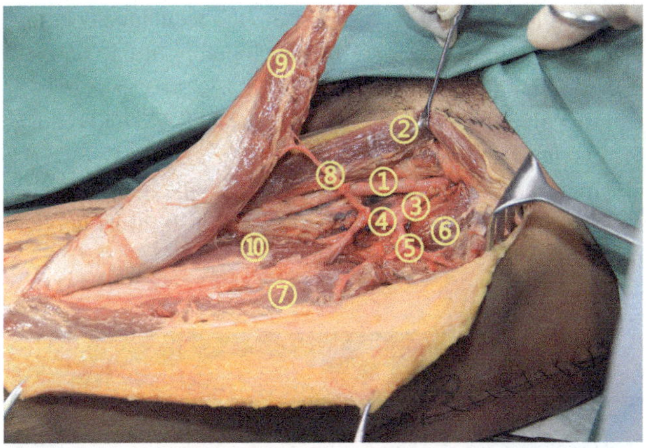

Fig. 1.6 Rectus femoris and its vascular pedicle. (1) Femoral artery; (2) Sartorius muscle; (3) Profunda femoral artery; (4) Descending branch of lateral femoral circumflex artery; (5) Transverse branch of lateral femoral circumflex artery; (6) Iliac muscle; (7) Lateral femoral muscle; (8) Descending branch of lateral circumflex femoral artery; rectus femoris muscle branch; (9) Rectus femoris; (10) Medial femoral muscle

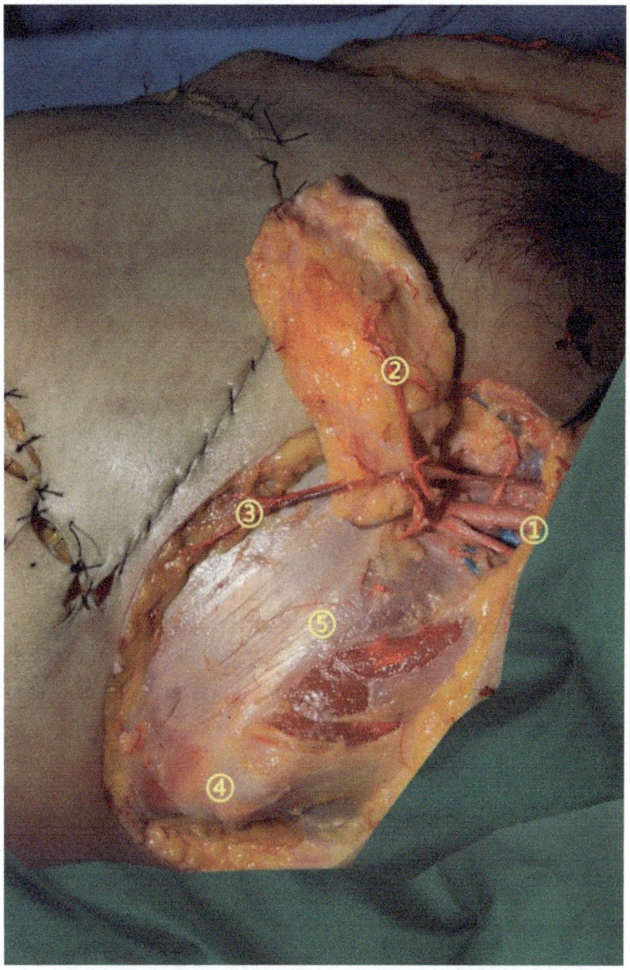

Fig. 1.7 Anatomy of ilioinguinal flap. (1) External iliac artery; (2) Superficial iliac circumflex artery; (3) Superficial abdominal artery; (4) Anterior superior iliac spine; (5) Inguinal ligament

have become the main methods of breast reconstruction in many hospitals.

Because it provides with reliability and aesthetics for plastic surgeons and patients [91].

1.7 Perforator Flap Base on the Deep Inferior Epigastric Artery

The perforator flap became popular in the 1990s, such as the perforator flap of deep inferior epigastric artery (DIEP).

This flap is considered to be an optimized technique to minimize donor site injury, preserve the integrity and function of rectus abdominis muscle, and thin waist shaping.

But it is technically more challenging and risky [102].

With better understanding of the anatomical structure of the abdominal wall, we realized that the successful removal of the abdominal wall flap does not necessarily sacrifice the rectus abdominis muscle.

In addition, pedicled TRAM flap is prone to subcutaneous fat necrosis in Area IV that is mostly blood perfusion insufficient.

Many people are actively looking for ways to improve flap perfusion and preserve muscle to replace TRAM flap for breast reconstruction.

In 1983, G. Ian Taylor [103] introduced an improved TRAM flap, namely, the extended lower abdominal artery perforator flap (DIEP), which is composed of the lower half of rectus abdominis muscle and the upper lateral extended fascia based on the perforator of the lower abdominal artery around the umbilicus.

Taylor GI described in this paper that the lower abdominal wall skin flap was composed of the lower end of rectus abdominis and the outward extension of the fascia above the umbilicus.

Super lateral fascia skin extension is based on periumbilical perforator.

This flap was large and could hide the donor site, which soon became popular [103] (Fig. 1.8).

Two years later, Friedman et al. [104] described an upper abdominal free flap for breast reconstruction. This report once again confirmed that the flap had the advantages of large caliber blood vessels, long vascular pedicle, and abundant soft tissue, which is exactly the flap required for breast reconstruction.

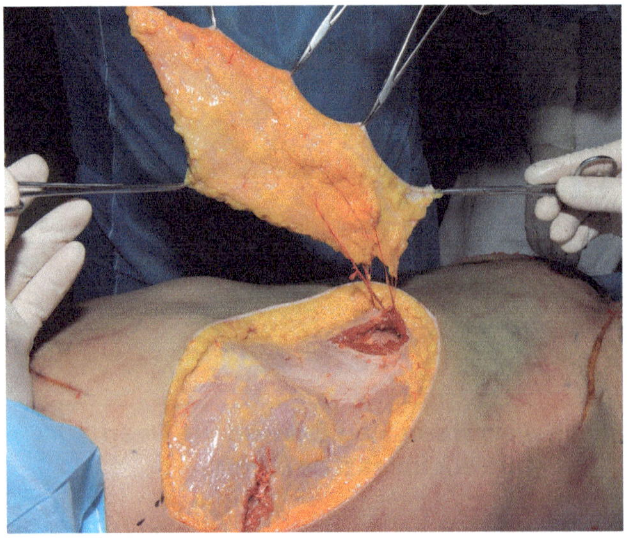

Fig. 1.8 Anatomy of perforator flap of inferior abdominal artery

Kroll reported the lumbar perforator flap in 1988 [105].

In 1986, a small study published by Onishi and Maruyama [106] provided an anatomical basis for the design of lower abdominal wall fascial flap based on perforator.

In 1989, Japanese surgeons Isao Koshima and Shugo SOEDA [107] described the ultra-thin paraumbilical perforator flap (PUP) based on the paraumbilical perforator of the inferior abdominal artery and used it for the reconstruction of contralateral inguinal and floor of mouth defects, respectively.

Noting the shortcomings of the myocutaneous flap at that time (i.e., sacrificing the main muscle tissue), Koshima and SOEDA [107] firstly introduced the technique of cutting the perforator flap of the inferior abdominal artery without sacrificing the rectus abdominis muscle at the international level.

They then renamed the same flap as the free thin periumbilical perforator flap and introduced its application in head and neck defects [68].

In September 1993, Phillip Blondeel, a Belgian plastic surgeon, who heard the publication of this achievement at the meeting of the American Society of plastic surgery (ASPS) in New Orleans, began to promote the use of DIEP flap in Belgium after the meeting, and then he was responsible for promoting it throughout Europe [108–111].

Allen RJ and Treece P [104] used this flap for breast reconstruction in 1994. They successfully reconstructed 15 breasts based on inferior abdominal vessels.

Before Allen RJ and Treece P discovered the DIEP flap and used it for breast reconstruction, the technique accumulated in plastic surgery and the development of flap had laid a solid foundation for this flap [104].

DIEP flap shares all the advantages of TRAM and reduces the extent of abdominal wall injury.

However, it is technically more challenging because changes in anatomy or vascular conditions limit its application (Fig. 1.9).

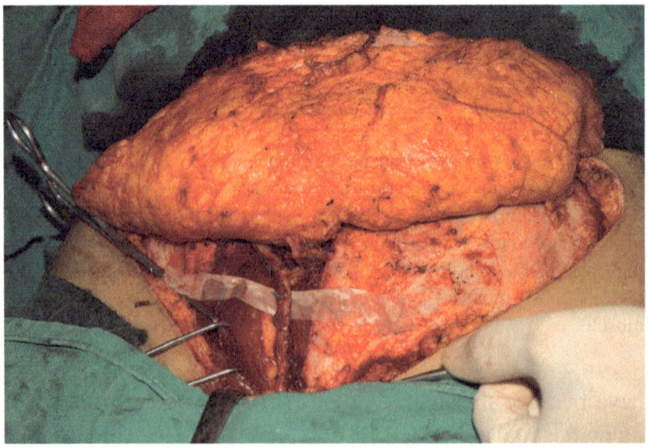

Fig. 1.9 Preparation of perforator flap of transverse inferior abdominal artery and separation of vascular pedicle

In the same year, Kroll et al. [112] and Mizgala et al. [112] found that the amount of sacrifice of rectus abdominis was directly proportional to the weakness of our abdominal wall.

In the application of these techniques, we still need to pay attention to maintaining abdominal wall strength [110].

In 1999, Blondeel [109, 110] made conclusions based on his experience of using 100 DIEP flaps (different from Hartrampf's statement on rectus abdominis flap): obese patients can benefit from this operation.

1.8 Other Abdominal Perforator Flaps

Later, two flaps from the abdomen were used for autologous breast reconstruction.

The first was the superficial epigastric artery (SIEA) flap.

After the first application of SIEA flap in breast reconstruction in 1989, Allen reported his first seven case series at the annual meeting of plastic surgery of southeast society in 1990.

Since then, in 1991, Grotting [113] reported a case report of using SIEA flap, and in 1999, Arnez et al. [114] also reported an example of applying SIEA flap to breast reconstruction.

The preparation of SIEA flap does not need to open the anterior sheath of rectus abdominis. Compared with pedicled or free TRAM flap with rectus abdominis or muscle sheath, SIEA flap reduces donor site complications.

In short, it provides with a large tissue flap that can be transferred for reconstruction.

Unfortunately, SIEA flap is not as anatomically stable as DIEP flap such as short pedicle length, small vascular diameter, and common deficiency [64, 115].

Taylor and Daniel [64] dissected 100 cadavers and found that 35% of the patients had no SIEA at all.

Elliott and Hartrampf [84] introduced the Rubens flap, which comes from the excess peri-iliac fat pad in the upper thigh and iliac crest area.

This flap is pedicled with the deep iliac circumflex artery (DCIA), which provides with a new choice for autologous breast reconstruction for women who have previously undergone abdominoplasty or abdominal TRAM flap [116].

The acquisition of this flap is cumbersome, and there is also risks of donor complications and hernia.

However, DCIA perforator flap can be combined with DIEP flap to form a larger flap based on DCIA perforator and DIEP perforator and their vascular pedicle [117].

1.9 Muscle Sparing Latissimus Dorsi (MSLD) Flap, Thoracodorsal Artery Perforator Flap, and Intercostal Artery Perforator Flap

We prefer to using extended MSLD flap combined with whole latissimus dorsi muscle for reconstruction for previously radiotherapy-treated tissues.

The thoracodorsal artery constitutes the main blood supply to the latissimus dorsi muscle, and other blood supply sources include intercostal arteries and lumbar arteries (Mathes and Nahai V-type circulation mode).

The thoracodorsal artery penetrates the latissimus dorsi muscle at 10–11 cm from the distal end of its own origin (Fig. 1.10).

In 1906, Tansini firstly described the application of LDMF in chest wall reconstruction. LDMF based on thoracic and dorsal vessels is one of the pedicled skin flaps widely used in breast reconstruction.

In 1912, d'Este firstly proposed the application of pedicled LDMF in reconstructing the defect after mastectomy.

In 1939, Hutchins recommended the use of LDMF to reconstruct the breast and reduce lymphedema after mastectomy.

In 1976, Nevin Olivari discovered that LDMF could be used for breast reconstruction and recommended its use in patients who had received radiotherapy [49].

In 1939, Hutchins suggested the use of LDMF for breast reconstruction to reduce post-mastectomy lymphedema.

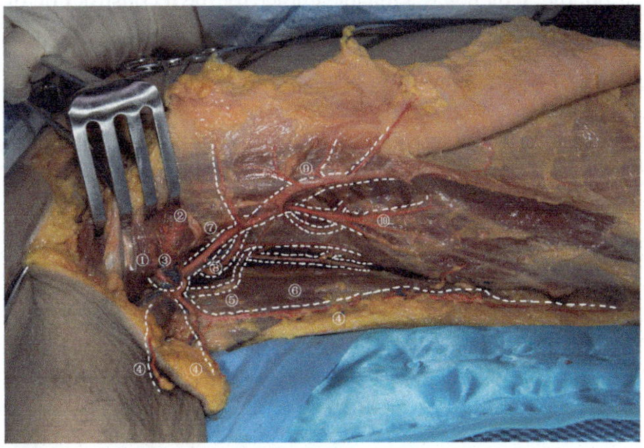

Fig. 1.10 Anatomy of thoracodorsal artery and its perforating branch. (1) Teres major; (2) Latissimus dorsi; (3) Circumflex scapular vessels; (4) Lateral thoracic artery (different sources); (5) Intercostal brachial nerve; (6) Pectoralis major; (7) thoracodorsal neurovascular bundle; (8) Long thoracic nerve; (9) Lateral branch of thoracodorsal artery and its perforating vessels; (10) Anterior serratus branch of thoracodorsal vessel

In 1987, Hawkin [118] described that the expanded LDF combined with lumbar fat, which can offer a greater amount of tissue for reconstruction.

However, the muscles with important functions are sacrificed if LDMF is used. Compared with LDMF, the other three perforator flaps obtained in the lateral chest are superior to LDMF because they do not need to sacrifice the latissimus dorsi muscle.

In 1985, Holmstrom and Lossing [119] introduced stage II breast reconstruction using the lateral thoracic fascia flap based on the same thoracic dorsal vascular pedicle combined with prosthesis.

Recently, the lateral thoracic flap has been proved to be a reliable option for immediate partial reconstruction of lateral breast defects [120, 121].

In 1995, Angrigiani [57] studied the muscle-free LDMF—the current thoracodorsal artery perforator flap (TDAPF)—in latex-perfused cadaver specimens.

In 2004, this vascular anatomy was further defined by Thomas et al. [122], and Hamdi et al. [123] further used intraoperative Doppler probe to identify more alternative perforator flaps based on intercostal artery system.

TDAP flap and intercostal artery perforator flap (ICAP) are large and reliable pedicled fascial flaps derived from the lateral thoracic region in addition to LDMF.

In 2008, Hamdi [124] proposed that the lateral intercostal artery perforator (LICAP) flap was a pedicled flap with reliable blood supply based on the posterior segment of the neurovascular bundle, which was a reliable choice for the reconstruction of complex lateral breast deformities (Fig. 1.11).

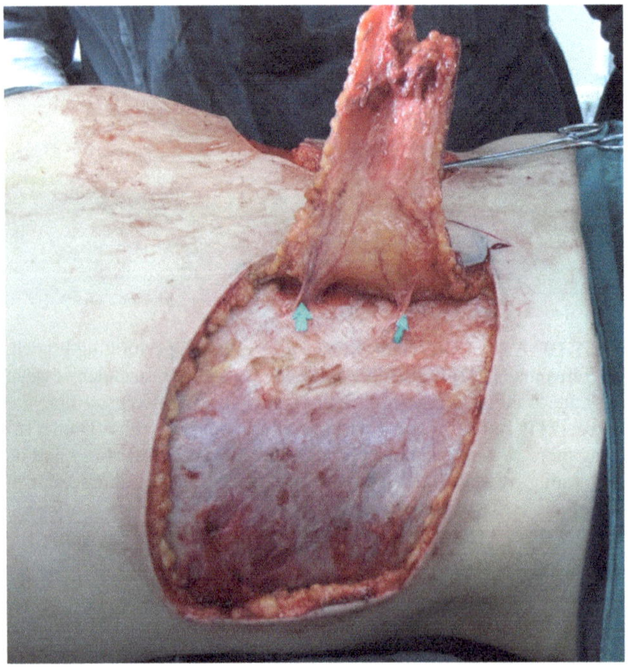

Fig. 1.11 Preparation of intercostal artery perforator flap

In addition, ICAP can also be based on the dorsal cutaneous branch of the posterior intercostal artery (dorsal intercostal artery perforator, DICAP) and the perforating branch of the anterior intercostal artery (anterior intercostal artery perforator, AICAP) [125].

However, compared with LICAP, these flaps cannot be widely used in breast reconstruction because of their short vascular pedicle and limited rotation arc [125] (Fig. 1.11).

1.10 Hip Flap

In 1973, Orticochea [126] harvested a pedicled gluteus maximus myocutaneous flap using the hip area as the donor area.

In 1975, Fujino [92] applied free superior gluteal artery myocutaneous flap for immediate reconstruction after mastectomy.

In 1989, Paletta, Bostwick, and Nahai applied inferior gluteal artery free flap to breast reconstruction [93].

In 1993, Allen [94] introduced the application of hip artery perforator flap (gluteal artery perforator, GAP) in breast reconstruction.

GAP flap is ideal for breast reconstruction in European and American women because they have more skin and fat in the hip than in the abdomen, and this flap is an important choice for breast reconstruction when the abdomen cannot be used as a donor area.

The amount of adipose tissue in GAP flap is relatively constant, and the harvested flap is often smaller than DIEP flap.

Similar to abdominal and superficial abdominal artery (SIEA) flaps, donor site complications of GAP flap were minimal without muscle sacrifice (Fig. 1.12).

However, Asian women often have small hips and are unable to provide with enough tissue, so gluteus maximus myocutaneous flap transplantation for breast reconstruction has not been popularized in Asia.

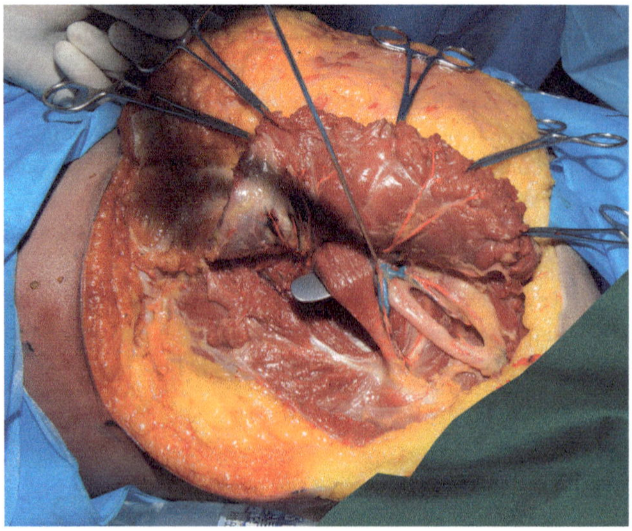

Fig. 1.12 The anatomy of gluteus maximus myocutaneous flap

GAP flap can be designed based on superior gluteal artery perforator (SGAP) or inferior gluteal artery perforator (IGAP) [127].

For the acquisition of SGAP skin island flap, it is recommended to carry out tissue resection while lifting the hip.

Proponents of this view believe that hip lifting can maintain the natural shape of hip donor area natural while leaving thick scars and obvious depressed hip contour [127].

IGAP made scar hidden in gluteal folding is possible. However, the hip contour may be obviously irregular if tissue obtained is excessive in SGAP or IGAP flaps.

In 2011, Tuinder et al. [123] applied the gluteal artery muscle septal perforator (sc-GAP) flap to breast reconstruction after mastectomy in a group of patients, and achieved good results.

This flap is based on the intermuscular septal perforators between gluteus maximus and gluteus medius, which is able to avoid intramuscular anatomy and increase the length of vascular pedicle.

However, the common disadvantage of all hip-derived flaps is that position change during operation is required [128].

1.11 Lumbar Artery Perforator Flap

In the initial description of a perforator flap in 1988, Kroll and Rosenfield [105] described a lumbar artery perforator (LAP) flap based on an unknown perforator in the midline of the lower back (Fig. 1.13).

LAP flap is a fascia flap supplied by the perforating branch of lumbar artery from the posterior midline to the anterior sheath of rectus abdominis and the vast skin area extending 10 cm above the anterior superior iliac spine (ASIS) [129] (Fig. 1.13).

LAP flap usually runs along ASIS and provides an alternative for autologous breast reconstruction in those unsuitable for DIEP flap [129, 130].

The advantage of this flap is that it can hide the scar well, and there is enough fat in the donor area for breast reconstruction. The disadvantage is the short length of vascular pedicle, which often requires simultaneous vein transplantation [131].

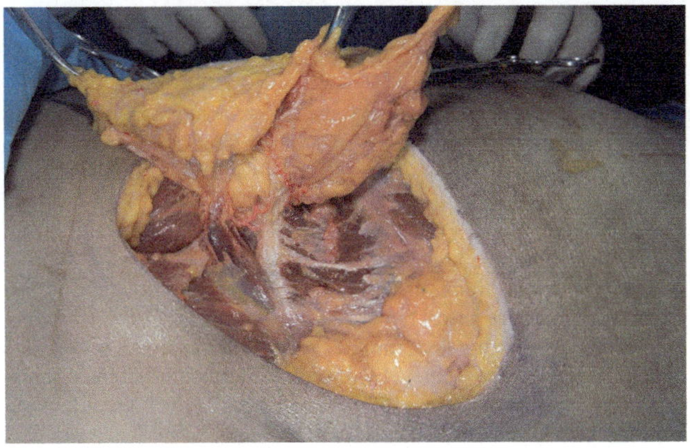

Fig. 1.13 Anatomy of lumbar artery perforator (LAP) flap

1.12 Thigh Flap

Hurwitz [132, 133] introduced the first posterior thigh flap based on inferior gluteal artery in 1980, and recorded the complete anatomy of the posterior thigh 1 year later (Fig. 1.14).

Hurteau et al. [134] described a case of repairing sciatic pressure ulcer using myocutaneous flap based on profunda femoral artery branch.

In 1983, Baek [135] firstly reported the lateral thigh flap based on the third perforator of profunda femoral vessels (Fig. 1.15).

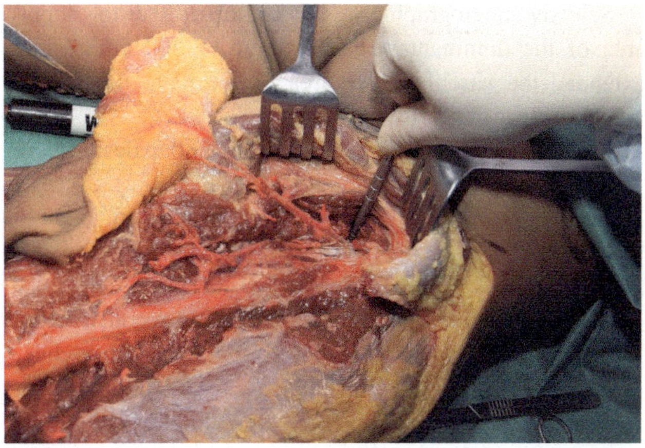

Fig. 1.14 Anatomy of posterior thigh flap based on inferior gluteal artery

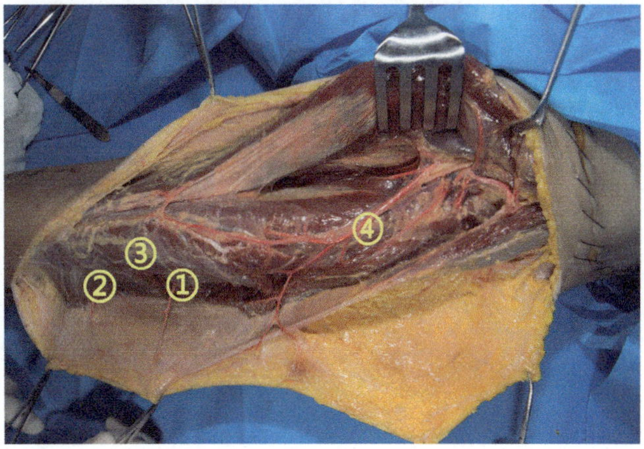

Fig. 1.15 Anatomical basis of lateral thigh flap pedicled with the third perforator of profunda femoral vessel. (1) The third perforating branch of profunda femoral artery; (2) Perforating branch of descending genicular artery; (3) Lateral femoral muscle; (4) Descending branch of lateral femoral circumflex artery

1.13 Transverse Upper Gracilis (TUG) Myocutaneous Flap

Transverse gracilis muscle, also known as transverse semilunar gracilis muscle (TUG), myocutaneous flap has been further found to be used in breast reconstruction since its anatomical structure was reported by Yousif et al. in 1992.

The gracilis muscle is a type II myocutaneous flap in the middle of the thigh (Mathes and Nahai). The dominant vascular pedicle comes from the profunda femoral artery and enters the deep surface of the gracilis muscle in the upper one-third segment, usually 9–12 cm below the pubic tubercle.

It is usually found that 2–3 vascular pedicles enter the muscle.

The skin island is often longitudinal so as to contain as many perforators as possible to guarantee blood perfusion to the distal end of the flap. Yousif et al. found that the perforators could distribute transversally, enabling safe removal of the skin island based on a different design.

Selective angiographic studies confirmed that the supply area of the dominant pedicle was up to 400 cm^2, which extended the vascular body area backward to the gracilis muscle [136] (Fig. 1.16).

Key points of vascular anatomy in TUG flap design:

1. For reconstruction for breast of small to medium volume.
2. The anatomy of vascular pedicle is constant.
3. The extended tug flap can optimize and reconstruct the subcutaneous tissue of the posterior and medial thighs.
4. The reorganization of subcutaneous tissue should be concentrated only on the surface of gracilis muscle and the posterior thigh.
5. The extension of the anterior skin island is limited because the perfusion of the anterior skin island is not very reliable, and patients generally do not accept the obvious scar left after the anterior skin island is cut.

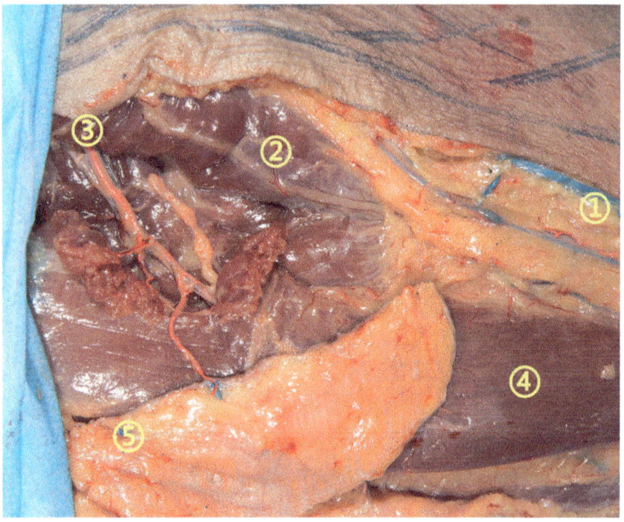

Fig. 1.16 Vascular anatomy of gracilis myocutaneous flap. (1) Great saphenous vein; (2) Adductor longus; (3) Gracilis muscle branch of profunda femoral artery; (4) Gracilis muscle; (5) PI island

1.14 Perforator Flap of Profunda Femoral Artery

The anatomy of the profunda femoral artery is complex, and the definition of the profunda femoral artery perforator flap has been confusing. Strictly speaking, the profunda femoral artery perforator flap should be named after where it is harvested, such as the medial femoral perforator flap pedicled with the profunda femoral artery, the lateral femoral perforator flap pedicled with the profunda femoral artery, and the posterior femoral perforator flap pedicled with the profunda femoral artery (Fig. 1.17).

In 1984, Song et al. [137] firstly introduced the posterior thigh free flap.

In 2001, Angrigiani et al. [138] described an adductor myocutaneous flap with the posterior and medial thigh skin based on the first musculocutaneous perforator of the profunda femoral artery.

The study of cadaver specimens conducted in 2007 confirmed that the source of blood vessels of this flap was the profunda femoral artery [139] (Fig. 1.18).

In the 13th International Conference in Mexico in 2010, Robert Allen proposed that the first profunda femoral artery perforator (PAP) flap could be used in breast reconstruction.

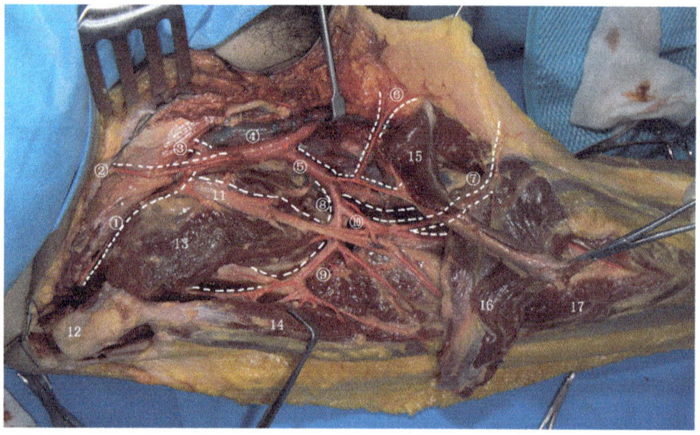

Fig. 1.17 Profunda femoral artery and related anatomy. (1) Deep iliac circumflex artery; (2) Superficial abdominal artery; (3) deep inferior epigastric artery; (4) Femoral artery and vein; (5) Profunda femoral artery; (6) Anteromedial femoral perforator (from sartorius branch of profunda femoral artery); (7) Anteromedial femoral perforator (from rectus femoris muscle branch of descending branch of lateral femoral artery); (8) Main trunk of lateral femoral circumflex artery; (9) Transverse branch of lateral femoral circumflex artery; (10) Descending branch of lateral femoral circumflex artery; (11) Femoral nerve; (12) Anterior superior iliac spine; (13) Iliopsoas muscle; (14) Tensor fascia lata; (15) Sartorius muscle; (16) Rectus femoris; (17) Lateral femoral muscle

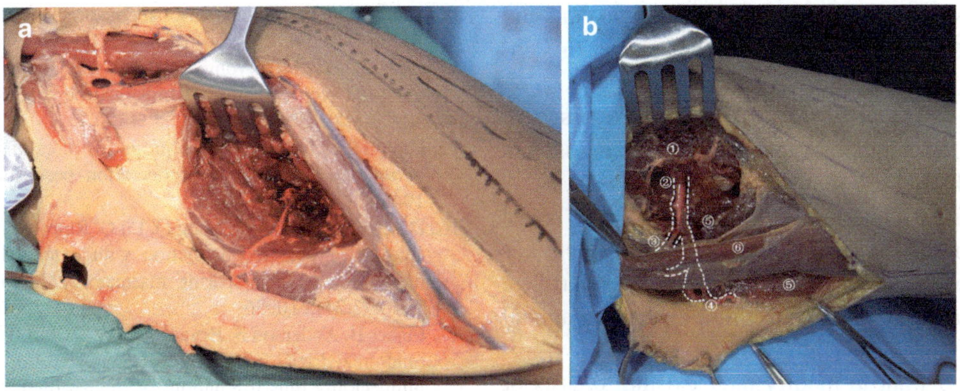

Fig. 1.18 Vascular anatomy of profunda femoral artery perforator flap (PAP) shows that the perforator arteries of muscle septum (**a**) and muscle skin (**b**) run in it. (1) Adductor longus; (2) Adductor major branch of profunda femoral artery; (3) Gracilis muscle branch from the great adductor branch; (4) The cutaneous branch from the great adductor branch; (5) Adductor major; (6) Gracilis muscle

In 2011, Allen et al. [140] reported the application of PAP flap in autologous breast reconstruction.

The advantages of this flap include unimportant function of donor area, concealed scar, long vascular pedicle, preserved muscle function, and easy shaping.

Similarly, the flap can be obtained at the lithotomy position, which enables the preparation of the vascular pedicle in the recipient area to be carried out at the same time (i.e., the patient does not need to change his position during the operation).

1.15 Progress of Breast Reconstruction

1.15.1 Autologous Fat Injection

The goal of breast reconstruction is to create a beautiful breast that matches the size and shape of the previous or contralateral breast. Autologous fat injection has been increasingly used to correct and improve the contour deformity of reconstructed breast [141].

The latest technique improves the methods of fat collection and handling as well as the survival rate of the autologous fat transplanted.

Among them, Roger Khouri's non-surgical Brava ultra-large volume autologous fat transplantation for breast augmentation has achieved impressive results.

However, autologous fat transplantation is usually not suitable for the reconstruction of the whole breast and can only be used for the reconstruction of partial breast defects [142].

Tissue regeneration and stem cell research are very popular in many disciplines.

In 2011, Morrison's team [143] published their adipose tissue engineered animal model and used the generated adipose tissue of large volume for breast reconstruction.

Adipose tissue derived from stem cell differentiation can produce new breast tissue, which may be a new frontier of breast reconstruction.

1.15.2 Upper Limb Lymphedema

Upper limb lymphedema is a serious complication of breast cancer treatment. We once thought it was not likely to be cured. Fortunately, the development of new microsurgery technique brings hope of success in surgical treatment of lymphedema.

Specifically, super-microsurgery (very small vascular anastomosis with a diameter of 0.5–0.8 mm) has been used for lymphatic venous anastomosis [144].

This technique has been shown to significantly improve the clinical effectiveness 10 years after operation over that of traditional lymphatic venous anastomosis [144, 145].

Other clinical studies have shown that transplantation of inguinal lymph nodes with autologous microvascular transplantation technique into the waist or armpit of breast cancer patients can alleviate their lymphedema [146, 147].

The concept of total breast anatomical repair (TBAR) was proposed by Jaume Masia. It is characterized by autologous breast reconstruction combined with biological lymphoid tissue pedicled with superficial iliac circumflex vessels and groin flap. It reconstructs breast tissue and upper limb lymphatic system that may be damaged in primary tumor resection or axillary lymph node dissection [148].

These clinical studies as well as better understanding of lymphangiogenesis at the molecular level may open a new chapter in the treatment of lymphedema, which was originally considered incurable.

1.16 The Future of Breast Reconstruction

There is no doubt that many significant and successful advances have been made in breast reconstruction.

Nevertheless, the current treatment is not perfect, so there is still room for improvement.

The progress of diagnostic radiology, treatment, and molecular genetics is helpful to develop better breast reconstruction technique in the future.

Since the breast is mainly composed of adipose tissue, in theory, the new regeneration of fat can adapt and adjust to a person's chest shape and volume.

The artificial cartilage may also play a role in breast reconstruction in the future. It is reported that progress has been made in the construction of human papillary cartilage slices by inoculating chondrocytes with polymers in animal models.

For those who want to modify their existing breasts or reconstruct breast(s) by surgery, the prospect of breast reconstruction seems bright.

Women in the twenty-first century have many choices, and the results are becoming more and more satisfactory.

Breast cancer is still the second leading cause of cancer death in women, and it continues to grow at a rate of 3–5% per year.

It is certain that plastic surgeons will continue to work with breast surgeons to create new management models and breast reconstruction techniques.

References

1. Wilkins EG, Cederna PS, Lowery JC, et al. Prospective analysis of psychosocial outcomes in breast reconstruction: one-year postoperative results from the Michigan Breast Reconstruction Outcome Study. Plast Reconstr Surg. 2000;106(5):1014–25; discussion 1026–7.
2. Al-Ghazal SK, Fallowfield L, Blamey RW. Comparison of psychological aspects and patient satisfaction following breast conserving surgery, simple mastectomy and breast reconstruction. Eur J Cancer. 2000;36(15):1938–43.
3. Stiefel M, Shaner A, Schaefer SD. The Edwin Smith Papyrus: the birth of analytical thinking in medicine and otolaryngology. Laryngoscope. 2006;116(2):182–8.
4. Vargas A, López M, Lillo C, Vargas MJ. [The Edwin Smith papyrus in the history of medicine]. Rev Med Chil. 2012;140(10):1357–62.
5. Bou KR, Richa S. When affective disorders were considered to emanate from the heart: the Ebers papyrus. Am J Psychiatry. 2014;171(3):275.
6. Wood WC. Progress from clinical trials on breast cancer. Cancer. 1994;74(9 Suppl):2606–9.
7. Wolfe JN. Breast cancer screening. A brief historical review. Breast Cancer Res Treat. 1991;18(Suppl 1):S89–92.
8. Teimourian B, Adham MN. Louis Ombredanne and the origin of muscle flap use for immediate breast mound reconstruction. Plast Reconstr Surg. 1983;72(6):905–10.
9. Halsted WS. I. The results of operations for the cure of cancer of the breast performed at the Johns Hopkins Hospital from June, 1889, to January, 1894. Ann Surg. 1894;20(5):497–555.
10. DE CHOLNOKY T. Late adverse results following breast reconstructions. Plast Reconstr Surg. 1963;31:445–52.
11. Halsted WS. I. The results of radical operations for the cure of carcinoma of the breast. Ann Surg. 1907;46(1):1–19.
12. Pennington DG. Breast reconstruction after mastectomy: current state of the art. ANZ J Surg. 2005;75(6):454–8.
13. Tajima T. [History of breast cancer surgery and its perspectives]. Nihon Geka Gakkai Zasshi. 2000;101(12):833–9.
14. Champaneria MC, Wong WW, Hill ME, Gupta SC. The evolution of breast reconstruction: a historical perspective. World J Surg. 2012;36(4):730–42.
15. Patey DH, Dyson WH. The prognosis of carcinoma of the breast in relation to the type of operation performed. Br J Cancer. 1948;2(1):7–13.
16. Du Z, Zhou Y, Chen J, Long Q, Lü Q. Retrospective observational study of breast reconstruction with extended latissimus dorsi flap following skin-sparing mastectomy. Medicine (Baltimore). 2018;97(31):e10936.
17. Fisher B, Anderson S, Bryant J, et al. Twenty-year follow-up of a randomized trial comparing total mastectomy, lumpectomy, and lumpectomy plus irradiation for the treatment of invasive breast cancer. N Engl J Med. 2002;347(16):1233–41.
18. Veronesi U, Cascinelli N, Mariani L, et al. Twenty-year follow-up of a randomized study comparing breast-conserving surgery with radical mastectomy for early breast cancer. N Engl J Med. 2002;347(16):1227–32.
19. Toth BA, Forley BG, Calabria R. Retrospective study of the skin-sparing mastectomy in breast reconstruction. Plast Reconstr Surg. 1999;104(1):77–84.
20. Carlson GW. Skin sparing mastectomy: anatomic and technical considerations. Am Surg. 1996;62(2):151–5.
21. Patani N, Mokbel K. Oncological and aesthetic considerations of skin-sparing mastectomy. Breast Cancer Res Treat. 2008;111(3):391–403.
22. Bartlett W. An anatomic substitute for the female breast. Ann Surg. 1917;66(2):208–11.
23. Uroskie TW, Colen LB. History of breast reconstruction. Semin Plast Surg. 2004;18(2):65–9.
24. Blichert-Toft M, Rose C, Andersen JA, et al. Danish randomized trial comparing breast conservation therapy with mastectomy: six years of life-table analysis. Danish Breast Cancer Cooperative Group. J Natl Cancer Inst Monogr. 1992;11:19–25.
25. Arriagada R, Lê MG, Rochard F, Contesso G. Conservative treatment versus mastectomy in early breast cancer: patterns of failure with 15 years of follow-up data. Institut Gustave-Roussy Breast Cancer Group. J Clin Oncol. 1996;14(5):1558–64.
26. van Dongen JA, Voogd AC, Fentiman IS, et al. Long-term results of a randomized trial comparing breast-conserving therapy with mastectomy: European Organization for Research and Treatment of Cancer 10801 trial. J Natl Cancer Inst. 2000;92(14):1143–50.
27. Poggi MM, Danforth DN, Sciuto LC, et al. Eighteen-year results in the treatment of early breast carcinoma with mastectomy versus breast conservation therapy: the National Cancer Institute Randomized Trial. Cancer. 2003;98(4):697–702.
28. Snyderman RK, Guthrie RH. Reconstruction of the female breast following radical mastectomy. Plast Reconstr Surg. 1971;47(6):565–7.
29. Sorta-Bilajac I, Muzur A. The nose between ethics and aesthetics: Sushruta's legacy. Otolaryngol Head Neck Surg. 2007;137(5):707–10.
30. Fredricks S. History of the American Society of Plastic and Reconstructive Surgeons. Plast Reconstr Surg. 1995;95(6):1135.
31. Ballard TN, Momoh AO. Advances in breast reconstruction of mastectomy and lumpectomy defects. Surg Oncol Clin N Am. 2014;23(3):525–48.
32. Jagsi R, Jiang J, Momoh AO, et al. Trends and variation in use of breast reconstruction in patients with breast cancer undergoing mastectomy in the United States. J Clin Oncol. 2014;32(9):919–26.
33. Saint-Cyr M, Dauwe P, Wong C, Thakar H, Nagarkar P, Rohrich RJ. Use of the serratus anterior fascia flap for expander coverage in breast reconstruction. Plast Reconstr Surg. 2010;125(4):1057–64.

34. Maxwell GP. Iginio Tansini and the origin of the latissimus dorsi musculocutaneous flap. Plast Reconstr Surg. 1980;65(5):686–92.
35. Gillies H. Surgical replacement of the breast. Proc R Soc Med. 1959;52:597–602.
36. Versaci AD. A method of reconstructing a pendulous breast utilizing the tissue expander. Plast Reconstr Surg. 1987;80(3):387–95.
37. Harris HI. Automammaplasty. J Int Coll Surg. 1949;12(6):827–39, illust.
38. Alexander JE, Block LI. Breast reconstruction following radical mastectomy. Plast Reconstr Surg. 1967;40(2):175–9.
39. Maliniac JW. Lessons of the postwar organization of plastic surgery in Europe. Plast Reconstr Surg (1946). 1950;6(1):38–40.
40. Yannilos HG. The use of composite tube pedicle in the reconstruction of breast defect with subsequent cosmetic repair of the donor breast. Plast Reconstr Surg (1946). 1950;6(5):396–9.
41. Holdsworth WG. A method of reconstructing the breast. Br J Plast Surg. 1956;9(2):161–2.
42. Millard DR. Breast reconstruction after a radical mastectomy. Plast Reconstr Surg. 1976;58(3):283–91.
43. Tai Y, Hasegawa H. A transverse abdominal flap for reconstruction after radical operations for recurrent breast cancer. Plast Reconstr Surg. 1974;53(1):52–4.
44. De Cholnoky T. Breast reconstruction after radical mastectomy: formation of missing nipple by everted navel. Plast Reconstr Surg. 1966;38(6):577–80.
45. McCraw JB. The recent history of myocutaneous flaps. Clin Plast Surg. 1980;7(1):3–7.
46. Davis HH, Tollman JP, Brush JH. Huge chondrosarcoma of rib, report of a case. Surgery. 1949;26(4):699–704.
47. Campbell DA. Reconstruction of the anterior thoracic wall. J Thorac Surg. 1950;19(3):456–61.
48. McCraw JB, Dibbell DG, Carraway JH. Clinical definition of independent myocutaneous vascular territories. Plast Reconstr Surg. 1977;60(3):341–52.
49. Olivari N. The latissimus flap. Br J Plast Surg. 1976;29(2):126–8.
50. Schneider WJ, Hill HL, Brown RG. Latissimus dorsi myocutaneous flap for breast reconstruction. Br J Plast Surg. 1977;30(4):277–81.
51. Mendelson BC, Masson JK. Treatment of chronic radiation injury over the shoulder with a latissimus dorsi myocutaneous flap. Plast Reconstr Surg. 1977;60(5):681–91.
52. Bostwick J, Jurkiewicz MJ. Recent advances in breast reconstruction: transposition of the latissimus dorsi muscle singly or with the overlying skin. Am Surg. 1980;46(10):537–47.
53. Bostwick J, Scheflan M. The latissimus dorsi musculocutaneous flap: a one-stage breast reconstruction. Clin Plast Surg. 1980;7(1):71–8.
54. Maxwell GP, Leonard LG, Manson PN, Hoopes JE. Craniofacial coverage using the latissimus dorsi myocutaneous Island flap. Ann Plast Surg. 1980;4(5):410–21.
55. Maxwell GP, McGibbon BM, Hoopes JE. Vascular considerations in the use of a latissimus dorsi myocutaneous flap after a mastectomy with an axillary dissection. Plast Reconstr Surg. 1979;64(6):771–80.
56. Elliott LF, Raffel B, Wade J. Segmental latissimus dorsi free flap: clinical applications. Ann Plast Surg. 1989;23(3):231–8.
57. Angrigiani C, Grilli D, Siebert J. Latissimus dorsi musculocutaneous flap without muscle. Plast Reconstr Surg. 1995;96(7):1608–14.
58. Hollos P. Breast augmentation with autologous tissue: an alternative to implants. Plast Reconstr Surg. 1995;96(2):381–4; discussion 385.
59. Hammond DC. Postmastectomy reconstruction of the breast using the latissimus dorsi musculocutaneous flap. Cancer J. 2008;14(4):248–52.
60. Milloy FJ, Anson BJ, Mcafee DK. The rectus abdominis muscle and the epigastric arteries. Surg Gynecol Obstet. 1960;110:293–302.
61. Scheflan M, Dinner MI. The transverse abdominal Island flap: part II. Surgical technique. Ann Plast Surg. 1983;10(2):120–9.
62. Bucky LP, May JW. Synthetic mesh. Its use in abdominal wall reconstruction after the TRAM. Clin Plast Surg. 1994;21(2):273–7.
63. Drever JM. Total breast reconstruction with either of two abdominal flaps. Plast Reconstr Surg. 1977;59(2):185–90.
64. Taylor GI, Daniel RK. The anatomy of several free flap donor sites. Plast Reconstr Surg. 1975;56(3):243–53.
65. Höhler H. [Carcinoma of the breast. Reconstructive surgery]. Langenbecks Arch Chir. 1977;345:78–86.
66. Brown RG, Fleming WH, Jurkiewicz MJ. An Island flap of the pectoralis major muscle. Br J Plast Surg. 1977;30(2):161–5.
67. Mathes SJ, Bostwick J. A rectus abdominis myocutaneous flap to reconstruct abdominal wall defects. Br J Plast Surg. 1977;30(4):282–3.
68. Koshima I, Moriguchi T, Soeda S, Tanaka H, Umeda N. Free thin paraumbilical perforator-based flaps. Ann Plast Surg. 1992;29(1):12–7.
69. Marshall DR, Anstee EJ, Stapleton MJ. Post-mastectomy breast reconstruction using a direct flap from an abdominal lipectomy. Br J Plast Surg. 1981;34(3):280–5.
70. Robbins TH. Rectus abdominis myocutaneous flap for breast reconstruction. Aust N Z J Surg. 1979;49(5):527–30.
71. Robbins TH. Post-mastectomy breast reconstruction using a rectus abdominis musculocutaneous Island flap. Br J Plast Surg. 1981;34(3):286–90.
72. Drever JM. The epigastric Island flap. Plast Reconstr Surg. 1977;59(3):343–6.
73. Hartrampf CR, Scheflan M, Black PW. Breast reconstruction with a transverse abdominal Island flap. Plast Reconstr Surg. 1982;69(2):216–25.
74. Grotting JC, Urist MM, Maddox WA, Vasconez LO. Conventional TRAM flap versus free microsurgical TRAM flap for immediate breast reconstruction. Plast Reconstr Surg. 1989;83(5):828–41; discussion 842–4.
75. Grotting JC. The free abdominoplasty flap for immediate breast reconstruction. Ann Plast Surg. 1991;27(4):351–4.
76. Allen RJ, Treece P. Deep inferior epigastric perforator flap for breast reconstruction. Ann Plast Surg. 1994;32(1):32–8.
77. Drever JM. Total breast reconstruction. Ann Plast Surg. 1981;7(1):54–61.
78. Marino H, Dogliotti P. Mammary reconstruction with bipedicled abdominal flap. Plast Reconstr Surg. 1981;68(6):933–6.
79. Semple JL. Retrograde microvascular augmentation (turbocharging) of a single-pedicle TRAM flap through a deep inferior epigastric arterial and venous loop. Plast Reconstr Surg. 1994;93(1):109–17.
80. Harashina T, Sone K, Inoue T, Fukuzumi S, Enomoto K. Augmentation of circulation of pedicled transverse rectus abdominis musculocutaneous flaps by microvascular surgery. Br J Plast Surg. 1987;40(4):367–70.
81. Codner MA, Bostwick J, Nahai F, Bried JT, Eaves FF. TRAM flap vascular delay for high-risk breast reconstruction. Plast Reconstr Surg. 1995;96(7):1615–22.
82. Moon HK, Taylor GI. The vascular anatomy of rectus abdominis musculocutaneous flaps based on the deep superior epigastric system. Plast Reconstr Surg. 1988;82(5):815–32.
83. Hartrampf CR, Bennett GK. Autogenous tissue reconstruction in the mastectomy patient. A critical review of 300 patients. Ann Surg. 1987;205(5):508–19.
84. Hartrampf CR, Noel RT, Drazan L, Elliott FL, Bennett GK, Beegle PH. Ruben's fat pad for breast reconstruction: a peri-iliac soft-tissue free flap. Plast Reconstr Surg. 1994;93(2):402–7.

85. Taylor GI, Townsend P, Corlett R. Superiority of the deep circumflex iliac vessels as the supply for free groin flaps. Plast Reconstr Surg. 1979;64(5):595–604.
86. Daniel RK, Taylor GI. Distant transfer of an Island flap by microvascular anastomoses. A clinical technique. Plast Reconstr Surg. 1973;52(2):111–7.
87. Taylor GI, Daniel RK. The free flap: composite tissue transfer by vascular anastomosis. Aust N Z J Surg. 1973;43(1):1–3.
88. Fujino T, Harasina T, Aoyagi F. Reconstruction for aplasia of the breast and pectoral region by microvascular transfer of a free flap from the buttock. Plast Reconstr Surg. 1975;56(2):178–81.
89. Fujino T, Harashina T, Enomoto K. Primary breast reconstruction after a standard radical mastectomy by a free flap transfer. Case report. Plast Reconstr Surg. 1976;58(3):371–4.
90. Elliott LF, Beegle PH, Hartrampf CR. The lateral transverse thigh free flap: an alternative for autogenous-tissue breast reconstruction. Plast Reconstr Surg. 1990;85(2):169–78; discussion 179–81.
91. Wei FC, Suominen S, Cheng MH, Celik N, Lai YL. Anterolateral thigh flap for postmastectomy breast reconstruction. Plast Reconstr Surg. 2002;110(1):82–8.
92. Fujino T, Abe O, Enomoto K. Primary reconstruction of the breast by free myocutaneous gluteal flap. Int Adv Surg Oncol. 1981;4:127–43.
93. Boustred AM, Nahai F. Inferior gluteal free flap breast reconstruction. Clin Plast Surg. 1998;25(2):275–82.
94. Allen RJ, Tucker C. Superior gluteal artery perforator free flap for breast reconstruction. Plast Reconstr Surg. 1995;95(7):1207–12.
95. Peek A, Müller M, Exner K. [The free gracilis perforator flap for autologous breast reconstruction]. Handchir Mikrochir Plast Chir. 2002;34(4):245–50.
96. Hartrampf CR, Elliott LF, Feldman S. A triceps musculocutaneous flap for chest-wall defects. Plast Reconstr Surg. 1990;86(3):502–9.
97. Harii K, Ohmori K, Torii S. Free gracilis muscle transplantation, with microneurovascular anastomoses for the treatment of facial paralysis. A preliminary report. Plast Reconstr Surg. 1976;57(2):133–43.
98. Serafin D, Georgiade NG. Transfer of free flaps to provide well-vascularized, thick cover for breast reconstructions after radical mastectomy. Plast Reconstr Surg. 1978;62(4):527–36.
99. Serafin D, Voci VE, Georgiade NG. Microsurgical composite tissue transplantation: indications and technical considerations in breast reconstruction following mastectomy. Plast Reconstr Surg. 1982;70(1):24–36.
100. Holmström H. The free abdominoplasty flap and its use in breast reconstruction. An experimental study and clinical case report. Scand J Plast Reconstr Surg. 1979;13(3):423–7.
101. Rizzuto RP, Allen RJ. Reconstruction of a partial mastectomy defect with the superficial deep inferior epigastric artery (SIEA) flap. J Reconstr Microsurg. 2004;20(6):441–5; discussion 446.
102. Granzow JW, Levine JL, Chiu ES, Allen RJ. Breast reconstruction with the deep inferior epigastric perforator flap: history and an update on current technique. J Plast Reconstr Aesthet Surg. 2006;59(6):571–9.
103. Taylor GI, Corlett R, Boyd JB. The extended deep inferior epigastric flap: a clinical technique. Plast Reconstr Surg. 1983;72(6):751–65.
104. Friedman RJ, Argenta LC, Anderson R. Deep inferior epigastric free flap for breast reconstruction after radical mastectomy. Plast Reconstr Surg. 1985;76(3):455–60.
105. Kroll SS, Rosenfield L. Perforator-based flaps for low posterior midline defects. Plast Reconstr Surg. 1988;81(4):561–6.
106. Onishi K, Maruyama Y. Cutaneous and fascial vasculature around the rectus abdominis muscle: anatomic basis of abdominal fasciocutaneous flaps. J Reconstr Microsurg. 1986;2(4):247–53.
107. Koshima I, Soeda S. Deep inferior epigastric artery skin flaps without rectus abdominis muscle. Br J Plast Surg. 1989;42(6):645–8.
108. Blondeel PN, Boeckx WD. Refinements in free flap breast reconstruction: the free bilateral deep inferior epigastric perforator flap anastomosed to the internal mammary artery. Br J Plast Surg. 1994;47(7):495–501.
109. Blondeel PN. One hundred free DIEP flap breast reconstructions: a personal experience. Br J Plast Surg. 1999;52(2):104–11.
110. Blondeel N, Vanderstraeten GG, Monstrey SJ, et al. The donor site morbidity of free DIEP flaps and free TRAM flaps for breast reconstruction. Br J Plast Surg. 1997;50(5):322–30.
111. Blondeel PN, Arnstein M, Verstraete K, et al. Venous congestion and blood flow in free transverse rectus abdominis myocutaneous and deep inferior epigastric perforator flaps. Plast Reconstr Surg. 2000;106(6):1295–9.
112. Kroll SS, Schusterman MA, Reece GP, Miller MJ, Robb G, Evans G. Abdominal wall strength, bulging, and hernia after TRAM flap breast reconstruction. Plast Reconstr Surg. 1995;96(3):616–9.
113. Mizgala CL, Hartrampf CR, Bennett GK. Abdominal function after pedicled TRAM flap surgery. Clin Plast Surg. 1994;21(2):255–72.
114. Arnez ZM, Khan U, Pogorelec D, Planinsek F. Breast reconstruction using the free superficial deep inferior epigastric artery (SIEA) flap. Br J Plast Surg. 1999;52(4):276–9.
115. Chevray PM. Breast reconstruction with superficial deep inferior epigastric artery flaps: a prospective comparison with TRAM and DIEP flaps. Plast Reconstr Surg. 2004;114(5):1077–83; discussion 1084–5.
116. Elliott LF, Hartrampf CR. The Rubens flap. The deep circumflex iliac artery flap. Clin Plast Surg. 1998;25(2):283–91.
117. Bergeron L, Tang M, Morris SF. The anatomical basis of the deep circumflex iliac artery perforator flap with iliac crest. Plast Reconstr Surg. 2007;120(1):252–8.
118. Hokin JA, Silfverskiold KL. Breast reconstruction without an implant: results and complications using an extended latissimus dorsi flap. Plast Reconstr Surg. 1987;79(1):58–66.
119. Holmström H, Lossing C. The lateral thoracodorsal flap in breast reconstruction. Plast Reconstr Surg. 1986;77(6):933–43.
120. Munhoz AM, Montag E, Arruda EG, et al. The role of the lateral thoracodorsal fasciocutaneous flap in immediate conservative breast surgery reconstruction. Plast Reconstr Surg. 2006;117(6):1699–710.
121. Yang JD, Ryu DW, Lee JW, et al. Usefulness of a lateral thoracodorsal flap after breast conserving surgery in laterally located breast cancer. Arch Plast Surg. 2013;40(4):367–73.
122. Thomas BP, Geddes CR, Tang M, Williams J, Morris SF. The vascular basis of the thoracodorsal artery perforator flap. Plast Reconstr Surg. 2005;116(3):818–22.
123. Hamdi M, Van Landuyt K, Monstrey S, Blondeel P. Pedicled perforator flaps in breast reconstruction: a new concept. Br J Plast Surg. 2004;57(6):531–9.
124. Hamdi M, Spano A, Van Landuyt K, D'Herde K, Blondeel P, Monstrey S. The lateral intercostal artery perforators: anatomical study and clinical application in breast surgery. Plast Reconstr Surg. 2008;121(2):389–96.
125. Hamdi M, Van Landuyt K, de Frene B, Roche N, Blondeel P, Monstrey S. The versatility of the inter-costal artery perforator (ICAP) flaps. J Plast Reconstr Aesthet Surg. 2006;59(6):644–52.
126. Orticochea M. Use of the buttock to reconstruct the breast. Br J Plast Surg. 1973;26(3):304–9.
127. Ahmadzadeh R, Bergeron L, Tang M, Morris SF. The superior and inferior gluteal artery perforator flaps. Plast Reconstr Surg. 2007;120(6):1551–6.
128. Tuinder S, Van Der Hulst R. Introducing the septocutaneous gluteal artery perforator flap: a simplified approach to microsurgical breast reconstruction. Plast Reconstr Surg. 2012;129(5):848e–9e; author reply 849e.

129. Kato H, Hasegawa M, Takada T, Torii S. The lumbar artery perforator based Island flap: anatomical study and case reports. Br J Plast Surg. 1999;52(7):541–6.
130. de Weerd L, Elvenes OP, Strandenes E, Weum S. Autologous breast reconstruction with a free lumbar artery perforator flap. Br J Plast Surg. 2003;56(2):180–3.
131. Ao M, Mae O, Namba Y, Asagoe K. Perforator-based flap for coverage of lumbosacral defects. Plast Reconstr Surg. 1998;101(4):987–91.
132. Hurwitz DJ. Closure of a large defect of the pelvic cavity by an extended compound myocutaneous flap based on the inferior gluteal artery. Br J Plast Surg. 1980;33(2):256–61.
133. Hurwitz DJ, Swartz WM, Mathes SJ. The gluteal thigh flap: a reliable, sensate flap for the closure of buttock and perineal wounds. Plast Reconstr Surg. 1981;68(4):521–32.
134. Jósvay J, Donáth A. Modified hamstring musculocutaneous flap for the coverage of ischial pressure sores. Plast Reconstr Surg. 1999;103(6):1715–8.
135. Baek SM. Two new cutaneous free flaps: the medial and lateral thigh flaps. Plast Reconstr Surg. 1983;71(3):354–65.
136. Song D, Li Z, Zhou X. Application of gracilis muscle flap combined with adductor magnus perforator flap in breast reconstruction. Chin J Reparat Reconstr Surg. 2018;32(06):707–13.
137. Song YG, Chen GZ, Song YL. The free thigh flap: a new free flap concept based on the septocutaneous artery. Br J Plast Surg. 1984;37(2):149–59.
138. Angrigiani C, Grilli D, Thorne CH. The adductor flap: a new method for transferring posterior and medial thigh skin. Plast Reconstr Surg. 2001;107(7):1725–31.
139. Ahmadzadeh R, Bergeron L, Tang M, Geddes CR, Morris SF. The posterior thigh perforator flap or profunda femoris artery perforator flap. Plast Reconstr Surg. 2007;119(1):194–200; discussion 201–2.
140. Allen RJ, Haddock NT, Ahn CY, Sadeghi A. Breast reconstruction with the profunda artery perforator flap. Plast Reconstr Surg. 2012;129(1):16e–23e.
141. Weichman KE, Broer PN, Tanna N, et al. The role of autologous fat grafting in secondary microsurgical breast reconstruction. Ann Plast Surg. 2013;71(1):24–30.
142. Uda H, Sugawara Y, Sarukawa S, Sunaga A. Brava and autologous fat grafting for breast reconstruction after cancer surgery. Plast Reconstr Surg. 2014;133(2):203–13.
143. Findlay MW, Dolderer JH, Trost N, et al. Tissue-engineered breast reconstruction: bridging the gap toward large-volume tissue engineering in humans. Plast Reconstr Surg. 2011;128(6):1206–15.
144. Koshima I, Nanba Y, Tsutsui T, Takahashi Y, Itoh S. Long-term follow-up after lymphaticovenular anastomosis for lymphedema in the leg. J Reconstr Microsurg. 2003;19(4):209–15.
145. Koshima I, Inagawa K, Urushibara K, Moriguchi T. Supermicrosurgical lymphaticovenular anastomosis for the treatment of lymphedema in the upper extremities. J Reconstr Microsurg. 2000;16(6):437–42.
146. Becker C, Assouad J, Riquet M, Hidden G. Postmastectomy lymphedema: long-term results following microsurgical lymph node transplantation. Ann Surg. 2006;243(3):313–5.
147. Lin CH, Ali R, Chen SC, et al. Vascularized groin lymph node transfer using the wrist as a recipient site for management of postmastectomy upper extremity lymphedema. Plast Reconstr Surg. 2009;123(4):1265–75.
148. Saaristo AM, Niemi TS, Viitanen TP, Tervala TV, Hartiala P, Suominen EA. Microvascular breast reconstruction and lymph node transfer for postmastectomy lymphedema patients. Ann Surg. 2012;255(3):468–73.

History of DIEP Flap in Breast and Chest Wall Reconstruction

2

Zan Li, Georgios Pafitanis, and Rene D. Largo

2.1 Background and Development of Inferior Abdominal Artery Perforator Flap for Breast Reconstruction and Chest Wall Reconstruction

The perforator vessels of deep inferior epigastric artery perforator (DIEP) flap start from the inferior deep abdominal artery and pass through the rectus abdominis muscle. This flap was firstly reported by Japanese doctor Hiroshima (Koshima) in 1989 and first used for breast reconstruction by American doctor Allen in 1994. It is the most widely used perforator flap in clinical research and application.

Among all types of autologous breast reconstruction, the current gold standard is to use perforator flap, especially DIEP flap for breast reconstruction.

Because of its long-lasting, natural, symmetrical, less complicated, and stable and reliable clinical effect, DIEP flap is widely popular in breast reconstruction [1] (Fig. 2.1).

By using abdominal skin and adipose tissue to reconstruct breast, DIEP flap plastic repair realizes the principle of "similarity and substitution."

After DIEP flap became the gold standard of autologous breast reconstruction, it was gradually accepted all over the world. In practice, we found that the success rate of free tissue flap transplantation was higher than that of other reconstruction techniques.

In more than 500 cases of DIEP flap transplantation, our success rate has exceeded 99%, and in the past 10 years, with the development of preoperative imaging technologies such as CTA and MRA, the operation time has been effectively shortened.

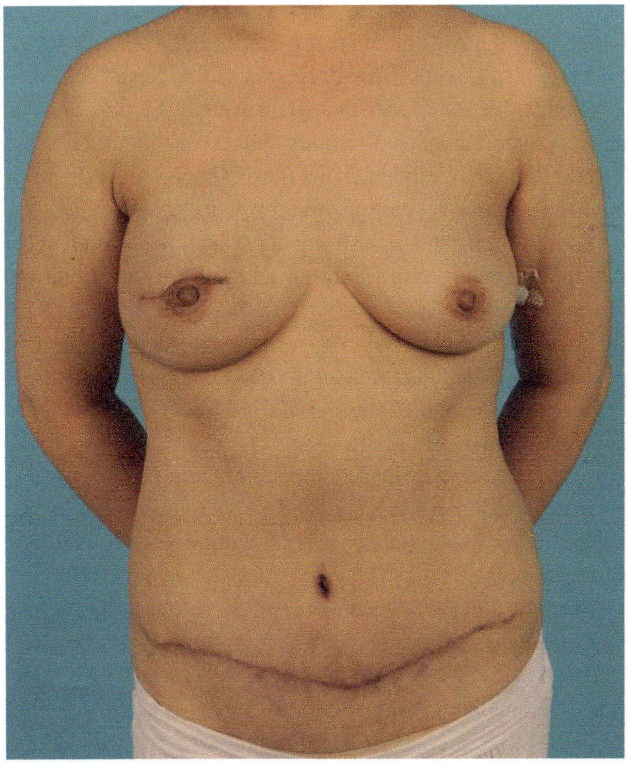

Fig. 2.1 The effect of breast reconstruction with DIEP flap is satisfactory

2.1.1 Advantages and Disadvantages

Since the first report and description, it has been proved that DIEP flap is a valuable and safe flap that can replace traditional TRAM as long as surgeons master the anatomy and anastomosis technique of perforating branches.

The choice of a traditional rectus abdominis flap or a muscle-containing flap or a real short pedicled perforator

Z. Li (✉)
Department of Oncology Plastic Surgery, Hunan Cancer Hospital, Changsha, Hunan, China

G. Pafitanis
Trauma, Orthoplastic, Lower Extremity and Head and Neck Reconstruction Center, London, UK

R. D. Largo
Department of Plastic Surgery, The University of Texas MD Anderson Cancer Center, Houston, TX, USA
e-mail: rdlargo@mdanderson.org

Z. Li, D. Song (eds.), *Oncoplastic Flap Surgery*, https://doi.org/10.1007/978-981-19-8926-1_2

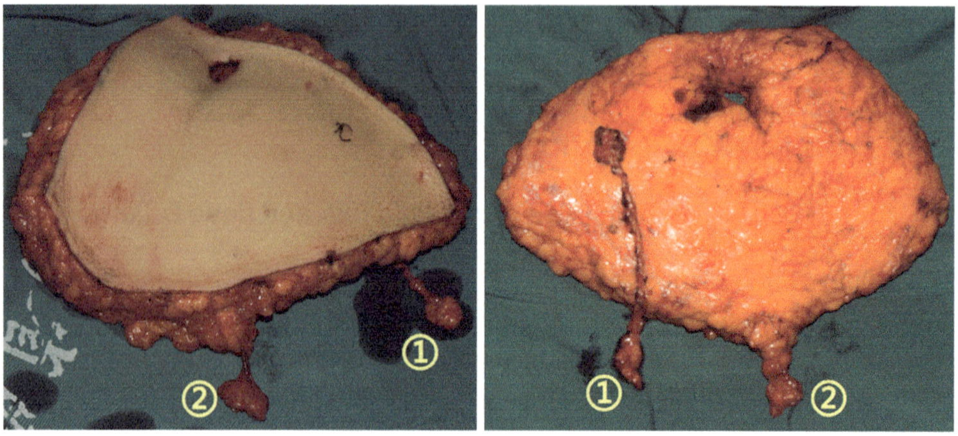

Fig. 2.2 Free DIEP flap with superficial abdominal vein

flap mainly depends on microsurgical skills, while other factors may also affect the final decision of flap type.

Blondeel et al. reported that when using DIEP flap, area IV had a greater incidence of venous obstruction than traditional TRAM flap. They explained that the drainage vein in this area mainly depended on the superficial venous system [2].

Therefore, if there is a strong superficial abdominal vein, they recommend establishing an additional venous anastomosis (Fig. 2.2).

Tran et al. established extra venous drainage in 5 of 100 consecutive DIEP flap grafts with good results [3].

Venous drainage in areas I–III is always completed by deep abdominal vein [2, 4].

If it is found that the accompanying vein in the vascular pedicle is extensively embolized, a venous bypass established by the ipsilateral superficial abdominal vein is a feasible choice [3].

Even if the main accompanying vein anastomosis has been unblocked, the superficial vein of the flap can be anastomosed with any vein in the chest wall to establish additional venous reflux pathway.

In addition, a countercurrent venous anastomosis can be established between the superficial abdominal vein and the inferior abdominal vein [5].

On the other hand, Cheng et al. found that Zone IV necrosis only happened in only one of the 74 flaps, but the incidence of fat necrosis was 13.5% [6].

Schaverien et al. used computed tomography angiography to observe DIEP flap on fresh cadavers. It showed that area IV was not perfused after the injection of contrast medium in the lateral row perforating branch, which suggested that the blood supply of Area IV was based on the medial row perforating branch [7].

In our clinical experience, we found that only in two cases can the single perforating branch of the lateral row provide blood supply for the whole lower abdominal flap (Figs. 2.3 and 2.4).

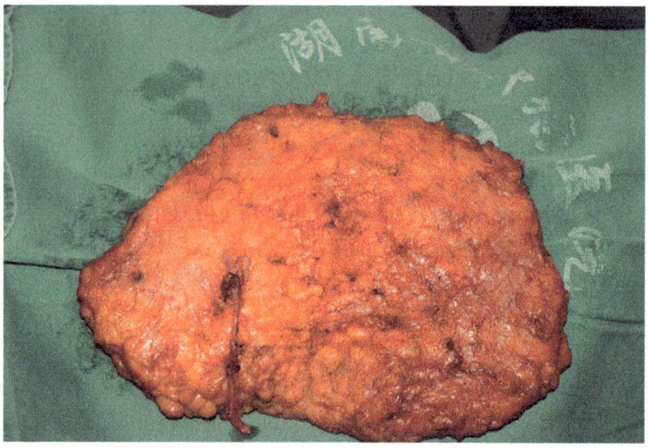

Fig. 2.3 In the first case, there is no large perforator vessel in the medial row, and the perforator vessel in the lateral row is relatively large. With it as the pedicle, the free DIEP flap can be safely cut

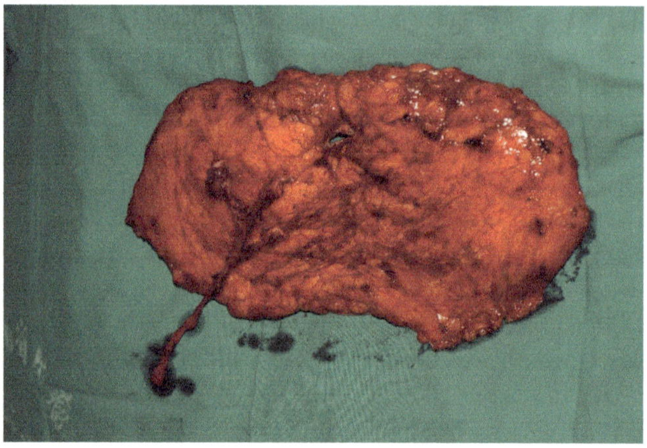

Fig. 2.4 In the second case, there are no large perforating vessels in the medial row, and there are multiple perforating vessels in the lateral row, but there is no dominant type. It is also safe to cut the free DIEP flap with multiple perforating vessels at the same time

Like anterolateral femoral perforator flap, preoperative imaging methods have also been used in the design of DIEP flap.

Rozen et al. found a good correlation between the detection results and intraoperative findings by CT angiography [8]. Blondeel and colleagues prefer to use color Doppler scanning for preoperative evaluation [9].

As an alternative to the commonly used horizontal design method, some experts put forward the idea of designing DIEP flap in the vertical direction, especially in patients with scar left in the abdominal midline, the length of the flap can be extended to 13 cm [10, 11] (Fig. 2.5).

By including sensory branches carrying segmental nerves accompanying perforator vessels, sensation can be reconstructed when the breast is reconstructed with perforator flap homograft.

After completing the nerve suture repair, compared with the flap without reconstructed sensation, the flap can restore the sense of temperature and pressure [12] (Fig. 2.6).

2.1.2 Indications

The most suitable population for breast reconstruction with DIEP flap is women who have enough abdominal fat, have no serious basic diseases, and have never received autologous tissue breast reconstruction before. Women with multiple pregnancies are best candidate.

The skin and fat of their abdomen have been naturally expanded many times, making their abdomen an ideal donor area for breast reconstruction with DIEP flap.

Another common indication for DIEP flap breast reconstruction is when prosthesis implantation fails [13].

About 20% of patients who underwent breast reconstruction with implant prosthesis suffer from implant-related problems including infection, capsule contracture, and prosthesis displacement. Patients with breast cancer undergoing postoperative radiotherapy are most vulnerable. Using self-tissue breast reconstruction can create a new and relatively natural breast for them (see typical cases in this chapter, Figs. 2.9, 2.10, 2.11, 2.12, 2.13, 2.14, 2.15, 2.16, 2.17, 2.18, and 2.19).

Therefore, we recommend autologous breast reconstruction.

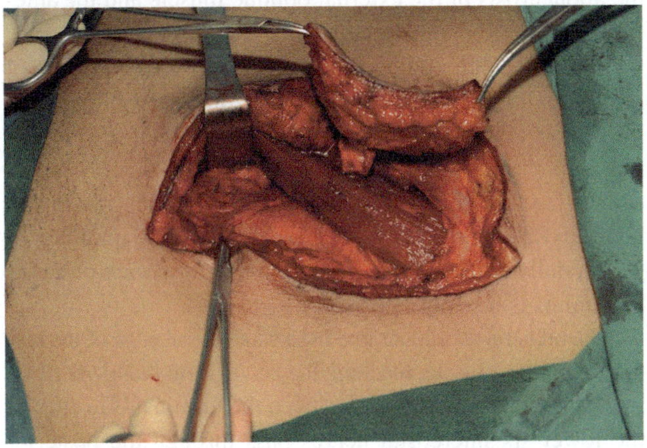

Fig. 2.5 DIEP flap is designed and cut in the vertical direction

2.1.3 Contraindication

The main contraindication of DIEP flap breast reconstruction is serious clinical basic diseases, such as serious cardiopulmonary diseases and other systemic diseases affecting the reconstruction operation.

Breast reconstruction is an option for patients, but even if it can benefit patients psychologically, attention should be paid to avoid affecting patients' quality of life.

Other risk factors to be considered include coagulation dysfunction, autoimmune diseases, obesity, history of abdominal surgery, and history of radiotherapy.

In addition, smoking is also significantly associated with the incidence of complications. Therefore, smoking cessation is required at least 4 weeks before operation.

For patients who may need radiotherapy after operation, tissue expander can be placed for delayed breast reconstruction to avoid the complications caused by radiotherapy.

Abdominal fat requires sufficient blood supply from the inferior abdominal artery. Therefore, women with a history of abdominal plastic surgery are not suitable for DIEP flap for breast reconstruction.

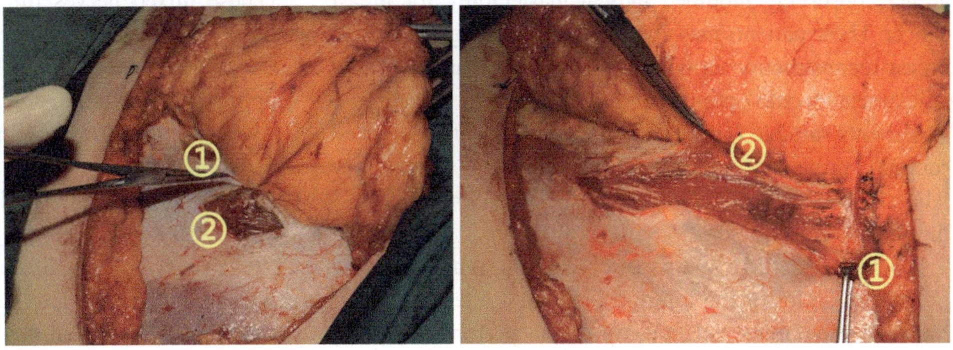

Fig. 2.6 DIEP flap with sensory branch of intercostal nerve was cut

Similarly, women who once received extensive abdominal surgery or gynecological pelvic organ resection should undergo imaging examination before DIEP flap breast reconstruction to ensure that the perforating branches of subabdominal vessels are still intact.

It is worth mentioning that although liposuction is not an absolute taboo for DIEP flap breast reconstruction, emaciated women with thin abdominal fat layer may not have enough subcutaneous tissue for surgeons to reconstruct a satisfactory breast.

For such women, we can choose thighs, back, and hips as donor areas for autologous breast reconstruction.

2.1.4 Preoperative Planning

All patients need to receive detailed preoperative talks to understand the surgical objectives, alternatives, expectations about postoperative effect, and possible complications.

Only in this way can patients actively participate in the process of surgical decision-making and the technical choice of breast reconstruction.

In the initial consultation stage, it is necessary to inform patients preparing for breast reconstruction with DIEP flap that they need to go through three steps.

The first step is DIEP flap breast reconstruction (for unilateral breast reconstruction, one-stage or two-stage contralateral breast lift, breast augmentation or breast reduction should also be considered.

The second stage is nipple reconstruction.

If the nipple is retained during mastectomy, trimming of the donor area, the reconstructed breast, and the contralateral breast is completed in the second step.

For example, excess tissue or necrotic fat in the donor area will be removed in this step.

The third step is to tattoo the nipple areola complex when nipple reconstruction is needed.

The first step requires hospitalization, and the average length of hospitalization is 7–14 days.

The second and third steps are generally carried out in the outpatient operating room.

At present, more and more patients are undergoing nipple-areola conserving modified radical mastectomy for breast cancer. These patients may complete the first stage DIEP flap breast reconstruction in only one step. Whereas sequential adjustments would optimize the final outlook.

Patients suitable for DIEP flap breast reconstruction need routine preoperative evaluation, including necessary laboratory examination and diagnostic research, and anesthesiologic consultation.

Using CTA or MRA, we can observe the running course of the perforator of the inferior abdominal artery and estimate the anatomical relationship of the perforator vessels required during the operation, so that there is no need to waste time in selecting the perforator vessels under general anesthesia.

In this way, surgeons can quickly identify the largest and most reliable perforating vessels, which significantly reduces the operation time and contributes to the safety and smooth recovery of patients.

In addition, imaging examination is not only used to locate the vessels in the recipient area, but also to estimate the volume of DIEP flap.

2.1.5 Anatomy

Rectus abdominis and external oblique abdominis together form the anterior abdominal wall; when the DIEP flap was cut, the rectus abdominis was almost completely unaffected.

Rectus abdominis muscle starts from the sixth, seventh, and eighth ribs and xiphoid cartilage. It is divided into four parts by tendon.

In about 80% of the population, the rectus abdominis is covered by the pyramidal muscle at its end of the pubis.

The muscle enters the rectus abdominis sheath and forms a white line without muscle surrounding at the midline.

The anterior sheath of rectus abdominis is composed of the aponeurosis of the external oblique muscle and the anterior layer of the aponeurosis of the internal oblique muscle.

Behind the rectus abdominis, the posterior sheath of rectus abdominis is formed by the internal oblique and transverse abdominal muscles in the far area of the arcuate line.

The arcuate lines on both sides protrude proximally between the anterior superior iliac spine and the midline.

Caudally to the arcuate line, the posterior sheath of rectus abdominis is missing.

The bilateral semilunar line marks the lateral edge of the rectus abdominis muscle, reaching the pelvis from the lower ribs.

Here, the segmental nerves from the terminal branches of the lower six intercostal nerves pass through the posterior sheath of rectus abdominis at the 3 cm plane inside the semilunar line to provide motor function for rectus abdominis and sensory innervation for abdominal skin.

These mixed nerves run between the rectus abdominis and the internal oblique abdominis.

According to Mathes and Nahai's classification, the blood supply type of abdominal skin and rectus abdominis is type III, which comes from the inferior epigastric artery (DIEA) and two accompanying veins running on the posterior surface of rectus abdominis in the rectus sheath (Fig. 2.7).

The DIEA runs proximally to the umbilicus and connects with the superior abdominal artery from the internal thoracic vessels; therefore, the deep superior epigastric artery (DSEA) can be another option of vessel pedicle [14].

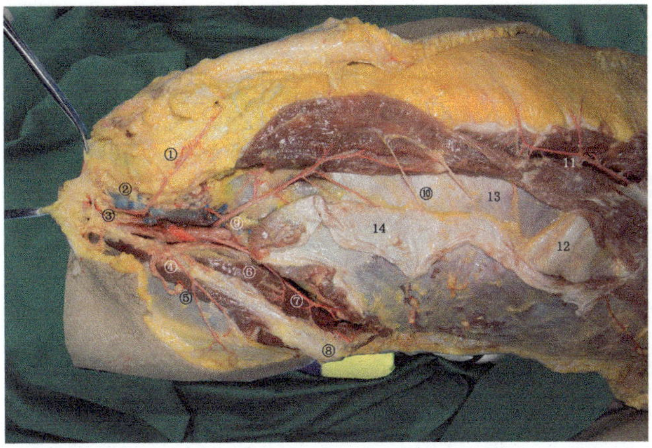

Fig. 2.7 Anatomy of rectus abdominis and its related tissues. (1) Superficial abdominal artery; (2) Femoral artery and vein; (3) Anterior femoral cutaneous artery; (4) Superficial iliac circumflex artery; (5) Sartorius muscle; (6) Iliopsoas muscle; (7) Deep iliac circumflex artery; (8) Anterior superior iliac spine; (9) deep inferior epigastric artery; (10) Segmental intercostal nerve; (11) Superior epigastric artery; (12) Costal arch; (13) Posterior sheath of rectus abdominis; (14) Anterior sheath of rectus abdominis

DIEA originates from the external iliac artery on the opposite side of the deep iliac circumflex artery (DCIA).

It runs toward the proximal midline outside the peritoneum, reaches the lateral edge of rectus abdominis, and passes through the transverse abdominal fascia 3–4 cm away from the arcuate line.

Blood vessels enter the rectus abdominis on the posterior surface of the rectus abdominis, in 78% of the cases at the lower one-third part of the rectus abdominis, in 17% of the cases at the distal end, and in 5% of the cases at the proximal end of the muscle [15].

The diameter of arteries and veins is large, ranging from 2 to 4.5 mm. The average length of blood vessels before entering the muscle is 10 cm.

In most cases, the veins merge before joining the external iliac vein.

Boyd and his colleagues have shown that the DIEAs dominates the blood supply of the anterior abdominal wall.

In addition to communicating with the superior epigastric artery (DSEA), DIEA vessels anastomose with the branches of intercostal arteries proximally and with the deep inferior epigastric artery (SIEA) laterally and distally.

The branches of the paraumbilical perforator diverge and distribute in all directions of the abdominal skin. Therefore, the flap can be cut in any direction of the abdominal skin.

However, according to Taylor's anatomical work, these branches predominantly distribute at an angle of 45° to horizontal level, which makes the design of oblique flap the most safe and reliable [16].

Based on the clinical experience of 16 single pedicled TRAM flaps, Hartrampf described four perfusion areas in the lower abdomen, which have been adopted by free rectus abdominis flap and perforator flap of inferior abdominal artery.

When a transverse flap is designed to be cut, it extends to both sides of the abdomen. Four flap areas are defined as: zone I is located in the ipsilateral rectus abdominis region, and zone III is the lateral region of the ipsilateral transverse semilunar line; The corresponding zones II and IV are located on the opposite side of the pedicle.

Studies on injection of contrast agents have confirmed that the blood supply of area IV is the poorest [17].

Using laser-induced fluorescence indocyanine green, Holm et al. found that there was little or no perfusion in zone IV, and the best perfusion areas were zones I and III [18].

In addition, selective dye injection showed that areas I–III were constantly supplied by a single perforating branch, while the fourth area was only partially stained or not stained at all [19].

Blondeel and his colleagues conducted detailed anatomical and blood flow studies on DIEA [20, 21].

They found that the DIEA was divided into two branches in about 75% of the subjects, of which the lateral branch was the dominant vessel (54%).

Eighteen percent of the medial branches have a larger diameter, but the blood flow through the perforating branches is the lowest in these examples.

According to the results, in 28% of the cases, there is only one accompanying vein to the DIEA and multiple collateral branches on the deep surface of the muscle.

Other clinical and anatomical results show that in 14% of the cases, the vascular pedicle can also be divided into three branches, so that the muscles can be separated without endangering the blood supply of each segment [22].

Therefore, the perforator can penetrate the muscle from the outside, inside, or center. It is often found that DIEA cutaneous perforators are most densely distributed around the umbilicus [23] (Fig. 2.8).

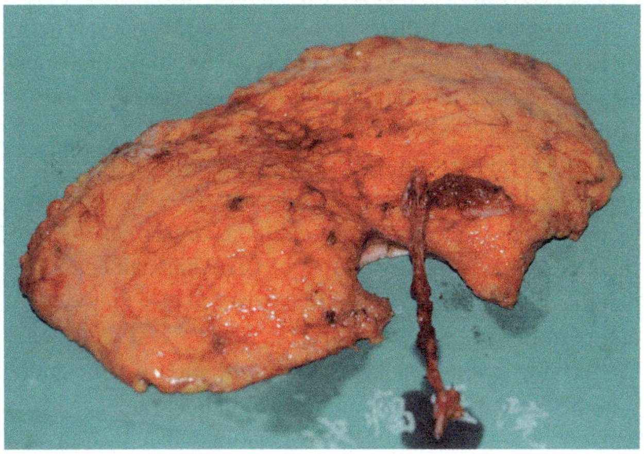

Fig. 2.8 DIEP flap was cut with paraumbilical perforator

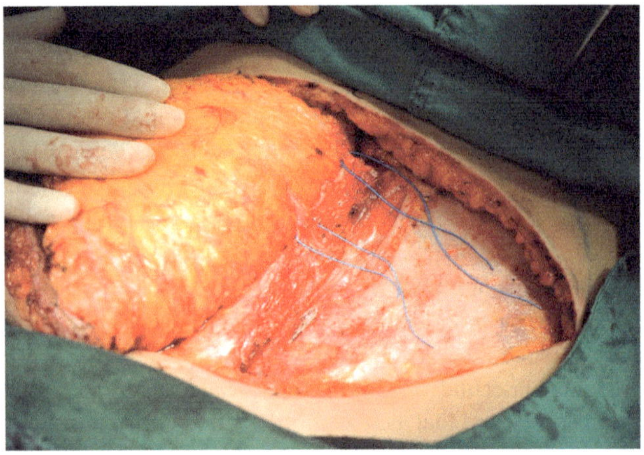

Fig. 2.9 Multiple perforators are located in the area 1–6 cm outside the rectus abdominis

The detailed anatomical study of Blondeel et al. showed that there were 2–8 perforators in each muscle, and the diameter of all perforators was at least 0.5 mm.

Most of these perforating branches are located in the area 1–6 cm outside the muscle, and the plane between 2 cm above the umbilicus and 6 cm below the umbilicus [9] (Fig. 2.9).

Vandevoort et al. described the course and distribution of perforating branches through rectus abdominis in 100 cases.

They found that in 65% of the cases, the perforating branch passed through the muscle with a short distance, while in 16% of the cases, the anatomy of perforators branch was complex making separation difficult.

Only in 9% of the cases, perforators were found to run a long intramuscular distance, which is the most difficult situation to harvest a free flap [24].

Munholz et al. published similar findings. It was found that 34% of the perforators were located in the lateral arch of rectus abdominis. In 79% of these perforators, the perforator ran in a straight line in the muscle, whereas only 18.2% medial perforators presented with similar distribution [25].

In the anatomical investigation of 329 DIEA perforators by Kikuchi et al., at least one "ideal" perforator with a diameter of at least 1 mm and parallel to the direction of muscle fibers existed [26].

These ideal perforating branches are located in the middle one-third area of rectus abdominis and 10–30 mm outside the umbilicus. Keller's theoretical model describes the arterial blood flow in the perforators of DIEP flap and concludes that the optimal flap would be that perfused by a major diameter perforator [27].

Carrying additional perforators will improve the blood flow of the flap, although donor site damage may increase and operation time extends. We assume that the adverse impact is minimal [28].

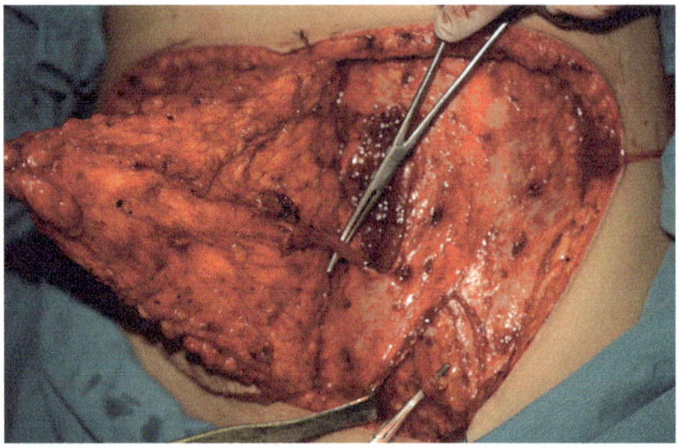

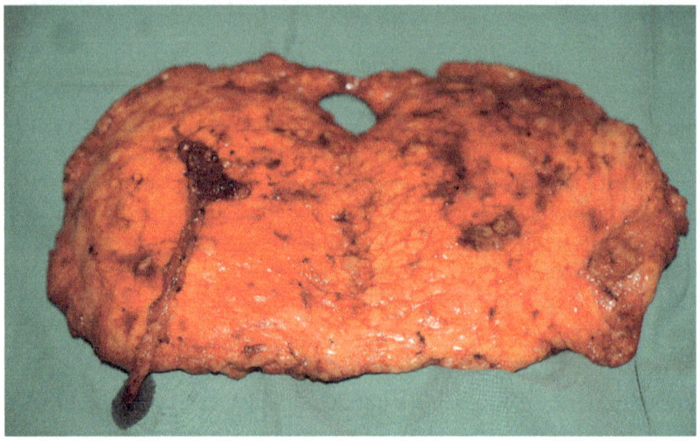

Fig. 2.10 A DIEP flap carrying the whole lower abdominal wall tissue was based on a single thick perforator as the pedicle

The importance of selecting a visible pulsating perforator with a diameter of at least 1 mm was emphasized by Kroll. He found that the fat necrosis rate of DIEP flap was very high among the initial unselected patients whose perforators were commonly small [29]. The report showed that the blood flow of the perforator was higher than that of the original artery and increased over time [30] (Fig. 2.10).

When a perforator flap with a long pedicle is selected, DSEA is an alternative to DIEA.

Mah et al. confirmed this technical point of view through anatomical and clinical studies. He used the superior epigastric artery perforator flap with long vascular pedicle for sternal reconstruction [31].

Understanding the route of inferior abdominal artery and vein and its perforators is the key to prepare a DIEP flap, which can be presented by preoperative CTA or MRA imaging.

Imaging examination will showcase the largest perforating vessel and mark it on the X-Y axis.

Without preoperative imaging, flaps with single perforator (commonly the lateral one) were used in only 20% of the cases; whereas the number reached about 70% when preoperative imaging was utilized and the medial perforators were preferred.

At the same time, in 8% of patients, we can find an intermuscular septal perforator, which passes by the medial edge of rectus abdominis without penetrating the muscle.

In this case, we can completely avoid muscle dissection and injury.

The best way to determine an intermuscular septal perforator is to depend on preoperative imaging. Generally, the most suitable perforator vessel is located around the umbilicus or slightly above.

Preoperative imaging examination can also find the thickest and best vascularized perforating vessels for the design of DIEP flap.

Interestingly, a 10-year retrospective study showed that before the era of preoperative imaging, the incidence of DIEP flap complications was related to the number of perforating vessels.

For example, through univariate analysis, some scholars found that partial necrosis of the flap was related to the selection of five perforators ($P < 0.05$).

In contrast, univariate and multivariate analysis showed that the complications of using single perforator were significantly reduced ($P < 0.05$).

In addition, the incidence of fat necrosis was positively correlated with the number of perforating branches ($P < 0.05$).

Therefore, as long as the largest and best single perforator is chosen, the single perforating DIEP flap is ideal theoretically.

This ideal perforator can be found and confirmed by preoperative imaging data combined with intraoperative identification [32].

However, in the accumulation of a large number of clinical cases, it is not found that increasing the number of perforators of the flap will increase the postoperative complications. On the contrary, carrying more perforator vessels can ensure the blood supply of the flap to a greater extent. Further detailed data statistics are being sorted out (Fig. 2.11).

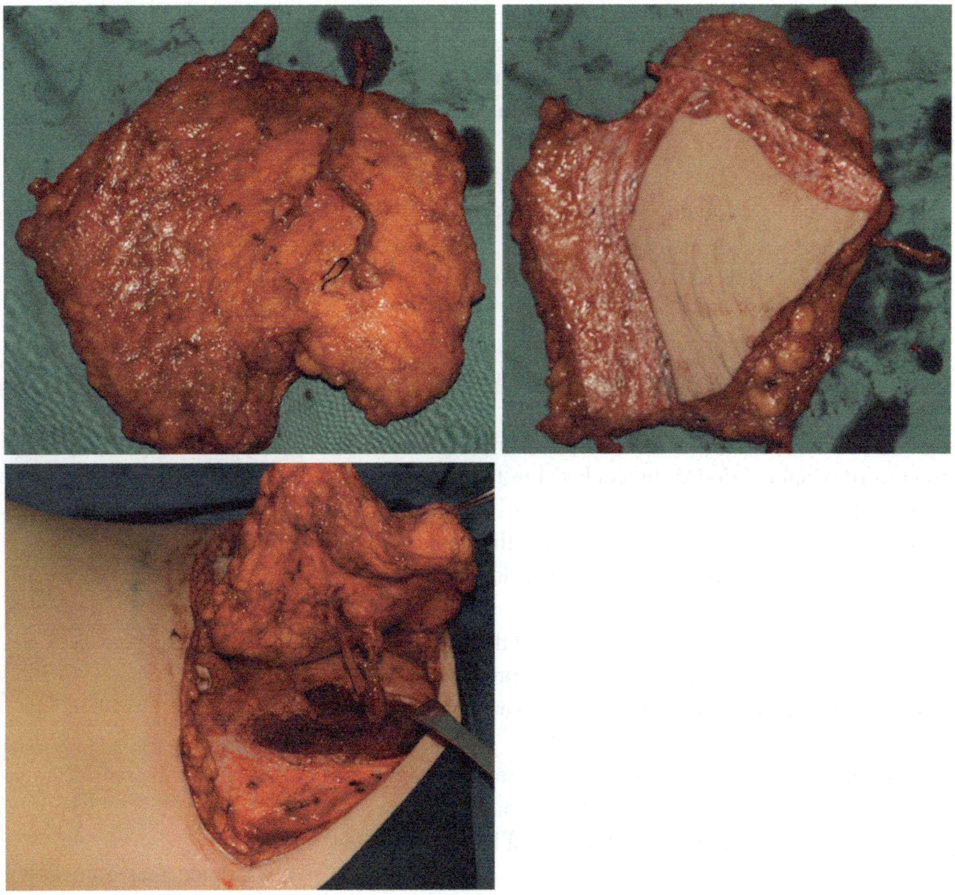

Fig. 2.11 Carrying multiple perforator vessels to ensure the blood supply of the flap to a greater extent

2.1.6 Surgical Technique

The penetrating branch of DIEP flap is based on the inferior abdominal artery and vein.

These perforating branches pass through or around the rectus abdominis and pass through the anterior sheath of rectus abdominis to provide blood supply to the skin and subcutaneous tissue.

To prepare a DIEP flap is to raise the lower abdominal soft tissue that is relying on one or more perforating branches.

Because the rectus abdominis is preserved on the abdomen, the length of DIEP vascular pedicle is longer than that of TRAM flap.

The longer the vascular pedicle is prepared, the easier would be for the DIEP flap to be mobilized on the chest wall and for the microvascular anastomosis.

In addition, we do not need to dissect below the external iliac vessels.

Flap designs were marked in the standing position before operation, and the anatomical marks of breast and abdomen were marked.

On the anterior chest wall, the boundary of bilateral breasts is marked. In the lower abdomen, mark the midline and around the umbilicus, and draw an oval flap outline in the lower abdomen.

Then, the patient takes the supine position and the position of important perforating branches is marked according to the results of CTA or MRA.

Hand-held Doppler can also be used to confirm the position of perforators.

At the same time, we need to move the tissue of the lower abdomen slightly upward to reduce the tension when closing the abdomen.

The abdominal wound is designed to be able to shift 7 cm downward when the donor site is closed in the second stage (Fig. 2.12).

The patient lies on his back on the operating table, and his arm can be abducted 60° or horizontally depending on the surgeon's preference.

Of course, it is generally necessary to abduct the patient's bilateral arms only when the breast surgeon needs bilateral sentinel lymph node biopsy and axillary lymph node dissection.

The preparation of abdominal flap and mastectomy were carried out simultaneously. Then, the internal thoracic arteries and veins were prepared and the medial breast was often used as the recipient area.

We generally expose the internal thoracic vessels in the second intercostal space between the second and third costal cartilage where the size of the vessels deems largest. If necessary, we can also remove part or all of the third costal cartilage (Fig. 2.13).

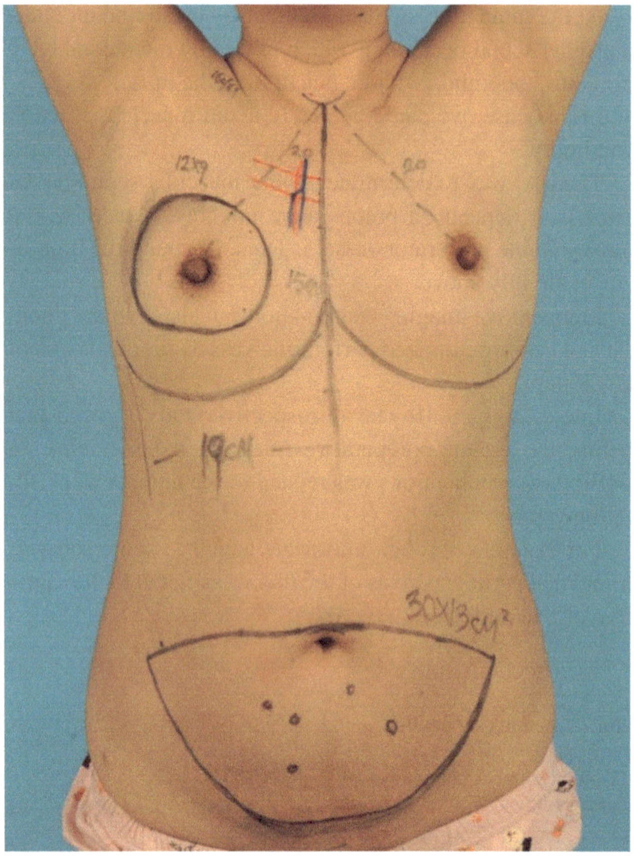

Fig. 2.12 Preoperative marking of perforator flap of inferior abdominal artery to mark the anatomical landmarks of the breasts and abdomen

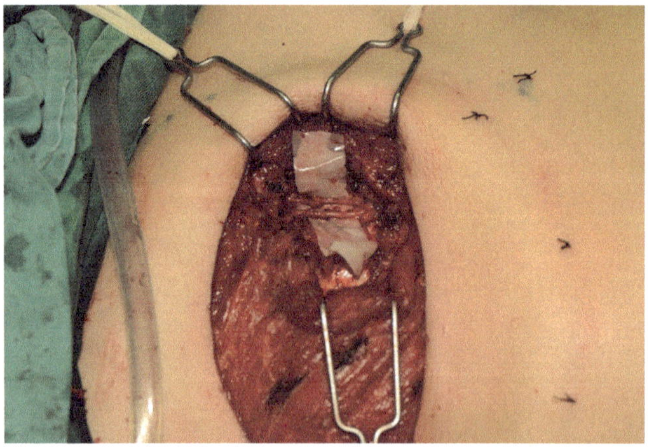

Fig. 2.13 The second intercostal space between the second and third costal cartilage is exposed, the blood vessels in the thorax are separated, and the third costal cartilage is removed

Vascular anastomosis without removing any ribs can be achieved in some cases. However, such large perforating vessels for anastomosis are rare in Asian women (Fig. 2.14).

If the surgical technique allows, try to preserve the ribs to protect the pectoralis major muscle and prevent chest wall deformity.

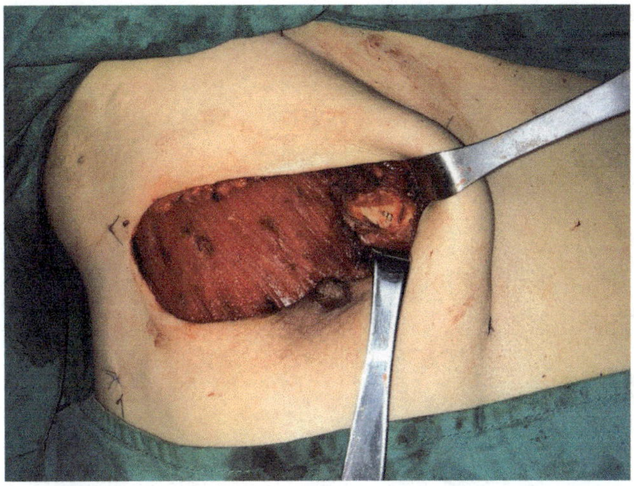

Fig. 2.14 In rare cases, the thick perforating branches of internal mammary vessels can be used as recipient vessels

In some cases, the perforating branches of the internal mammary vessels are big enough for revascularization, which spares dissecting the deeper internal mammary vascular system in the intercostal space.

In addition, in nipple sparing mastectomy, preserving these perforations can preserve skin sensation and provide blood supply for nipple areola complex.

More and more microsurgeons routinely determine the perforators of subabdominal blood vessel through preoperative CTA or MRA, which enables them to accurately evaluate the size and route of the perforators.

We often use hand-held Doppler probe to confirm the selected perforator vessels before operation, and then pinpoint that perforator in flap preparation and perforator isolation.

The first step of raising the flap is to make an incision on the marked line, open the full abdominal wall until the anterior fascia, and then turn up the flap.

At this time, if the perforator vessel has been confirmed by preoperative image, the selected perforator can be dissected directly.

If bilateral DIEP flaps are used, a midline incision can be made first.

If the medial or intermuscular septal perforators are chosen, the perforator vessels should be dissected before opening the lateral edge of the abdominal flap.

Once the largest perforator vessel is clearly located, it will be more convenient and fast to open the flap from the lower rectus abdominis fascia surface.

It should be noted that except the dominant perforating branches, the remaining perforators are scattered, hence caution should be paid to finding the superficial blood vessels in the abdominal wall at the lower edge of the incision, especially in preparation of a DIEP flap with predominant superficial venous drainage, where it is particularly important to preserve the superficial abdominal vein.

The DIEP flap was separated under magnifying glasses. The first step was to open the anterior sheath of rectus abdominis around the selected perforator.

Some surgeons often retain a 1–2 mm wide sheath around the perforator, which is normally unnecessary. However, when the surrounding tissues are seriously adhered and the perforator vessels are poor, do not peel off the tissues excessively, which can improve the safety of the operation.

Microscissors or bipolar electrocoagulation can be used to carefully separate or electrocoagulate all small branches along the rectus abdominis muscle.

It is noteworthy that if second or third level perforating branches have been selected, we must pay attention to its continuity with the source perforator.

Similarly, preoperative imaging is also very helpful in determining blood vessels.

During dissection, the muscle was cut along the direction of the muscle fiber, all intercostal nerves that did not cross the two perforators were retained, and finally the severed nerves between the two perforators were repaired (Fig. 2.15).

The perforating vessel was then separated downward to the communicating point with the main trunk of deep inferior epigastric vessels.

The optimal length of vascular pedicle is 8–10 cm.

The deep inferior epigastric artery and 1–2 accompanying veins were severed respectively to complete the preparation of DIEP flap.

It is helpful to apply methylene blue to the surface of blood vessels before disconnection.

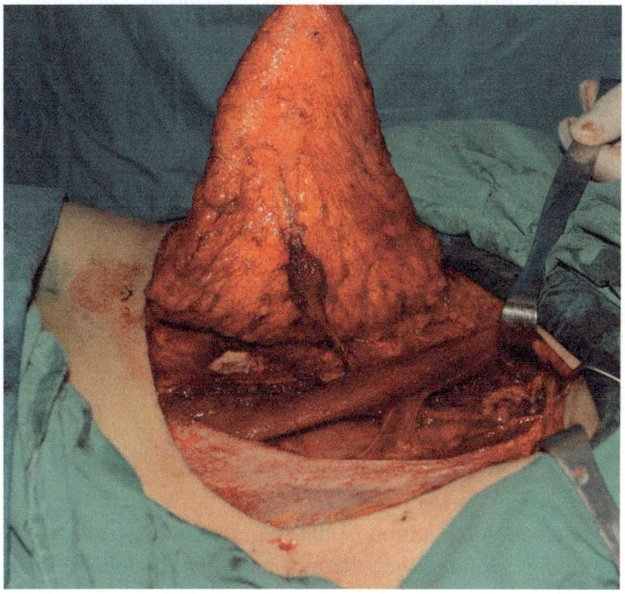

Fig. 2.15 Minimize the injury to rectus abdominis and intercostal nerves during the separation of vascular pedicle

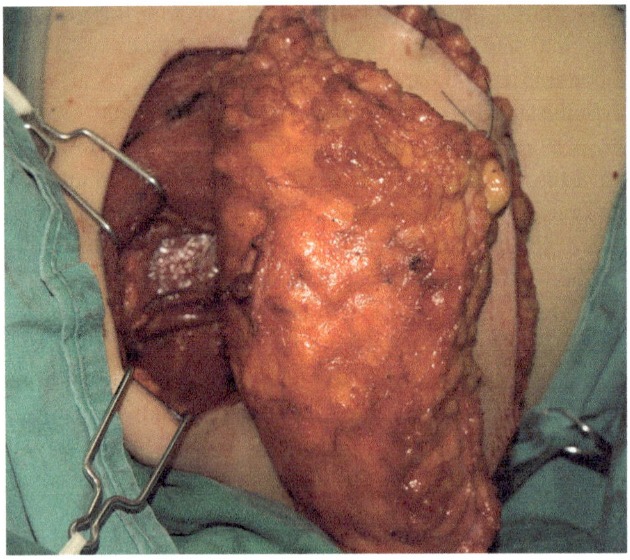

Fig. 2.16 The flap is transferred to and temporarily fixed on the chest wall

In addition, smaller accompanying veins can be removed and only larger accompanying veins and arteries can be reserved for anastomosis.

How much flap tissue is required comprehensively determined by the size of the removed breast tissue or implant. After preparation, the flap is transferred to and temporarily fixed on the chest wall (Fig. 2.16).

Next, the microscope is in place above the receiving area for vascular anastomosis. Vascular distortion should be cautious with.

The end-to-end anastomosis of vein can be performed by microvascular coupler, while the end-to-end anastomosis of artery needs to be manually sutured with 9-0 nylon thread (Fig. 2.17).

We can adjust the thickness and contour of the DIEP flap and fill tissue to achieve an ideal breast size and shape.

After mastectomy, the skin envelope is filled with the de-epithelized flap that is fixed on flap sides in a suitable position using absorbable suture. The vascular pedicle is also needed to be with absorbable suture.

Three closed drainage devices are placed through the edge of the primary incision or additional incisions.

When shaping is finished, the subcutaneous and skin layers are sutured.

Some microsurgeons use Doppler blood flow coupler or directly place Doppler needles into the anastomotic end of arteriovenous anastomosis for postoperative monitoring. Instead, reserving a skin island for observation is simple and practical (Fig. 2.18).

After the preparation of the flap, it is transferred to the receiving area, and then the incision of the abdominal wall can be closed.

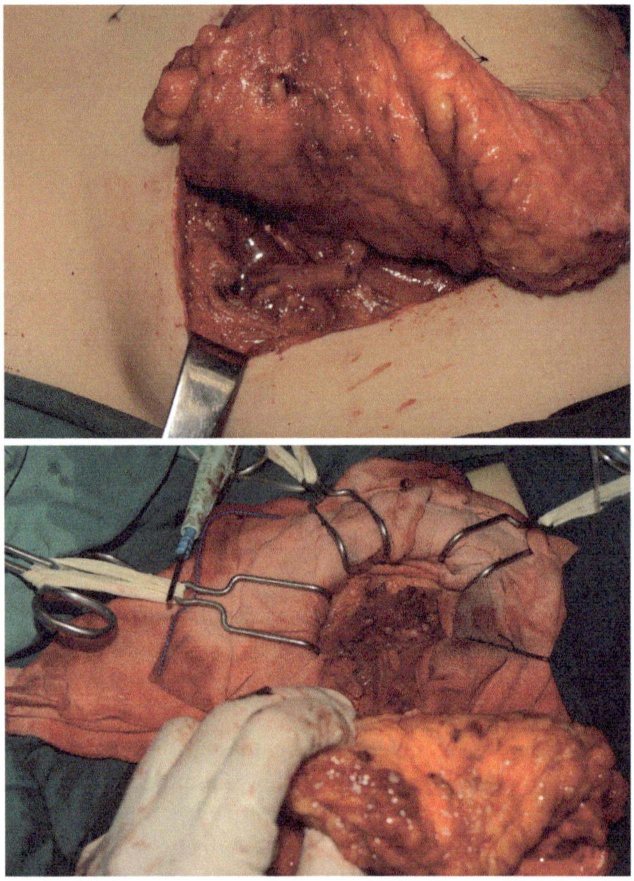

Fig. 2.17 Attention should be paid to avoid vascular distortion during vascular anastomosis

The anterior sheath of rectus abdominis was closed with two-layer barbed suture or 7# silk thread. Mesh is not needed if the anterior sheath defect is small.

A dorsal elevated position is usually required for tension-free closure of the abdominal wall in Asian women due to insufficient subcutaneous fat on the abdomen.

The subcutaneous tissue and skin of abdominal wall are closed layer by layer. Scarpa's fascia is sutured with double-armed 2-0 absorbable thread or barbed thread, and finally the subcutaneous and skin layer are sutured.

Two closed drainage tubes are placed on both sides of the abdominal incision and led out through the side incision.

The umbilicus is pulled out through an oval opening where the umbilicus shadows vertically on the abdominal wall, and it is fixed it with 4-0 absorbable sutures in semi buried mattress way (Fig. 2.18) (see this chapter for details and operation drawings).

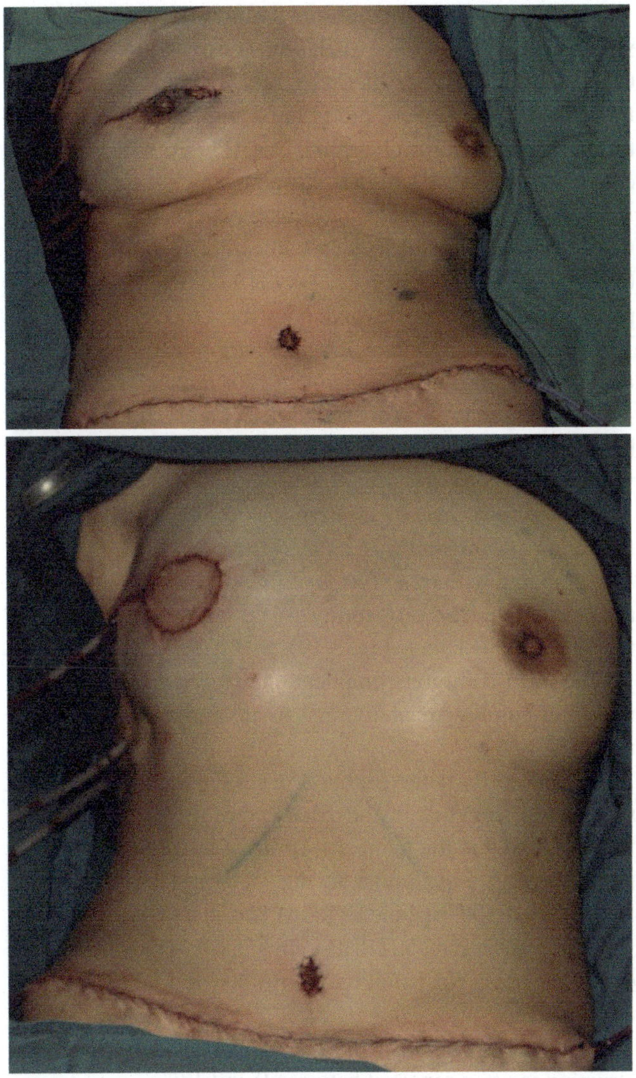

Fig. 2.18 Further shaping after flap placement, flap shaping and vacuum-assisted drainage were performed, and a skin island was reserved as postoperative observation window

2.1.7 Postoperative Management

The patient will be observed in the resuscitation room for 1–2 h.

During this period, the flap will be examined every 15–30 min, including the evaluation of skin color, temperature, capillary response, and Doppler signal.

Then the patient is transferred to the general ward for flap examination every 2–4 h.

During hospitalization, anticoagulation, prevention of deep venous thrombosis, and continuous vacuum suction are required.

Patients can resume normal diet the next day and ambulation 3–4 days after operation.

During hospitalization, the flap should be examined every 4 h, and the patient can usually be discharged 3 or 4 days after operation.

Four weeks after discharge, patients were encouraged to resume preoperative activity as soon as possible.

Nowadays, the importance of postoperative flap monitoring is being strengthened and valued.

According to a 7-year retrospective study of 400 patients with breast free flap reconstruction in Tisch Hospital of New York University, 4 patients were re-operated: 2 patients had venous crisis that happened early in the post-anesthesia care unit (PACU) which was solved by building superficial venous drainage, and the other 2 patients had flap problems after discharge with one flap failure and the other almost wholly necrotic.

Flap failure after discharge is usually irreparable, hence postoperative flap monitoring during hospitalization is very important.

2.1.8 Complications

The authoritative comments of Hofer et al. on perioperative complications found that the complication rate was as high as 40% in the first 30 DIEP cases.

The following studies showed that the perioperative complication rate of the subsequent 144 flaps were reduced to 13% with only one flap completely necrotic [33].

The donor site complications of DIEP flap are reported to be lower than that of TRAM flap [1, 32, 34–36], but the number may increase in female patients with pregnancy scars. The specific data are being counted [37].

In addition, when using DIEP flap for breast reconstruction in overweight or obese female patients, the occurrence of abdominal wall relaxation and hernia or abdominal wall bulging is rare, which is not statistically different from that of normal weight patients [38].

On the other hand, Vyas et al. found that obesity was an important risk factor for donor site complications, and in their study, there was no significant increase in donor site complications who underwent previous abdominal surgery [39].

Bajaj et al. found no difference in donor site complications between DIEP and muscle sparing TRAM flap.

Therefore, they advocated the most rapid and reliable flap based on the vascular anatomy of the DIEP system [21].

Schaverien et al. found that there was no difference in subjective function limitation of daily activities between patients receiving unilateral DIEP flap and TRAM flaps [40].

Bonde and colleagues objectively evaluated the abdominal wall strength after cutting DIEP flap and muscle preserving TRAM flap.

Statistically significant clinical advantage was observed in the DIEP group when measuring eccentric muscle strength [41].

In order to minimize the loss of abdominal donor area, Wu proposed a skin flap based on superficial vascular system (SIEA) to replace DIEP and muscle preserving TRAM skin flap. The skin flap based on superficial abdominal artery is a method to minimize injury and muscle injury is zero [42].

However, this alternative approach is largely not feasible among Asian women.

DIEP flap is a significant progress in autologous breast reconstruction.

Different from pedicled or free TRAM flap, DIEP flap retains rectus abdominis muscle, which can maintain sufficient abdominal wall strength and reduce the risk of abdominal bulging or hernia.

In addition, the preservation of rectus abdominis not only reduces the incidence of abdominal wall complications but also improves the shape of abdominal wall. As a result, the application of DIEP flap for breast reconstruction contributes to less postoperative pain, shorter hospital stay, and faster recovery.

In addition, a long vascular pedicle is good for flap mobility and the beauty of the reconstructed breast.

DIEP flap has become the gold standard of breast reconstruction because it minimizes adverse impact of surgery on daily life, ensures patients' quality of life, and maximizes the cosmetic effect.

Compared with patients reconstructed with pedicled TRAM flap, patients reconstructed with DIEP flap have less postoperative pain and faster recovery. This is agreed by patients, nurses, and surgeons.

Studies have confirmed that DIEP flap surgery caused light postoperative pain and was not anesthesia demanding. Patients may satisfy with oral painkillers early after operation, recover faster, and have shorter hospital stay. They can often be discharged from the hospital 3–4 days after operation.

In 2001, a comparative study of breast reconstruction with DIEP flap and TRAM flap hosted by M.D. Anderson Cancer Center showed that after breast reconstruction with DIEP flap, the dosage of morphine could be reduced by half through patient-controlled analgesia (PCA), which significantly shortened the length of hospital stay.

We found that 10.3% of DIEP flap patients had abdominal wound non-healing; the incidence of complications was higher than expected in those with a history of smoking, hypertension, previous radiotherapy, and high body mass index (BMI).

Re-operation rate due to early complications was 4% including 2% venous embolism and 2% hematoma.

We found that the probability of vascular exploration can be further reduced using vascular anastomosis device, which was not necessary for arterial anastomosis.

The necrosis rate of the flap was 0.3%, and the partial failure rate of the flap was 2.7%.

Compared with other forms of free flap breast reconstruction technique, the probability of the above complications for DIEP flap is lower (Fig. 2.19).

The most common complication after breast reconstruction with autologous abdominal tissue transplantation is fat necrosis.

It is generally believed that it occurs in the area of perfusion deprivation, that is, the distal end of the flap.

We found that the fat necrosis rate of DIEP flap for breast reconstruction was similar to that of free TRAM flap, but lower than that of pedicled TRAM flap.

Fat necrosis rate of DIEP flap is 14%, which is significantly related to smoking, previous radiotherapy, and chemotherapy.

Similarly, the fat necrosis rate of free TRAM flap reconstruction is often reported between 0 and 13%.

Studies of pedicled TRAM flap reconstruction showed that the fat necrosis rate varied from 11 to 25%. We had similar findings. Modified surgical technique could only mitigate rather than prevent fat necrosis since this is determined by the anatomy.

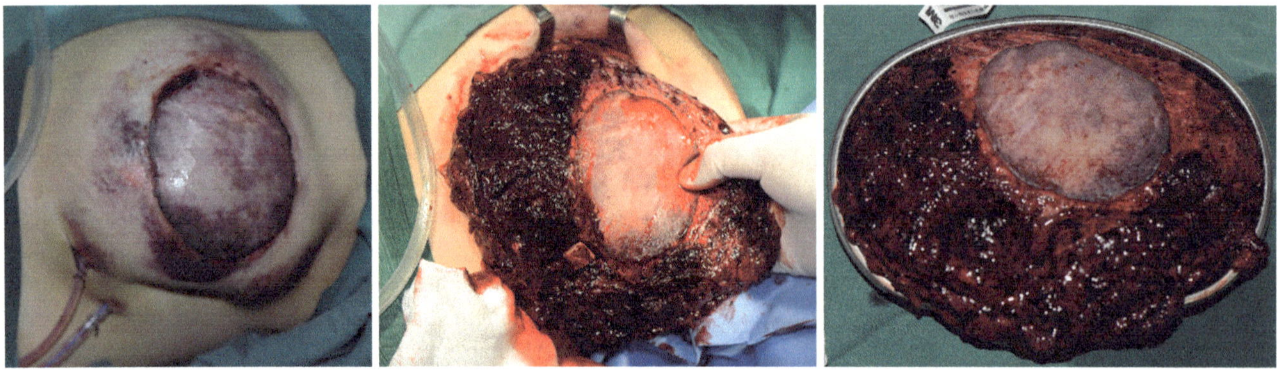

Fig. 2.19 Venous crisis occurred in the flap after operation, resulting in extensive hematoma, flap necrosis, and operation failure

The late complications of DIEP flap included 0.5% of the postoperative flap bloated rate, which was significantly lower than the pedicle TRAM flap in a cohort of the same sample size, with a 9% incidence rate.

It has been reported that free TRAM flap has a higher incidence of abdominal wall swelling and hernia, which is generally between 1 and 15%, and sometimes it can be as high as 82%.

A considerable advantage of DIEP flap reconstruction is that it can avoid mesh implantation, which is routinely needed in pedicled and free TRAM reconstruction.

Because of its prolonged anesthesia time, some opponents of perforator flap still oppose to the inclusion of DIEP flap in routine use.

However, after the initial learning stage, microsurgeons who committed to breast reconstruction with perforator flap can complete unilateral reconstruction in as short as 3 h and bilateral reconstruction in 4 h.

This is equivalent to the time consumed for pedicled TRAM flap and prosthesis implantation.

In addition, it can be said that the breast reconstruction with DIEP flap is actually easier and safer than the TRAM flap regarding muscle preservation. In particular, after the use of preoperative imaging, the selected sites of perforating vessels are fully visible in the anatomical process, which avoids unnecessary injury during the operation.

To sum up, modern microsurgery has gradually developed into a period in which high failure rate and long operation time will be eliminated.

Compared with pedicled TRAM myocutaneous flap, free DIEP flap is more difficult, time-consuming, and has longer operator training cycle. However, considering its advantages and disadvantages systematically, free DIEP flap is still the best choice for breast reconstruction with autologous tissue transplantation.

The application of DIEP flap technique has expanded the range of people suitable for autologous breast reconstruction. Obese patients or patients with a history of abdominal surgery can now receive autologous breast reconstruction.

With the increasing use of preoperative imaging, the operation time is gradually reduced, and the operation procedure itself becomes safer and more predictable.

DIEP flap breast reconstruction is especially suitable for women who need manual labor, radiotherapy, and bilateral reconstruction. In addition, DIEP flap reconstruction can also be used in patients who are contraindicated, cautious, or inappropriate in other reconstruction methods.

DIEP flap is the most advanced technique representing breast reconstructing using abdominal autologous tissue, which can provide the best long-term aesthetic effect. With further popularization of microsurgical technique, DIEP flap transplantation that minimizes donor damage and maximizes patient satisfaction will be accepted by the public.

2.1.9 Summary

Unilateral DIEP flap may not provide enough tissue to reconstruct one side of the breast. Therefore, it can achieve better results by using bilateral DIEP flap to reconstruct one side of the breast.

In the past decade, the rate of bilateral mastectomy has greatly increased. In the final analysis, most people believe that the reason is genetic testing.

At the same time, the increase of double mastectomy rate and the rise of nipple preserving mastectomy have greatly stimulated the improvement of breast reconstruction. Now, bilateral breast reconstruction is becoming more and more common, and the application of two flaps is often better than that of single flap for unilateral breast repair.

References

1. Blondeel N, Vanderstraeten GG, Monstrey SJ, et al. The donor site morbidity of free DIEP flaps and free TRAM flaps for breast reconstruction. Br J Plast Surg. 1997;50(5):322–30.
2. Blondeel PN, Arnstein M, Verstraete K, et al. Venous congestion and blood flow in free transverse rectus abdominis myocutaneous and deep inferior epigastric perforator flaps. Plast Reconstr Surg. 2000;106(6):1295–9.
3. Tran NV, Buchel EW, Convery PA. Microvascular complications of DIEP flaps. Plast Reconstr Surg. 2007;119(5):1397–405; discussion 1406–8.
4. Carramenha e Costa MA, Carriquiry C, Vasconez LO, Grotting JC, Herrera RH, Windle BH. An anatomic study of the venous drainage of the transverse rectus abdominis musculocutaneous flap. Plast Reconstr Surg. 1987;79(2):208–17.
5. Liu TS, Ashjian P, Festekjian J. Salvage of congested deep inferior epigastric perforator flap with a reverse flow venous anastomosis. Ann Plast Surg. 2007;59(2):214–7.
6. Cheng MH, Robles JA, Ulusal BG, Wei FC. Reliability of zone IV in the deep inferior epigastric perforator flap: a single center's experience with 74 cases. Breast. 2006;15(2):158–66.
7. Schaverien M, Saint-Cyr M, Arbique G, Hatef D, Brown SA, Rohrich RJ. Three- and four-dimensional computed tomographic angiography and venography of the anterolateral thigh perforator flap. Plast Reconstr Surg. 2008;121(5):1685–96.
8. Rozen WM, Ribuffo D, Atzeni M, et al. Current state of the art in perforator flap imaging with computed tomographic angiography. Surg Radiol Anat. 2009;31(8):631–9.
9. Blondeel PN, Beyens G, Verhaeghe R, et al. Doppler flowmetry in the planning of perforator flaps. Br J Plast Surg. 1998;51(3):202–9.
10. Santanelli F, Paolini G, Renzi L. Preliminary experience in breast reconstruction with the free vertical deep inferior epigastric perforator flap. Scand J Plast Reconstr Surg Hand Surg. 2008;42(1):23–7.
11. Tan O. Versatility of the vertical designed deep inferior epigastric perforator flap. Microsurgery. 2009;29(4):282–6.
12. Blondeel PN, Demuynck M, Mete D, et al. Sensory nerve repair in perforator flaps for autologous breast reconstruction: sensational or senseless. Br J Plast Surg. 1999;52(1):37–44.
13. Levine SM, Lester ME, Fontenot B, Allen RJ. Perforator flap breast reconstruction after unsatisfactory implant reconstruction. Ann Plast Surg. 2011;66(5):513–7.
14. Hallock GG. The superior epigastric(RECTUS ABDOMINIS) muscle perforator flap. Ann Plast Surg. 2005;55(4):430–2.

15. Milloy FJ, Anson BJ, Mcafee DK. The rectus abdominis muscle and the epigastric arteries. Surg Gynecol Obstet. 1960;110:293–302.
16. Taylor GI, Daniel RK. The anatomy of several free flap donor sites. Plast Reconstr Surg. 1975;56(3):243–53.
17. Kaufman T, Hurwitz DJ, Boehnke M, Futrell JW. The microcirculatory pattern of the transverse-abdominal flap: a cross-sectional xerographic and CAT scanning study. Ann Plast Surg. 1985;14(4):340–5.
18. Keller A. Perfusion zones of the DIEP flap revisited: a clinical study. Plast Reconstr Surg. 2006;118(4):1076–7; author reply 1077.
19. Heitmann C, Felmerer G, Durmus C, Matejic B, Ingianni G. Anatomical features of perforator blood vessels in the deep inferior epigastric perforator flap. Br J Plast Surg. 2000;53(3):205–8.
20. Blondeel PN, Boeckx WD. Refinements in free flap breast reconstruction: the free bilateral deep inferior epigastric perforator flap anastomosed to the internal mammary artery. Br J Plast Surg. 1994;47(7):495–501.
21. Bajaj AK, Chevray PM, Chang DW. Comparison of donor-site complications and functional outcomes in free muscle-sparing TRAM flap and free DIEP flap breast reconstruction. Plast Reconstr Surg. 2006;117(3):737–46; discussion 747–50.
22. Sadove R, Merrell JC. The split rectus abdominis free muscle transfer. Ann Plast Surg. 1987;18(2):179–81.
23. Boyd JB, Taylor GI, Corlett R. The vascular territories of the superior epigastric and the deep inferior epigastric systems. Plast Reconstr Surg. 1984;73(1):1–16.
24. Vandevoort M, Vranckx JJ, Fabre G. Perforator topography of the deep inferior epigastric perforator flap in 100 cases of breast reconstruction. Plast Reconstr Surg. 2002;109(6):1912–8.
25. Munhoz AM, Ishida LH, Sturtz GP, et al. Importance of lateral row perforator vessels in deep inferior epigastric perforator flap harvesting. Plast Reconstr Surg. 2004;113(2):517–24.
26. Harii K, Ohmori K, Sekiguchi J. The free musculocutaneous flap. Plast Reconstr Surg. 1976;57(3):294–303.
27. Kikuchi N, Murakami G, Kashiwa H, Homma K, Sato TJ, Ogino T. Morphometrical study of the arterial perforators of the deep inferior epigastric perforator flap. Surg Radiol Anat. 2001;23(6):375–81.
28. Patel SA, Keller A. A theoretical model describing arterial flow in the DIEP flap related to number and size of perforator vessels. J Plast Reconstr Aesthet Surg. 2008;61(11):1316–20; discussion 1320.
29. Kroll SS. Fat necrosis in free transverse rectus abdominis myocutaneous and deep inferior epigastric perforator flaps. Plast Reconstr Surg. 2000;106(3):576–83.
30. Figus A, Ramakrishnan V, Rubino C. Hemodynamic changes in the microcirculation of DIEP flaps. Ann Plast Surg. 2008;60(6):644–8.
31. Mah E, Rozen WM, Ashton MW, Flood S. Deep superior epigastric artery perforators: anatomical study and clinical application in sternal reconstruction. Plast Reconstr Surg. 2009;123(6):1719–23.
32. Gill PS, Hunt JP, Guerra AB, et al. A 10-year retrospective review of 758 DIEP flaps for breast reconstruction. Plast Reconstr Surg. 2004;113(4):1153–60.
33. Hofer SO, Damen TH, Mureau MA, Rakhorst HA, Roche NA. A critical review of perioperative complications in 175 free deep inferior epigastric perforator flap breast reconstructions. Ann Plast Surg. 2007;59(2):137–42.
34. Zoghbi Y, Gerth DJ, Tashiro J, Golpanian S, Thaller SR. Deep inferior epigastric perforator versus free transverse rectus abdominis myocutaneous flap: complications and resource utilization. Ann Plast Surg. 2017;78(5):516–20.
35. Krishnan NM, Purnell C, Nahabedian MY, et al. The cost effectiveness of the DIEP flap relative to the muscle-sparing TRAM flap in postmastectomy breast reconstruction. Plast Reconstr Surg. 2015;135(4):948–58.
36. Hamdi M, Weiler-Mithoff EM, Webster MH. Deep inferior epigastric perforator flap in breast reconstruction: experience with the first 50 flaps. Plast Reconstr Surg. 1999;103(1):86–95.
37. Parrett BM, Caterson SA, Tobias AM, Lee BT. DIEP flaps in women with abdominal scars: are complication rates affected. Plast Reconstr Surg. 2008;121(5):1527–31.
38. Garvey PB, Buchel EW, Pockaj BA, Gray RJ, Samson TD. The deep inferior epigastric perforator flap for breast reconstruction in overweight and obese patients. Plast Reconstr Surg. 2005;115(2):447–57.
39. Vyas RM, Dickinson BP, Fastekjian JH, Watson JP, Dalio AL, Crisera CA. Risk factors for abdominal donor-site morbidity in free flap breast reconstruction. Plast Reconstr Surg. 2008;121(5):1519–26.
40. Schaverien MV, Perks AG, McCulley SJ. Comparison of outcomes and donor-site morbidity in unilateral free TRAM versus DIEP flap breast reconstruction. J Plast Reconstr Aesthet Surg. 2007;60(11):1219–24.
41. Bonde CT, Lund H, Fridberg M, Danneskiold-Samsoe B, Elberg JJ. Abdominal strength after breast reconstruction using a free abdominal flap. J Plast Reconstr Aesthet Surg. 2007;60(5):519–23.
42. Wu LC, Bajaj A, Chang DW, Chevray PM. Comparison of donor-site morbidity of SIEA, DIEP, and muscle-sparing TRAM flaps for breast reconstruction. Plast Reconstr Surg. 2008;122(3):702–9.

3 The Importance of Preserving Intercostal Nerves

Zan Li and Jie Ma

The deep inferior epigastric artery perforator (DIEP) flap is the most commonly used method for autologous breast reconstruction. It is significantly advantageous over the rectus abdominis flap in retaining the rectus abdominis muscle, which can maintain sufficient abdominal wall strength and reduce the risk of abdominal bulging or hernia [1, 2].

Many studies have confirmed the importance of preserving the muscle and fascia integrity in reducing donor site injury [3–5] (Figs. 3.1 and 3.2).

At the same time, many studies have shown that the injury of intercostal nerve in rectus abdominis muscle will lead to complications such as abdominal wall hernia and abdominal wall bulging.

When cutting DIEP flap, it is important not only to preserve the integrity of the rectus abdominis muscle, but also to preserve its vegetative nerve (Fig. 3.3).

The seventh to eleventh intercostal nerves and subcostal nerves enter the rectus abdominis sheath laterally to the rectus abdominis.

As the DIEPs intersect with the intercostal nerve branches, the separation should be careful.

Careful manipulation in isolating the perforators can preserve both the blood supply and innervation of muscles to a greatest extent [5–9].

Figure 3.3, it was shown that the vascular pedicle is separated bit by bit on the premise of preserving the integrity of the intercostal nerve. In this way, all intercostal nerve branches innervating the rectus abdominis are completely preserved

Rozen et al. found that 4–7 nerve branches entered the lateral boundary or posterior surface of rectus abdominis and accompanied with the lateral branch of DIEA and its perfo-

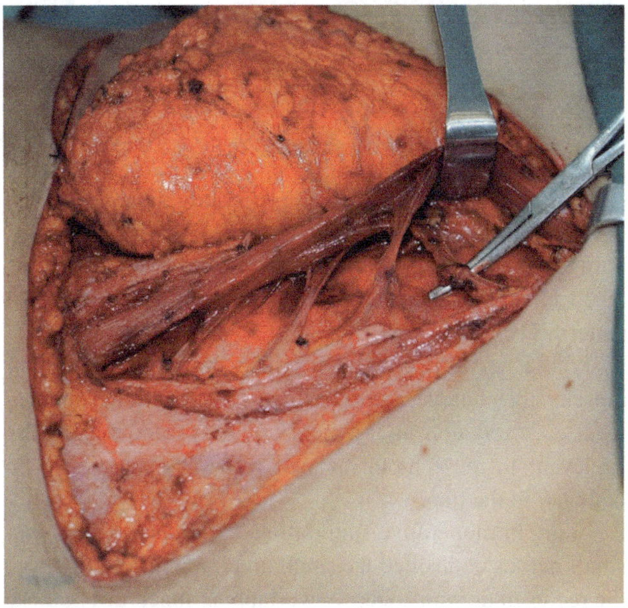

Fig. 3.1 Preservation of rectus abdominis integrity after removal of DIEP flap

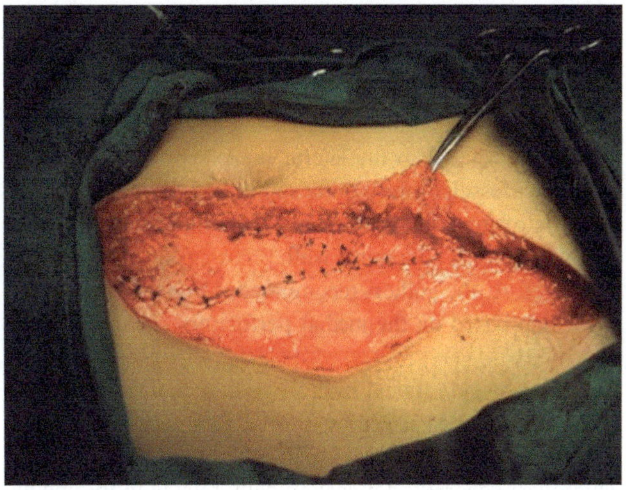

Fig. 3.2 Preservation of the integrity of the anterior sheath of rectus abdominis in the donor area where the DIEP flap was harvested

Z. Li (✉)
Department of Oncology Plastic Surgery, Hunan Cancer Hospital, Changsha, Hunan, China

J. Ma
Department of Breast Surgery, Tangshan People's Hospital, Tangshan, HeBei, China

Z. Li, D. Song (eds.), *Oncoplastic Flap Surgery*, https://doi.org/10.1007/978-981-19-8926-1_3

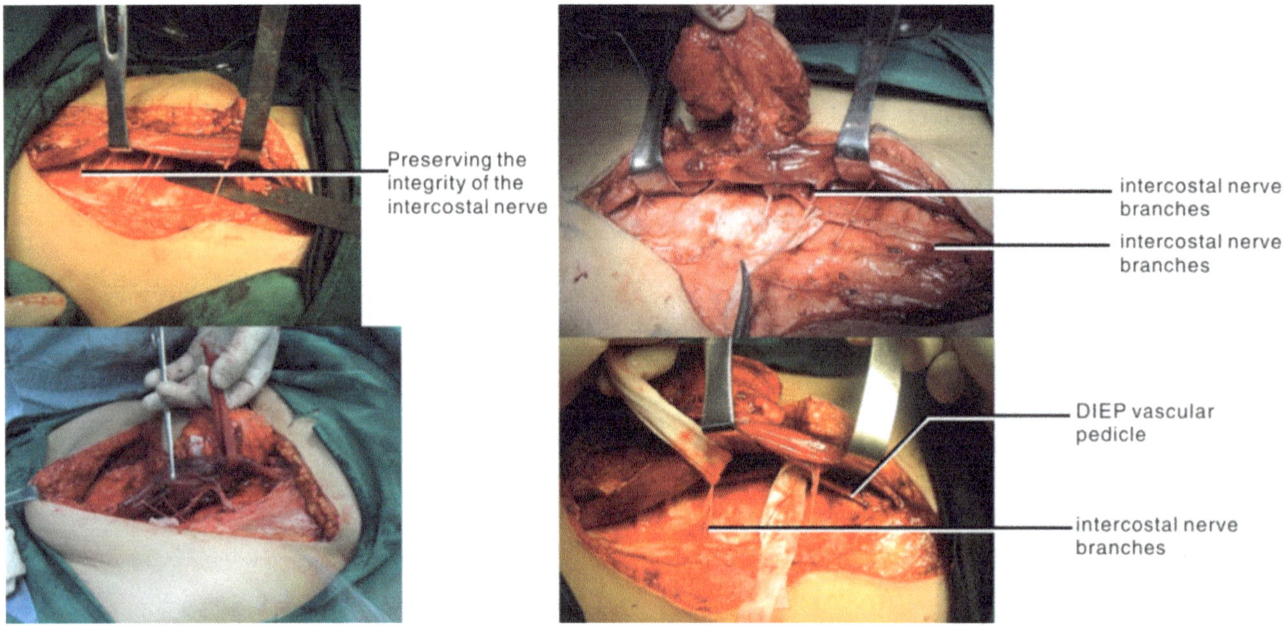

Fig. 3.3 Intercostal nerve branches are completely preserved

rating branches. They firstly reported that rectus abdominis received segmental innervation that were divided into two patterns [10, 11].

Type I nerves were small, which innervated the small muscle fiber bundles, yet no significant functional impairment occurred after injury; therefore, the medial perforators irrelevant to these motor nerves were very suitable to be included in the flap.

Using intraoperative stimulation, the authors found that small nerves controlled the small and long muscle fibers of the rectus abdominis. Due to overlapping innervation, these small nerves could be sacrificed without functional damage.

Type II nerves were important and located on the level of the arcuate line. These nerves entered the medial part of muscles and dominated the entire rectus abdominis muscle, it should be extra careful in maintaining nerve continuity while seperating vessels.

The rectus abdominis is dominated by type II nerves that are closely related to the lateral branches of deep inferior epigastric vessels. Injury to these nerves will lead to extensive loss of innervation of rectus abdominis and a series of complications of abdominal wall.

Therefore, the authors recommended that the harvest of a DIEP flap based on the medial perforators should be given priority to.

Anatomy and clinical practice further confirmed that the segmental intercostal nerves formed a nerve plexus around the lateral perforators of the deep inferior epigastric vessels, which was generally not anatomically related to the medial perforators [12].

Therefore, from the perspective of anatomy, taking the medial perforator vessels as the pedicle to cut the flap will reduce the occurrence of abdominal hernia and abdominal wall protrusion.

Avoiding motor nerve injury during perforator separation can also reduce muscle injury.

Sacrificing the larger nerve innervating the full width of rectus abdominis at the level of the arcuate line may lead to increased donor site injury [13].

If myofascial folding and abdominoplasty are used immediately after flap resection, the appearance of DIEP donor area can be significantly improved [14].

In the real sense, the deep inferior epigastric artery perforator flap retains the rectus abdominis muscle together with the integrity of intercostal nerves to the greatest extent, which not only reduces the incidence of abdominal wall complications but also improves the appearance of abdominal wall. Patients with DIEP flap for breast reconstruction can benefit with less postoperative pain, shorter hospital stay, and faster recovery.

Because the adverse effects of surgery on daily life are minimized, the quality of life is guaranteed, and the cosmetic effect is improved to the greatest extent, the DIEP flap is considered to be the gold standard for breast reconstruction with autologous tissue transplantation.

Note: We do not recommend cutting the unilateral DIEP flap with both the lateral and medial perforators, which will cause great damage to the donor area and prolong anesthesia time. If required, the contralateral DIEP or superficial epigastric vessels can be used to provide additional blood supply for the flap.

3.1 Process Steps of Actual Surgical Separation of Intercostal Nerves (Figs. 3.4, 3.5, 3.6, 3.7, 3.8, and 3.9)

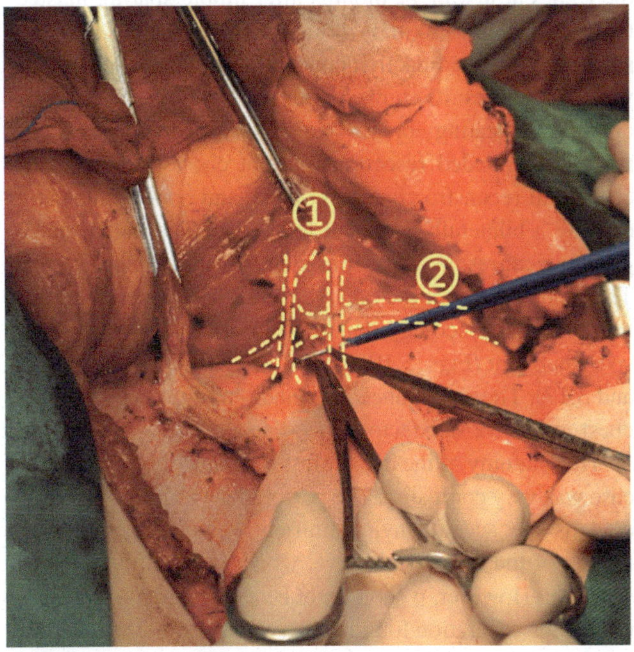

Fig. 3.4 Lifting the rectus abdominis muscle from outside to inside to expose the intercostal nerves and vascular pedicle. (1) Intercostal nerves; (2) Deep inferior epigastric vascular pedicle

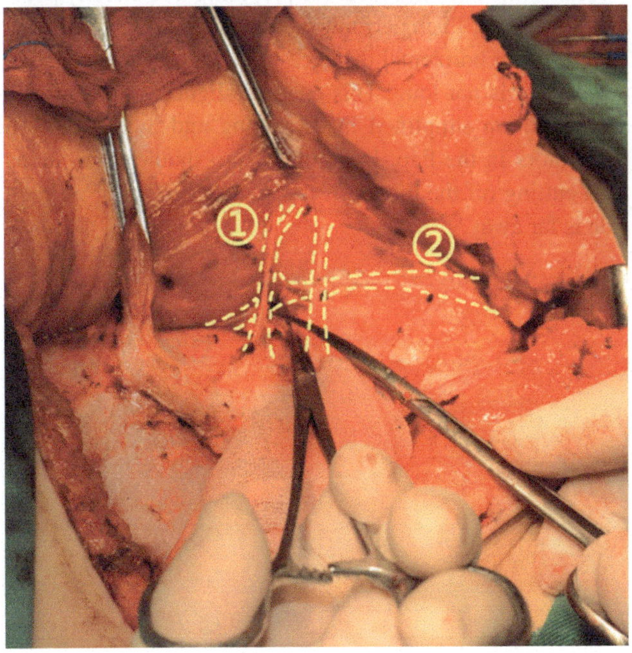

Fig. 3.5 Anterograde separation of vascular pedicle and preservation of intercostal nerves along the way. (1) Intercostal nerves; (2) Deep inferior epigastric vascular pedicle

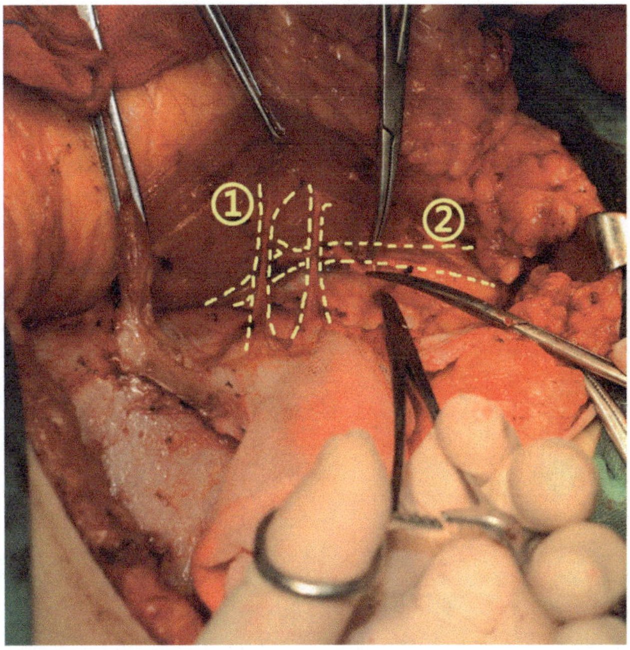

Fig. 3.6 Deep inferior epigastric vessels are often divided into internal and external branches as well as multiple muscular and cutaneous branches that need to be carefully separated and ligated one by one. (1) Intercostal nerves; (2) Deep inferior epigastric vessels

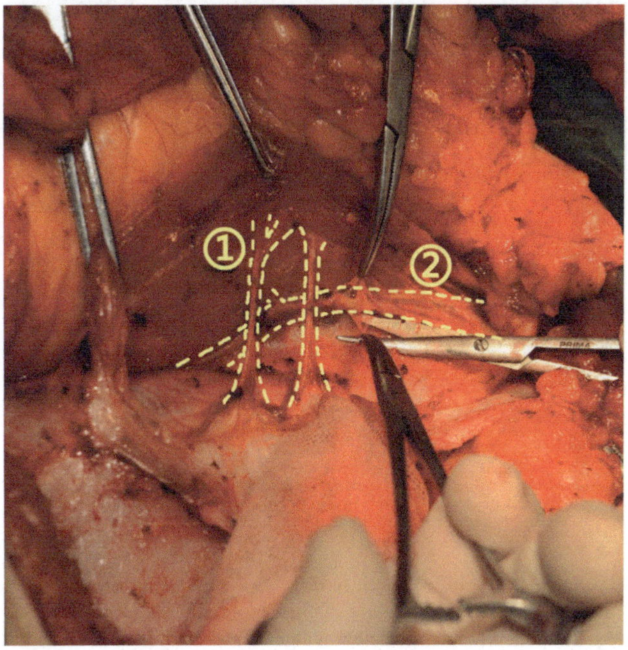

Fig. 3.7 The vascular pedicle was completely separated from the intercostal nerves. (1) Intercostal nerves; (2) Deep inferior epigastric vessels

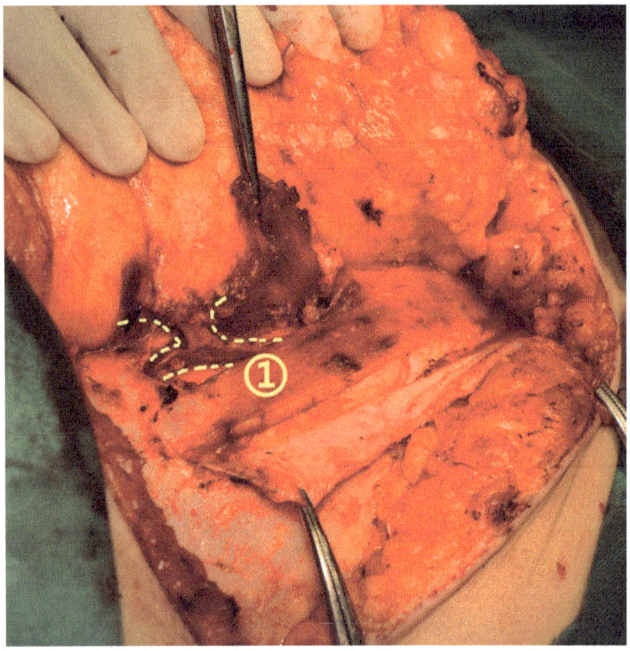

Fig. 3.8 The vascular pedicle was freed in a rendezvous method. (1) The trunk of the deep inferior epigastric vessels

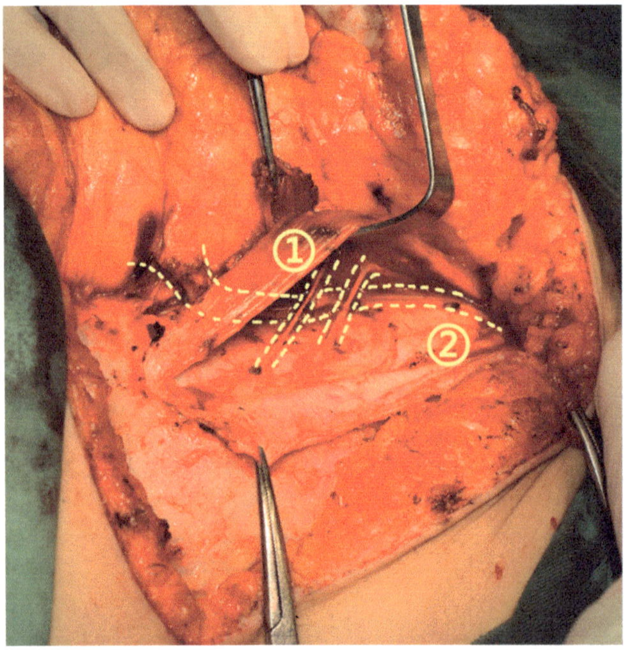

Fig. 3.9 The vascular pedicle was ligated and disconnected from the proximal plane and extracted retrogradely through the rectus abdominis tunnel. (1) Intercostal nerves; (2) The trunk of the deep inferior epigastric vessels

3.1.1 Case 1: Preserving the Intercostal Nerves When Separating the DIEPs

A 31-year-old woman presented with a tumor reoccurring on the right chest wall 71 months after nipple sparing mastectomy (NSM) plus axillary lymph node dissection. PET-CT showed a high radioactive concentration on the right chest wall. Biopsy results showed poorly differentiated adenocarcinoma indicating breast cancer relapse. The patients received expanded resection of right chest wall mass and chest wall reconstruction using mesh and bone cement covered by a bilaterally pedicled DIEP flap. The postoperative pathological results were consistent with the biopsy results. The blood supply of the flap was good. The patient was then transferred to oncology department for further comprehensive treatment (Figs. 3.10, 3.11, 3.12, 3.13, 3.14, 3.15, 3.16, and 3.17). The appearance and function of the reconstructed chest wall were satisfactory.

The anatomy of the deep inferior epigastric vessels in this case was very confusing. The perforator was initially considered as the accompanying nutrient vessel of the sensory branch of the intercostal nerve, which is a common clinical situation. However, it should not be easily damaged. Careful retrograde separation found that it was a perforator at a lower level crisscrossing the sensory branch of the intercostal nerve crosses before they penetrated the subcutaneous tissue concomitantly. This situation is especially suitable for the preparation of sensory subabdominal artery perforator flap.

This is the anatomy ideal for preparing a bilaterally pedicled DIEP flap. Each perforator of corresponding DIEA was large and the horizontal distance between perforators above the muscle is not long. This enabled slight muscle damage and operation simplified in separating and including both perforators in the flap. In contrast, one should be cautious with cutting off the muscle if the chosen perforator on each side is far away.

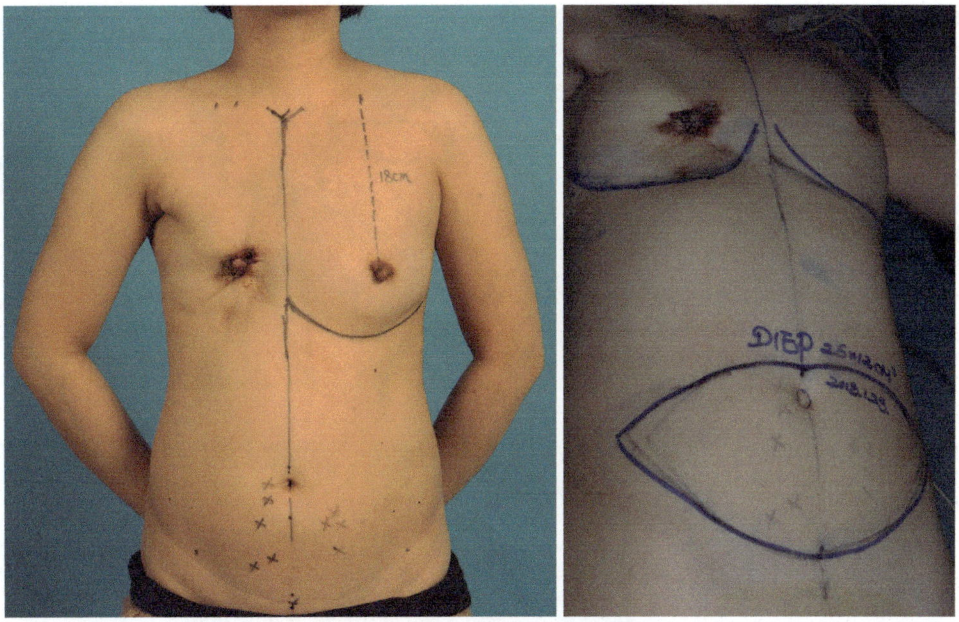

Fig. 3.10 Preoperative appearance and surgical design

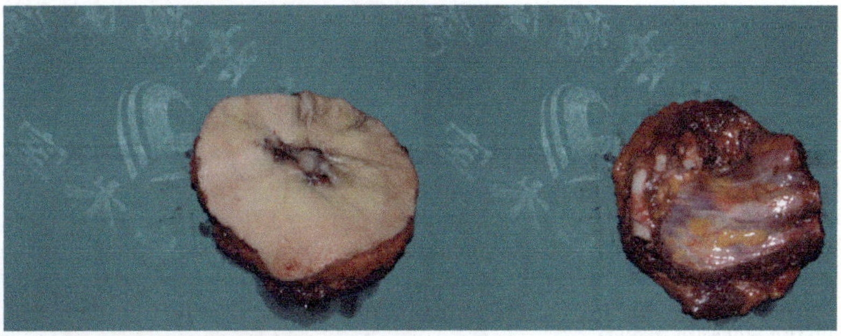

Fig. 3.11 The entire lesion was removed and found infiltrating the full thickness of the chest wall

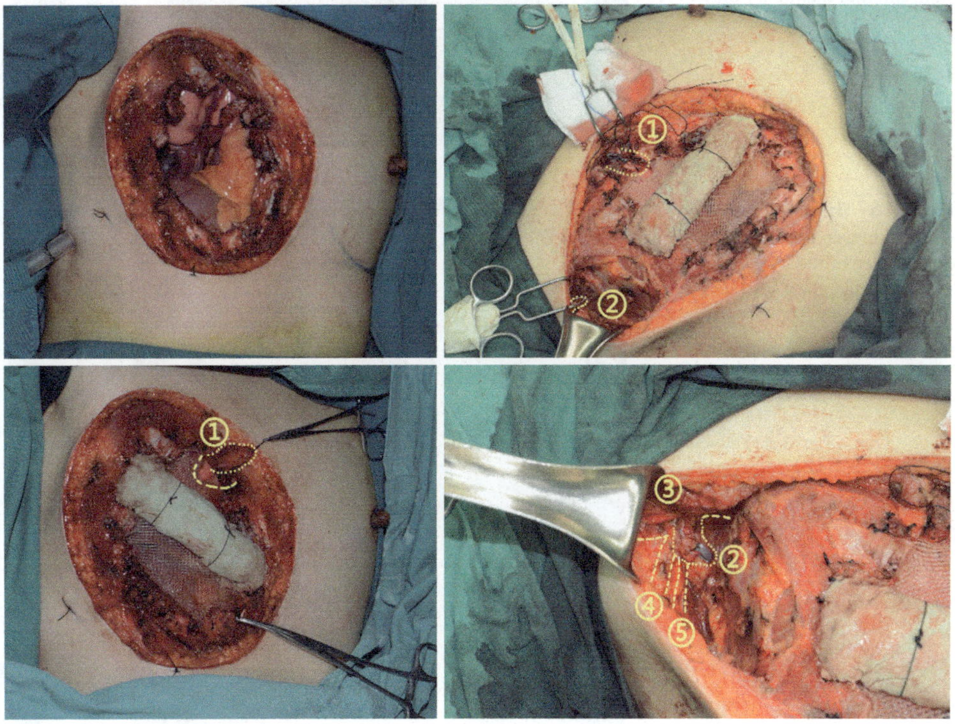

Fig. 3.12 When the tumor was removed, the huge defect of the chest wall was repaired using a mesh and bone cement, recipient vessels were also prepared. (1) Proximal end of right internal mammary vessel; (2) Right lateral thoracic artery and vein; (3) The right axillary vein; (4) The right thoracodorsal vessels; (5) The right thoracodorsal nerve

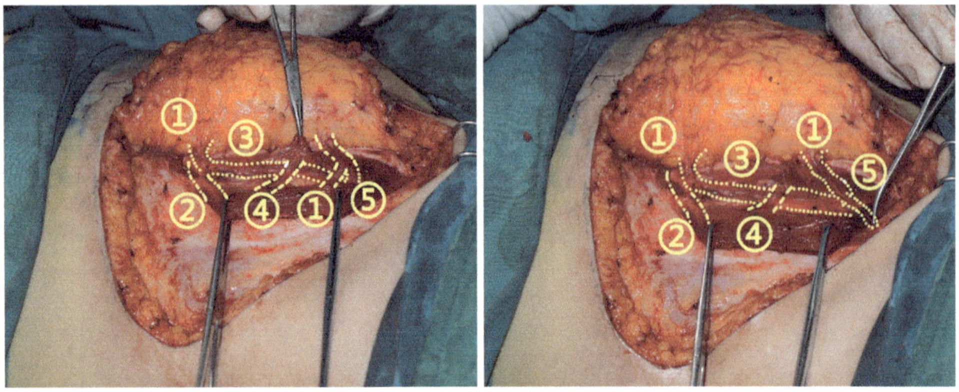

Fig. 3.13 Exposure and separation of the right DIEP. (1) Right DIEPs; (2) Right tendon scratch of the rectus abdominus; (3) Right deep inferior epigastric vessels; (4) Motor branch of right intercostal nerve; (5) Sensory branch of right intercostal nerve

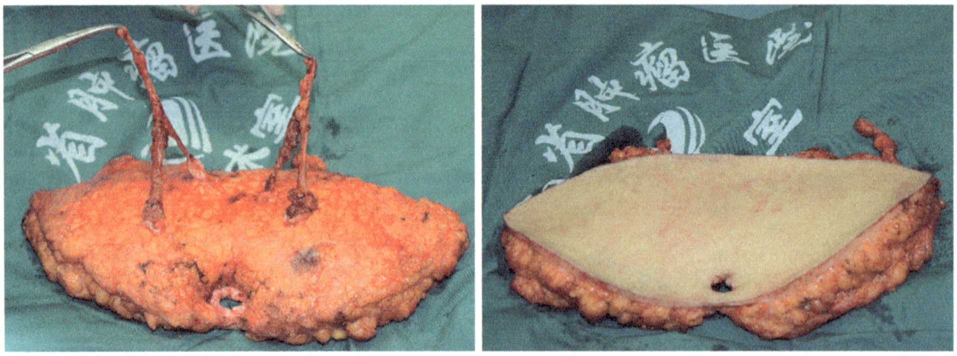

Fig. 3.14 Preparation of DIEP flap pedicled with bilateral vessels

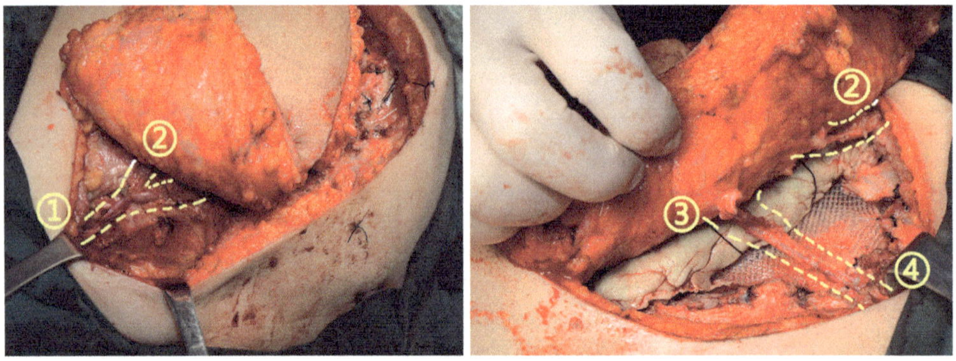

Fig. 3.15 The left deep inferior epigastric vessels were connected with the right lateral thoracic vessels (A: $V = 1:1$) and the right deep inferior epigastric vessels with the proximal ends of the right internal mammary blood vessels (A: $V = 1:1$)

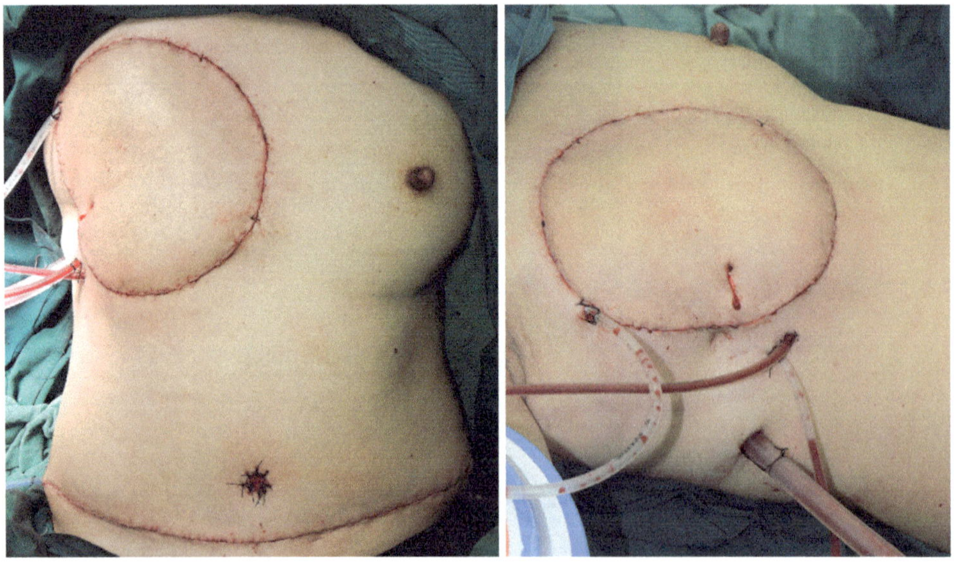

Fig. 3.16 The blood supply of the flap was good and the appearance of the reconstructed chest wall was satisfactory

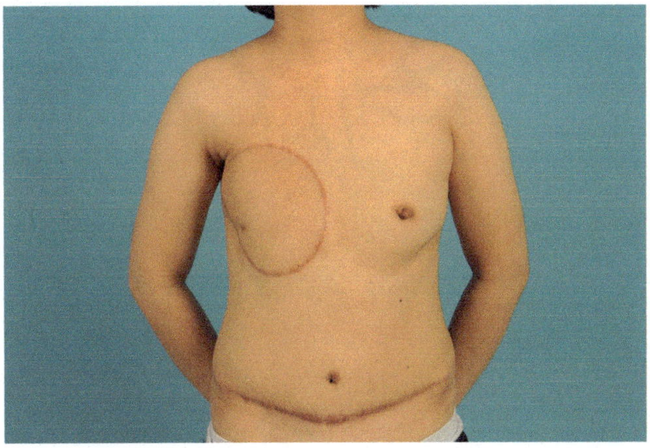

Fig. 3.17 The appearance of reconstructed chest wall was satisfactory at 16 months of follow-up

References

1. Nahabedian MY, Dooley W, Singh N, Manson PN. Contour abnormalities of the abdomen after breast reconstruction with abdominal flaps: the role of muscle preservation. Plast Reconstr Surg. 2002;109(1):91–101.
2. Nahabedian MY, Momen B, Galdino G, Manson PN. Breast reconstruction with the free TRAM or DIEP flap: patient selection, choice of flap, and outcome. Plast Reconstr Surg. 2002;110(2):466–75; discussion 476–7.
3. Bajaj AK, Chevray PM, Chang DW. Comparison of donor-site complications and functional outcomes in free muscle-sparing TRAM flap and free DIEP flap breast reconstruction. Plast Reconstr Surg. 2006;117(3):737–46; discussion 747–50.
4. Selber JC, Serletti JM. The deep inferior epigastric perforator flap: myth and reality. Plast Reconstr Surg. 2010;125(1):50–8.
5. Man LX, Selber JC, Serletti JM. Abdominal wall following free TRAM or DIEP flap reconstruction: a meta-analysis and critical review. Plast Reconstr Surg. 2009;124(3):752–64.
6. Nahabedian MY, Tsangaris T, Momen B. Breast reconstruction with the DIEP flap or the muscle-sparing (MS-2) free TRAM flap: is there a difference. Plast Reconstr Surg. 2005;115(2):436–44; discussion 445–6.
7. Gill PS, Hunt JP, Guerra AB, et al. A 10-year retrospective review of 758 DIEP flaps for breast reconstruction. Plast Reconstr Surg. 2004;113(4):1153–60.
8. Allen RJ. DIEP versus TRAM for breast reconstruction. Plast Reconstr Surg. 2003;111(7):2478.
9. Vega S, Smartt JM, Jiang S, et al. 500 consecutive patients with free TRAM flap breast reconstruction: a single surgeon's experience. Plast Reconstr Surg. 2008;122(2):329–39.
10. Rozen WM, Ashton MW, Murray AC, Taylor GI. Avoiding denervation of rectus abdominis in DIEP flap harvest: the importance of medial row perforators. Plast Reconstr Surg. 2008;122(3):710–6.
11. Rozen WM, Ashton MW, Kiil BJ, et al. Avoiding denervation of rectus abdominis in DIEP flap harvest II: an intraoperative assessment of the nerves to rectus. Plast Reconstr Surg. 2008;122(5):1321–5.
12. Rozen WM, Tran TM, Barrington MJ, Ashton MW. Avoiding denervation of the rectus abdominis muscle in DIEP flap harvest III: a functional study of the nerves to the rectus using anesthetic blockade. Plast Reconstr Surg. 2009;124(2):519–22.
13. Rozen WM, Tran TM, Ashton MW, Barrington MJ, Ivanusic JJ, Taylor GI. Refining the course of the thoracolumbar nerves: a new understanding of the innervation of the anterior abdominal wall. Clin Anat. 2008;21(4):325–33.
14. Munhoz AM, Sturtz G, Montag E, et al. Clinical outcome of abdominal wall after DIEP flap harvesting and immediate application of abdominoplasty techniques. Plast Reconstr Surg. 2005;116(7):1881–93.

Raising the DIEP Flap on Cadaver

4

Zan Li and Jianghua Ou

4.1 Introduction

Our clinical experience is consistent with the report of Bernard et al. [1] that the anatomy of the DIEPs varies greatly. This makes it challenging to balance the sufficient blood supply of the flap and minimize the muscle and nerve injury in the donor area. The wide application of DIEP flap cannot accurately reflect the technical improvements such as the reduction of the degree of injury in the donor area.

The anatomy of perforating vessels plays a decisive role in the degree of donor area injury. According to the extent of donor area damage in clinical practice, the technique of DIEP separation is divided into three categories: (1) zero injury to rectus abdominis muscle and its vegetative nerves; (2) segmental nerve injury with little damage to the muscle; and (3) the medial and lateral perforators of the deep inferior epigastric vessels are both harvested with segmental nerve injury and serious muscle damage (Figs. 4.1, 4.2, 4.3, 4.4, and 4.5).

In recent years, we have performed over 500 cases of breast and chest wall reconstruction using DIEP flap in the Oncoplastic Surgery Department of Hunan Cancer Hospital. During the same period, we carried out anatomical research aiming to simulate the process of raising DIEP flaps; we have documented anatomical data in detail and hence accumulated some experience (see below).

- The lateral perforators runs a very short distance inside the muscle making separation relatively simple, while the medial perforators are closer to the center of the flap harboring larger vascular body area.

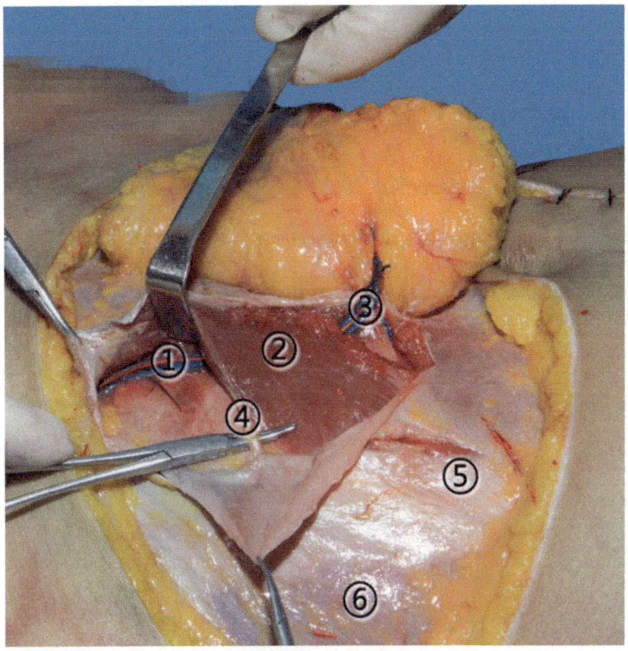

Fig. 4.1 The trunk of deep inferior epigastric vessels and the rectus abdominis muscle was exposed and segmental intercostal nerves along the way were preserved. (1) Deep inferior epigastric vessels; (2) Rectus abdominis; (3) Perforating branch of inferior abdominal wall; (4) Intercostal nerve; (5) Anterior sheath of rectus abdominis; (6) Aponeurosis of external oblique abdominal muscle

- The accompanying veins of the lateral perforating arteries are smaller. It probably requires double veins for revascularization when a DIEP flap pedicled with lateral perforators is used.
- The anatomy of the right perforators above refers to Category 3 aforementioned, which will yield great damage to the rectus abdominis and intercostal nerves. These perforating branches of deep inferior epigastric artery came from internal and external row, respectively. Not only the muscle in between but also the segmental intercostal nerve must be cut off [2–4], which will cause great damage to the donor area.

Z. Li (✉)
Department of Oncology Plastic Surgery, Hunan Cancer Hospital, Changsha, Hunan, China

J. Ou
Department of Breast Surgery, Plastic and Reconstructive Surgery, The Affiliated Tumor Hospital of Xinjiang Medical University, Urumqi, Xinjiang, China

Z. Li, D. Song (eds.), *Oncoplastic Flap Surgery*, https://doi.org/10.1007/978-981-19-8926-1_4

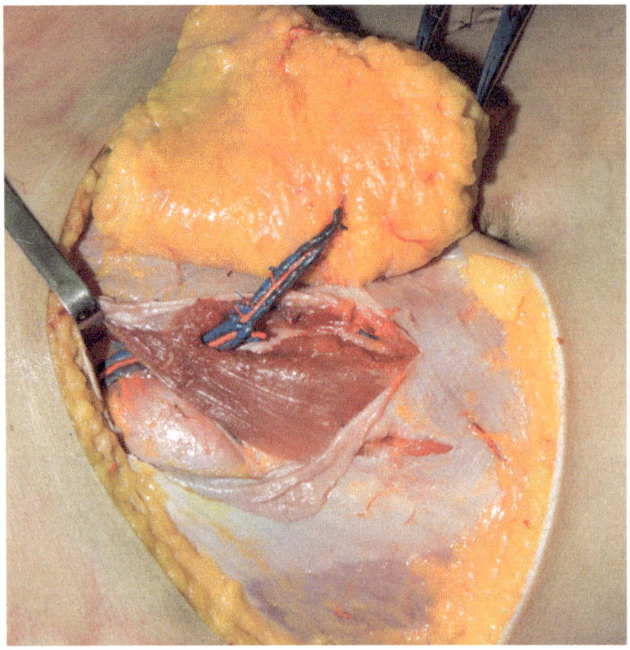

Fig. 4.2 Intramuscular retrograde separation of the perforators and trunk till the surface of posterior sheath of rectus abdominis. The two perforating vessels on the left were close above the muscle. This pertains to category 2

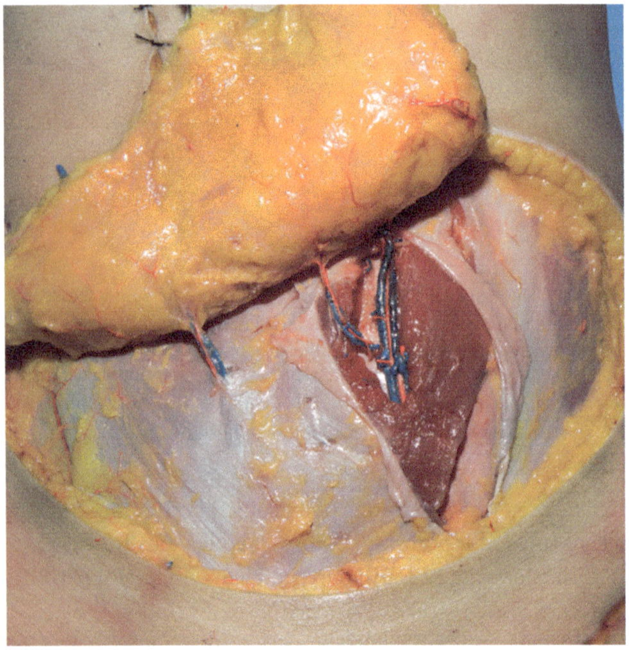

Fig. 4.3 Flip over the flap to expose the contralateral perforating vessels

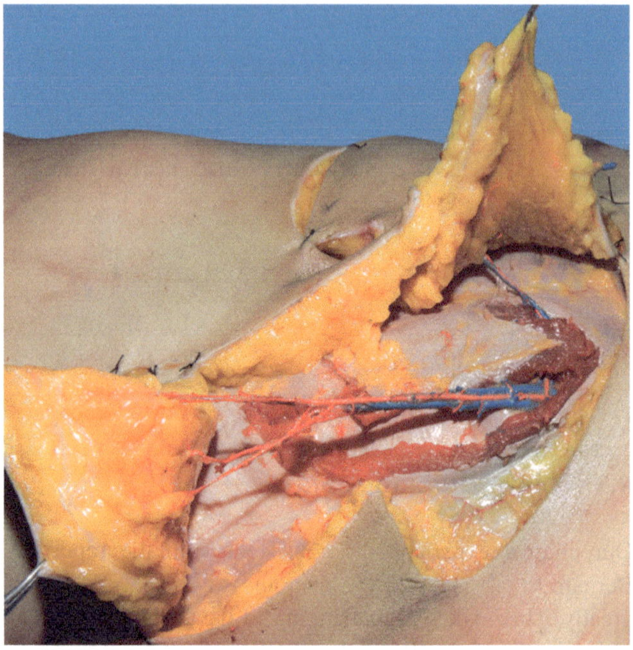

Fig. 4.4 The vascular pedicle was isolated by the rendezvous method and was retrogradely extracted from the intramuscular tunnel after ligation and disconnection from the issuing plane

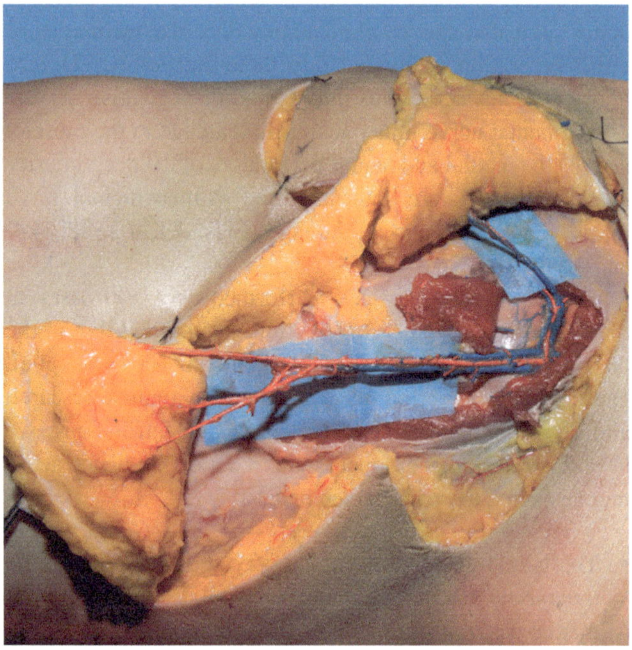

Fig. 4.5 Two right perforating branches were exposed and found to respectively derive from the internal and external branches of the deep inferior epigastric blood vessels after intramuscular dissection. The rectus abdominis muscle between the two perforating branches was cut off and the vascular pedicle was separated to the emitting plane

4.2 Steps of a DIEP FLAP Raising on Cadaver

Schematic diagram of simulated specimen operation (Figs. 4.6, 4.7, 4.8, 4.9, 4.10, 4.11, and 4.12).

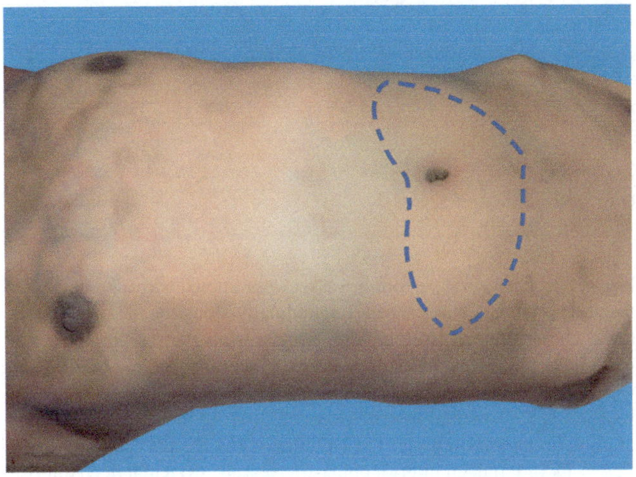

Fig. 4.6 Flap design and marking. A DIEP flap was cut transversely on the right and obliquely on the left

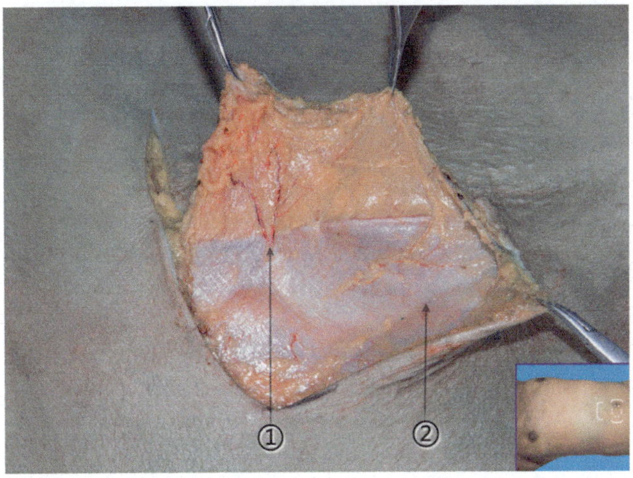

Fig. 4.7 The first step was to cut the right DIEP flap, next to lift the flap from the aponeurosis surface of the external oblique muscle along the design line inward the anterior sheath of the rectus abdominis to expose the perforator vessel. (1) Perforating vessels; (2) Aponeurosis of external oblique abdominal muscle

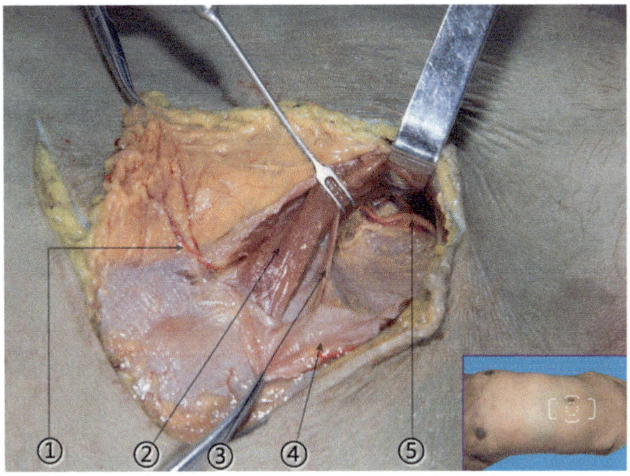

Fig. 4.8 We opened the anterior sheath of rectus abdominis longitudinally outside of the perforating vessel, exposed the perforator and the deep inferior epigastric vascular pedicle, and carefully preserved the terminal branch of intercostal nerves crossing with the vascular pedicle on the way. (1) Perforating vessels; (2) Rectus abdominis; (3) Intercostal nerve branch; (4) Anterior sheath of rectus abdominis; (5) Deep inferior epigastric vessels

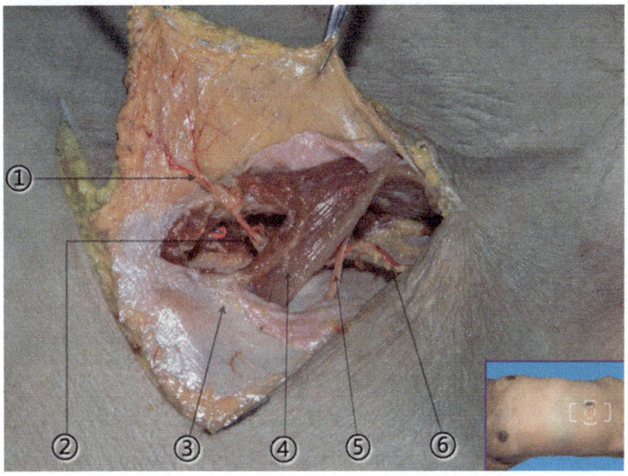

Fig. 4.9 Separation of perforator vessel and deep inferior epigastric vessel pedicle by rendezvous method. Type I perforator, single and thick perforator. (1) Perforating vessels; (2) Distal end of the deep inferior epigastric vessels; (3) Anterior sheath of rectus abdominis; (4) Rectus abdominis; (5) Intercostal nerve branch; (6) Proximal end of deep inferior epigastric vessels

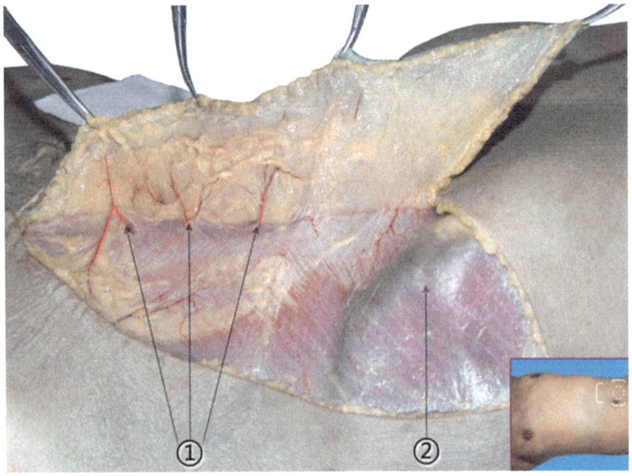

Fig. 4.10 We lifted the left DIEP flap obliquely from the aponeurosis surface of the external oblique muscle inward the anterior sheath surface of rectus abdominis to expose three large perforator vessels. (1) Perforating vessels; (2) Aponeurosis of external oblique abdominal muscle

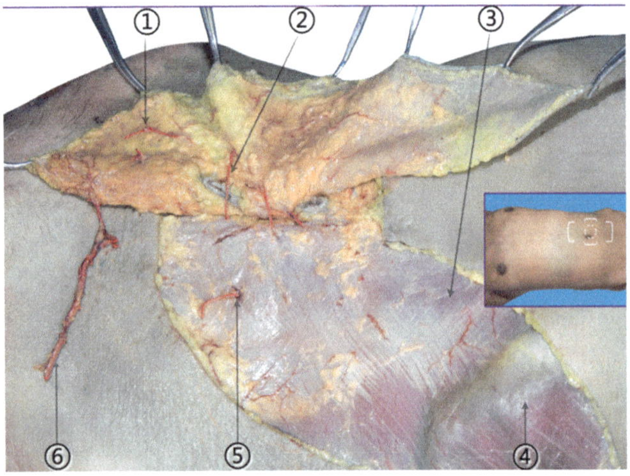

Fig. 4.11 The left perforators were found to contain lateral and medial branches. (1) Right perforator vessel; (2) Left medial perforator vessel; (3) Aponeurosis of external oblique abdominal muscle; (4) Costal arch; (5) Left lateral perforator; (6) Right deep inferior epigastric vascular pedicle

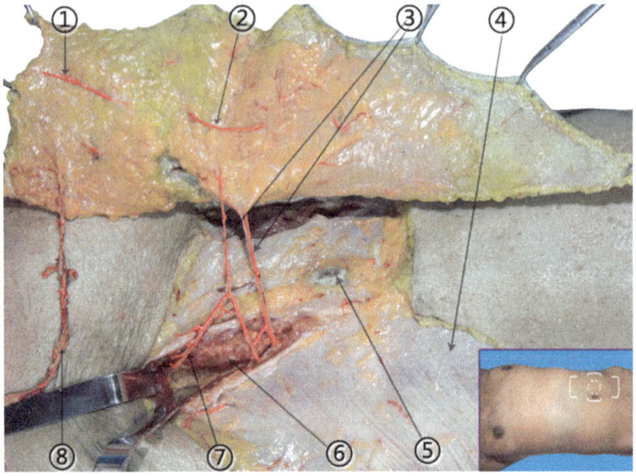

Fig. 4.12 The lateral perforator vessel was retained with a great length, the anterior sheath was opened longitudinally along the medial perforator, each perforator vessel and the vascular trunk were separated retrogradely in the rectus abdominis, now a bilaterally pedicled DIEP flap was prepared. (1) Right perforator vessel; (2) Left lateral perforator vessel; (3) Left medial perforator vessel; (4) Aponeurosis of external oblique abdominal muscle; (5) Umbilicus; (6) Rectus abdominis; (7) The trunk of left deep inferior epigastric vessels; (8) Right deep inferior epigastric vascular pedicle

Key Points of Flap Design

- Because the cutting plane of the flap completely depends on the position of the perforating branch selected, the final design of the flap can only be determined after exposing the thick pulsating perforating branch.
- The most suitable perforator can usually be found at 10–30 mm lateral to the umbilicus at the level of one-third of the rectus abdominis muscle. Because the perforator supports the dense subcutaneous vascular network which communicates with vessels outside the flap, the skin island can be designed in any direction as long as the flap contains a thick periumbilical perforator.
- To ensure blood supply, the range of flap resection should not extend to Area IV which is lateral to the contralateral semilunar line. If an oblique design is adopted on the ipsilateral side, the flap can reach the rib edge.
- The flap design corresponds to the main origin direction of the subcutaneous vascular network. According to the abdominal skin relaxation degree and the direction of the flap axis, the flap can be as wide as more than 10 cm.
- The subcutaneous vascular network is primarily at an angle of 45° to the horizontal level, and densely distributed DIEPs can be found around the umbilicus. Therefore, the oblique design of the flap around the umbilicus is the most reliable.
- The oblique skin flap near the umbilicus is generally safe. In this area, it can be found that the perforating branches from the inferior abdominal artery are densely distributed.
- Doppler detection of perforator position before operation is helpful to flap design.

- The flap should be separated from the outside to the umbilicus, which makes it easy to dissect and find the perforator.
- The deep inferior epigastric artery can always be located when the perforator is separated retrograde, so it is not necessary to look for and separate the pedicle alone.
- Pulling up the deep inferior epigastric artery is helpful to locate the branch. The branch must be carefully ligated and disconnected. The posterior sheath of rectus abdominis cannot be opened.
- There is no need to free the deep inferior abdominal artery to the external iliac artery. Generally, the vascular pedicle is long enough.
- The superior epigastric artery can also be used as a source vessel.

- Cut the subcutaneous tissue of the skin open to the anterior sheath of rectus abdominis muscle. Based on preoperative Doppler imaging, at least one perforator was included in the flap. The medial edge of the flap was located on the midline, and the lateral pole of the flap can reach the costal arch.
- Starting from the lateral edge, lift the flap in the plane above the fascia and separate the flap to the semilunar line. The first perforating branch can be exposed within a few centimeters of the semilunar line, and its thickness and pulsation can be observed.
- Continue to separate the flap on the superficial surface of the anterior sheath of rectus abdominis, and expose the second thick perforator around the umbilicus. Two perforations were included in the flap.
- Carefully lift the flap to fully expose the anterior sheath of rectus abdominis for further dissection of blood vessels. In thinner patients, the DIEA is faintly visible as soon as the flap is slightly lifted upward.
- Carefully dissect the anterior sheath of rectus abdominis around the first perforating branch. If the accompanying sensory nerve is found, cut it off.

Key Points of Operation

- Continue to open the fascia around the second perforating branch, bluntly separate muscle fibers, and expose the deep inferior epigastric blood vessels.
- The deep inferior epigastric vascular pedicle was isolated in a circular pattern. Vascular suspenders were used to expose and facilitate ligating the muscular branches.
- The deep inferior epigastric vessel was freed caudally by blunt dissociation of the muscle fibers instead of removing them. The posterior sheath of rectus abdominis was not damaged.
- The deep inferior epigastric vessels were retrogradely separated to the origin from the external iliac artery without extending the skin incision.
- The deep inferior epigastric vascular pedicle was ligated and cut off at the origin with its perforator perfusing the flap.
- Now the flap was ready for transfer. If necessary, the flap can be thinned by removing excess adipose tissue, leaving only the tissue around the subcutaneous vascular plexus, and perforating branches. Suture rectus abdominis and the anterior sheath, indwell drainage tube. Finally, close the skin opening.
- According to the literature, the anatomy of perforators above was classified in Category 2. The emitting points of the two perforating branches were basically located on the same level of the rectus abdominis muscle bundle, where the muscle damage was not severe, yet the segmental intercostal nerve between perforators had to be cut off.

References

1. Lee BT, Chen C, Nguyen MD, Lin SJ, Tobias AM. A new classification system for muscle and nerve preservation in DIEP flap breast reconstruction. Microsurgery. 2010;30(2):85–90.
2. Rozen WM, Ashton MW, Murray AC, Taylor GI. Avoiding denervation of rectus abdominis in DIEP flap harvest: the importance of medial row perforators. Plast Reconstr Surg. 2008;122(3):710–6.
3. Rozen WM, Ashton MW, Kiil BJ, et al. Avoiding denervation of rectus abdominis in DIEP flap harvest II: an intraoperative assessment of the nerves to rectus. Plast Reconstr Surg. 2008;122(5):1321–5.
4. Rozen WM, Tran TM, Barrington MJ, Ashton MW. Avoiding denervation of the rectus abdominis muscle in DIEP flap harvest III: a functional study of the nerves to the rectus using anesthetic blockade. Plast Reconstr Surg. 2009;124(2):519–22.

The DIEA Branching Pattern and Its Relationship to Perforators

5

Zan Li and Yiyin Tang

The deep inferior epigastric vessels constantly originate from the external iliac vessels, yet how the vessels travel and branch is highly variable and complicated. This needs to be discussed systematically regarding each variation.

5.1 The Number of Perforating Branches of Deep Inferior Epigastric Vessels

Boyd firstly described the anatomy of deep inferior epigastric vascular bifurcation in 1984 that the vascular trunk was divided into two to three main branches [1].

Since then, disparity regarding the branching patterns of DIEP was reported in subsequent studies [2, 3]. In 1988, Moon and Taylor firstly proposed a classification system [4], namely, single perforator pattern (Fig. 5.1), dual perforator pattern, and triple perforator pattern [3, 5].

The classification was based on the size of perforators and how the perforators communicated with the supraumbilical and superior epigastric arteries [6].

Further studies emphasized that this classification system was based on the size of the certainly existing paraumbilical branches which were either the medial small branches from single or dual perforator(s) or a member of the triple perforators [4].

In plain view, harvesting a DIEP flap based on single perforator brings little damage to the donor area, but in practice, it is commonly found that the perforator and vascular pedicle travel a long distance in the muscle (as shown in Figs. 5.2 and 5.3). Great damage to the donor area is inevitable especially when the vessels run in an oblique direction.

It was reported that when a DIEP flap based on single perforator was chosen for breast reconstruction, a large enough perforator with simple anatomical relationship was preferred so that the ischemic time and the incidence of venous complications could be minimized (as shown in Figs. 5.4 and 5.5) [7].

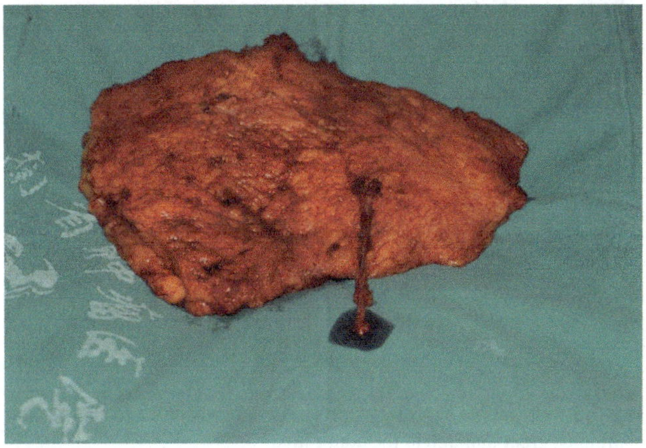

Fig. 5.1 A DIEP flap based on single perforator blood supply

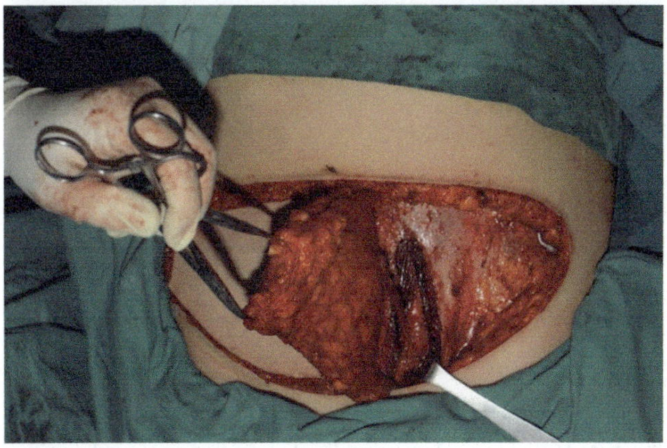

Fig. 5.2 The single vascular pedicle keeps running inside the muscle resulting in extensive muscle separation and great damage

Z. Li (✉)
Department of Oncology Plastic Surgery, Hunan Cancer Hospital, Changsha, Hunan, China

Y. Tang
Department of Breast Surgery, Yunnan Cancer Hospital, Kunming, Yunnan, China

Z. Li, D. Song (eds.), *Oncoplastic Flap Surgery*, https://doi.org/10.1007/978-981-19-8926-1_5

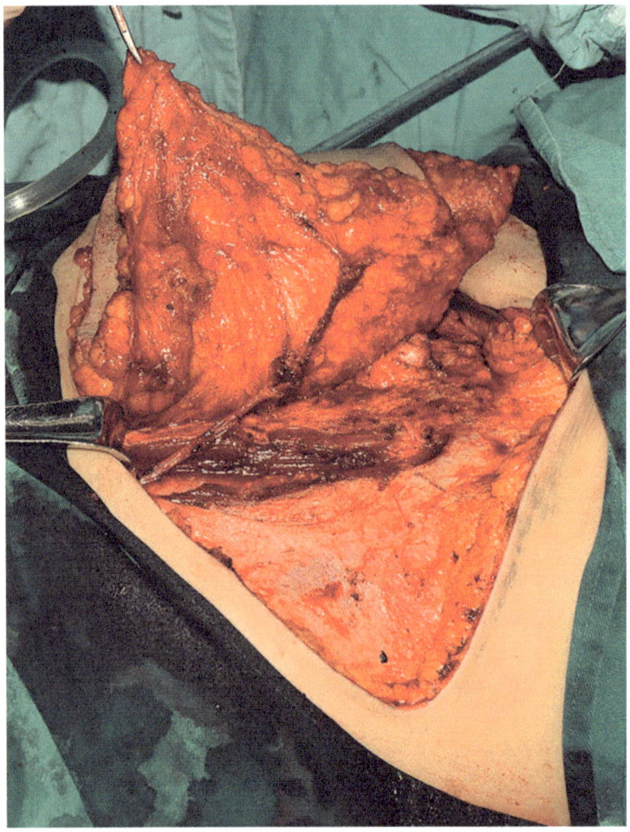

Fig. 5.3 The single perforator traveled a long distance in the muscle leading to great damage to the donor area

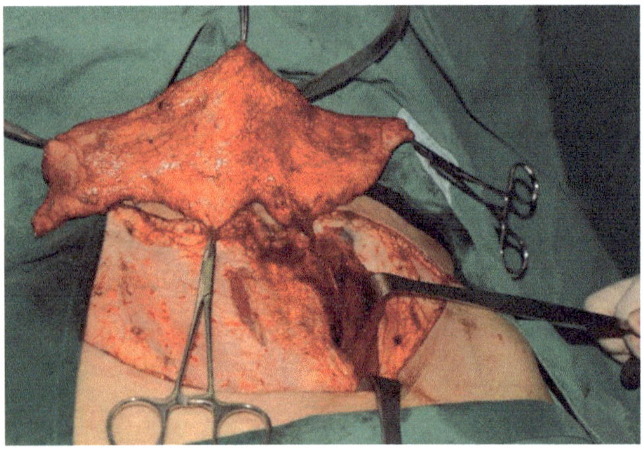

Fig. 5.4 None but single paraumbilical perforator was found on either side and retrograde separation showed that there were no other branches of deep inferior epigastric vessels

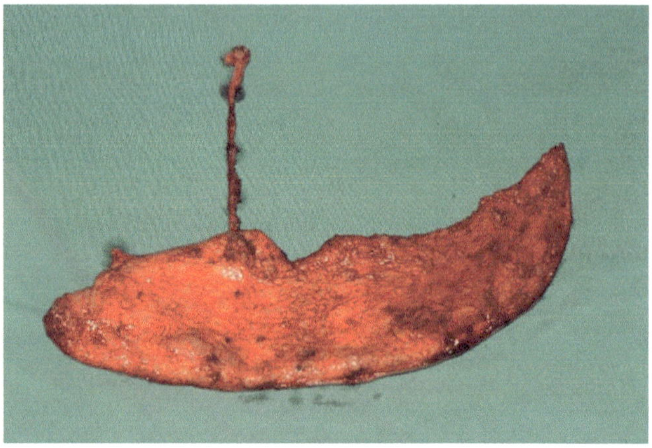

Fig. 5.5 Good blood circulation in area IV. The dual-perforator pedicle is divided into the medial row and lateral row

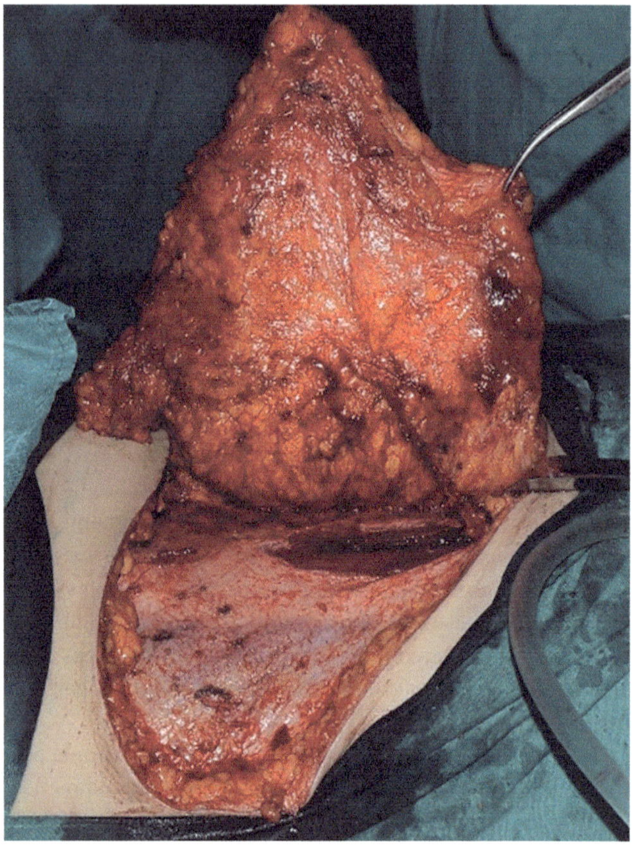

Fig. 5.6 Perforating branch of the medial row

Studies have proved that the medial perforators of deep inferior epigastric vessels deliver blood for a larger area than the lateral ones [8].

Using a flap pedicled with a dominant medial perforator is beneficial for unilateral breast reconstruction especially in reconstructing a large breast (as shown in Figs. 5.6, 5.7, 5.8, and 5.9). In general, the single lateral perforator pedicle mainly supplies blood to the ipsilateral abdominal wall, and its blood supply capacity to the contralateral abdominal wall crossing the midline is limited (as shown in Fig. 5.10) [9].

A DIEP flap with dual or triple perforators should be based on the premise of reliable blood supply of the flap. So far, we have not harvested a triple-perforator flap. In our opinion, a single pedicle containing two perforators or bilateral pedicles, by reasonable design and skillful dissection, is

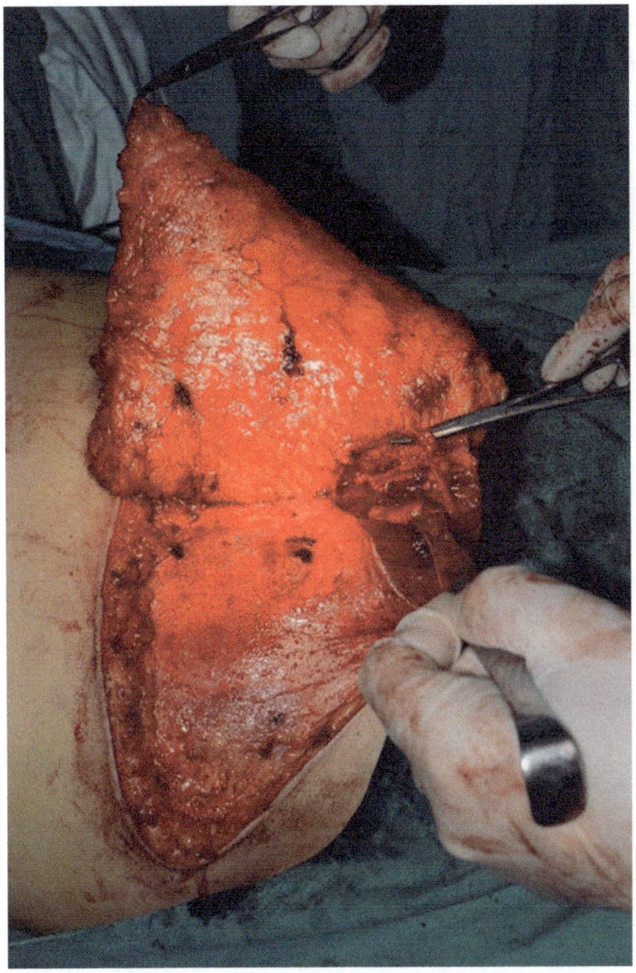

Fig. 5.7 Intramuscular retrograde separation of the medial perforator and vascular pedicle

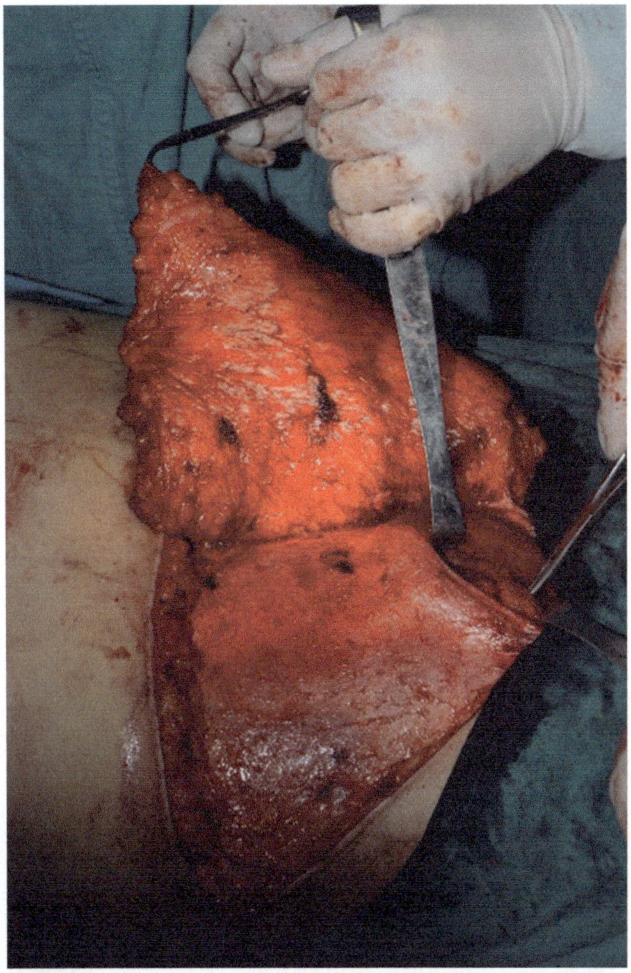

Fig. 5.8 The proximal end of vascular pedicle was exposed from the lateral edge of rectus abdominis, and the morbidity of rectus abdominis and intercostal nerve was minimized

far enough for flap blood supply, even if the whole lower abdominal flap is used.

Trying to make a single pedicled flap with three perforating branches will lead to excessive damage to the flap donor area. Furthermore, it is difficult to accurately estimate whether multiple perforating branches share a common stem during the operation; if it happens, then a rectus abdominis-containing flap is suggested (as shown in Figs. 5.11, 5.12, and 5.13).

5.1.1 Case 1: Anatomical Type of Perforating Branch

In this case, a DIEP flap with bilateral vascular pedicles was used for breast reconstruction. The anatomical types of the perforators on both sides were different (as shown in Figs. 5.14, 5.15, 5.16, 5.17, 5.18, and 5.19).

Key points:(1) This perforator pattern is vulnerable to be injured by mistake in clinical practice when the vessel travels

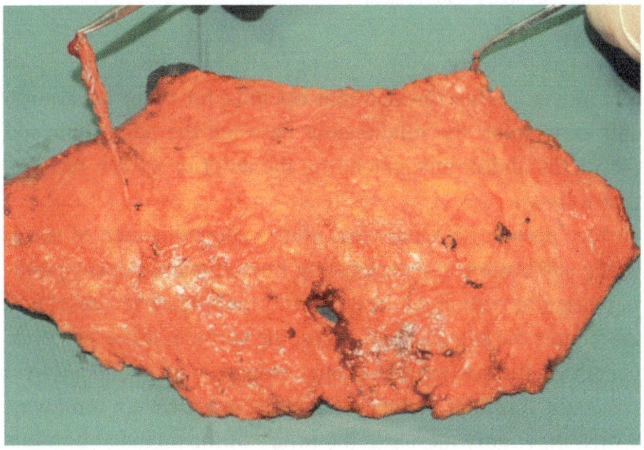

Fig. 5.9 Dual perforators offered reliable blood supply to Area IV

a long distance underneath the anterior sheath or on the surface of the muscle. To avoid this, we advise to make a small opening 0.5 cm away from where the perforator comes out of

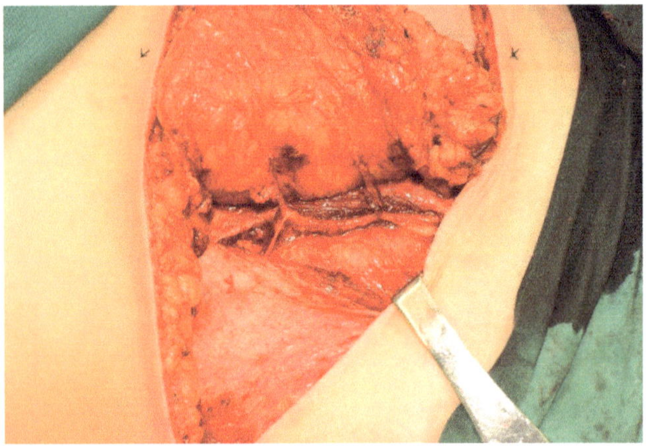

Fig. 5.10 The lateral branch of deep inferior epigastric vessel, vertically sending out two perforators, was used as pedicle to ensure the blood supply of the flap

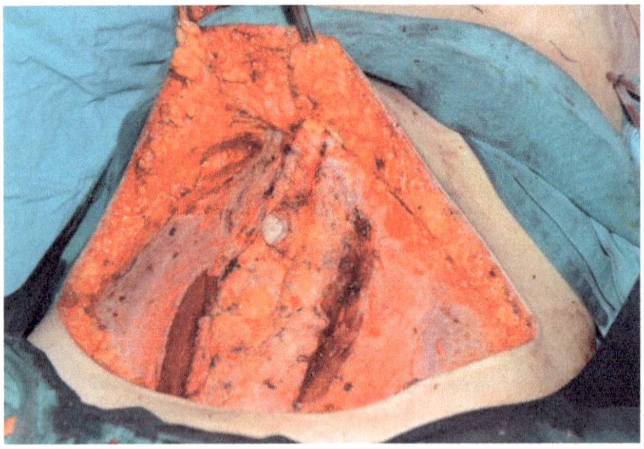

Fig. 5.11 Bilateral vascular pedicle flaps can still preserve the integrity of bilateral donor anterior sheath and rectus abdominis, and minimize the damage of donor area

the anterior sheath at first; the next step is to insert the tip of a hemostat clamp through that opening for blunt separation and understand the relationship between the perforator and the rectus abdominis, extending the anterior sheath incision that follows.

Key points: (2) Generally, after a short distance of retrograde separation, the perforating branch and its corresponding vascular pedicle of the deep inferior epigastric vessel will then enter the muscle and run on the surface of the posterior sheath of the rectus abdominis. However, in many clinical cases, the vascular pedicle runs in the muscle for a long way, which inevitably increases the injury of the rectus abdominis and the difficulty of operation.

Pressure equilibrium law: The normal blood supply of a specific skin area is basically stable, and its supporting blood vessels are compensatory to each other in terms of caliber and interval. If the caliber of one blood vessel is small, the caliber of the adjacent blood vessel is correspondingly large, or the spacing is correspondingly shortened.

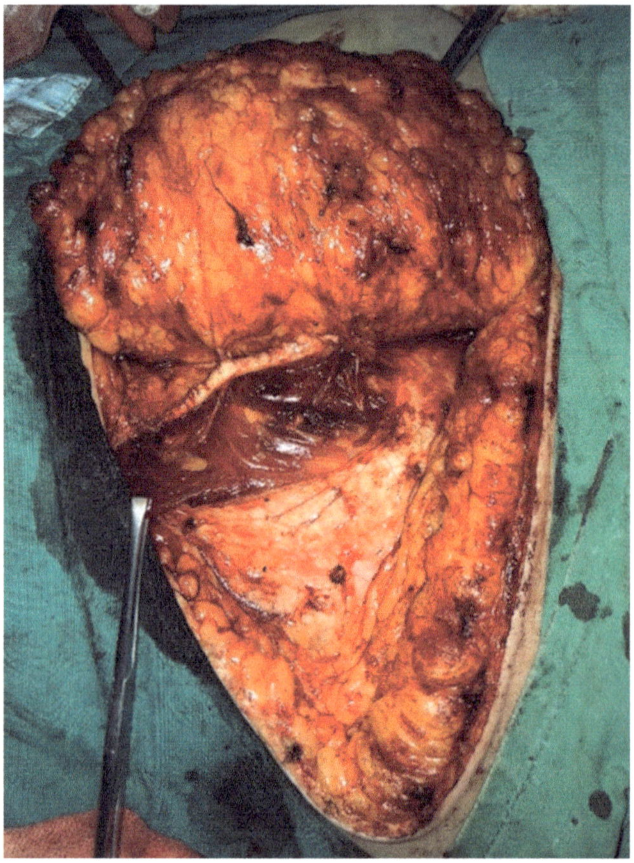

Fig. 5.12 The three perforating branches were widely distributed, and the injury of rectus abdominis was extensive

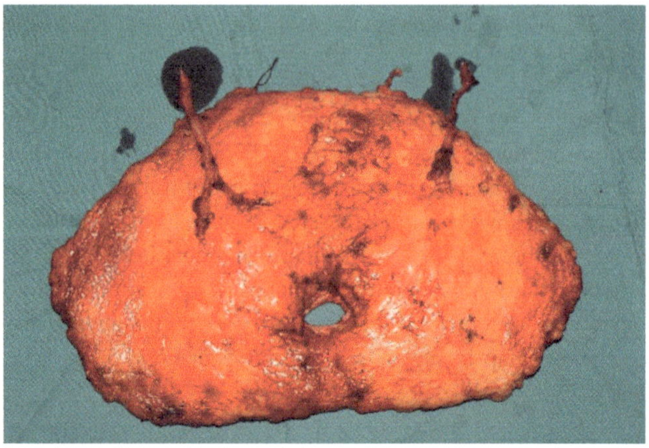

Fig. 5.13 A DIEP flap with bilateral pedicles. Both pedicles were the lateral branch of corresponding deep inferior epigastric vessels. The left pedicle included one perforator and the right pedicle contained three perforators, yet to reduce muscle damage, only two perforators were selected

5.1.2 Case 2: Multiple Perforator Pattern

A 20-year-old female was hospitalized and diagnosed as a giant phyllode tumor of the right breast with extensive skin invasion. After admission, right mastectomy and DIEP flap for breast reconstruction were performed.

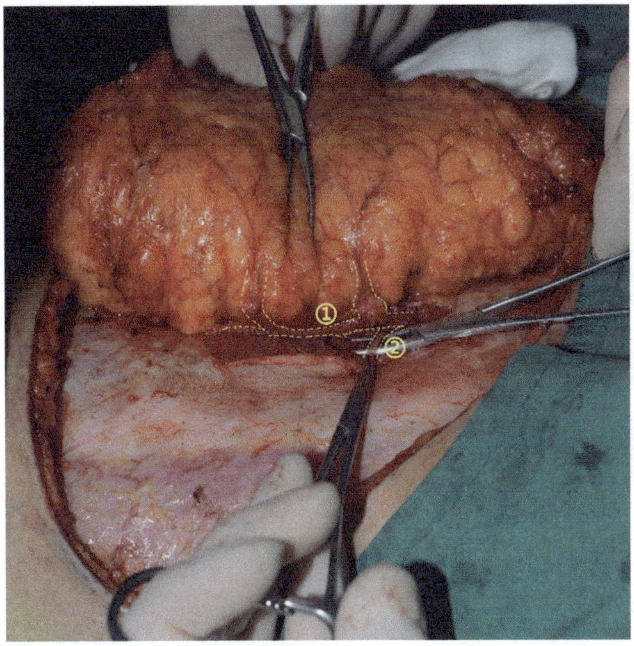

Fig. 5.14 The right DIEP was exposed and the intercostal nerve that crisscrossed with the right DIEP was preserved. (1) Inferior abdominal vascular pedicle; (2) Intercostal nerve

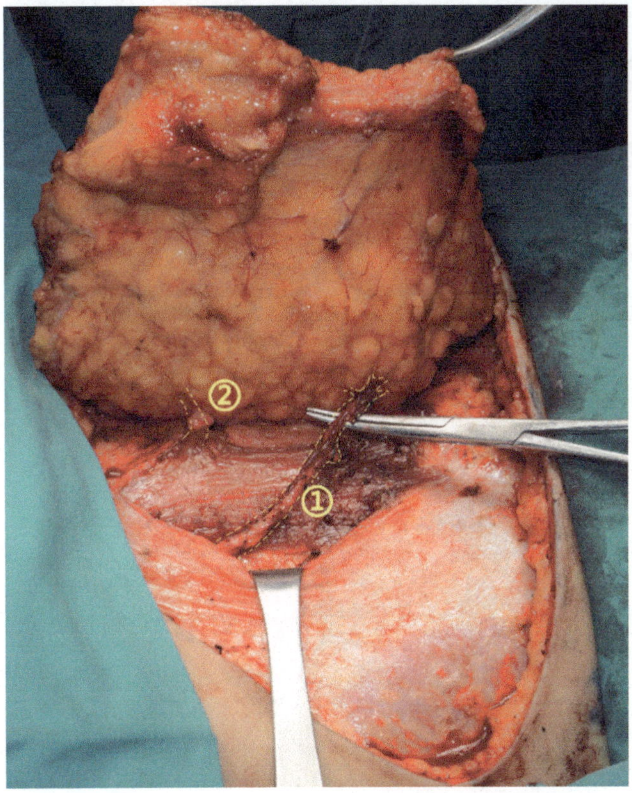

Fig. 5.15 Further separation found that the left lateral perforator traveled a long distance on the surface of the rectus abdominis and penetrated from the outer edge of the muscle. (1) Lateral perforator; (2) Medial perforator

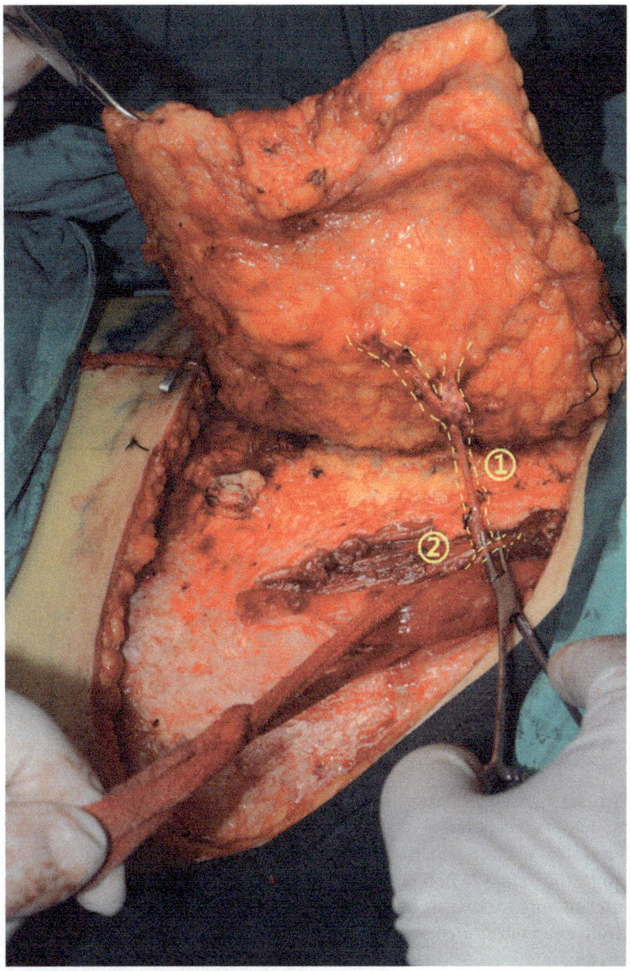

Fig. 5.16 A long segment of the perforator and the trunk of the right epigastric vessel runs inside the rectus abdominis muscle. (1) Deep inferior epigastric vascular pedicle; (2) Intercostal nerve

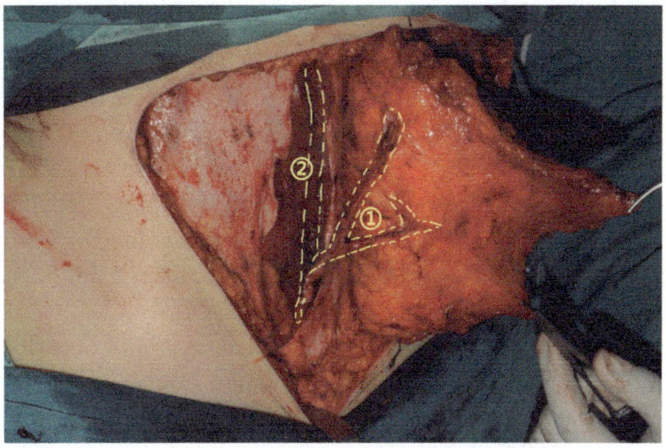

Fig. 5.17 A long segment of the vessel pedicle ran in the muscle. Along the way, it was necessary to carefully ligate small branches and protect intercostal nerve branches. The operation was difficult, the operation time was significantly prolonged, and the degree of injury in the donor area was increased. (1) Deep inferior epigastric vascular pedicle; (2) The gap left after the rectus abdominis was dissected

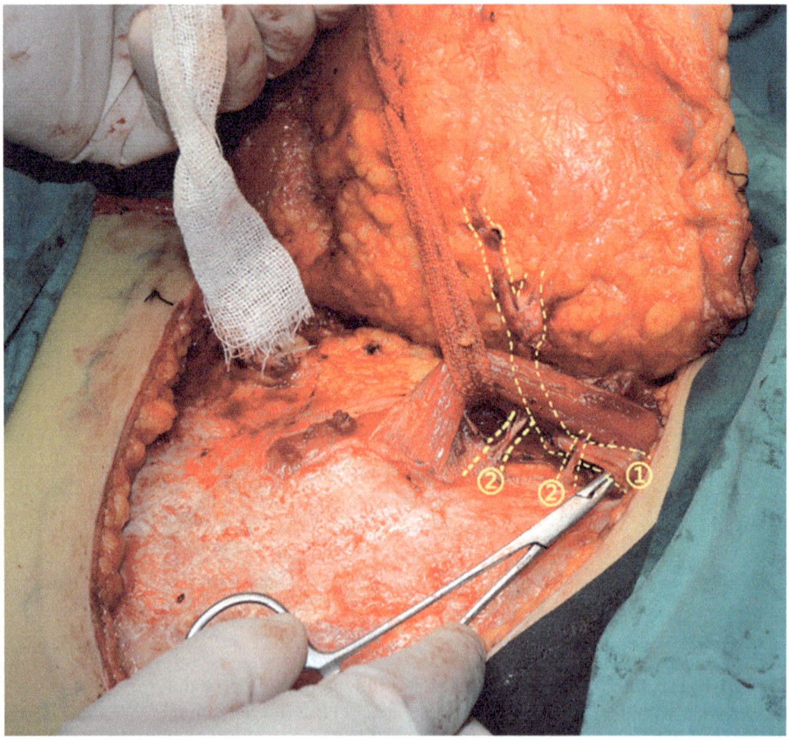

Fig. 5.18 The vascular pedicle was isolated at the posterior space of the rectus abdominis muscle and the integrity of segmental intercostal nerve was preserved. (1) Deep inferior epigastric vascular pedicle; (2) Intercostal nerve

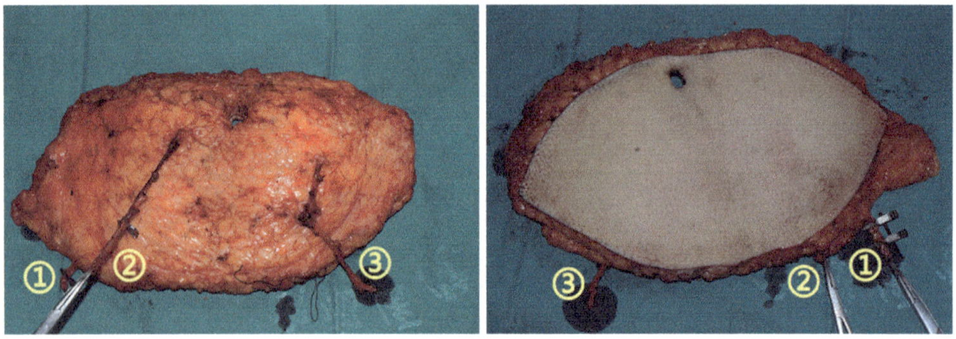

Fig. 5.19 A DIEP flap with bilateral pedicles was harvested. (1) Left superficial epigastric vein; (2) Left deep inferior epigastric vessel; (3) Right deep inferior epigastric vessel

During the operation, the right DIEP flap was used and the tissue in Area IV and part of Area III of the flap were removed.

The right internal thoracic vessels were anastomosed with the right inferior epigastric vessels of the flap (A: v = 1:2).

The flap survived completely after operation, and the shape and function of the reconstructed breast were satisfactory (as shown in Figs. 5.20, 5.21, 5.22, 5.23, 5.24, 5.25, 5.26, 5.27, 5.28, 5.29, 5.30, and 5.31).

The key of flap harvest is to select an appropriate perforating branch. The selected perforating artery should be accompanied by vein, with appropriate size and diameter ≥ 0.5 mm.

There are many tricks as to separating and exposing the perforating vessels, for example, after finding the lateral perforating vessels; if it is necessary to further understand the condition of the medial perforators, it is better to look for them from the inferior margin of the flap toward the superior margin, so as not to damage the paraumbilical perforating vessels and be disturbed by the lateral perforating vessels.

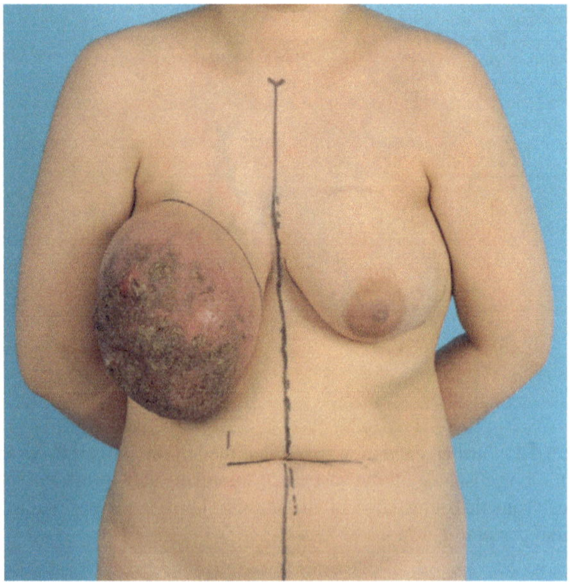

Fig. 5.20 Preoperative conditions

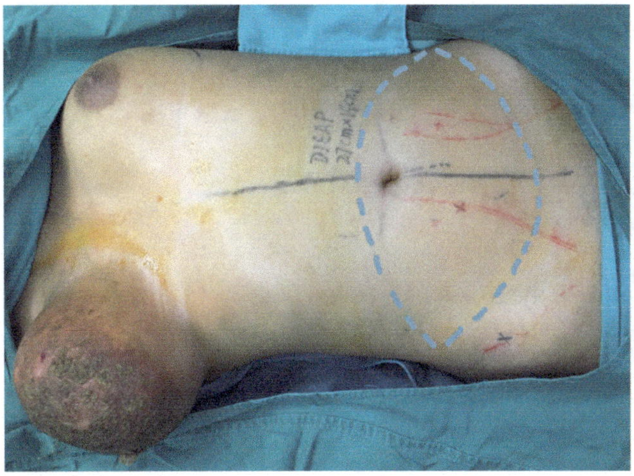

Fig. 5.21 Intraoperative flap design

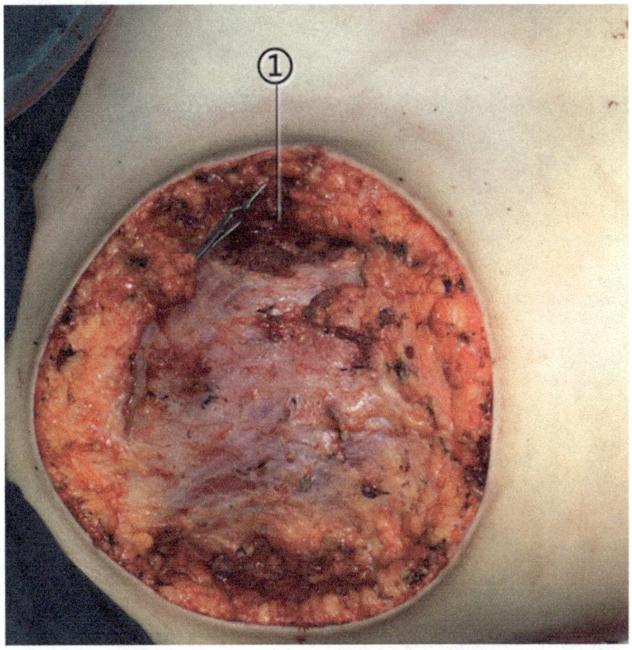

Fig. 5.22 Separation and exposure of internal mammary vessels after extended mastectomy on the right side. (1) Internal thoracic vessels

This was a type 1 perforator pattern where no obvious branches were found in the deep inferior epigastric vessels, yet the perforator and the corresponding vascular pedicle trunk ran obliquely in the rectus abdominis for a long distance. The manipulation is far from easy and the resulting injury to the rectus abdominis is also greater than that of the typical type 1 perforator pattern.

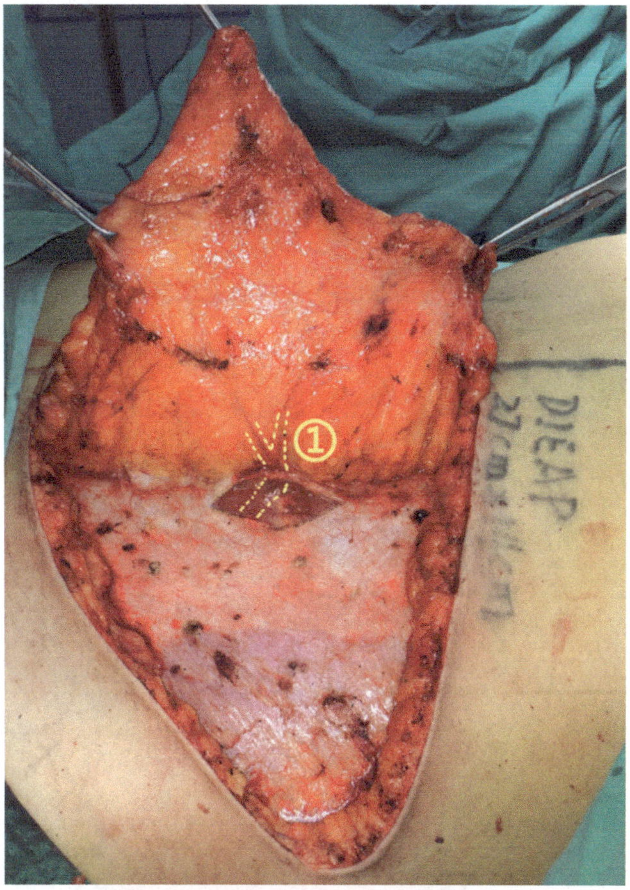

Fig. 5.23 Lift the left abdominal flap, make an incision on the anterior sheath when the perforator was spotted and expose the hidden perforator and vascular pedicle.(1) Deep inferior epigastric vessels

The anatomical classification of deep inferior epigastric vessels should not only be based on their branching pattern, but also on their intramuscular running and running direction (as shown in Fig. 5.32).

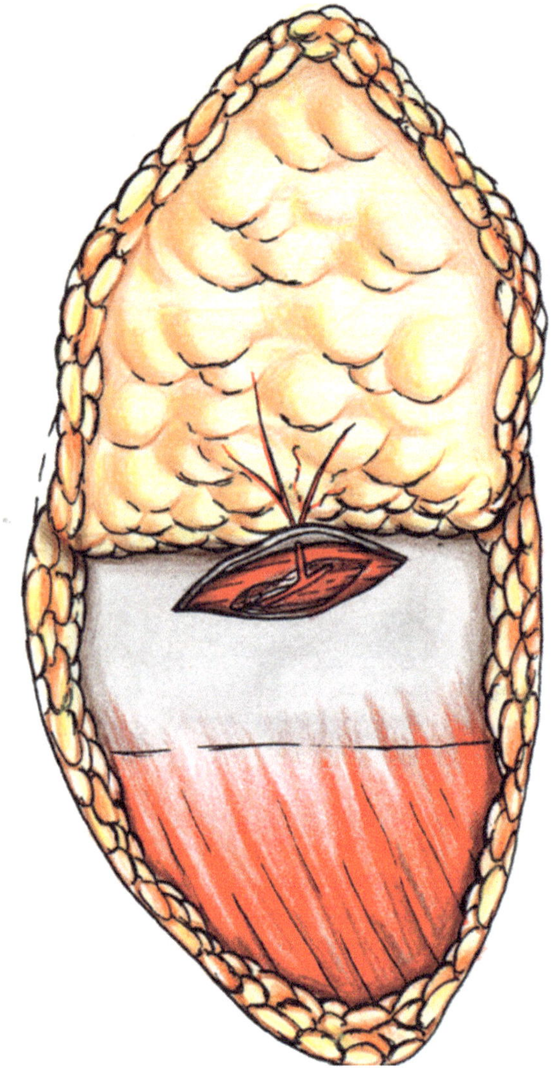

Fig. 5.24 The perforating branch traveled in a horizontal oblique way. Consistent with the literature, this anatomical pattern of the perforating vessels was commonly seen with the lateral branch of the deep inferior epigastric vessels, which significantly increased the damage to the donor site

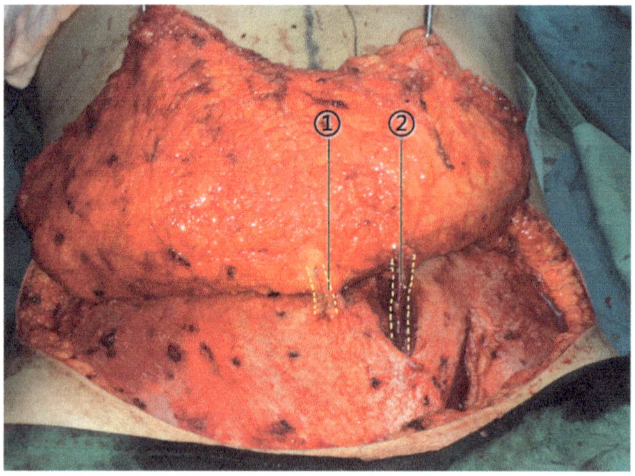

Fig. 5.25 Further separate revealed another thick perforating vessel on the inner side that was considered the medial branch from the deep inferior epigastric vessel and maintained for the time being. (1) Medial branch of deep inferior epigastric vessel; (2) Lateral branch of deep inferior epigastric vessel

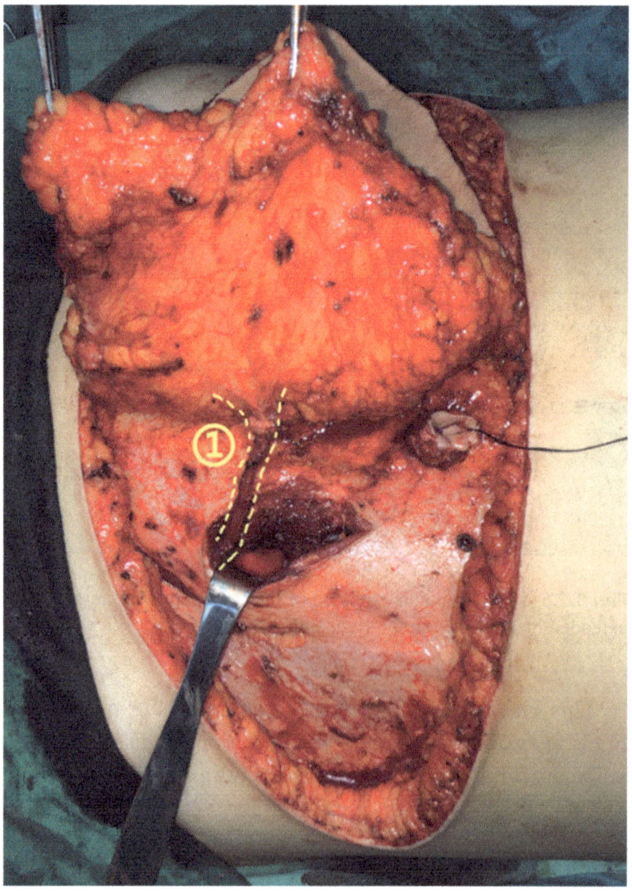

Fig. 5.26 The vascular pedicle was not oblique outward, instead vertically penetrating the muscle and running a long distance inside the rectus abdominis. (1) Deep inferior epigastric vessels

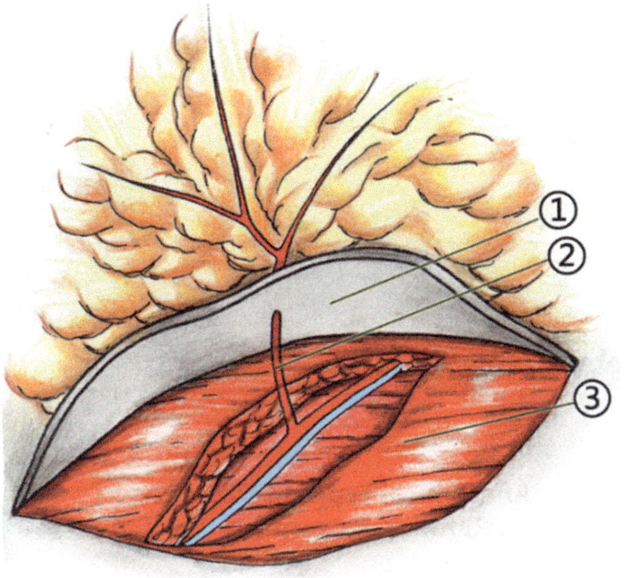

Fig. 5.27 The anatomical structure of a perforator branch. (1) Anterior sheath of rectus abdominis; (2) Perforating vessels; (3) Rectus abdominis

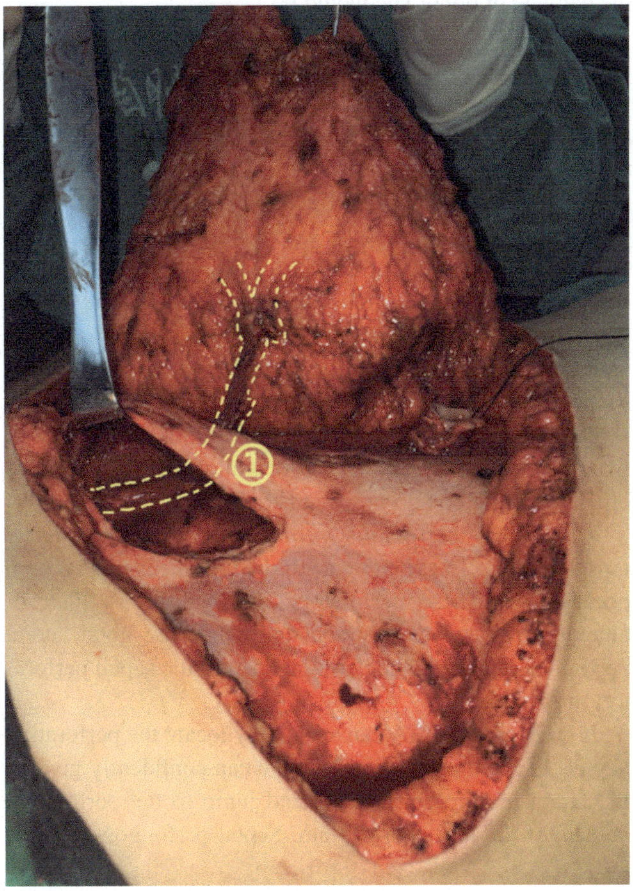

Fig. 5.28 A modified method for dissecting the entire vascular pedicle to preserve the integrity of anterior sheath and rectus abdominis to the greatest extent. (1) Deep inferior epigastric vessels

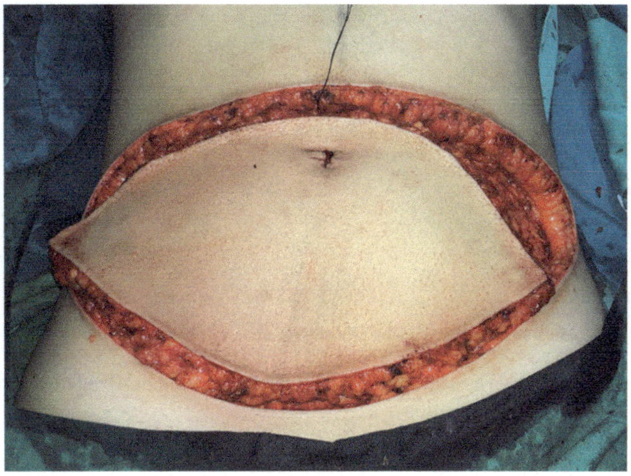

Fig. 5.29 Flap dissection completed

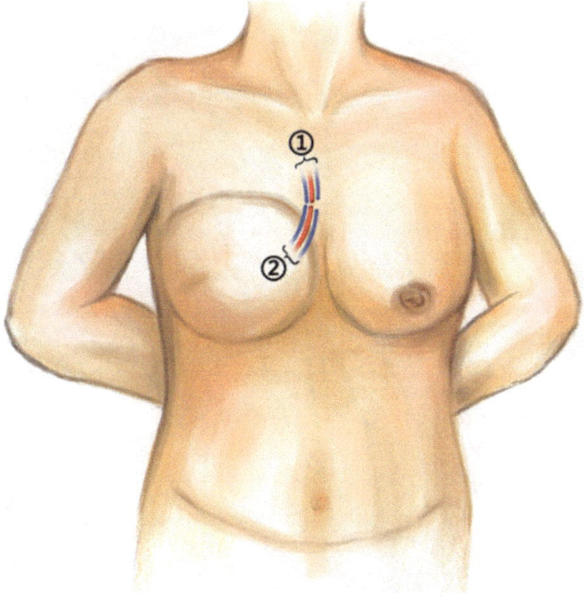

Fig. 5.30 Revascularization mode: the right deep inferior epigastric vessels were anastomosed with the right internal thoracic vessels (A: v = 1:2). (1) Right internal mammary vessels; (2) Right deep inferior epigastric vessel

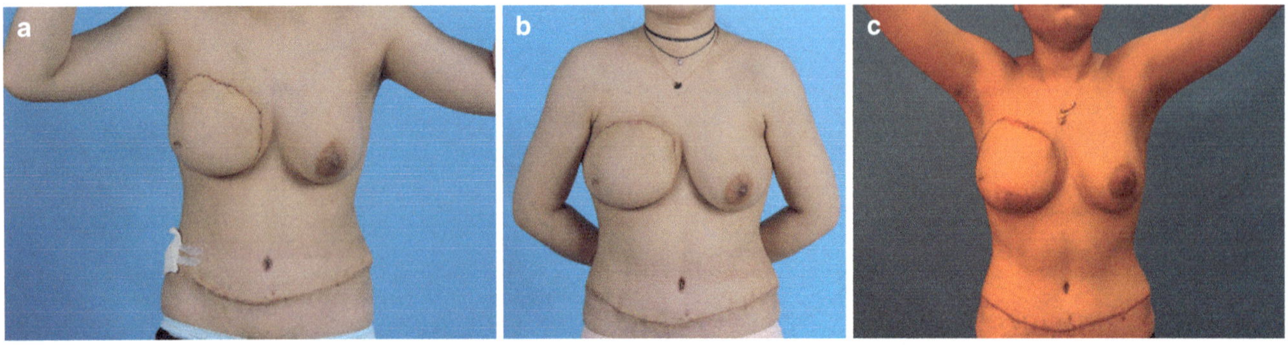

Fig. 5.31 (**a**) The appearance 1 month after operation. (**b**) The appearance 6 months after operation. (**c**) The patients were followed up for 12 months after operation

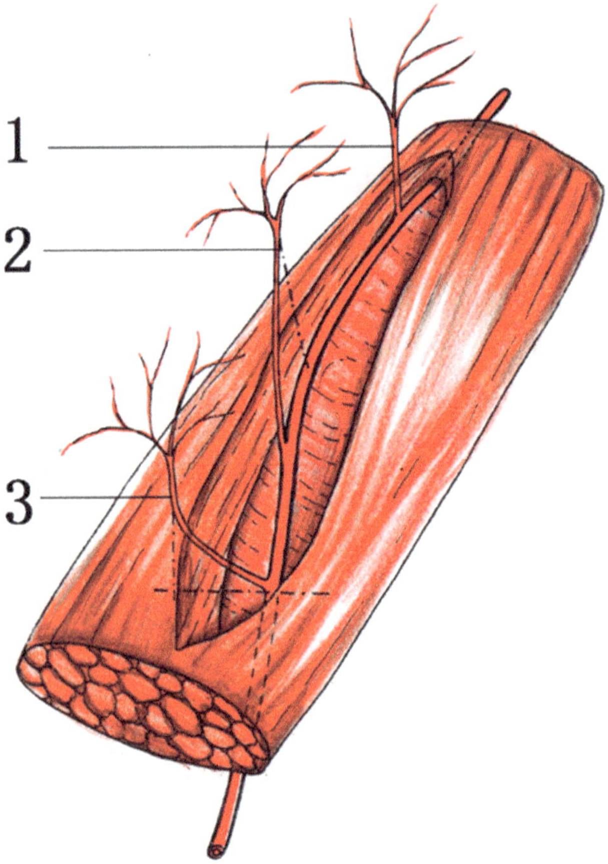

Fig. 5.32 According to the direction of the perforating branch in the rectus abdominis, the perforating branch is divided into three types: (1) Vertical perforating branch: the perforator rises vertically from the deep inferior epigastric vessel and passes through the rectus abdominis; (2) Vertical oblique perforator: after the perforator is sent out, it penetrates the rectus abdominis perpendicular to the longitudinal level; (3) Horizontal oblique perforator: after the perforator is sent out, it penetrates the rectus abdominis transversely parallel to the horizontal level

5.2 Anatomical Types of DIEPs Based on Running Pattern

Further anatomical and clinical studies found that the branches of the deep inferior epigastric artery were related to the intramuscular course of the perforators [5].

In the process of separating perforator vessels, the greater the extent of transverse muscle disconnection is, the greater the damage of donor site would be.

The range of triple perforators through the muscle is significantly wider than that of dual perforators, especially when the dual perforators of the lateral branch are selected, the sacrificed muscle is significantly less than that of the triple perforators, in other words, the muscle injury is reduced. This has been confirmed in clinical work [6].

Based on the clinical findings, we summarized three common anatomical types of DIEPs regarding the running patterns as follows: (1) musculocutaneous perforator; (2) perforating branch of tendon; (3) septal perforator.

It is difficult to separate the perforating branch of tendon scratch. If required, it is recommended to carry appropriate tendon scratch tissue around the perforating branch vessel, which can not only reduce the operation risk but also the operation duration (as shown in Fig. 5.33).

Thick septal perforators medial to the rectus abdominis muscle (about 8%) right beneath the umbilicus can be seen occasionally. These perforators can be used as Plan B, although they are usually abandoned because good lateral perforators are already determined before the septal perforators are reached.

If preoperative CTA can accurately locate the perforating vessels of the muscular septum, we can confidently give up the lateral perforating vessels and jump to the perforating vessels of the muscular septum. Septal perforators of large

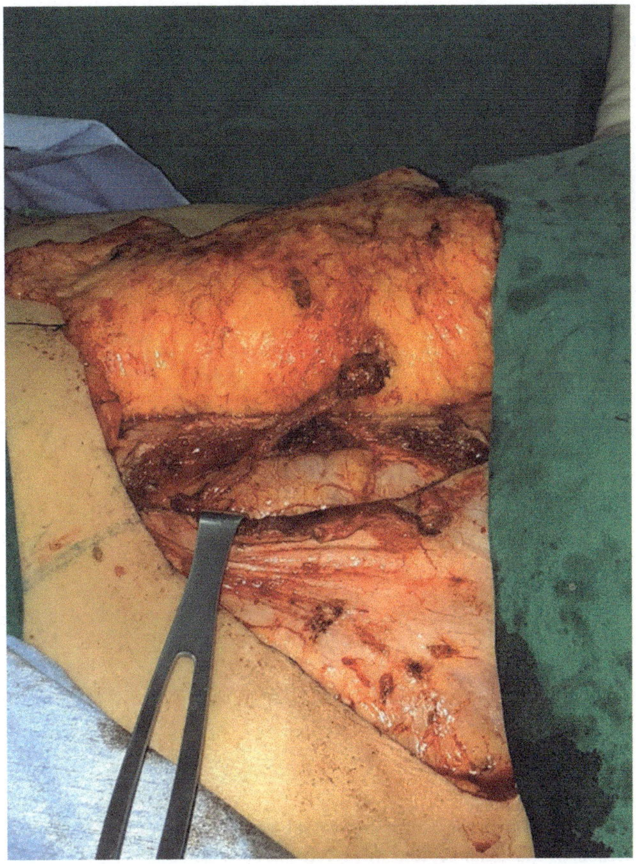

Fig. 5.33 A small amount of muscle and tendon scratch tissue were preserved together with the perforator of tendon scratch

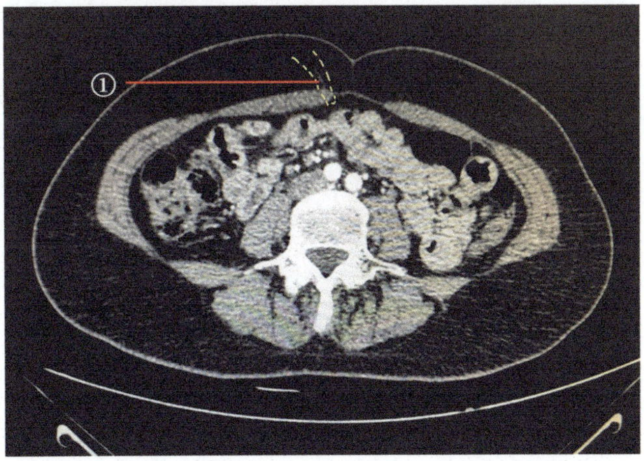

Fig. 5.34 Preoperative abdominal CTA showed a septal perforator on the medial rectus abdominis muscle on the right side. (1) Septal perforator

caliber are able to adequately deliver blood supply to bilateral flaps (as shown in Figs. 5.34 and 5.35).

Circumferential branch of musculocutaneous artery, also known as "direct cutaneous branch of muscular vessels," was

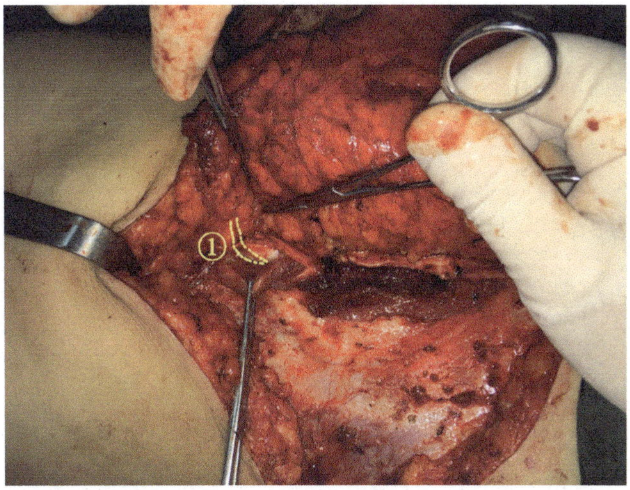

Fig. 5.35 The septal perforator from the medial edge of rectus abdominis. (1) Perforating vessels of muscular septum

proposed in 1984 by Zhong Shizhen, a Chinese anatomist. It refers to the artery that comes out from the trunk of musculocutaneous artery and does not penetrate into the muscle parenchyma, instead it enters the skin from the edge of the muscle.

5.2.1 Case 3: Muscular Septal Perforating Branch of Deep Inferior Epigastric Artery

A 41-year-old female presented with a right breast mass found for half a year. Preoperative biopsy indicated right breast ductal carcinoma in situ. The patient received right mastectomy plus right sentinel lymph node biopsy plus reconstruction with DIEP flap.

The left deep inferior epigastric artery and veins were anastomosed end-to-end with the right internal thoracic artery and vein (1A2V).

The tumor was diagnosed on postoperative pathological examination as a high grade intraductal carcinoma with nuclear Grade II, consisting of mostly comedo-carcinoma and partly papillary carcinoma; the patient was staged pTisN0M0; no cancer involvement was found in skin, basal margin, and nipple; no cancer metastasis was found in the right axillary sentinel lymph node.

The flap survived smoothly after operation, and the shape and function of the flap were satisfactory during follow-up (as shown in Figs. 5.36, 5.37, 5.38, 5.39, 5.40, 5.41, 5.42, 5.43, 5.44, 5.45, and 5.46).

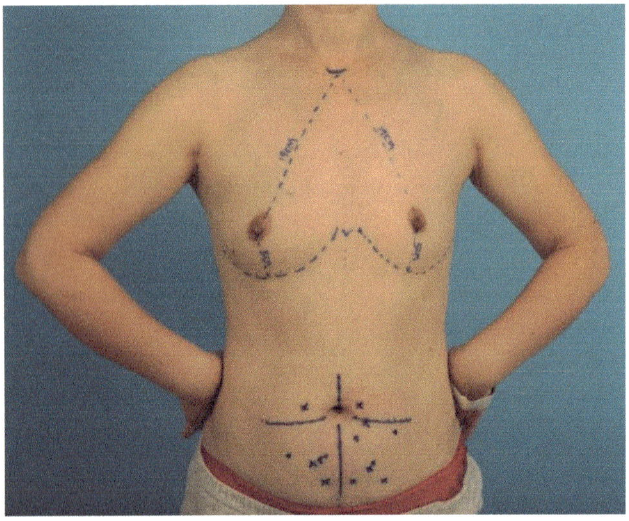

Fig. 5.36 Preoperative design

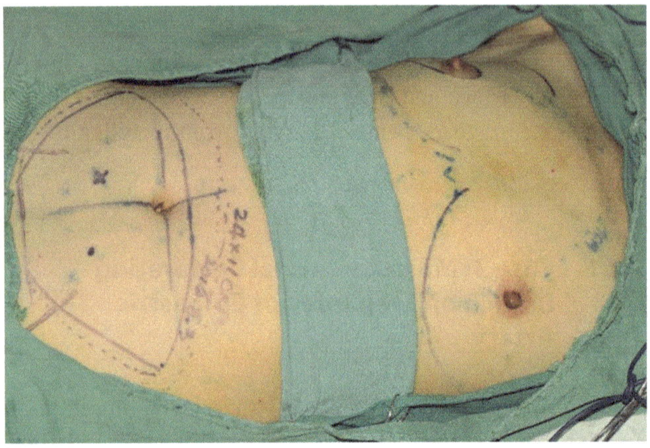

Fig. 5.37 Intraoperative design

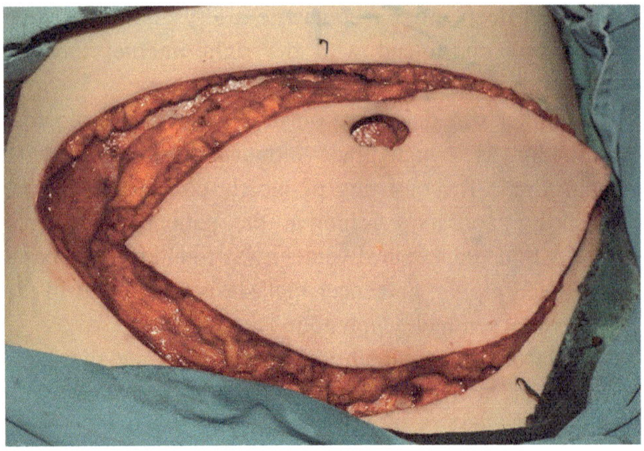

Fig. 5.38 The flap was disconnected from the abdominal wall

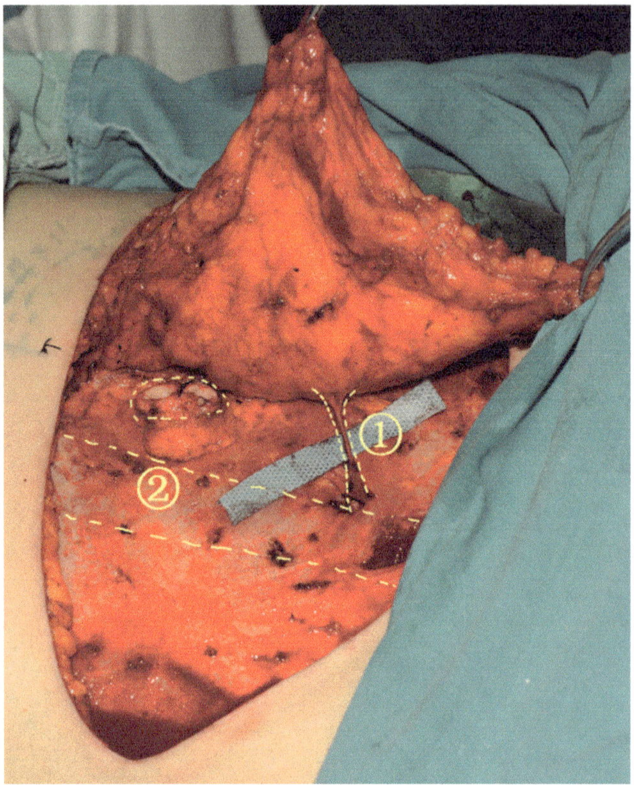

Fig. 5.39 The right perforator vessel was unveiled. (1) Perforating vessels of muscular septum; (2) Rectus abdominis

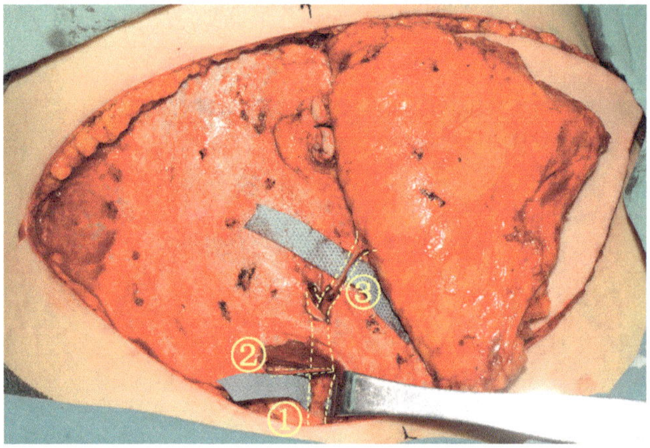

Fig. 5.40 The vascular pedicle was separated through an auxiliary incision, and a septal perforator medial to the muscle was found. (1) Deep inferior epigastric vessels; (2) Intercostal nerve; (3) Perforating vessels of muscular septum

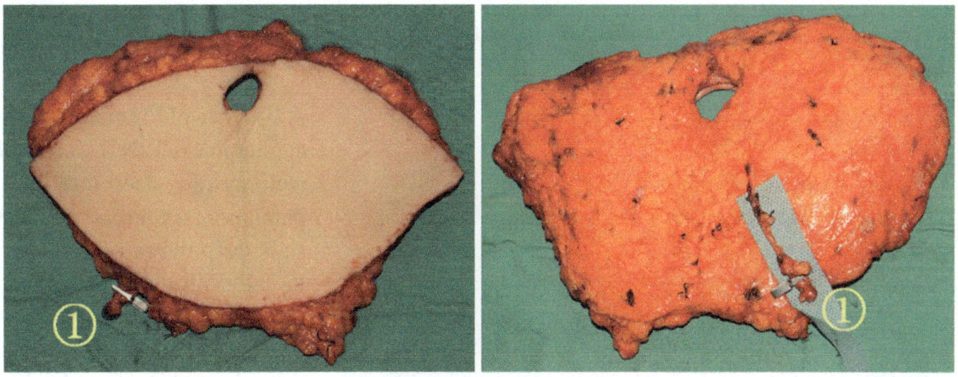

Fig. 5.41 The flap was cut off. (1) Deep inferior epigastric vessels

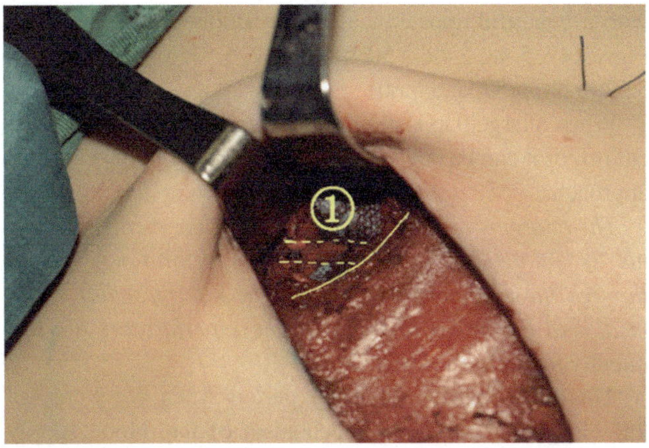

Fig. 5.42 The vascular pedicle in the receiving area is ready. (1) Lateral thoracic vessels

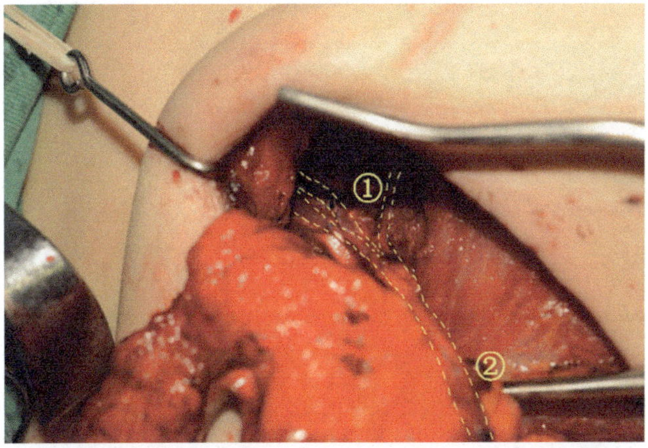

Fig. 5.43 Anastomosis of inferior epigastric vessels and lateral thoracic vessels. (1) Lateral thoracic vessels; (2) Deep inferior epigastric vessels

Although it is the type of muscular septum, the operation time is not significantly shortened due to the medial position of perforating vessels and the time-consuming exposure and separation.

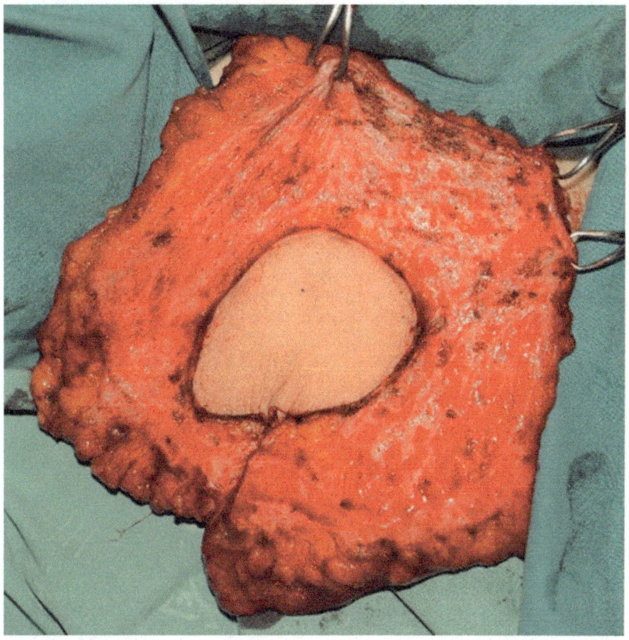

Fig. 5.44 Most of the skin islands were de-epithelized and the skin flap shaping was completed

Septocutaneous vessels feed the skin through the fascia space between muscles. These vessels pass through the connective tissue space between the left and right rectus abdominis muscles. They may also develop muscular branches on the way to the deep fascia. The branches of the septocutaneous vessels then enter the subcutaneous tissue and skin. It was proposed by Zhong Shizhen, a Chinese anatomist, in 1983.

Even if the perforating branch of the muscular septum is not thick, it can still support a large area of the flap because of its middle position.

By adjusting the thickness and contour trimming of the flap as well as tissue filling, a rebuilt breast with ideal size and shape can be achieved.

The flap was placed into the skin envelope with the de-epithelized tissue covered by the spared breast skin. The flap

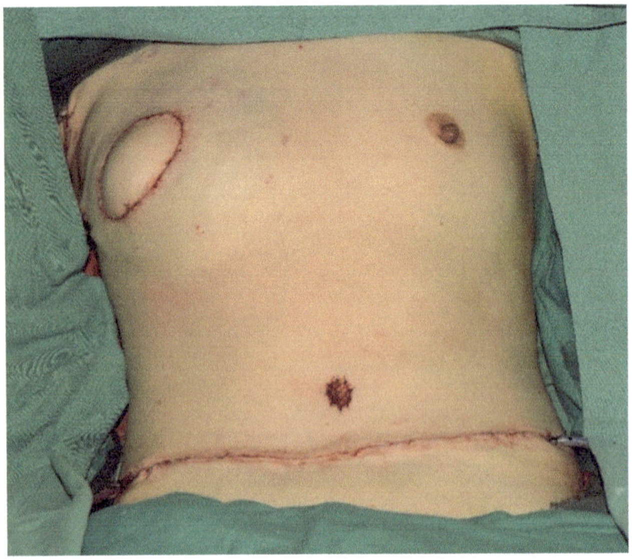

Fig. 5.45 The appearance of the reconstructed breast immediately after operation when the patient was seated at 60°

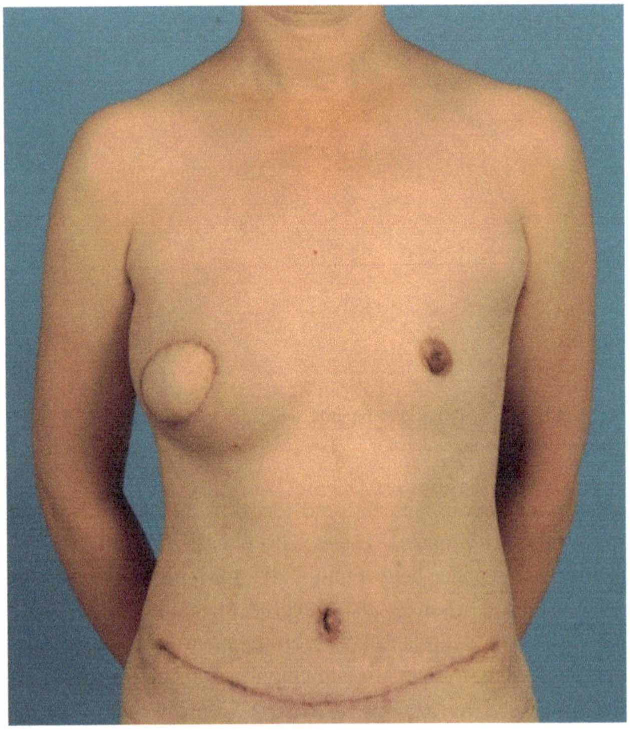

Fig. 5.46 The appearance of 6-month follow-up after operation

along with the pedicle were fixed in an appropriate position using absorbable sutures. Place a closed drainage device through the edge of the original incision or an individual incision. When the flap is shaped, the subcutaneous and skin layers are sutured.

5.2.2 Case 4: Muscular Septal Perforating Branch of Inferior Epigastric Artery

A 35-year-old female was admitted for left breast invasive carcinoma (cT2N1M0,IIb). The left modified radical mastectomy plus deep inferior epigastric perforator flap transplantation for breast reconstruction were performed. The right deep inferior epigastric vessels were anastomosed end-to-end with the anterior serratus muscle branch of the left thoracodorsal vessel (1A2V).

The flap survived completely without obvious complications. It was transferred to internal medicine for further comprehensive treatment. The reconstructed breast presented with a beautiful appearance during follow-up (as shown in Figs. 5.47, 5.48, 5.49, 5.50, 5.51, 5.52, 5.53, 5.54, 5.55, 5.56, 5.57, 5.58, 5.59, and 5.60).

When a large flap is required, the skin to the fascia can be cut off, or it can be cut step by step according to the standard approach.

The anatomy of perforators bypassing the rectus abdominis is relatively simple, including perforators passing through the tendinous scratch and the intermuscular space medial to the rectus abdominis. These perforators are frequently found to run vertically.

This was done at the early period when we were not knowledgeable about the mechanism of flap blood supply and hence uncertain whether the medial or lateral perforator that were equally large should be chosen. Finally, both perforators were harvested, resulting in extensive muscle discon-

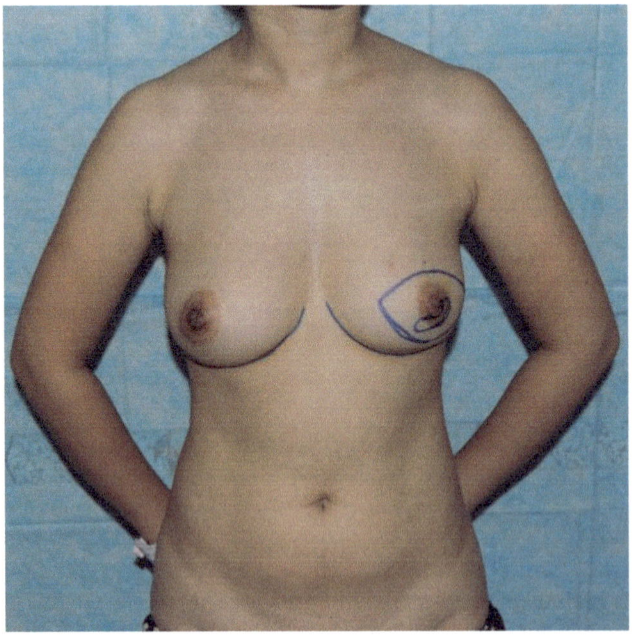

Fig. 5.47 Preoperative design

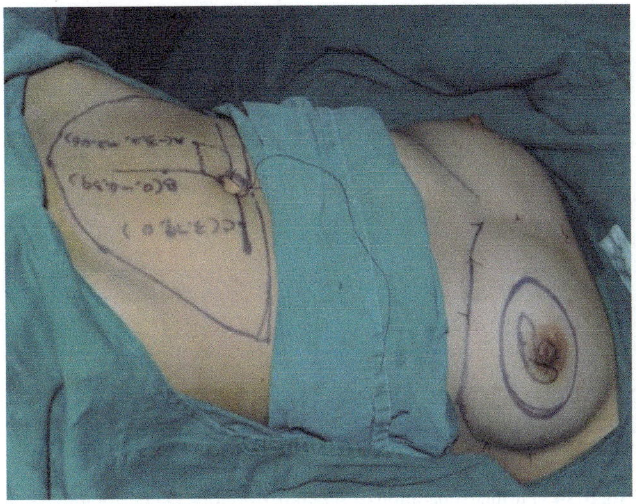

Fig. 5.48 Intraoperative design was determined according to the number and position of perforations located by CTA before operation

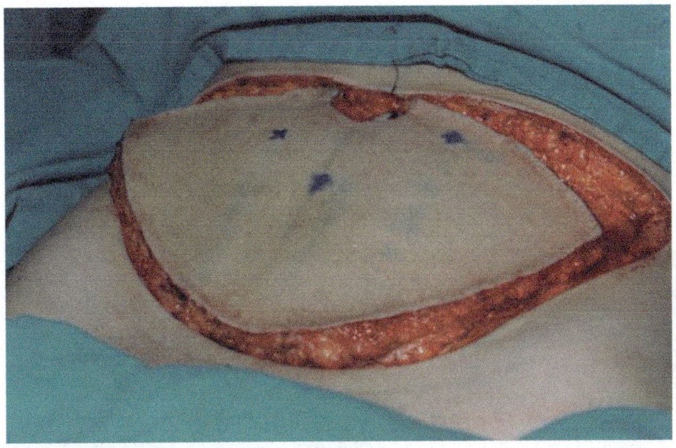

Fig. 5.49 The whole skin edge of the flap was cut open

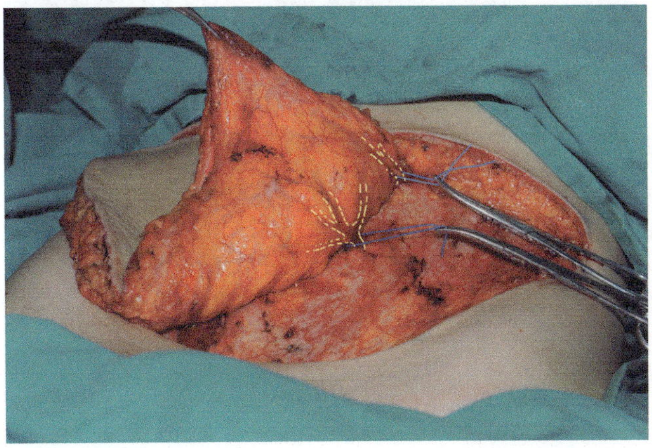

Fig. 5.50 It showed two perforating branches of the left lower abdomen

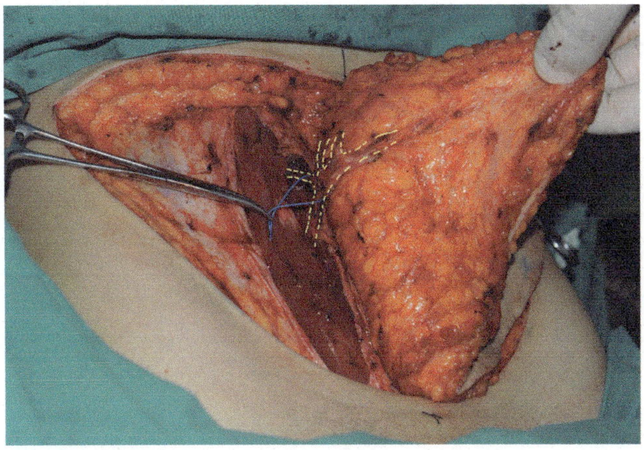

Fig. 5.51 Expose the right medial rectus abdominis perforator

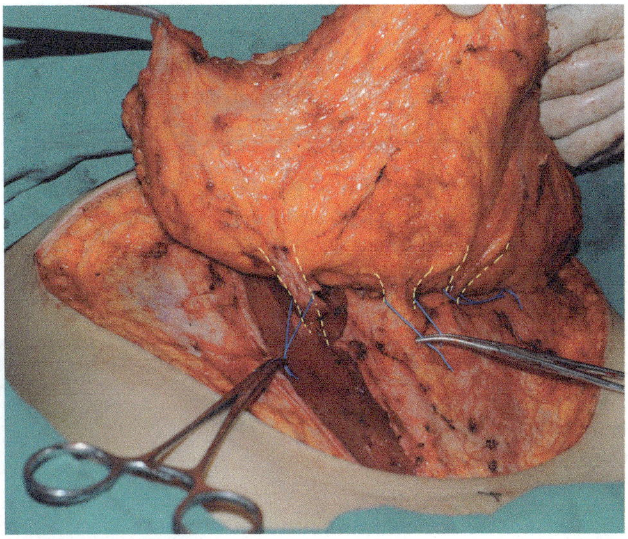

Fig. 5.52 To separate the perforator and determine that it was the septal perforator medial to the rectus abdominis

nection and increased donor site damage on the right lower abdomen. As the learning curve improved, when similar circumstance was encountered, we were confident that the medial paraumbilical perforators were powerful enough for blood supply for an entire DIEP flap.

5.2.3 Case 5: Superficial Medial Vascular Branch of Deep Inferior Epigastric Artery

The patient was 44 years old at admission and received left modified radical mastectomy 5 years ago. The scar of the left chest wall was removed and breast reconstruction using DIEP

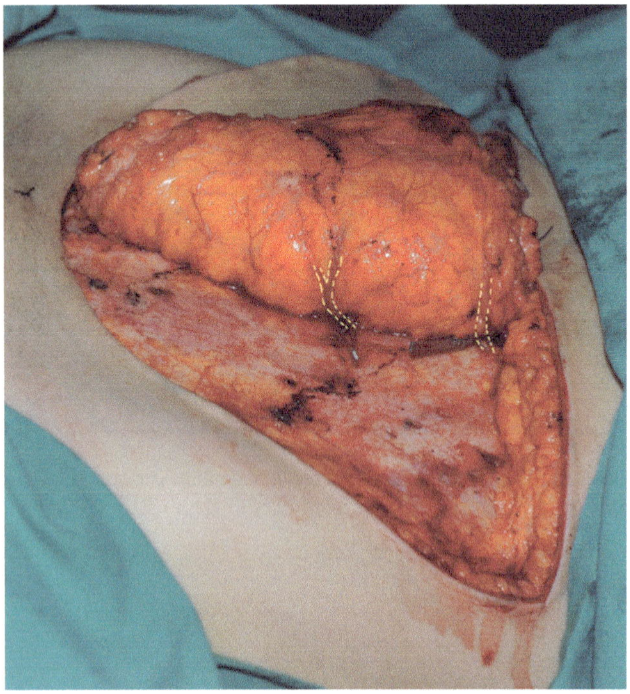

Fig. 5.53 By clamping the left perforator temporarily, it was determined that the flap was with good blood supply by the right perforator, then cut off the right perforator

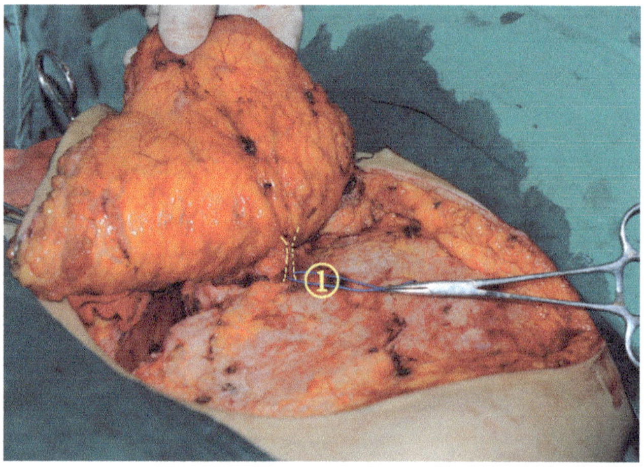

Fig. 5.54 Further separation of septal perforators. (1) Perforating vessels of muscular septum

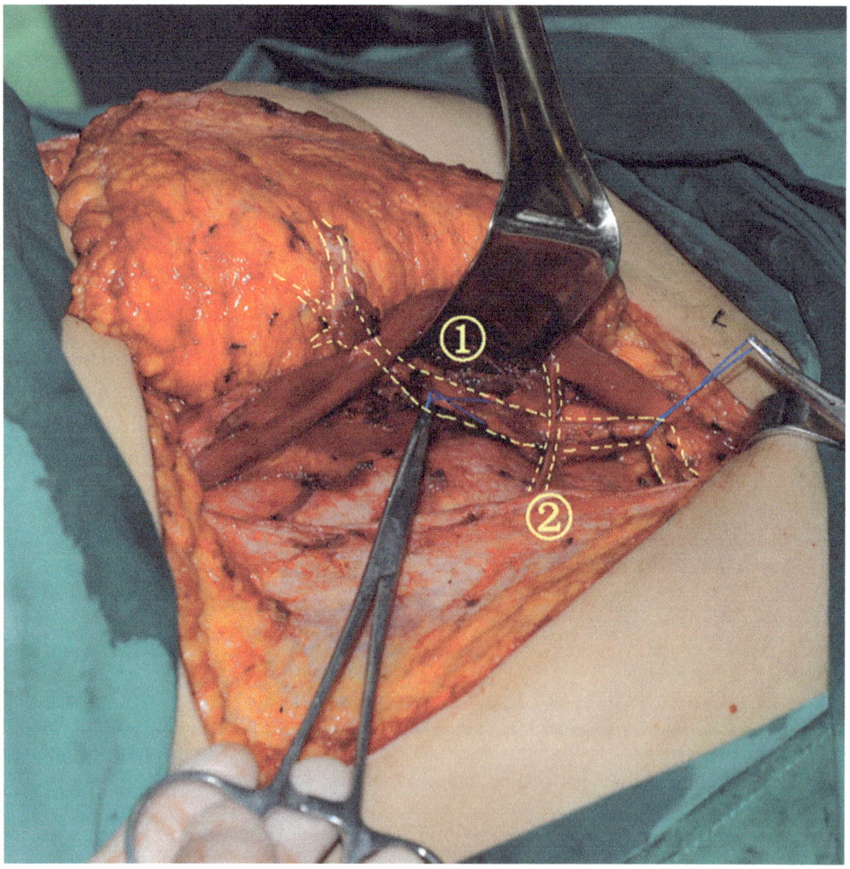

Fig. 5.55 Separate the right vascular pedicle and carefully protect the intercostal nerve branch. (1) Deep inferior epigastric vessels; (2) Intercostal nerve branch

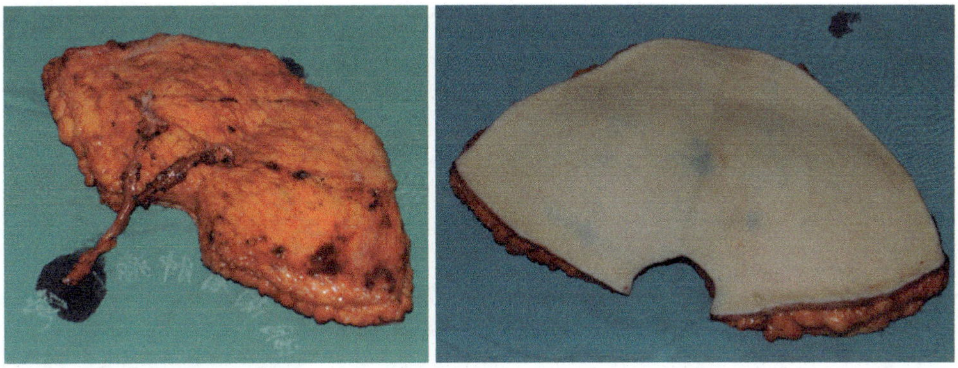

Fig. 5.56 End-to-end anastomosis was performed between the right lateral perforator vessel and the distal end of ipsilateral deep inferior epigastric vascular pedicle (A: V = 1:1). After confirming that the flap blood supply was good, the flap was cut off

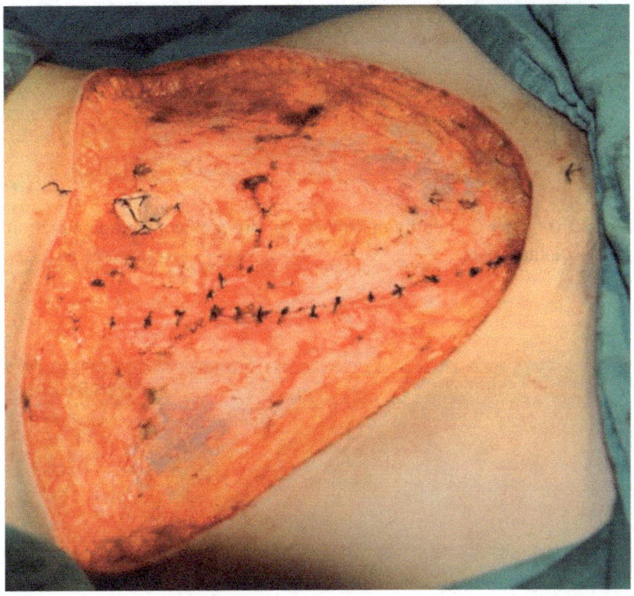

Fig. 5.57 Tension-free closure of anterior sheath of rectus abdominis

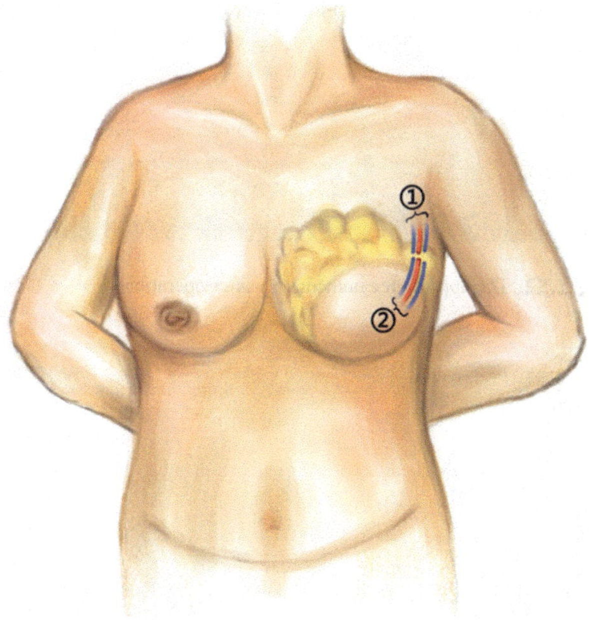

Fig. 5.58 Revascularization: right deep inferior epigastric vessels to left anterior serratus branch of thoracodorsal vessel. (1) Anterior serratus branch of left thoracodorsal vessel; (2) Right deep inferior epigastric vessel

flap was performed. After operation, the flap owned good blood circulation and the appearance of the reconstructed breast was satisfactory (Figs. 5.61, 5.62, 5.63, 5.64, and 5.65).

5.2.4 Case 6: DIEP Flap Containing Both the Medial and Lateral Perforating Branches

A 42-year-old female patient was hospitalized for finding a right breast mass for half a year.

Color Doppler ultrasound showed a hypoechoic mass on the right breast classified BI-RADS 4b. Right breast invasive ductal carcinoma of histological grade II was confirmed by biopsy. Immunohistochemistry findings were ER (−), PR (−), C-erbB2 (1 +), low expression of p53, and Ki-67 value was 70%.

Nipple-areola sparing mastectomy plus axillary lymph node dissection and breast reconstruction using DIEP flap transplantation were performed. The intraoperative frozen section showed that the right areola and nipple were free of tumor. The results of routine pathological examination were as follows: (1) (right breast) Invasive ductal carcinoma, grade II–III, with a mass size of about 6.5 cm × 6 cm × 3 cm; (2) 2/17 of right axillary lymph nodes showed cancer metastasis; (3) No cancer was found in the areola, subpapillary margin, skin, and basal margin. Pathological stage was pT3N1M0 stage IIIA, immunohistochemistry: ER (weak, about 2%), PR (−), CerbB (1 +), and Ki-67 of about 60%.

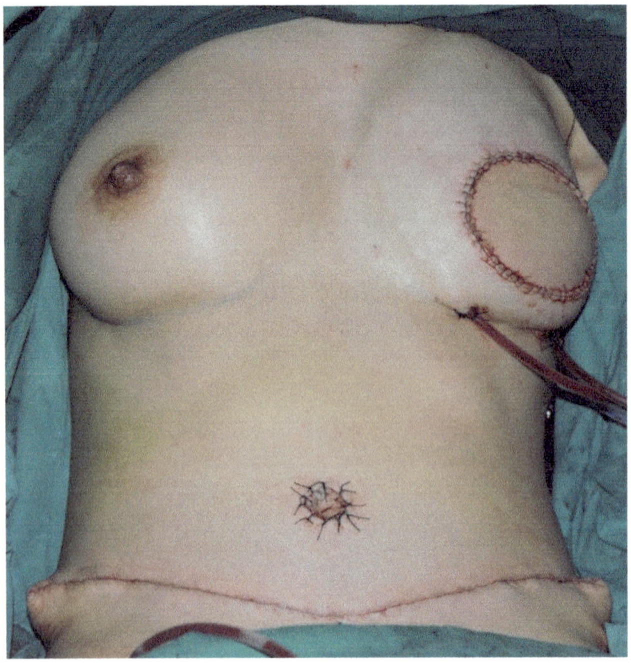

Fig. 5.59 The appearance immediately after operation

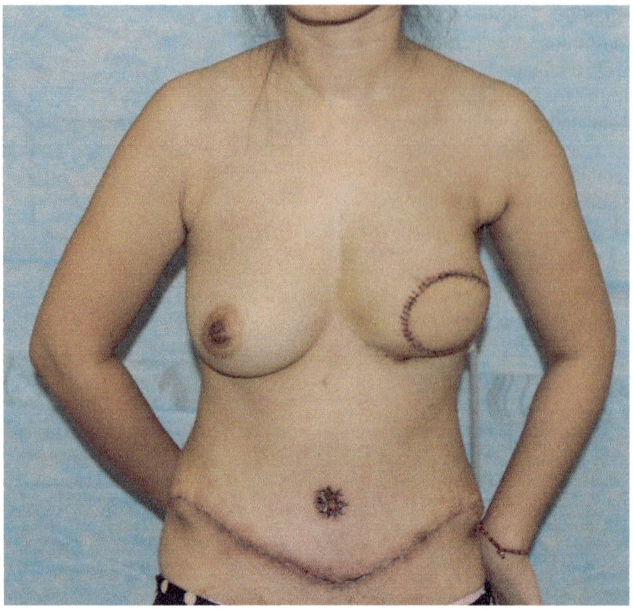

Fig. 5.60 After 2 months of follow-up, the appearance and function were satisfactory

Fig. 5.61 Preoperative conditions

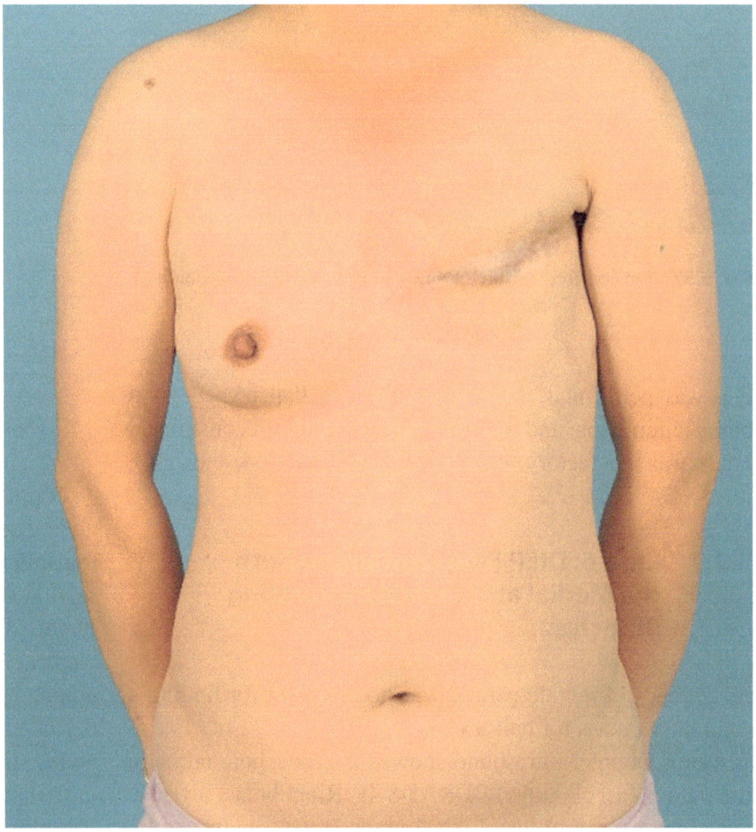

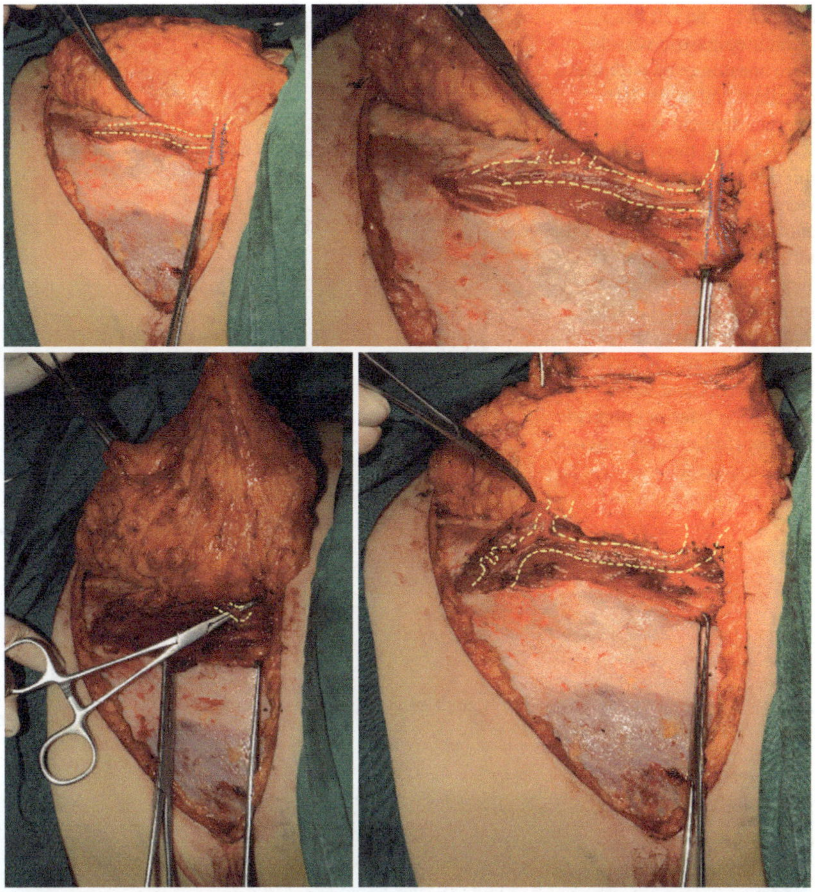

Fig. 5.62 The perforating vessels in the lower abdomen were explored during the operation. The medial bifurcation of deep inferior epigastric vessel was found of large diameter and travelling a long distance on the surface of the rectus abdominis, which was very likely to be injured by mistake

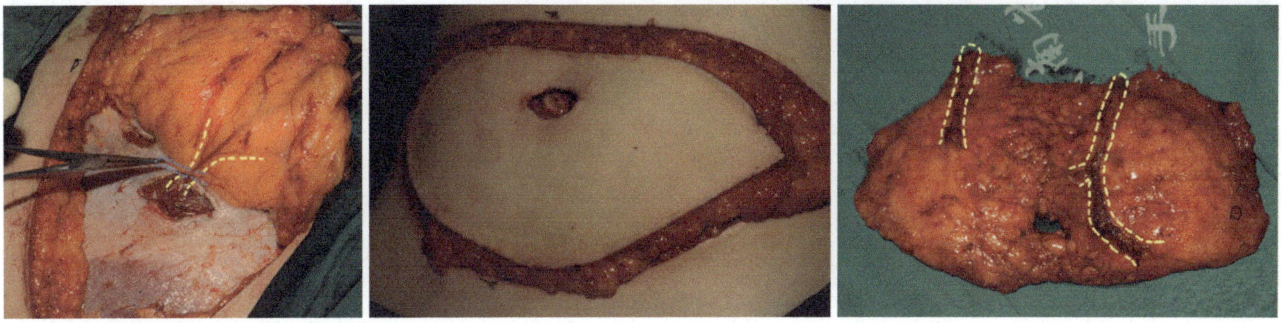

Fig. 5.63 Clamping test showed that the left perforator vessel alone was not enough to supply the blood supply of the whole flap. A DIEP flap with bilateral pedicles was finally cut

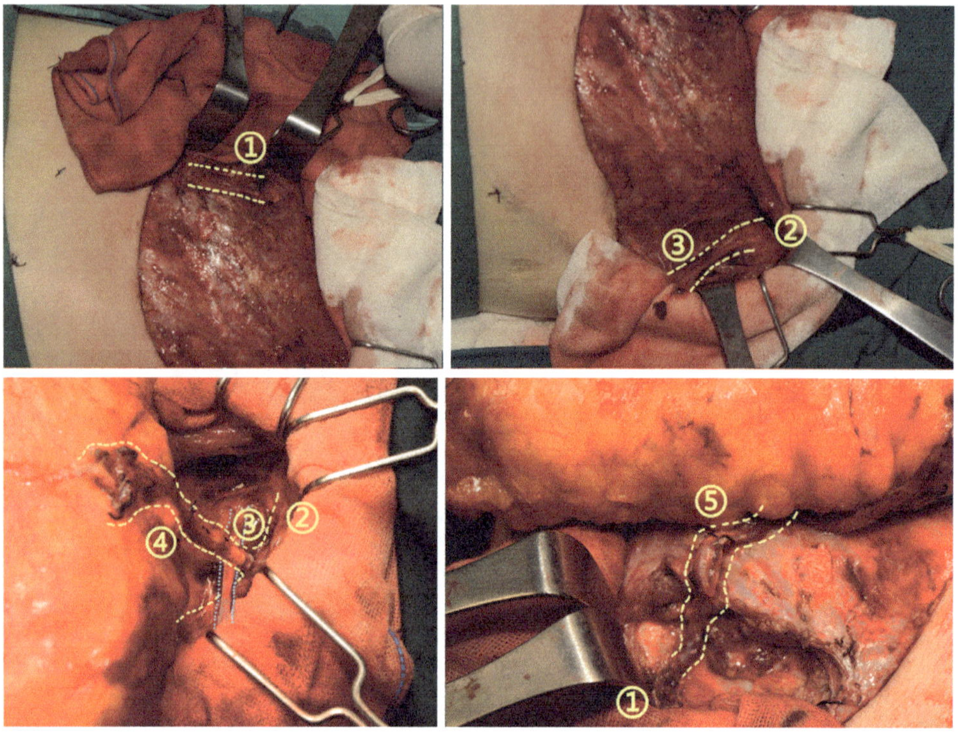

Fig. 5.64 The left deep inferior epigastric vessels were anastomosed with the proximal end of the left internal thoracic vessels (A: $V = 1{:}1$), and the right deep inferior epigastric vessels were anastomosed with the anterior serratus branch of the left thoracodorsal vessel (A: $V = 1{:}2$). (1) Left internal mammary vessel; (2) Left thoracodorsal vessels; (3) Anterior serratus branch of left thoracodorsal vessel; (4) Right deep inferior epigastric vessels; (5) Left deep inferior epigastric vessel

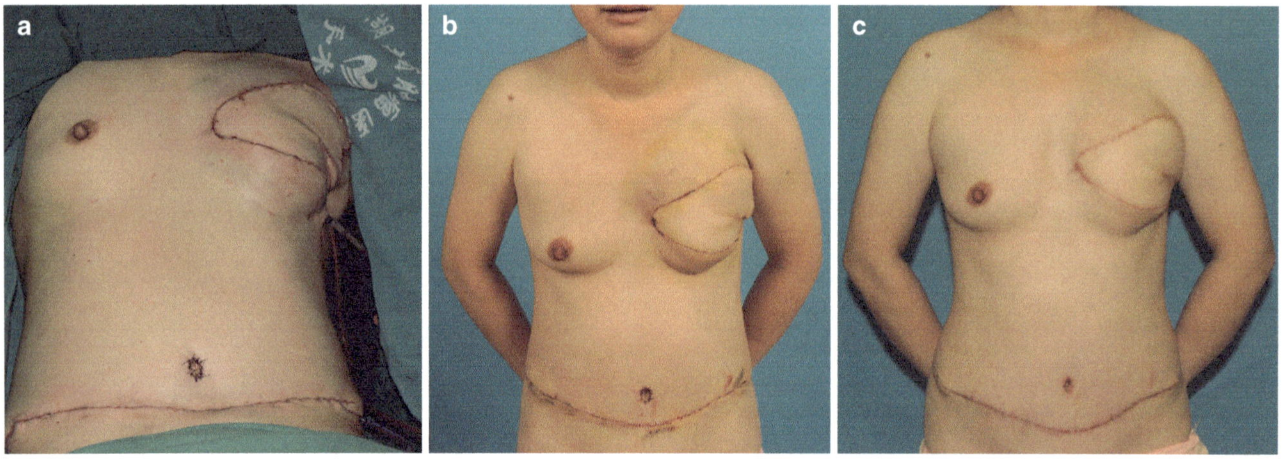

Fig. 5.65 (**a**) Immediate after operation; (**b**) Discharge 1 week after operation; (**c**) The patients were followed up for 2 months after operation

The patient was then transferred to internal medicine for further radiotherapy and chemotherapy, and the appearance and function of the reconstructed breast were satisfactory during follow-up (as shown in Figs. 5.66, 5.67, 5.68, and 5.69).

In rare cases, the medial perforators from the lateral branch of the deep inferior epigastric vessels neither run on the superficial surface of the muscle nor on the deep surface of the muscle, instead they repeatedly penetrate the superficial part of the muscle. This situation is difficult to predict before operation. Such perforators and the pedicle are very likely to be injured, when the anterior sheath is cut longitudinally on the lateral side of the perforating vessels (as shown in Figs. 5.70, 5.71, and 5.72).

Only has the perforator leaving the rectus abdominis muscle and entering the anterior sheath been determined, further steps can be continued. First, make a small opening on the anterior sheath with a scalpel or the tip of sharp scissors—do not cut it all at once, otherwise it is easy to damage the blood vessels underneath. Then, expand the opening and explore the location and running course of the perforator. Finally, separate the anterior sheath from the muscle bluntly to further free the perforating vessels.

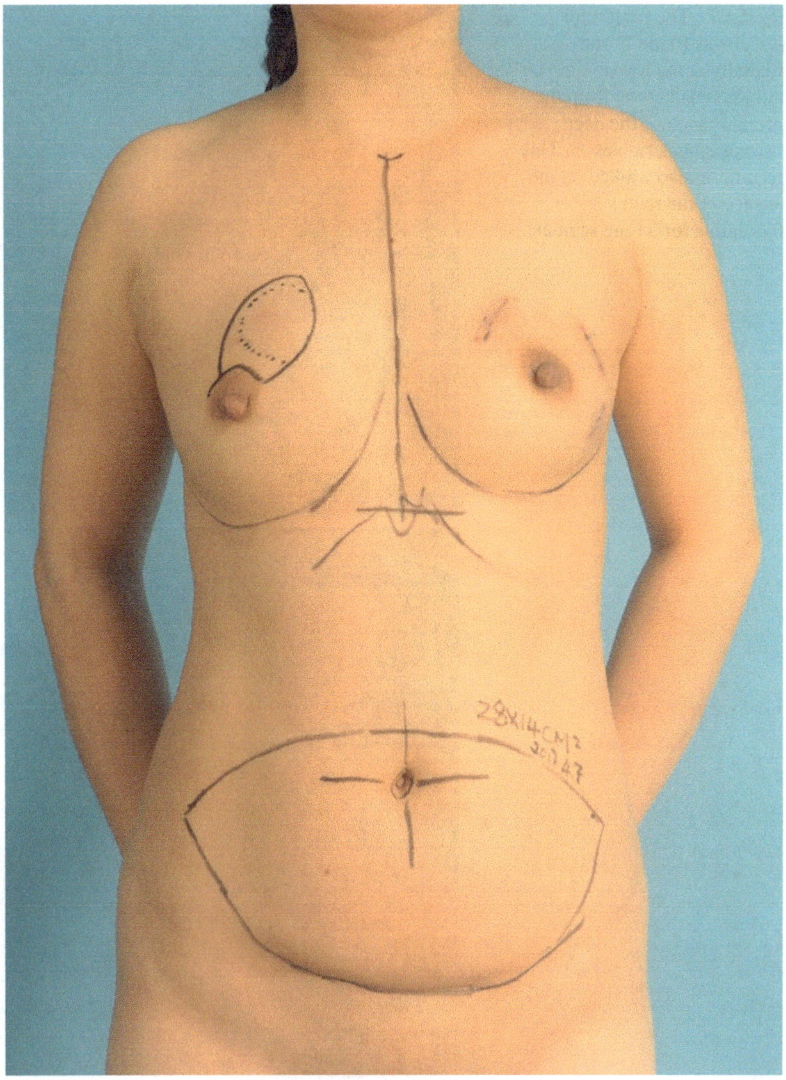

Fig. 5.66 Preoperative situation and design

In 2003, CT angiography was used to evaluate perforators in DIEP flaps. The emergence of this technology triggered a revolution in this field.

CT angiography is now a common imaging technique used by most surgeons before performing DIEP flap harvest.

It is very valuable in helping us understand the previously unknown vascular and pathophysiological problems of the abdominal flap.

CT angiography can be used to help us evaluate the vascular course of abdominal flap before operation and select the perforating artery that can best nourish the flap.

It provides comprehensive information about the superficial and deep branches of the superior epigastric artery, as well as the location, diameter, and course of the dominant perforating artery.

When studying these features, CT angiography can detect the presence of the septal perforator artery beside the muscle.

These vessels are considered as ideal perforator arteries in DIEP flap because their myometrial walking characteristics can avoid the risk of damaging perforator arteries during cumbersome muscle stripping.

The deep branch of the deep inferior epigastric artery contains many terminal branches which are all paramuscular perforating arteries.

They are large and located in the midline of the abdomen, and provide excellent blood supply to the flap.

In addition, septal perforators are absent of intramuscular travelling. The characteristics aforementioned make this perforator artery easy to be separated from the rest of the tissue, an ideal perforator option for skin flap in breast reconstruction.

Therefore, if a paramuscular perforator is found by CT angiography, it can be selected as the vascular pedicle of the flap.

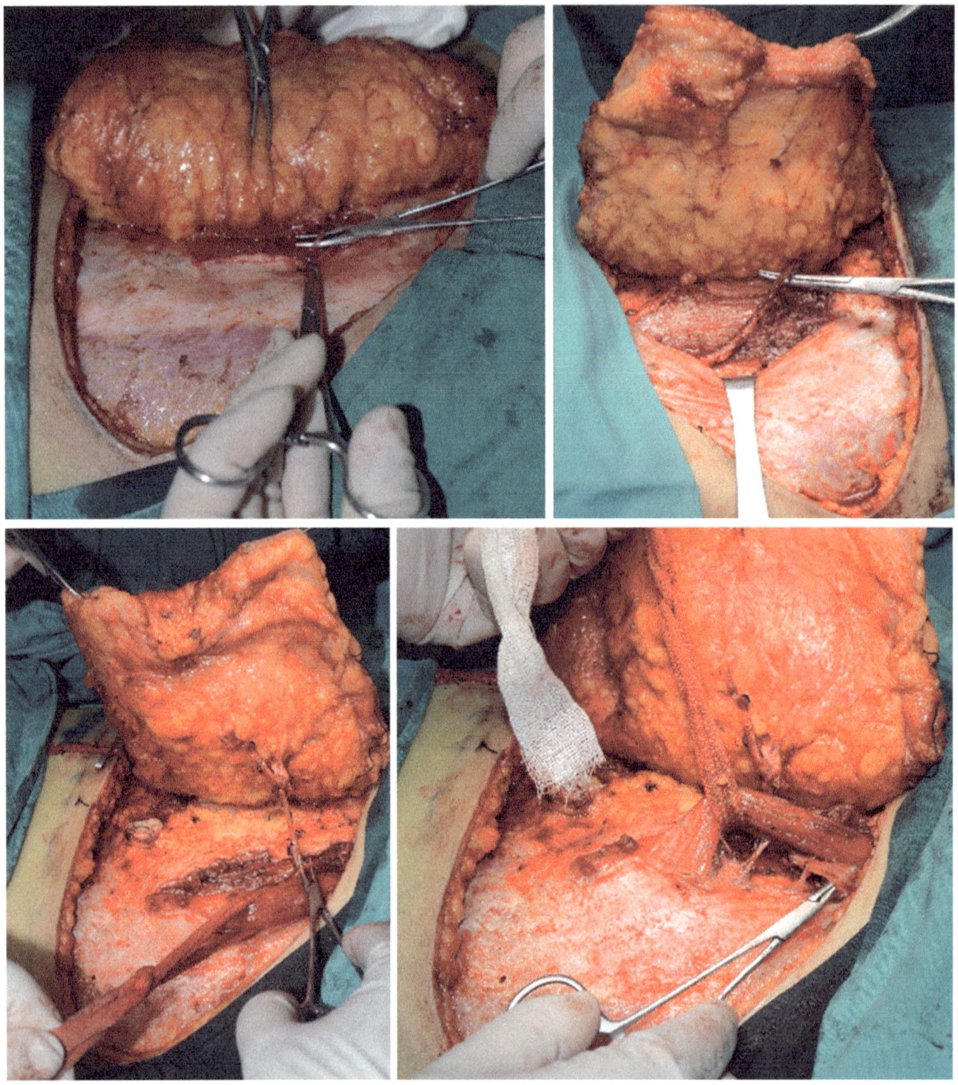

Fig. 5.67 The perforator vessel was found to run medially at the lower abdomen and come from the lateral branch of the deep inferior epigastric vessel. This perforator also walked on the surface of the rectus abdominis for a long segment

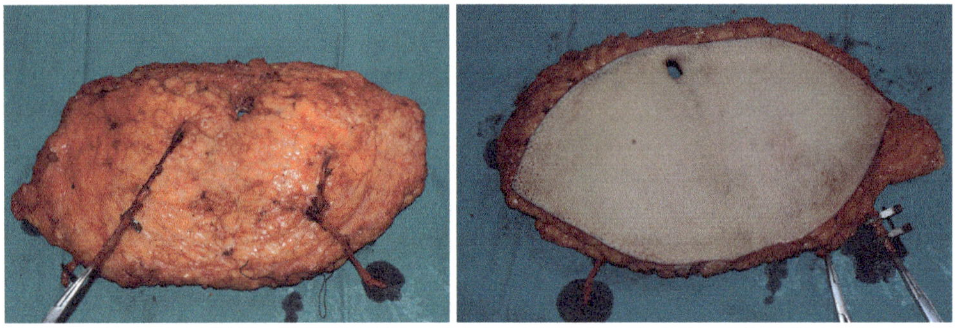

Fig. 5.68 A DIEP flap pedicled with bilateral blood vessels was cut off

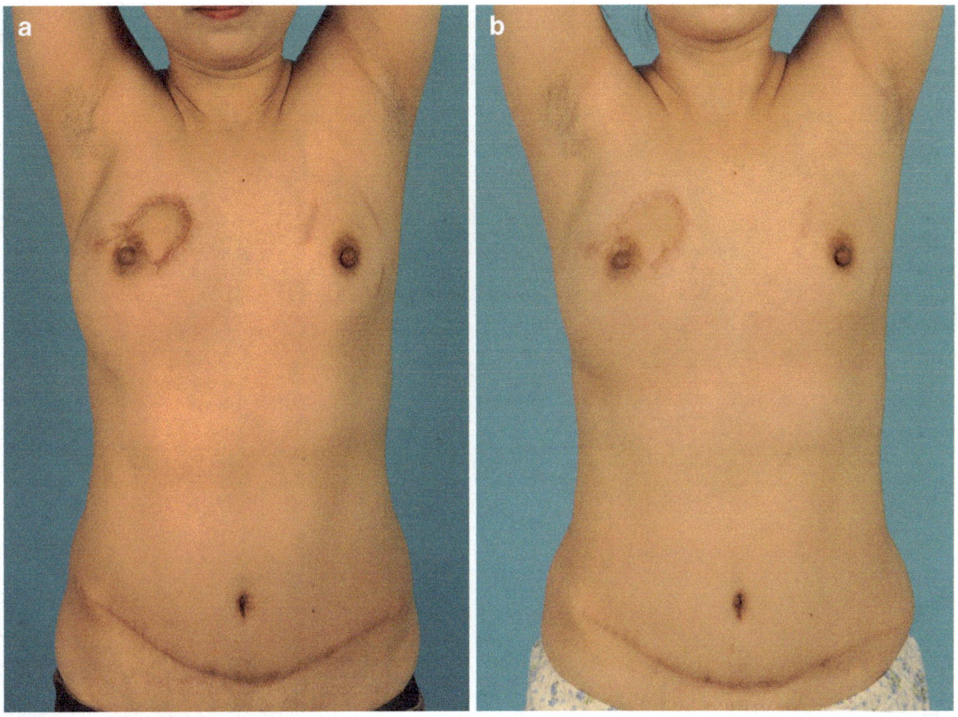

Fig. 5.69 (**a**) Functional appearance after 9 months of follow-up. (**b**) The appearance and function recovered satisfactorily 18 months after operation

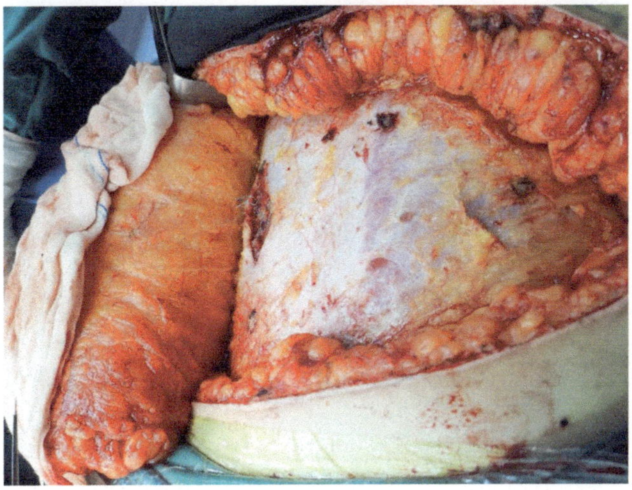

Fig. 5.70 After a longitudinal incision of the anterior sheath along the lateral side of the perforating vessel was made, it was found to run in the deep surface of the anterior sheath, which was a very complex condition

Preoperative CT angiography is performed to evaluate the vascular course of abdominal flap.

First, the superficial branches of the deep inferior epigastric artery are evaluated to determine the possibility of performing SIEA-based flap.

Then, the deep branches from the deep inferior epigastric artery are studied.

The location, diameter, course, and cutaneous branch (axial) of the selected perforator vessel were evaluated.

This information should be directly marked on the surface of abdominal skin before operation.

The operation began by dissecting the superficial branch of the deep inferior epigastric vein.

This vein should be retained as a life-saving straw to prevent complications.

Then dissect from the outside to the inside along the fascia of the flap until it reaches the midline and locate the paramuscular perforator.

Since it is known in advance about whether the selected vessel is the main perforator vessel or not, the remaining perforator vessels can be discarded and ligated.

Once the paramuscular perforator vessel is located, if the fascial space has been exposed, it can be dissected through it or through its wrapped tunnel.

After opening the fascia, the perforating vessels will be unveiled on the inner side of the rectus abdominis.

When turning up this muscle, we can observe the course of the reverse branch of this muscle branch, and some muscle branches must be removed until the deep branch of the deep inferior epigastric vessel is found.

Sometimes, the intermuscular perforator vessels send some branches to the diaphragm and peritoneum that require ligation.

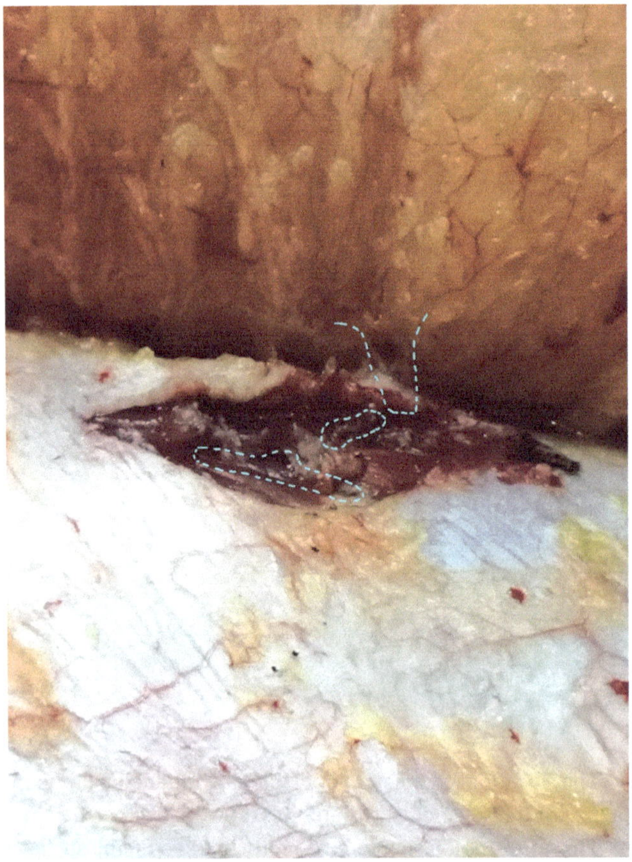

Fig. 5.71 It was identified that the deep inferior epigastric vessel traveled in the shallow muscle fibers and sent out a perforator toward the medial side. The perforator entered the muscle after leaving the vascular trunk and traveled for a short distance, and then ran at the muscle surface for a certain distance; after that, it entered the muscle again and moved inward, and finally vertically escaped the rectus abdominis and penetrated the anterior sheath

Special attention must be paid to the confluence of the medial branch and the lateral branch of the deep branch of the deep inferior epigastric vessel, especially if the lateral branch has an intramuscular course, the pedicle of the flap may be attached to the posterior edge of the rectus abdominis muscle.

In this case, it is necessary to ensure good exposure and carefully separate the collateral branches in order to use the vascular clamp and separate it from the main pedicle of the flap.

When the diameter of the artery and vein of the deep branch of the deep inferior epigastric vessel at the anastomosis of the pedicle is quite large, the flap can be cut at this time.

Because the perforator vessel of the paramuscular septum is a large vessel without intramuscular walking process (the caliber is 1.0–2.8 mm), it is easier to dissect and faster than the intramuscular perforator vessel.

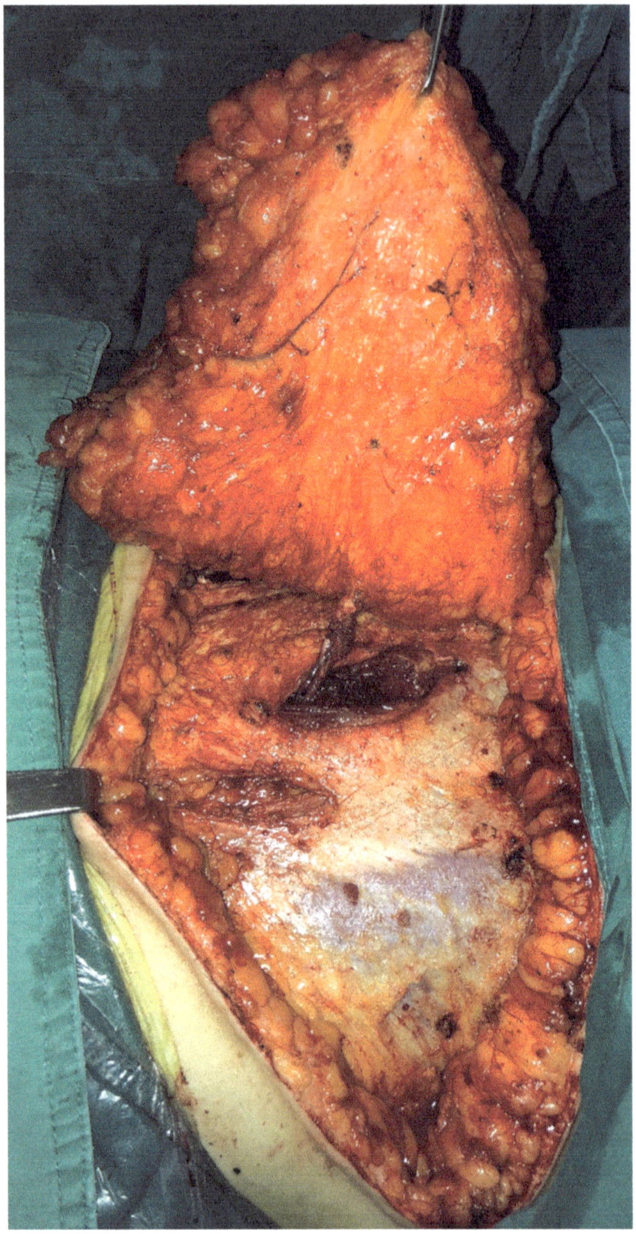

Fig. 5.72 Once the position and level of perforator vessel and vascular pedicle are determined, it will not be too difficult to cut the flap

Nevertheless, in some cases, the dissection of the paramuscular perforator vessels is more tedious than usual, especially when the posterior part of the perforator is close to the posterior abdominal fascia in the abdominal white line layer.

In this case, more detailed manipulation is required.

What we are most concerned about is the location of the main perforator vessels in the abdominal perforator flap.

Fortunately, with the help of CT angiography, this problem has been solved.

Using this technique, the best perforator vessel of abdominal flap can be located, selected, and dissected as the pedicle of flap, so as to provide as good blood supply as possible.

The application of this imaging technology has significantly reduced the incidence of complications.

Ideally, the best perforator vessel of the flap should have a large diameter, be located in the center of the flap, and present the best subcutaneous branch pattern and the smallest intramuscular route.

Once the perforating vessel is selected, the physician team will face the most challenging and critical step: intramuscular dissection. Precise anatomical techniques are essential and care should be taken in this step to prevent perforator injury or vasospasm.

It should be borne in mind that the shorter the intramuscular route is, the lower the risk of injury will be.

The information collected by CT angiography is used to determine the paramuscular perforator.

The main advantage of these perforating vessels is the lack of intramuscular walking process, which can reduce the risk of damaging the vascular pedicle when dissecting them.

In addition, since the perforating vessels do not coincide with the motor nerve at any point, the risk of damaging the function of rectus abdominis is very small.

In fact, the paramuscular perforator vessels can be considered to support more blood supply area of the flap than the musculocutaneous perforator vessels, because they directly nourish the abdominal flap from the deep branches of the deep inferior epigastric vessels without passing through the rectus abdominis.

According to the information provided by CT angiography, there are paramuscular perforators in a considerable number of patients, and the reported number is 8–15.8%.

Its morphological characteristics, location, and no intramuscular running give this perforator vessel priority in being the pedicle for a DIEP flap, because they can be obtained in a faster, simpler, and safer way.

References

1. Boyd JB, Taylor GI, Corlett R. The vascular territories of the superior epigastric and the deep inferior epigastric systems. Plast Reconstr Surg. 1984;73(1):1–16.
2. Itoh Y, Arai K. The deep inferior epigastric artery free skin flap: anatomic study and clinical application. Plast Reconstr Surg. 1993;91(5):853–63; discussion 864.
3. El-Mrakby HH, Milner RH. The vascular anatomy of the lower anterior abdominal wall: a microdissection study on the deep inferior epigastric vessels and the perforator branches. Plast Reconstr Surg. 2002;109(2):539–43; discussion 544–7.
4. Moon HK, Taylor GI. The vascular anatomy of rectus abdominis musculocutaneous flaps based on the deep superior epigastric system. Plast Reconstr Surg. 1988;82(5):815–32.
5. Rozen WM, Ashton MW, Pan WR, Taylor GI. Raising perforator flaps for breast reconstruction: the intramuscular anatomy of the deep inferior epigastric artery. Plast Reconstr Surg. 2007;120(6):1443–9.
6. Rozen WM, Palmer KP, Suami H, et al. The DIEA branching pattern and its relationship to perforators: the importance of preoperative computed tomographic angiography for DIEA perforator flaps. Plast Reconstr Surg. 2008;121(2):367–73.
7. Garvey PB, Salavati S, Feng L, Butler CE. Abdominal donor-site outcomes for medial versus lateral deep inferior epigastric artery branch perforator harvest. Plast Reconstr Surg. 2011;127(6):2198–205.
8. Wong C, Saint-Cyr M, Arbique G, et al. Three- and four-dimensional computed tomography angiographic studies of commonly used abdominal flaps in breast reconstruction. Plast Reconstr Surg. 2009;124(1):18–27.
9. Schaverien M, Saint-Cyr M, Arbique G, Brown SA. Arterial and venous anatomies of the deep inferior epigastric perforator and superficial deep inferior epigastric artery flaps. Plast Reconstr Surg. 2008;121(6):1909–19.

Adjustment of Vascular Body Area of DIEP Flap

6

Zan Li and Zhuangqing Yang

When selecting the DIEP flap and muscle-sparing TRAM for breast reconstruction, a perfect balance can be achieved between ensuring sufficient blood supply of the flap and minimizing abdominal wall injury [1].

Although the lower abdominal wall has become the best choice for autologous tissue transplantation in breast reconstruction, its tissue texture and volume are still unsatisfactory [2].

In many cases, the DIEP flap cannot make full use of abdominal tissue, especially in areas with poor blood supply, which has been reported in detail [3–5].

In order to improve the safety of flap blood supply, scholars have been trying to establish zoning standards for the blood supply of lower abdominal flap.

The zoning standard was first reported by Scheflan and Dinner on the application of unilateral pedicled transverse rectus abdominis myocutaneous flap [6].

Scheflan divided the flap into four areas according to his clinical experience in flap blood perfusion [7].

The establishment and modification process of the zoning system was complex, and it has been improving in the process of self-verification and continuously being overthrown.

One year later, Dinner made further research and observation on this, exchanging the previously defined zones II and III, making all scholars change the concept of zoning standard [8].

Nevertheless, when Hartrampf finally developed a recognized zoning standard, it was determined according to what was originally described by Scheflan [9].

After Holm et al. applied the experimental perfusion technique, the exchange of areas II and III in the classical Hartrampf zoning standard were confirmed [10].

Z. Li (✉)
Department of Oncology Plastic Surgery, Hunan Cancer Hospital, Changsha, Hunan, China

Z. Yang
Department of Mammary Surgery, The Third Affiliated Hospital of Kunming Medical University (Yunnan Cancer Hospital, Yunnan Cancer Center), Kunming, Yunnan, China

The establishment of this zoning standard confirmed that the blood flow of vascular pedicle preferentially perfused ipsilateral flap before passing through the midline of abdominal wall.

In 2008, Wong et al. used scanning technology to determine that the vascular body areas of the perforators varied, and re-evaluated the perfusion zoning according to their research results [11].

In our clinical work, the measurement results showed that there was no significant difference in blood perfusion between zone II and zone III.

In further anatomical study, we confirmed the blood supply pattern of flap depended on the perforators.

Therefore, how much and which part of the harvested flap are required should not only be based on the zoning standard, but it should also be personalized and flexibly adjusted according to the size, character, position, and quantity of perforating branches [12].

It is generally believed that the key to the success of breast reconstruction with deep inferior epigastric artery perforator flap is to select the largest perforator pedicle, no matter it comes from the medial or lateral branch.

Professor Kohima firstly reported that the dominant perforator vessel of a DIEP flap came from the medial branch of the deep inferior epigastric artery [13–16].

Further research demonstrated that the dominant perforator of deep inferior epigastric artery in the medial row provided sufficient blood supply for zones I and II, while zones III and IV were slightly poor in perfusion [17].

On this anatomical basis, some scholars reported that half of area III and all of area IV should be removed to avoid the risk of partial necrosis and fat liquefaction of the flap (Fig. 6.1) [17].

The blood supply range of the medial perforators of the DIEP flap is wide, but these perforators are not adjacent to areas III and IV, which impairs the blood supply to these areas.

Z. Li, D. Song (eds.), *Oncoplastic Flap Surgery*, https://doi.org/10.1007/978-981-19-8926-1_6

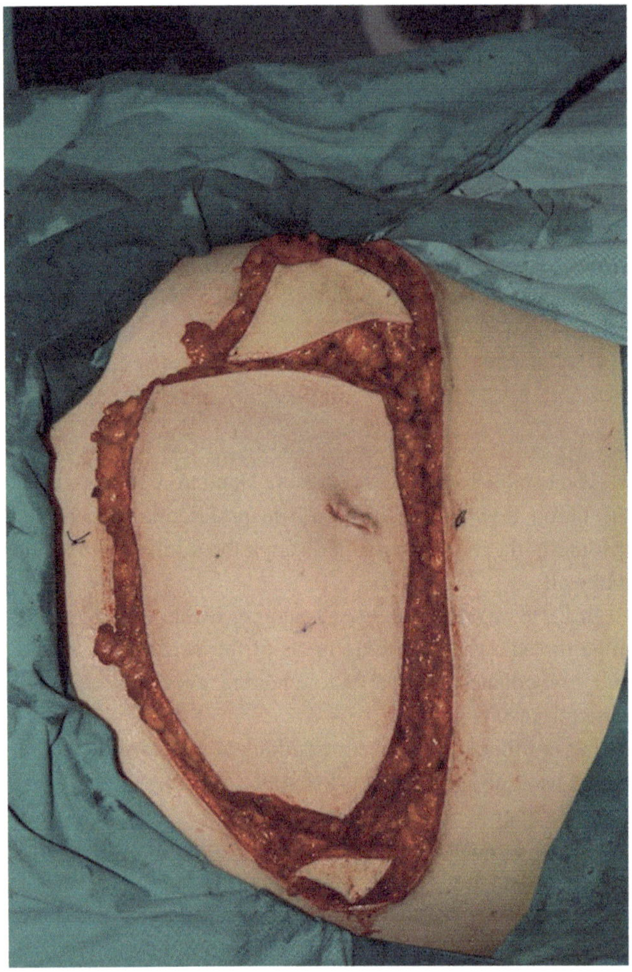

Fig. 6.1 Most of area IV and part of area III was removed

This is of great clinical significance. In a large number of clinical cases, it was found that almost all flap partial necrosis or fat liquefaction occurred in the distal end of zone III and zone IV.

The perfusion mode of the single dominant perforator of the medial branch is also of great significance for choosing unilateral or bilateral pedicled flap for breast reconstruction. A clear understanding of their situation is helpful to predict the surgical design and safety.

Preoperative evaluation of deep inferior epigastric vascular branches is very useful for flap resection, because the use of medial perforating branches is associated with less damage to the donor area than the lateral perforating branches [18].

The injury of donor area will also have an impact on the full utilization of the vascular body area of the flap, and hence it should be considered in the separation of perforating branches. The injury of the donor area as well as the blood supply of the flap need to be well balanced.

The anatomical basis that a single dominant medial perforator can provide sufficient blood supply for zone I, zone II, and part of zone III are as follows (Fig. 6.2):

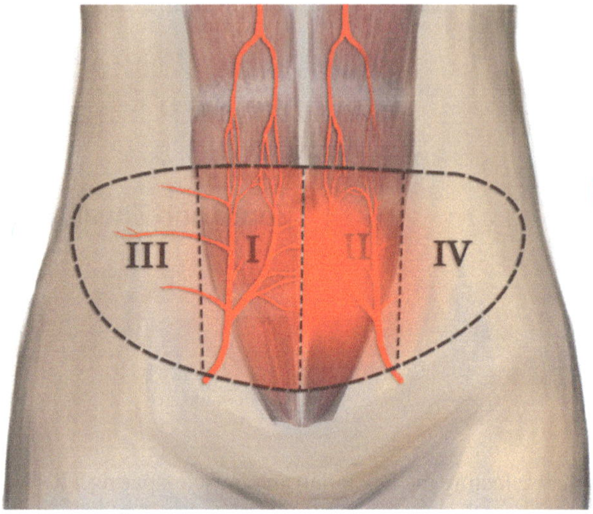

Fig. 6.2 Schematic diagram of blood supply area of the single dominant medial perforator

1. The single dominant medial perforator vessel can generally cross the midline and communicate with the contralateral medial perforator vessel through the subdermal vascular network.
2. The contralateral medial perforator vessels can be connected with the ipsilateral lateral perforator vessels through direct and indirect vascular anastomosis system.
3. The single dominant medial perforator vessel also links with other perforator vessels that share the same pedicle.

The safety of vascular body area should be considered in the flap shaping. If it is necessary to harvest abdominal tissue as much as possible, it is important to locate the perforating vessel before operation. Try to locate the perforating point near the central area of the flap.

If the blood supply area of a single perforator is insufficient, the number of perforators should be increased. To cut a perforator flap pedicled with bilateral deep inferior epigastric vessels using the turbocharged or supercharged method is reliable for blood supply. However, it is not recommended to cut the flap supplied with the medial and lateral perforator branches from the same deep inferior epigastric vessel, because the damage to the donor area is great and it is no better than to raise a muscle-sparing TRAM flap.

6.1 Case 1: Adjustment of Vascular Body Area of DIEP Flap

A 31-year-old female patient was admitted with "a left breast tumor found for 2 months." Left breast cancer (cT2N1M0, IIb) was diagnosed by preoperative biopsy and imaging examination. The location of the tumor was shown in photograph (Fig. 6.3).

The patient received modified radical mastectomy plus free DIEP flap transplantation for breast reconstruction, and the size of the flap was designed to be about 24 cm × 14 cm.

The left deep inferior epigastric artery and veins were anastomosed end-to-end with the branches of lateral thoracic artery and vein (1A2V). Postoperative routine pathological examination showed that the left breast invasive ductal carcinoma was grade III, and the mass size was 5 cm × 4.5 cm × 2.5 cm, no cancer invasion was found in the skin, basal margin, and nipple, a little cancer invasion was found in the adipose tissue between the pectoral muscles, and cancer metastasis was found in 3/23 of the left axillary lymph nodes.

Pathological stage was pT3N1M0 IIIA, immunohistochemical results: ER60% +, PR60% +, Cerb-2 (1 +), Ki-67% (40%). The patients were treated with adjuvant chemotherapy using regime EC-T followed by radiotherapy and endocrine therapy (Figs. 6.3, 6.4, 6.5, 6.6, 6.7, 6.8, 6.9, and 6.10).

The patient was supine on the operating table, and her arms were abducted 60–90 ° depending on the surgeon's preference.

Bilateral arm abduction is required only when the breast surgeon needs bilateral sentinel lymph node biopsy and axillary lymph node dissection.

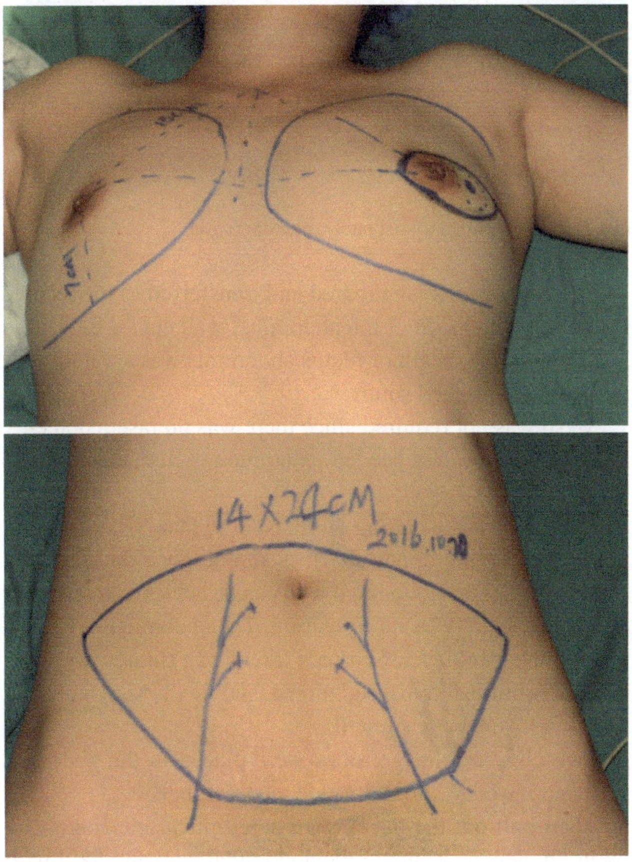

Fig. 6.3 Intraoperative design

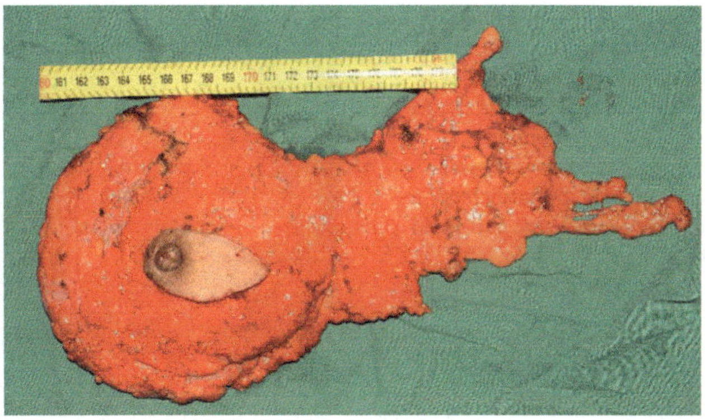

Fig. 6.4 Completion of modified radical mastectomy for breast cancer

Determine the blood supply of the flap tissue farthest from the perforator vessel and remove the part with poor blood supply.

- *Cutaneous angiosome: The largest anatomical area that can be reached by a skin vessel and its branches in morphology, and its corresponding surgical concept is the maximum range of the flap that the vessel can support. The concept of flap blood vessel was proposed by Australian physician Taylor in 1986.*

6.1.1 Anatomical Territory

In anatomical morphology, the range of vascular branches is the most basic vascular donor area. It is the first level of skin vascular donor division by British anatomist Cormack in 1984.

6.1.2 Hemodynamic Donor Territory

On the junction line of adjacent donor areas, when decreased blood flow pressure due to unilateral vascular blockage occurs, the other side of the blood vessel will provide additional blood flow to the donor area and expand the donor area to that side. It is the second level of skin vascular donor division by British anatomist Cormack.

6.1.3 Potential Territory

The donor area is expanded by human intervention (such as delayed surgery, drug delayed, etc.). If extended flap harvest is required for defect repair, extension could go beyond hemodynamic donor area and even reach adjacent donor site without compromising the flap. It is the third level of skin vascular donor division by British anatomist Cormack.

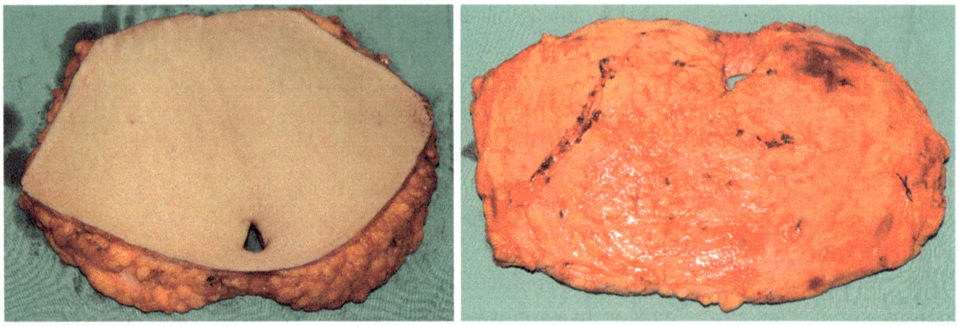

Fig. 6.5 The single pedicled DIEP flap was cut off. Clamping test confirmed that even if a large flap was cut, as long as the appropriate dominant perforator vessel was selected, the sufficient blood supply of the flap could be ensured

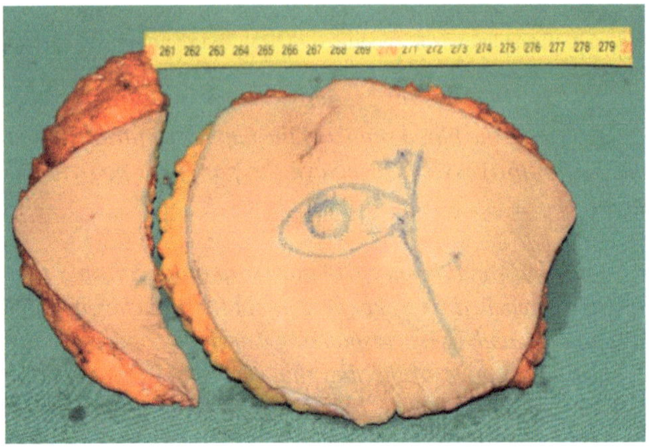

Fig. 6.6 Resection of the contralateral Zone IV tissue

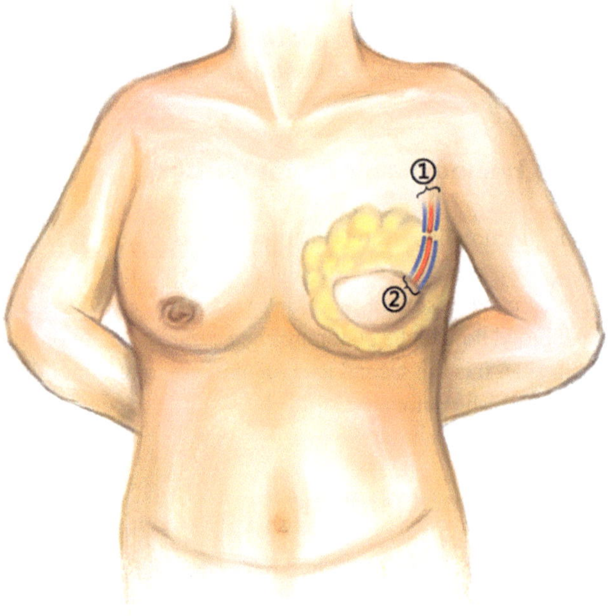

Fig. 6.7 Pattern of revascularization: left deep inferior epigastric vessels + left lateral thoracic vessels (1A2V). (1) Left lateral thoracic vessels; (2) Left deep inferior epigastric vessel

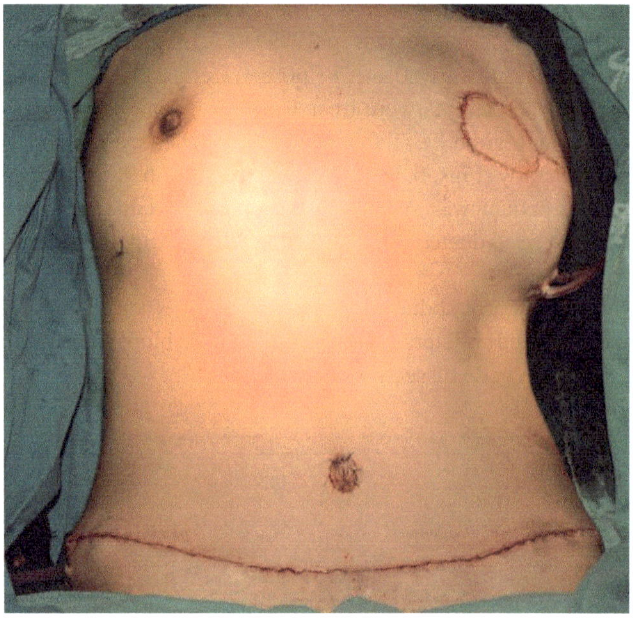

Fig. 6.8 Appearance immediately after operation

When the flap was prepared and transferred to the receiving area, the incision of the abdominal wall can be closed.

The anterior sheath of rectus abdominis was sutured with two layers of barbed suture.

Mesh was not required since there was no fascia defect.

Where suture was needed, continuous suture can be used for repair.

Generally, if the cutting width is more than 8 cm, it is difficult to close the donor site in a supine position. Tension-free closure of the abdominal wall can be achieved by placing the patient in a “V” shape position. The abdominal wall was sutured layer by layer, Scarpa’s fascia was sutured with 2-0 absorbable thread or barbed thread, and finally subcutaneous and skin layers were sutured.

Two closed drainage tubes were placed in the abdomen wall and introduced out through a lateral incision.

Then pull out the navel from an elliptical incision made on its shadowing point on the abdominal wall and fix it with 4-0 absorbable suture in semi-buried mattress method.

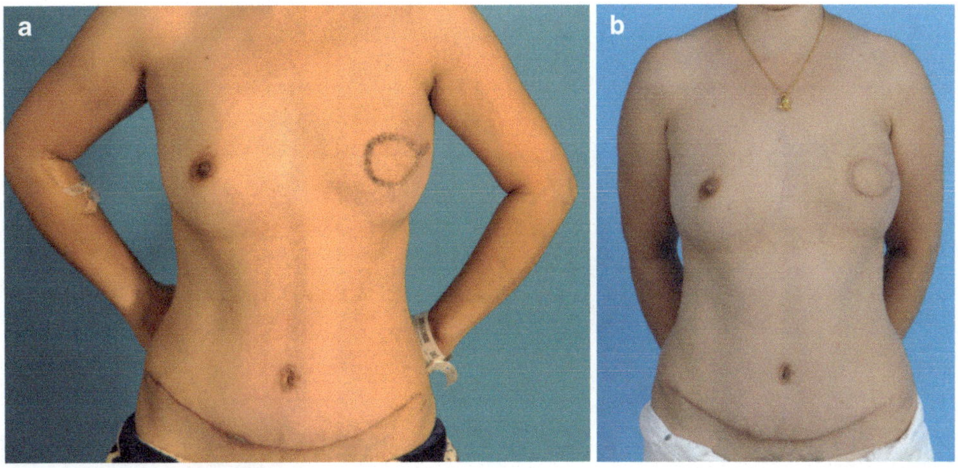

Fig. 6.9 (**a**) 3-month follow-up after operation. (**b**) The patients were followed up for 24 months

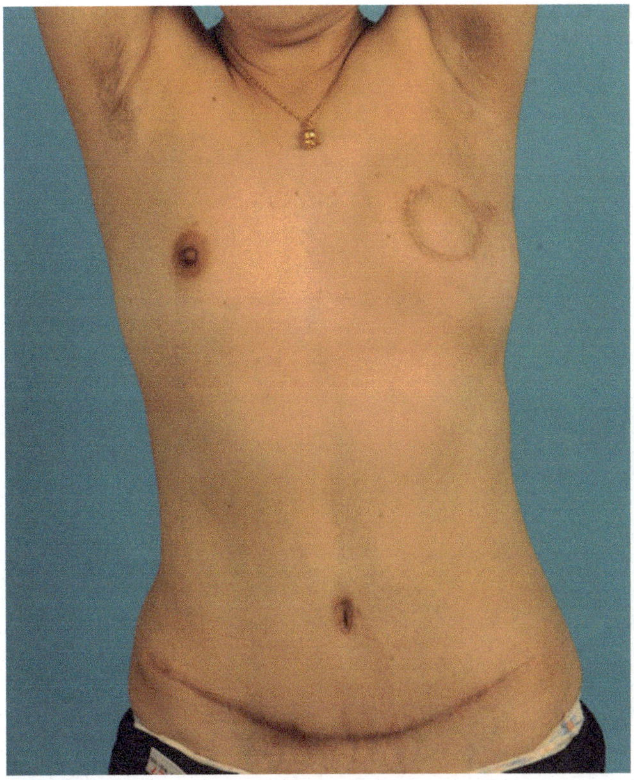

Fig. 6.10 36-month follow-up after operation

6.2 Case 2: A DIEP Flap Pedicled with a Paraumbilical Perforator of the Lateral Branch

A 40-year-old female received modified radical mastectomy in the local hospital 15 months ago and recovered uneventfully.

The postoperative pathological results were "right breast invasive ductal carcinoma (pT2N0M0,IIa) of histological grade II-III, positive lymphatic-vascular invasion and the size of the mass was about 2.7 cm × 1.5 cm × 1.5 cm, no metastatic cancer was found in the right axillary lymph node(0/13); ER70%, PR70%, HER2(2+), Ki67 50%, FISH negative."

Six cycles of chemotherapy with "FEC" regimen were given after operation, and endocrine therapy with tamoxifen 60 mg QD X5yr was followed.

The patient underwent right chest wall scar reduction + FREE DIEP flap transplantation for breast reconstruction under general anesthesia in our hospital. Postoperative pathological examination showed that the right chest wall scar was free of tumor. The patient had good blood supply of the flap, and satisfactory appearance and function of the reconstructed breast during follow-up (Figs. 6.11, 6.12, 6.13, and 6.14).

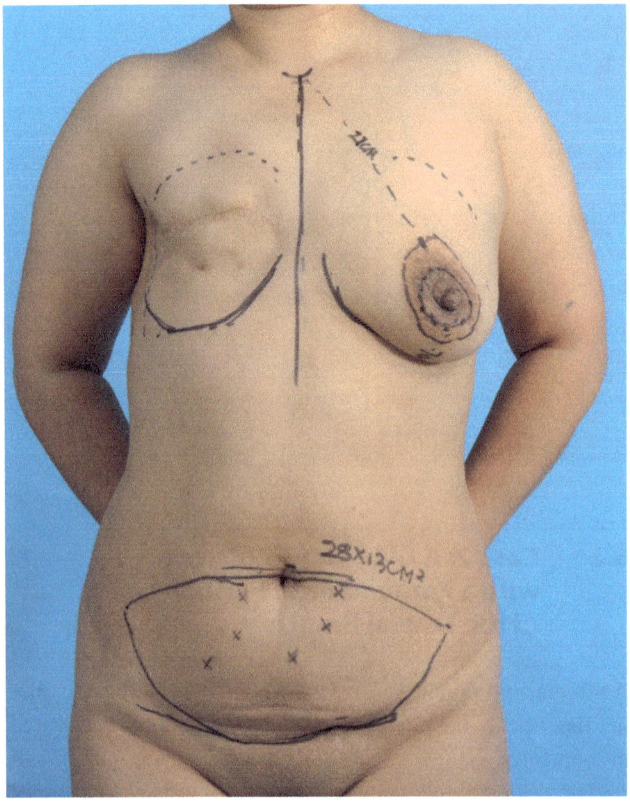

Fig. 6.11 Preoperative findings

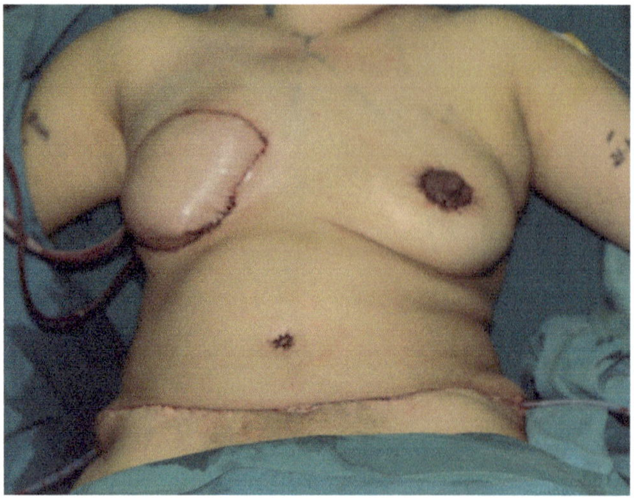

Fig. 6.13 Appearance immediately after breast reconstruction during operation

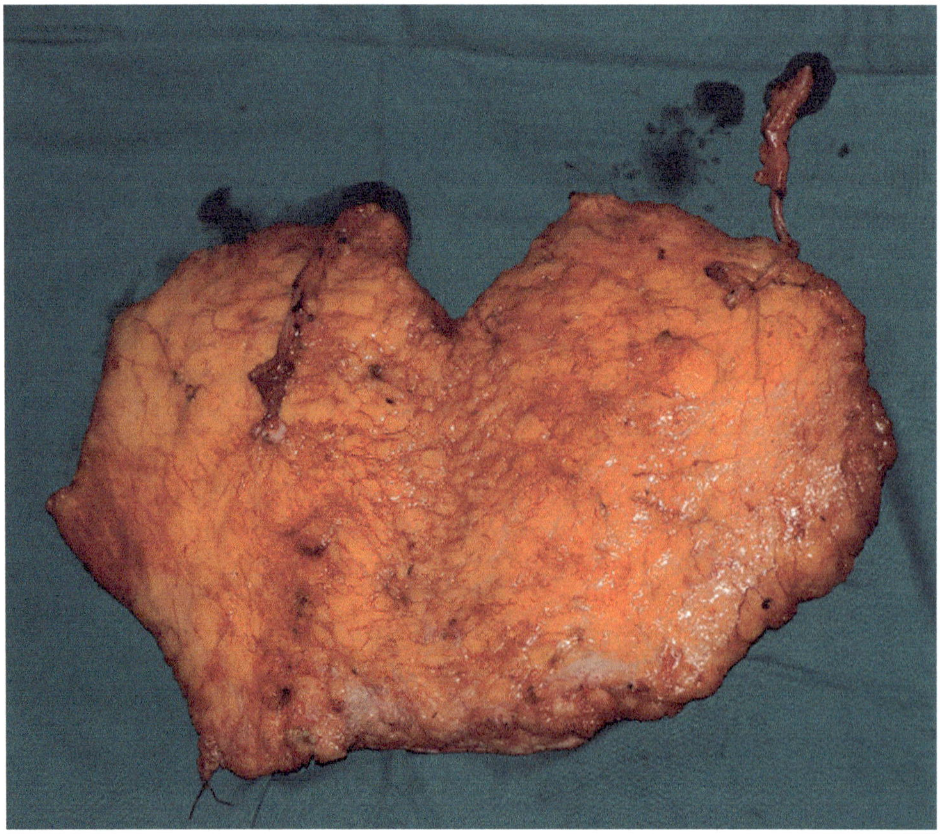

Fig. 6.12 Intraoperative exploration of perforating vessels of bilateral inferior abdominal arteries found that the skin entry point of the right perforating vessel was in the umbilical plane and came from the lateral row of inferior abdominal vessels. The position of the left perforating vessel was lower and also from the lateral row. Considering that the patient's breast was large and required much tissue, the perforating vessels on both sides came from the lateral row and were not located in the central area of the flap, it was decided to harvest a DIEP flap with bilateral vascular pedicles

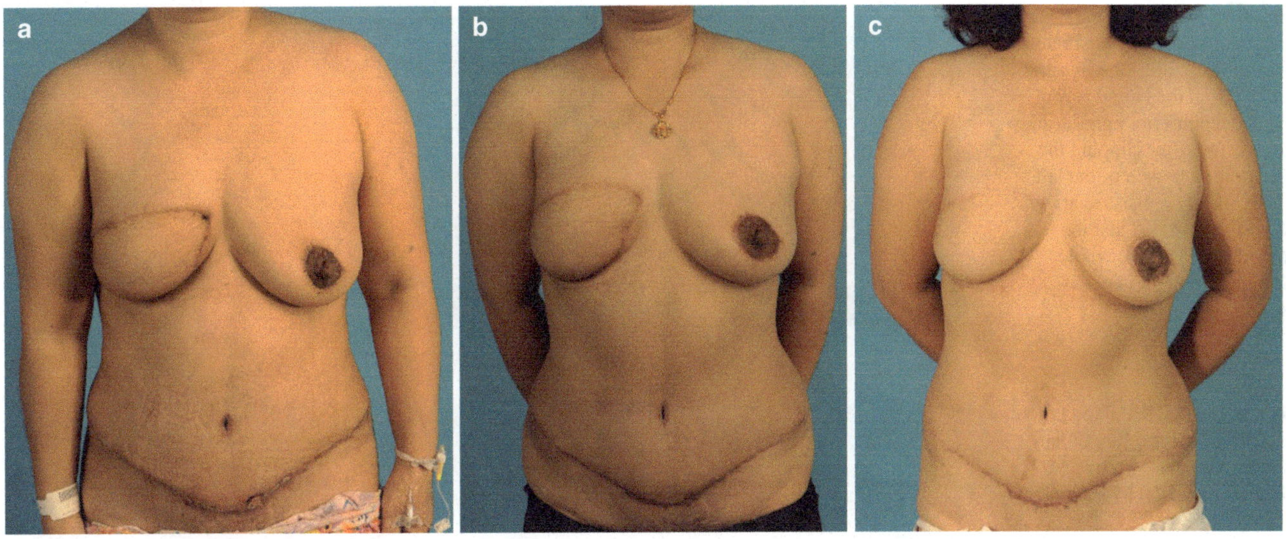

Fig. 6.14 (**a**) Appearance and function of the reconstructed breast after discharge 2 weeks after operation; (**b**) The function and appearance of reconstructed breast and flap donor area were followed up 6 months after operation; (**c**) The patients were followed up 12 months after operation

6.3 Case 3: A DIEP Flap Pedicled with Perforators of the Lateral Branch

The patient, a 47-year-old female, complained that she accidentally found a right nipple mass with itching nipple without pain or nipple discharge 2 months ago.

She received right breast mass resection and sentinel lymph node biopsy at local a hospital. Intra-operative frozen section showed that the right breast tumor was low-grade intraductal carcinoma and the margins and the sentinel lymph node were clear of tumor cells. Breast conserving surgery was performed. However, postoperative pathological examination found cancer cells at the medial margin. The patient came to our hospital for further treatment. Pathological re-evaluation of the surgical specimen was performed and the conclusions were as follow: high grade intraductal carcinoma of the right breast (cribriform type, partly comedo-type), co-existing with invasive tubular carcinoma (size: 0.3 cm × 0.2 cm), no LVI, clear superior and basal margins, cancer cells found at the medial margin, negative sentinel lymph nodes (0/4). Immunohistochemistry findings: right breast invasive carcinoma: ER90%, PR95%, CerbB-2 (+/−). Right sentinel lymph node biopsy + right mastectomy + breast reconstruction with free inferior abdominal artery perforator flap transplantation were performed. The blood supply of the flap was satisfactory and the patient was transferred to internal medicine for further comprehensive treatment.

The appearance and function of reconstructed breast were satisfactory during follow-up. Nipple reconstruction was performed 12 months after operation (Figs. 6.15, 6.16, 6.17, 6.18, and 6.19).

Most literature reports and most clinical examples have proved that the lateral perforating branch of unilateral deep inferior epigastric vessel used as pedicle cannot provide reliable blood supply for the IV area of the flap, but it is not necessary to routinely adopt bilateral vascular pedicles. The safety of using unilateral perforator as flap pedicle can be assessed by clamping the contralateral perforators and ICG angiography. Moreover, the amount of flap tissue is usually reduced for flap shaping which will improve the likelihood of success. According to our clinical experience, obstructed venous drainage is the most common reason for flap failure, which can be solved by revascularization of ipsilateral superficial epigastric veins.

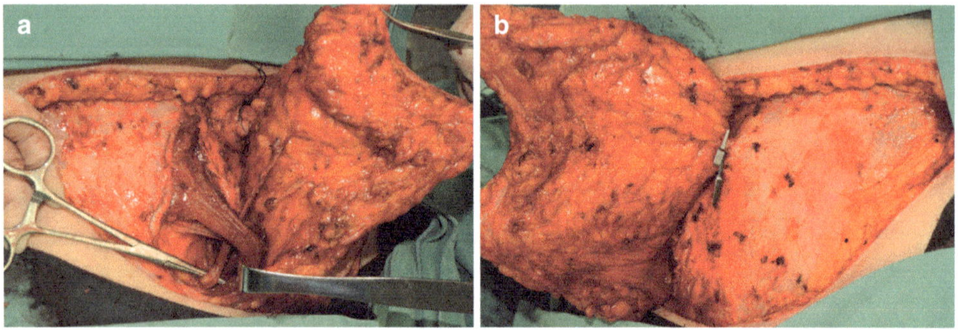

Fig. 6.15 (**a**) Double perforator pedicled perforator flap of deep inferior epigastric artery from the lateral row of right deep inferior epigastric artery; (**b**) After clipping the perforating branch of the left deep inferior epigastric artery, it was determined that the blood supply of the whole lower abdominal flap was good

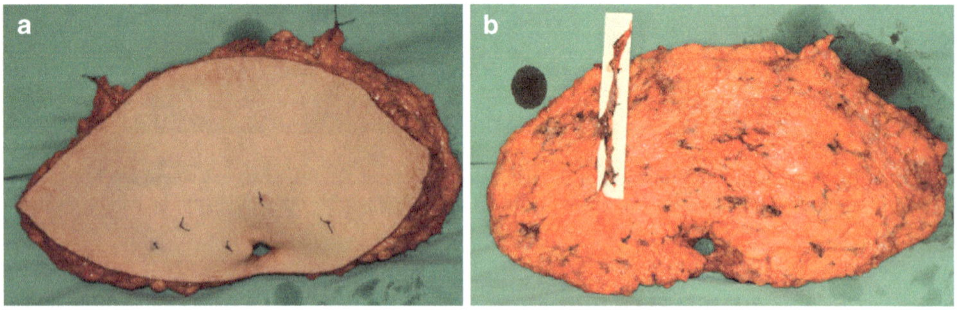

Fig. 6.16 A DIEP flap carrying bilateral superficial epigastric veins was cut. (**a**) Lateral view; (**b**) Medial view

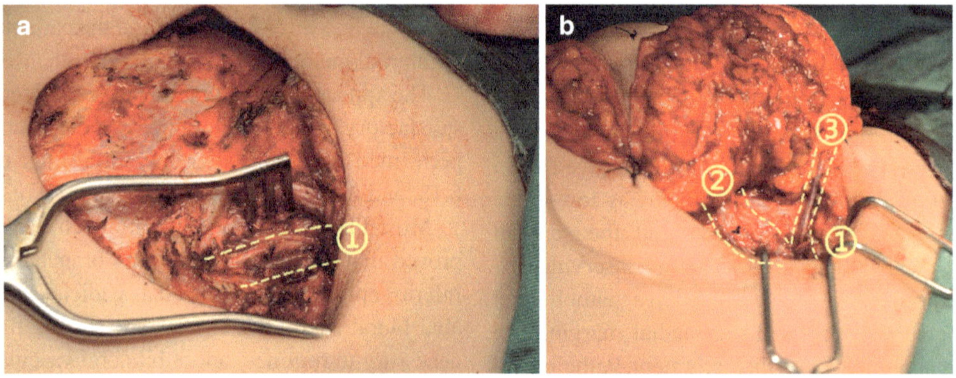

Fig. 6.17 (**a**) The blood vessels in the right thorax of the receiving area were ready. (**b**) The right deep inferior epigastric vessel was anastomosed with the proximal end of the right internal mammary vessel (A: V = 1:1); the right superficial epigastric vein was anastomosed with the distal end of the right internal thoracic vein (A: V = 1:1). (1) Right internal mammary vessels; (2) Right deep inferior epigastric vessels; (3) Right superficial epigastric vein

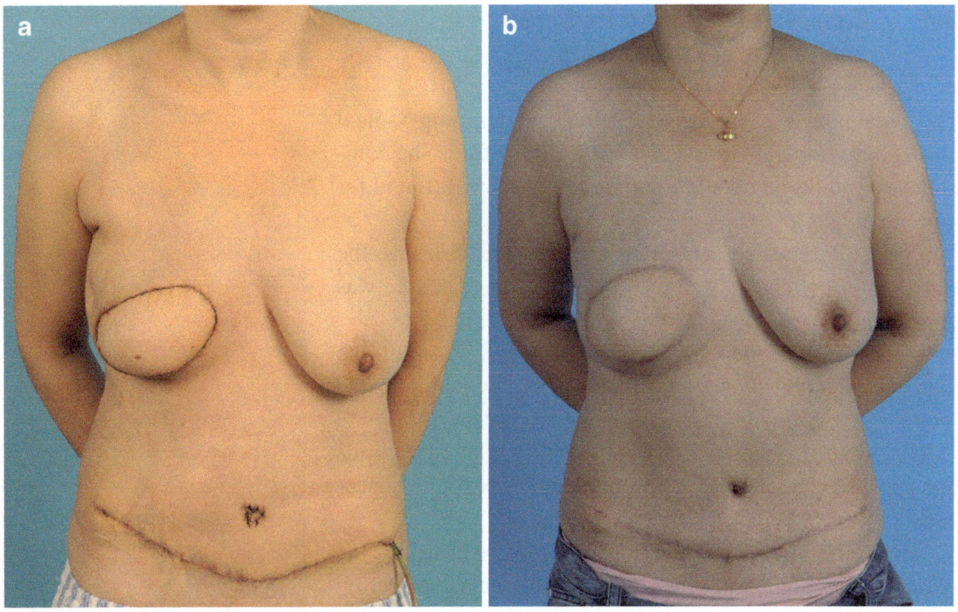

Fig. 6.18 (**a**) The appearance 10 days at discharge after DIEP breast reconstruction; (**b**) Follow-up of appearance and function 12 months after DIEP breast reconstruction

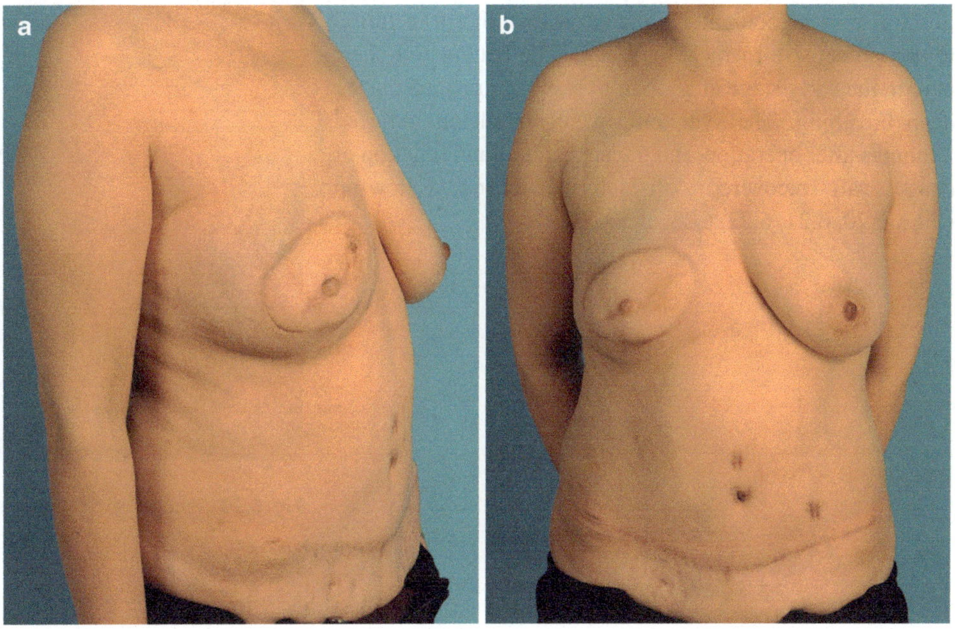

Fig. 6.19 (**a**) 18 months after DIEP breast reconstruction and 6 months after right nipple reconstruction; (**b**) 24 months after DIEP breast transplantation and 12 months after right nipple reconstruction

6.4 Case 4: A DIEP Flap Pedicled with Lateral Perforators

The patient was a 35-year-old female undergoing radical mastectomy for right breast cancer 6 years before. She complained of multiple nodules on the right chest wall found for more than half a year.

Chest CT revealed several subcutaneous nodules on the right anterior chest wall, and metastatic disease was considered.

Breast color Doppler ultrasound showed multiple hypoechoic nodules on the right chest wall, which indicated recurrence and no obvious mass in the left breast.

No enlarged lymph nodes were found in bilateral armpits and supraclavicular areas. Chest nodule biopsy found cancer cells.

After admission, the patient underwent removal of the tumor lesions and chest skin plus partial sternal rib resection + thoracotomy plus chest wall reconstruction using mesh and bone cement plus DIEP flap transfer. The blood supply of the flap was good and the patient was further transferred to comprehensive medical treatment. The patient felt chest pain in the early stage after operation and aggravated during deep breathing. The symptoms were completely relieved 2 months after operation, and the appearance and function of chest wall recovered satisfactorily during follow-up (Figs. 6.20, 6.21, 6.22, 6.23, and 6.24).

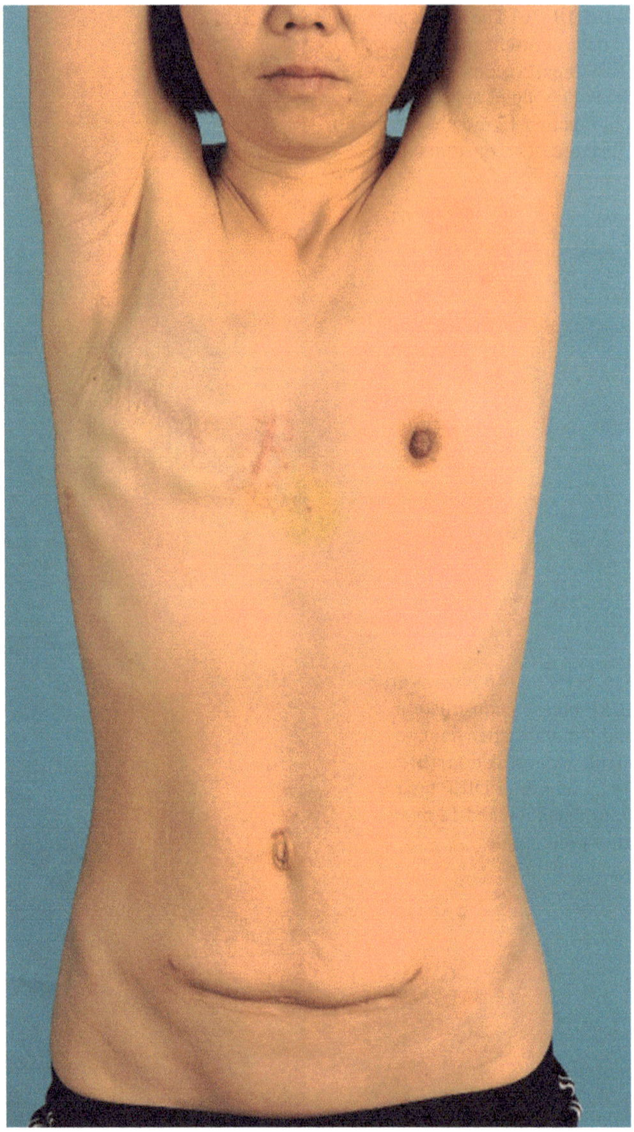

Fig. 6.20 Preoperative conditions

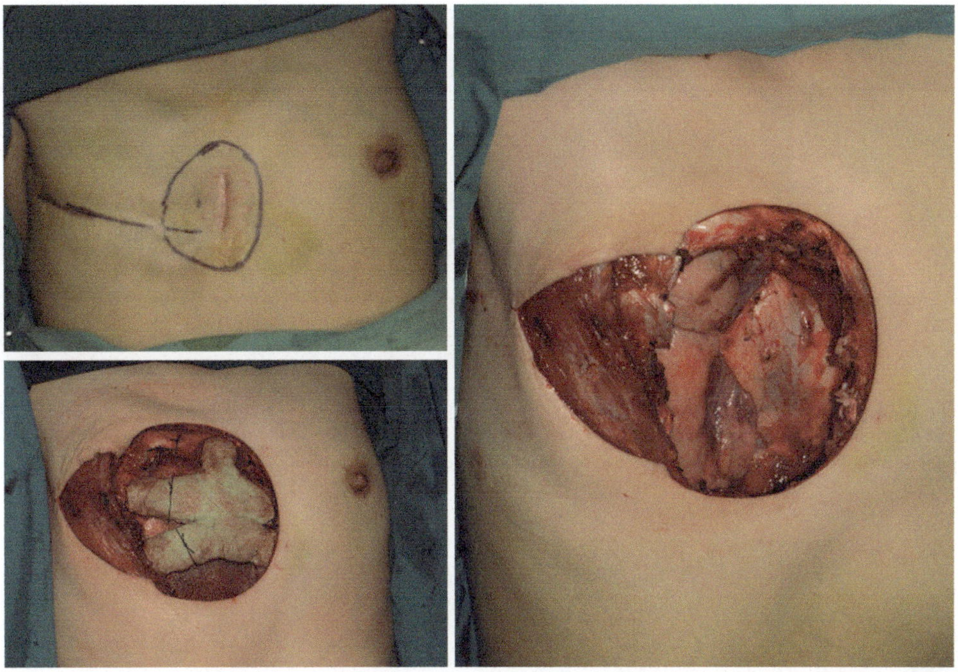

Fig. 6.21 A massive chest defect was left after right chest lesion removed and reconstructed with mesh and bone cement scaffold

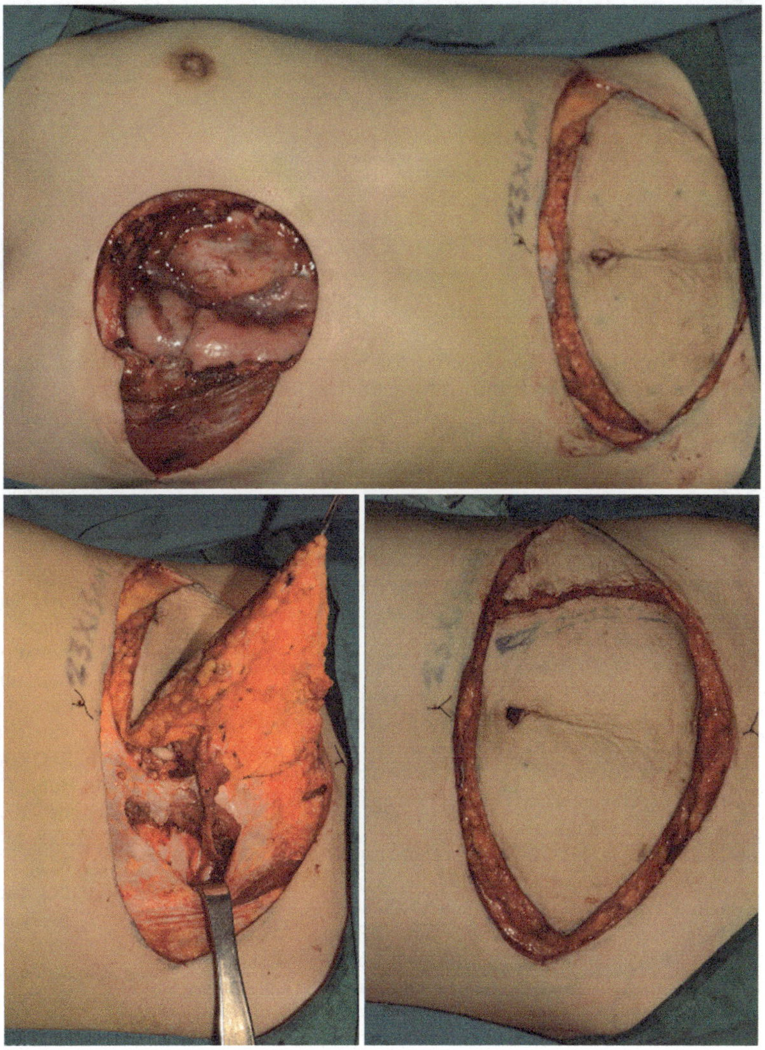

Fig. 6.22 The right DIEP flap was used for transplantation. The perforator comes from the lateral branch of the right deep inferior epigastric artery. Remove area IV, which appeared to be poorly perfused

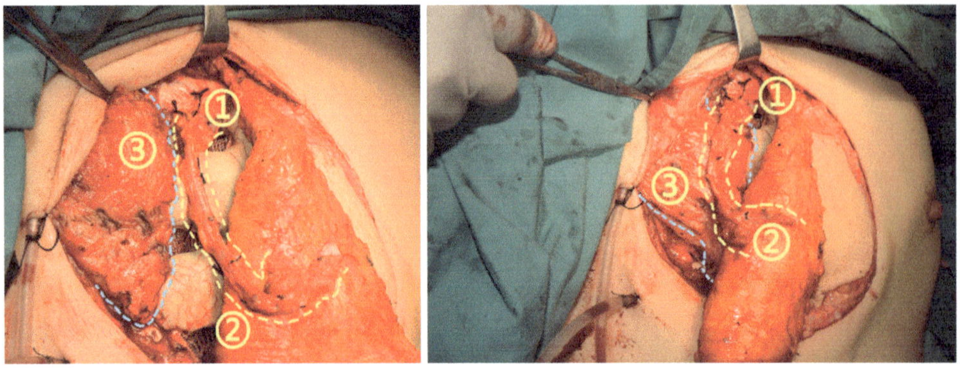

Fig. 6.23 Revascularization of the right deep inferior epigastric vessel and the right internal mammary blood vessel (A: $V = 1{:}1$). The vascular pedicle was cushioned by a local pectoralis major muscle flap to prevent vascular spasm and embolism induced by direct contact with the cement. (1) Proximal end of right internal mammary vessel; (2) Right deep inferior epigastric vessels; (3) Right pectoralis major muscle flap

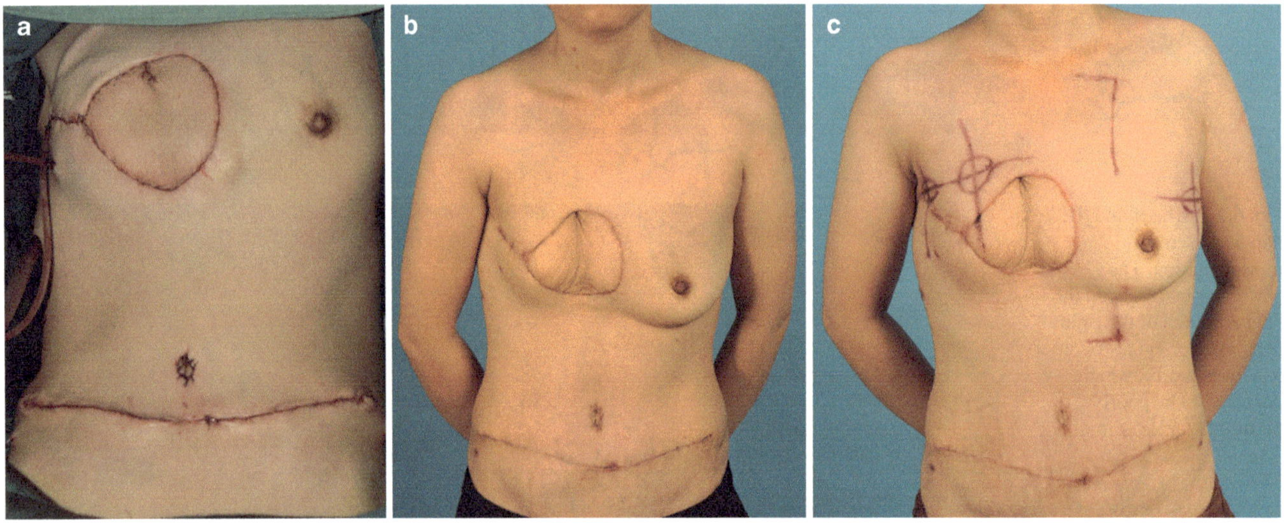

Fig. 6.24 (**a**) The blood supply of the flap was determined to be good during the operation; (**b**) Follow-up 2 months after operation; (**c**) The patients were followed up 4 months after operation

References

1. Granzow JW, Levine JL, Chiu ES, Allen RJ. Breast reconstruction with the deep inferior epigastric perforator flap: history and an update on current technique. J Plast Reconstr Aesthet Surg. 2006;59(6):571–9.
2. Chevray PM. Breast reconstruction with superficial deep inferior epigastric artery flaps: a prospective comparison with TRAM and DIEP flaps. Plast Reconstr Surg. 2004;114(5):1077–83; discussion 1084–5.
3. Taylor GI, Palmer JH. The vascular territories (angiosomes) of the body: experimental study and clinical applications. Br J Plast Surg. 1987;40(2):113–41.
4. Moon HK, Taylor GI. The vascular anatomy of rectus abdominis musculocutaneous flaps based on the deep superior epigastric system. Plast Reconstr Surg. 1988;82(5):815–32.
5. Ingvaldsen CA, Tønseth KA, Pripp AH, Tindholdt TT. Microcirculatory evaluation of the abdominal skin in breast reconstruction with deep inferior epigastric artery perforator flap. Plast Reconstr Surg Glob Open. 2016;4(2):e616.
6. Scheflan M, Dinner MI. The transverse abdominal Island flap: part II. Surgical technique. Ann Plast Surg. 1983;10(2):120–9.
7. Scheflan M, Dinner MI. The transverse abdominal Island flap: part I. Indications, contraindications, results, and complications. Ann Plast Surg. 1983;10(1):24–35.
8. Dinner MI, Dowden RV, Scheflan M. Refinements in the use of the transverse abdominal Island flap for postmastectomy reconstruction. Ann Plast Surg. 1983;11(5):362–72.
9. Hartrampf CR, Scheflan M, Black PW. Breast reconstruction with a transverse abdominal Island flap. Plast Reconstr Surg. 1982;69(2):216–25.
10. Holm C, Mayr M, Höfter E, Ninkovic M. Perfusion zones of the DIEP flap revisited: a clinical study. Plast Reconstr Surg. 2006;117(1):37–43.
11. Wong C, Saint-Cyr M, Arbique G, et al. Three- and four-dimensional computed tomography angiographic studies of commonly used abdominal flaps in breast reconstruction. Plast Reconstr Surg. 2009;124(1):18–27.
12. Rozen WM, Whitaker IS, Ashton MW. A combined anatomical and clinical study for quantitative analysis of the microcirculation in the

classic perfusion zones of the deep inferior epigastric artery perforator flap. Plast Reconstr Surg. 2011;128(3):821–2; author reply 822–3.
13. Koshima I, Moriguchi T, Fukuda H, Yoshikawa Y, Soeda S. Free, thinned, paraumbilical perforator-based flaps. J Reconstr Microsurg. 1991;7(4):313–6.
14. Koshima I, Moriguchi T, Soeda S, Tanaka H, Umeda N. Free thin paraumbilical perforator-based flaps. Ann Plast Surg. 1992;29(1):12–7.
15. Koshima I, Inagawa K, Urushibara K, Moriguchi T. Paraumbilical perforator flap without deep inferior epigastric vessels. Plast Reconstr Surg. 1998;102(4):1052–7.
16. Koshima I, Inagawa K, Yamamoto M, Moriguchi T. New microsurgical breast reconstruction using free paraumbilical perforator adiposal flaps. Plast Reconstr Surg. 2000;106(1):61–5.
17. Bailey SH, Saint-Cyr M, Wong C, et al. The single dominant medial row perforator DIEP flap in breast reconstruction: three-dimensional perforasome and clinical results. Plast Reconstr Surg. 2010;126(3):739–51.
18. Garvey PB, Salavati S, Feng L, Butler CE. Abdominal donor-site outcomes for medial versus lateral deep inferior epigastric artery branch perforator harvest. Plast Reconstr Surg. 2011;127(6):2198–205.

Various Forms of DIEP Flaps

7

Zan Li and Huaihua Qi

The deep inferior epigastric artery perforator flap is considered to be the gold standard for breast reconstruction with autologous tissue transplantation. However, with the popularization and in-depth study of clinical application, it is found that the classical deep inferior epigastric artery perforator flap still has some limitations [1].

In recent years, on the basis of adhering to the core concept of perforator flap, the operation of deep inferior epigastric artery perforator flap has been continuously developed, not only because of its large vascular body area, long vascular pedicle, and rich tissue volume, but also according to the advantages of its anatomical basis, different types of tissue flaps can be designed to meet different clinical needs.

To conform with the defect of the recipient area, the DIEP flap can be placed transversely, obliquely, vertically, and so on. To conserve the main recipient vessels, vascular bridging can be used on the flap. To avoid the bloated flap, thinning under microscope is applied. To repair the super large wound, joined DIEP flap is developed. To repair multiple wounds, segmented DIEP flap based on one pedicle is created. To achieve three-dimensional aesthetic repair of breast chest wall defect combined with deep muscle tissue defect, chimeric DIEP flap is innovated [2].

The emergence and development of these special forms of DIEP flap enrich the connotation of and expand the indications of DIEP flap.

Z. Li (✉)
Department of Oncology Plastic Surgery, Hunan Cancer Hospital, Changsha, Hunan, China

H. Qi
Department of Breast Surgery, Tangshan People's Hospital, Tangshan, Hebei, China

7.1 Transverse Perforator Flap of Deep Inferior Epigastric Artery

The perforator flap of the transverse inferior abdominal artery is the most commonly used design for breast reconstruction. It includes areas I–IV of the lower abdomen. The advantages of this flap include a large amount of tissue, flexible placement and shaping of the flap, and basically unrestricted placement of the vascular pedicle [3].

7.1.1 Case 1: Transverse Perforator Flap of Deep Inferior Epigastric Artery

The patient was a 52-year-old female with clinical manifestations: right breast mass was found in physical examination for 10 days.

After admission, right skin nipple and areola sparing mastectomy plus right sentinel lymph node biopsy plus free transverse DIEP flap transplantation for breast reconstruction were performed.

The perforator flap of deep inferior epigastric artery was pedicled with the left deep inferior epigastric artery. Flap tissue in Area IV and part of Area III was removed, and the deep inferior epigastric artery and veins were anastomosed with the internal thoracic artery and vein (1A2V). The postoperative pathological examination results showed that: (1) The histology of right breast invasive ductal carcinoma was Grade II, and the maximum diameter of the tumor was 1 cm; (2) No cancer was found at the posterior margin of nipple areola; (3) No cancer metastasis (0/4) was found in the right axillary sentinel lymph node, and the pathological stage was T1bN0M0 stage I.

Immunohistochemistry: ER (strong, 90%), PR (medium, 90%), CerbB-2 (0), Ki-67 (+, 30%).

After the operation, the flap survived uneventfully. The patient was transferred to internal medicine for further comprehensive treatment. The patients were followed up with satisfactory sensory function and appearance of reconstructed

Z. Li, D. Song (eds.), *Oncoplastic Flap Surgery*, https://doi.org/10.1007/978-981-19-8926-1_7

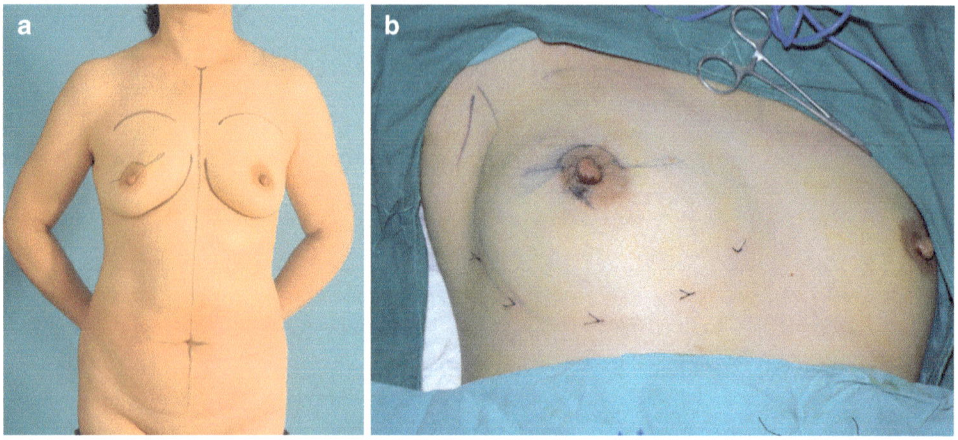

Fig. 7.1 (**a**) Preoperative design. (**b**) Intraoperative incision and separation range design

breast (Figs. 7.1, 7.2, 7.3, 7.4, 7.5, 7.6, 7.7, 7.8, 7.9, 7.10, 7.11, 7.12, 7.13, 7.14, and 7.15).

We usually expose the intrathorax vessels at the second intercostal space where the vessels harbor the greatest caliber. If necessary, we would remove part or all of the third costal cartilage. In fortunate cases, vascular anastomosis can be conducted without removing any ribs.

If the surgical technique allows, try to preserve the ribs to protect the pectoralis major muscle and prevent chest wall deformity.

In some cases, the internal mammary blood vessels will be divided into perforating branches with a diameter suitable for direct anastomosis, which can save the operation steps of dissecting the deeper internal mammary vascular system in the costal space.

In addition, in nipple sparing mastectomy, preserving these perforations can preserve skin sensation and provide necessary blood supply for nipple areola complex.

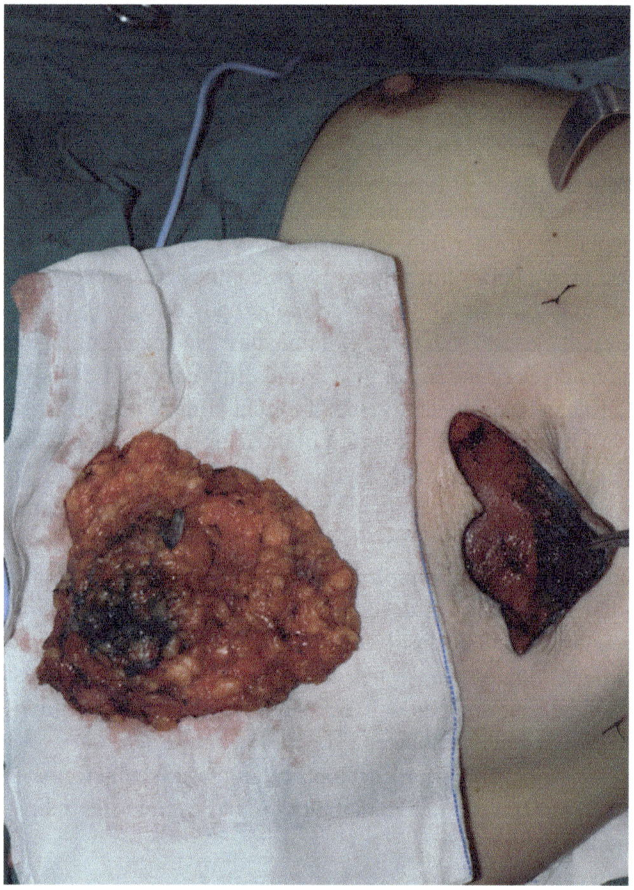

Fig. 7.2 The right breast tissue was removed

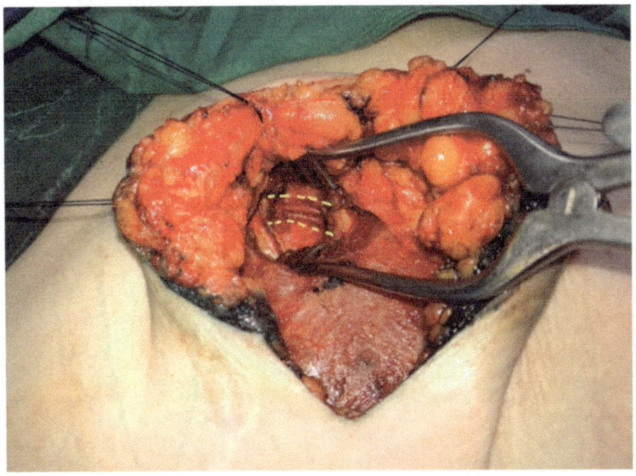

Fig. 7.3 The blood vessels in the thorax were ready

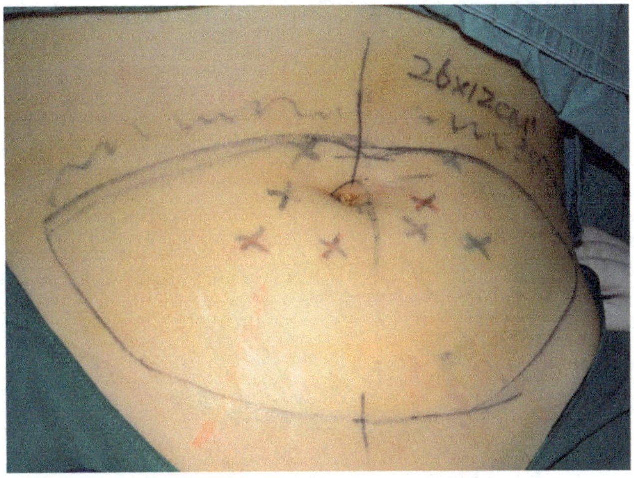

Fig. 7.4 Flap design

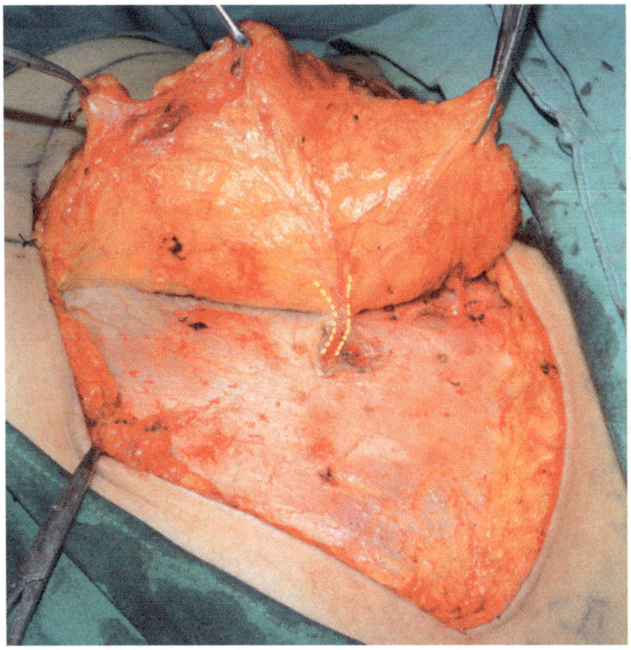

Fig. 7.5 The left deep inferior epigastric perforator

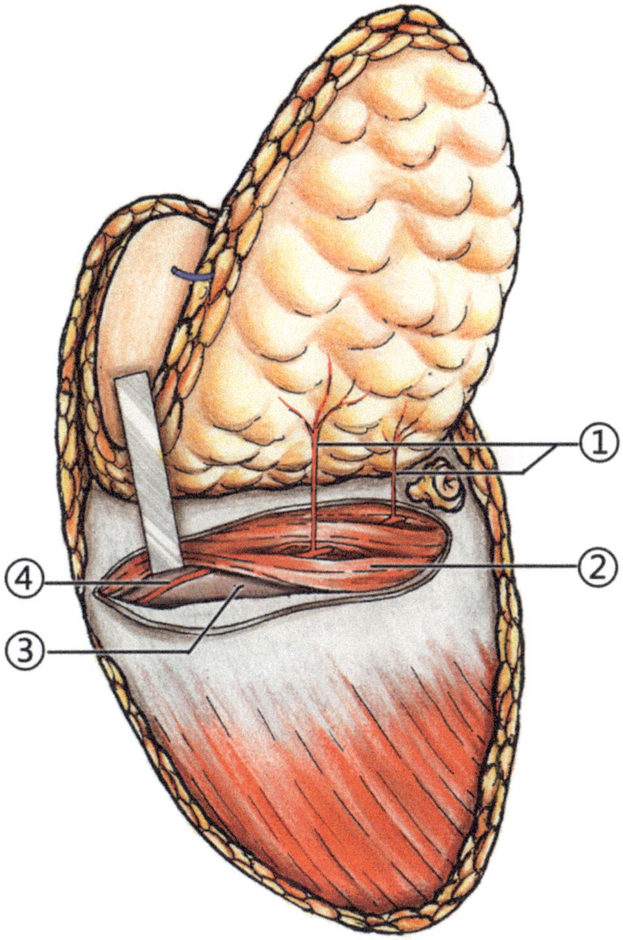

Fig. 7.6 Determine the course of perforator and vascular pedicle. (1) Perforating vessels; (2) Rectus abdominis; (3) Posterior sheath of rectus abdominis; (4) Deep inferior epigastric vessels

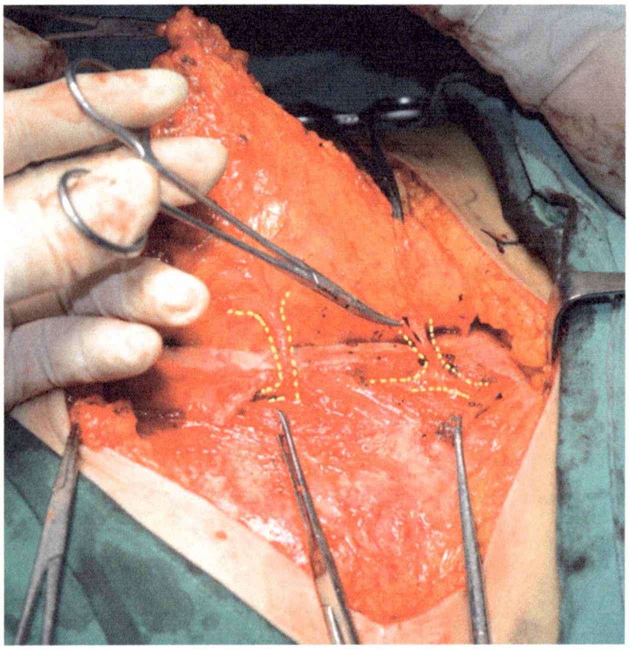

Fig. 7.7 Intramuscular separation of left vascular pedicle

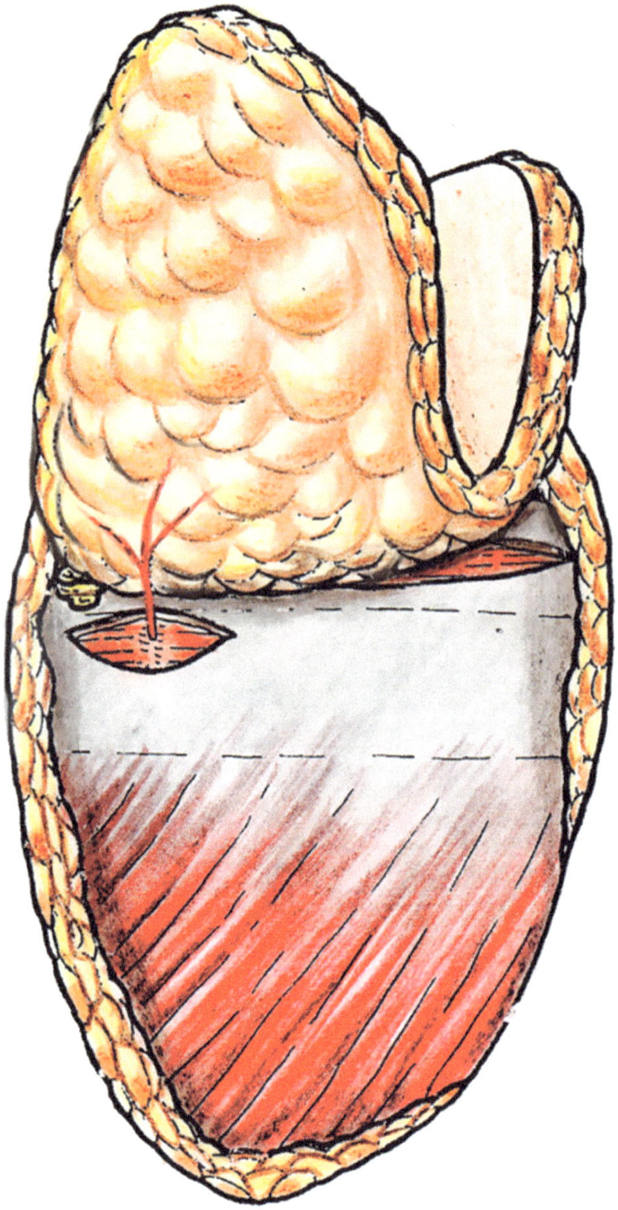

Fig. 7.8 The right deep inferior epigastric perforator

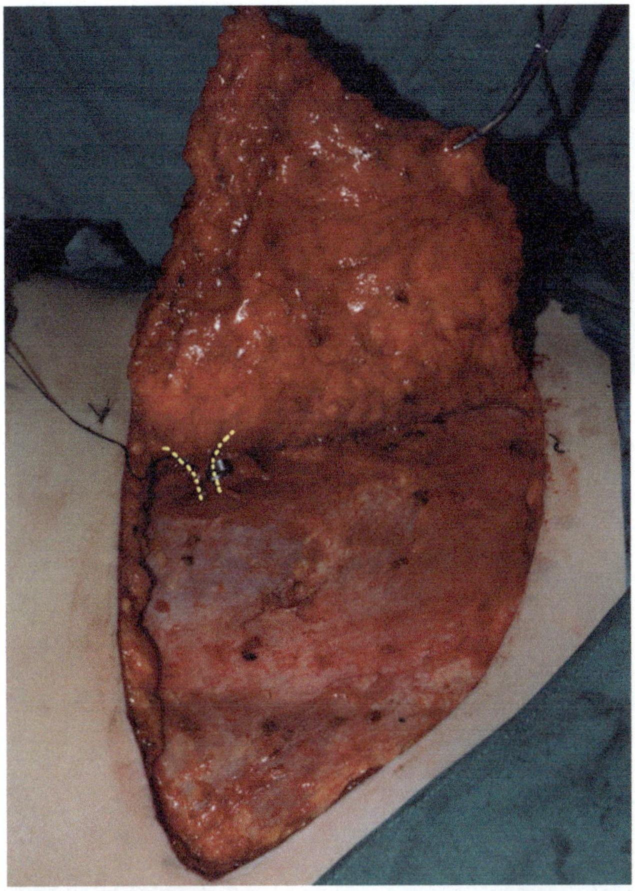

Fig. 7.9 Clamping test showed blood supply of the whole flap was good with only the left perforator and hence the right perforator vessel could be disconnected

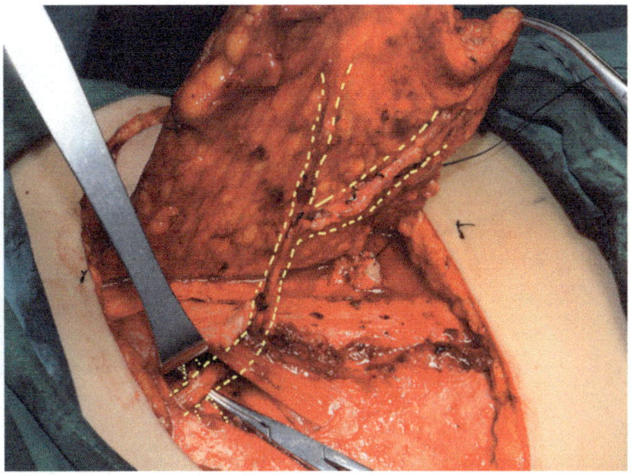

Fig. 7.10 The proximal end of vascular pedicle was exposed outside rectus abdominis

Fig. 7.11 The right perforator vessel was ligated and disconnected after the clamping test confirming that the blood supply of the flap was safe. (1) Right deep inferior epigastric vascular pedicle

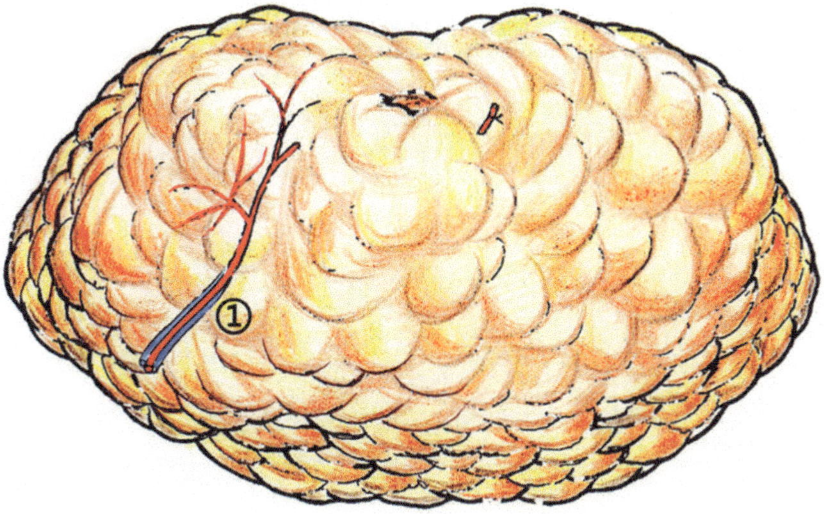

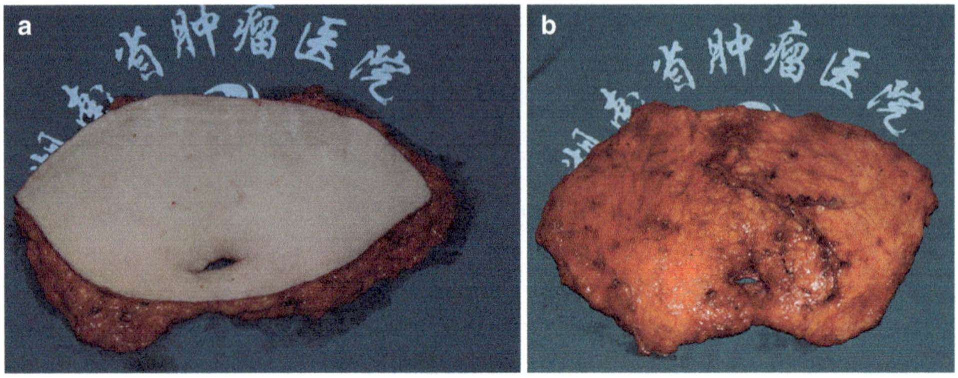

Fig. 7.12 The flap was prepared. (**a**) front view; (**b**) back view

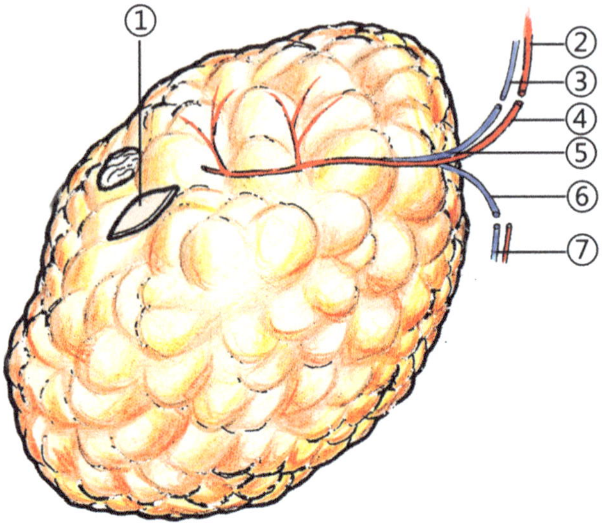

Fig. 7.13 Revascularization mode. (1) The skin island for observation; (2) Proximal internal thoracic artery; (3) Proximal internal thoracic vein; (4) Deep inferior epigastric artery; (5) Deep inferior epigastric vein 1; (6) Deep inferior epigastric vein 2; (7) Distal thoracic vessels

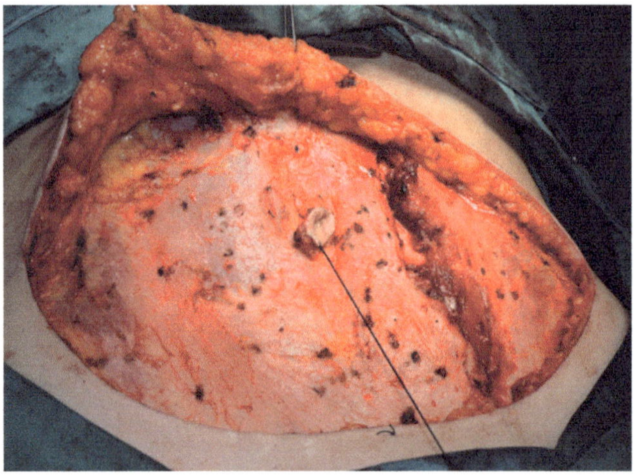

Fig. 7.14 The rectus abdominis was intact and umbilicus was in situ

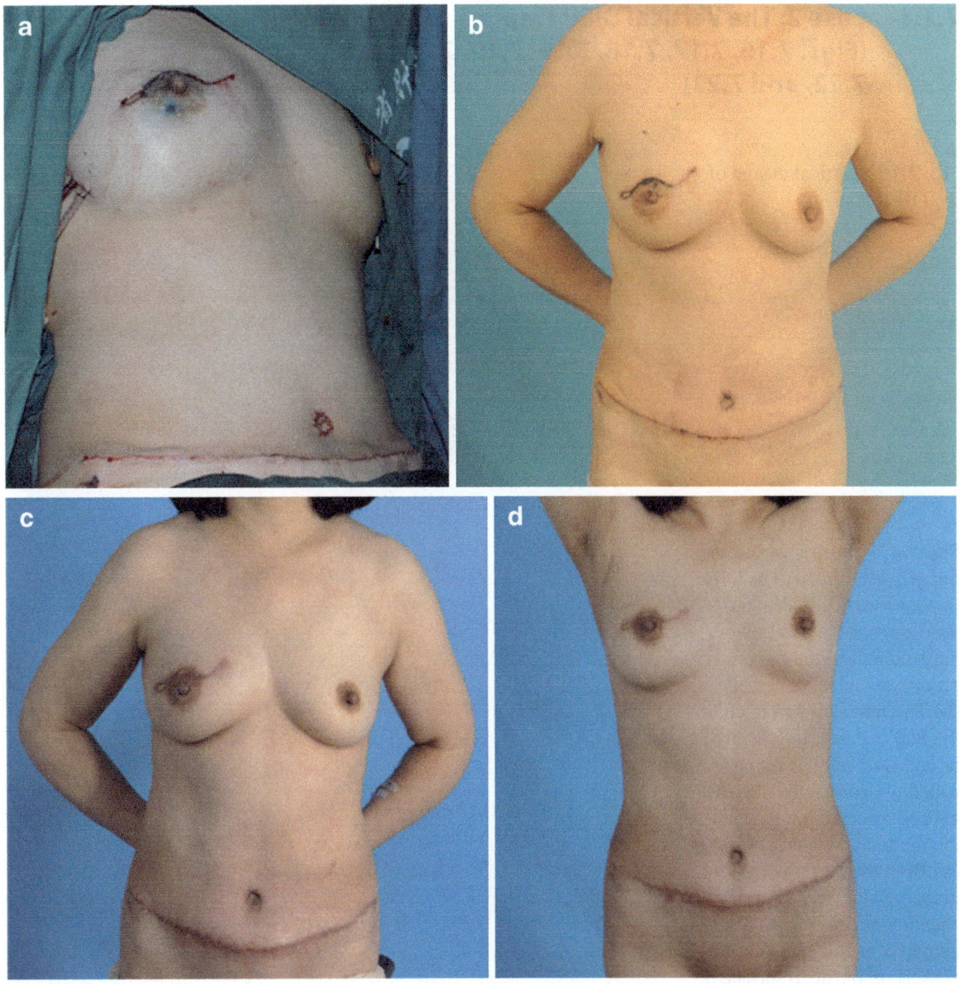

Fig. 7.15 (**a**) Appearance immediate after operation. (**b**) The appearance 2 weeks after operation. (**c**) The appearance 3 months after operation. (**d**) The appearance 12 months after operation

7.2 Vertical DIEP Flap

The DIEP flap for breast reconstruction is typically designed horizontally. However, if a transverse flap is used to repair small and medium-sized soft tissue defects, it will carry undue tissue, extend the donor scar, reduce the blood supply of the flap, and prolong the operation time.

In particular, the transverse design will damage the contralateral abdominal perforating vessels, which cannot be used as a backup scheme for future treatment.

Large flap cutting area may also lead to insufficient blood supply of the flap, and remarkable scar of the donor area. When the defect of the recipient area is small, it is not necessary to routinely use a transverse abdominal flap.

The vertical design of DIEP flap can minimize the amount of flap tissue and realize "make up as much as you need."

The advantages of vertical design of a DIEP flap include [4]:

1. The flap can be accurately cut according to the required tissue volume, and the contralateral abdominal tissue can be completely preserved and used as a backup.
2. The DIEP flap with vertical design is free of blood supply obstruction because the traditional flap division that is poor in perfusion is not involved. Common causes of poor skin flap blood flow include diabetes, peripheral vascular disease, aging, and smoking history. In clinical practice, we found that the blood supply of such flaps was so rich that it would not be impaired by trimming, thinning, or de-epithelization.
3. The vertical flap significantly reduces the time for anesthesia especially that for donor site closure since the flap is not extensive.
4. For patients with a history of abdominal surgery, especially with vertical incision of Cesarean section, vertical incision of flap is more advantageous.
5. The scar of the flap donor area was shorter and the injury of the donor area was significantly reduced.

However, because the shape of the flap donor area may be greatly affected, the vertical DIEP flap is just suitable used to reconstruct a medium-sized breast.

7.2.1 Case 2: The Vertical DIEP Flap (Figs. 7.16, 7.17, 7.18, 7.19, 7.20, 7.21, 7.22, and 7.23)

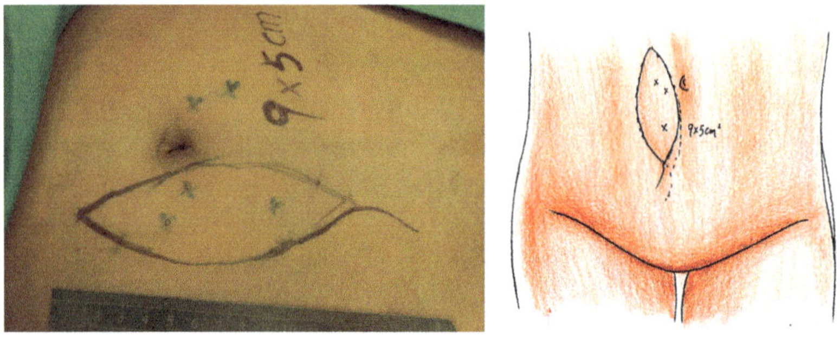

Fig. 7.16 Vertical design of the DIEP flap

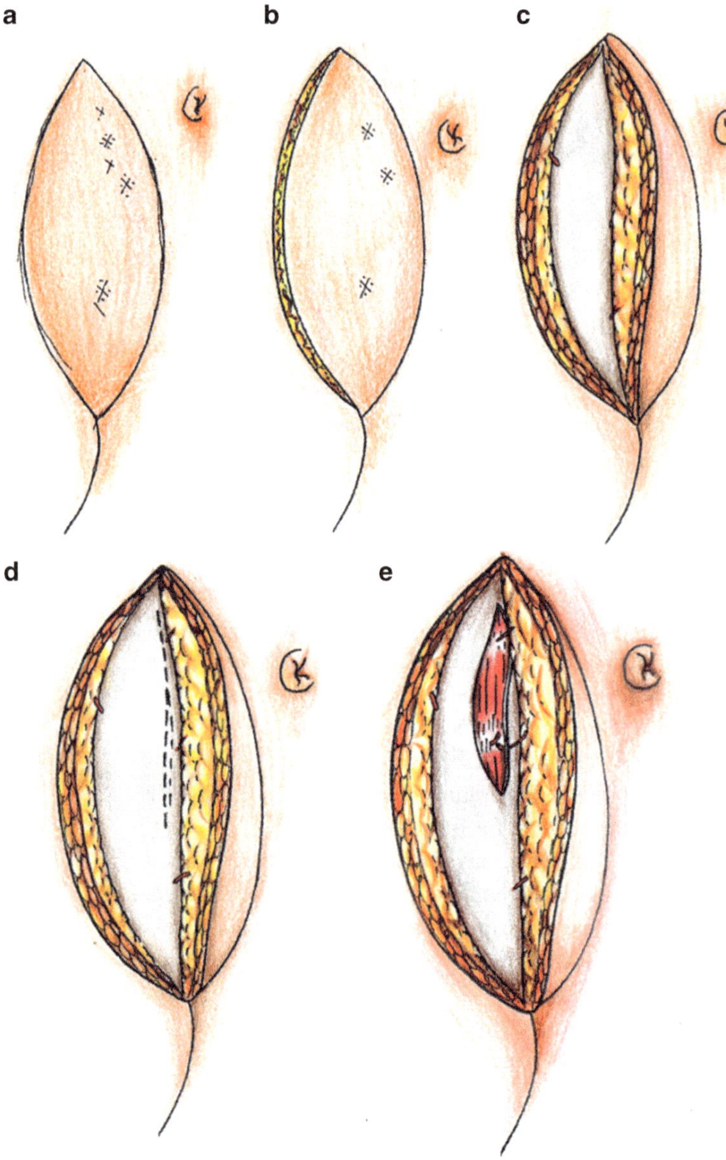

Fig. 7.17 Illustrations of the flap perforators. (**a**) The DIEP flap was vertically designed according to the position of perforators located by preoperative Doppler probe. (**b**) The first step was to cut the flap open starting from the lateral side. (**c**) The flap was rolled up from both sides to expose a perforator each on the medial and lateral sides. (**d**) Both the perforators were preserved and the anterior sheath was opened. (**e**) The course of medial perforating vessels on the deep surface of anterior sheath was examined

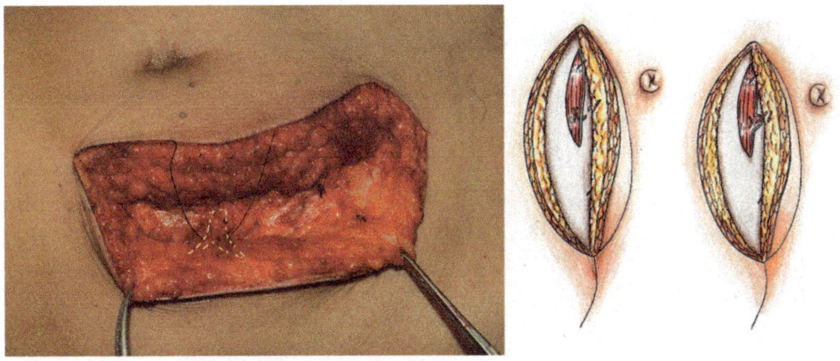

Fig. 7.18 The medial perforator vessel was small, a tendinous inscription perforator, not candidate for flap pedicle

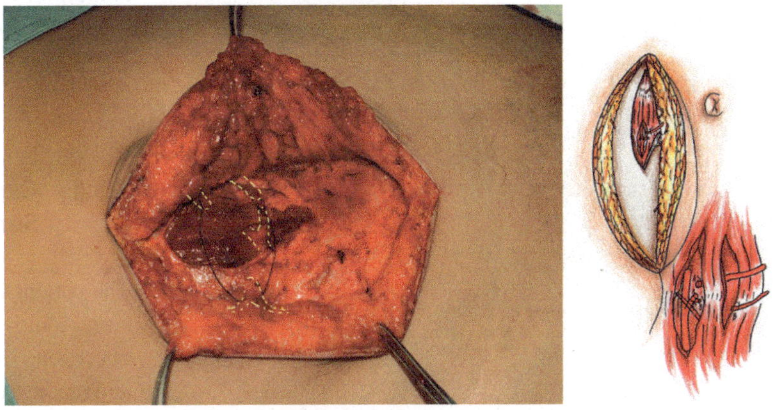

Fig. 7.19 Further examination showed that the anatomic relationship between the medial branch of the deep inferior epigastric vessel and the intercostal nerve branch was complex. In order to avoid excessive damage to the donor area, the perforating vessel was ligated and discarded

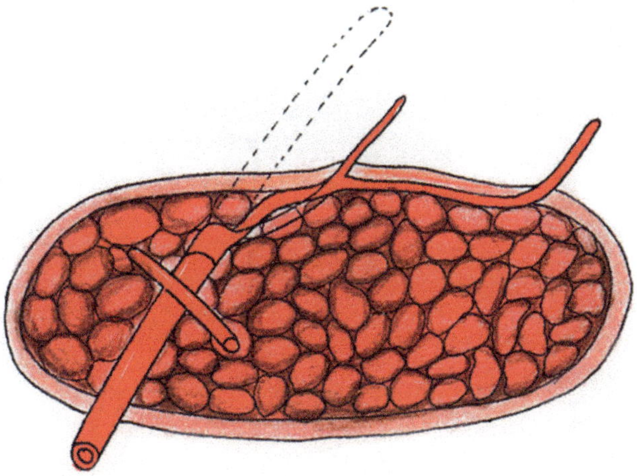

Fig. 7.20 Cross-section illustration of the relationship of the medial perforator and the intercostal nerve

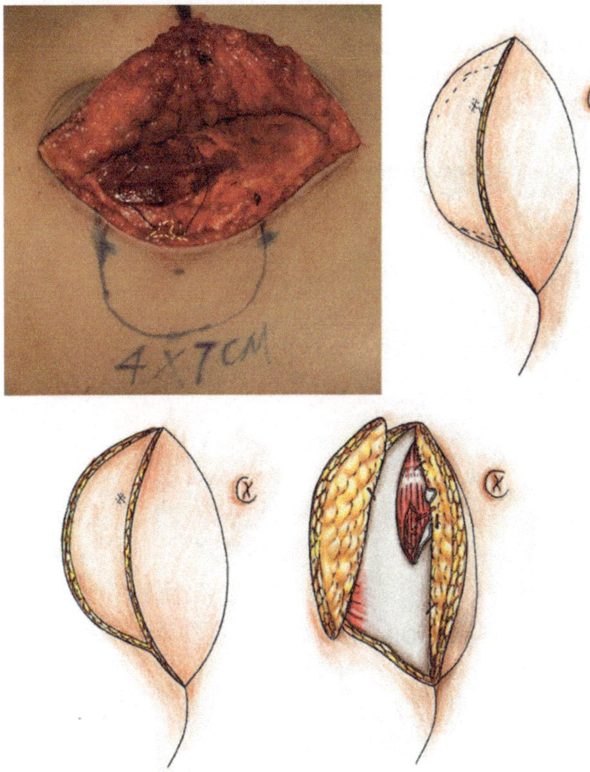

Fig. 7.21 The flap was designed with the lateral perforator as the pedicle. The subcutaneous tissue of the flap was cut and the lateral flap was free

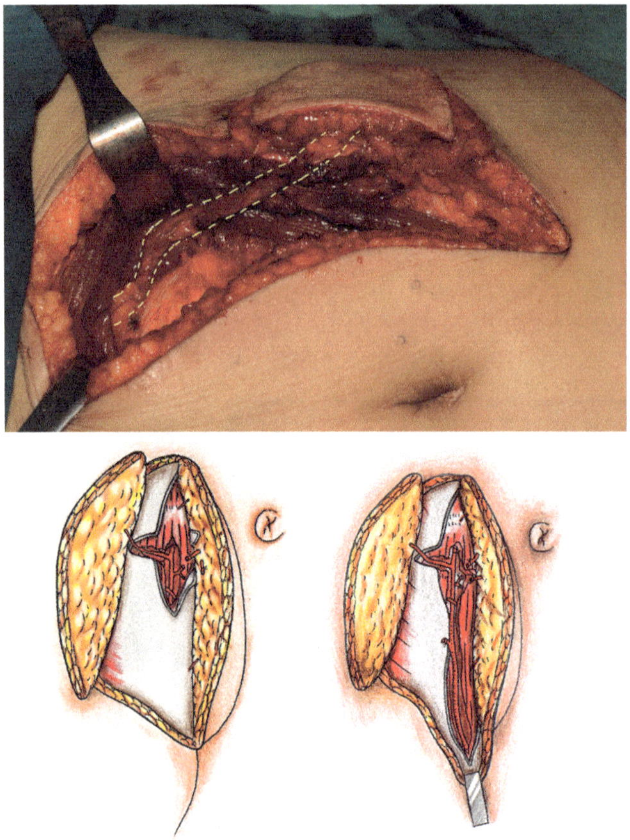

Fig. 7.22 The lateral perforating vessels in the rectus abdominis was isolated in rendezvous method and the whole deep inferior epigastric vessel was revealed

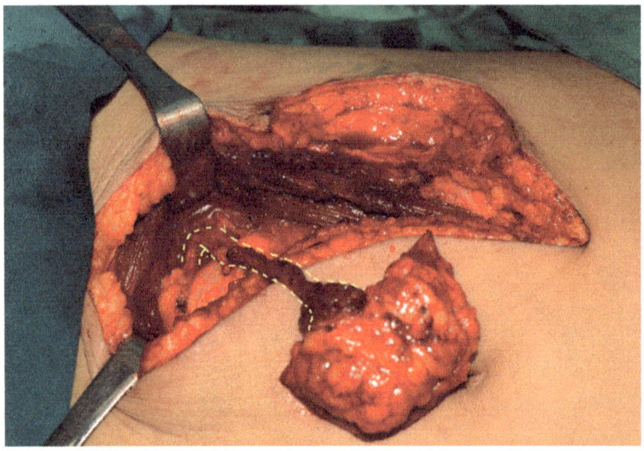

Fig. 7.23 The vertical DIEP flap was prepared

7.3 Oblique Design of DIEP Flap

In 1998, Kostakoglu and Kecik [5] applied oblique DIEP flaps in 14 patients, and entire flap necrosis and distal flap necrosis occurred in 2 cases.

The oblique DIEP flap bears a certain risk of distal necrosis, but for slim patients, especially children, the oblique DIEP flap is one of the few alternative repair methods. It can repair large recipient area defect with the minimum donor area defect. The oblique flap carries a narrower and longer skin island than the transverse flap and contains larger amount of tissue than the vertical flap [6].

Steps of raising an oblique DIEP flap (Figs. 7.24, 7.25, 7.26, 7.27, 7.28, 7.29, 7.30, 7.31, 7.32, 7.33, and 7.34).

7.3.1 Case 3: An Oblique DIEP Flap with Sensation

The patient was a 39-year-old female. She had chest fibrosarcoma removed 1 year ago and tumor relapse 6 months after operation. Upon admission, she received extended resection and reconstruction using an oblique DIEP flap with sensation. The blood supply of the flap was good and the shape of the chest wall was satisfactory (Figs. 7.35, 7.36, 7.37, 7.38, and 7.39).

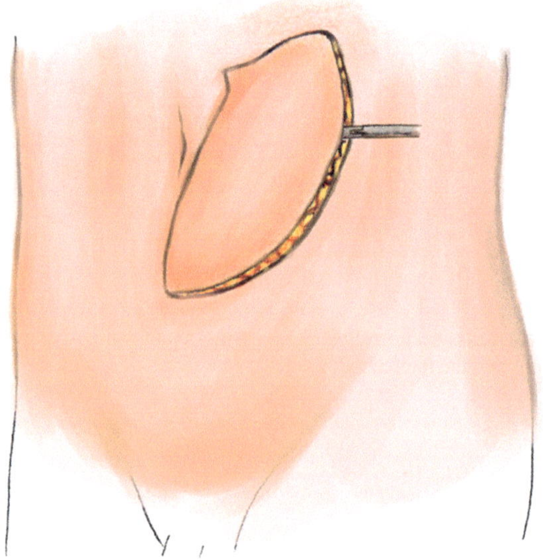

Fig. 7.24 Started with cutting open the skin at the lateral line of the flap till the aponeurosis surface of external oblique muscle was seen

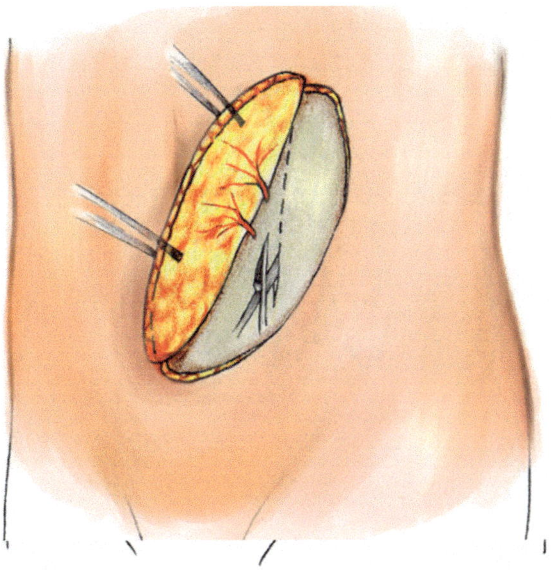

Fig. 7.25 Then the flap was sharply separated from outside to inside and two perforators were unveiled with the large one beyond the umbilicus and the other on the umbilical level. Cut the anterior sheath longitudinally along the lateral edge of the two perforating branches

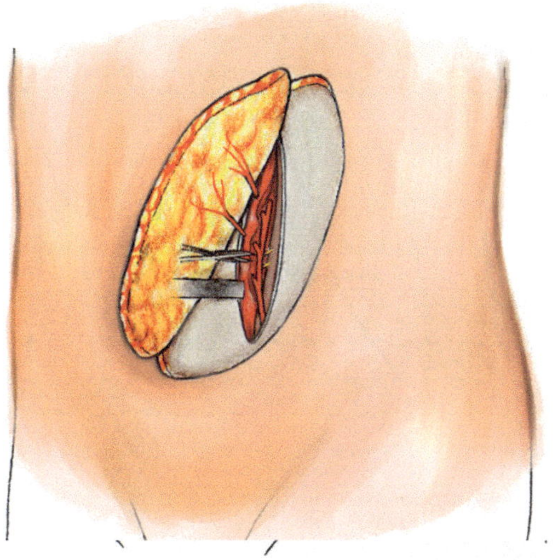

Fig. 7.27 Anterograde intramuscular separation along the lateral branch was performed till the distal end of the perforators and the vascular trunk were clearly visible. The two intercostal nerve branches along the way were required to be conserved

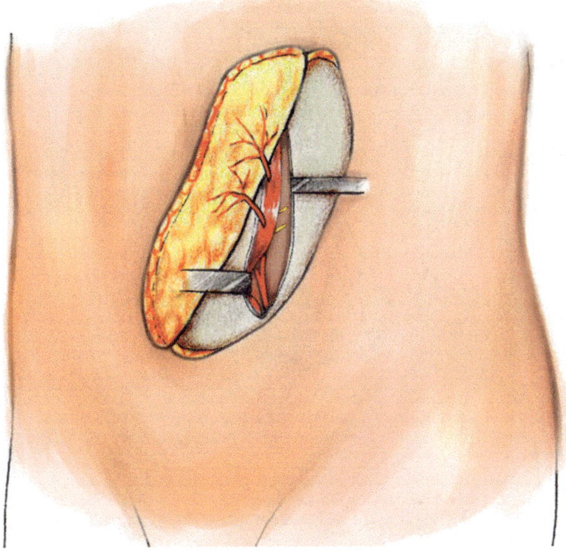

Fig. 7.26 Pull open the anterior sheath, determine the muscle piercing position of the two perforating branches on the surface of the rectus abdominis, pull the distal end of the rectus abdominis inward, and expose the trunk of deep inferior epigastric vessel and its thick lateral branch and medial branch dividing at a proximal position

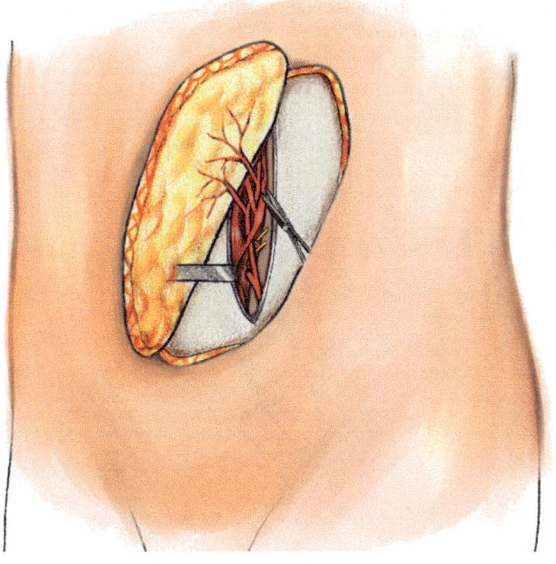

Fig. 7.28 Retrograde intramuscular separation along the two perforators. The whole segment of the two perforators from the surface of the rectus abdominis to the issuing plane of the perforator on the deep surface of the muscle was separated in rendezvous method. The muscle was separated parallel to the direction of the rectus abdominis fiber to minimize muscle damage. Due to the different perforator planes, the separated rectus abdominis fiber will be cut off

This patient had a long history of anti-hepatitis B treatment (not specified). The deep inferior epigastric artery was good and the concomitant veins were large, yet the venous wall was extremely thin (probably drug-induced) making separation impossible under microscope when the veins were shrunken. To solve this problem, the arterial anastomosis was performed first and venous separation and connection followed when the blood filled the veins.

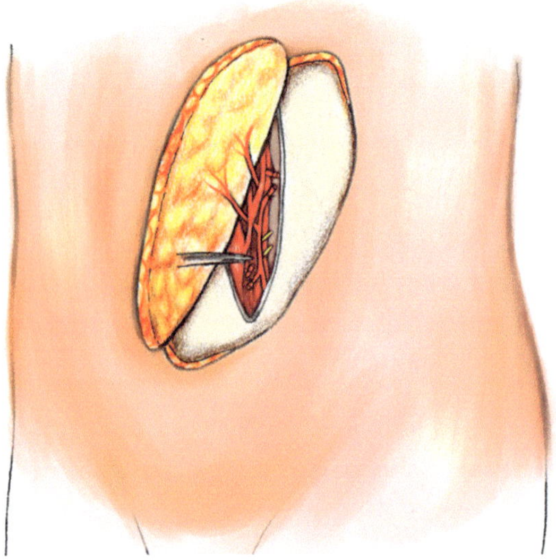

Fig. 7.29 The whole lateral branch of deep inferior epigastric vessel was completely dissociated retrograde. Further separate the small intercostal nerve branch and its nutrient vessels on the way. If it is closely connected with the vascular pedicle and cannot be separated, cut it off. Retrograde further separate the vascular pedicle to close to the emitting plane, and ligate the medial branch of the lower abdominal wall blood vessel at a low position

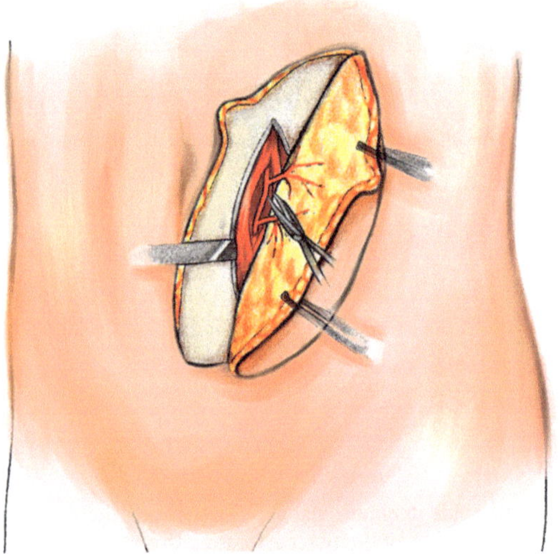

Fig. 7.30 Cut open the flap at the medial margin till the anterior sheath, sharply separate the flap from the inside to the outside, ligate and disconnect the small perforating branches along the way, and separate the flap near the main perforating branches

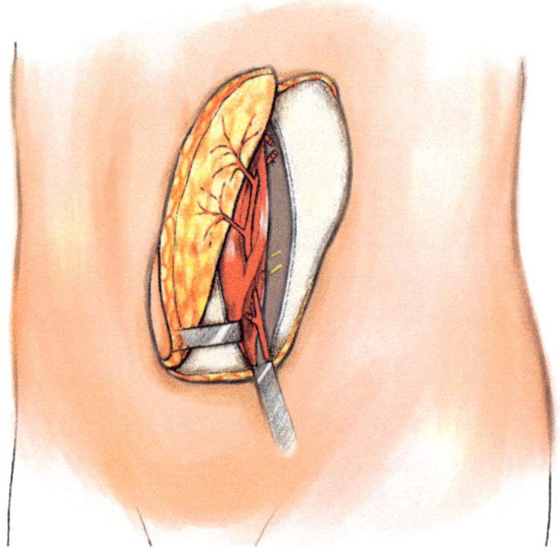

Fig. 7.31 The anterior sheath was extended caudally, a sufficient length of the inferior epigastric vessel was revealed in retrograde way, and then the vascular trunk was ligated and disconnected the vascular trunk

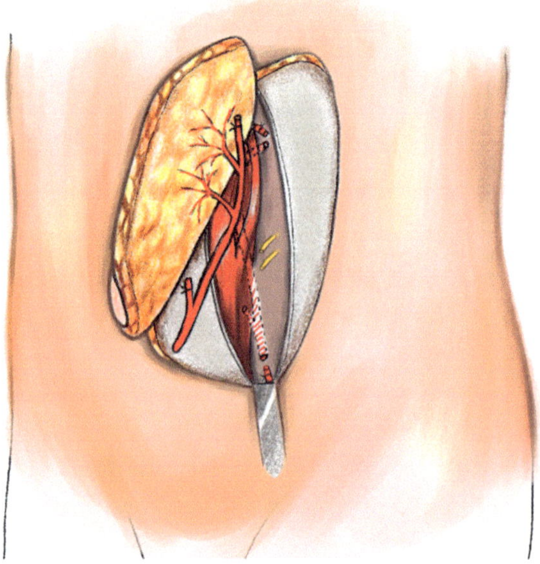

Fig. 7.32 Extract the vascular pedicle from the intramuscular tunnel

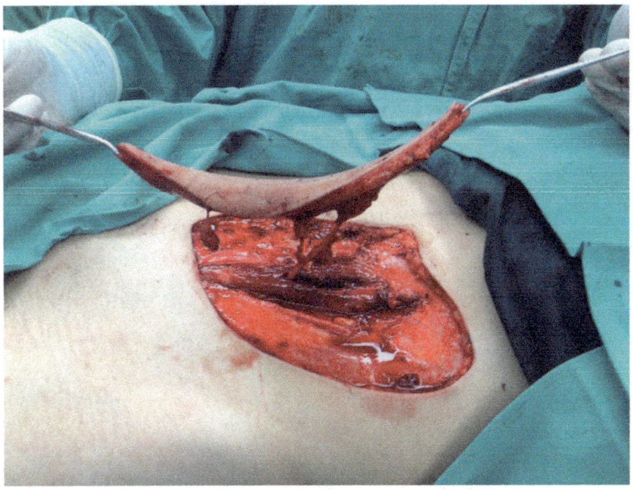

Fig. 7.33 Retrograde extraction of vascular pedicle trunk from rectus abdominis tunnel with separated perforating branches

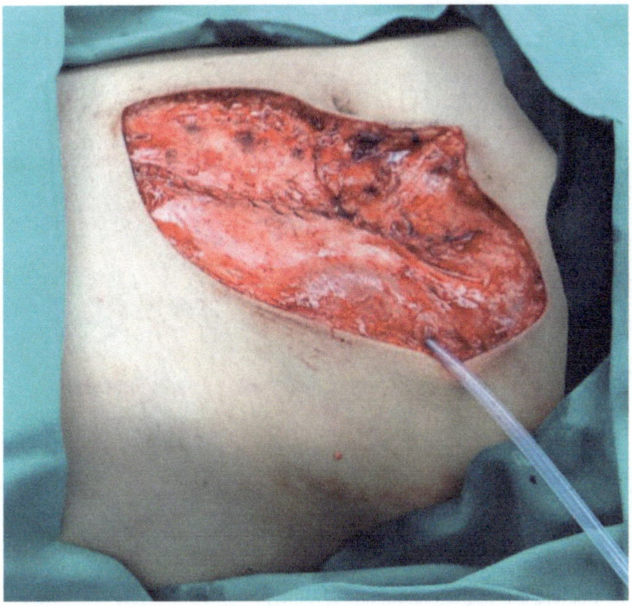

Fig. 7.34 Direct closure of anterior sheath of rectus abdominis

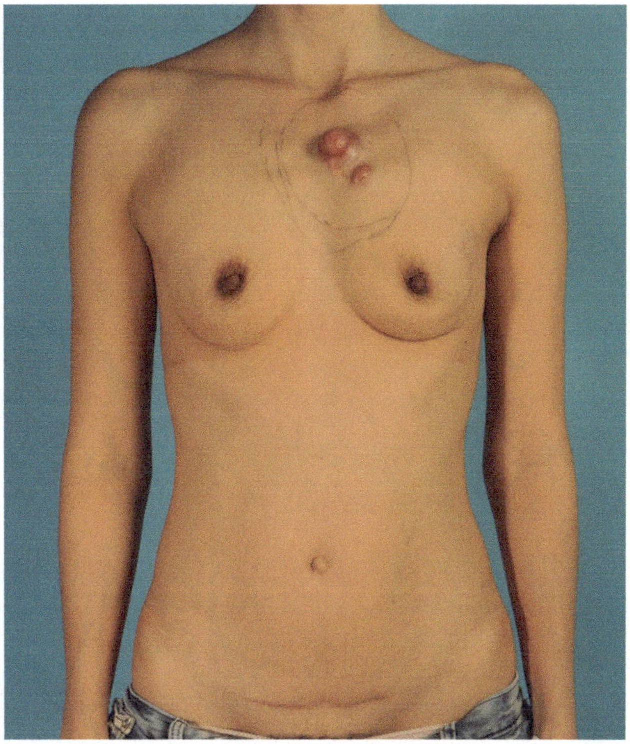

Fig. 7.35 Preoperative conditions

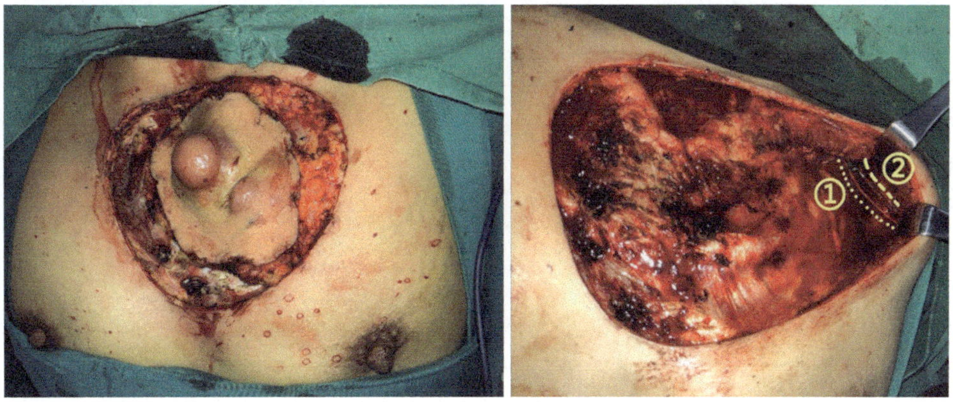

Fig. 7.36 Extended resection of chest wall mass, leaving the pectoralis major muscle branch of the left thoracoacromial vessel as the recipient vessel, preserving the integrity of the nutrient nerve of the pectoralis major muscle. (1) The muscular branch of pectoralis major of the left thoracodorsal frontal vessel; (2) Pectoralis major nutrient nerve

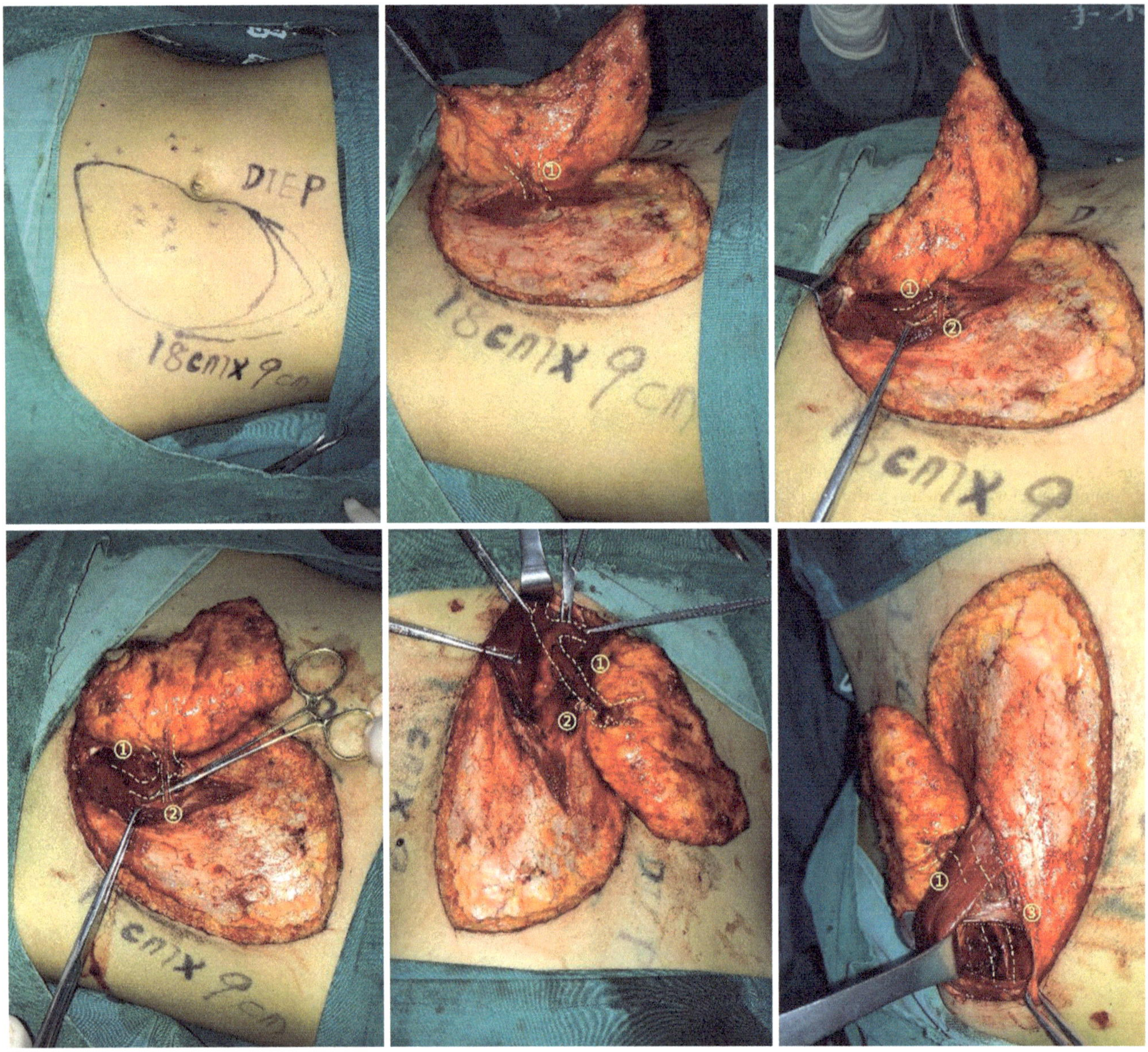

Fig. 7.37 The amount of tissue in the patient's lower abdomen was insufficient. Pinch test determined that and oblique DIEP flap was the optimal option. The perforator was found to go through the tendinous inscription and then enter the flap together with the sensory branch of intercostal nerve. Both the perforator and the sensory nerve branch were included in the flap. Retrograde separation showed that most of the pedicle ran in the medial and middle part of the muscle and hence a great length of muscle was required to be cut open for isolating the pedicle. To minimize muscular injury, dissection should be aligned with the direction of the muscle fibers and large muscular branch of the intercostal nerve should be conserved. (1) Deep inferior epigastric vascular perforator; (2) Rectus abdominus; (3) Intercostal nerve

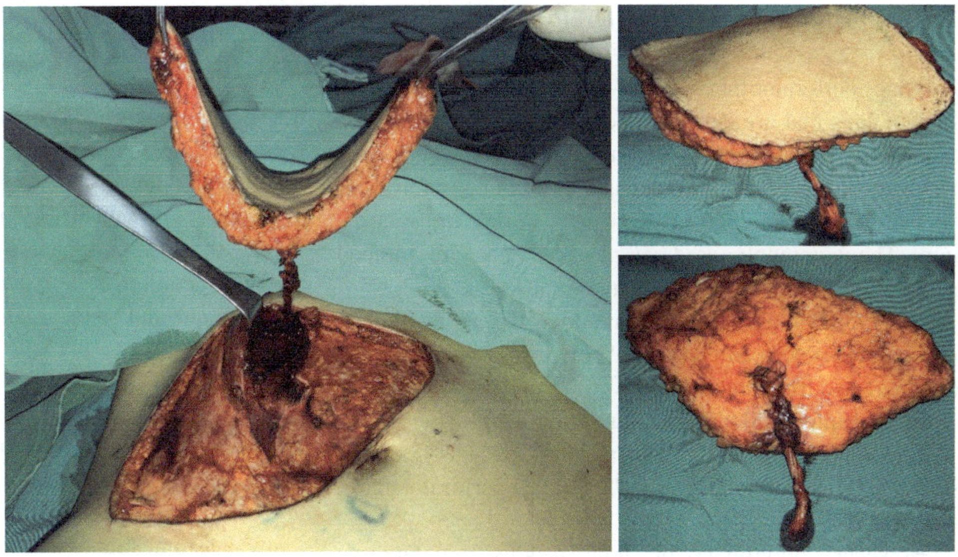

Fig. 7.38 The oblique deep inferior epigastric artery perforator flap with sensation was prepared

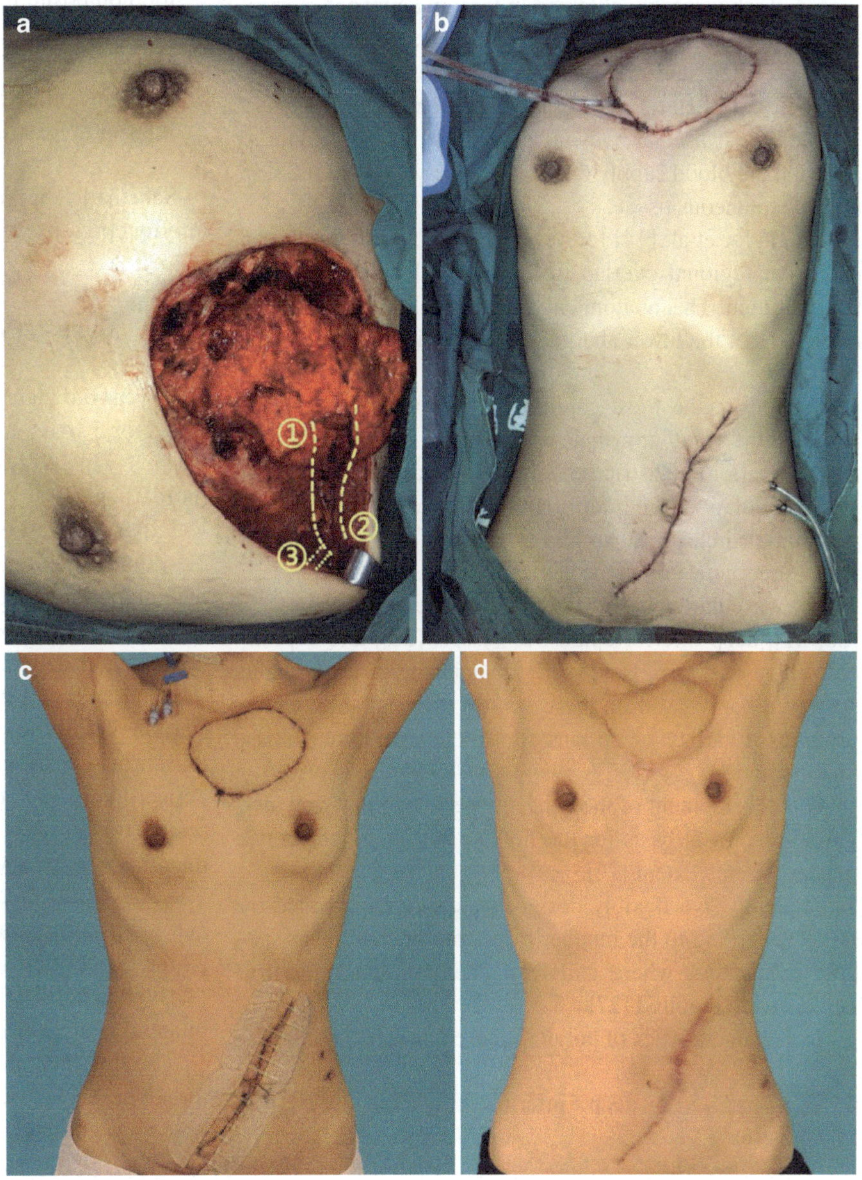

Fig. 7.39 (**a**) The left deep inferior epigastric vessels were anastomosed with the pectoralis major muscle branch of the left thoraco-acromial vessels (A: $V = 1{:}2$). The nerve included in the flap was anastomosed with the third intercostal nerve on the left chest wall to preserve the integrity of the nutritional nerve of the pectoralis major muscle. Two vacuum-assisted drainage tubes were respectively reserved in the donor and recipient areas, and the wound margin was sutured by layers. (1) Left deep inferior epigastric vessel; (2) The pectoralis major branch of the left thoraco-acromial vessel; (3) Pectoralis major nutrient nerve. (**b**) Immediate intraoperative look. (**c**) Discharge 8 days after operation. (**d**) The results were reviewed 3 months after operation

7.4 Polyflaps Based on DIEP

Polyflaps perforator flap: it refers to two or more similar perforator flaps that are cut from the same vascular body area (donor area), and the blood circulation of these perforator flaps can be reconstructed by anastomosing only one vascular pedicle (i.e., mother blood vessels) during transplantation. The commonly used surgical methods are bilobed perforator flap and trilobed perforator flap.

In 1993, Belousov et al. [7] reported the application of multiple lobes flap. At that time, "polyflaps" was used to be distinguished from "monoflaps."

Later, Hallock [8] also mentioned "polyflaps."

Now it is increasingly called "paddles," such as "Double-skin paddle perforator flap" or "2 paddles perforator flap," etc. [9–12].

However, "polyfoliate" or "multi paddle" is commonly used in Chinese when translated in to English [12], in vice versa, which is rarely expressed in foreign countries.

When reconstructing bilateral breasts, bilateral DIEP flaps are often selected, which is based on the anatomical symmetry of bilateral sides of the abdomen [13].

The term "vascular body area" was first used by Taylor to describe the blood supply range of source vessels to the skin and subcutaneous tissue.

Ian Taylor et al. [14] further confirmed that there was an extensive regional overlap in the bilateral perforasome of the abdomen. This anatomical discovery allowed the perforator flaps of the lower abdomen to be cut in different forms [15, 16].

Previously, the most commonly used vascular pedicles included the vascular pedicle of transverse rectus abdominis flap—superior epigastric vessel [17], the vascular pedicle of free DIEP flap—deep inferior epigastric vessel [18], and the vascular pedicle of superficial epigastric artery perforator flap—superficial epigastric vessel [19].

The vascular body areas of superior epigastric vessels [20, 21], deep inferior epigastric vessels [22], and superficial epigastric vessels [23–25] coincide with each other. Any free flaps based on these vessels are available, which provides a variety of options for autologous tissue breast reconstruction.

The development of the concept "perforasome" provided more anatomical basis for the flexible cutting of perforator flap to extreme extent [26].

Clinically, we flexibly designed the polyflaps based on DIEP according to the number of perforators and other specific conditions, where unilateral deep inferior epigastric vessels were required [27].

The characteristics of polyflaps based on DIEP include:

1. The trunk of deep inferior epigastric vessel is "must-have."
2. When polyflaps are used to repair wide wounds, skin grafting in the lower abdominal donor area can be avoided and the effect would be better.
3. The premise of successful transplantation of polyflaps DIEP flaps is that the two or more perforators share the same original vessel and enter the skin at a certain distance. If there is no satisfactory perforator found in clinical practice, the operation scheme and design need to be adjusted.
4. The operation is demanding in design, dissection, and technique and bears great surgical risk.

Notes:

1. When perforators are found to originate from different vessels during operation, it can be changed to combined perforator flaps to reconstruct the blood supply of the flap by anastomosing two or more groups of vessels.
2. In case of accidental injury of perforator or small perforator, composite tissue flap or chimeric perforator flap can be used.
3. It is recommended to perform CTA before operation to determine the trunk and perforating branches of deep inferior epigastric vessels.

Schematic diagram of cutting process of bilobed deep inferior epigastric artery perforator flap (Figs. 7.40 and 7.41).

7.4.1 Case 4: Polyflaps Based on DIEP

A 43-year-old male patient presented with a chest wall mass found for 5 years. Chest enhanced CT showed a sternal neoplasm which was considered myxochondrosarcoma (borderline).

Expanded resection plus chest reconstruction using 3D-printed titanium sternum and ribs, prolene mesh, greater omentum plus free DIEP flap were performed.

The mass was about 15 cm × 17 cm in size, hard, unclear boundary, closely related to muscle.

The tumor and the tissue 2 cm away from the tumor, the sternum below the sternal manubrium, the rib cartilage from the third to costal arch, the adhesive tissue in front of the pericardium, and the adhesive mediastinal pleura were removed altogether. The proximal ends of bilateral internal mammary vessels were preserved and marked with threads. The chest wall reconstruction was undertaken using mesh and 3D-printing titanium alloy bracket, which was covered by the greater omentum.

Bilobed DIEP flaps with partial rectus abdominis and bilateral pedicles were taken.

The free flap was transferred to cover the greater omentum. The deep inferior epigastric artery was anastomosed with the right internal thoracic artery, and the two accompa-

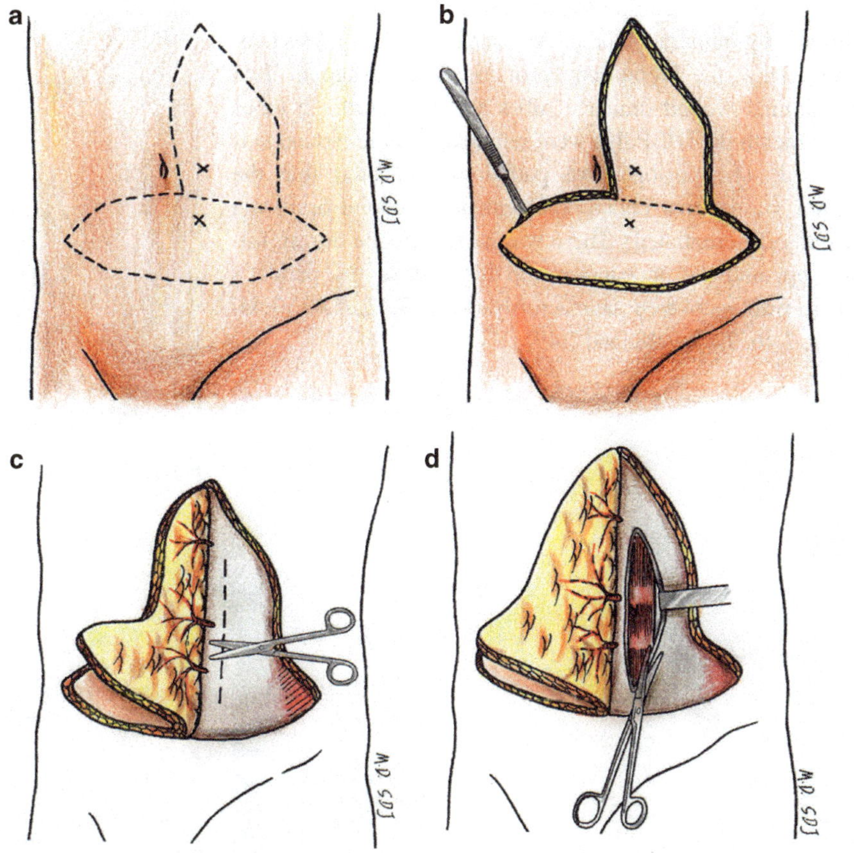

Fig. 7.40 Schematic diagram of polyflaps DIEP flap with unilateral vascular pedicle. (**a**) Flap design. (**b**) Cut the whole skin and subcutaneous tissue of the flap. (**c**) Lift the flap from outside to inside to expose the number and location of perforating vessels. (**d**) Open the anterior sheath along the outer edge of the perforating branch, and expose the rectus abdominis muscle in a long segment

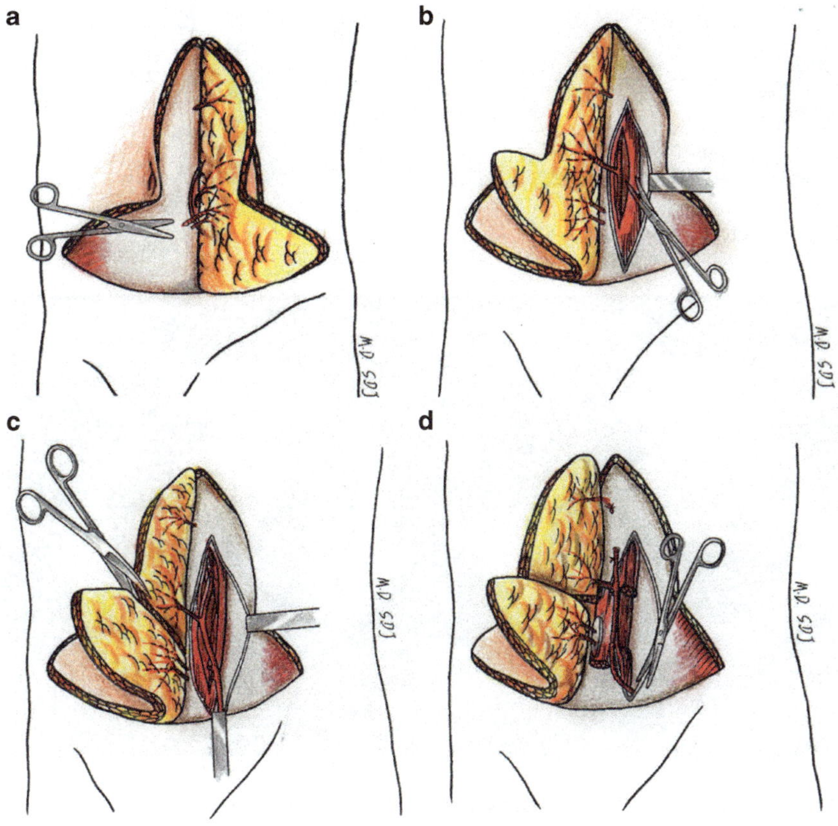

Fig. 7.41 Schematic diagram of polyflaps DIEP flap with unilateral vascular pedicle. (**a**) The flap was lifted from the opposite side till the perforator vessel was seen, and the additional perforators were retained. (**b**) A long segment of the vascular pedicle was separated inside the muscle. (**c**) The vascular pedicle was free and the flap was further cut along the design line. (**d**) The vascular pedicle was further separated retrograde and the surrounding muscle can be conserved to damage the perforator

nying veins were anastomosed with the proximal ends of the left and right internal thoracic veins, respectively. It was confirmed that the blood supply of the flap was good. Two abdominal wound drainage tubes and two drainage tubes underneath the DIEP flap were retained, and the wound was sutured. The postoperative pathology indicated that the tumor was sternal chondroma with focal chondrosarcoma (highly differentiated). There was no recurrence during follow-up, and the appearance and function of the patient's chest wall recovered satisfactorily (Figs. 7.42, 7.43, 7.44, 7.45, 7.46, 7.47, 7.48, and 7.49).

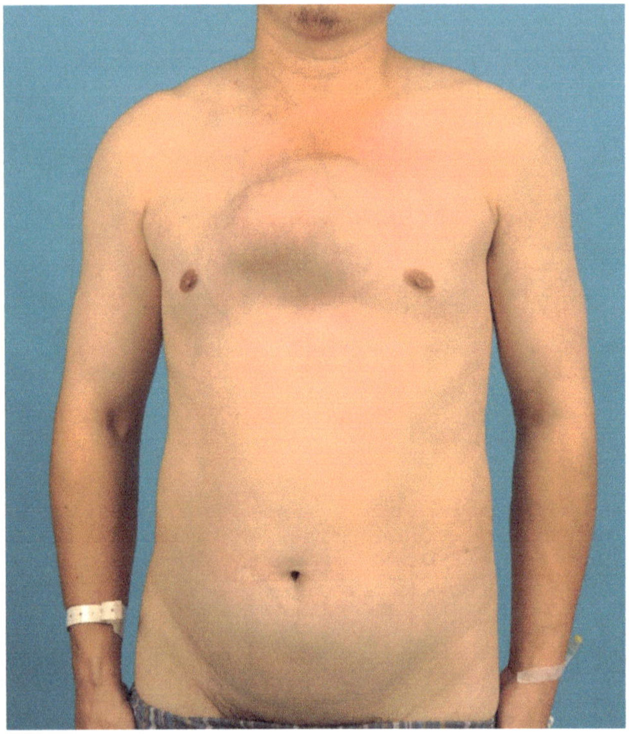

Fig. 7.42 Preoperative findings

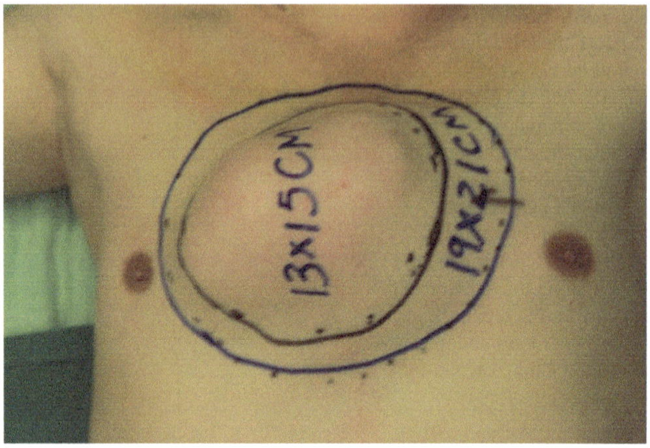

Fig. 7.44 The cutting extent decided before operation

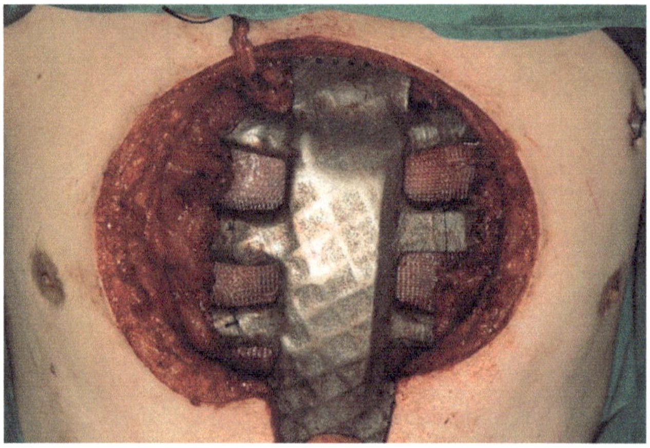

Fig. 7.45 After expanded resection, the defect was repaired with mesh covered by 3D-printed titanium alloy bracket to reconstruct the chest wall

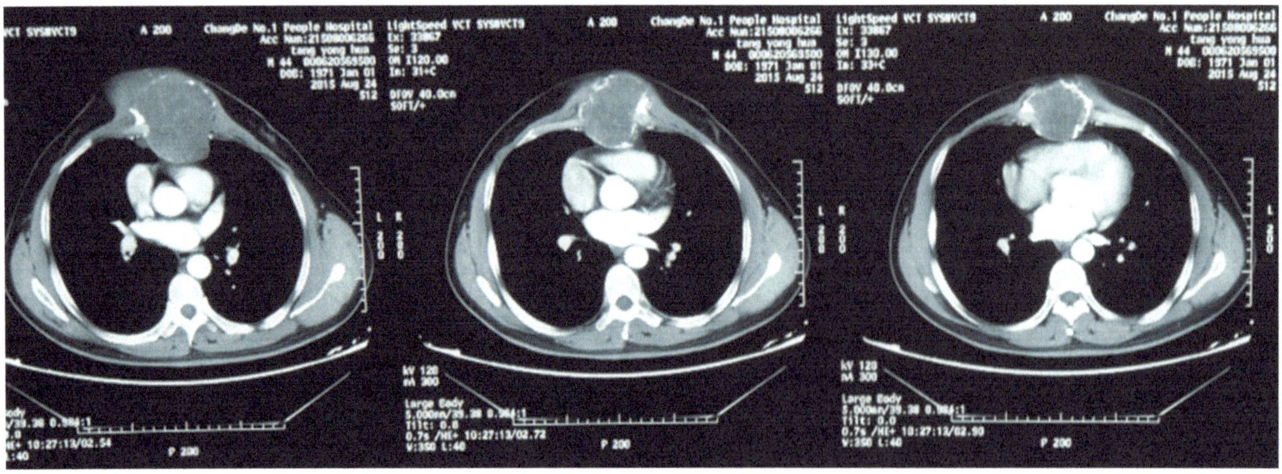

Fig. 7.43 Preoperative chest CT showed the location, size, and extent of the mass

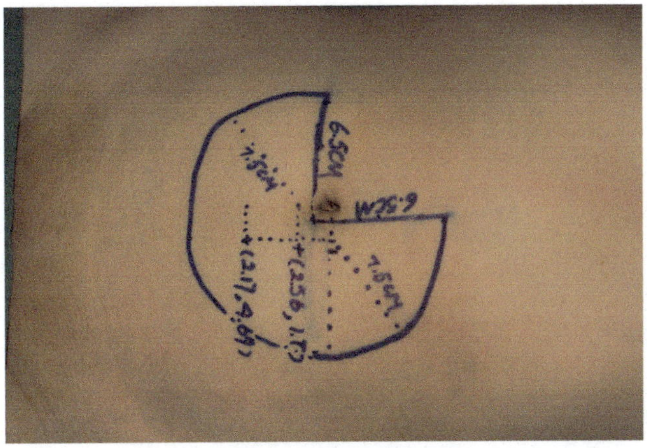

Fig. 7.46 The design of bilobed DIEP flaps

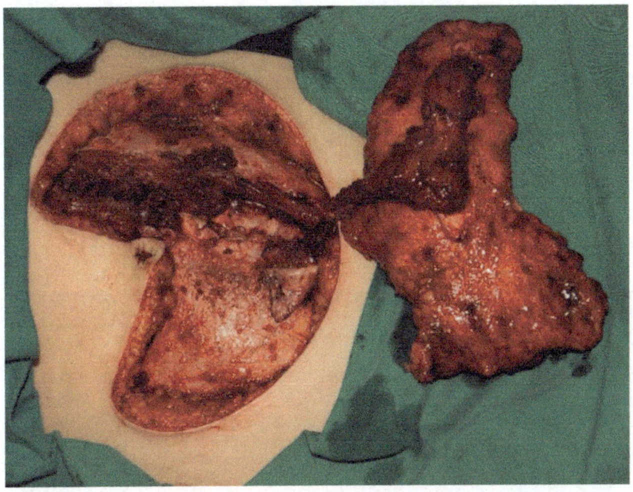

Fig. 7.47 In order to protect the vascular pedicle, part of rectus abdominis was carried on the flap

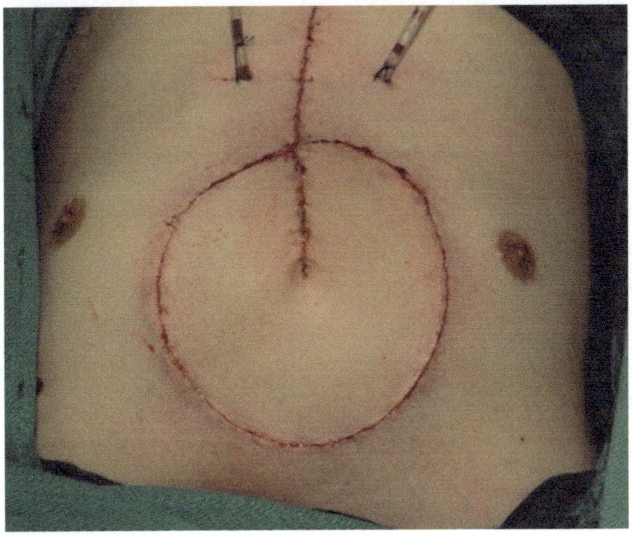

Fig. 7.48 Immediate view of intraoperative repair

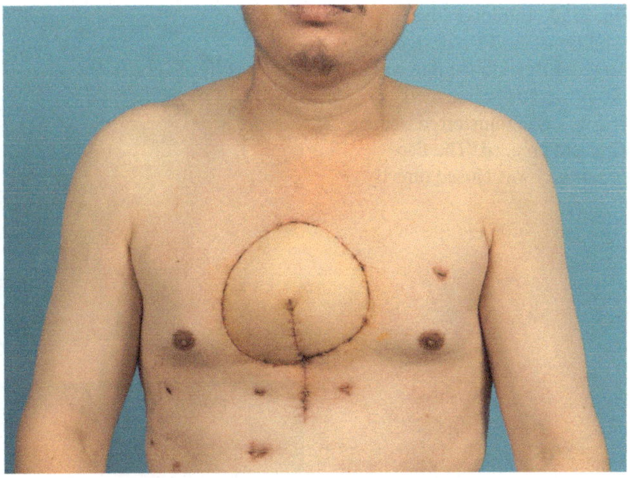

Fig. 7.49 Two-month follow-up after operation

7.4.2 Case 5: Polyflaps DIEP Flap

The patient, a 32-year-old male, was admitted to the hospital due to left hand machine strangulation and compression injury combined with multiple skin and soft tissue defects of the hand. After debridement, he underwent free transplantation of left lower abdominal lobulated DIEP flap (Fig. 7.50).

Lobed perforator flap refers to two or more similar perforator flaps that are cut from the same vascular body area (donor area), and the blood circulation of these perforator flaps can be reconstructed by anastomosing only one vascular pedicle (i.e., mother blood vessels) during transplantation. It is suitable for the repair of large and wide wounds, multiple wounds, and penetrating defects.

7.4.3 Case 6: Lobed DIEP Flap

A 4-lobe flap was microdissected thin (Figs. 7.51, 7.52, and 7.53).

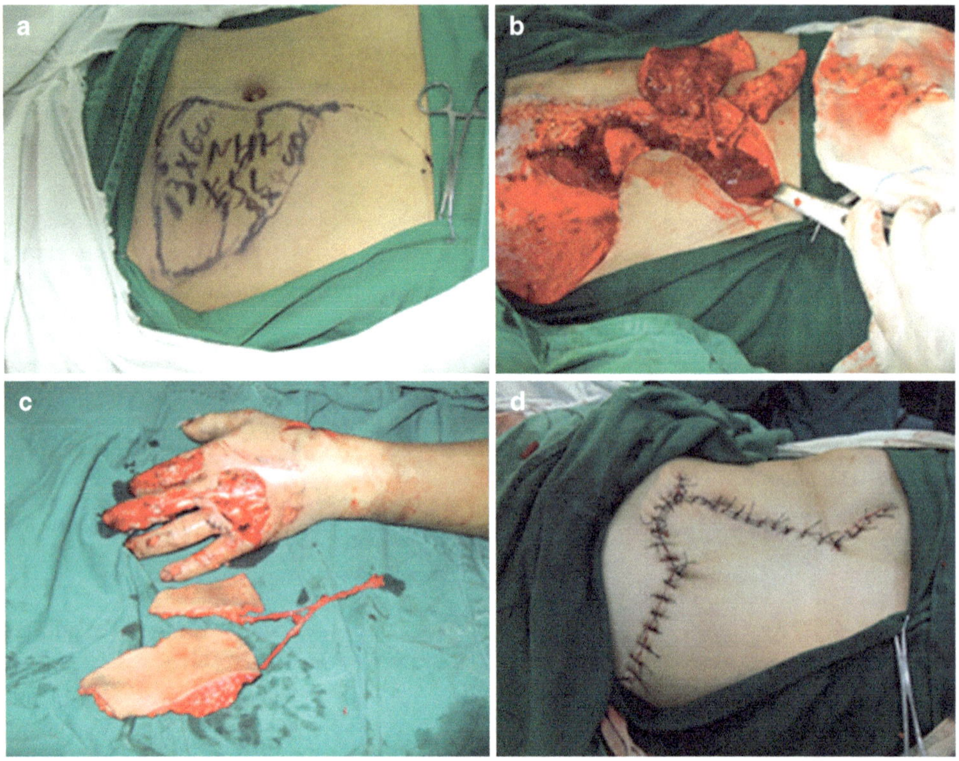

Fig. 7.50 Intraoperative conditions. (**a**) Flap design. (**b**) After the bilobed flap was cut, it was further thinned. (**c**) The flap was transferred to the recipient area. (**d**) The flap donor area was closed directly

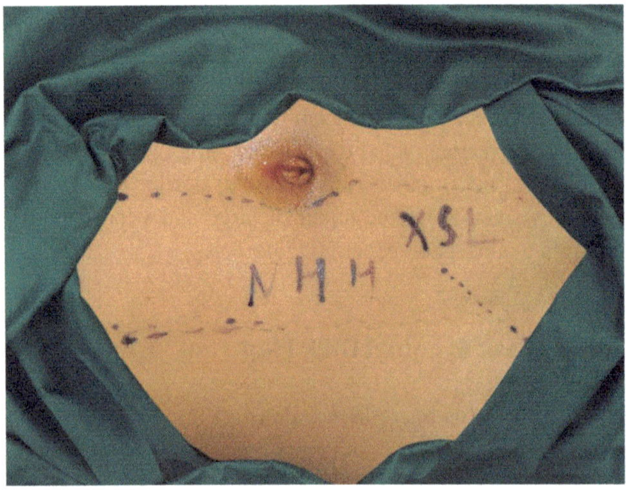

Fig. 7.51 Flap design

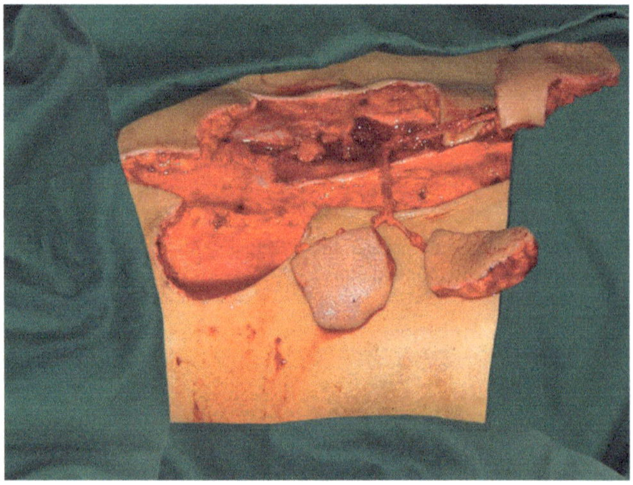

Fig. 7.52 A 4-lobe DIEP flap was harvested

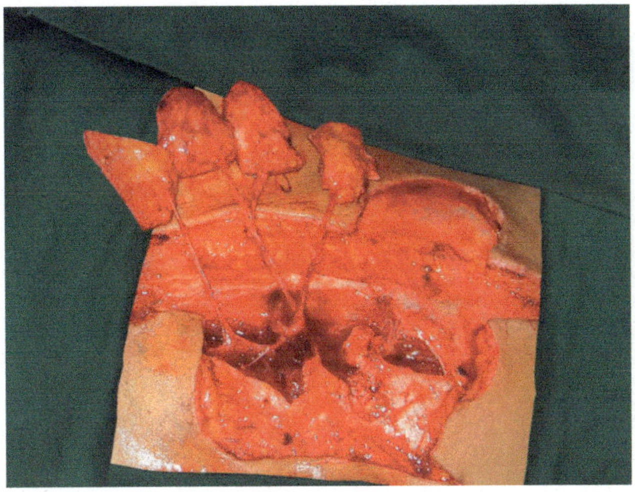

Fig. 7.53 The flap was debulked

7.5 Microsurgical Debulking of the DIEP Flap

Microdissected thin perforator flap: it refers to the perforator flap that retains the perforator vessels and their branches in the superficial fascia and the subdermal vascular network with most of the superficial fascia fat removed under the microscope (or magnifying glasses) with microsurgical instruments.

The core of this operation is to extend the dissection of the perforating branch from the intramuscular part and deep fascia to the superficial fascia layer. The flap does not carry muscle or deep fascia or most of the adipose tissue in the superficial fascia layer.

Clodius et al. [28] and Ohmori et al. [29] reported the application advantages of thin skin flap in 1973 and in 1976, respectively. However, at that time, the skin flaps selected were thin themselves, such as the dorsalis pedis flap [30].

In the early 1990s, Koshima et al. [31, 32] and Kimura et al. [33] successfully applied supermicrosurgery to thin the skin flap.

In 2002, Kimura et al. [34–38] reported consecutive successful cases of microdissected thin perforator flaps. From then on, the thin perforator flap had been widely popularized [39–45].

"Thinned flap" is prepared under the microscope by completely removing the excess fat of the flap, making the flap more beautiful and avoiding multiple operations, especially suitable for the repair of thin areas such as hands and feet [46].

The additional advantages of microdissected thin perforator flap include: (1) to reduce donor site damage; (2) to provide flexible flaps; (3) to cover a wound of large size.

Tips for preparing thin perforator flap of deep inferior epigastric artery:

1. The thinning of the flap should be completed before the pedicle is disconnected when the perforating vessels are well filled. By doing so, the perforator is not likely to be damaged during dissection and thorough hemostasis can be achieved to avoid the occurrence of postoperative hematoma and vascular crisis.
2. The thinning of the flap can be performed from the periphery of the flap toward where the perforator enters the flap or vice versa.
3. To prepare a flap with sensory nerve for sensory reconstruction, the abundant anastomosis between perforator vessels and sensory branches of intercostal nerve needs to be preserved, and the thinning extent in this area should be conservative.
4. The thinning around the place where the perforator penetrates the flap should be cautious and inclined outward. The thinning extent depends on the branching of perforator vessels while the integrity of subdermal vascular network must be preserved.

7.5.1 Case 7: Microdissected Thin DIEP Flap with Multiple Perforators

The patient was a 32-year-old male with crush injury of the right foot. After debridement, the right DIEP flap containing multiple perforators was used for repair. After immediate thinning, it was transplanted to repair the wound of the right foot. The flap survived smoothly, the foot was not swelling, and the appearance and function recovered satisfactorily (Figs. 7.54, 7.55, 7.56, 7.57, and 7.58).

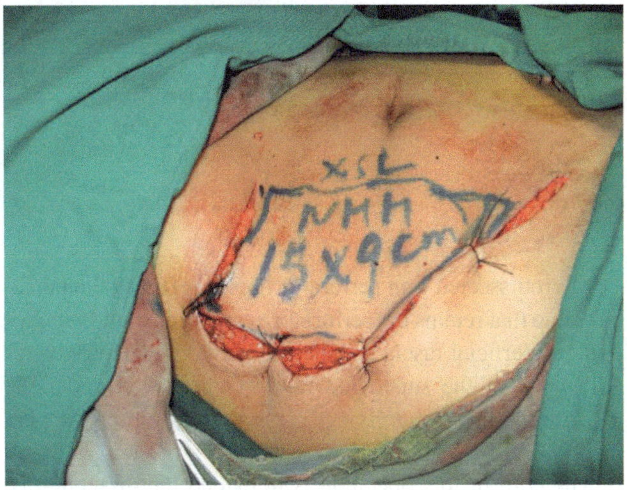

Fig. 7.54 Flap design

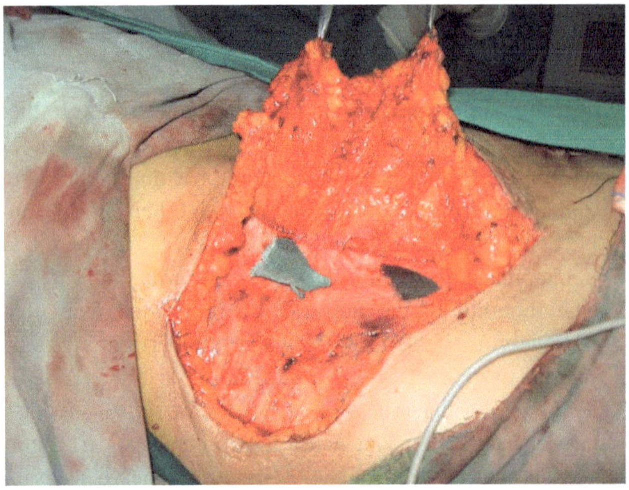

Fig. 7.55 Exposure of perforating vessels

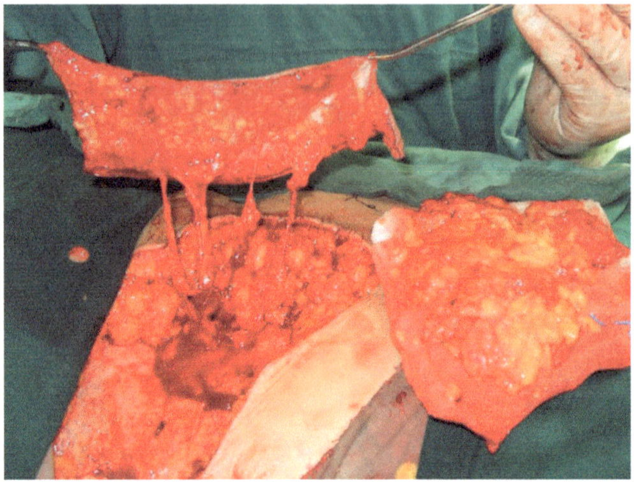

Fig. 7.56 The flap was pedicled with multiple perforating branches and further thinned

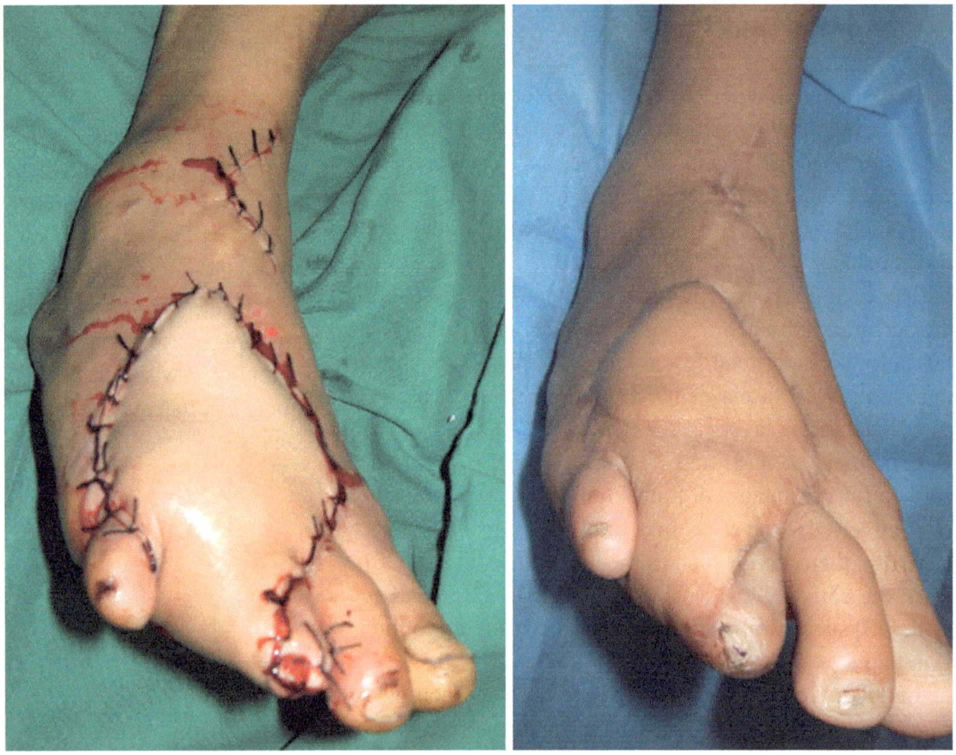

Fig. 7.57 The foot wound was covered with a thinned flap. The postoperative follow-up showed that the flap was not bulky

Microdissected thin perforator flap: it refers to the perforator flap that retains the perforator vessels and their branches in the superficial fascia and the subdermal vascular network with most of the superficial fascia fat removed under the microscope (or magnifying glasses) with microsurgical instruments.

The core of this operation is to extend the dissection of the perforating branch from the intramuscular part and deep fascia to the superficial fascia layer. The flap does not carry muscle or deep fascia or most of the adipose tissue in the superficial fascia layer.

Subdermal vascular plexus flap, also known as "super thin flap," is formed by removing most of the subcutaneous fat of traditional free-styled or axial flaps with just a thin layer of fat underneath the dermal vascular network reserved. This flap derived from the free skin with subdermal vascular plexus and was first introduced by Chinese doctor Situ Pu in 1986.

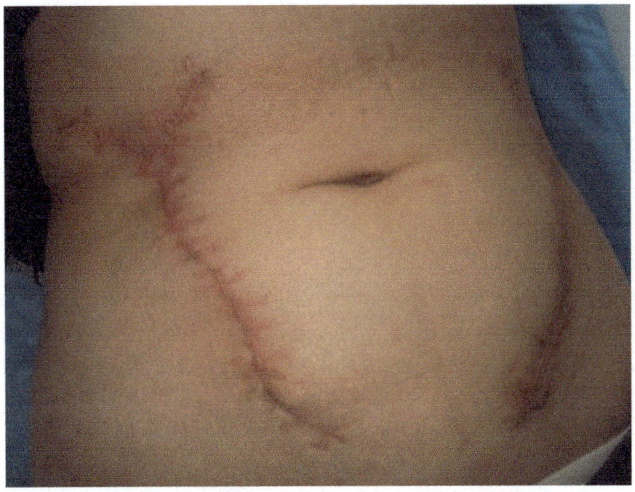

Fig. 7.58 Only linear scar was left in the donor area

7.5.1.1 Super-Thin Perforator Flap

It pertains to the skin flap with subdermal vascular plexus supplied by perforating vessels. It was first reported by Japanese doctor Koshima in 1992. It is mainly used for the repair of facial and hand wounds to meet the needs of its thin shape and function.

7.6 De-epithelized DIEP Flap

The de-epithelized DIEP flap is often used for immediate breast reconstruction after skin sparing modified radical mastectomy and to reconstruct the plump shape of the breast [47, 48].

The know-how of de-epithelization is easy, however, special attention should be paid to complete hemostasis to avoid hematoma formation [49].

7.6.1 Case 8: De-epithelized DIEP Flap

The patient was a 41-year-old female. She complained of a left breast mass found more than 2 months ago. Left breast invasive carcinoma was confirmed on biopsy. After admission, NSM and breast reconstruction with a free DIEP flap were performed.

The right deep inferior epigastric artery and one accompanying vein were end-to-end anastomosed with the left lateral thoracic artery and vein, and the other accompanying vein was end-to-end anastomosed with another lateral thoracic vein with a vascular coupler (1A2V).

Postoperative pathological examination report was as follows: (1) (left breast) Invasive ductal carcinoma, histological grade II–III, containing high-grade intraductal carcinoma, LVI tested positive, and the mass was about 3 cm × 3 cm × 2 cm in size; (2) No cancer metastasis was found in left axillary lymph node 0/13; (3) No cancer invasion was found in the nipple, areola complex, skin, and basal margin; (4) Intraductal carcinoma: ER (−) PR (−) CerbB-2 (3 +) Ki-67 60%; invasive carcinoma: ER (−) PR (−) CerbB-2 (3 +) Ki-67 60%.

TNM staging: pT2N0M0 IIA. The patients were treated with adjuvant chemotherapy combined with targeted therapy (Figs. 7.59, 7.60, 7.61, 7.62, 7.63, 7.64, 7.65, 7.66, 7.67, 7.68, 7.69, 7.70, and 7.71).

The appearance and function of reconstructed breast were satisfactory.

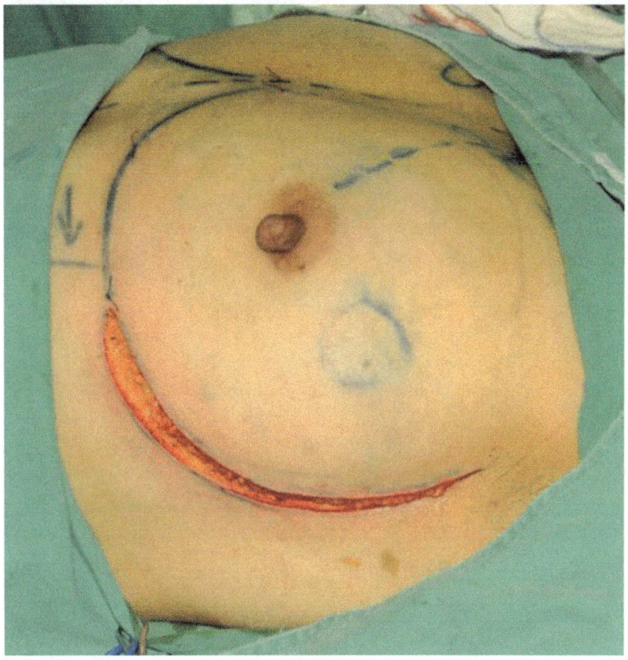

Fig. 7.59 Incision design and proposed resection range

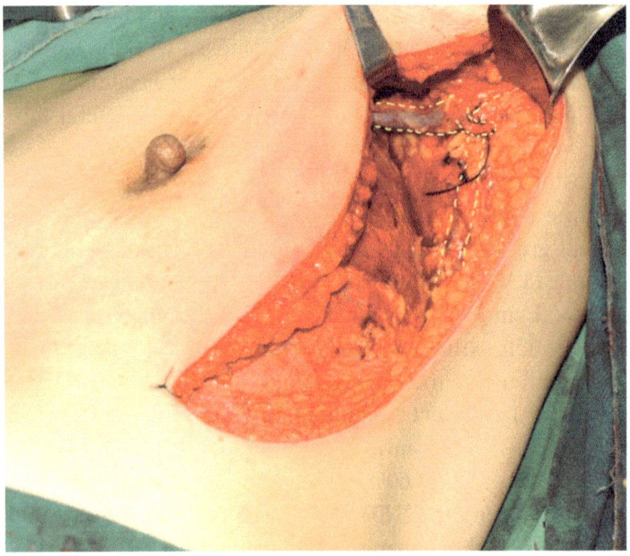

Fig. 7.60 The lateral thoracic vessels in the receiving area were prepared

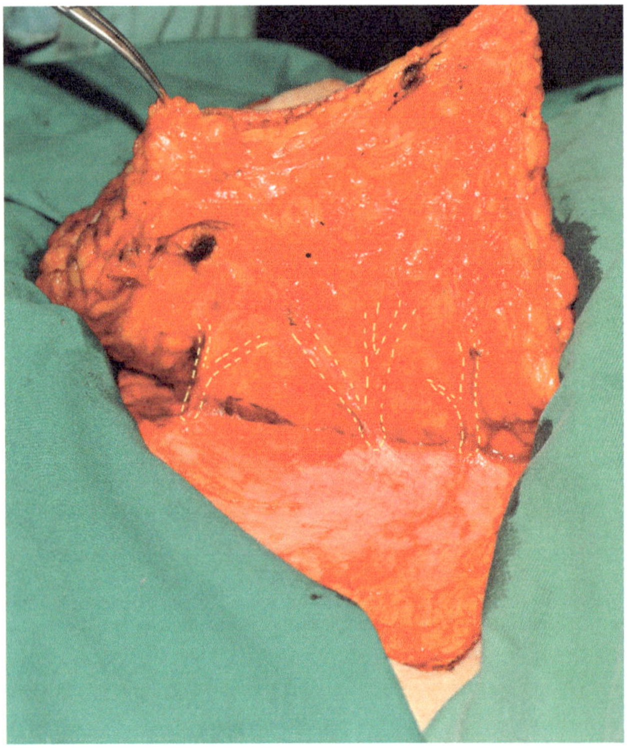

Fig. 7.61 The flap was lifted to expose the perforating vessels of the right lower abdomen

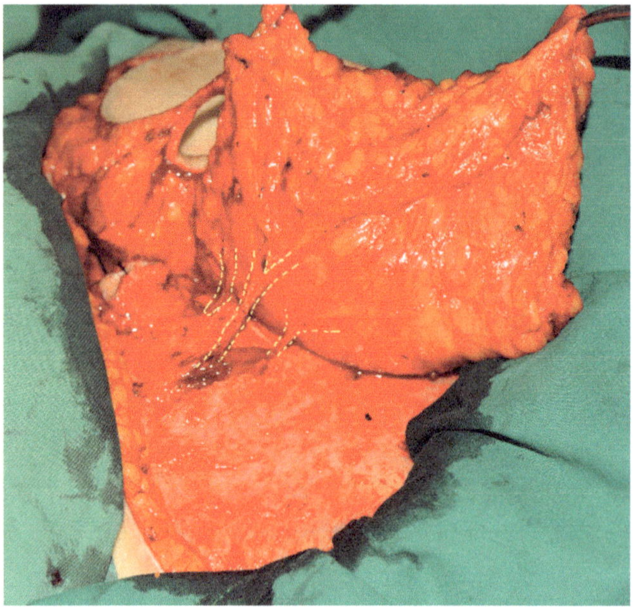

Fig. 7.62 The anterior sheath was cut open to expose the underlying right perforator

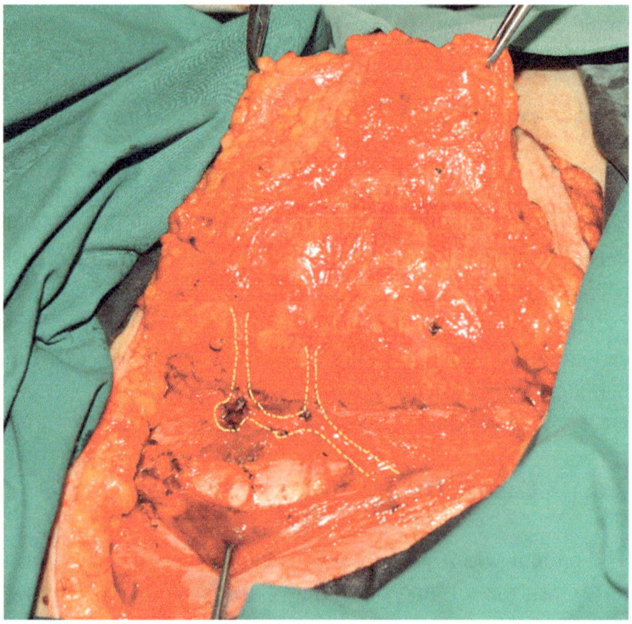

Fig. 7.63 Separation of right perforator vessel and main pedicle in rectus abdominis muscle

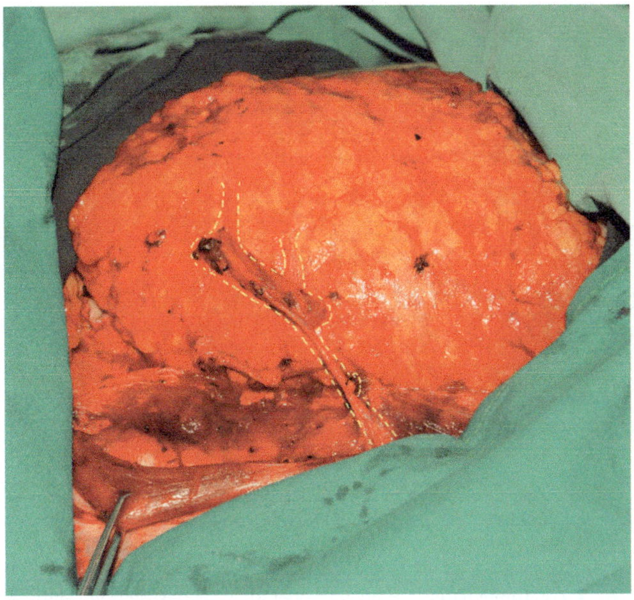

Fig. 7.64 The integrity of rectus abdominis and intercostal nerve was preserved

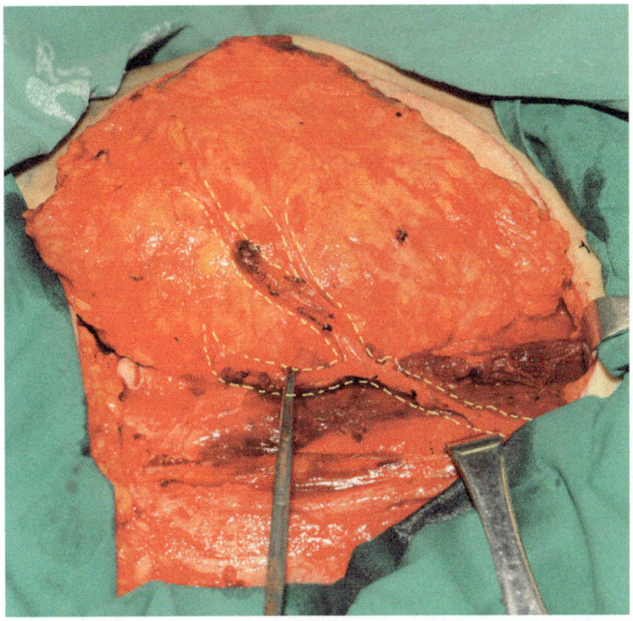

Fig. 7.65 The perforating branch and vascular pedicle of the right deep inferior epigastric vessel are unveiled

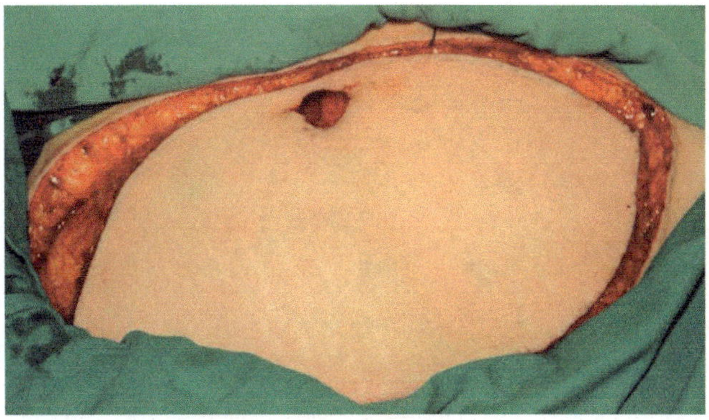

Fig. 7.66 The flap was prepared

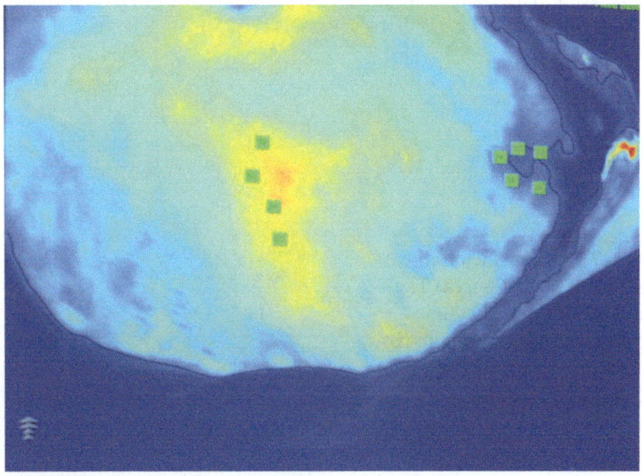

Fig. 7.67 ICG (indocyanine green) angiogram showed that the blood supply of the flap was good

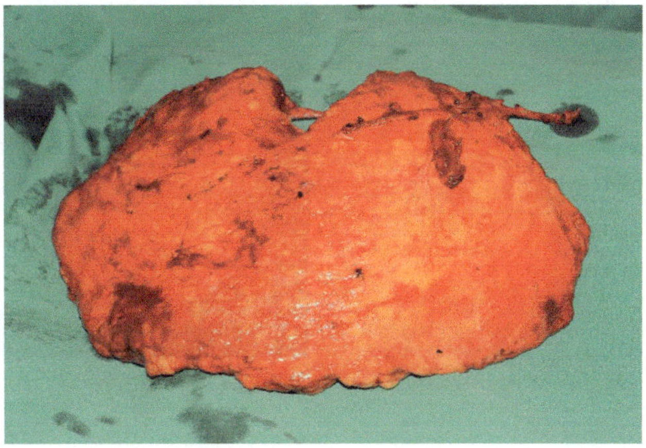

Fig. 7.68 De-epithelization was performed over the whole skin flap

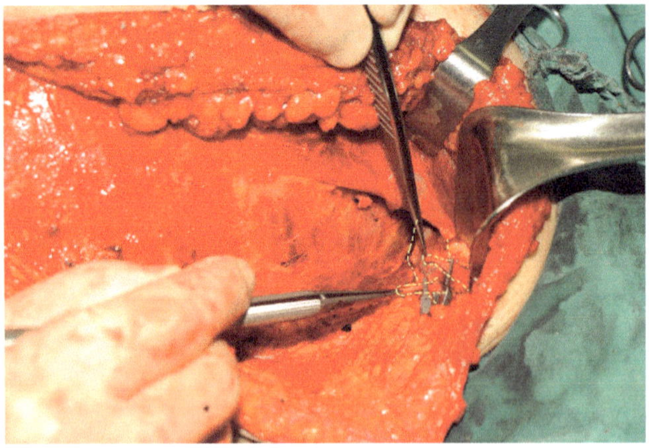

Fig. 7.69 The right deep inferior epigastric vessels were anastomosized with the left lateral thoracic vessels (1A2V)

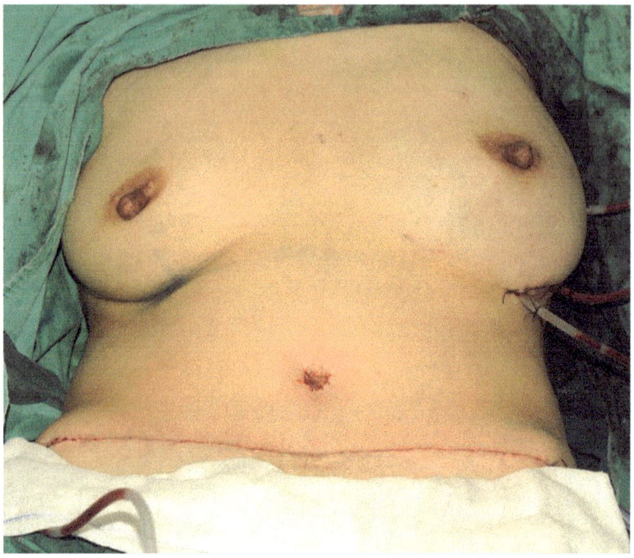

Fig. 7.70 Immediately after intraoperative reconstruction, only a small skin island was reserved as the observation window

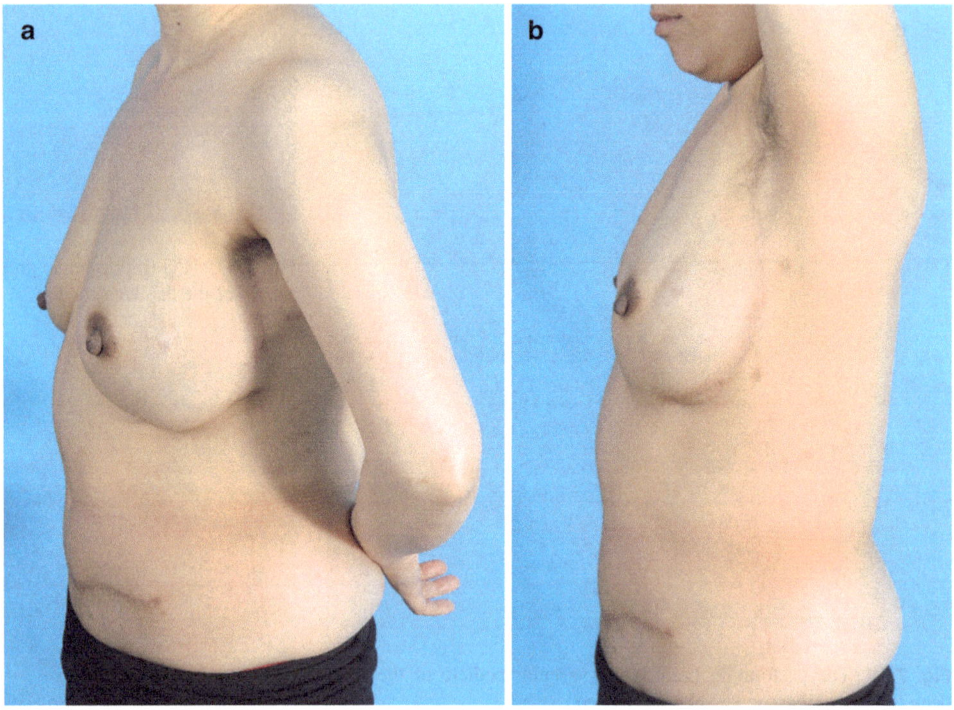

Fig. 7.71 Satisfactory breast shape and function. (**a**) The appearance at follow-up 5 months after operation. (**b**) Function was at follow-up 5 months after operation

7.7 Chimeric DIEP Flap

Chimeric perforator flap: it refers to two or more independent tissue flaps of different types (such as skin flaps, fascia flaps, muscle flaps, bone flaps, etc.) harvested from the same vascular body area (donor area). These independent tissue flaps contain at least one perforator flap, and the nutrient vessels originate from the same primary source vessels which are used for anastomosis to provide blood supply to the independent flaps.

Chimerism includes skin flap and muscle flap [50, 51], skin flap and bone flap [46, 52, 53], skin flap and fascia flap [10], skin flap plus muscle flap plus bone flap, and other forms.

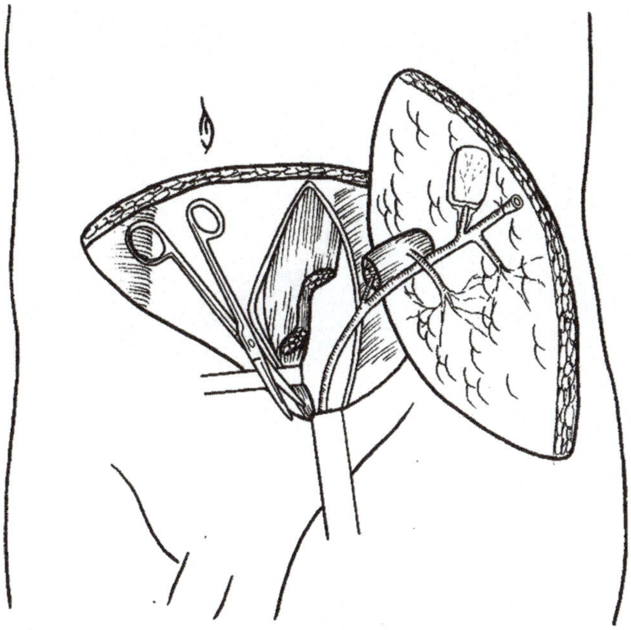

Fig. 7.72 Schematic diagram of chimeric DIEP flap

In 1993, Koshima et al. [54] reported about the chimeric perforator flap. This flap shares the common upsides with the musculocutaneous flap and the osteocutaneous flap in terms of good blood supply and strong resistance to infection, realizing three-dimensional repair of wound (Fig. 7.72) [55].

The advantages of the chimeric perforator flap include:

1. The defect can be repaired in one stage.
2. To accord with the principle of supplying the shortage and avoid bulking.
3. To avoid unnecessary waste of tissue on donor site.
4. High flap mobility and flexible repair.
5. It can repair the defects of different tissues in different areas.
6. Reliable blood supply.
7. It can avoid poor blood supply and even necrosis of tissue flap caused by compression.

Existing problems and precautions:

1. The design and cutting of chimeric perforator flap need to be imagined in three-dimension and are technically demanding.
2. When fixing the chimeric flap, we must pay attention to protect the perforating vessels to avoid accidental injury.

A chimeric flap consisting of a DIEP skin flap and rectus abdominis muscle flap bearing a vascular pedicle can be used to repair the skin and soft tissue defect with the skin flap and to fill the deep cavity with the muscle flap [56].

A DIEP flap featured by thick subcutaneous tissue is suitable to fill large and deep defect, flap thinning is generally not necessary. The postoperative appearance of the donor site in patients receiving DIEP flap is much better than in those undergoing TRAM flap transfer. Nonetheless, the donor site damage aggravates as the amount of muscle harvested increases. When there are other better choices for harvesting a chimeric myocutaneous flap, it is better not to first consider the lower abdomen as the donor area.

7.7.1 Case 9: Chimeric DIEP Flap with Muscle Flap (Figs. 7.73, 7.74, 7.75, 7.76, and 7.77)

Composite tissue flap: it refers to a living tissue flap with multiple tissue structures and its own blood circulation system. From the perspective of blood supply, it can be divided into two categories: simple composite flap supported by single vascular pedicle and combined flap supported by multiple vascular pedicles.

Composite skin flap: it refers to a flap containing a variety of different tissue structures supported by a single vascular pedicle. These tissue structures are dependent on each other and inseparable. Composite skin flap with single pedicle, such as musculocutaneous flap, teno-cutaneous flap, and osteocutaneous flap, which are used to fill large defects or to repair multiple tissue defects. In clinical practice, the composite skin flap often refers to the skin flap containing bone tissue, such as fibular skin flap, iliac skin flap, scapular skin flap, and so on.

Musculocutaneous flap: it refers to a composite tissue flap containing layers of skin, superficial fascia, deep fascia, and muscle tissue. It contains a complete arterial and venous system. The viability of the skin depends on the muscle, and the

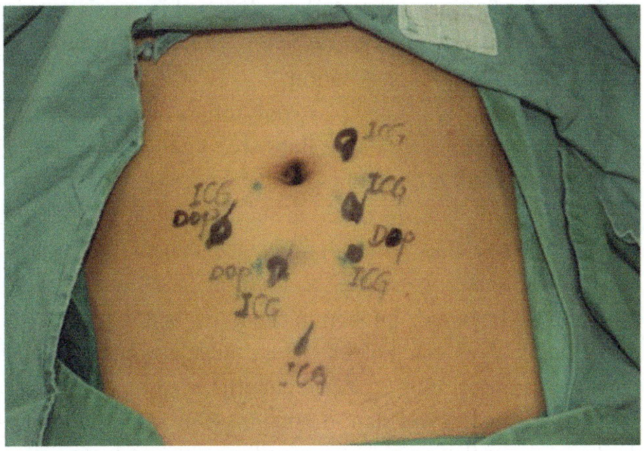

Fig. 7.73 Location of perforator by CTA before operation

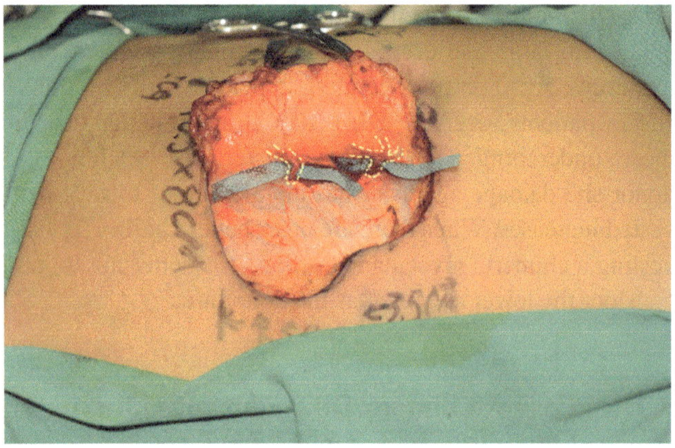

Fig. 7.74 Exposure of perforating vessels

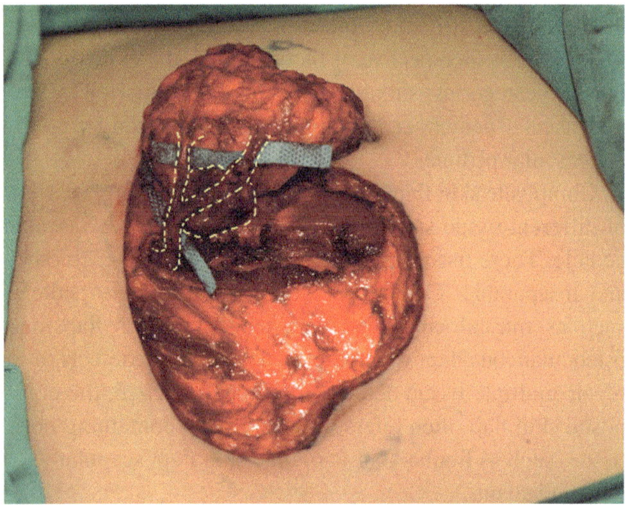

Fig. 7.75 Simultaneous removal of skin flap and muscle flap

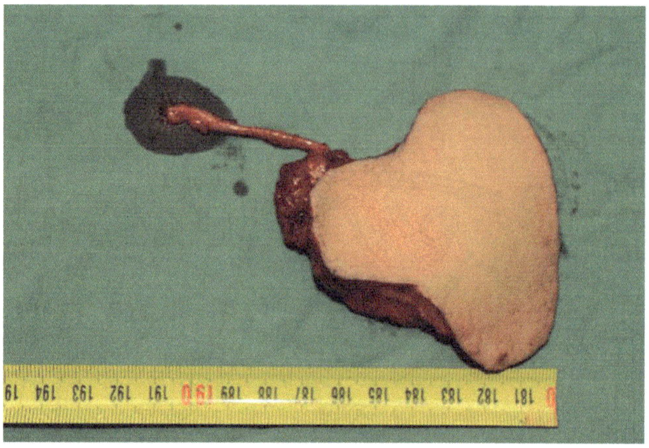

Fig. 7.76 Dorsal view of flap

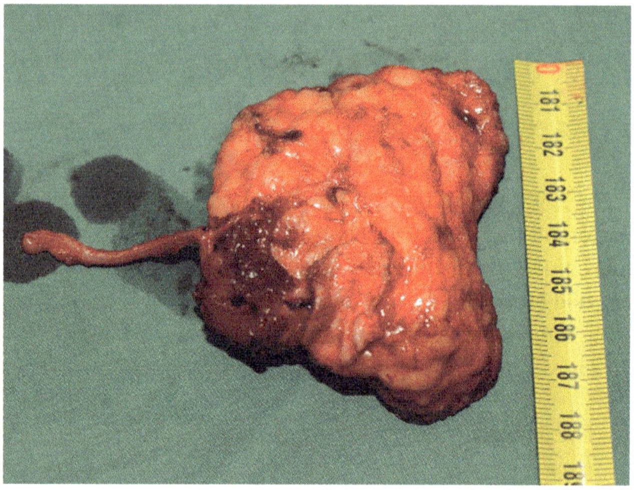

Fig. 7.77 Ventral view of flap

muscle in the deep layer must be included in the flap. This flap is large and can be used to fill deep tissue defects; it has strong anti-infection ability and can be used to repair osteomyelitis wounds; if innervation is preserved, it can be used for motor function reconstruction.

Chimeric flap: also known as "polyfoliate flap," it consists of multiple independent tissue flaps sharing the same vascular body area and a common "mother" pedicle. These flaps are independent in terms of blood supply, indicating that the viability of one flap does not influence that of the others. Flaps of the same types (such as multiple skin flaps or multiple muscle flaps, i.e., bilobed flap and trilobed flap) or flaps of different types (such as skin flap, muscle flap, and bone flap) constitute various chimeric patterns.

Chimeric perforator flap: it contains a group of independent perforator flaps which are raised from the same vascular body area and share a common major vascular pedicle. The application of a chimeric perforator flap is suitable when the blood supply of muscle comes from a main blood vessel pedicle (Mathes Types I, II, V). It is necessary to confirm that these perforators originate from the same "mother" pedicle of muscle, if not, extra vascular anastomosis is required.

Compared with the traditional composite tissue flap and combined flap, the chimeric perforator flap has great advantages.

Chimeric perforator flap refers to two or more independent tissue flaps of different types (skin, fascia, tendon, muscle, bone, etc.) cut in the same vascular unit. These independent tissue flaps contain at least one perforator flap, and the nutrient vessels originate from the same primary source vessels that are used for anastomosis to distribute blood among the tissue flaps.

Illustrations of transplantation of a chimeric flap including a DIEP flap, a rectus sheath fascia flap, and a rectus abdominis muscle flap (Figs. 7.78, 7.79, and 7.80).

No matter what form of DIEP flap is used, key details always need to be followed:

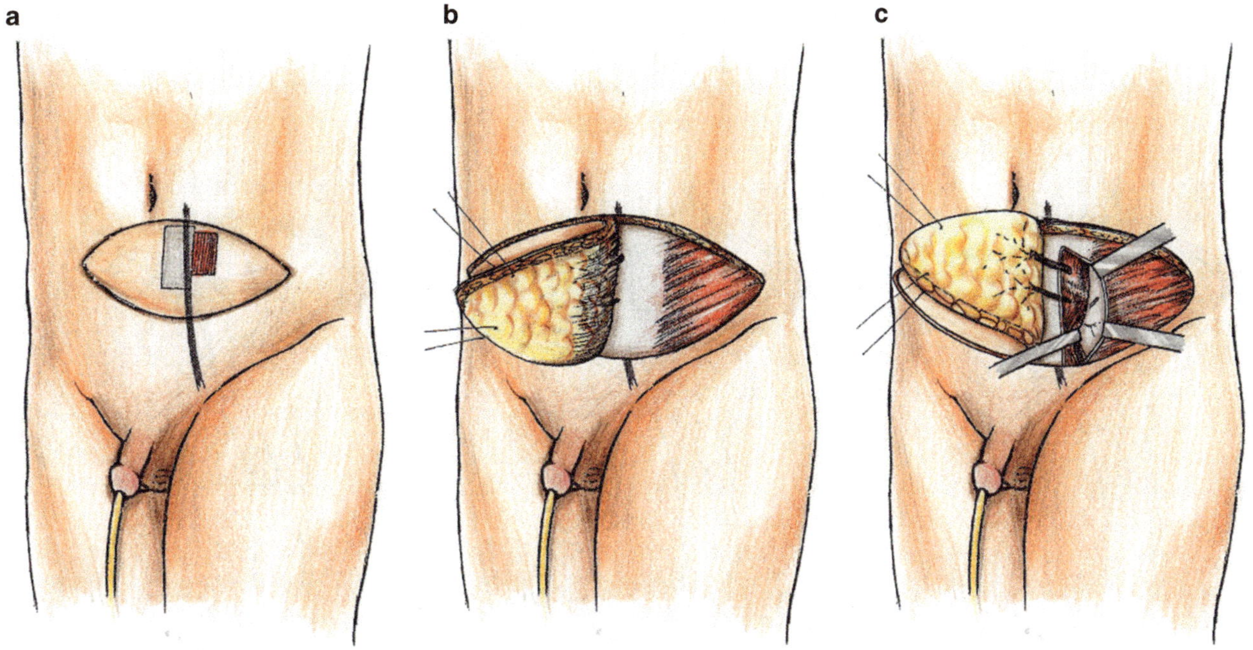

Fig. 7.78 Schematic diagrams of raising a chimeric flap including a DIEP flap, a rectus sheath fascia flap, and a rectus abdominis muscle flap. (**a**) Flap design. The skin and subcutaneous tissue was cut open along the annular lining. (**b**) The flap was lifted from the outside to the inside on the aponeurosis surface of the external oblique muscle to expose a perforator at the umbilical level and a perforator below the umbilicus. The anterior sheath lateral to the perforators was opened longitudinally using a scalpel or scissors. (**c**) The rectus abdominis muscle was pulled medially to expose the entire motor branch of intercostal nerve and a major accompanying nutrient vessel. The trunk of deep inferior epigastric vessel was found caudally

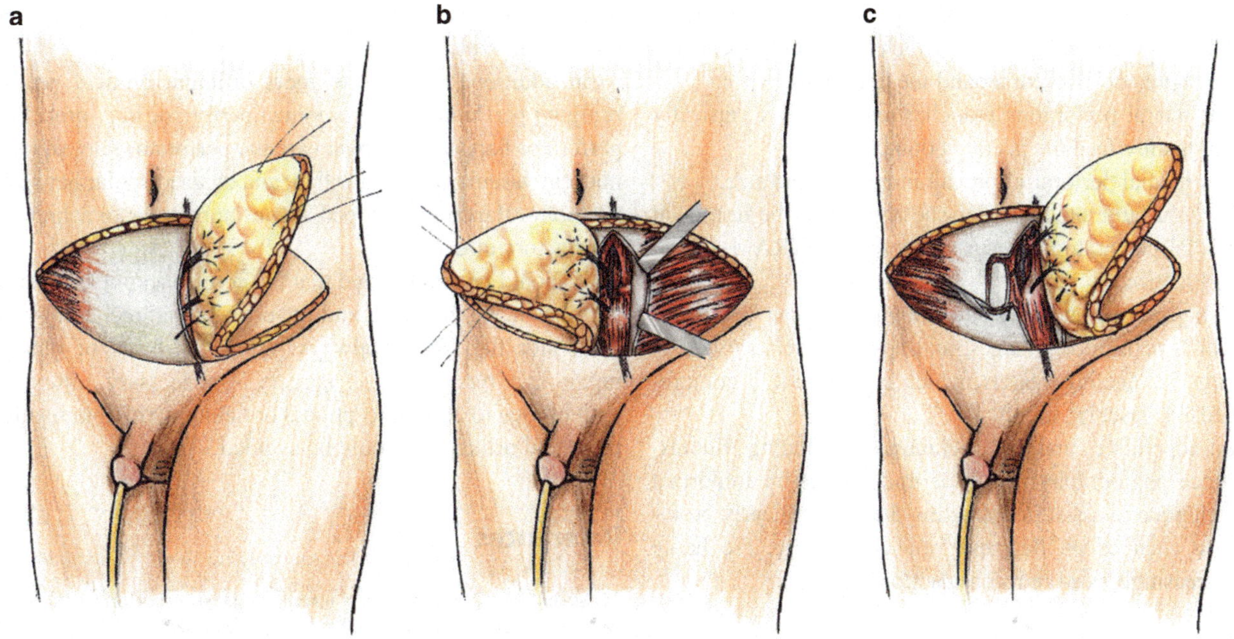

Fig. 7.79 Schematic diagrams of raising a chimeric flap including a DIEP flap, a rectus sheath fascia flap, and a rectus abdominis muscle flap. (**a**) The flap was raised from inside to outside till the perforators were revealed. Another small perforator below the umbilicus was found and ligated. (**b**) The anterior sheath between the perforator and the incision was cut horizontally. A fascia branch proximal to the upper perforator was found underlying the anterior sheath and preserved. That upper perforator was separated retrograde inside the muscle toward the branching level deep to the muscle. The lower perforator was small yet completely isolated. (**c**) The fascia flap based on the anterior sheath branch of the upper perforator was used

a b c

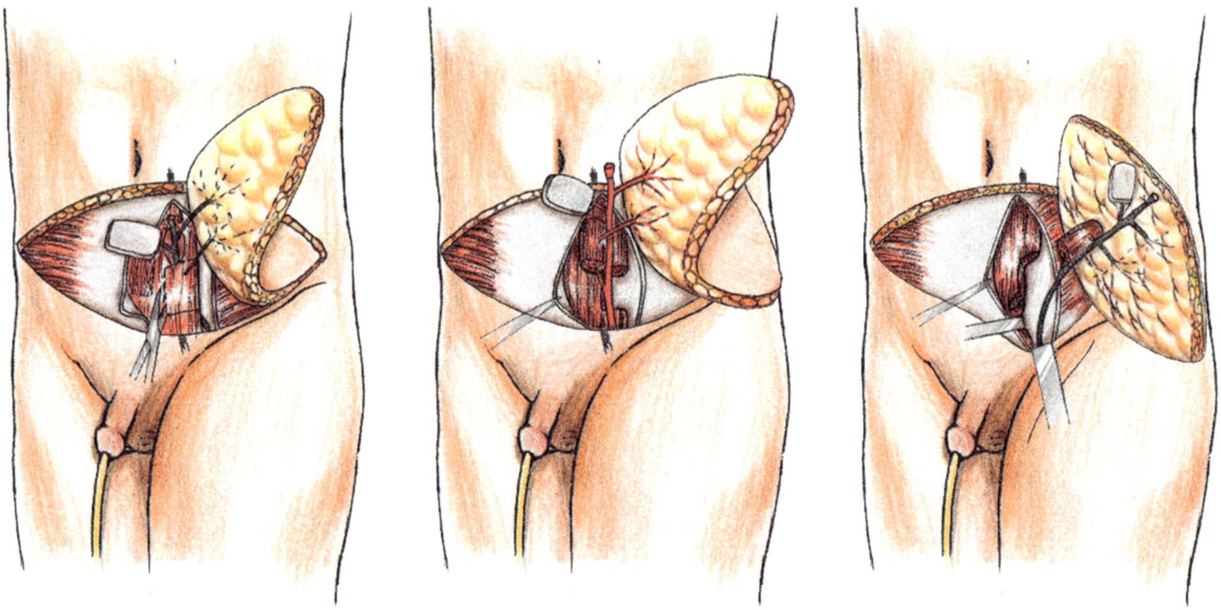

Fig. 7.80 Schematic diagrams of raising a chimeric flap including a DIEP flap, a rectus sheath fascia flap, and a rectus abdominis muscle flap. (**a**) The rectus abdominis muscle flap was pedicled with the lower perforator. The muscle flap was split along the medial design line. The entire deep inferior epigastric vessel was separated anterograde and the bifurcating level of the lower perforator was exposed. The lower perforator was small and intramuscular separation was not performed. (**b**) The deep inferior epigastric vessel was ligated at the proximal end distanced from the upper perforator, here, the chimeric flap was connected to the donor area by the distal vascular pedicle alone. (**c**) The blood supply of the flap was examined good. High ligation of the deep inferior epigastric vessel was not performed until the pedicle was dissected retrograde to a sufficient length

1. The feeding vessel of DIEP flap should be the largest dominant perforating vessel, which is generally located at the "hot spot" 3–5 cm around the umbilicus.
2. The lateral perforating branches tend to travel vertically and mainly feed the lateral abdomen.
3. The medial perforators prevail in number and size.
4. When a large amount of tissue is needed, the dominant medial perforators or muscle preserving TRAM should be preferred.
5. Using preoperative CTA technology, we can determine which perforator is largest and how it travels as well as large connecting vessels, which can provide a comprehensive vascular supply.
6. Intraoperative imaging techniques, including fluorescence angiography and laser imaging, as an important technique to assist in evaluating the effect of early perfusion changes on flap and venous drainage, are being increasingly used in reconstruction surgery.

With the continuous development of the concept and technique of perforator flap, the form of perforator flap is becoming more and more abundant, and its scope of application is also expanding. The perforator flap can be thinner and larger, and can repair various complex defects. The sensory function of the flap and various tissue structures can be reconstructed and the damage to the donor area minimized.

In addition, in order to meet different clinical needs, bridging perforator flap, conjoined perforator flap, propeller perforator flap, neurotrophic vascular perforator flap, venous nutrient vascular perforator flap, and chain vascular network perforator flap are developed accordingly, so as to achieve a satisfactory effect.

It should be emphasized that the core concept of flap surgery has never changed, and the concept and technology of perforator flap should always follow the basis of plastic repair and reconstruction surgery. Unnecessary injury to patients due to being exceptional or flaunting or violating the treatment principles should be avoided.

References

1. Allen RJ, Treece P. Deep inferior epigastric perforator flap for breast reconstruction. Ann Plast Surg. 1994;32(1):32–8.
2. Xiao Zhou, Dajiang Song, Zan Li. The development of perforator flap and its application in oncoplastic surgery. Chin J Aesthet Plast Surg2017. 28(2): 69–72.
3. Pont LP, Marcelli S, Robustillo M, et al. Immediate breast reconstruction with abdominal free flap and adjuvant radiotherapy, evaluation of quality of life and outcomes. Plast Reconstr Surg. 2017;140:681.

4. Tan O. Versatility of the vertical designed deep inferior epigastric perforator flap. Microsurgery. 2009;29(4):282–6.
5. Kostakoğlu N, Keçik A. Deep inferior epigastric artery (DIEA) skin flap: clinical experience of 15 cases. Br J Plast Surg. 1998;51(1):25–31.
6. Tang J, Fang T, Song D, Liang J, Yu F, Wang C. Free deep inferior epigastric artery perforator flap for reconstruction of soft-tissue defects in extremities of children. Microsurgery. 2013;33(8):612–9.
7. Belousov AE, Kishemasov SD, Kochish AY, Pinchuk VD. A new classification of vascularized flaps in plastic and reconstructive surgery. Ann Plast Surg. 1993;31(1):47–52; discussion 52–3.
8. Hallock GG. Further clarification of the nomenclature for compound flaps. Plast Reconstr Surg. 2006;117(7):151e–60e.
9. Loeffelbein DJ, Hölzle F, Wolff KD. Double-skin paddle perforator flap from the lateral lower leg for reconstruction of through-and-through cheek defect—a report of two cases. Int J Oral Maxillofac Surg. 2006;35(11):1016–20.
10. Tang L, Pafitanis G, Yang P, et al. Combined multi-lobed flaps: a series of 39 extensive hand and multi-digit injuries one-staged reconstructions using modified designs of ALT, DPA and chimeric linking flaps. Injury. 2017;48:1527.
11. Chi Z, Yang P, Song D, et al. Reconstruction of totally degloved fingers: a novel application of the bilobed spiraled innervated radial artery superficial palmar branch perforator flap design provides for primary donor-site closure. Surg Radiol Anat. 2017;39(5):547–57.
12. Li KW, Song DJ, Liu J, Xie SL. Tripaddle posterior interosseous artery flap design for 3-finger defects: an evaluation of 3 surgical approaches. Ann Plast Surg. 2016;77:406.
13. Smith ML, Gandolfi BM, Dayan E, et al. Bilateral breast reconstruction from a single hemiabdomen using angiosome-based flap design. Plast Reconstr Surg. 2013;132(2):291–4.
14. Taylor GI, Palmer JH. The vascular territories (angiosomes) of the body: experimental study and clinical applications. Br J Plast Surg. 1987;40(2):113–41.
15. Keller A. Perfusion zones of the DIEP flap revisited: a clinical study. Plast Reconstr Surg. 2006;118(4):1076–7; author reply 1077.
16. Rozen WM, Ashton MW, Le RCM, Pan WR, Corlett RJ. The perforator angiosome: a new concept in the design of deep inferior epigastric artery perforator flaps for breast reconstruction. Microsurgery. 2010;30(1):1–7.
17. Taylor GI, Corlett RJ, Dhar SC, Ashton MW. The anatomical (angiosome) and clinical territories of cutaneous perforating arteries: development of the concept and designing safe flaps. Plast Reconstr Surg. 2011;127(4):1447–59.
18. Schaverien M, Saint-Cyr M, Arbique G, Brown SA. Arterial and venous anatomies of the deep inferior epigastric perforator and superficial deep inferior epigastric artery flaps. Plast Reconstr Surg. 2008;121(6):1909–19.
19. Spiegel AJ, Khan FN. An intraoperative algorithm for use of the SIEA flap for breast reconstruction. Plast Reconstr Surg. 2007;120(6):1450–9.
20. Kundu N, Chopra K, Morales R, Djohan R, Chung T, Gastman BR. Superior epigastric artery perforator (SEAP) flap: a novel approach to autologous breast reconstruction. J Plast Reconstr Aesthet Surg. 2015;68(4):519–24.
21. Hamdi M, Craggs B, Stoel AM, Hendrickx B, Zeltzer A. Superior epigastric artery perforator flap: anatomy, clinical applications, and review of literature. J Reconstr Microsurg. 2014;30(7):475–82.
22. Boyd JB, Taylor GI, Corlett R. The vascular territories of the superior epigastric and the deep inferior epigastric systems. Plast Reconstr Surg. 1984;73(1):1–16.
23. Fukaya E, Kuwatsuru R, Iimura H, Ihara K, Sakurai H. Imaging of the superficial deep inferior epigastric vascular anatomy and preoperative planning for the SIEA flap using MDCTA. J Plast Reconstr Aesthet Surg. 2011;64(1):63–8.
24. Holm C, Mayr M, Höfter E, Raab N, Ninkovic M. Interindividual variability of the SIEA Angiosome: effects on operative strategies in breast reconstruction. Plast Reconstr Surg. 2008;122(6):1612–20.
25. Holm C, Mayr M, Höfter E, Ninkovic M. The versatility of the SIEA flap: a clinical assessment of the vascular territory of the superficial epigastric inferior artery. J Plast Reconstr Aesthet Surg. 2007;60(8):946–51.
26. Schmidt M, Tinhofer I, Duscher D, Huemer GM. Perforasomes of the upper abdomen: an anatomical study. J Plast Reconstr Aesthet Surg. 2014;67(1):42–7.
27. Gilmour A, Mackay IR. Bilateral deep inferior epigastric perforator flaps based on unilateral perforators. J Plast Reconstr Aesthet Surg. 2013;66(6):848–50.
28. Clodius L, Smahel J. Thin and thick pedicle flap. Acta Chir Plast. 1972;14(1):30–5.
29. Ohmori K, Harii K. Free dorsalis pedis sensory flap to the hand, with microneurovascular anastomoses. Plast Reconstr Surg. 1976;58(5):546–54.
30. Thomas CV. Thin flaps. Plast Reconstr Surg. 1980;65(6):747–52.
31. Koshima I, Moriguchi T, Soeda S, Tanaka H, Umeda N. Free thin paraumbilical perforator-based flaps. Ann Plast Surg. 1992;29(1):12–7.
32. Koshima I, Moriguchi T, Fukuda H, Yoshikawa Y, Soeda S. Free, thinned, paraumbilical perforator-based flaps. J Reconstr Microsurg. 1991;7(4):313–6.
33. Kimura N, Satoh K, Hasumi T, Ostuka T. Clinical application of the free thin anterolateral thigh flap in 31 consecutive patients. Plast Reconstr Surg. 2001;108(5):1197–208; discussion 1209–10.
34. Kimura N. A microdissected thin tensor fasciae latae perforator flap. Plast Reconstr Surg. 2002;109(1):69–77; discussion 78–80.
35. Kimura N, Satoh K. Consideration of a thin flap as an entity and clinical applications of the thin anterolateral thigh flap. Plast Reconstr Surg. 1996;97(5):985–92.
36. Kimura N, Satoh K, Hosaka Y. Microdissected thin perforator flaps: 46 cases. Plast Reconstr Surg. 2003;112(7):1875–85.
37. Kimura N, Saitoh M. Free microdissected thin groin flap design with an extended vascular pedicle. Plast Reconstr Surg. 2006;117(3):986–92.
38. Kimura N, Saito M, Itoh Y, Sumiya N. Giant combined microdissected thin thigh perforator flap. J Plast Reconstr Aesthet Surg. 2006;59(12):1325–9.
39. Dabernig J, Sorensen K, Shaw-Dunn J, Hart AM. The thin circumflex scapular artery perforator flap. J Plast Reconstr Aesthet Surg. 2007;60(10):1082–96.
40. del Piñal F, Garcia-Bernal FJ, Studer A, Ayala H, Cagigal L, Regalado J. Super-thinned iliac flap for major defects on the elbow and wrist flexion creases. J Hand Surg Am. 2008;33(10):1899–904.
41. Akizuki T, Harii K, Yamada A. Extremely thinned inferior rectus abdominis free flap. Plast Reconstr Surg. 1993;91(5):936–41.
42. Kim DY, Jeong EC, Kim KS, Lee SY, Cho BH. Thinning of the thoracodorsal perforator-based cutaneous flap for axillary burn scar contracture. Plast Reconstr Surg. 2002;109(4):1372–7.
43. Rajacic N, Gang RK, Krishnan J, Lal BR. Thin anterolateral thigh free flap. Ann Plast Surg. 2002;48(3):252–7.
44. Nojima K, Brown SA, Acikel C, et al. Defining vascular supply and territory of thinned perforator flaps: part II. Superior gluteal artery perforator flap. Plast Reconstr Surg. 2006;118(6):1338–48.
45. Yang WG, Chiang YC, Wei FC, Feng GM, Chen KT. Thin anterolateral thigh perforator flap using a modified perforator microdissection technique and its clinical application for foot resurfacing. Plast Reconstr Surg. 2006;117(3):1004–8.
46. Song D, Deng X, Chen Y, Xie S, Zhou X. Thinned chimeric radial collateral artery perforator flap in complex distal thumb reconstruction. Arch Orthop Trauma Surg. 2015;135(11):1623–31.
47. Lai YL, Yu YL, Centeno RF, Weng CJ. Breast augmentation with bilateral deepithelialized TRAM flaps: an alternative approach to

breast augmentation with autologous tissue. Plast Reconstr Surg. 2003;112(1):302–8; discussion 309–11.
48. Allen RJ, Heitland AS. Autogenous augmentation mammaplasty with microsurgical tissue transfer. Plast Reconstr Surg. 2003;112(1):91–100.
49. Kim EK, Suh YC, Maldonado AA, Yun J, Lee TJ. Patients' aesthetic concerns after horizontally placed abdominal free flap breast reconstruction. Aesthet Plast Surg. 2015;39(5):686–93.
50. Dajiang Song, Zan Li, Xiao Zhou. Clinical application of free medial femoral chimeric perforator myocutaneous flap in the repair of defects after tongue cancer surgery. Chin J Otorhinolaryngol Head Neck Surg2017. 52(4): 278–282.
51. Dajiang Song, Zan Li, Xiao Zhou. Observation of curative effect of different forms of free profunda femoral artery pedicle chimeric perforator myocutaneous flap in the repair of defects after tongue cancer surgery. Chin J Reparat Reconstr Surg2017. 31(06): 696–701.
52. Song D, Xu J, Lv H, Liu J, Li J. Wraparound chimeric radial collateral artery perforator flap for reconstruction of thumb loss. J Reconstr Microsurg. 2015;31(2):95–101.
53. Liu J, Song D, Li J, Xu J, Lv H. Modified osteomyocutaneous iliac crest flaps transplantation. J Plast Surg Hand Surg. 2015;49(2):102–6.
54. Koshima I, Yamamoto H, Hosoda M, Moriguchi T, Orita Y, Nagayama H. Free combined composite flaps using the lateral circumflex femoral system for repair of massive defects of the head and neck regions: an introduction to the chimeric flap principle. Plast Reconstr Surg. 1993;92(3):411–20.
55. Sano K, Hallock GG, Hamazaki M, Daicyo Y. The perforator-based conjoint (chimeric) medial Sural(MEDIAL GASTROCNEMIUS) free flap. Ann Plast Surg. 2004;53(6):588–92.
56. Hallock GG. An introduction to the chimeric deep inferior epigastric artery perforator (DIEP)-rectus abdominis muscle flap. Ann Plast Surg. 2008;61(5):580–3.

Modified Auxiliary Incision for Flap Removal

8

Zan Li and Wuping Zheng

The vascular pedicle separation of the DIEP flap is mainly divided into two cases:

1. The vascular pedicle keeps running on the deep and medial side of the rectus abdominis muscle. The rectus abdominis muscle on the surface of the vascular pedicle must be separated and pulled longitudinally along the fiber direction, and the segmental intercostal nerve must be protected at the same time.
2. The vascular pedicle runs from the outside to the inside on the deep surface of the rectus abdominis. The traditional method is to extend the anterior sheath of the rectus abdominis obliquely outward and downward to the lateral edge of the rectus abdominis, and then lift the rectus abdominis from the outside to expose the vascular pedicle. The pedicle is freed in rendezvous method (Fig. 8.1).

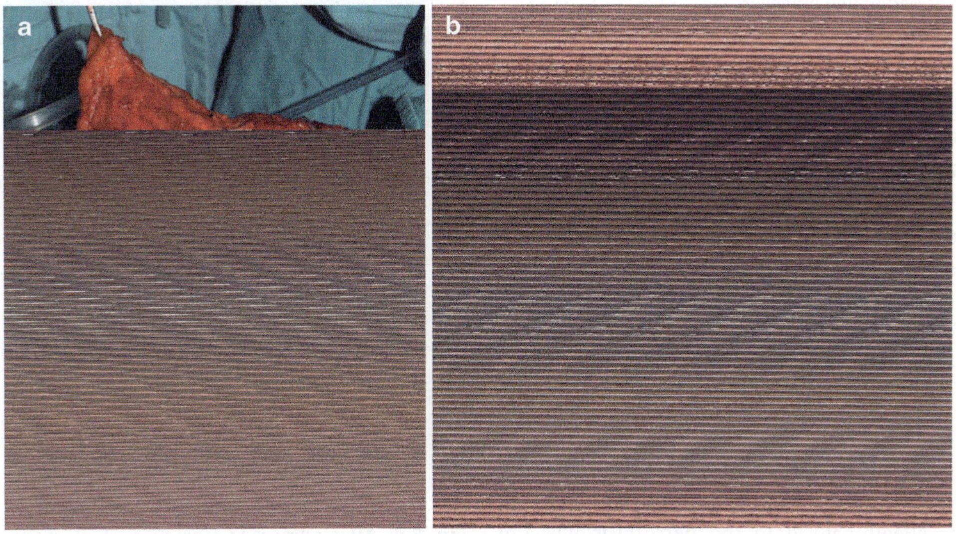

Fig. 8.1 (**a**) The first case: the vascular pedicle keeps running on the deep and medial side of the rectus abdominis. The rectus abdominis on the surface of the vascular pedicle must be separated and pulled longitudinally along the fiber direction, and the segmental intercostal nerve must be protected at the same time. (**b**) The second situation: the vascular pedicle runs from the outside to the inside on the deep surface of the rectus abdominis. The traditional method is to extend the anterior sheath of the rectus abdominis obliquely outward and downward to the lateral edge of the rectus abdominis, and then lift the rectus abdominis from the outside to expose the vascular pedicle under the abdominal wall for separation

Z. Li (✉)
Department of Oncology Plastic Surgery, Hunan Cancer Hospital, Changsha, Hunan, China

W. Zheng
Department of Breast and Thyroid Surgery at the Second Affiliated Hospital of Hainan Medical College, Haikou, Hainan Province, China

Z. Li, D. Song (eds.), *Oncoplastic Flap Surgery*, https://doi.org/10.1007/978-981-19-8926-1_8

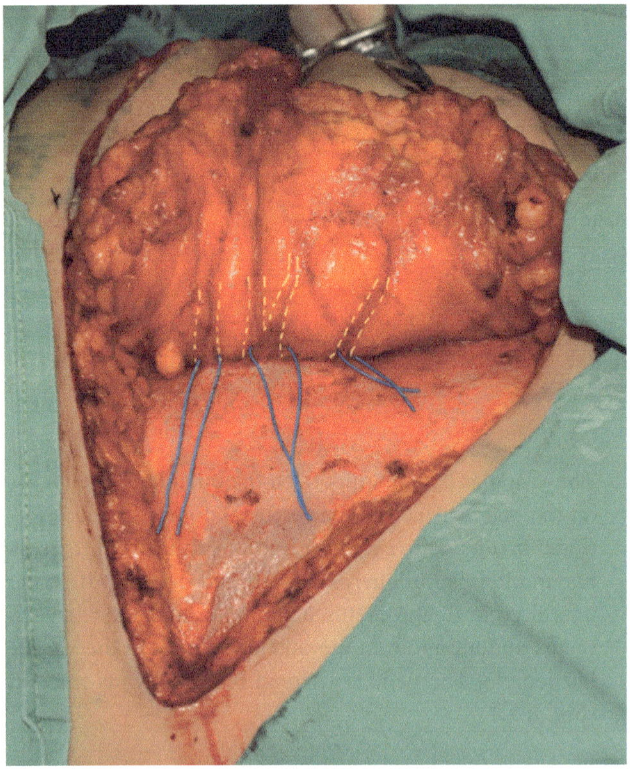

Fig. 8.2 Exposure of perforating branches

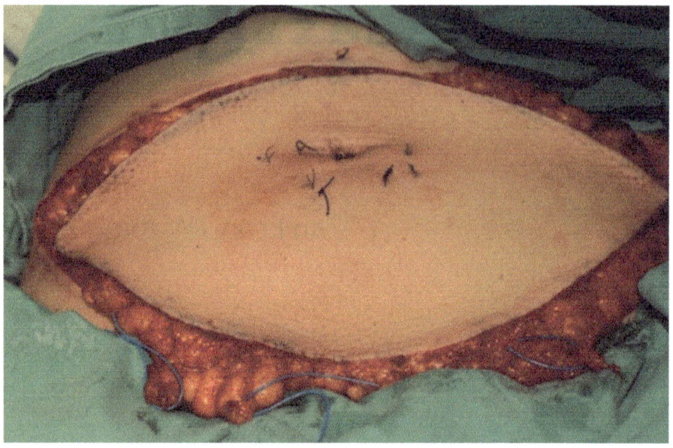

Fig. 8.3 Bilateral superficial deep inferior epigastric veins were preserved on the flap, and the position of perforating vessels were marked by suture

As shown in Fig. 8.1, the conventional method of vascular pedicle separation requires long-section incision of rectus abdominis and anterior sheath. Through continuous clinical practice, we designed and improved the method of auxiliary incision to cut the perforator flap of deep inferior epigastric artery, which can minimize the damage of rectus abdominis and anterior sheath. Although the surgical field is slightly limited, it is still safe and reliable.

Specific steps of the modified perforator flap of deep inferior epigastric artery (Figs. 8.2, 8.3, and 8.4):

1. Flap design.
2. Preserve superficial epigastric vein.
3. Lift the flap to expose the appropriate perforator.
4. The anterior sheath lateral to the perforator was cut open, and the perforator was confirmed to go through the tendinous inscription, making separation difficult.
5. The muscle fibers were dissected layer by layer, and the perforator and DIEA trunk were separated.
6. The distal end of DIEA trunk was ligated and disconnected at a suitable plane.
7. The DIEA trunk was separated retrogradely toward its proximal end from intramuscular space to the surface of the posterior sheath, and the medial or lateral branches of DIEA along the way were ligated.
8. It has been difficult in separating the perforator from posterior tissue because small muscular branches from the DIEA may be encountered. Therefore, the posterior tissue can be cut off in stratification after being cauterized by bipolar electrocoagulation.
9. An auxiliary longitudinal incision was made distal to the lateral side of the rectus abdominis to avoid excessive stripping of the anterior sheath. The disadvantages are that the rectus abdominis cannot be fully pulled open,

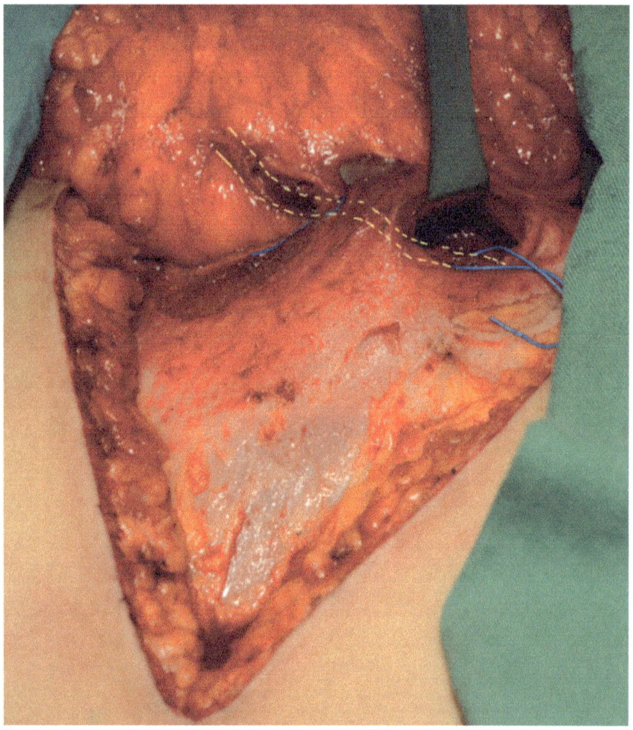

Fig. 8.4 After retrograde separation of the perforator and vascular pedicle, the pedicle was revealed and further separated by lifting the rectus abdominis muscle from the outside with an auxiliary incision. The anterior sheath of rectus abdominis and intercostal nerve were preserved to the greatest extent

the operation field is narrow, and accidental injury is likely to happen.

10. It is difficult to locate the lateral incision of rectus abdominis, especially for patients with repeated chemotherapy whose rectus abdominis, anterior sheath, and posterior sheath are prone to be thinner, subjecting the peritoneum to damage and even access into the abdominal cavity.

Exposing the rectus abdominis muscle and determining its lateral edge is convenient to further expose the vascular pedicle at the emitting plane.

The modified incision can minimize the damage to the rectus abdominis and its anterior sheath, but it is technically demanding for the operator. This incision is neither suitable when a long segment of the vascular pedicle runs in the muscle nor when the pedicle keeps traveling medially behind the rectus abdominis.

8.1 Case 1: Modified Auxiliary Incision for Raising a DIEP Flap

The patient was a female, 59 years old. She had found a mass on the left breast for 2 years. Angiogenic tumor of the left breast, probably well-differentiated angiosarcoma was pathologically considered on core needle biopsy. On admission, the patient received left total mastectomy plus unilateral TRAM flap plus contralateral free DIEP flap for chest wall reconstruction.

The left deep inferior epigastric artery and vein were anastomosed with the left lateral thoracic artery and vein (1A2V).

The flap and wounds healed well after operation, and postoperative routine pathological examination was consistent with that before operation. The patient was transferred to internal medicine for comprehensive treatment.

The shape and function of chest wall were satisfactory during follow-up, and there was no recurrence (Figs. 8.5, 8.6, 8.7, 8.8, 8.9, 8.10, 8.11, 8.12, 8.13, and 8.14).

When separating the perforators, it is recommended to adopt the standard manipulation such as sharp separation using scissors, bipolar coagulation, or microvascular clamp to avoid thermal damage caused by ultrasonic scalpel and unipolar electro cauterizer.

Although there are many advantages regarding this modified method, it is not suitable when the vascular pedicle keeps running in the medial area of rectus abdominis, where the dissection of vascular pedicle can be achieved through a single incision (as shown in Fig. 8.1a).

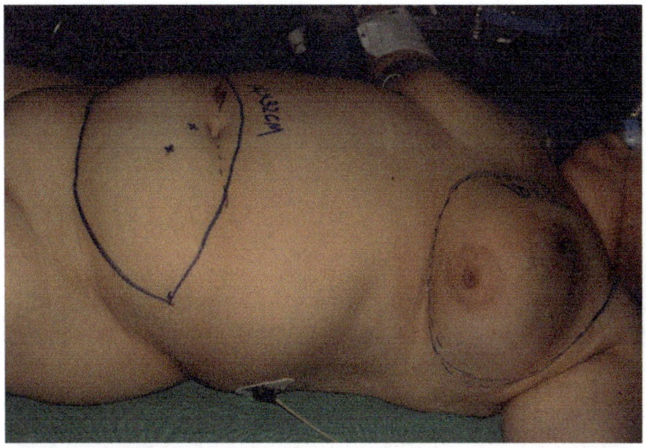

Fig. 8.5 Flap design

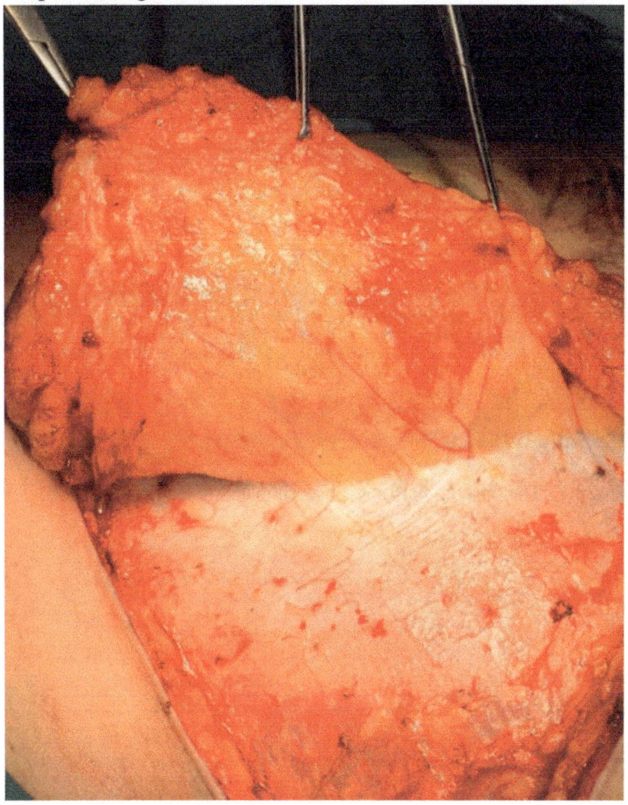

Fig. 8.6 The flap was lifted from the surface of the anterior sheath of rectus abdominis to preserve the superficial epigastric vein

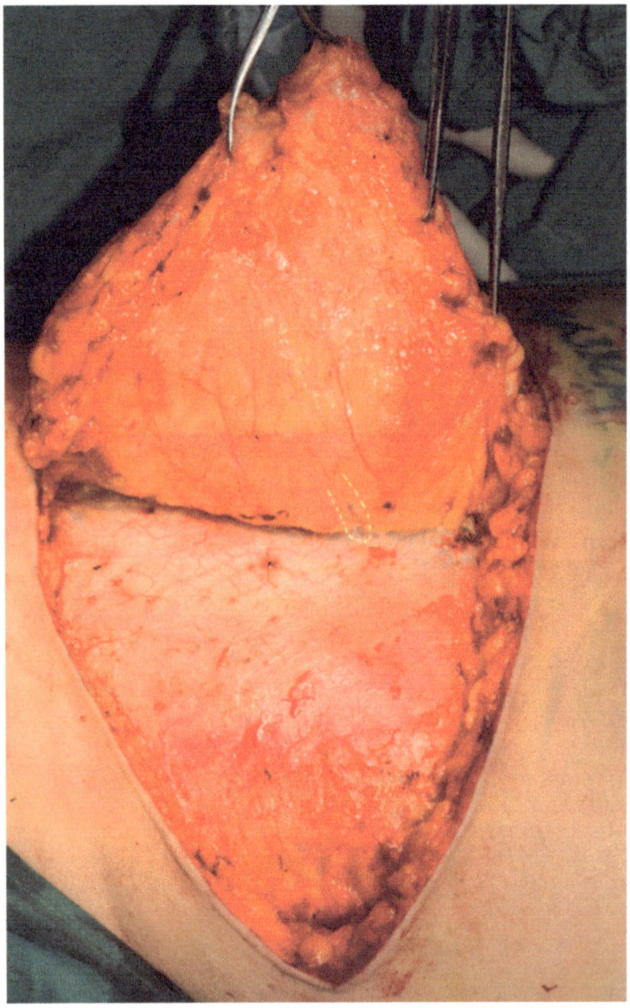

Fig. 8.7 The obscure perforator was shown

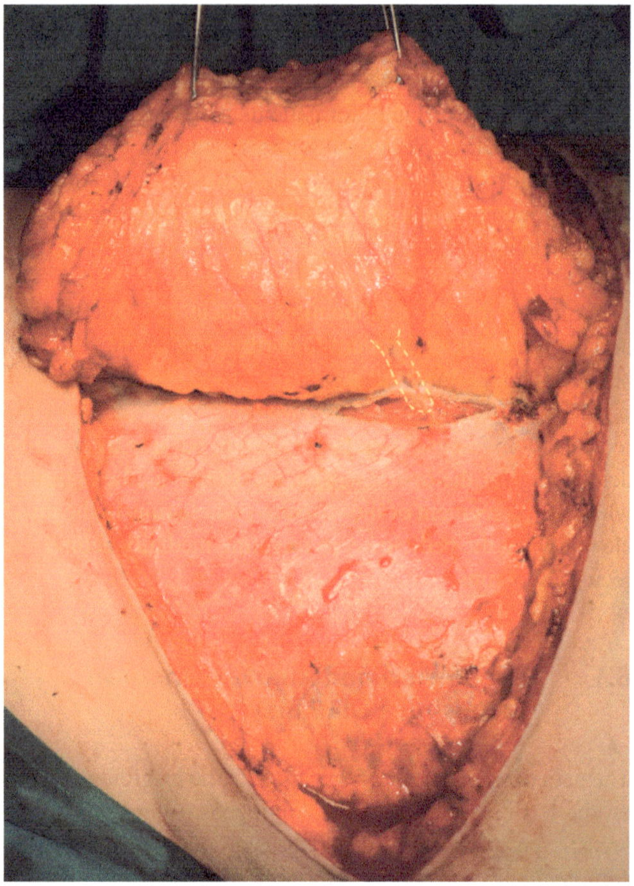

Fig. 8.8 The anterior sheath longitudinally was cut open lateral to the perforator that was found to be running through the tendinous inscription

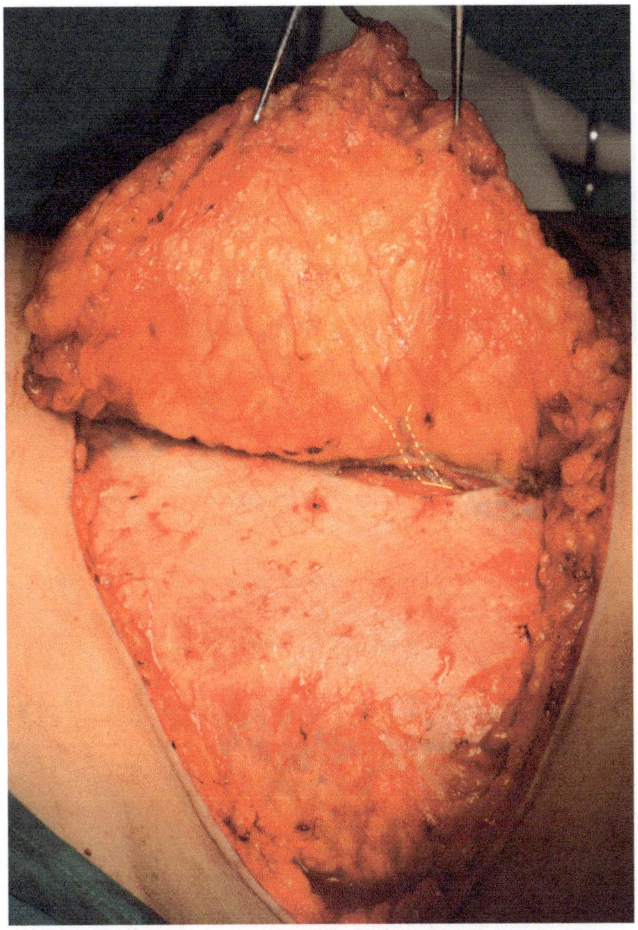

Fig. 8.9 The tendinous inscription on the surface of the perforator was removed bit by bit to unveil the underlying vessel

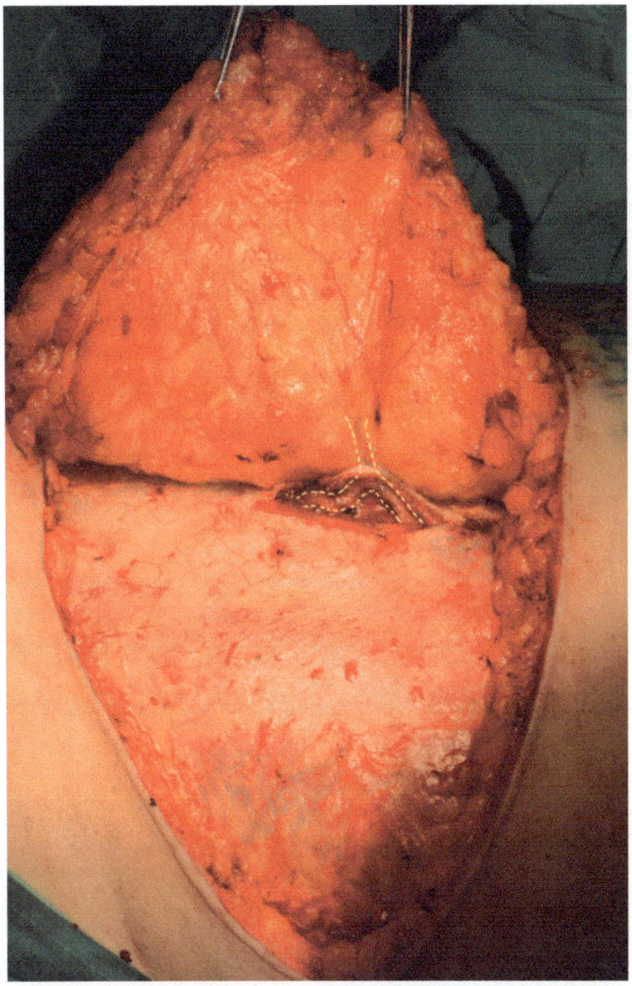

Fig. 8.10 Retrograde dissection of rectus abdominis muscle on the deep surface of anterior sheath was performed to completely expose the perforating vessel and the inferior epigastric vessels

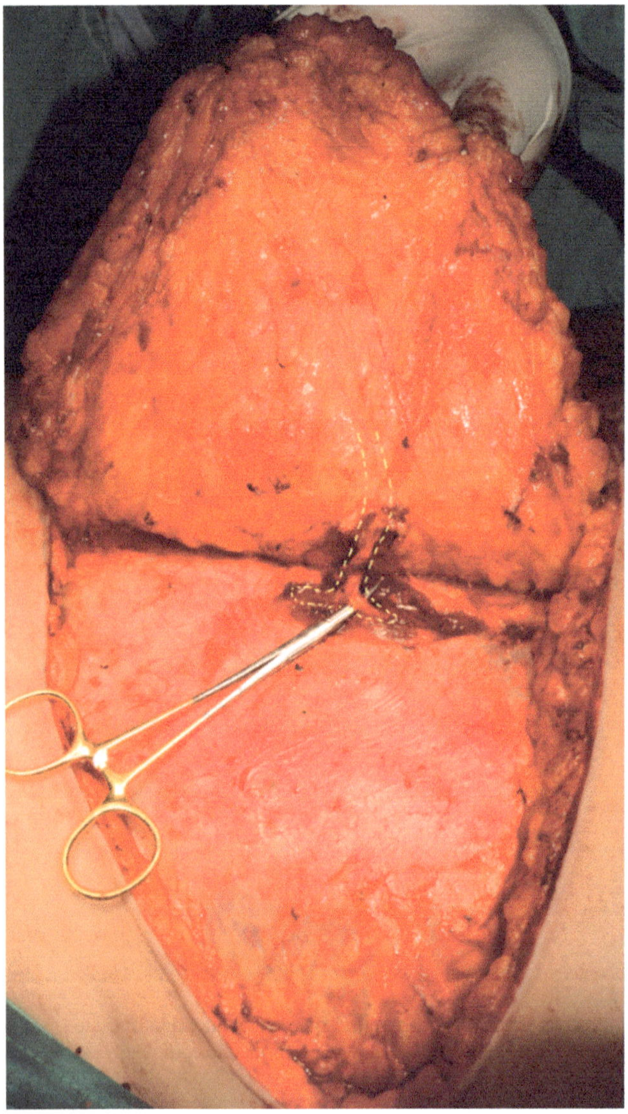

Fig. 8.11 The distal end of the deep inferior epigastric vessels was ligated away from the perforator

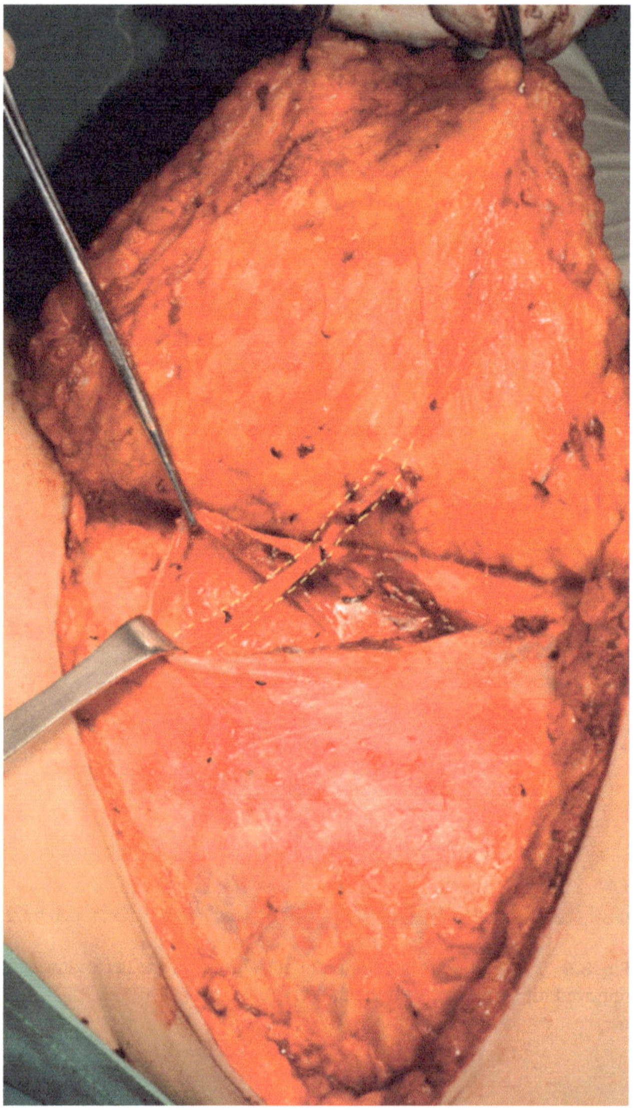

Fig. 8.12 The vascular pedicle was dissected retrogradely from intramuscular space to the deep surface of the rectus abdominis where the pedicle ran on the surface of the posterior sheath

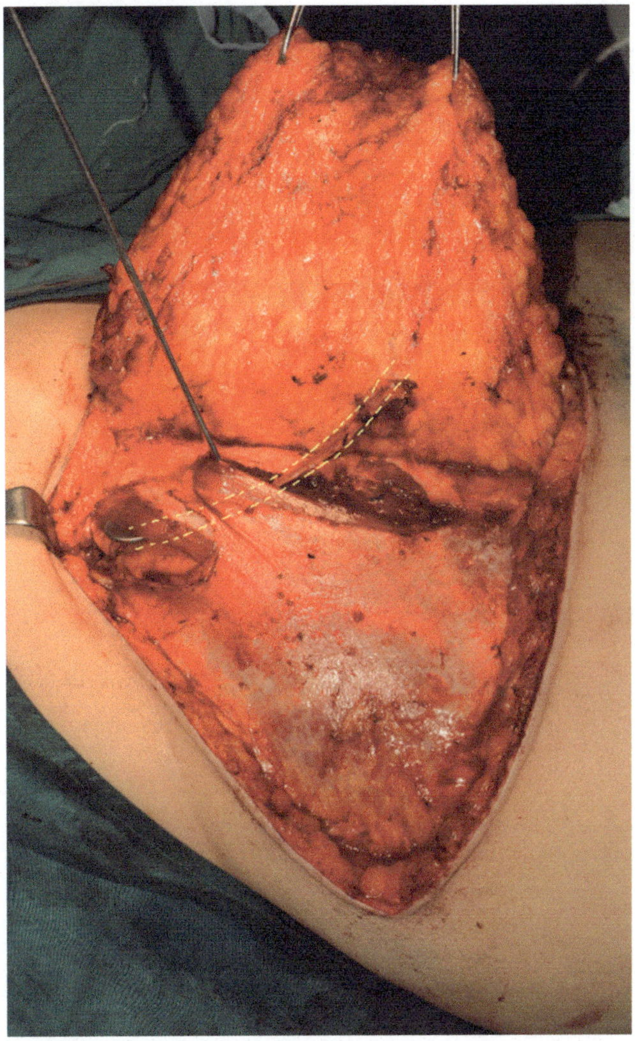

Fig. 8.13 An auxiliary incision was made longitudinally at the lateral edge of the ending plane of rectus abdominis, which was lifted and pulled inward to expose the proximal end of the deep inferior epigastric vessels

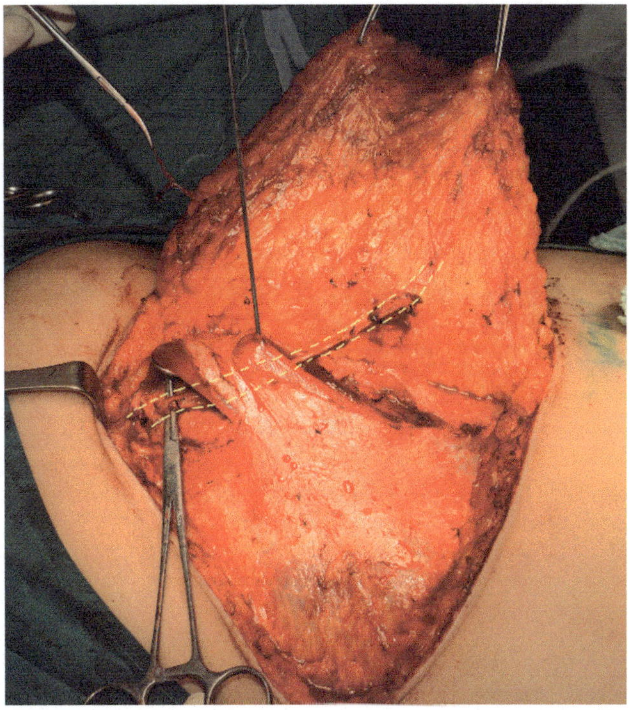

Fig. 8.14 The vascular pedicle was completely freed in the space posterior to the rectus abdominis muscle

9 Unilateral Pedicled TRAM Flap Plus Contralateral Free DIEP Flap

Zan Li and Haiyan Gao

To ensure sufficient blood supply of a unilateral pedicled rectus abdominis flap, the contralateral deep inferior epigastric vessels can be revascularized. Many reports have introduced the specific methods [1].

The classic pedicled rectus abdominis myocutaneous (RAM) flap contains a large amount of tissue that can be used to fill the subclavian vacancy and reconstruct the anterior axillary fold. The scar of the abdominal wall donor area is hidden, and abdominoplasty can also be achieved.

The pedicled RAM flap has been widely used in breast reconstruction because it is neither complex in procedure nor demanding in hardware or technique, and postoperative outcome is good.

However, the incidence of complications is high. About 10% of single-pedicled rectus abdominis myocutaneous flaps occur with blood supply disorder, resulting in partial necrosis or fat liquefaction of the flap [2, 3].

For patients with large breast on the unaffected side and extensive skin defect to be repaired due to radiation ulcer and scar on the affected chest wall, if the single-pedicled RAM flap is used, partial or total necrosis of the flap is likely to happen due to insufficient blood supply, here a double-pedicled abdominal flap would be better [4].

However, due to the limitation of early technology and equipment, operators can only use bilateral pedicled rectus abdominis myocutaneous flap, which would seriously impair flap transfer and the abdominal wall function [5].

The operation of the classic free deep inferior epigastric artery perforator flap is relatively cumbersome, which requires the operator to have high competency in oncoplastic surgery. The operation anesthesia time is long, and it is easy to damage the perforator vessels during vascular dissection, especially when the perforator is skeletonized, which significantly increases the probability of flap failure [6–10].

When using the double pedicled perforator flap of inferior abdominal artery, two vascular pedicles from the donor site are required at the same time, which significantly increases the operation anesthesia time and the operation risk and difficulty [11].

Furthermore, most patients once received radiotherapy and chemotherapy, which may bring the systemic and local blood vessels into poor condition, that is, the perforating vessels in the lower abdomen are often atrophic with narrow lumen and easy-to-tear wall. In many cases, it is difficult to harvest bilateral vascular pedicles [12–16].

In addition, the choices of vessels in the receiving area of phase II breast reconstruction are often limited. In patients with previous mastectomy, the lateral thoracic vessels and the anterior serratus branches of the thoracodorsal vessels are generally unavailable. The trunk of the thoracodorsal vessels is better to be the last to resort to. In practice, the first choice is the internal thoracic vessels. The leading disadvantage of these vessels is that the venous wall is very thin. If chest radiotherapy was once given, the vascular properties of the internal thoracic arteries and veins on the affected side would further deteriorate, where the use of double-pedicled rectus abdominis myocutaneous flap will be of great risk. Similarly, neither the proximal nor the distal thoracic vessels is suitable for revascularization with the bilateral vascular pedicles of a free DIEP flap.

In these cases, a pedicled rectus abdominis flap combined with a free perforator flap of deep inferior epigastric artery is undoubtedly the best choice [14].

The application of a pedicled rectus abdominis flap combined with a free deep inferior epigastric artery perforator flap for breast reconstruction shares the advantages of each flap yet overcomes the shortages of either the pedicled RAM flap or the free DIEP flap, improving the tissue utilization rate and viability of the flap to the greatest extent as well as avoiding the dysfunction of the donor area after flap transplantation.

Z. Li (✉)
Department of Oncology Plastic Surgery, Hunan Cancer Hospital, Changsha, Hunan, China

H. Gao
Department of Breast Surgery, Changzhou Tumor Hospital, Changzhou, P. R. China

Z. Li, D. Song (eds.), *Oncoplastic Flap Surgery*, https://doi.org/10.1007/978-981-19-8926-1_9

This combined flap is characterized with reliable blood supply, abundant tissue, directly closed donor area, and being shaping friendly. Moreover, in patients with a median surgical incision scar on the midline in the lower abdominal wall, this method can also avoid the great impact on abdominal wall function caused by double pedicled rectus abdominis myocutaneous flap and reduce the great surgical risk of bilateral free deep inferior epigastric artery perforator flap [12].

9.1 Combined Flap

It is a flap assembled by multiple independent mono-flaps containing poly flap ranges (or structures). Each single flap retains its own independent blood supply source. According to the different combination patterns, it can be divided into three categories: combined flap, lobed flap, and serial flap.

9.2 Siamese Flap

It is also known as the "conjoined flap." The transferred flaps are continuous in structure yet the flap area exceeds the support range of any of the included vascular pedicles. Therefore, auxiliary blood supply, that is, improving blood flow by anastomosing the distal or contralateral vascular end is a must to ensure the viability of the flap. Clinically, this is usually used for mega flap covering a wide range. The vascular pedicle at one end (side) is often retained and the distal end (opposite side) is cut off to obtain a large rotating arc. It is necessary to reconstruct the auxiliary blood supply of the distal part of the tissue flap.

9.3 Case 1: Pedicled RAM Flap Combined with Free DIEP Flap with the Lateral Thoracic Vessels as Recipient Vessels

The patient, 38 years old, was admitted to our hospital for right breast cancer (pre-treatment situation shown in Fig. 9.1).

Preoperative pathological examination showed that it was invasive carcinoma of the right breast (cT4N2M0, stage IIIB) with ER (0), PR (0), CerbB-2 (3 +) ki67.50%. The patient was treated with neoadjuvant EC-THP regimen. The tumor retreated significantly.

The right modified radical mastectomy was performed and pedicled rectus abdominis myocutaneous flap combined with free deep inferior epigastric perforator flap was used to repair the chest wall defect. The right chest wall defect was about 26 cm × 24 cm in size.

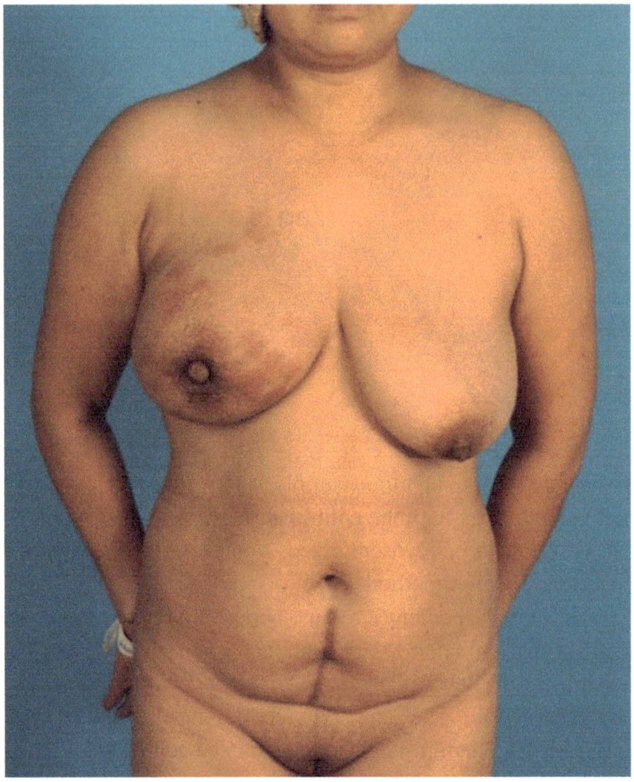

Fig. 9.1 Preoperative findings

The left TRAM flap pedicled with the left rectus abdominis muscle and the right perforator flap pedicled with the deep inferior epigastric artery were harvested. The prepared flap was transferred to the right chest wall through the subcutaneous tunnel to the right chest wall.

The right deep inferior epigastric artery and veins were anastomosed end-to-end with the lateral thoracic artery and vein (1A2V).

Pathological examination results were as follows: (1) (right breast) invasive lobular carcinoma (pT4N0M0, stage IIIa); (2) absent metastasis in (axillary) lymph nodes (0/15); (3) nipple invasion positive; (4) no tumor on skin and basal margins; IHC: ER (0), PR (0), CerbB-2 (3 +) Ki67 about 20%.

The flap survived well without obvious complications.

The patient was then transferred to internal medicine department for comprehensive treatment, and the reconstructed chest wall was followed up with satisfactory reconstruction function and appearance (Figs. 9.1, 9.2, 9.3, 9.4, 9.5, 9.6, 9.7, 9.8, 9.9, 9.10, 9.11, 9.12, and 9.13).

When free deep inferior epigastric artery perforator flap combined with pedicled rectus abdominis myocutaneous flap is considered, the internal mammary blood vessels in the receiving area have to be determined in good condition.

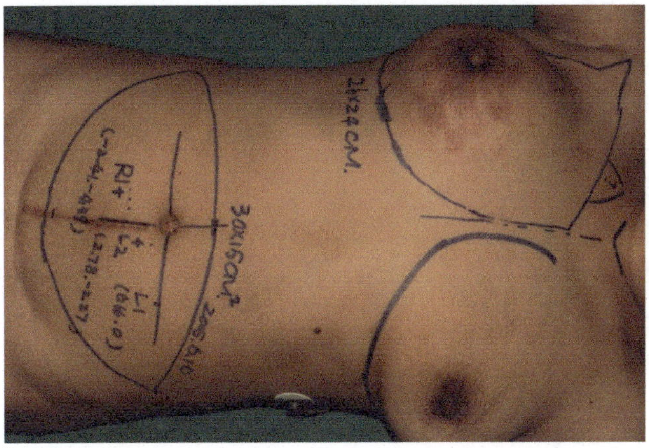

Fig. 9.2 Intraoperative design

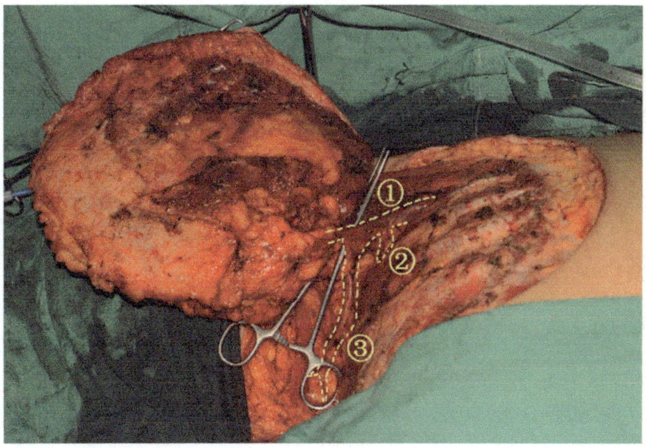

Fig. 9.3 After the lesion was completely removed, the lateral thoracic vessels and the thoracic acromial vessels were prepared as recipient vessels. (1) Axillary vein; (2) Thoracic acromial vessels; (3) Lateral thoracic vessels

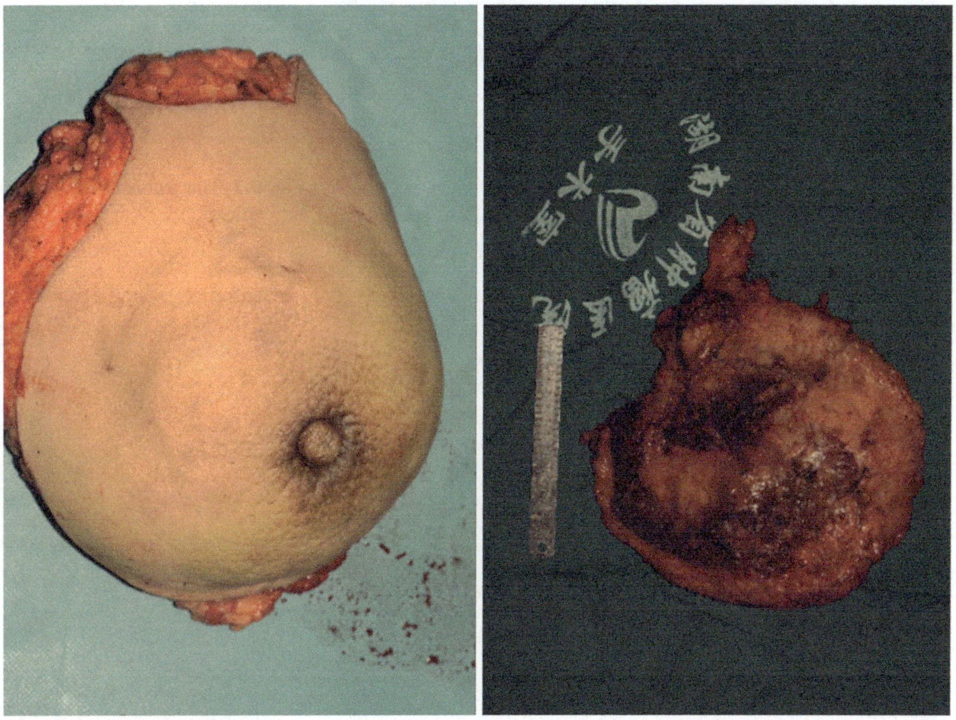

Fig. 9.4 Lesion resection completed

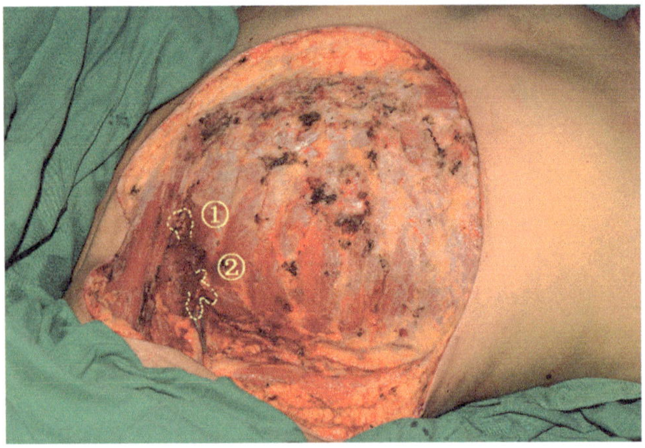

Fig. 9.5 The lateral thoracic artery and vein and thoracic acromial artery and vein in the receiving area were prepared. (1) Thoracoacromial vessels; (2) Lateral thoracic vessels

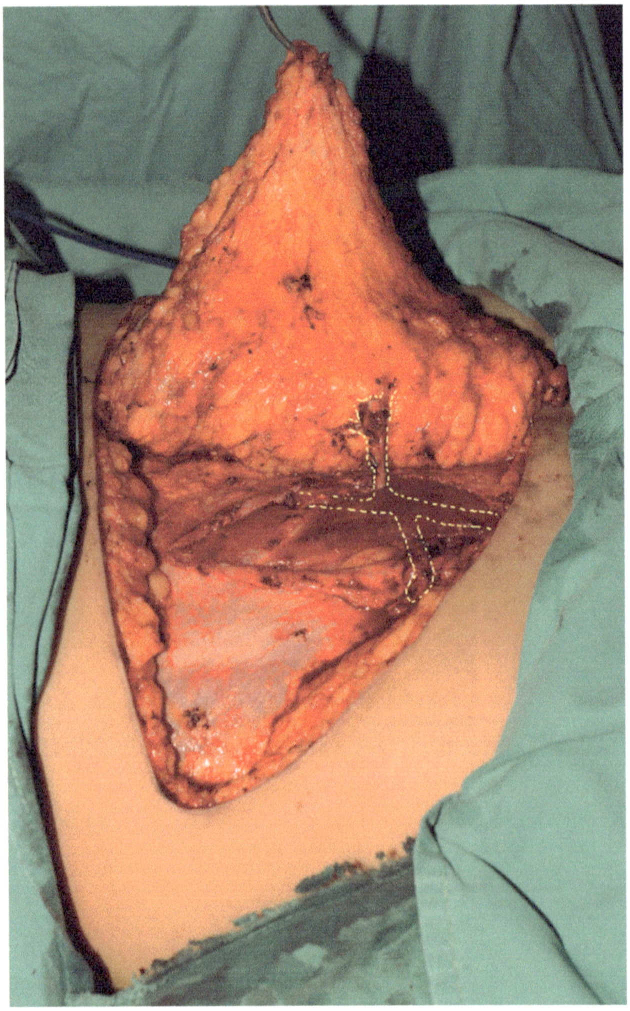

Fig. 9.6 The right deep inferior epigastric perforator vessel was revealed

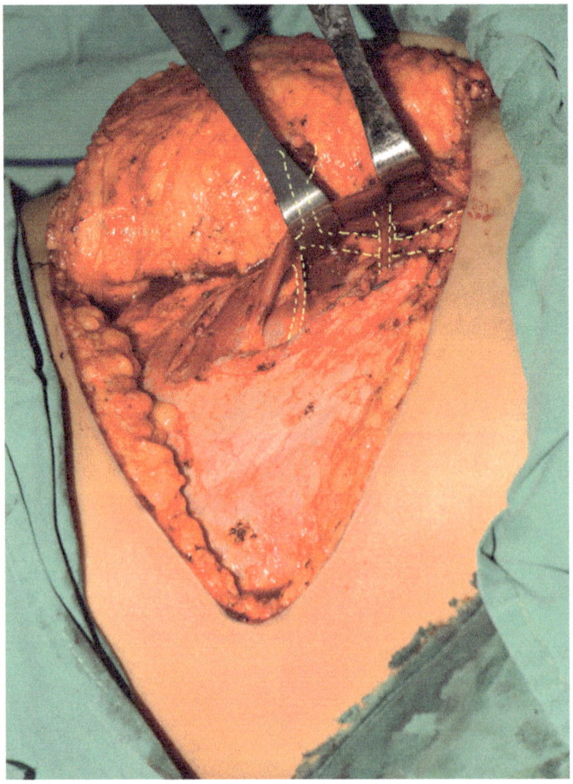

Fig. 9.7 The rectus abdominis muscle was lifted to expose the vascular pedicle

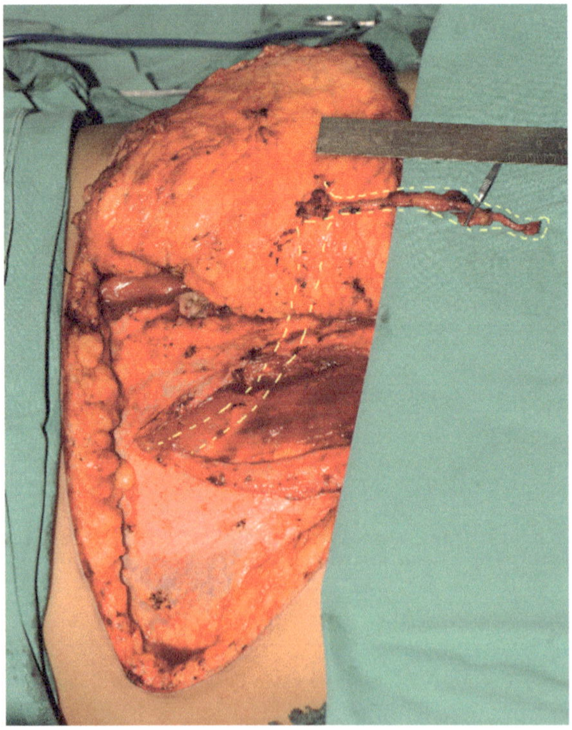

Fig. 9.8 The vascular pedicle was extracted from the rectus abdominis tunnel

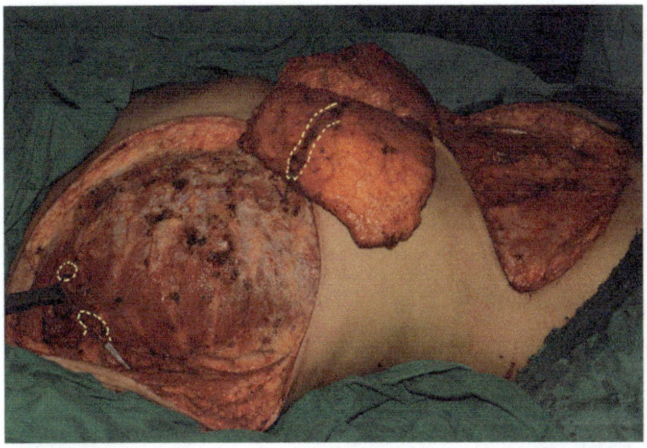

Fig. 9.9 The combined flap pedicled with the left rectus abdominis muscle was transferred from the upper abdominal subcutaneous tunnel to the chest wall defect area

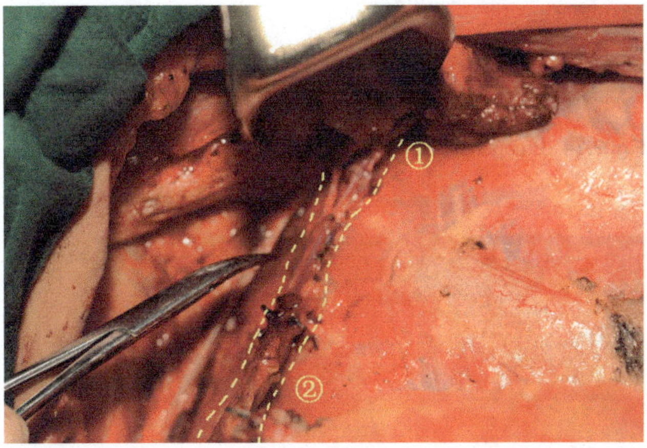

Fig. 9.10 The right deep inferior epigastric artery and vein carried by the flap were anastomosed with the right lateral thoracic artery and vein. (1) Lateral thoracic vessels; (2) Deep inferior epigastric vessels

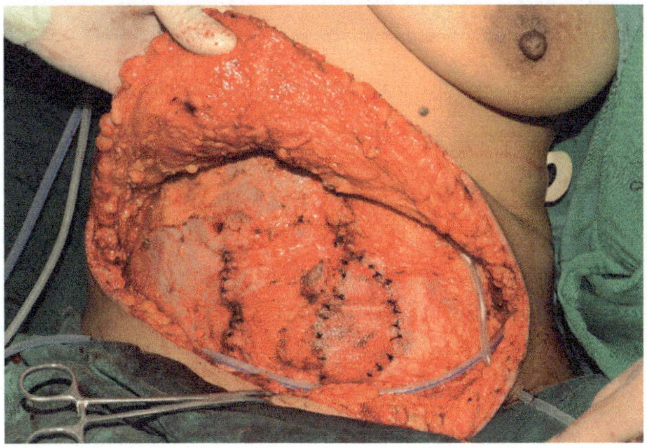

Fig. 9.11 The left rectus abdominis anterior sheath defect was covered with mesh in abdominal donor area

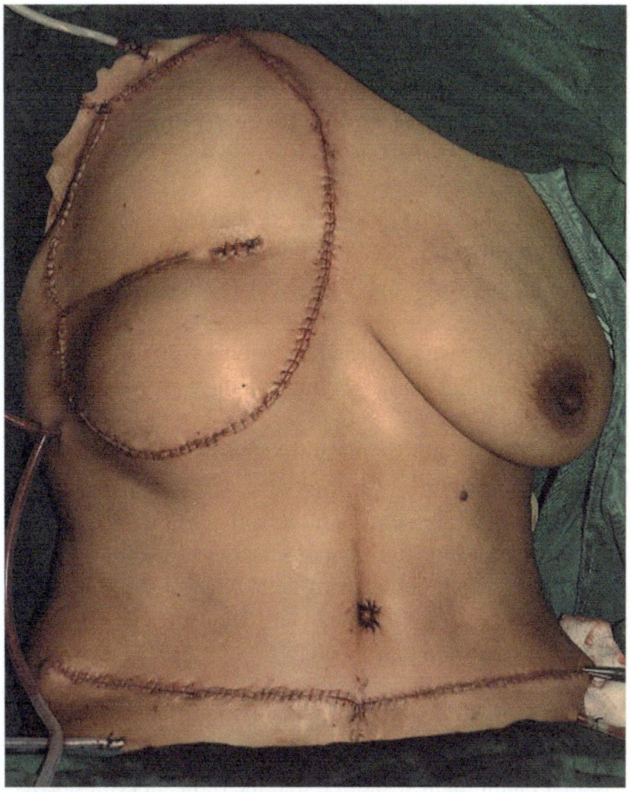

Fig. 9.12 Immediate intraoperative observation

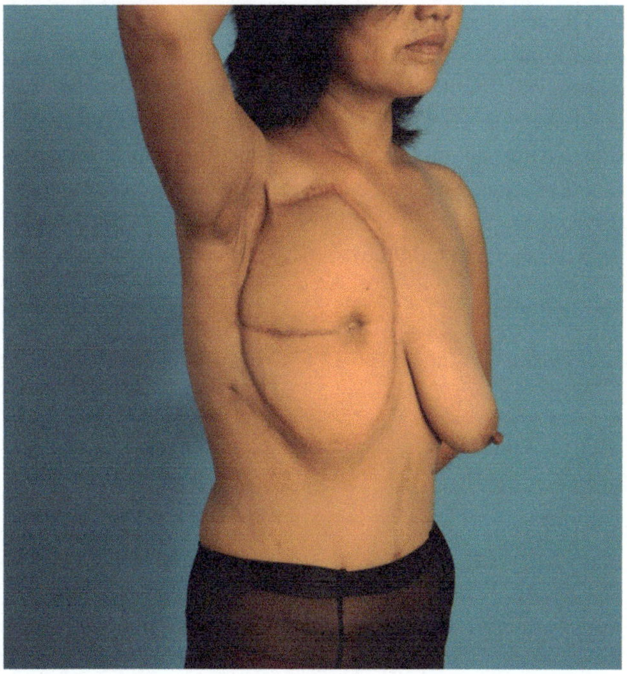

Fig. 9.13 Appearance and function after 16 months of follow-up

9.4 Case 2: Pedicled Rectus Abdominis Flap Combined with Free Perforator Flap of Deep Inferior Epigastric Artery: The Thoracoacromial Vessels as Recipient

The patient was a 44-year-old female and found a right breast mass 14 months ago. The mass had been growing rapidly for 12 months since she applied herbal medicine on the right breast skin.

Right breast invasive ductal carcinoma with cancer metastasis to ipsilateral axillary lymph node was confirmed on biopsy.

The tumor shrunk significantly after neoadjuvant chemotherapy. The response was evaluated as PR and the patient was hospitalized for surgical treatment.

After admission, right breast cancer radical mastectomy plus breast reconstruction using right rectus abdominis myocutaneous flap combined with left deep inferior epigastric perforator flap were performed.

The size of the flap was about 28 cm x 14 cm. After the right TRAM flap was prepared, the perforating vessels of the left deep inferior epigastric artery were further exposed. The vascular clamping test showed that the right superior epigastric vessels alone were not able to bring sufficient blood supply to the whole flap, which was then transferred to the right chest defect through the subcutaneous tunnel.

The left deep inferior epigastric vessels and the thoracoacromial artery and vein were anastomosed end to end, respectively (A: $V = 1{:}1$). The blood supply of the flap was good, and the defect area and flap donor area healed in one stage. After 24 months of follow-up, the appearance and function were excellent, and there was no tumor recurrence (Figs. 9.14, 9.15, 9.16, 9.17, 9.18, 9.19, 9.20, 9.21, 9.22, 9.23, 9.24, 9.25, and 9.26).

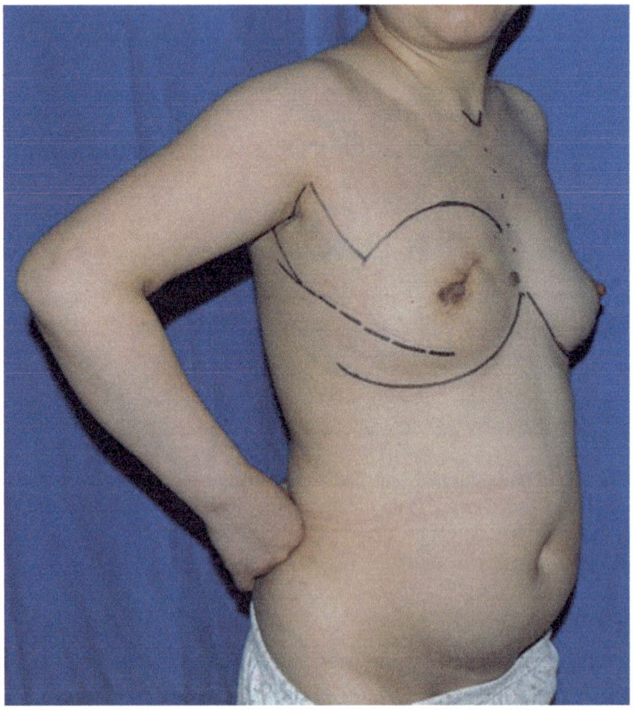

Fig. 9.14 Preoperative findings

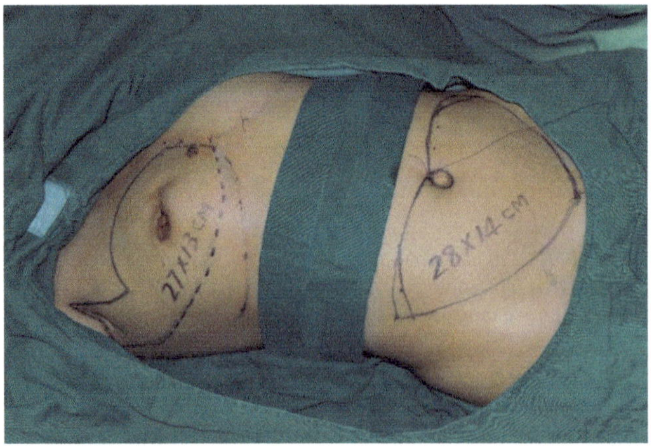

Fig. 9.15 Intraoperative marking of right mastectomy range and flap design

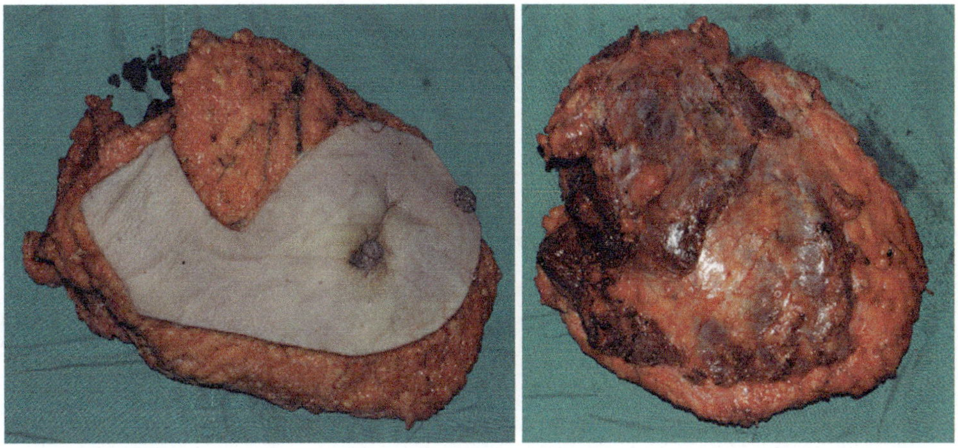

Fig. 9.16 The breast lesions were removed

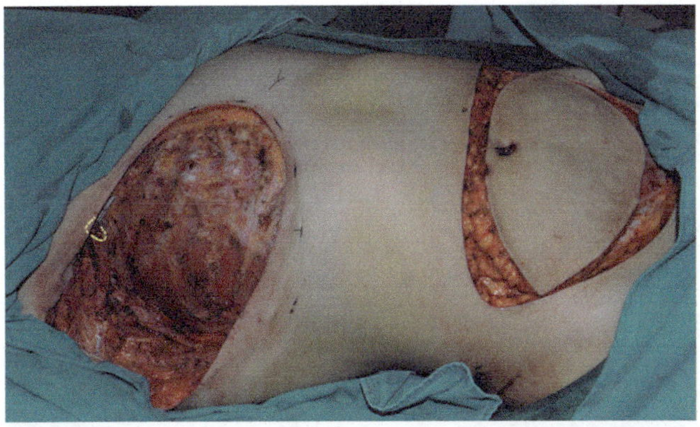

Fig. 9.17 Right chest defect. The thoracic acromial vessels were prepared as recipient vessels, and the flap margins were completely cut open

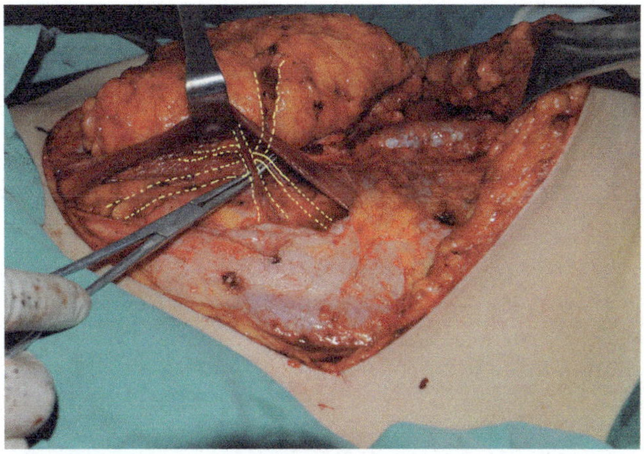

Fig. 9.19 The left epigastric vascular pedicle was dissected

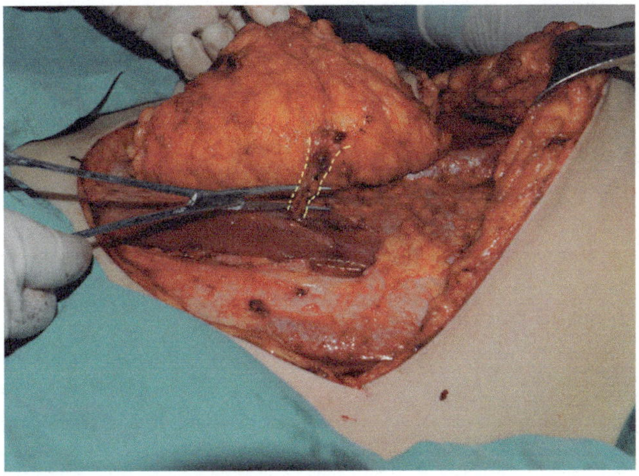

Fig. 9.18 The left deep inferior epigastric perforator was unveiled and separated

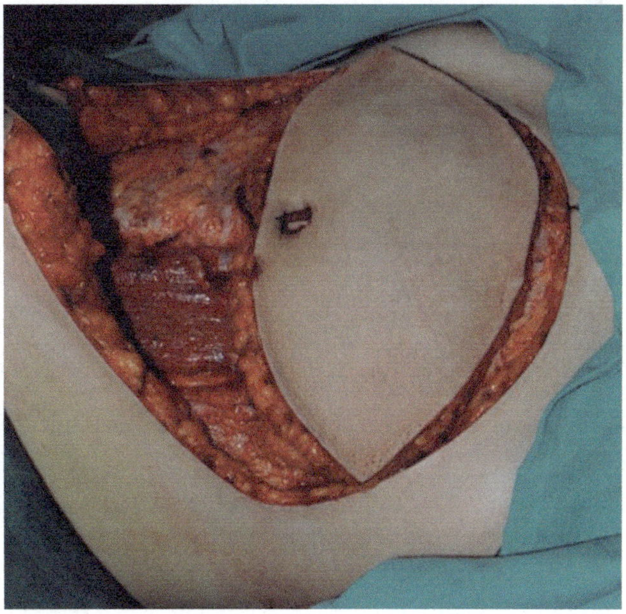

Fig. 9.20 The subcutaneous tunnel of the upper abdomen and the right muscle pedicle were all prepared

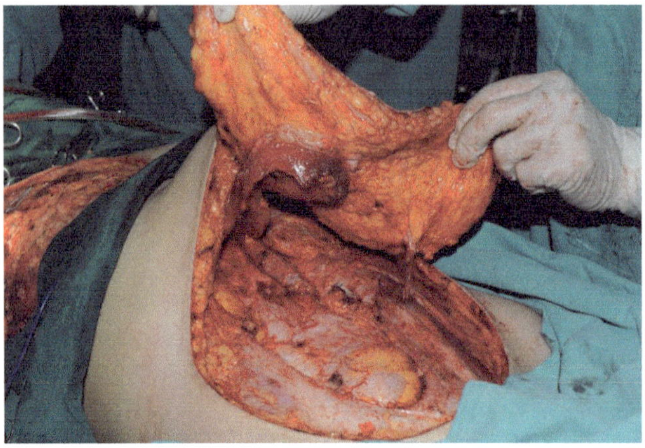

Fig. 9.21 The combined flap was cut and ready to be transferred to the right chest wall defect area

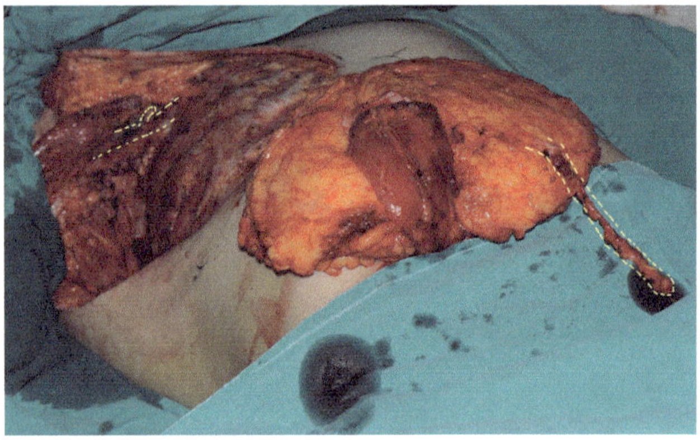

Fig. 9.22 The combined flap was ready to be transferred to the right chest wall defect area through the tunnel, and the vascular pedicle of the flap and the recipient vascular pedicle were prepared

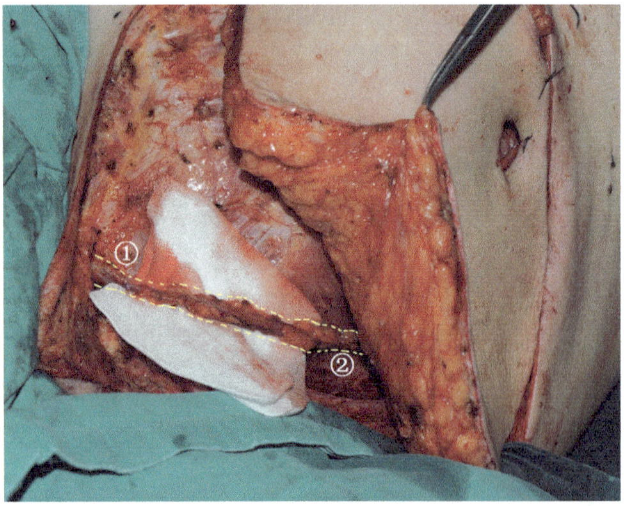

Fig. 9.23 Anastomosis between the left deep inferior epigastric vessels and the right thoracoacromial vessels were made (1A2V). (1) Thoracic acromial vessels; (2) Deep inferior epigastric vessels

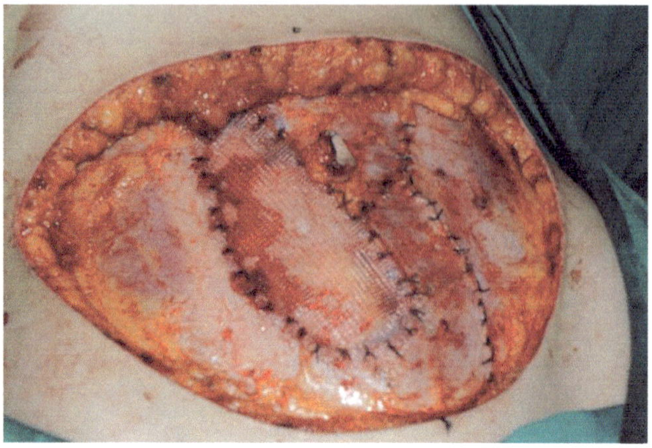

Fig. 9.24 The anterior sheath of rectus abdominis was repaired with mesh

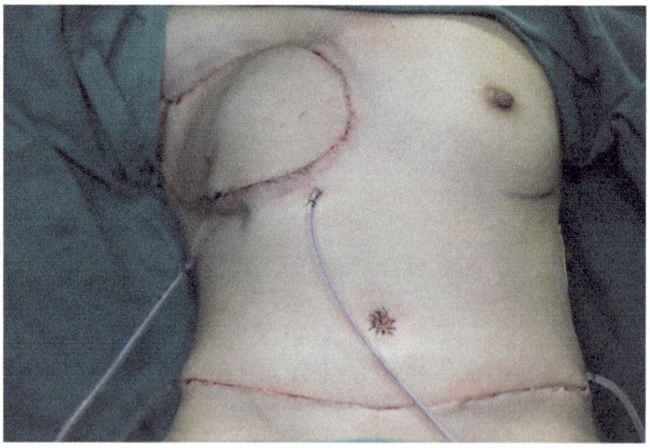

Fig. 9.25 Immediate view of chest wall reconstruction during operation

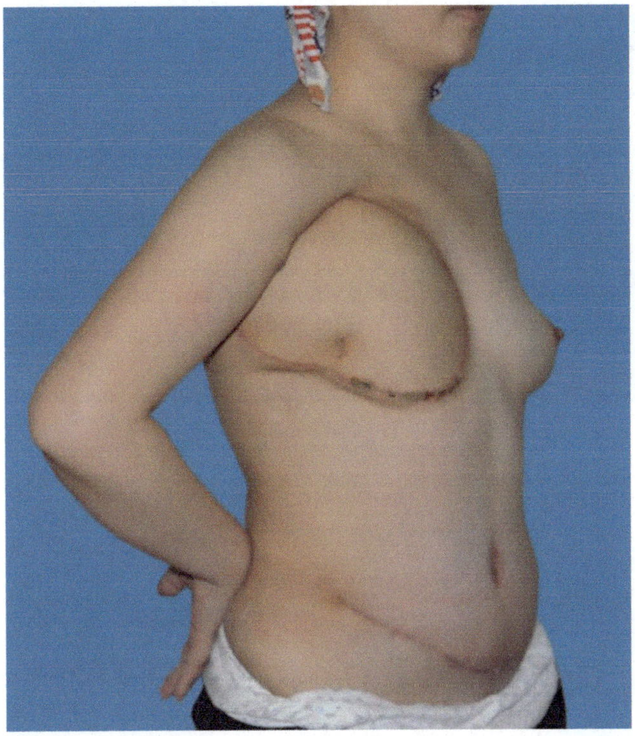

Fig. 9.26 At 24 months of follow-up, the appearance and function were good, and there was no tumor recurrence

9.5 Case 3: Pedicled Rectus Abdominis Flap Combined with Free Perforator Flap of Deep Inferior Epigastric: An Anterior Serratus Branch of the Thoracodorsal Vessels as Recipient

The patient was a 47-year-old female who was admitted for a huge tumor on the left breast. The diagnosis of left breast cancer (cT4cN2M0, IIIB) was made on biopsy and the immunohistochemistry results were ER (about 50%), PR (medium strength, about 70%), CerbB-2 (2+, FISH test was suggested), positive HER2 amplification on FISH, KI-67 (+, about 45%), CK5/6 (−), P63 (−), EGFR (−), (+). EC2w followed by PHw was given as neoadjuvant therapy.

The tumor showed great response to neoadjuvant therapy and partial remission was determined by physical examination and imaging evaluation.

After adequate preoperative preparation, left radical mastectomy and chest wall reconstruction using free deep inferior epigastric perforator flap combined with pedicled rectus abdominis myocutaneous flap were performed.

The deep inferior epigastric vessels were anastomosed with the left lateral thoracic artery and vein (1A2V). The flap was in good viability after operation, and the incision in the donor area healed well. The results of routine pathological examination showed that only very little residual cancer degeneration were found in the left breast, and no cancer was found at the cutting edge or in the axillary lymph nodes (0/13).

Radiotherapy and adjuvant systematic treatment followed, the flap survived completely, and the follow-up was satisfactory (Figs. 9.27, 9.28, 9.29, 9.30, 9.31, 9.32, 9.33, 9.34, 9.35, and 9.36).

When the conditions of donor and recipient areas are ideal, bilateral free deep inferior epigastric artery perforator flap can be selected for breast reconstruction.

If the blood vessels in the receiving area have been damaged by radiotherapy and the patients have medical diseases at the same time, the transplantation of pedicled rectus abdominis myocutaneous flap combined with free perforator flap of deep inferior epigastric artery is an ideal method of breast reconstruction.

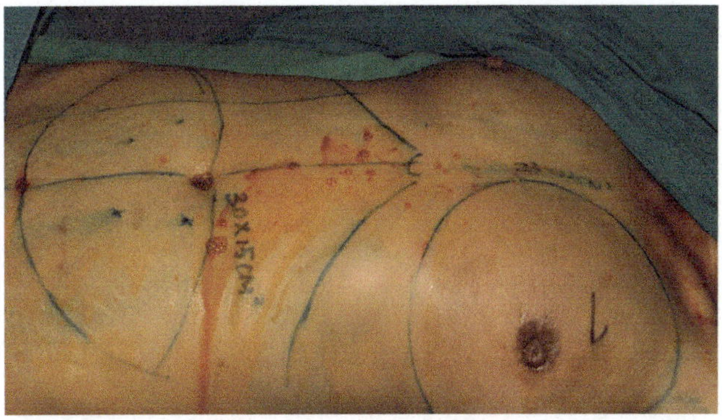

Fig. 9.27 Preoperative design

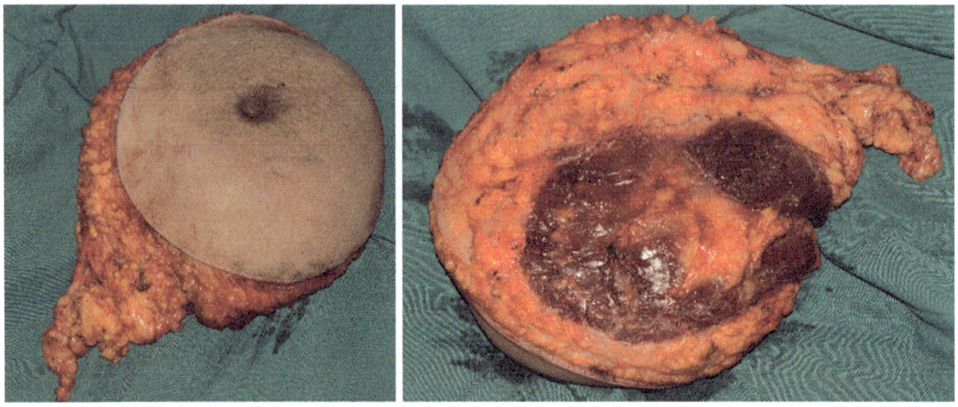

Fig. 9.28 The lesion was completely removed

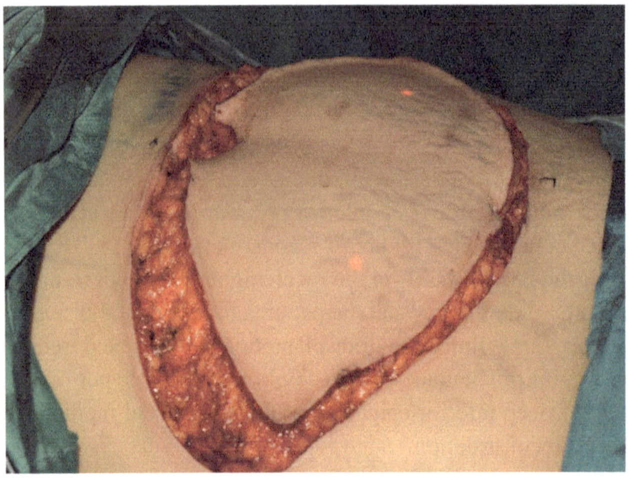

Fig. 9.29 The flap margins were all incised

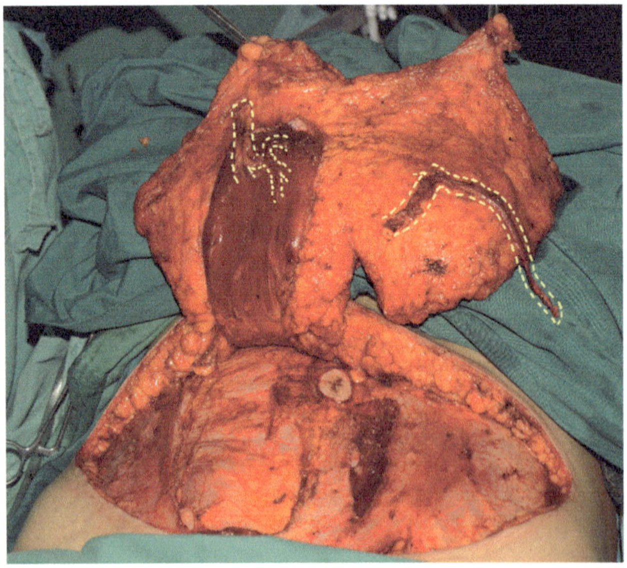

Fig. 9.30 The combined flap was harvested

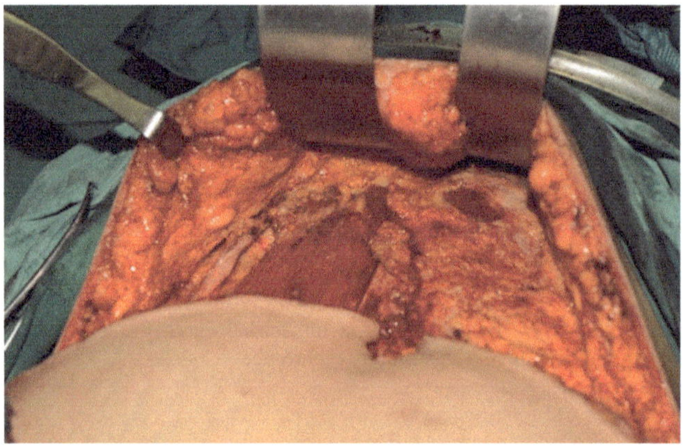

Fig. 9.31 Subcutaneous tunnel was made

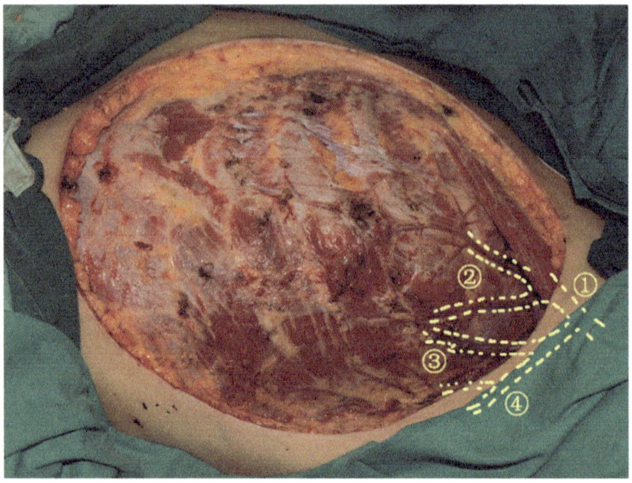

Fig. 9.32 The anterior serratus branch of thoracodorsal vessels played a recipient role. (1) Axillary vessels; (2) Lateral thoracic vessels; (3) Anterior serratus branch of thoracodorsal vessels; (4) Thoracodorsal vessels

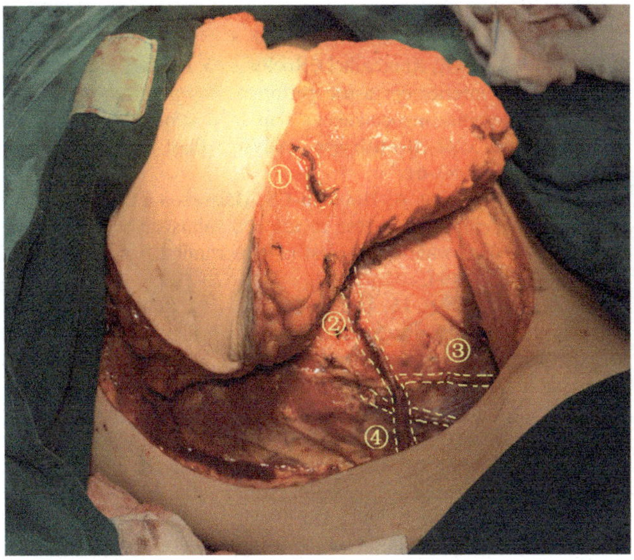

Fig. 9.33 Anastomosis of left deep inferior epigastric vessels with left anterior serratus muscle branch was conducted (1A2V). (1) Superficial epigastric vein; (2) Deep inferior epigastric vessels; (3) Lateral thoracic vessels; (4) Anterior serratus branch of thoracodorsal vessel

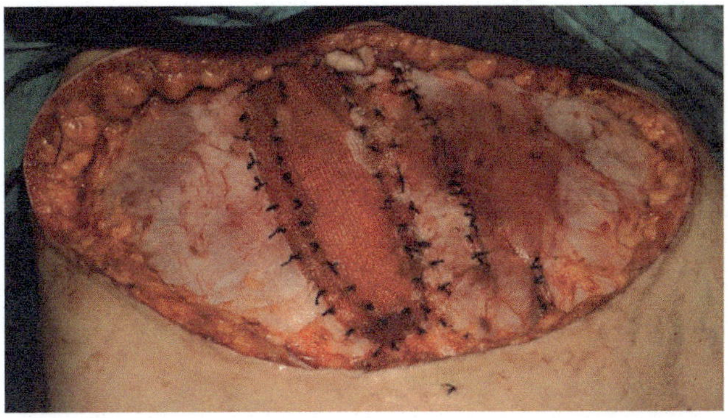

Fig. 9.34 The anterior sheath of rectus abdominis was repaired with mesh

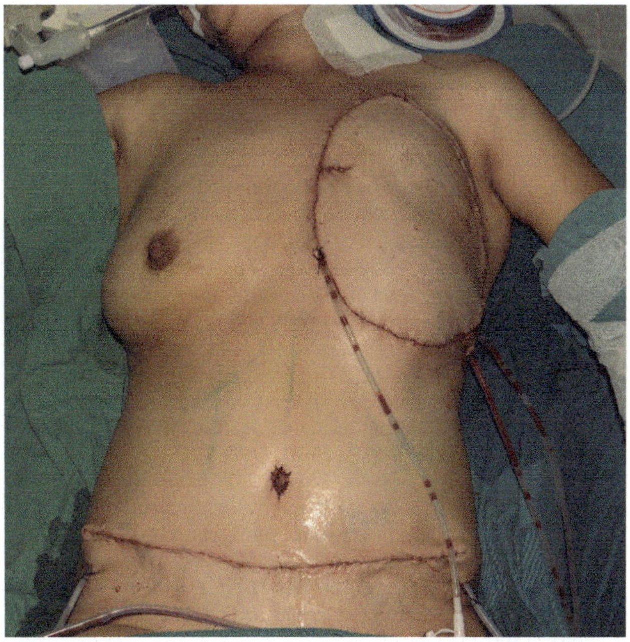

Fig. 9.35 Immediate intraoperative appearance

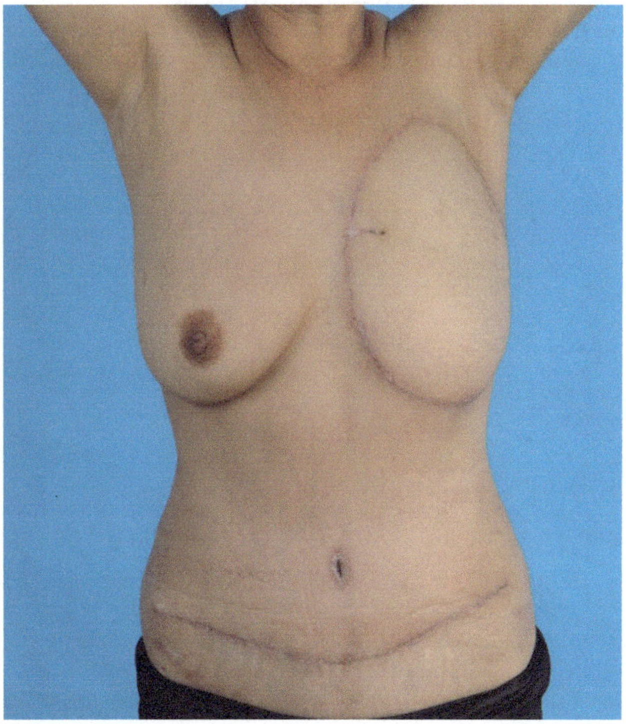

Fig. 9.36 Functional appearance after 6 months of follow-up

References

1. Berrino P, Casabona F, Adami M, Muggianu M. The "parasite" TRAM flap for autogenous tissue breast reconstruction in patients with vertical midabdominal scars. Ann Plast Surg. 1999;43(2):119–26.
2. Blondeel N, Vanderstraeten GG, Monstrey SJ, et al. The donor site morbidity of free DIEP flaps and free TRAM flaps for breast reconstruction. Br J Plast Surg. 1997;50(5):322–30.
3. Selber JC, Nelson J, Fosnot J, et al. A prospective study comparing the functional impact of SIEA, DIEP, and muscle-sparing free TRAM flaps on the abdominal wall: part I. Unilateral reconstruction. Plast Reconstr Surg. 2010;126(4):1142–53.
4. Ascherman JA, Seruya M, Bartsich SA. Abdominal wall morbidity following unilateral and bilateral breast reconstruction with pedicled TRAM flaps: an outcomes analysis of 117 consecutive patients. Plast Reconstr Surg. 2008;121(1):1–8.
5. Chun YS, Sinha I, Turko A, Lipsitz S, Pribaz JJ. Outcomes and patient satisfaction following breast reconstruction with bilateral pedicled TRAM flaps in 105 consecutive patients. Plast Reconstr Surg. 2010;125(1):1–9.
6. Gill PS, Hunt JP, Guerra AB, et al. A 10-year retrospective review of 758 DIEP flaps for breast reconstruction. Plast Reconstr Surg. 2004;113(4):1153–60.
7. Knox AD, Ho AL, Leung L, et al. Comparison of outcomes following autologous breast reconstruction using the DIEP and pedicled TRAM flaps: a 12-year clinical retrospective study and literature review. Plast Reconstr Surg. 2016;138(1):16–28.
8. Saulis AS, Mustoe TA, Fine NA. A retrospective analysis of patient satisfaction with immediate postmastectomy breast reconstruction: comparison of three common procedures. Plast Reconstr Surg. 2007;119(6):1669–76; discussion 1677–8.
9. Thoma A, Veltri K, Khuthaila D, Rockwell G, Duku E. Comparison of the deep inferior epigastric perforator flap and free transverse rectus abdominis myocutaneous flap in postmastectomy reconstruction: a cost-effectiveness analysis. Plast Reconstr Surg. 2004;113(6):1650–61.
10. Tong WM, Bazakas A, Hultman CS, Halvorson EG. The transition from pedicle transverse rectus abdominis myocutaneous to perforator flap: what is the cost of opportunity. Ann Plast Surg. 2012;68(5):489–94.
11. Cheng MH, Robles JA, Ulusal BG, Wei FC. Reliability of zone IV in the deep inferior epigastric perforator flap: a single center's experience with 74 cases. Breast. 2006;15(2):158–66.
12. Atisha D, Alderman AK. A systematic review of abdominal wall function following abdominal flaps for postmastectomy breast reconstruction. Ann Plast Surg. 2009;63(2):222–30.
13. Feingold RS. Improving surgeon confidence in the DIEP flap: a strategy for reducing operative time with minimally invasive donor site. Ann Plast Surg. 2009;62(5):533–7.
14. Chun YS, Sinha I, Turko A, et al. Comparison of morbidity, functional outcome, and satisfaction following bilateral TRAM versus bilateral DIEP flap breast reconstruction. Plast Reconstr Surg. 2010;126(4):1133–41.
15. Venkat R, Lee JC, Rad AN, Manahan MA, Rosson GD. Bilateral autologous breast reconstruction with deep inferior epigastric artery perforator flaps: review of a single surgeon's early experience. Microsurgery. 2012;32(4):275–80.
16. Lindsey JT. Integrating the DIEP and muscle-sparing (MS-2) free TRAM techniques optimizes surgical outcomes: presentation of an algorithm for microsurgical breast reconstruction based on perforator anatomy. Plast Reconstr Surg. 2007;119(1):18–27.

Strategies for Improving Venous Drainage in DIEP Flap for Chest Wall and Breast Reconstruction

10

Zan Li and Georgios Pafitanis

10.1 Introduction

Venous congestion is caused by the inconsistence between the blood output and the total blood input of the flap that cannot be fully compensated.

Common causes include insufficient perfusion of the venous network, tension of the recipient area, postoperative swelling of the flap, thrombosis, and vascular pedicle compression or vascular pedicle spasm.

Venous problems are still a common vascular complication in breast reconstruction using free tissue transplantation [1].

It is reported that the incidence of venous congestion of DIEP flap is about 4–20%, in the early stage, flap congestion is caused by the venous system overburden by blood input from the artery.

As the congestion problem persists, the arterial pressure rises beyond the normal capillary pressure causing the capillaries to bleed, making the flap look purple, yet the flap is still probably viable [2].

Blondeel et al. [3] reported serial cases of DIEP flap failure that were all caused by venous reflux disorder.

Many other scholars have also made many similar reports in this regard [4].

In nine patients with venous congestion at our center, 60% occurred before the disconnection of the vascular pedicle, and the other 40% occurred after microsurgical anastomosis or even after the completion of the operation.

In the process of cutting the perforator flap of the deep inferior epigastric artery, the function of the severed superficial venous system cannot be fully compensated by the deep venous system, resulting in venous congestion of the flap [5].

Z. Li (✉)
Department of Oncology Plastic Surgery, Hunan Cancer Hospital, Changsha, Hunan, China

G. Pafitanis
Trauma, Orthoplastic, Lower Extremity and Head and Neck Reconstruction Center, London, UK

Studies have shown that venous congestion has a greater impact on the effective flap area than arterial perfusion. Therefore, some scholars have proposed that dissecting the bilateral venous system in the early stage can significantly improve the viability rate [6, 7].

Different methods of anastomosing additional blood vessels to promote venous reflux are applied. Specific options include:

1. The concomitant vein of ipsilateral deep inferior epigastric artery [8, 9].
2. The concomitant vein of contralateral deep inferior epigastric artery [10].
3. Ipsilateral superficial epigastric vein [6].
4. Contralateral superficial epigastric vein [4].

The basis for deciding whether to use additional venous anastomosis to improve venous reflux for the flap includes:

1. Whether there is a suitable vein in the recipient area to match the vein in the flap.
2. Whether the superficial subcutaneous vein retained on the flap before the pedicle disconnection was enlarged or overfilled.
3. Whether there is obvious venous congestion after flap vascular anastomosis [11].

In order to increase the operation safety, reduce the operation risk and complications, and shorten the operation duration, whether and which of the superficial epigastric vein should be reserved for additional anastomosis should be considered in the preoperative design and during operation.

It is preferred to anastomose the contralateral superficial epigastric vein; if it is absent, the ipsilateral superficial epigastric vein can also be used [11].

The lateral thoracic vein, anterior serratus branch of thoracodorsal vein or distal thoracic acromial vein, and internal thoracic vein are common recipient vessels. A reasonable

Z. Li, D. Song (eds.), *Oncoplastic Flap Surgery*, https://doi.org/10.1007/978-981-19-8926-1_10

plan of flap venous augmentation requires little additional time and no additional auxiliary incision.

In addition, the placement and length of vascular pedicle also needs to be considered. Generally, when the internal thoracic vessels are connected with the flap pedicle, the anastomosis between the superficial epigastric vein and the lateral thoracic vein or the anterior serratus branch of the thoracodorsal vein or the thoracoacromial vein is relatively easy; when the lateral thoracic vessels are connected with the flap pedicle, the anastomosis between the superficial epigastric vein and all the internal and external veins in the recipient area is feasible.

In some extreme cases, when bilateral superficial epigastric veins are required, vascular bridging can be used to make up for the insufficiency in the vascular pedicle length [12].

10.2 Anatomy Essentials

There are some important steps that can help prevent venous congestion in the process of cutting the flap, and can also deal with the flap congestion at later stage.

The deep venous drainage system of the DIEP flap lies above the Scarpa's fascia and 4–6 cm lateral to the ventral midline. It is composed of the deep venous system including deep inferior epigastric veins (DIEV) and the concomitant veins of the arterial pedicle and the superficial venous system including the superficial deep inferior epigastric vein (SIEV).

Soon after flap raising is started, the superficial deep inferior epigastric vein should be seriously taken care of.

As soon as the flap skin is cut open, carefully identify the SIEVs in the subcutaneous fat layer.

Blood vessels with a diameter of 1–3 mm and a length of 7–10 cm can be dissected downward in the area where operation has not been performed before.

The SIEV should be separated till the maximum diameter and length of the vessel is obtained. If necessary, venous grafting can be used to improve venous drainage.

Next, the operator needs to carefully identify a perforator of appropriate size and protect the vascular pedicle that includes the deep inferior epigastric vein (DIEV).

The DIEV should be harvested as long as possible just in case it is needed in supercharge or to communicate the SIEV and recipient vein.

When the superficial epigastric vein is prepared, the subsequent steps are equal to that of a DIEP flap raising.

10.3 Preoperative Management

For any operation, the selection of appropriate patients is key.

In the process of asking the medical history, we should ask in advance whether there is a history of existing lower abdominal scar, and make sure that the scar is located in the midline, paramedian, or transverse scar, so as to prevent the need to switch to the application of superficial abdominal vein. The history and position (midline, paramedian, or transverse) of lower abdominal scar should be investigated before operation to evaluate the utility of SIEV.

In theory, previous abdominal scar may either lead to "delayed viability" of the flap or improve blood supply.

The previous transverse incision left after caesarean section might compromise bilateral SIEV, so patients with this scar are not suitable candidates for SIEV flap.

In addition, understanding the feasibility of other potential recipient vessels, such as thoracodorsal vessels, will be conducive to intraoperative decision-making.

Finally, it is also important to understand any coagulation problems that may affect the reconstruction of free flap before operation.

Informed consent is required for all candidates, including from after they are fully informed, including consent to vein grafting and additional donor incision and scar that may appear if additional recipient veins are needed to be communicated with.

At the same time, patients should be informed that if complications occur during recovery, the time for accomplishing breast reconstruction will be extended.

Finally, patients are informed that perioperative blood transfusion is likely required especially when reducing flap congestion without microsurgery.

10.4 Intraoperative Management

Early manifestations of venous congestion must be paid attention to. Microsurgeons should be highly alert to and identify flap crisis as early as possible because local ischemia is crucial to the viability of transplanted tissue.

Arterial ischemia and venous congestion will affect the flap viability. Abnormal changes of flap should be identified in the early stage.

After the separation of the vascular pedicle, do not hurry to ligate and disconnect it. First evaluate the arterial blood supply and venous drainage before jumping to disconnect the freed vascular pedicle, and then decide in advance whether to anastomose other veins to promote the flap reflux.

Injury to vascular pedicle and ignorance of small branches must be identified and handled in time.

Venous reflux disorder of flap is solved by combing and problem-shooting.

Choosing the vein most capable of drainage for anastomosis is particularly important for large flap.

In fact, in most cases, the manifestations regarding poor venous drainage can be easily identified during the operation (Fig. 10.1) [13]. If it is hard to tell, temporary switch-off of surgical light can be helpful (Fig. 10.2).

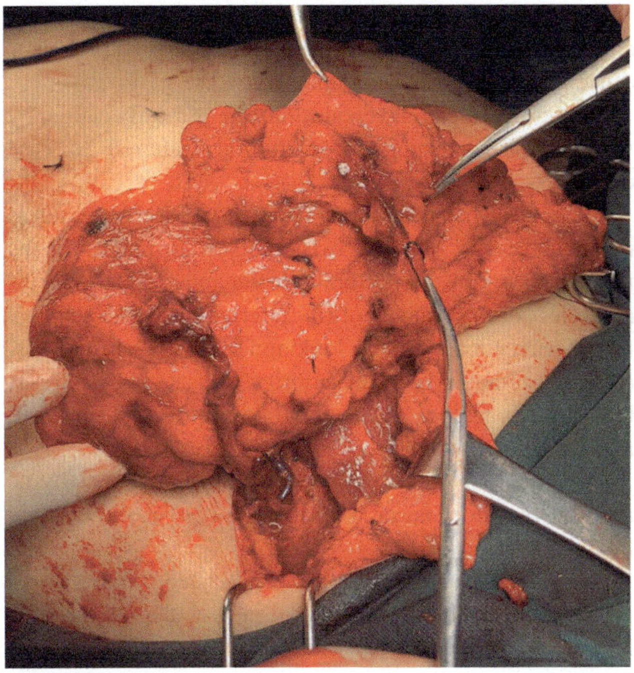

Fig. 10.1 When the vascular pedicle of DIEP flap was revascularized, blood input of the flap overwhelmed output, which was represented by overfilled and enlarged superficial epigastric veins

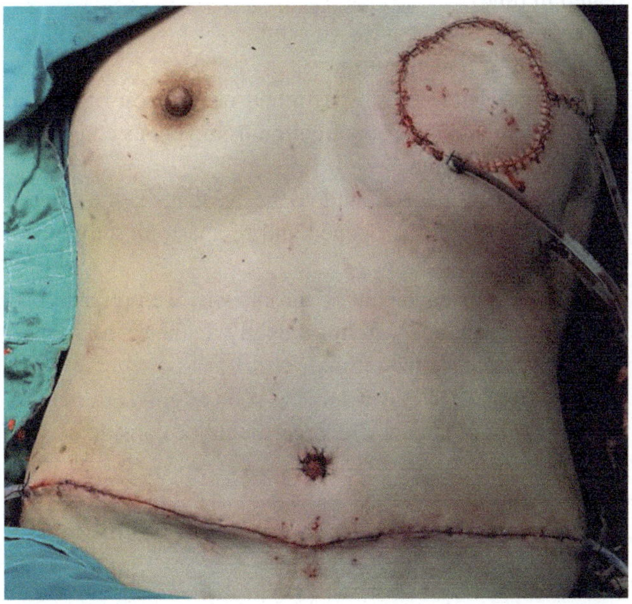

Fig. 10.2 Appearance of venous congestion during operation with surgical light off

In Cheng's study, signs of venous congestion were present in all of ten patients with venous congestion during operation.

We can perform auxiliary examination by removing the surgical light from the operation area. During the cutting process, the damaged vascular pedicle must be identified and repaired.

The vein good at drainage is the best candidate for anastomosis.

A large vein is usually responsible for blood output of an extensive tissue area. This anatomical basis is particularly critical when using the larger deep inferior epigastric artery perforator flap in the contralateral medial and lateral area.

When the vascular pedicle is freed yet disconnected from the donor area, looking for early signals of venous congestion of the flap can remind doctors of venous exploration. When conservative treatment and surgical exploration do not work, the flap should be abandoned and resort to other methods.

10.5 Management of Venous Congestion

This section systematically introduces and summarizes the continuous steps to solve the problem of venous congestion of flap.

10.5.1 Microscopic Exploration

The reason of venous congestion is the key to solve the problem with appropriate strategies.

Surgical exploration is crucial for revealing the causes of venous congestion unless flap crisis related to blood supply takes place. Given that flap congestion is basically by surgical manipulation, it generally requires surgery [2].

The best timing for surgical intervention is during the same operation. Previous reports have proved that the incidence of complications is greatly reduced in cases handled during operation rather than those after operation [13] (Fig. 10.3).

10.5.2 Pressure Reduction

Increased venous pressure and crisis caused by hematoma can be found early in operation.

Even hematoma near the drainage tube within a closed wound is likely to cause flap crisis that should be addressed in time.

Vascular pedicle compression is likely to occur when a large DIEP flap is placed on the stone-hard chest wall or inside a highly tense chest skin envelope due to radiotherapy in patients receiving delayed breast reconstruction.

10.5.3 Flap Trimming

If the flap size is significantly larger than that of the removed breast, excessive tension induced by direct closure can also

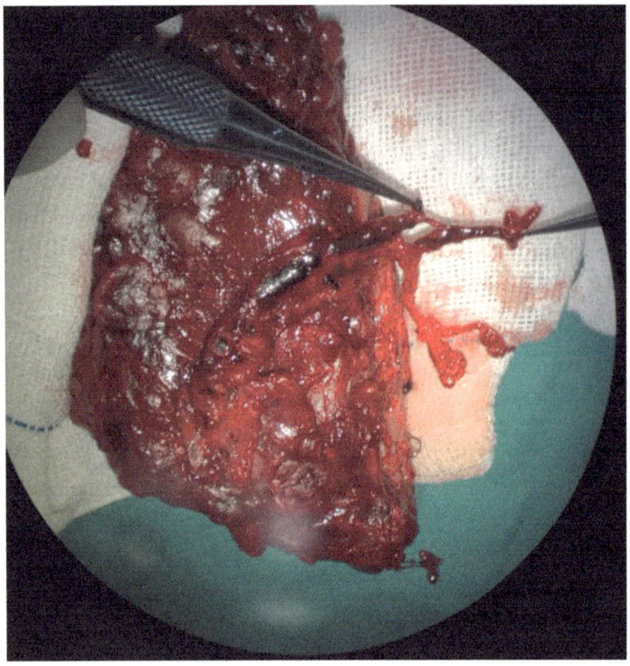

Fig. 10.3 Immediate intraoperative exploration found that the vein responsible for venous drainage of the flap was not completely isolated and compressed, resulting in congestion

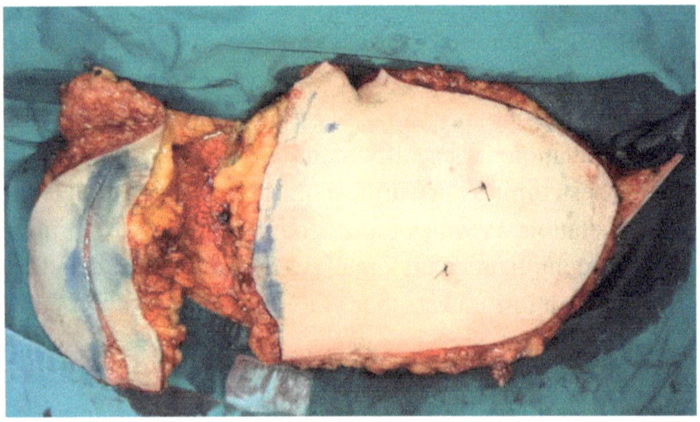

Fig. 10.4 Before the vascular pedicle was broken off, the congestion part of the flap identified by fluorescence angiography as light-dark appearance was removed

cause flap crisis. This can be settled by reducing the amount of flap tissue before placement.

The congested area of the flap can be evaluated by ICG fluorography. When congestion appearing in Area IV or contralateral lateral area, it can be solved by removal, resulting with reduced venous load and improved blood circulation of the whole flap (Fig. 10.4). Refer to the DIEP + SIEAPF case example.

10.5.4 Replacement of Vascular Pedicle

When vascular anastomosis is completed, the blood flow patency test should be carried out at the proximal and distal ends of veins and arteries to verify the anastomotic patency.

Although the free vascular pedicle is very fragile, it usually becomes the most stable part after vascular anastomosis, especially when vascular coupler is used.

Therefore, impaired venous drainage is mostly caused by vascular pedicle injury or distortion (referred to case examples).

However, when the internal mammary vessels are used as recipient vessels, vascular twist is likely to happen at the junction between the pectoralis major muscle and the ribs regardless of the removal of rib (referred to case examples). Under such circumstances, looking for the presence of vascular twist should be given priority. Repeated anastomosis before verifying the cause will not be helpful, instead it will make the situation worse.

If vasospasm occurs during operation, it can usually be relieved by lidocaine or by removing part of the external fiber.

Venous congestion can also be mitigated by injecting a great quantity of heparinized saline into the flap venous pedicle to dilate the venous network and rebuild venous drainage.

The operator should try these treatments immediately to restore the natural physiological state of the flap.

At the same time, arterial crisis must be identified and treated in time.

In arterial crisis, excessive outflow of blood flow is not related to insufficient inflow.

But once there is vasospasm and obstruction of arterial inflow, we should shift our attention from venous congestion to anastomotic stoma.

If venous reflux is found to be weakened, the arterial anastomosis should be opened and re-anastomosed with or without venous grafting.

Regarding management of thrombosis, we prefer to perform thrombectomy without Fogarty catheter assistance, which may damage the intima.

Venous drainage may resume as soon as good arterial perfusion is built, if not, supercharge should be considered.

10.5.5 Selection and Preparation of Recipient Vessels

The addition of a vessel candidate in the recipient area increases blood output of a DIEP flap and further improves the venous drainage [14] (Fig. 10.5).

First, it is necessary to determine the patency and viability of the proximal and distal internal thoracic vein (IMV). If it is in good condition, the distal vein can be used to improve the flap reflux (Fig. 10.6). In contrast, we need to look for other vessel candidates for revascularization aiming to guarantee the vascular patency of the flap (Fig. 10.7).

If the blood vessels in the receiving area are in poor condition, a pedicled TRAM flap with supercharged venous

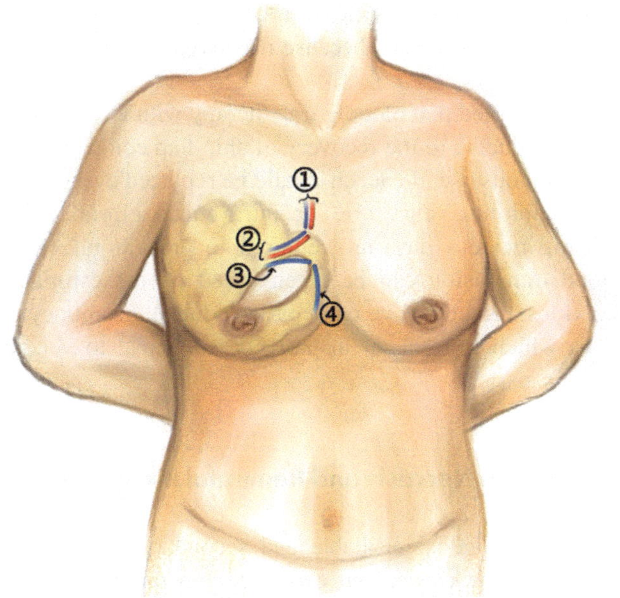

Fig. 10.5 Venous reflux is improved by anastomosis of the accompanying vein of the deep inferior epigastric artery with the distal end of the internal thoracic vein. (1) Proximal end of internal thoracic artery and vein; (2) Deep inferior epigastric artery and accompanying vein; (3) The other concomitant vein of deep inferior epigastric artery; (4) Distal internal thoracic vein

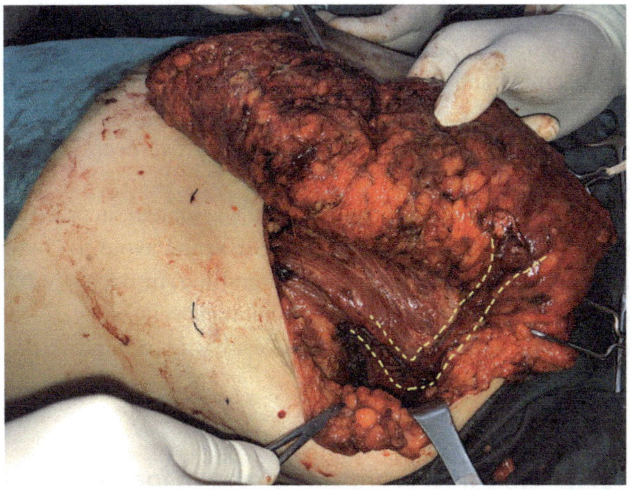

Fig. 10.7 Insufficient venous drainage was improved by additional vascular anastomosis using thoracoacromial vein

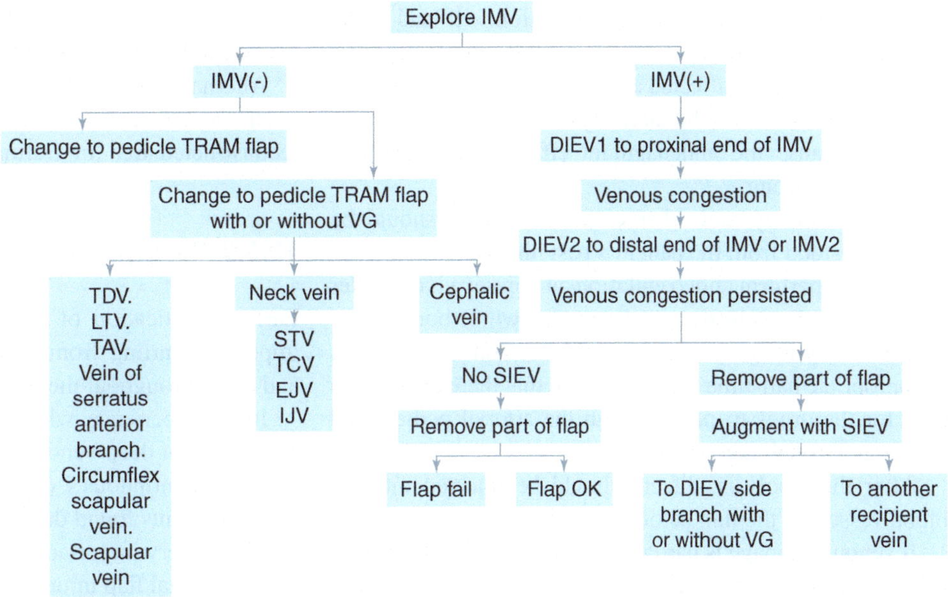

Fig. 10.6 The decision-making process of treating venous congestion of DIEP flap. *DIEP* deep inferior epigastric artery, *DIEV* deep inferior epigastric vein, *EJV* external jugular vein, *IJV* internal jugular vein, *Ima* internal thoracic artery, *IMV* internal thoracic vein, *SIEA* superficial epigastric artery, *SIEV* superficial epigastric vein, *STV* superior thyroid vein, *TCV* transverse jugular vein, *TDV* thoracodorsal vein, *TRAM* transverse rectus abdominis, *VG* venous grafting. (Reprinted from Perforator Flaps for Breast Reconstruction)

drainage using superficial epigastric vein rather than a DIEP flap is recommended [13].

In addition, repair with the pedicled latissimus dorsi flap is commonly used for salvage in breast reconstruction, besides, the thoracodorsal vessel is an alternative recipient vessel to improve the blood supply of the flap.

10.5.6 Flexible Application of Superficial Epigastric Vein

The addition of a vein from the donor site to increase flap blood outflow can effectively improve the venous drainage [15].

Studies have confirmed that the superficial venous system composed of superficial epigastric veins is critical in the management and prevention of venous congestion, which is better solved by anastomosing SIEV than by connecting a second concomitant vein of DIEA to improve deep venous reflux [9, 10, 14, 16].

When the number of recipient veins is limited, in order to make up for the limited length of SIEV and avoid the prolonged anesthesia time due to vein grafting, turbocharge by communicating SIEV with a concomitant vein of DIEA in end-to-side pattern is a simple and easy way to improve the venous reflux of the flap [17].

Another method is to leave a vein open, yet this is not routinely recommended because it is easy to cause serious blood loss.

It is reported that bloodletting therapy with leech can be more conducive to the recovery of skin flap congestion; if in continuous use, the leech should be replaced every hour, and antibiotics (e.g., oral or intravenous ciprofloxacin 500 mg twice a day) are required to prevent infection. Blood transfusion can be given based on the estimated blood loss. Keep an eye on heparin-induced thrombocytopenia which is frequent in patients subjective to venous thrombosis.

10.5.7 Non-microsurgical Approach for Flap Salvage

If flap crisis cannot be settled by microsurgical approach, non-microsurgical methods should be attempted before giving up the flap.

Thrombolytic therapy is indicated when thrombus occurs in branches distal to the vascular pedicle of the flap beyond resection. This thrombus can occur in different levels of vascular branches, including those constituting microcirculation.

In addition, persistent venous congestion will lead to the arterial crisis, which can progress to flap crisis requiring intervention with the affected artery.

The indications must be carefully evaluated before thrombolysis, because the anticoagulant effect of thrombolytic drugs is very strong.

Medical allergy and other contraindications should be well understood from the patient's past history.

We often perform anticoagulation on flaps ex vivo to deter thrombolytic drugs from spreading to the whole body.

Thrombolytic agents such as urokinase and streptokinase of appropriate half-time period are used that there are enough time for the drugs to pass through the arterial pedicle and discharge through the venous pedicle.

After thrombolysis, diluent should be injected into the blood vessels of the flap before re-anastomosis.

If venous drainage is partially restored, the venous flow in the congested flap can be improved by the de-epithelized skin island.

A week later, compensatory vessels grow and introduce congested blood out slowly through the microcirculatory vein to improve the flap congestion.

If bloodletting therapy from the margins of the de-epithelized flap or with leech is used, it is required to wipe the skin with heparin-soaked gauze at bedside every hour after operation to prevent blood coagulation and ensure continuous venous outflow.

10.5.8 Flap Necrosis and Remedial Measures

If flap abortion is inevitable and secondary operation is expected to be carried out early after operation, vacuum-assisted cleaner (VAC) is an option to cover the wound for temporary purpose.

A large skin island is required for wound closure and avoids contraction of the wound edge and the expansion of the defect.

However, if the latissimus dorsi flap is planned to be used for repair in the later stage, VAC is generally not considered, because it needs to cut a skin island as large as the DIEP flap making it difficult to close the donor area.

Alternatively, the skin can be taken from the necrotic flap itself or the contralateral abdominal flap in the non-reconstructed area for grafting.

10.5.9 Postoperative Management

Early identification of venous obstruction is always very important starting from vessel separation and anastomosis and even throughout the postoperative recovery period.

In our experience, when heparin is used for treatment and prevention of deep venous thrombosis, the treatment will be given for continuous 7 days postoperatively in patients with vascular events found during the operation.

This is very important for preventing potential hematoma and accidental flap injury.

In addition, squeezing the flap must be avoided when placing the dressing and abdominal restraint.

Once venous obstruction is suspected, primary measures include removing the suture and adjusting the flap position and patient position.

Generally speaking, once venous congestion is suspected, emergency surgical exploration should be considered without hesitation (Fig. 10.8).

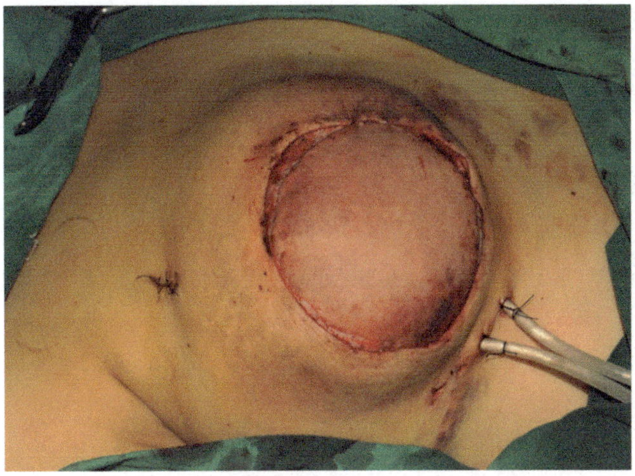

Fig. 10.8 Venous congestion occurred in the perforator flap of inferior abdominal artery after operation and was solved by emergency surgical exploration

Transplantation of perforator flap of deep inferior epigastric artery with increasing flow of superficial vein on the contralateral epigastric wall typical Case 1.

10.6 Case 1: A DIEP Flap Supercharged Using Ipsilateral Superficial Epigastric Vein

A 41-year-old female patient with right breast mass found for more than 10 days was admitted.

Pathological examination of the excised tumor showed that the histological grade of invasive ductal carcinoma (right breast) was grade II–III with regional invasive lobular carcinoma (as shown in Fig. 10.9).

The patient underwent right modified radical mastectomy plus breast reconstruction using free DIEP flap. The size of the flap was about 36 cm × 13 cm in size (as shown in Fig. 10.10).

The right superficial epigastric vein at a length of about 7 cm was retained.

The left deep inferior epigastric vessels were anastomosed end-to-end with the right thoracoacromial arteriovenous branches (1A2V).

Postoperative pathological results: (1) No residual cancer was found in the right breast; (2) No cancer metastasis was found in 13 right axillary lymph nodes. (3) No cancer was found in skin margins, nipple, and basal margin.

Pathological stage pT2N0M0 IIA.

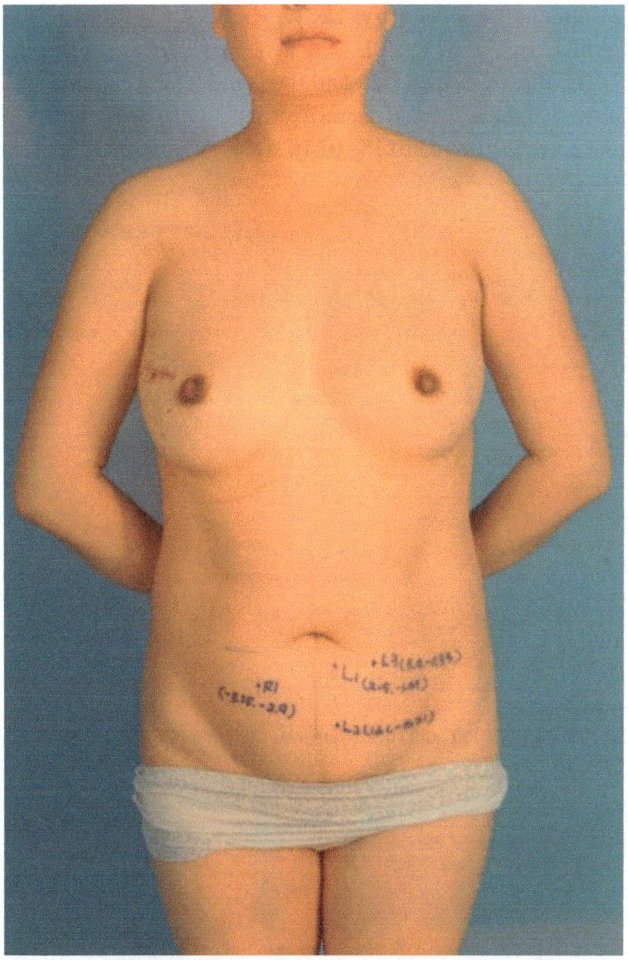

Fig. 10.9 Pre-operation viewing

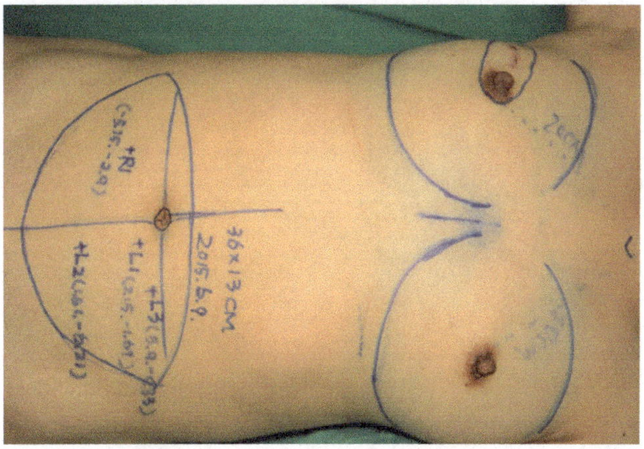

Fig. 10.10 The flap was designed based on the number and position of perforating branches in lower abdomen according to preoperative CTA

Immunohistochemistry: ER (2 +, 30%), PR (2 +, 35%), CerbB-2 (−), Ki67 (10%).

The flaps survived well and the patients' appearance and function recovered satisfactorily (Figs. 10.9, 10.10, 10.11, 10.12, 10.13, 10.14, 10.15, 10.16, 10.17, and 10.18).

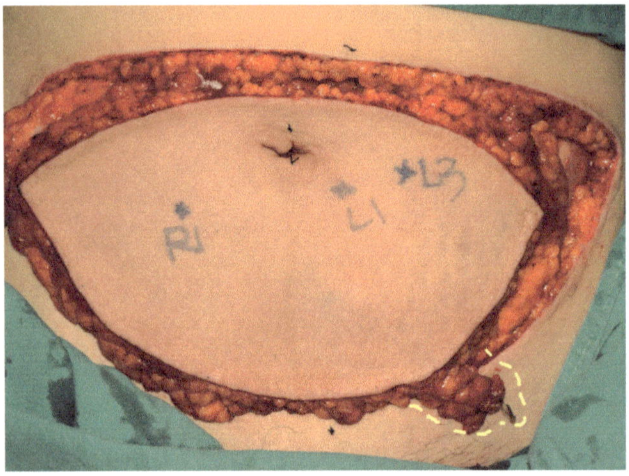

Fig. 10.11 The left superficial vein was included in the flap

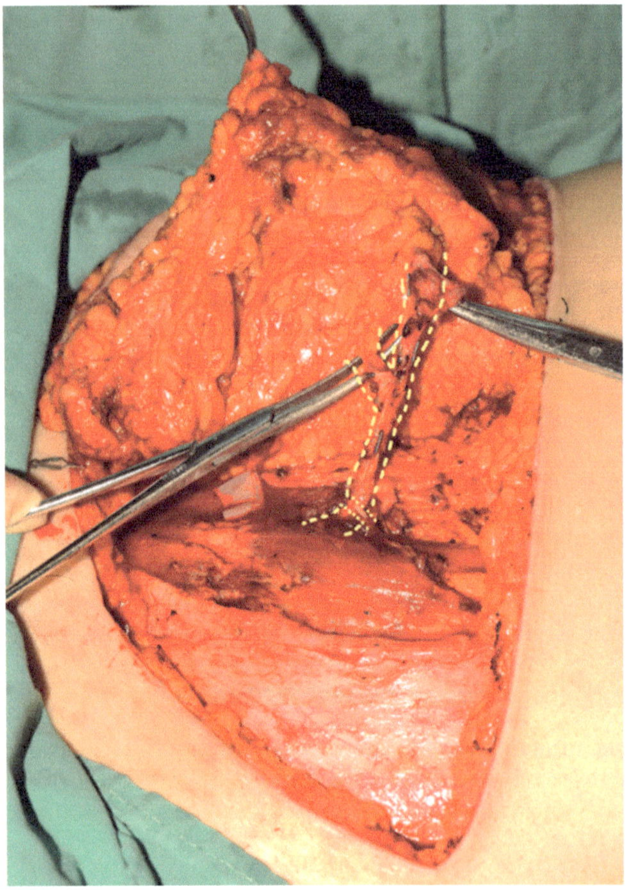

Fig. 10.12 A long segment of the left epigastric perforator and vascular pedicle was separated

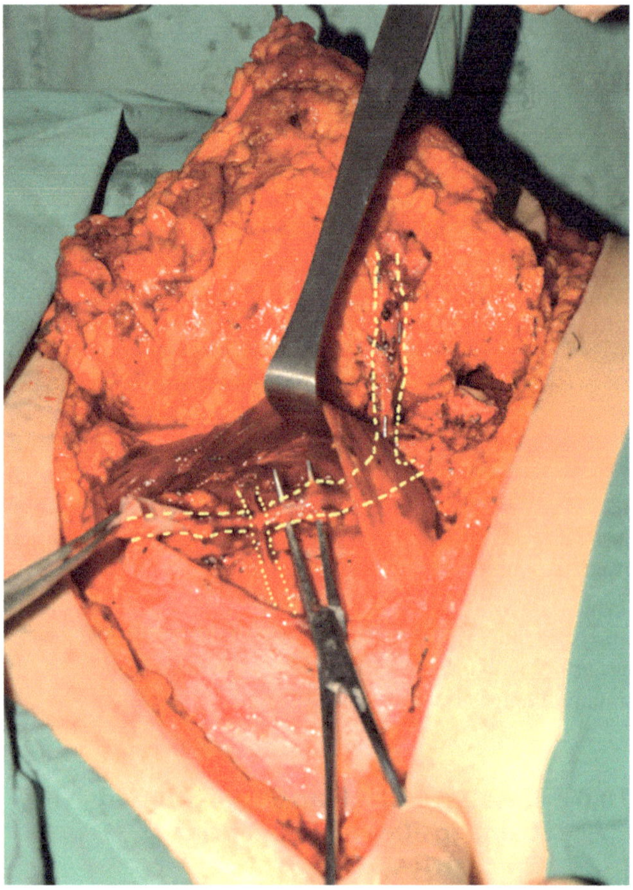

Fig. 10.13 The left vascular pedicle was separated to the greatest extent and the integrity of intercostal nerve was preserved

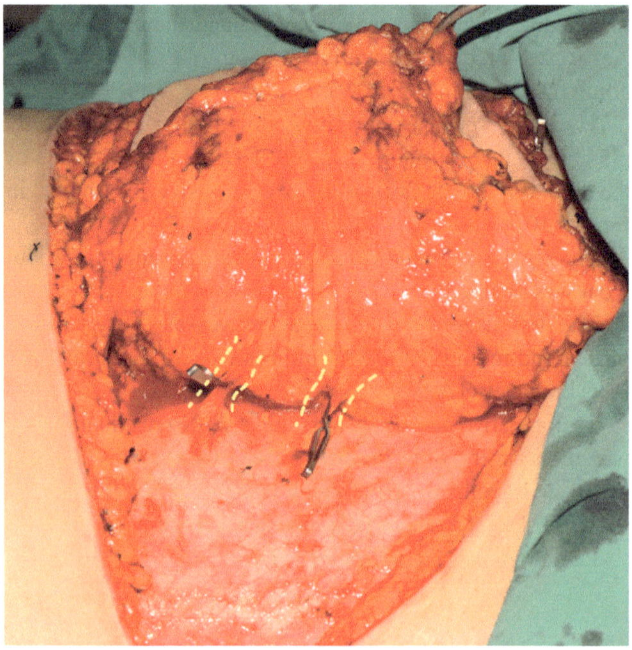

Fig. 10.14 The right perforator was exposed. Clamping test confirmed that the blood supply of the flap was reliable. The right perforator was ligated and disconnected

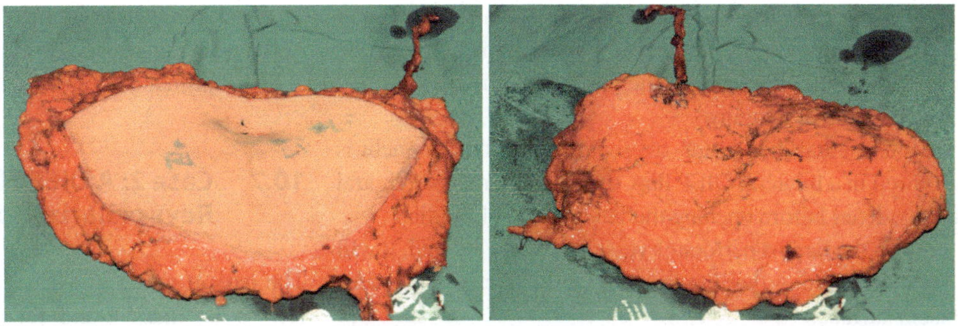

Fig. 10.15 Flap harvest was finished

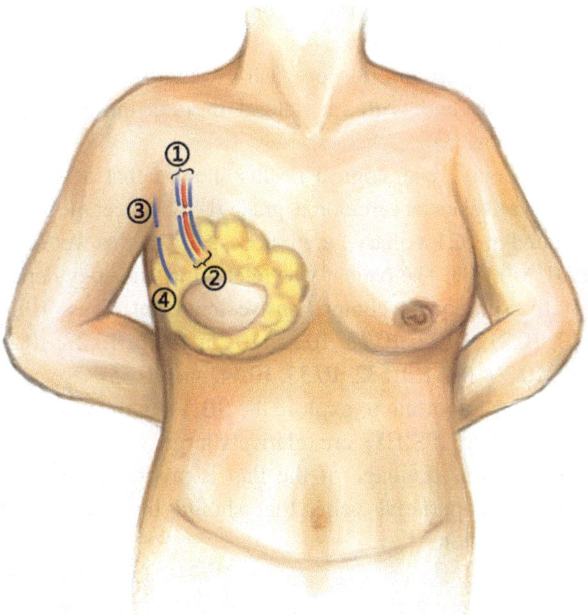

Fig. 10.16 End-to-end anastomosis (1A2V) was performed between the left deep inferior epigastric vessels and the right thoracoacromial arteriovenous branch. After vascular anastomosis, the flap was significantly perfused, and the left superficial epigastric vein was anastomosed with the left lateral thoracic vein. (1) Thoracic acromial vessels; (2) Deep inferior epigastric vessels; (3) Lateral thoracic vein; (4) Superficial epigastric vein

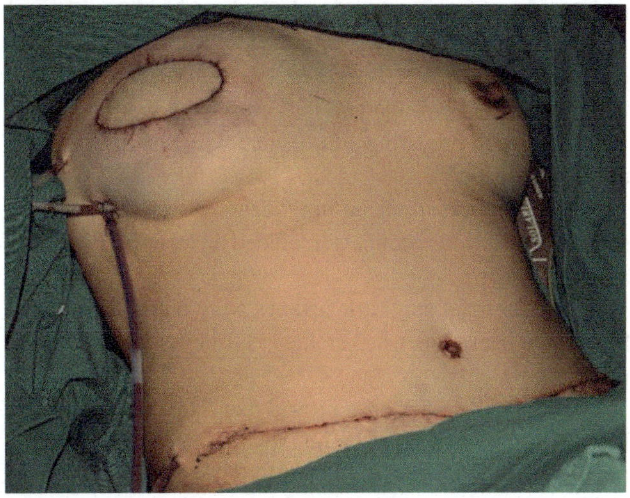

Fig. 10.17 Immediately after operation

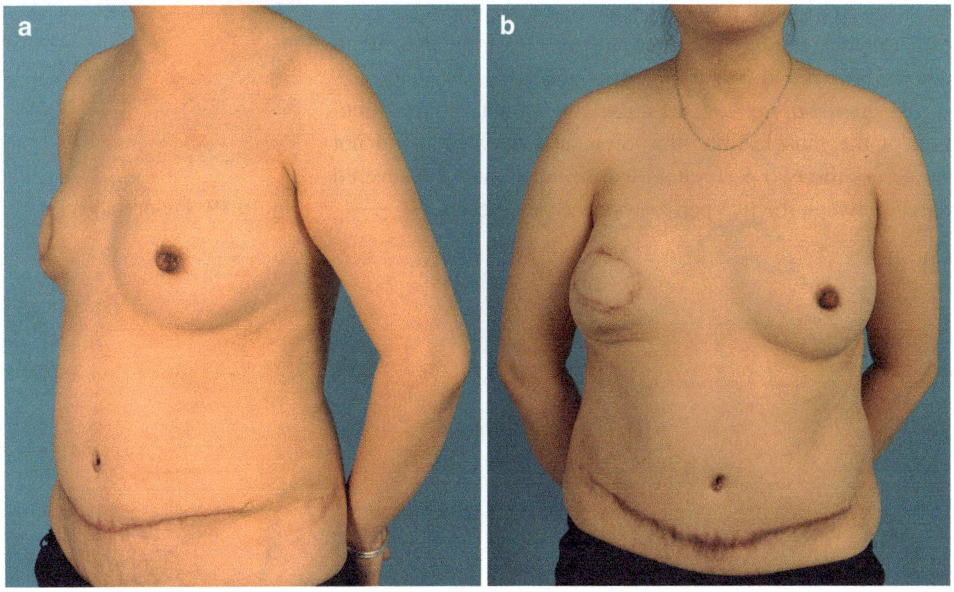

Fig. 10.18 (**a**) 6-month follow-up; (**b**) 24-month follow-up

The first step of preparing the flap is to make an incision along the marked line, cut the skin open till the anterior fascia, and lift the flap. Dissect the perforator if it is confirmed by preoperative imaging.

If a medial perforator or septal cutaneous branch is required in a bilateral DIEP flap, the perforator vessel should be dissected before opening the lateral edge of the flap.

Once the largest perforator vessel is clearly located, it will facilitate opening the flap from the lower rectus abdominis fascia surface.

It should be noted that perforating branches except the main perforator are scattered, which should be kept in mind in finding the superficial epigastric vessels beneath the incision.

It is particularly important to preserve the superficial epigastric veins in preparing a DIEP flap with venous drainage dominated by SIEV.

Although the superficial epigastric vessels are not constant, it should be routinely included in planning a lower abdominal flap.

The superficial epigastric arteries were dissected prior to SIEVs to determine whether they can be used as vascular pedicle [18].

Anatomical studies have proved that the venous reflux of the lower abdomen is predominantly delivered by the superficial veins; based on this, bilateral SIEVs should be carried routinely in the flap [2].

The perforator is separated under magnifying glasses. The first step is to open the anterior sheath of rectus abdominis around the selected perforator.

Some surgeons often retain a 1–2 mm wide sheath around the perforating branch.

Then, all small branches were carefully separated or electrocoagulated along the rectus abdominis muscle by micro scissors or bipolar electrocoagulation.

It is especially important to note that if the second- or third-level perforating branches are selected, we must pay attention to its continuity with the source perforator.

Similarly, preoperative imaging is also very helpful in determining blood vessels.

During the dissection, the muscle was cut along the direction of the muscle fiber, the intercostal nerve that did not crisscross the two perforators was retained, and the severed nerve between the two perforators was repaired.

Separation was continued downward until the main trunk of the deep epigastric vessels were unveiled.

The optimal length of vascular pedicle is 8–10 cm.

10.7 Case 2: A DIEP Flap with SIEV Revascularization

The patient was a 37-year-old female who complained of a left breast mass found for 2 years. It was diagnosed on lumpectomy as invasive carcinoma of left breast.

Left modified radical mastectomy plus breast reconstruction using free DIEP flap.

The left deep inferior epigastric vessels were anastomosed end-to-end with the lateral thoracic arteriovenous branches (1A2V).

Postoperative pathological results showed that it was left breast invasive ductal carcinoma, grade II–III; cancer metastasis was found in 1/21 axillary lymph nodes; all margins were clear (pT2N1M0,IIB). The patient was referred to oncology department for subsequent comprehensive treatment (Figs. 10.19, 10.20, 10.21, 10.22, 10.23, 10.24, 10.25, 10.26, 10.27, 10.28, 10.29, 10.30, 10.31, 10.32, 10.33, 10.34, and 10.35).

It is very important to explore the SIEVs in the process of cutting the flap. If SIEVs are relatively large, which indicates that the venous drainage of the flap is predominantly performed by superficial veins that should be prepared for revascularization.

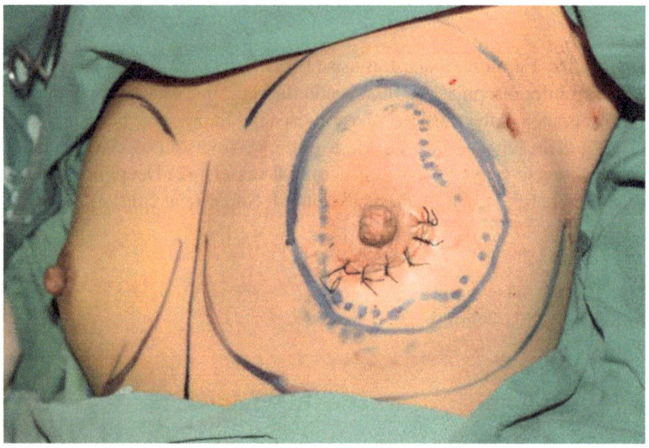

Fig. 10.19 Pre-operation

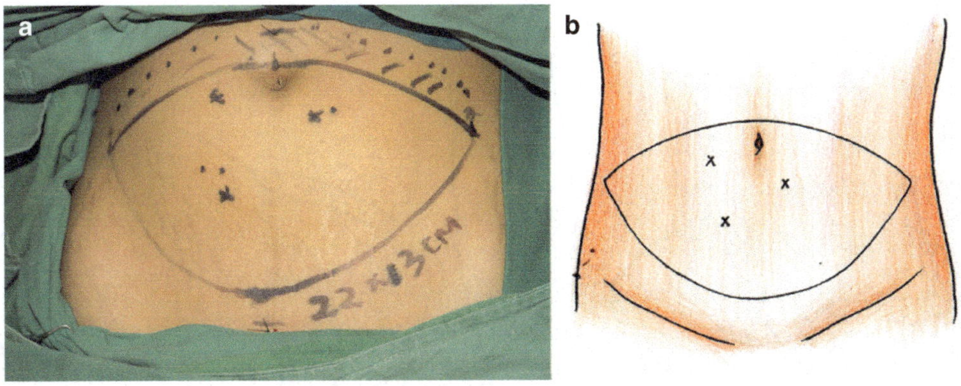

Fig. 10.20 (a, b) Design of a DIEP flap. "X" stands for the perforator position determined by preoperative Doppler probe

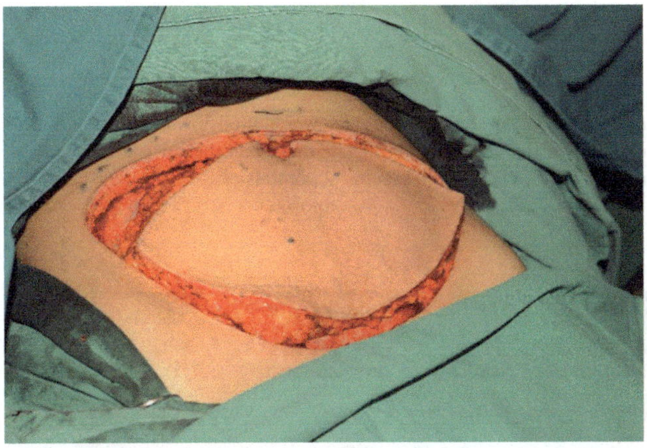

Fig. 10.21 The margin of the flap was cut

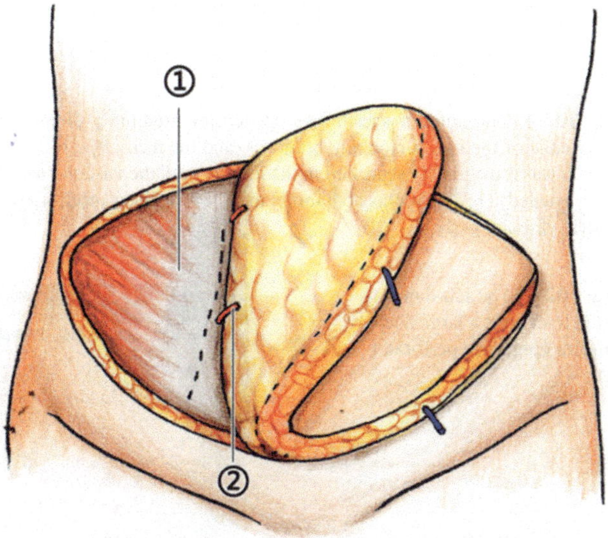

Fig. 10.23 The right flap was lifted from the aponeurosis surface of external oblique abdominal muscle to expose the two perforating branches on the surface of anterior sheath of rectus abdominis muscle. (1) Aponeurosis of external oblique abdominal muscle; (2) Perforating vessels

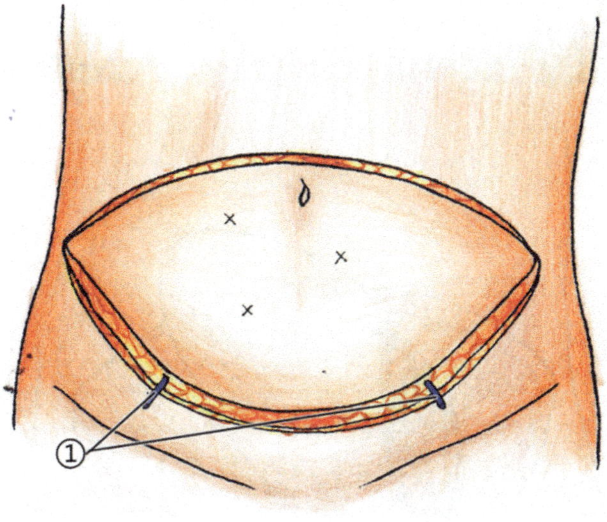

Fig. 10.22 Bilateral SIEVs were carefully separated and carried in the flap. (1) SIEVs

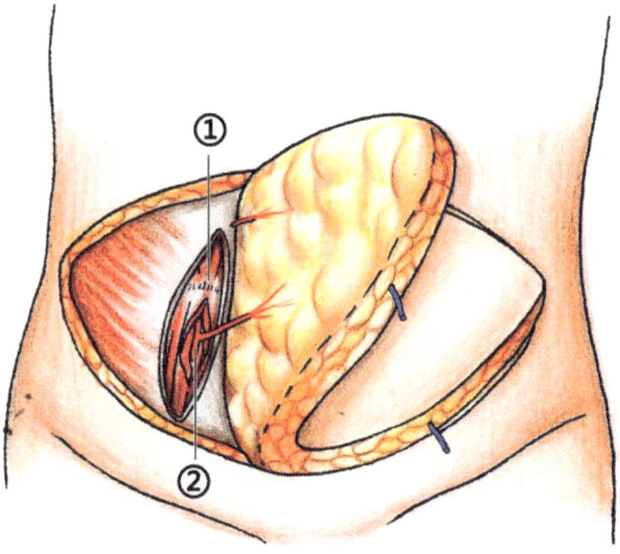

Fig. 10.24 The anterior sheath was opened longitudinally along the outer edge of the two perforating branches, and the medial perforating branch was retrogradely separated in the muscle until the vascular trunk was revealed; (1) The rectus abdominis muscle; (2) Deep inferior epigastric vascular pedicle

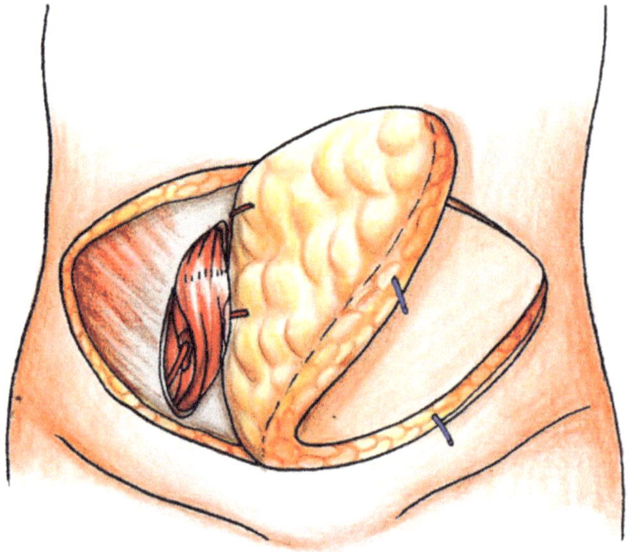

Fig. 10.25 The rectus abdominis was pulled toward the midline to expose and free the vascular pedicle that lay at the surface of the posterior sheath of the proximal rectus abdominis

Fig. 10.26 The left flap was lifted to expose a large deep inferior epigastric perforator

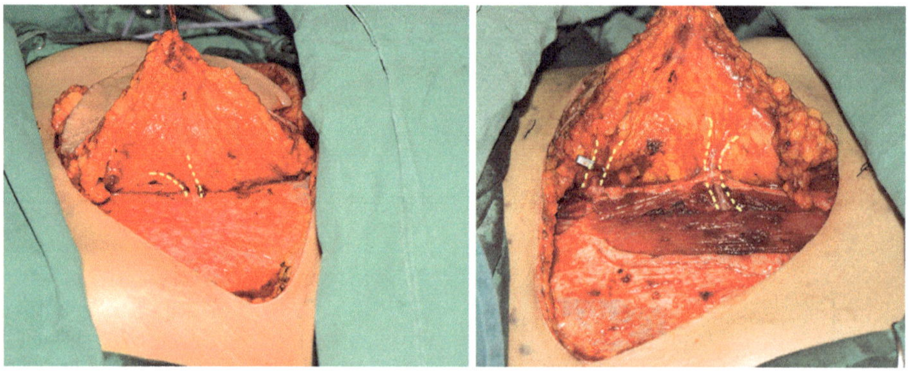

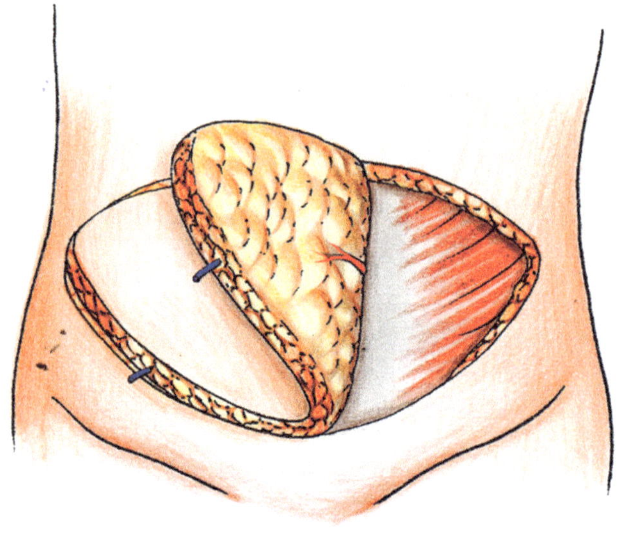

Fig. 10.27 The left flap is raised from the aponeurosis surface of the external oblique muscle

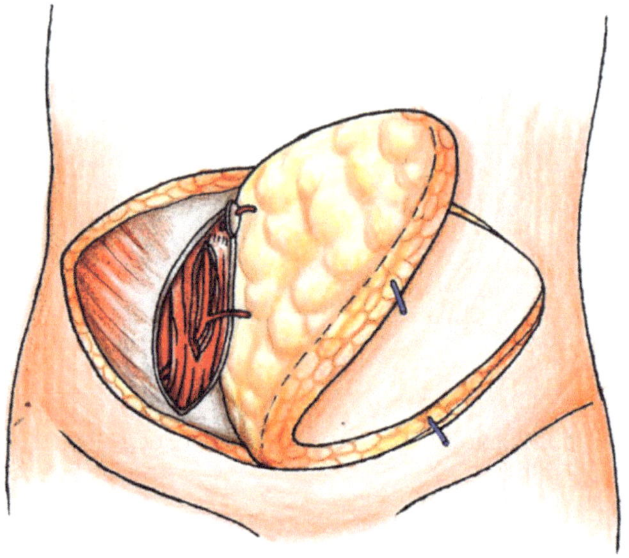

Fig. 10.28 The right paraumbilical perforator was freed with muscle reserved

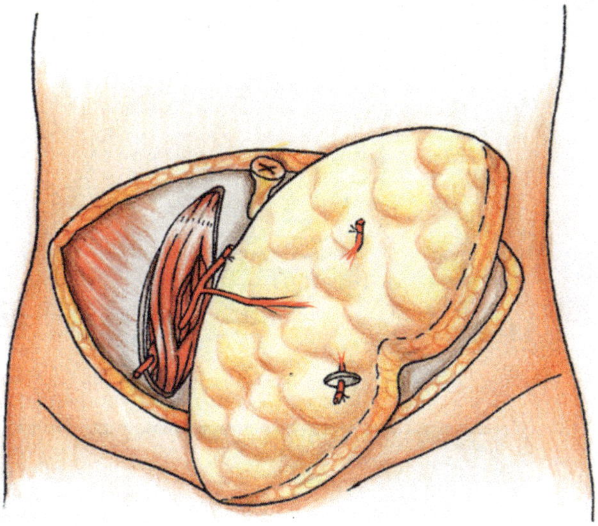

Fig. 10.29 The right paraumbilical perforator and the left large perforator were clamped, blood supply was found to be good based on the right medial perforator alone. The flap was finally pedicled with the right medial perforator

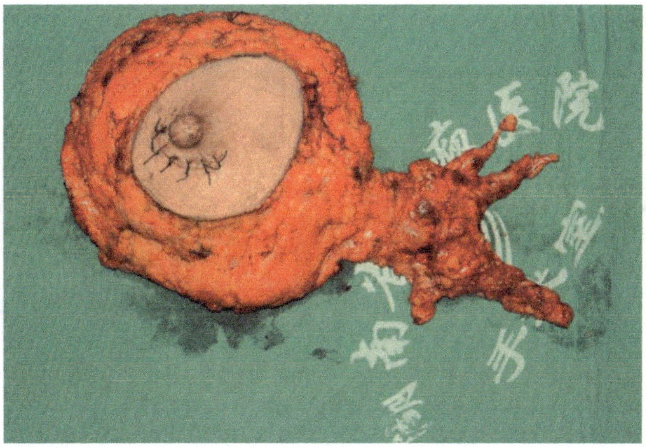

Fig. 10.30 Mastectomy was finished

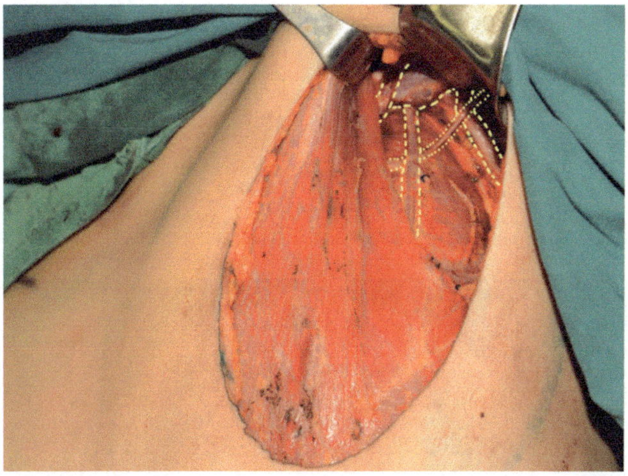

Fig. 10.31 Recipient vessels (lateral thoracic artery and vein) were prepared

Fig. 10.32 (**a**) Back view of the flap; (**b**) The flap was transferred to the receiving area and de-epithelized according to the actual skin defect area

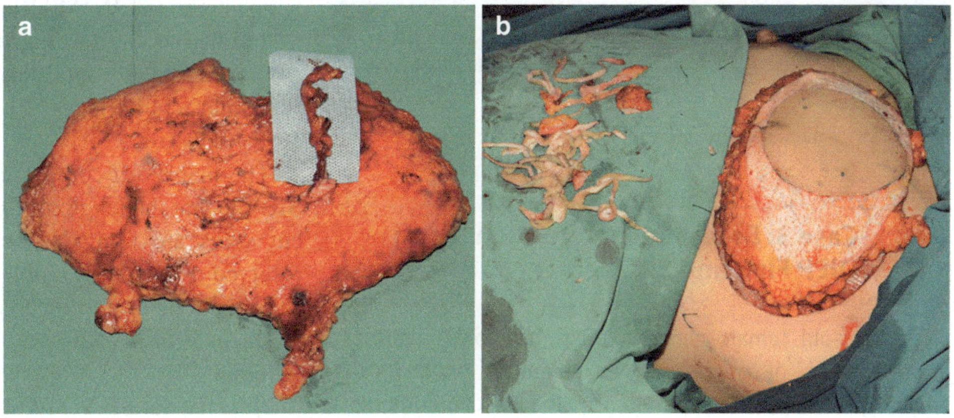

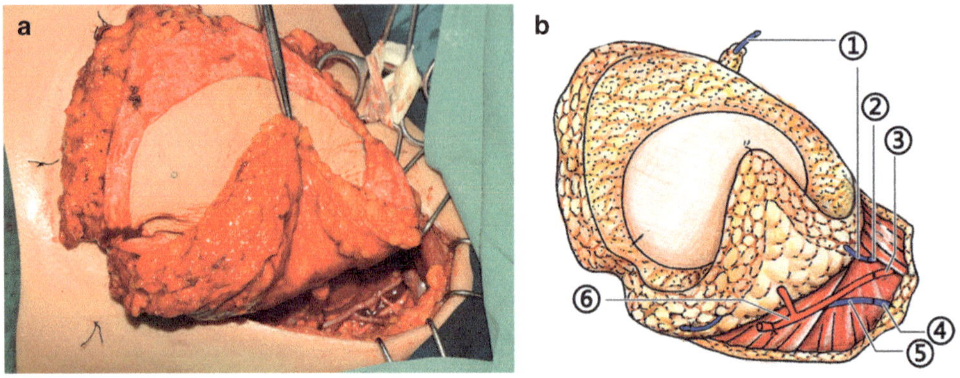

Fig. 10.33 Vascular anastomosis. (**a**) Vascular anastomosis was completed. (**b**) Revascularization illustration. (1) SIEV; (2) Lateral thoracic vein; (3) Lateral thoracic artery; (4) Lateral thoracic vein; (5) Deep inferior epigastric vein; (6) Deep inferior epigastric artery

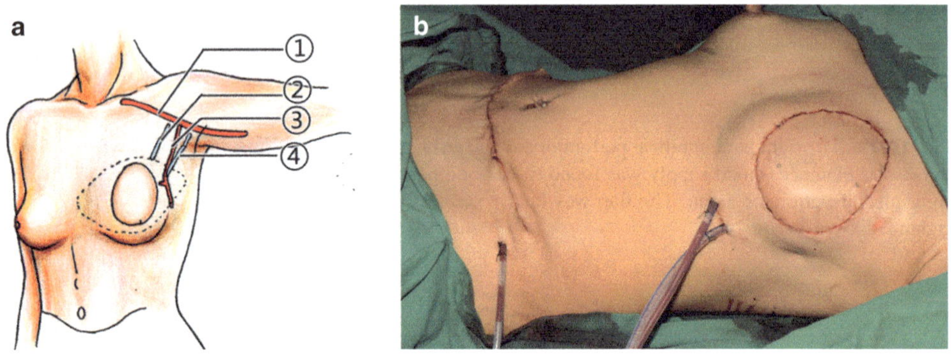

Fig. 10.34 (**a**) Revascularization illustration. (1) Axillary artery; (2) Lateral thoracic vein; (3) Lateral thoracic artery; (4) Deep inferior epigastric vein. (**b**) Immediate after reconstruction

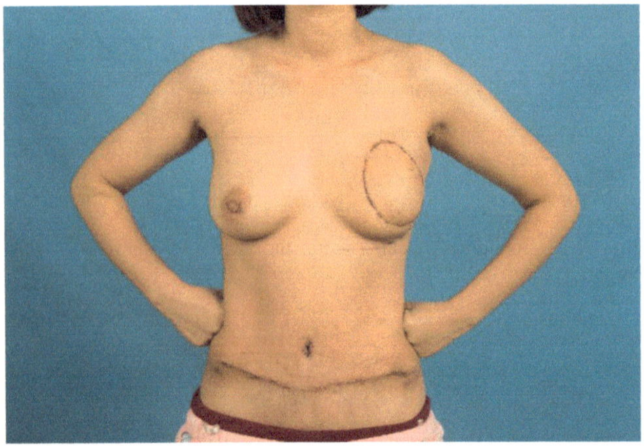

Fig. 10.35 2-month follow-up

10.8 Case 3: Breast Reconstruction Using DIEP Flap and SIEV

A 55-year-old female patient with right subaxillary mass after 4 years of operation was diagnosed with locally advanced breast cancer 1 month after the last chemotherapy.

The patient received right radical mastectomy plus reconstruction using free DIEP flap. The flap size was about 33 cm × 17 cm. The length of bilateral SIEVs was about 7 cm.

The right deep inferior epigastric artery and vein were anastomosed end-to-end with the right internal thoracic artery and vein, and the right SIEV was anastomosed end-to-end with the branch of the right lateral thoracic vein (1A3V).

Pathological results: invasive micro-papillary carcinoma of the right breast, cancer tissue, and tumor thrombus in vessels were seen in the dermis of the cutting edge, cancer was seen in the fat and skeletal muscle tissue of the chest wall, and a little cartilage was also seen. The cancer tissue was close to the cartilage.

Cancer metastasis was seen in 3/17 of the right axillary lymph nodes (pT3N1M0,IIIa).

The flap survived well. After further comprehensive treatment, the patient's appearance and sensory function recovered satisfactorily (Figs. 10.36, 10.37, 10.38, 10.39, 10.40, 10.41, and 10.42).

The major difficulty in cutting a DIEP flap containing SIEV is that the length of SIEVs and the number of recipient veins are limited. Therefore, the SIEVs should be reserved as long as possible. It is best to determine which SIEV is to be used prior to operation. The selection of the recipient vein is also very important, and alternatives are required.

If ipsilateral SIEV of DIEA is chosen, the proximal and distal ends of the internal mammary vessels can be used for anastomosis. The contralateral SIEV, if utilized, can be anastomosized with the internal mammary vessels and lateral thoracic vessels, respectively, or the lateral thoracic vessels, thoracodorsal vessels, or anterior serratus branches.

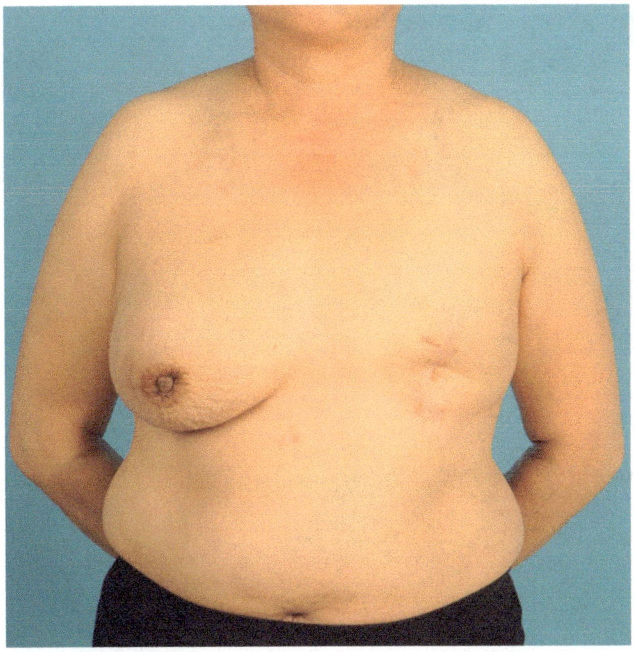

Fig. 10.36 Pre-operation viewing

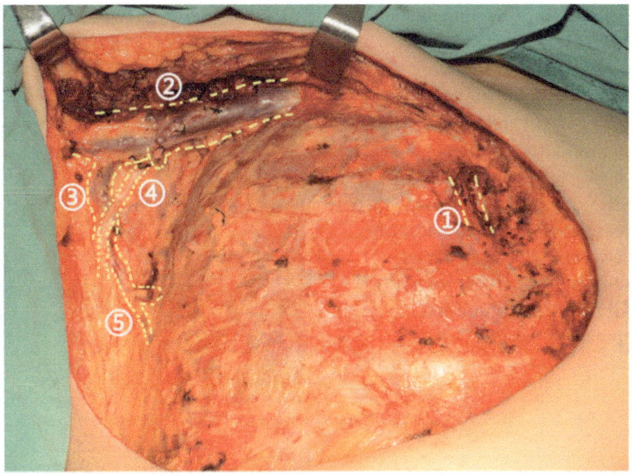

Fig. 10.38 The right lateral thoracic artery and vein were prepared after complete resection of the lesion. (1) Internal mammary vessels; (2) Axillary vein; (3) Thoracodorsal vessels; (4) Thoracodorsal nerve; (5) Lateral thoracic vessels

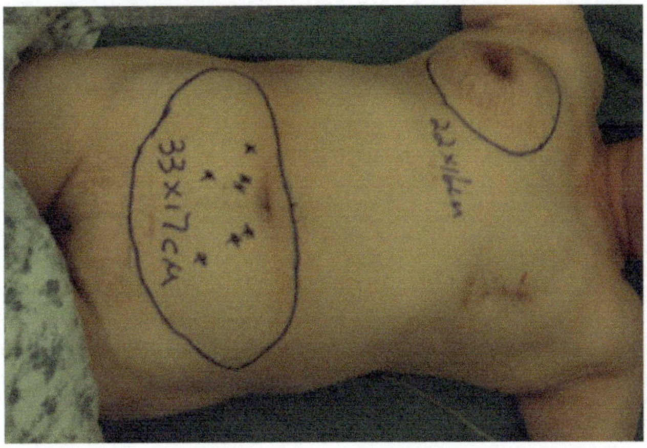

Fig. 10.37 Flap design

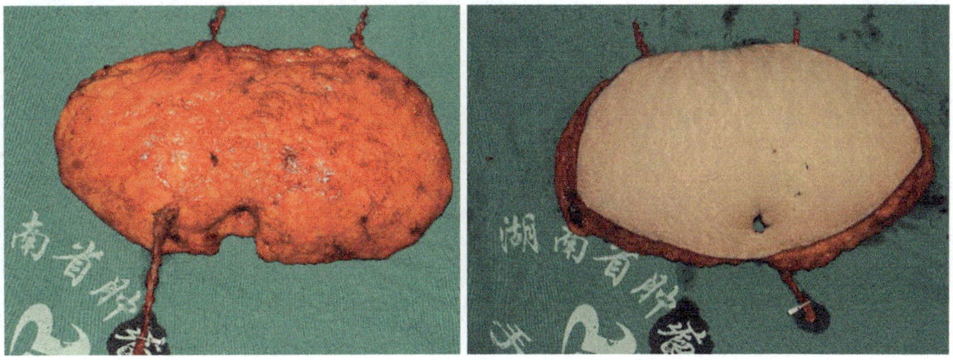

Fig. 10.39 The flap was harvested

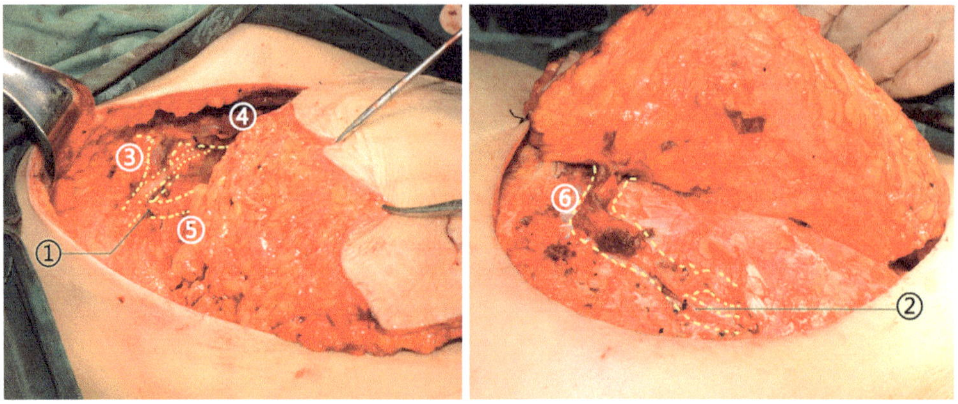

Fig. 10.40 The right deep inferior epigastric vessels were communicated with the right internal mammary vessels (A: $V = 1{:}1$). The right lateral thoracic vein was anastomosed with the left SIEV. (1) Lateral thoracic vessels; (2) Internal mammary vessels; (3) Thoracodorsal vessels; (4) Axillary vein; (5) SIEV; (6) Deep inferior epigastric vessels

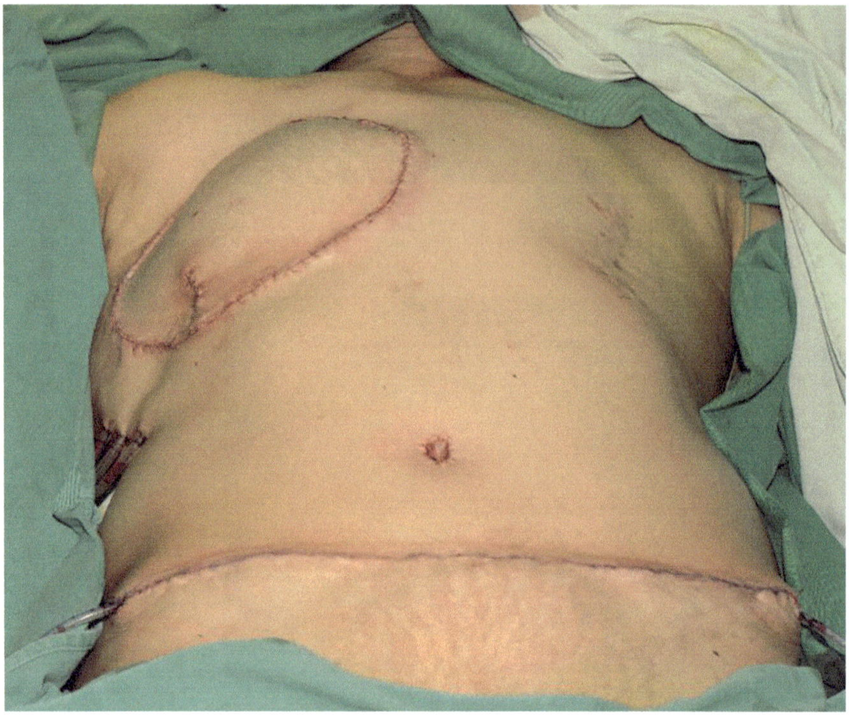

Fig. 10.41 Immediate viewing after operation

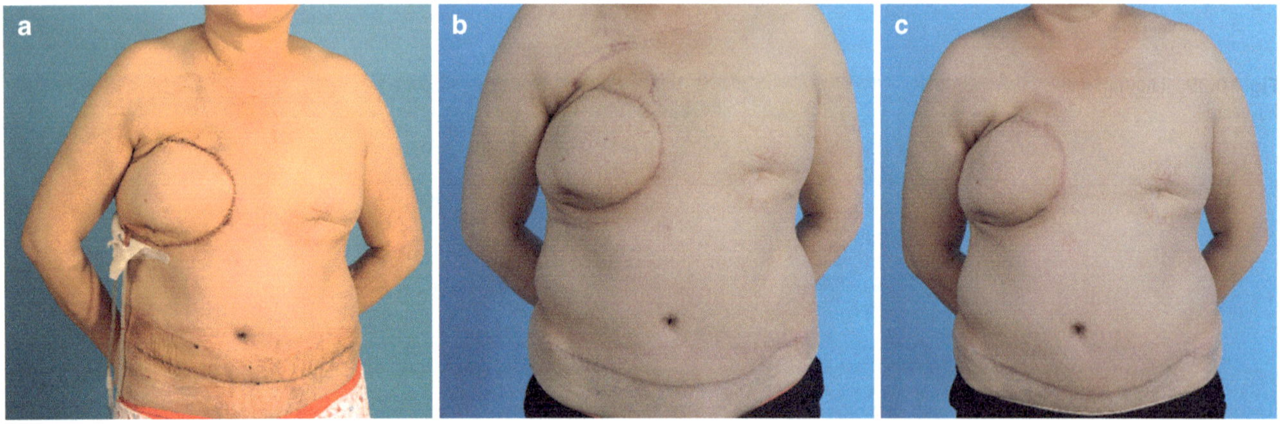

Fig. 10.42 Satisfactory appearance and function during postoperative follow-up. (**a**) 2 weeks after operation. (**b**) 3 months after operation. (**c**) 9 months after operation

10.9 Case 4: DIEP Flap Including SIEV for Reconstruction

The patient, a 49-year-old female, received right radical mastectomy 7 years ago.

She underwent right chest wall scar excision, axillary scar disconnection, and breast reconstruction with free DIEP flap.

The scar on the right chest wall was completely removed, leaving a huge defect of about 16 cm × 10 cm in size.

The third costal cartilage at a length of 3 cm was excised near the right sternum, and the perichondrium and intercostal muscle were removed to expose the internal thoracic vessels.

The size of DIEP flap was about 26 cm × 12 cm.

The right deep inferior epigastric artery and vein and the left deep inferior epigastric artery and vein were anastomosed with the proximal and distal ends of the right internal thoracic artery and vein, respectively.

Flap congestion persisted even when bilateral vascular pedicles were revascularized, yet it improved immediately when the reserved SIEV was communicated with the lateral thoracic vein. The flap was in good viability and the patient recovered uneventfully. The sensory function and appearance of the rebuilt breast were satisfactory (Figs. 10.43, 10.44, 10.45, 10.46, 10.47, 10.48, 10.49, and 10.50).

Second staged breast reconstruction requires complete removal of scar tissue in order to free the skin envelope and facilitate breast shaping. The removed scar tissue must be sent for pathological examination [19].

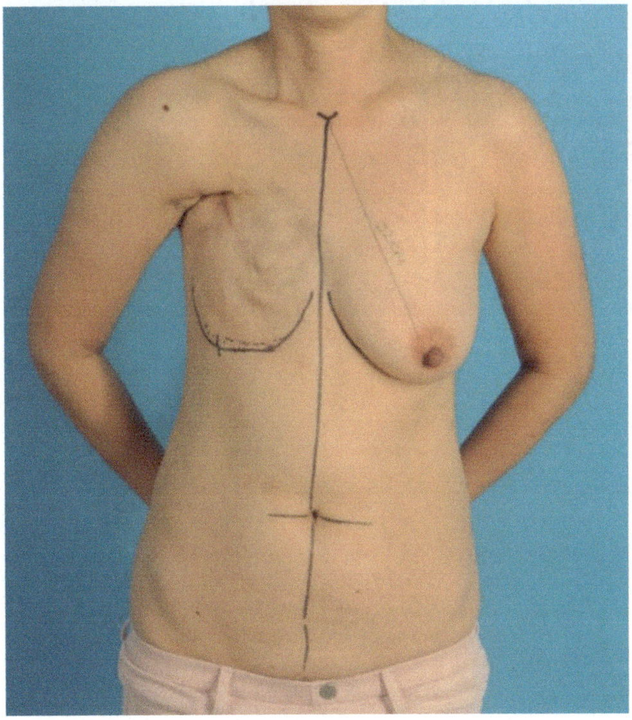

Fig. 10.43 Pre-operation viewing

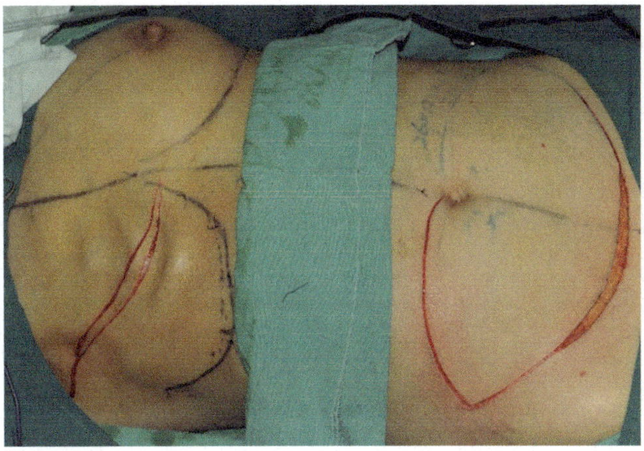

Fig. 10.44 During operation protocol

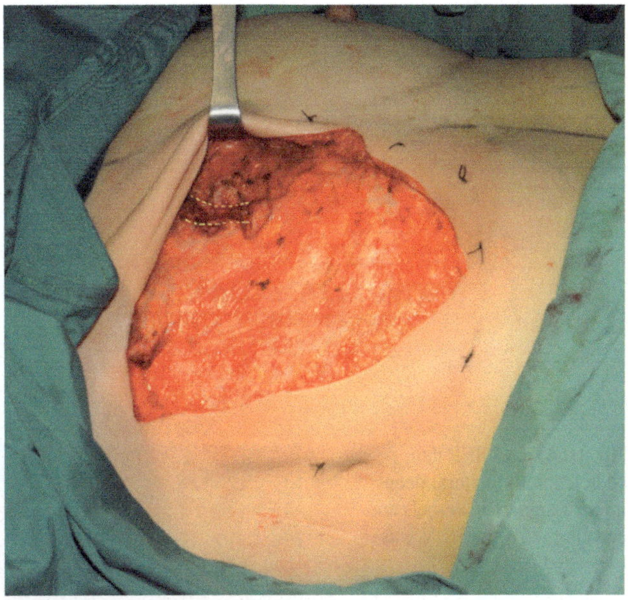

Fig. 10.45 The skin envelope was completely freed, the right internal mammary vessel was prepared

Flap shaping is the most important step in breast reconstruction, which needs to be completed in a sitting position. On the one hand, it is necessary to reshape the beauty of the breast, on the other hand, it is also necessary to consider the safety of the vascular pedicle. Where and how of multiple drainage tubes are placed is also required with care.

The medial and lower edges of the flap are most vulnerable to necrosis, hence sufficient blood supply should be guaranteed.

1. Firstly, the flap was fixed on the chest wall by intermittent suture, and the shape of the flap was observed from multiple angles.
2. De-epithelization of the flap was performed according to the actual size of the required skin island.

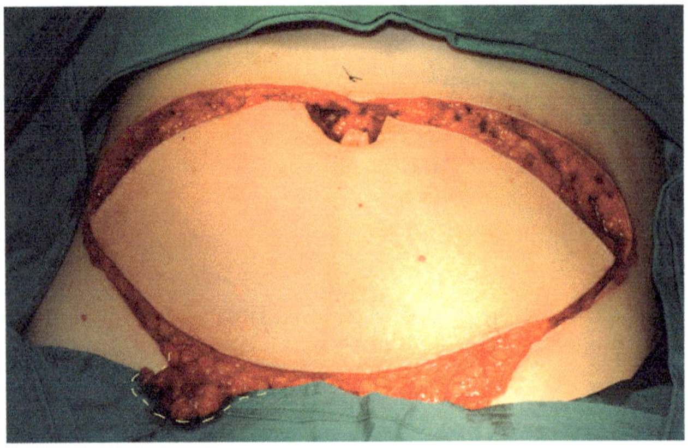

Fig. 10.46 The right SIEV is included in the flap

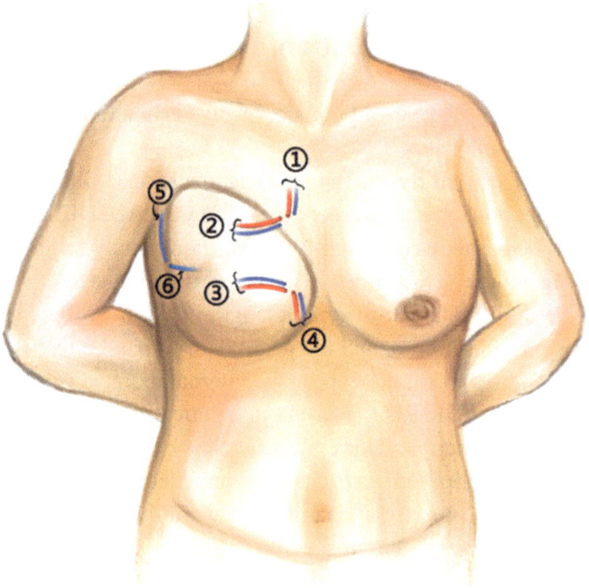

Fig. 10.48 The right deep inferior epigastric artery and vein were anastomosed with the proximal end of the right internal mammary artery and vein (1A1V), the left deep inferior epigastric artery and vein were anastomosed with the distal end of the right internal mammary artery and vein (1A1V), and the right SIEV was anastomosed with the accompanying vein of the anterior serratus branch of the right thoracodorsal artery. (1) Proximal end of internal mammary vessels; (2) Right deep inferior epigastric vessels; (3) Left deep inferior epigastric vessel; (4) Distal end of internal mammary vessels; (5) The accompanying vein of the anterior serratus branch of the right thoracodorsal artery; (6) Right SIEV

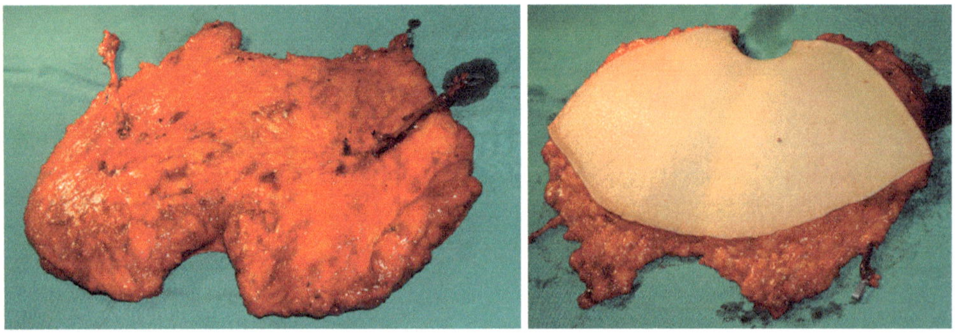

Fig. 10.47 A DIEP flap pedicled with bilateral deep inferior epigastric vessels and carrying the right SIEV was harvested

3. During the shaping process, twisting and compression of the vascular pedicle should always be cautious while mobilizing the flap.

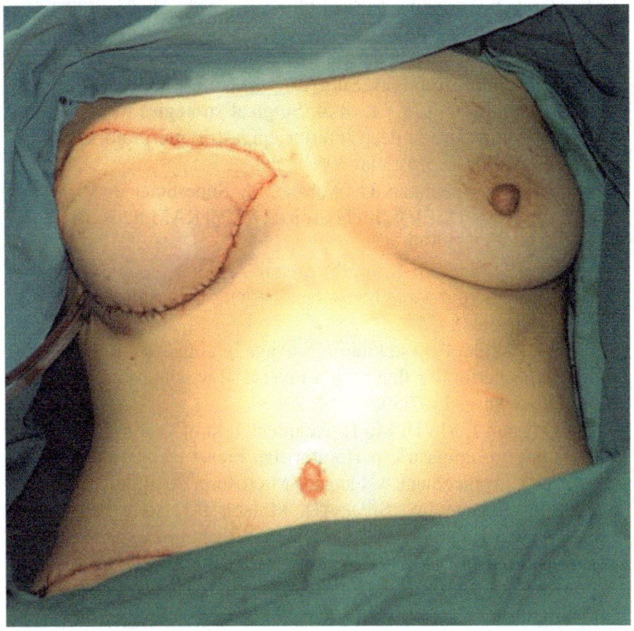

Fig. 10.49 Immediate after operation

4. The drainage tubes should be placed and distributed away from the vascular pedicle while effective drainage is achieved.

In the utilization of DIEP flap, the prevention and treatment of venous congestion should begin with preoperative planning and risk assessment.

The perforator flap of deep inferior epigastric artery is the gold standard for autologous breast reconstruction, but early identification of venous congestion is also crucial.

If venous congestion is noted, intraoperative intervention brings about the best outcome. There should be an effective solution to any suspected venous outflow problems before the patient leaves the operating room.

At the same time, the right microsurgical and non-microsurgical methods are selected according to the causes of venous congestion.

In conclusion, the standard process of rescuing the flap combined with the surgeon's experience can optimize the vein management and make the perforator flap of deep inferior epigastric artery safe and reliable in breast reconstruction [20].

Fig. 10.50 6 months at follow-up

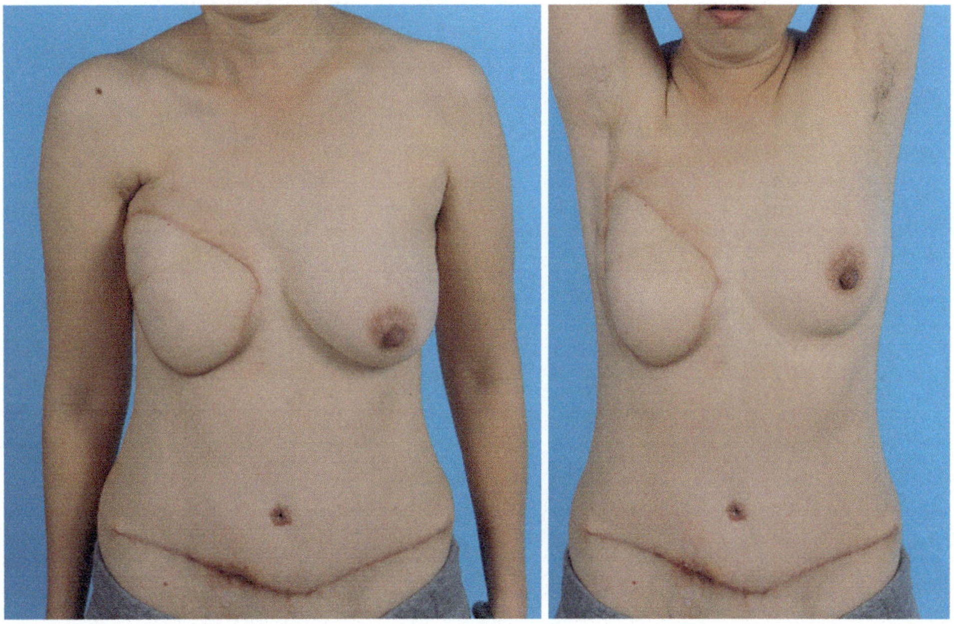

References

1. Tran NV, Buchel EW, Convery PA. Microvascular complications of DIEP flaps. Plast Reconstr Surg. 2007;119(5):1397–405; discussion 1406–8.
2. Blondeel PN, Arnstein M, Verstraete K, et al. Venous congestion and blood flow in free transverse rectus abdominis myocutaneous and deep inferior epigastric perforator flaps. Plast Reconstr Surg. 2000;106(6):1295–9.
3. Blondeel PN. One hundred free DIEP flap breast reconstructions: a personal experience. Br J Plast Surg. 1999;52(2):104–11.
4. Wechselberger G, Schoeller T, Bauer T, Ninkovic M, Otto A, Ninkovic M. Venous superdrainage in deep inferior epigastric perforator flap breast reconstruction. Plast Reconstr Surg. 2001;108(1):162–6.
5. Sadik KW, Pasko J, Cohen A, Cacioppo J. Predictive value of SIEV caliber and superficial venous dominance in free DIEP flaps. J Reconstr Microsurg. 2013;29(1):57–61.
6. Nedomansky J, Nickl S, Radtke C, Haslik W, Schroegendorfer KF. Venous superdrainage in DIEP flap breast reconstruction: the impact of superficial deep inferior epigastric vein dissection on abdominal seroma formation. Plast Reconstr Surg. 2018;141(2):206e–12e.
7. Enajat M, Rozen WM, Whitaker IS, Smit JM, Acosta R. A single center comparison of one versus two venous anastomoses in 564 consecutive DIEP flaps: investigating the effect on venous congestion and flap survival. Microsurgery. 2010;30(3):185–91.
8. Marck KW, van der Biezen JJ, Dol JA. Internal mammary artery and vein supercharge in TRAM flap breast reconstruction. Microsurgery. 1996;17(7):371–4.
9. Tutor EG, Auba C, Benito A, Rábago G, Kreutler W. Easy venous superdrainage in DIEP flap breast reconstruction through the intercostal branch. J Reconstr Microsurg. 2002;18(7):595–8.
10. Blondeel PN. Venous augmentation of the free TRAM flap. Br J Plast Surg. 2002;55(1):87.
11. Boutros SG. Double venous system drainage in deep inferior epigastric perforator flap breast reconstruction: a single-surgeon experience. Plast Reconstr Surg. 2013;131(4):671–6.
12. Ayestaray B, Yonekura K, Motomura H, Ziade M. A comparative study between deep inferior epigastric artery perforator and thoracoacromial venous supercharged deep inferior epigastric artery perforator flaps. Ann Plast Surg. 2016;76(1):78–82.
13. Ali R, Bernier C, Lin YT, et al. Surgical strategies to salvage the venous compromised deep inferior epigastric perforator flap. Ann Plast Surg. 2010;65(4):398–406.
14. Villafane O, Gahankari D, Webster M. Superficial deep inferior epigastric vein (SIEV): 'lifeboat' for DIEP/TRAM flaps. Br J Plast Surg. 1999;52(7):599.
15. Mehrara BJ, Santoro T, Smith A, et al. Alternative venous outflow vessels in microvascular breast reconstruction. Plast Reconstr Surg. 2003;112(2):448–55.
16. Liu TS, Ashjian P, Festekjian J. Salvage of congested deep inferior epigastric perforator flap with a reverse flow venous anastomosis. Ann Plast Surg. 2007;59(2):214–7.
17. Xin Q, Luan J, Mu H, Mu L. Augmentation of venous drainage in deep inferior epigastric perforator flap breast reconstruction: efficacy and advancement. J Reconstr Microsurg. 2012;28(5):313–8.
18. Park JE, Shenaq DS, Silva AK, Mhlaba JM, Song DH. Breast reconstruction with SIEA flaps: a single-institution experience with 145 free flaps. Plast Reconstr Surg. 2016;137(6):1682–9.
19. Warner RM, Wallace DL, Ferran NA, et al. Mastectomy scars following breast reconstruction: should routine histologic analysis be performed. Plast Reconstr Surg. 2009;123(4):1141–7.
20. Lee KT, Mun GH. Benefits of superdrainage using SIEV in DIEP flap breast reconstruction: a systematic review and meta-analysis. Microsurgery. 2017;37(1):75–83.

Bipedicled Turbocharged DIEP Flaps for Unilateral Breast Reconstruction

11

Zan Li and Rene D. Largo

11.1 Introduction

In 1994, Allen first reported about the application of the deep inferior epigastric perforator flap to breast reconstruction [1], which has the advantage of being the most common method for breast reconstruction after breast cancer [2].

However, the perforator flap of deep inferior epigastric artery still has some shortcomings and disputes. In some cases, it may do more harm than good.

It bears the risks of flap necrosis, poor venous reflux, and fat liquefaction necrosis [3–5], which are closely related to the insufficient blood supply of the flap.

One of the solutions to improve the blood supply of the perforator flap is to use the conjoined perforator flap [6].

In 1982, Song et al. [7] successfully applied conjoined frontal flap for nasal reconstruction. At that time, it was named the "conjoined" frontal flap. Later, some scholars reported cases of "conjoined twins" [8].

Hallock [9, 10] successfully introduced this method into the field of perforator flap.

After the flap is combined, a perforator flap can repair a large wound and reduce the damage of the flap donor area.

Conjoined perforator flap refers to a special perforator flap containing two or more perforator flaps with the skin and superficial fascia structures continuous, while the length of the flap exceeds any vascular body area of each perforator. It is necessary to rebuild perforator vessels in other vascular body areas at the distal or proximal end of the flap to ensure the viability of the flap.

Conjoined perforator flap with two perforators and conjoined perforator flap with three perforators are commonly used in clinic.

Z. Li (✉)
Department of Oncology Plastic Surgery, Hunan Cancer Hospital, Changsha, Hunan, China

R. D. Largo
Department of Plastic Surgery, The University of Texas MD Anderson Cancer Center, Houston, TX, USA
e-mail: rdlargo@mdanderson.org

Ng made a summary about breast reconstruction with bilateral vascular pedicle rectus abdominis myocutaneous flap. They believe that using bilateral vascular pedicle technique for unilateral breast reconstruction can ensure reliable blood supply of tissue flap and reduce incidence of complications in donor area [11].

The conjoined flap technique with bilateral vascular pedicle has also been reported and applied to increase the blood supply of the flap, especially for patients with large breast, slim figure, or abdominal surgery history [12–14].

With the improvement of microsurgical technique, the lower abdominal tissue flap is increasingly used for the perforator flap of the inferior abdominal artery over the rectus abdominis flap. In our clinical work, we have a deeper understanding that it is very important to the whole lower abdominal tissue, including Areas I–IV, which is required to reconstruct a large breast or repair a large chest wall defect. Otherwise, the reconstructed breast may be asymmetric or topically depressed due to insufficient flap tissue, which requires the use of conjoined flap technique.

Although there have been many reports on breast reconstruction with bilateral pedicle conjoined rectus abdominis myocutaneous flap to improve the blood supply of the flap [15–19], the application of bilateral pedicle rectus abdominis myocutaneous flap for breast reconstruction will cause serious damage to the patient's donor area. These problems can be perfectly solved by utilizing pure perforator skin flap.

Pennington [17] first reported that the blood supply of the contralateral part of the rectus abdominis flap can be improved by anastomosing the distal end of the deep inferior epigastric vessels and the contralateral periumbilical perforator vessels.

In fact, this flap was pedicled with classic deep inferior epigastric artery perforator flap on one side and the periumbilical perforator on the other side. The flap was not split. It was an improved form of the traditional deep inferior epigastric artery perforator flap, which reduced the damage of the donor area and preserved the integrity of rectus abdominis to the greatest extent [20, 21].

Z. Li, D. Song (eds.), *Oncoplastic Flap Surgery*, https://doi.org/10.1007/978-981-19-8926-1_11

Although Nahabedian et al. reported that bilateral pedicled perforator flap of deep inferior epigastric artery would cause more donor site complications than unilateral pedicled flap [22–24], other scholars such as Kroll [25] and Ascherman [26] did not find significant differences in donor site injury and complications between bilateral and unilateral perforator flap of deep inferior epigastric artery [3, 4, 23, 27–31].

It is reported that the complete recovery of rectus abdominis innervation can be observed 6 months after a DIEP flap harvest. Therefore, as long as the damage is minimized during the cutting process, there is no need to worry that the perforator flap of the deep inferior epigastric artery will have a significant impact on the donor area of the abdominal wall [32].

It is also reported that [33] there is no significant difference between bilateral or unilateral DIEP flaps regarding the abdominal donor site injury, but how much the anterior sheath and rectus abdominis muscle has been preserved is associated with the incidence of donor site complications; the donor site injury of a DIEP flap with bilateral vascular pedicles is significantly lower than that of bilateral rectus abdominis muscle flap.

However, cutting the perforator flap of the deep inferior epigastric artery does not mean that the injury of the donor area will be absolutely reduced. Only when the medial or lateral perforators are carried on each side of a DIEP flap, the injury of the abdominal donor area will be significantly reduced. In Case 3, complete separation of the perforator and vessel pedicle is bound to increase the injury of the donor area.

Our statistical results also showed that the incidence of complications in the donor area in patients with a DIEP flap with bilateral pedicles prepared according to the non-invasive standard technique did not significantly increase, yet the operation time was significantly prolonged [34].

Many methods have been reported for preparing a DIEP flap with bilateral vascular pedicles, each has its own advantages and disadvantages [12–14].

Anastomosis of bilateral vascular pedicles of the flap and two sets of vascular pedicles in the recipient area are most frequently used, but in many cases, it is difficult to find two sets of suitable recipient vessels.

Regarding the recipient vessels, the internal mammary vessels come first [10, 35] and the thoracodorsal vessels follow [36, 37].

However, using thoracodorsal vessels for anastomosis will bring great damage to the donor area and it is technically demanding due to narrow space [37].

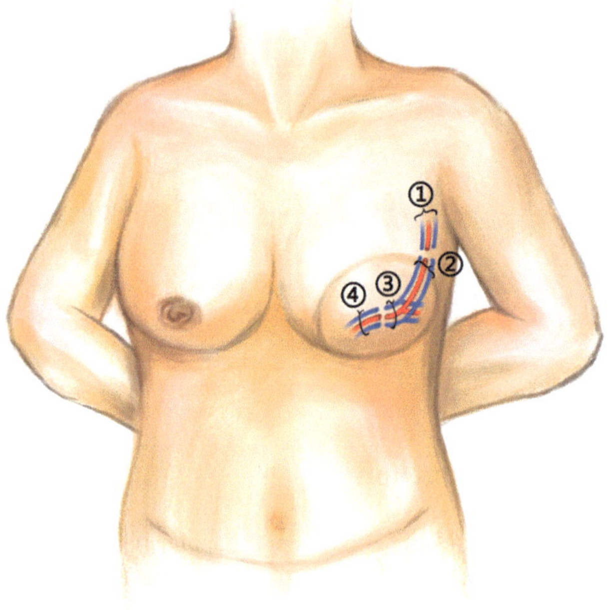

Fig. 11.1 Schematic diagram of revascularization for turbocharge: left deep inferior epigastric vessels to the distal end of right deep inferior epigastric vessels (1A2V); proximal end of right deep inferior epigastric vessel to lateral thoracic vessels (1A2V)

In clinical practice, we often use lateral thoracic vessels as recipient vessels to minimize donor injury (as shown in Fig. 11.1).

11.1.1 Turbocharge

The distal vascular pedicle is anastomosed with another branch of its own vascular pedicle of the flap in establishing contralateral (or distal) auxiliary blood circulation for a super conjoined flap.

Flow-through perforator flap: where the proximal end (primary source blood vessel yet not vascular trunk, such as the descending branch of the lateral femoral circumflex artery) and distal end of the source blood vessel of the perforator flap is respectively anastomosed with the proximal end and distal end of the main blood vessel (such as the radial artery) in the receiving area to rebuild blood circulation of the flap without compromising (or reconstructing) the continuity of the recipient vascular trunk.

This perforator flap can also be used in combined flap transplantation, that is, the distal end of its primary source vessel is used to reconstruct the blood flow of another tissue flap.

11.2 The Indications and Advantages of Turbocharge

There are indications and strengths of turbocharged flow-through perforator flap. Soutar et al. [38] reported in 1983 that when the radial artery flap was used to repair head and neck defects, the radial artery was bridged with the external carotid artery and facial artery. Firstly, the concept of flow through flap was proposed.

Subsequently, Foucher et al. [39] applied it to repair the soft tissue defect of limbs and reconstruct the main blood vessel defect at the same time in 1984.

In 1999, Koshima et al. [40] reported "blood flow bridging thin latissimus dorsi perforator flap," which introduced the blood flow bridging method into the field of perforator flap.

There are many forms of turbocharged flow-through DIEP flap [13, 19]. At present, the common ways of turbocharge include: (1) anastomosis of periumbilical perforator vessel and the distal end of contralateral deep inferior epigastric vessel pedicle; (2) anastomosis of periumbilical perforating vessels with the large contralateral DIEP; (3) anastomosis of periumbilical perforator vessels and the branches of equal level to the contralateral deep inferior epigastric vascular pedicle.

Schoeller reported that turbocharge was completed by anastomosis of the contralateral periumbilical perforator and the distal superior epigastric of ipsilateral vascular pedicle [41].

However, perforator–perforator anastomosis alone has many limitations, including short perforator vascular pedicle and small vascular diameter. Therefore, we generally perform turbocharge by end-to-end anastomosis between bilateral vascular pedicles. In this way, the surgical difficulty is reduced to the greatest extent and has become our first choice.

The five commonly used forms of turbocharge flow-through in DIEP flaps are as follows (Figs. 11.2, 11.3, 11.4, 11.5, and 11.6):

1. The proximal ends of the contralateral deep inferior epigastric vessels is anastomosed with the distal end of the ipsilateral deep inferior epigastric vessel (Fig. 11.3).
2. The proximal end of the contralateral deep inferior epigastric vessel is anastomosed with the muscular branch of the ipsilateral deep inferior epigastric vessel (Fig. 11.4).
3. The proximal end of the contralateral deep inferior epigastric vessel is anastomosed with the medial branch of the ipsilateral deep inferior epigastric vessel (Fig. 11.5).
4. The proximal end of the contralateral deep inferior epigastric vessel is anastomosed with the lateral branch of the ipsilateral deep inferior epigastric vessel (Fig. 11.5).

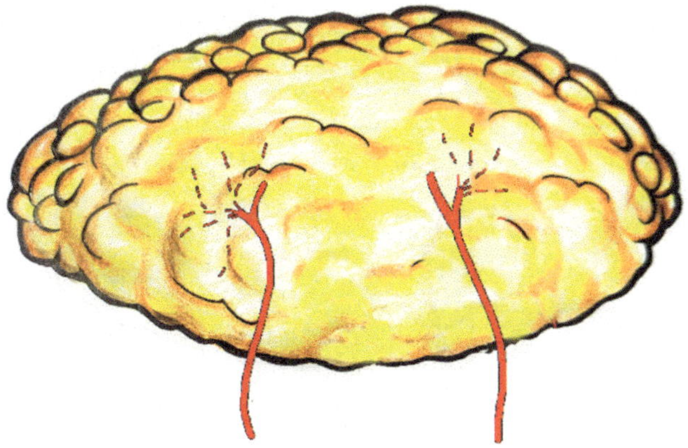

Fig. 11.2 A bilaterally pedicled DIEP flap was prepared

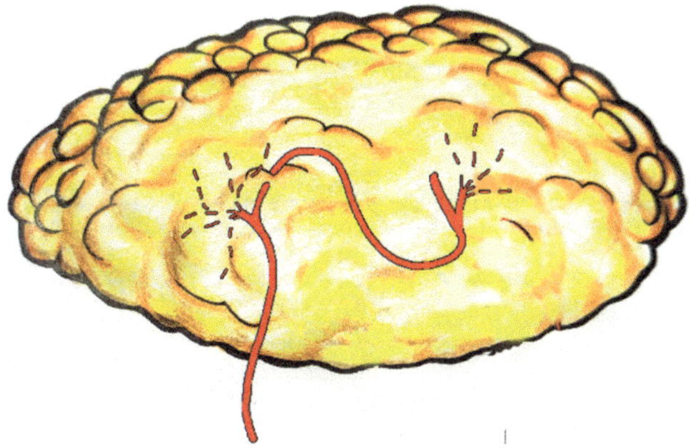

Fig. 11.3 Turbocharge by end-to-end anastomosis between unilateral deep inferior epigastric vascular pedicle and the distal end of the contralateral vascular pedicle

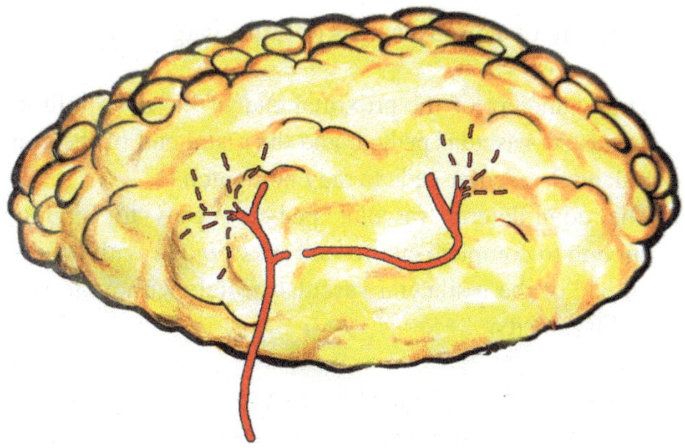

Fig. 11.4 Turbocharge by end-to-end anastomosis of the unilateral deep inferior epigastric vessel with the muscular branch of the contralateral deep inferior epigastric vessel

5. The perforating branch of the contralateral deep inferior epigastric vessel is anastomosed with the distal end of the ipsilateral deep inferior epigastric vessel (Fig. 11.6).

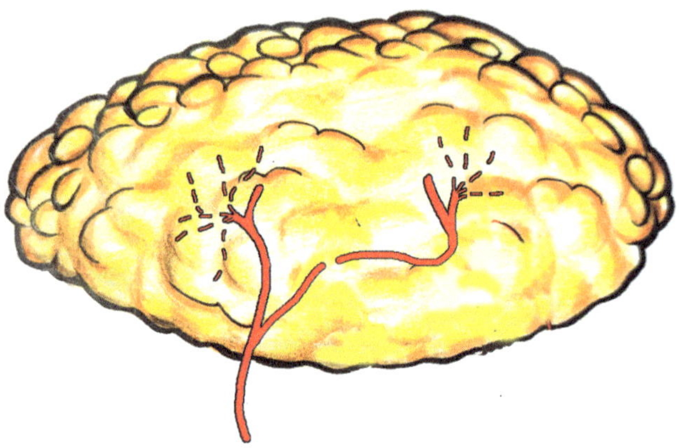

Fig. 11.5 Turbocharge by end-to-end anastomosis of unilateral deep inferior epigastric vascular pedicle and the main branch of the contralateral deep inferior epigastric vessel

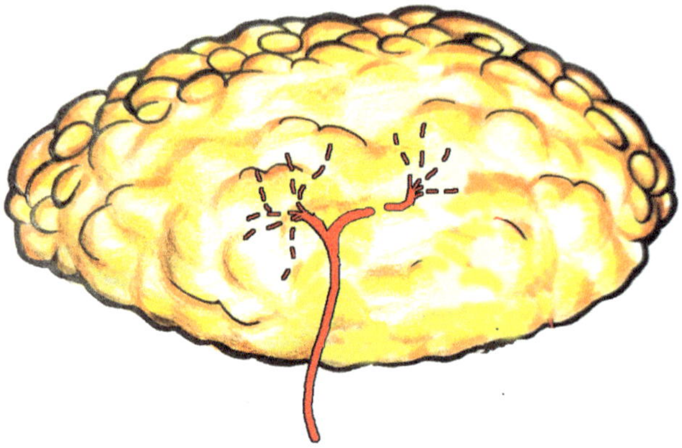

Fig. 11.6 Turbocharge by anastomosis of the perforator of contralateral deep inferior epigastric vessel and the distal end of ipsilateral deep inferior epigastric vessel

There are two disadvantages of turbocharge form one:

1. The diameters of the proximal end of the deep inferior epigastric vascular pedicle and the distal end of the contralateral vascular pedicle may not match.
2. The contralateral vascular pedicle needs to be long enough to complete end-to-end anastomosis with the distal end of the ipsilateral vascular pedicle without torsion and tortuosity.

This should be performed by an experienced and skillful operator. On the contralateral side, short vascular pedicle harbors a suitable caliber for anastomosis, paradoxically a long vessel pedicle facilitates anastomosis yet the vessel is commonly at large caliber.

Unfavorable anatomical situation should be always considered in preoperative design and during operation, flexible adjustment is required according to real conditions.

In clinical practice, it is found that the vascular pedicle in most cases does not contain a suitable collateral branch for turbocharge anastomosis. Our statistics showed that only 38% of cases were anatomically suitable candidates for turbocharge. Turbocharge forms 2–4 are not applicable to every patient. All branches of vascular pedicle found during operation should be carefully identified, if appropriate; they should be separated as far as possible to reserve an appropriate vascular length for revascularization.

Different from the traditional turbocharge methods, we often practice turbocharge by anastomosis of bilateral vascular pedicle trunk and branches. Although the damage to the donor area will inevitably increase, continuous improvement in surgical method can minimize the damage to the rectus abdominis itself and its blood supply, greatly improve the safety of the operation, and significantly shorten surgical duration. In this way, the clinical risk and high technical requirements of revascularization based on perforator–perforator anastomosis can be avoided.

11.3 Case 1: Turbocharge

The patient was a 45-year-old female who had found a left breast mass for 1 month.

The breast mass was diagnosed on biopsy as intraductal carcinoma with focal infiltration.

At admission, left modified radical mastectomy was performed and a free deep inferior epigastric perforator flap (containing the right SIEV at a length of about 7 cm) was used to reconstruct the left breast.

The left deep inferior epigastric artery and vein were anastomosed end-to-end with the branches of the lateral thoracic artery and vein (1A1V). Yet the venous reflux of the flap was poor, and it was improved by communicating the right SIEV with the thoracodorsal vein.

The postoperative pathological examination results showed that: (1) invasive ductal carcinoma (left breast), grade III, LVI positive, and the size of the mass was about 3 cm × 3 cm × 2 cm; (2) no cancer invasion was found in skin, basal margin, and nipple; (3) no cancer metastasis was found in axillary lymph nodes 0/33 (pT2N0M0, stage IIa).

Immunohistochemical results: ER (<1%), PR (<1%), CerbB-2 (3 +), and Ki-67 index about 50%.

The regimen of EC2w-TH was given as adjuvant therapy. The flap was in good viability without any complications. The sensory function and appearance of the reconstructed breast were satisfactory (Figs. 11.7, 11.8, 11.9, 11.10, 11.11, 11.12, 11.13, 11.14, 11.15, 11.16, 11.17, 11.18, and 11.19).

Preoperative Doppler probe and intra-operative clamping test are good means to determine the optimal perforators.

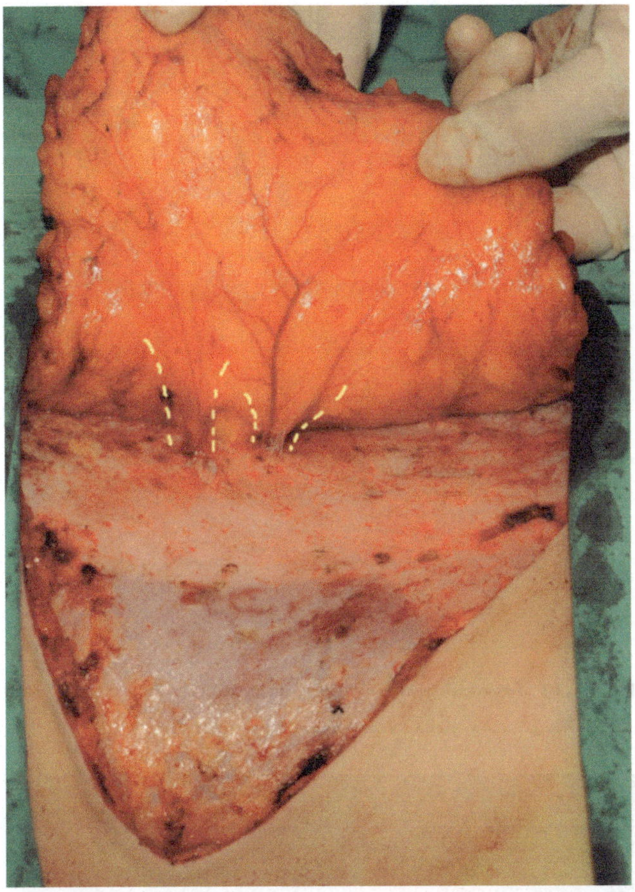

Fig. 11.7 The left perforator

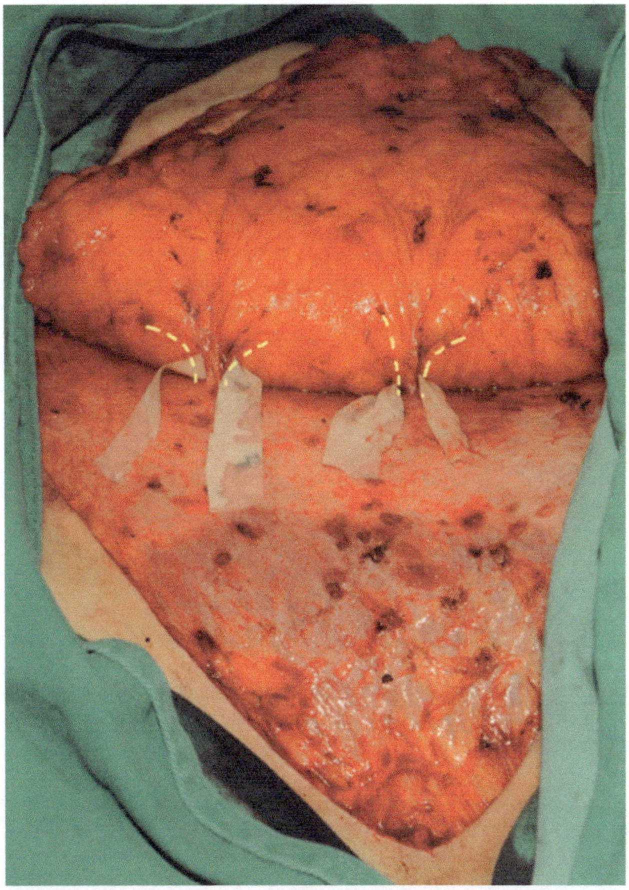

Fig. 11.8 The left perforator was exposed and freed

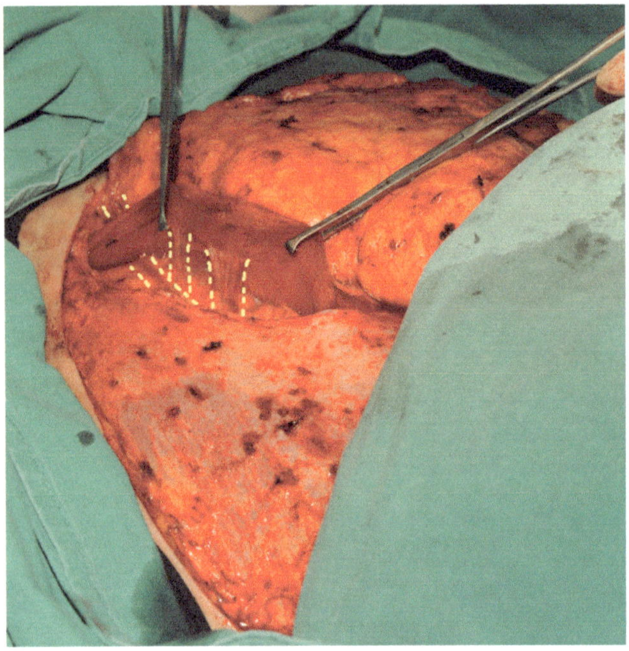

Fig. 11.9 The anterior sheath of the left rectus abdominis was opened, the rectus abdominis was lifted to expose the main left deep inferior epigastric vessels

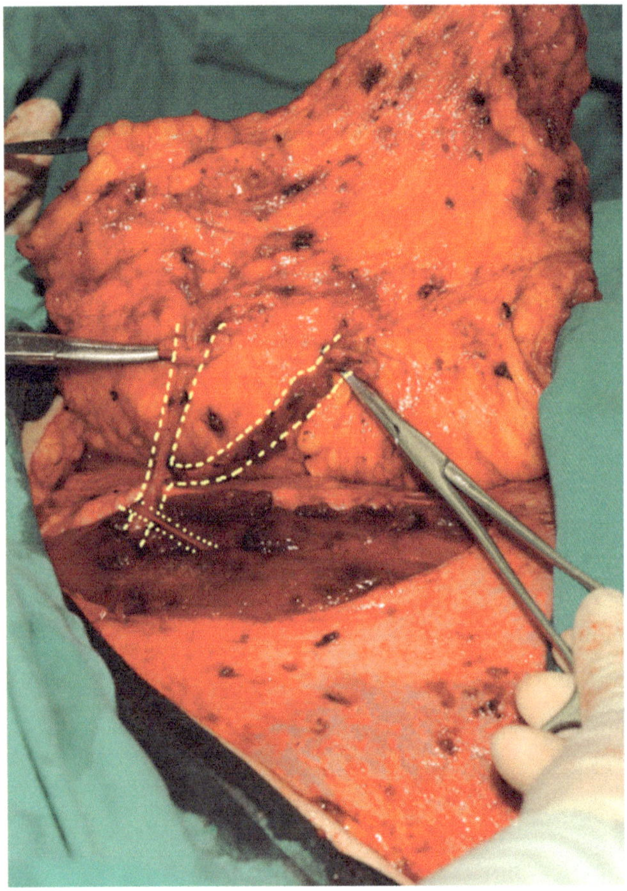

Fig. 11.10 Intramuscular separation of perforator and vascular pedicle

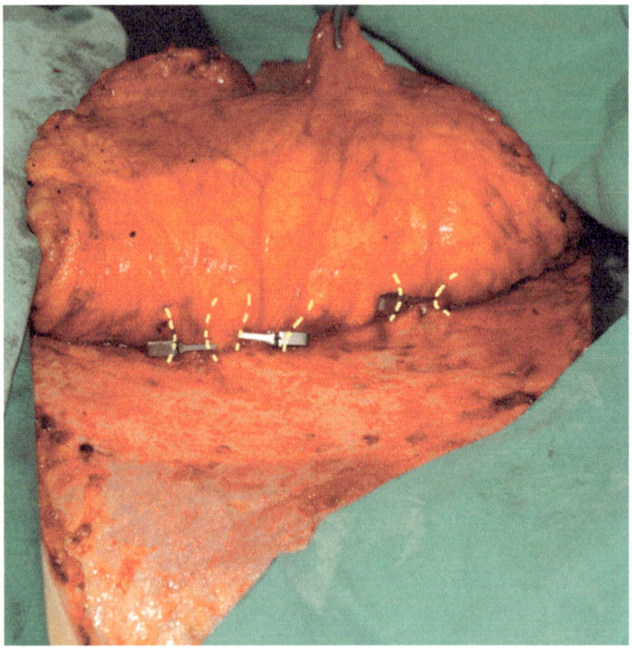

Fig. 11.11 Exposure of the right perforator vessel

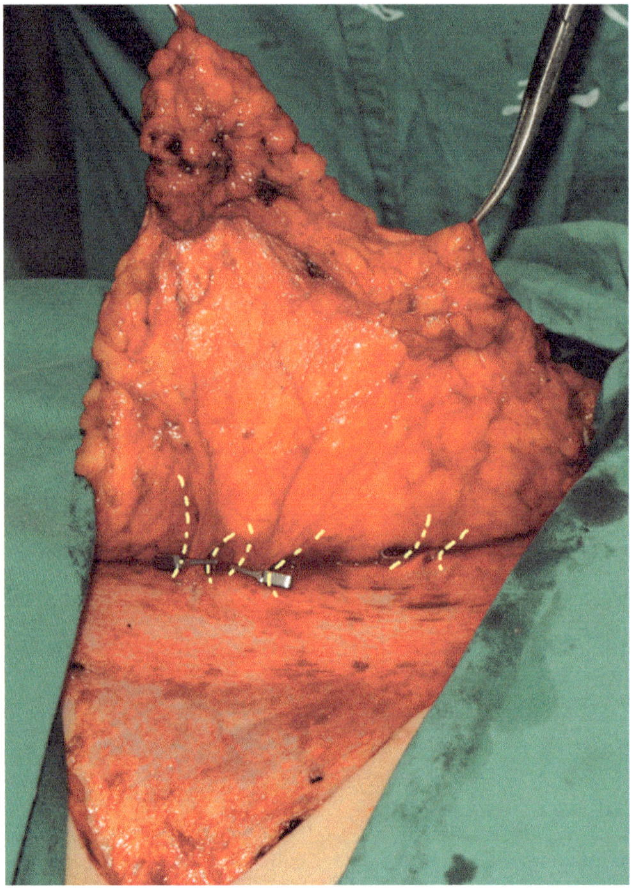

Fig. 11.12 It was suggested that venous congestion occurred when the right perforator was clamped. SIEVs were not available and the right deep inferior epigastric artery and its perforating branch were prepared

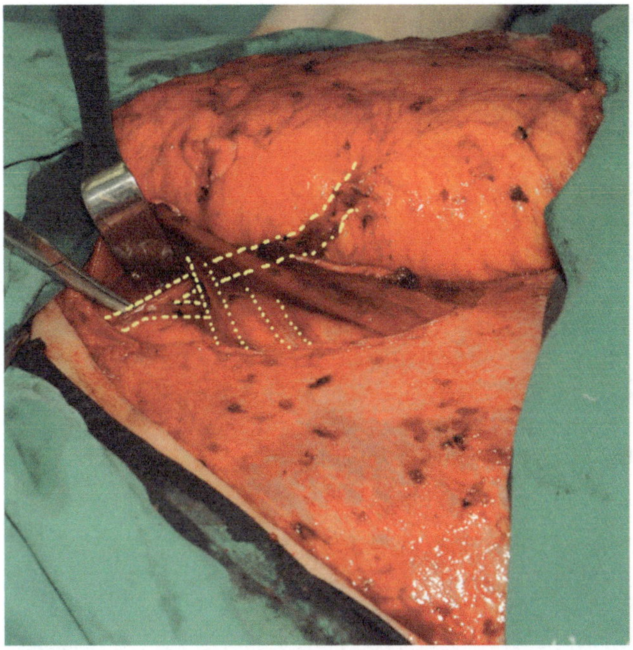

Fig. 11.13 The left vascular pedicle was separated till it was close to the issuing plane where it was ligated and disconnected, and then it was withdrawn retrogradely from the rectus abdominis tunnel

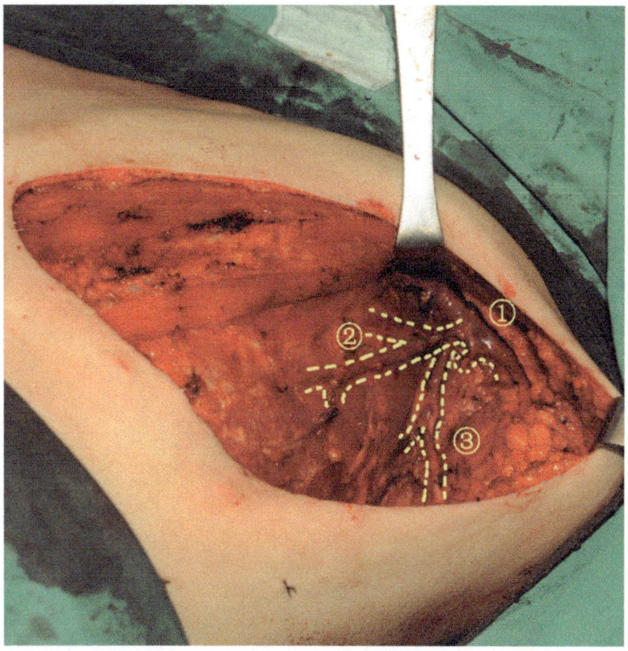

Fig. 11.14 The lateral thoracic vessels and the thoracodorsal vessels in the receiving area were prepared. (1) Axillary vein; (2) Lateral thoracic vessels; (3) Thoracodorsal vessels

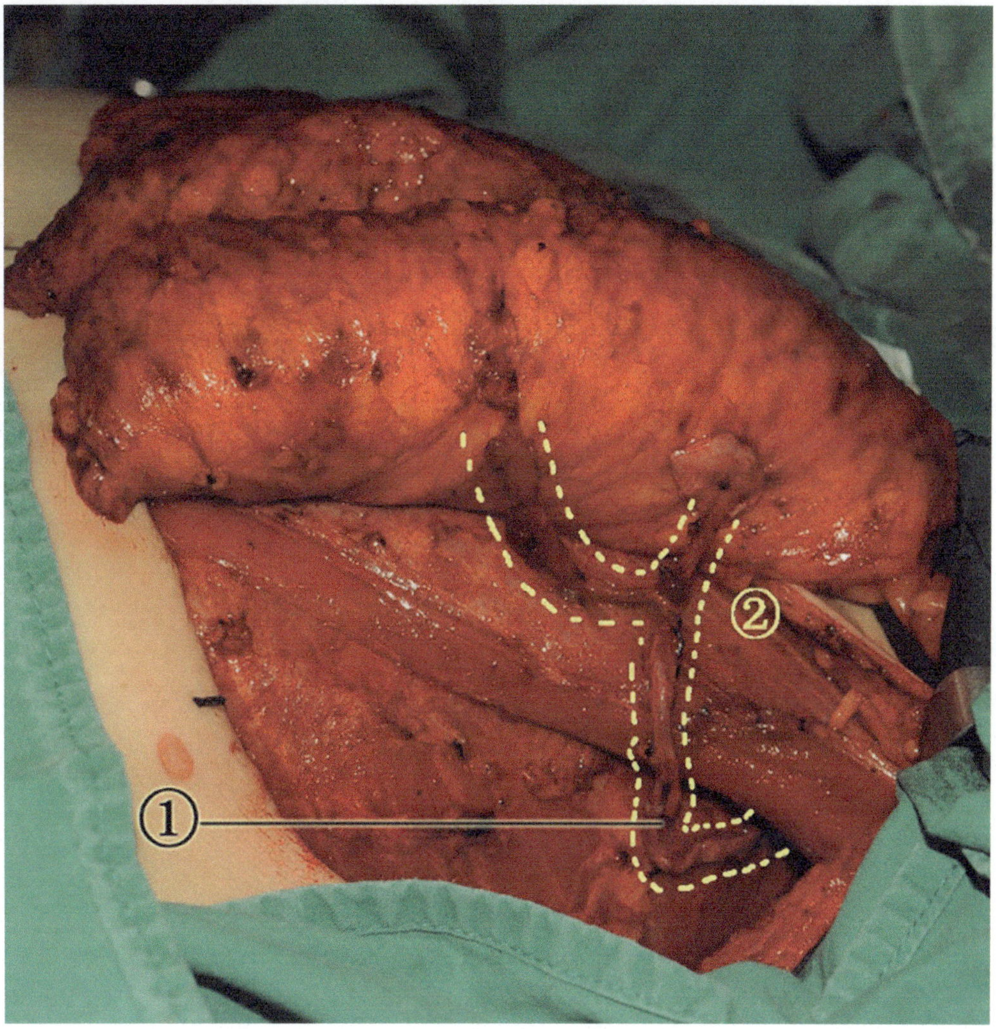

Fig. 11.15 The left lateral thoracic artery and vein were anastomosed with the proximal end of the left deep inferior epigastric artery and vein. (1) Lateral thoracic vessels; (2) Left deep inferior epigastric vessels

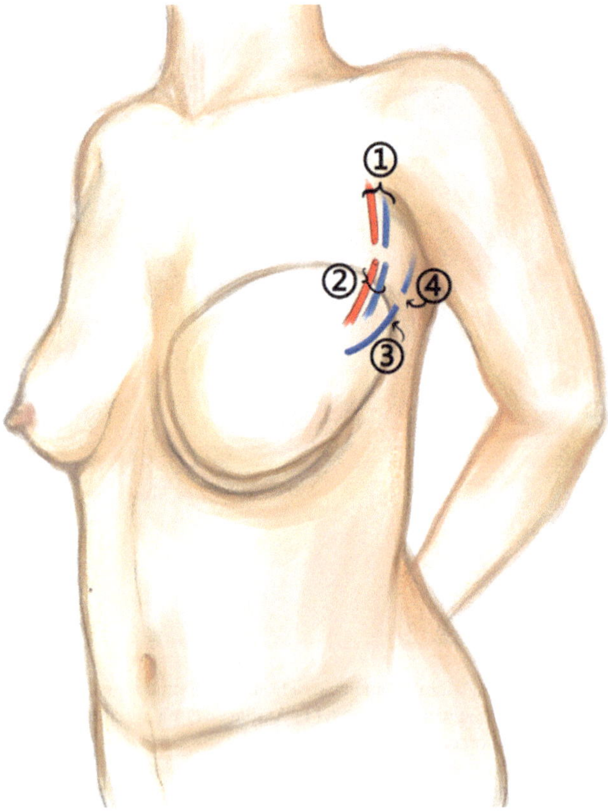

Fig. 11.16 The venous drainage of the flap was poor, which was settled by communicating the concomitant vein of the right deep inferior epigastric artery with the left thoracodorsal vein. The blood supply of the flap was satisfactory. Revascularization pattern. The left deep inferior epigastric artery and vein were anastomosed end-to-end with the left lateral thoracic artery and vein (1A1V), and the accompanying vein of the right deep inferior epigastric artery was anastomosed with the left thoracodorsal vein. (1) Left lateral thoracic artery and vein; (2) Left deep inferior epigastric artery and vein; (3) Right deep inferior epigastric artery with vein; (4) Left thoracodorsal vein

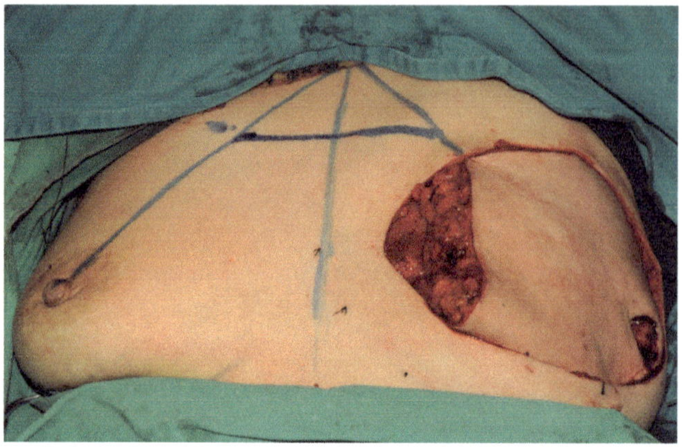

Fig. 11.17 Intraoperative flap shaping

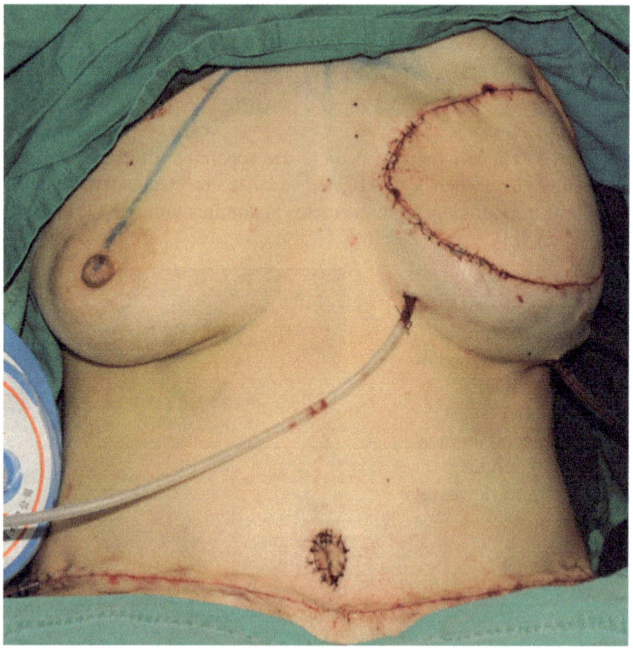

Fig. 11.18 Intraoperative view immediately after reconstruction

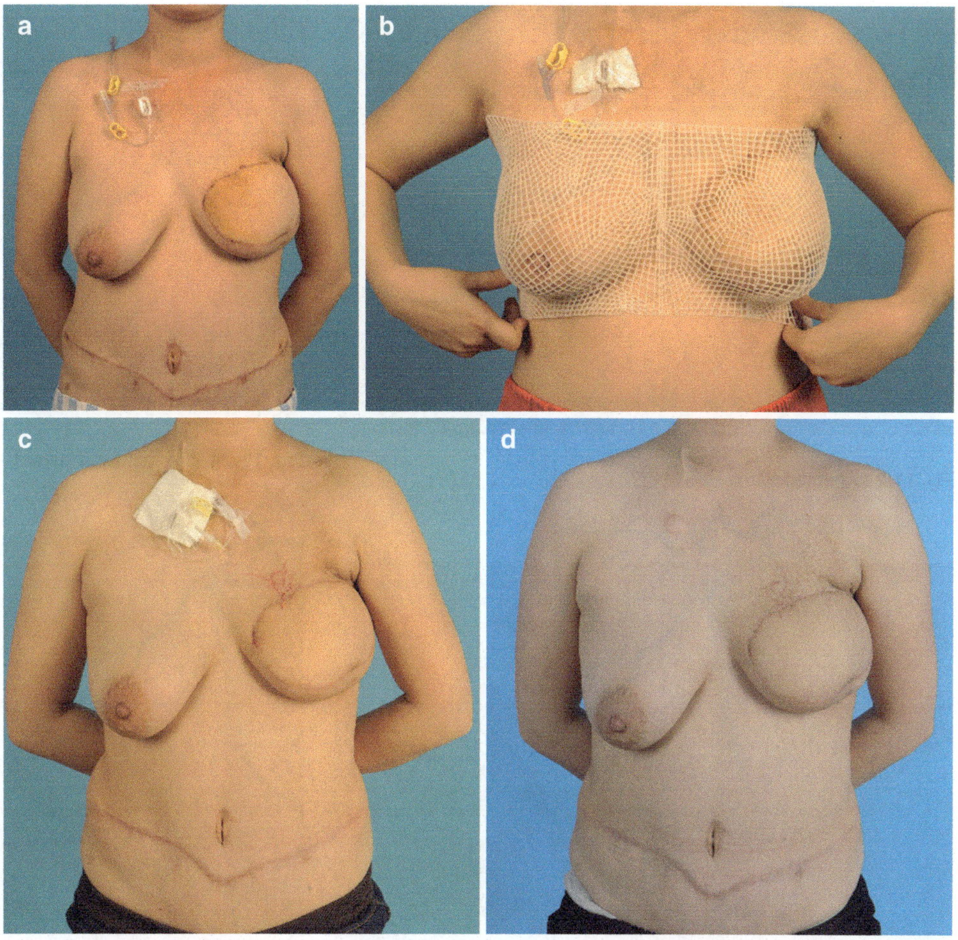

Fig. 11.19 (**a**) 2 months after operation; (**b**) 3 months after operation; (**c**) 6 months after operation; (**d**) 12 months after operation

11.4 Case 2: Turbocharged DIEP Flap

The patient was a 42-year-old female who received modified radical mastectomy for left breast cancer 5 years ago.

The patient received chest scar removal and breast reconstruction using a free deep inferior epigastric artery perforator flap.

The left internal thoracic artery and its accompanying vein were prepared for anastomosis. The size of the flap was about 24 cm × 11 cm, end-to-end anastomosis (1A2V) was performed between the right deep inferior epigastric artery and vein and the distal end of the left deep inferior epigastric artery and vein to form a turbocharged DIEP flap.

The left deep inferior epigastric artery and vein were anastomosed with the internal mammary artery and vein in end-to-end pattern.

The flap survived without any complications. The sensory function and appearance of the reconstructed breast were satisfactory (Figs. 11.20, 11.21, 11.22, 11.23, 11.24, 11.25, 11.26, 11.27, 11.28, 11.29, 11.30, 11.31, 11.32, 11.33, and 11.34).

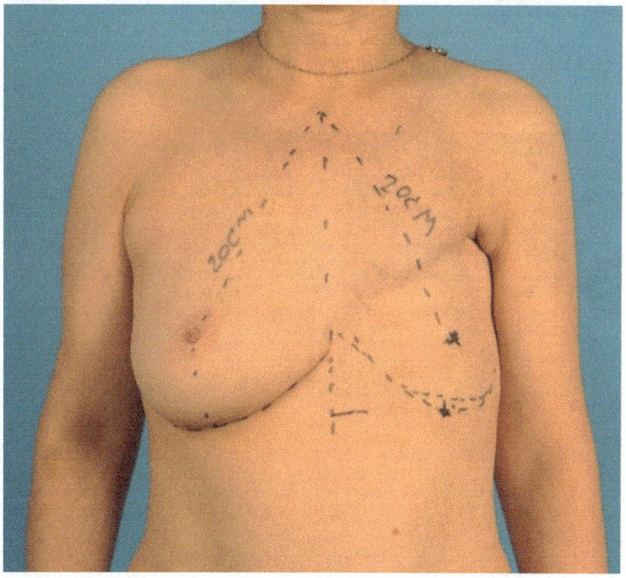

Fig. 11.20 Preoperative view

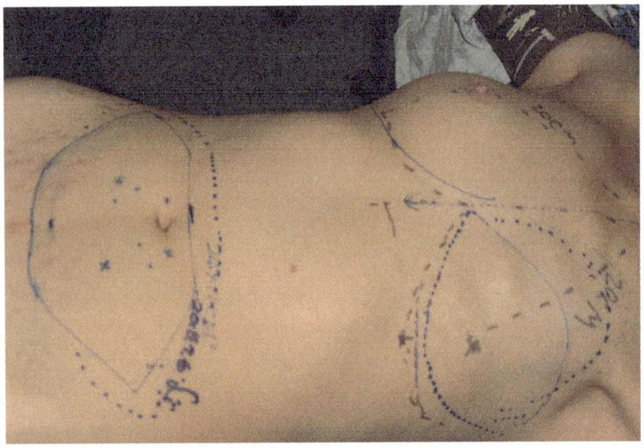

Fig. 11.21 Intraoperative design

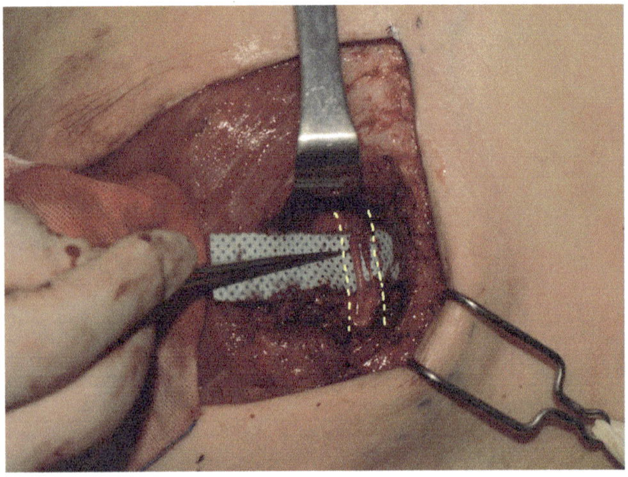

Fig. 11.22 The internal mammary vessel was prepared

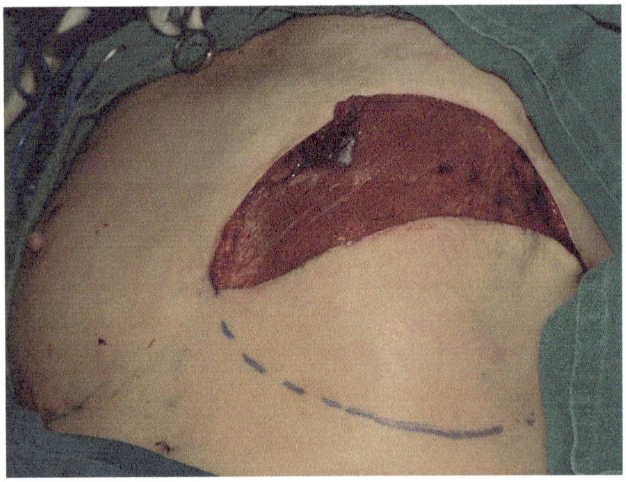

Fig. 11.23 Chest skin envelope was separated

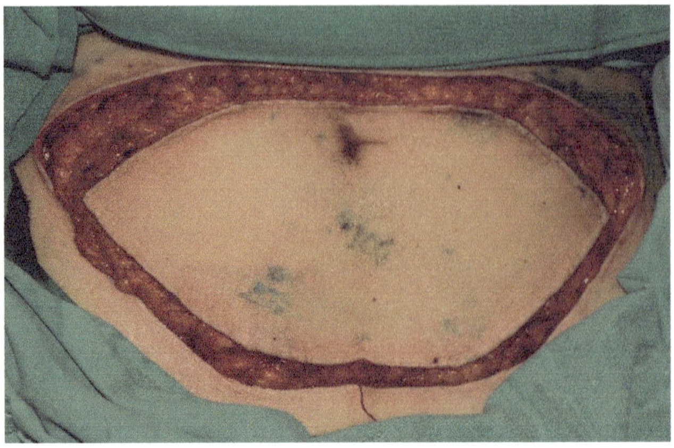

Fig. 11.24 The flap was incised

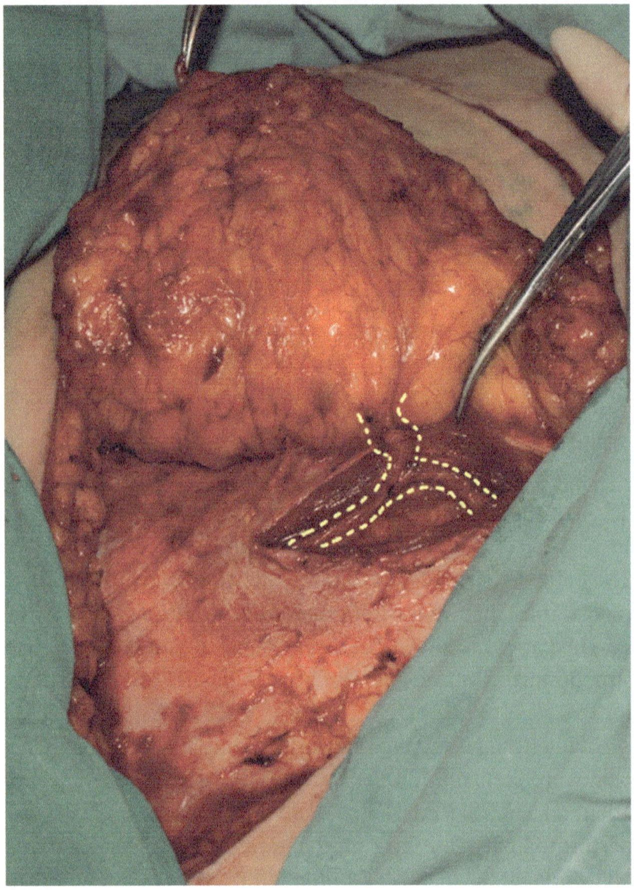

Fig. 11.25 Expose the right perforator vessel, open the anterior sheath, and separate the perforator and the main vascular pedicle in the rectus abdominis muscle

It is very important to mark the bilateral inframammary fold in the patient's sitting position before operation. The separation of the inferior skin envelope ended at the level

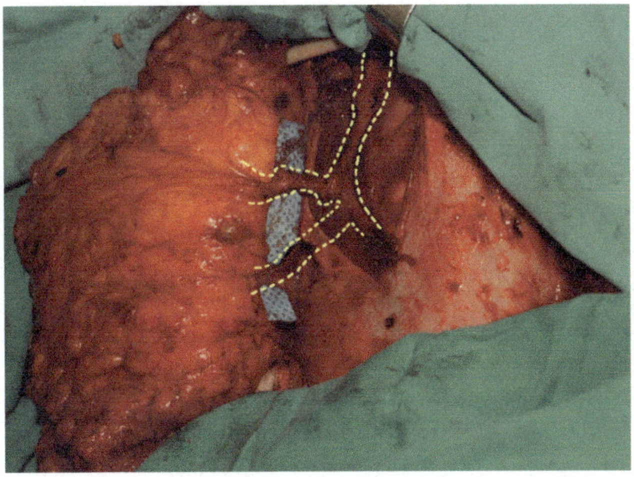

Fig. 11.26 The vascular pedicle was separated till it was close to its emitting plane

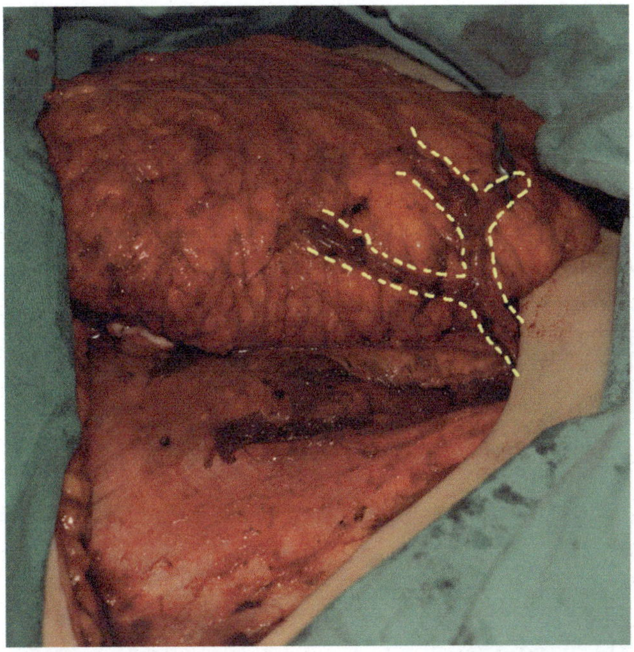

Fig. 11.27 When the flap was lifted medially, another large perforator was found and carried in the flap

1–2 cm above the marked inframammary fold, because ultimately the reconstructed fold will be pulled downward when the abdominal donor area is closed.

The patient was in the supine position, and the affected limb was abducted by 80°, so as to avoid brachial plexus injury caused by extreme abduction.

The patient's hip joint was placed on the flexible plane of the operating table to facilitate the closure of the abdominal donor area and flap shaping in a sitting position.

The patient had a longitudinal scar on the lower abdomen left after a previous surgery and unilateral flap was not large

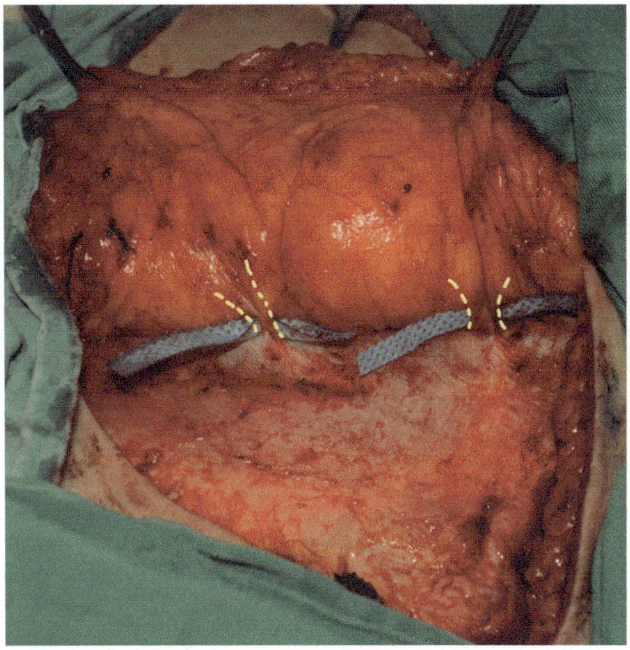

Fig. 11.28 The left perforator was exposed

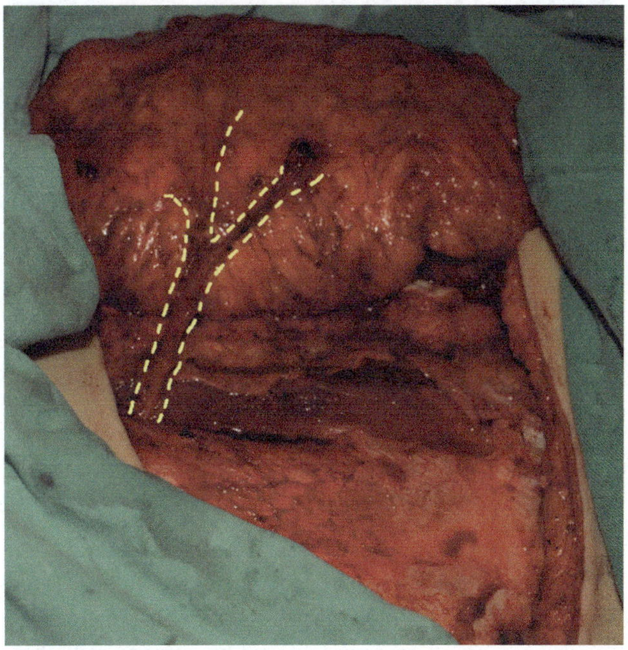

Fig. 11.29 The left perforator and vascular pedicle was separated until it was close to the emitting plane

enough to build a satisfactory breast, therefore, a bilaterally pedicled DIEP flap was used.

Before disconnecting the vascular pedicle of the flap, we must fully evaluate the reliability of the vessels in the recipient area in terms of vascular pulsation and size, vascular wall thickness, as well as the length of the vascular pedicle.

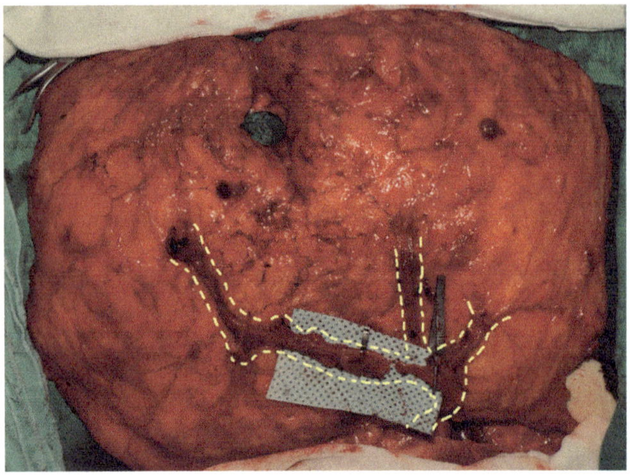

Fig. 11.30 End-to-end anastomosis (1A2V) was performed between the proximal ends of the right deep inferior epigastric artery and vein and the distal ends of the left deep inferior epigastric artery and vein to form turbocharge

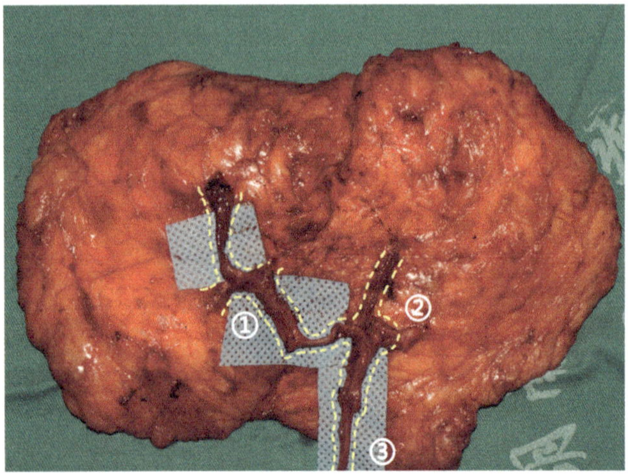

Fig. 11.31 The left deep inferior epigastric artery and vein were end-to-end anastomosed with the internal mammary artery and vein to form turbocharge. (1) The proximal end of the right deep inferior epigastric vessels; (2) Left deep inferior epigastric vessel; (3) Internal mammary vessels

This is particularly important in secondary breast reconstruction, because the blood vessels in the recipient area may have been exposed or even damaged by surgery, radiotherapy, and chemotherapy.

In separating the main vascular pedicle, a segment of vascular pedicle distal to the perforator, a branch of the vascular pedicle or a large muscle branch was harvested to communicate with the contralateral deep inferior epigastric vessels to prepare a turbocharged flap or serial flap.

Notes:

1. Preoperative abdominal CTA angiography and Doppler probing are required to evaluate the perforating vessels and vascular pedicle.

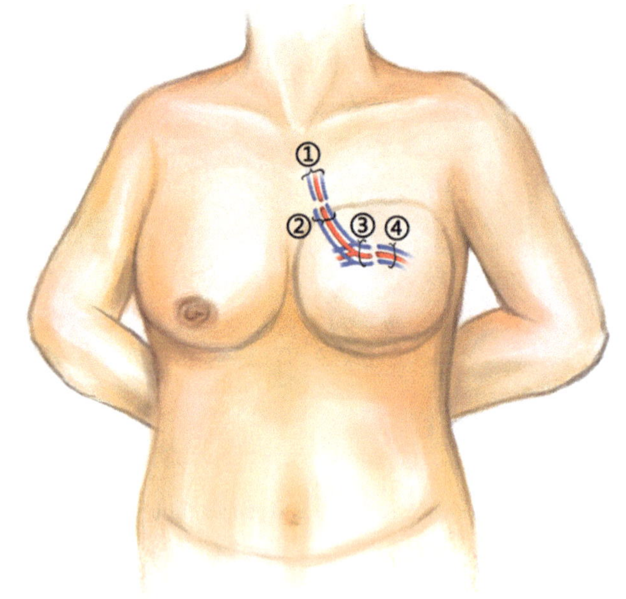

Fig. 11.32 Pattern of revascularization: End-to-end anastomosis (1A2V) were performed between the right deep inferior epigastric artery and vein and the distal ends of the left deep inferior epigastric artery and vein to form turbocharge. The left deep inferior epigastric artery and vein were anastomosed with the internal mammary artery and vein in end-to-end pattern. (1) Internal mammary vessels; (2) The proximal ends of the left deep inferior epigastric vessels; (3) Distal ends of left deep inferior epigastric vessels; (4) Proximal ends of the right deep inferior epigastric vessels

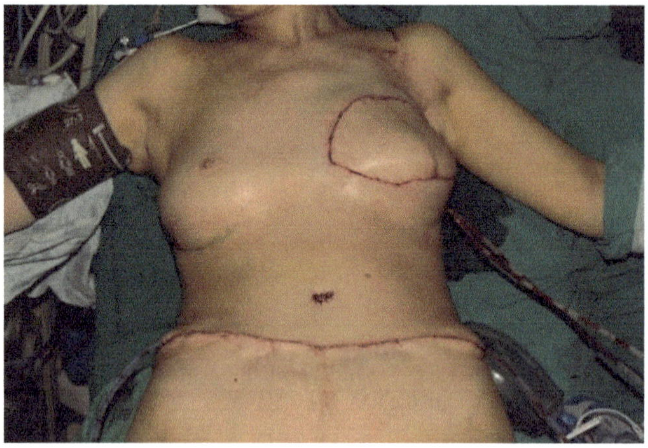

Fig. 11.33 Immediate intraoperative view

2. Turbocharge requires anastomosis of additional arteries and veins, which can effectively avoid venous crisis and guarantee the viability of the flap.
3. Bipedicled turbocharged DIEP flaps can solve some clinical difficulties that are hardly overcome using experience alone. However, it should be noted that good blood supply of the flap simply represented by marginal bleeding is unreliable, yet partial necrosis of the flap may occur after operation.

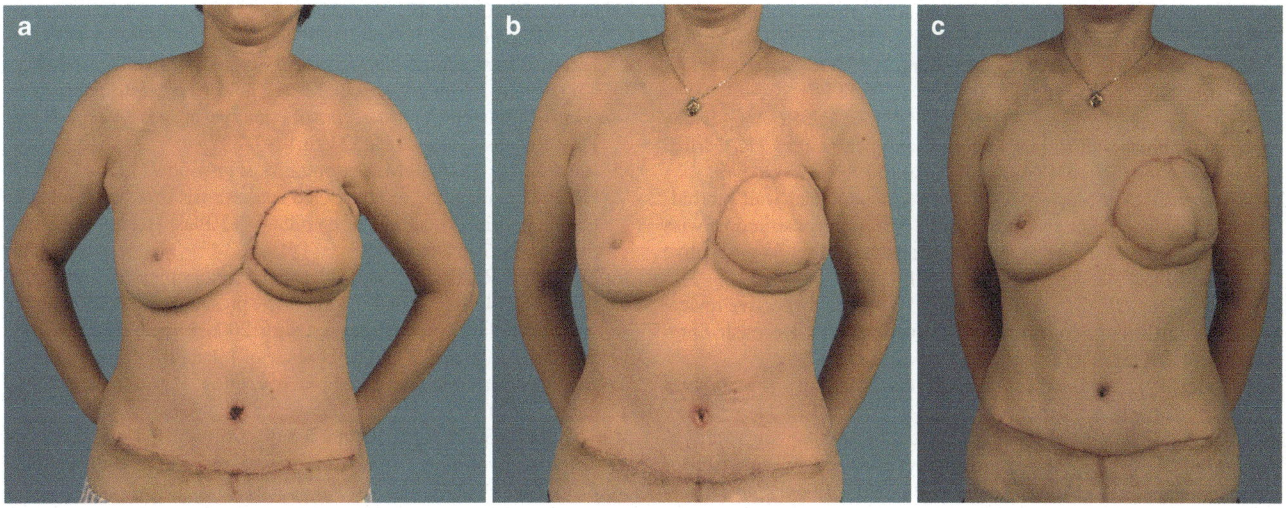

Fig. 11.34 (**a**) 1 month after operation; (**b**) 6 months after operation; (**c**) 12 months after operation

4. Bipedicled turbocharged DIEP flaps for breast or chest wall reconstruction are highly demanding for the operator and the team. It does not need to be selected as a routine operation. It should be carried out only when the indications are clear.

References

1. Allen RJ, Treece P. Deep inferior epigastric perforator flap for breast reconstruction. Ann Plast Surg. 1994;32(1):32–8.
2. Hartrampf CR. The transverse abdominal Island flap for breast reconstruction. A 7-year experience. Clin Plast Surg. 1988;15(4):703–16.
3. Nahabedian MY, Momen B, Galdino G, Manson PN. Breast reconstruction with the free TRAM or DIEP flap: patient selection, choice of flap, and outcome. Plast Reconstr Surg. 2002;110(2):466–75; discussion 476–7.
4. Kroll SS. Fat necrosis in free transverse rectus abdominis myocutaneous and deep inferior epigastric perforator flaps. Plast Reconstr Surg. 2000;106(3):576–83.
5. Blondeel PN, Arnstein M, Verstraete K, et al. Venous congestion and blood flow in free transverse rectus abdominis myocutaneous and deep inferior epigastric perforator flaps. Plast Reconstr Surg. 2000;106(6):1295–9.
6. Blondeel PN, Boeckx WD. Refinements in free flap breast reconstruction: the free bilateral deep inferior epigastric perforator flap anastomosed to the internal mammary artery. Br J Plast Surg. 1994;47(7):495–501.
7. Song R, Ling Y, Wang G, Yang R. One-stage reconstruction of the nose. The Island frontal flap and the "conjoined" frontal flap. Clin Plast Surg. 1982;9(1):37–44.
8. Zuker RM, Filler RM, Lalla R. Intra-abdominal tissue expansion: an adjunct in the separation of conjoined twins. J Pediatr Surg. 1986;21(12):1198–200.
9. Hallock GG. The complete nomenclature for combined perforator flaps. Plast Reconstr Surg. 2011;127(4):1720–9.
10. Hallock GG. Branch-based conjoined perforator flaps. Plast Reconstr Surg. 2008;121(5):1642–9.
11. Ng RL, Youssef A, Kronowitz SJ, Lipa JE, Potochny J, Reece GP. Technical variations of the bipedicled TRAM flap in unilateral breast reconstruction: effects of conventional versus microsurgical techniques of pedicle transfer on complications rates. Plast Reconstr Surg. 2004;114(2):374–84; discussion 385–8.
12. Ali RS, Garrido A, Ramakrishnan V. Stacked free hemi-DIEP flaps: a method of autologous breast reconstruction in a patient with midline abdominal scarring. Br J Plast Surg. 2002;55(4):351–3.
13. Hamdi M, Khuthaila DK, Van Landuyt K, Roche N, Monstrey S. Double-pedicle abdominal perforator free flaps for unilateral breast reconstruction: new horizons in microsurgical tissue transfer to the breast. J Plast Reconstr Aesthet Surg. 2007;60(8):904–12; discussion 913–4.
14. Agarwal JP, Gottlieb LJ. Double pedicle deep inferior epigastric perforator/muscle-sparing TRAM flaps for unilateral breast reconstruction. Ann Plast Surg. 2007;58(4):359–63.
15. Ishii CH, Bostwick J, Raine TJ, Coleman JJ, Hester TR. Double-pedicle transverse rectus abdominis myocutaneous flap for unilateral breast and chest-wall reconstruction. Plast Reconstr Surg. 1985;76(6):901–7.
16. Arnez ZM, Scamp T. The bipedicled free TRAM flap. Br J Plast Surg. 1992;45(3):214–8.
17. Pennington DG, Nettle WJ, Lam P. Microvascular augmentation of the blood supply of the contralateral side of the free transverse rectus abdominis musculocutaneous flap. Ann Plast Surg. 1993;31(2):123–6; discussion 126–7.
18. Semple JL. Retrograde microvascular augmentation (turbocharging) of a single-pedicle TRAM flap through a deep inferior epigastric arterial and venous loop. Plast Reconstr Surg. 1994;93(1):109–17.
19. Lam TC, Sellars GD. Free perforator crossover TRAM flap for breast reconstruction. Ann Plast Surg. 2003;50(2):126–31.
20. Koshima I, Inagawa K, Yamamoto M, Moriguchi T. New microsurgical breast reconstruction using free paraumbilical perforator adiposal flaps. Plast Reconstr Surg. 2000;106(1):61–5.
21. Schoeller T, Bauer T, Gurunluoglu R, et al. Modified free paraumbilical perforator flap: the next logical step in breast reconstruction. Plast Reconstr Surg. 2003;111(3):1093–8; discussion 1099–1101.
22. Nahabedian MY, Dooley W, Singh N, Manson PN. Contour abnormalities of the abdomen after breast reconstruction with abdominal flaps: the role of muscle preservation. Plast Reconstr Surg. 2002;109(1):91–101.
23. Vyas RM, Dickinson BP, Fastekjian JH, Watson JP, Dalio AL, Crisera CA. Risk factors for abdominal donor-site morbidity in free flap breast reconstruction. Plast Reconstr Surg. 2008;121(5):1519–26.

24. Nahabedian MY, Tsangaris T, Momen B. Breast reconstruction with the DIEP flap or the muscle-sparing (MS-2) free TRAM flap: is there a difference. Plast Reconstr Surg. 2005;115(2):436–44; discussion 445–6.
25. Kroll SS, Schusterman MA, Reece GP, Miller MJ, Robb G, Evans G. Abdominal wall strength, bulging, and hernia after TRAM flap breast reconstruction. Plast Reconstr Surg. 1995;96(3):616–9.
26. Ascherman JA, Seruya M, Bartsich SA. Abdominal wall morbidity following unilateral and bilateral breast reconstruction with pedicled TRAM flaps: an outcomes analysis of 117 consecutive patients. Plast Reconstr Surg. 2008;121(1):1–8.
27. Gill PS, Hunt JP, Guerra AB, et al. A 10-year retrospective review of 758 DIEP flaps for breast reconstruction. Plast Reconstr Surg. 2004;113(4):1153–60.
28. Blondeel PN. One hundred free DIEP flap breast reconstructions: a personal experience. Br J Plast Surg. 1999;52(2):104–11.
29. Uda H, Kamochi H, Sarukawa S, Sunaga A, Sugawara Y, Yoshimura K. Clinical and quantitative isokinetic comparison of abdominal morbidity and dynamics following DIEP versus muscle-sparing free TRAM flap breast reconstruction. Plast Reconstr Surg. 2017;140(6):1101–9.
30. Nahabedian MY, Momen B. Lower abdominal bulge after deep inferior epigastric perforator flap (DIEP) breast reconstruction. Ann Plast Surg. 2005;54(2):124–9.
31. Hamdi M, Weiler-Mithoff EM, Webster MH. Deep inferior epigastric perforator flap in breast reconstruction: experience with the first 50 flaps. Plast Reconstr Surg. 1999;103(1):86–95.
32. Uda H, Tomioka YK, Sarukawa S, et al. Abdominal morbidity after single- versus double-pedicled deep inferior epigastric perforator flap use. J Plast Reconstr Aesthet Surg. 2016;69(9):1178–83.
33. Chang EI, Chang EI, Soto-Miranda MA, et al. Comprehensive analysis of donor-site morbidity in abdominally based free flap breast reconstruction. Plast Reconstr Surg. 2013;132(6):1383–91.
34. Xu H, Dong J, Wang T. Bipedicle deep inferior epigastric perforator flap for unilateral breast reconstruction: seven years' experience. Plast Reconstr Surg. 2009;124(6):1797–807.
35. Barabás AG, Shafighi M, Sassoon EM, Haywood RM. The bilateral DIEP flap: a method of bipedicled anastomosis to a single internal mammary artery and venae comitantes. J Plast Reconstr Aesthet Surg. 2008;61(10):1249–51.
36. Das-Gupta R, Busic V, Begic A. Deep inferior epigastric perforator flap (DIEP) breast reconstruction in the presence of a midline vertical scar. J Plast Reconstr Aesthet Surg. 2006;59(6):675–6.
37. Beahm EK, Walton RL. The efficacy of bilateral lower abdominal free flaps for unilateral breast reconstruction. Plast Reconstr Surg. 2007;120(1):41–54.
38. Soutar DS, Scheker LR, Tanner NS, McGregor IA. The radial forearm flap: a versatile method for intra-oral reconstruction. Br J Plast Surg. 1983;36(1):1–8.
39. Foucher G, van Genechten F, Merle N, Michon J. A compound radial artery forearm flap in hand surgery: an original modification of the Chinese forearm flap. Br J Plast Surg. 1984;37(2):139–48.
40. Koshima I, Saisho H, Kawada S, Hamanaka T, Umeda N, Moriguchi T. Flow-through thin latissimus dorsi perforator flap for repair of soft-tissue defects in the legs. Plast Reconstr Surg. 1999;103(5):1483–90.
41. Schoeller T, Wechselberger G, Roger J, Hussl H, Huemer GM. Management of infraumbilical vertical scars in DIEP-flaps by crossover anastomosis. J Plast Reconstr Aesthet Surg. 2007;60(5):524–8.

Bipedicled Supercharged DIEP Flap for Unilateral Breast Reconstruction

12

Zan Li and Xiaomin Yang

The lower abdominal tissue is an ideal donor for autologous breast reconstruction.

In patients with insufficient abdominal fat, however, a unilateral flap pedicled with ipsilateral DIEP is usually unable to provide as much tissue amount for breast reconstruction as that of the contralateral breast.

Transplantation along with contralateral pedicled abdominal perforator flap is an optimal way to increase the amount of fat and skin tissue.

We found that a large bipedicled flap was adequate to reconstruct a symmetric and ptotic breast. Patients with significant chest defects after radiotherapy or a large and ptotic breast on the contralateral side or requiring delayed breast reconstruction are best candidates for breast reconstruction using a bipedicled abdominal flap.

Arnez and Scamp [1] firstly reported the application of double pedicled free rectus abdominis myocutaneous flap in unilateral breast reconstruction in two patients with abdominal midline scar.

Since then, a variety of methods have been used to expand the blood supply of the free tissue flap [2–4].

A bipedicled supercharged DIEP flap is not prepared simply by addition of an abdominal perforator flap, and a second vascular pedicle would exponentially complicate reconstruction.

The increased technical difficulties of microsurgery include the placement of flap and that the dual blood supply of flap must be considered in postoperative monitoring.

The complex operation of double pedicled deep inferior epigastric perforator flap makes it more challenging in manipulation than that of unilateral abdominal perforator flap.

Moreover, the flap size is determined based on flap viability and donor site morbidity as well as required tissue amount [5, 6].

The inclusion of a second vascular pedicle also indicates the need to further separate and dissect the vessels in the recipient area at the same time [7], and if turbocharge is required, an appropriate branch of the first vascular pedicle must also be considered.

When cutting the free perforator flap of deep inferior epigastric artery, we should always weigh the donor area injury against flap blood supply.

Especially when a large defect needs to be reconstructed, the actual operation would be more complex.

However, these obstacles can be foreseen and overcome as long as adequate preoperative preparation is made [8].

The goal of reasonable flap selection and technical improvement is that the reconstructed breast has a symmetrical appearance, donor area injury is minimized, and the postoperative functional recovery of patients is not impaired [9, 10].

There are many ways of revascularization of bilateral vascular pedicles, and bilateral vascular pedicles anastomosed with two vascular pedicles in the receiving area is most commonly used, that is, bipedicled supercharge DIEP flap [8].

12.1 Indications

The bilateral pedicled DIEP flap in breast reconstruction is mainly indicated for patients with large breast and a small amount of abdominal tissue.

Abundant tissue can ensure the symmetry and beauty of the reconstructed breast, and avoid prosthesis implantation and contralateral breast reduction.

Many patients have a history of abdominal surgery. The residual scar will prevent unilateral perforator from offering blood supply to the contralateral flap, limit the size of reconstructed breast, and increase the difficulty of breast reconstruction with abdominal flap transplantation. However, if

Z. Li (✉)
Department of Oncology Plastic Surgery, Hunan Cancer Hospital, Changsha, Hunan, China

X. Yang
Department of Breast Surgery, Tumor Hospital of Shaanxi Province, Xi'an, Shaanxi, China

Z. Li, D. Song (eds.), *Oncoplastic Flap Surgery*, https://doi.org/10.1007/978-981-19-8926-1_12

the donor site can provide enough tissue for breast reconstruction, the history of previous abdominal wall surgery is not an absolute contraindication.

12.2 Surgical Methods and Imaging Features of Double Pedicled Perforator Flap of Deep Inferior Epigastric Artery

The evaluation of blood vessels by preoperative magnetic resonance angiography (MRA) or CTA is of great significance to maximize the success rate of surgery and reduce the time of anesthesia.

The first step of MRA or CTA is to determine the optimal perfusion perforator on one side.

Usually, the deep inferior epigastric blood vessels are the first choice because they are large in diameter, and where they breed contains a thicker fat layer in the central area of the lower abdomen.

Other alternative vessels are the superficial deep inferior epigastric vessels and the superficial circumflex iliac vessels.

The second step is to accurately estimate the difficulty of vascular pedicle anastomosis of bilateral abdominal valves, which can be achieved by locating along the vascular pedicle.

In addition, we need to evaluate how the bilateral deep inferior epigastric vessels bifurcate and whether the large branch is matched in size with the distal end of the perforator distal to the vascular pedicle. If bilateral vascular candidates vary greatly in diameter, supercharged rather than turbocharged vascular anastomosis is favored.

The superficial epigastric artery also needs to be evaluated.

The intraoperative anatomical approach should also be considered when evaluating the anatomy of blood vessels.

If the best perforator of the flap is on the medial side that cannot be approached using a medial incision, a lateral incision is required and cutting off the lateral perforators is inevitable. Raising a bilateral DIEP flap usually starts from the lateral side or from the proximal end to the distal end, and we do not prefer a midline incision on the abdominal wall.

If there is a more suitable vessel on the medial side (visible in MRA or CTA), the lateral perforator may be sacrificed, but in some cases, even if it is confirmed that there is a large perforator on the medial side, the lateral perforator can be retained.

In addition, the perforator can be directly selected by analyzing the MRA or CTA images, or dissecting the contralateral medial perforator when separation of unilateral deep inferior epigastric vascular pedicle using rendezvous method is completed.

A long vascular pedicle is conducive to provide more alternatives for flap vascular anastomosis, and facilitates the placement of flap.

There are two main points in dissecting the deep inferior epigastric vascular pedicle:

1. If anastomosis between unilateral pedicle to contralateral pedicle is planned, a sufficient length of the cephalic end of one pedicle is required.
2. When dissecting the vascular pedicle caudally, it should be cut off where it is close to the external celiac vessels.

The freed vascular pedicle >8 cm in length is helpful to place the flap and reduce the tension during microvascular anastomosis. In our clinical practice, we can harvest a vascular pedicle as long as at least 12–14 cm (Figs. 12.1, 12.2, 12.3, 12.4, and 12.5).

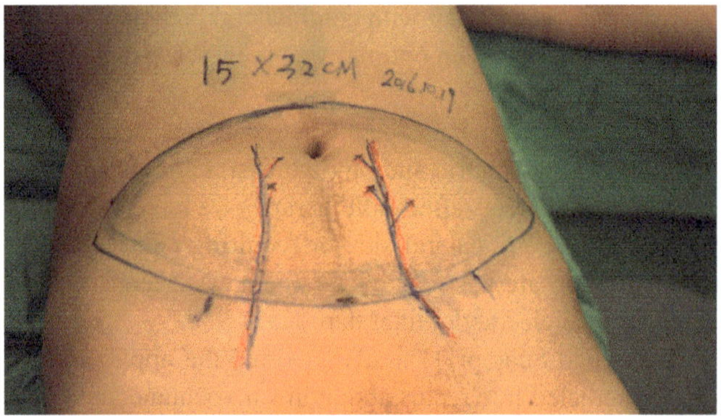

Fig. 12.1 Flap design. A longitudinal Cesarean section incision was seen in the abdominal wall, and a perforator flap of deep inferior epigastric artery with bilateral vascular pedicles was designed

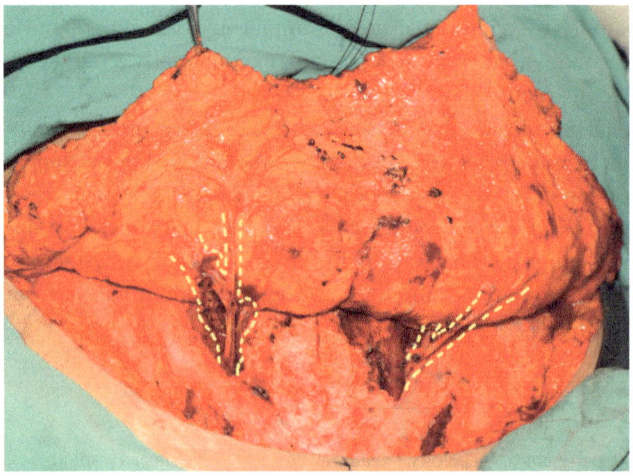

Fig. 12.2 A perforator flap with bilateral epigastric vascular pedicles was harvested

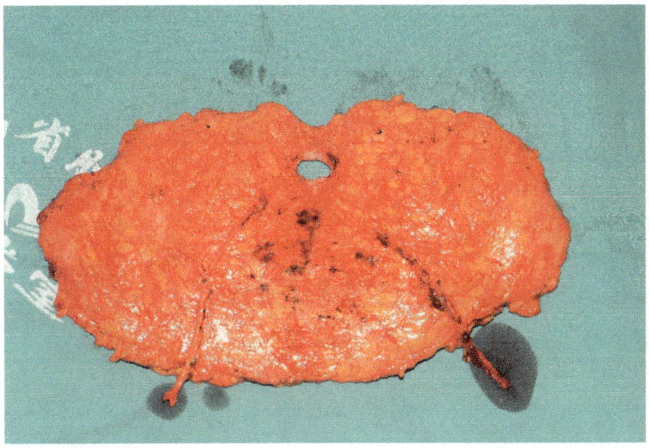

Fig. 12.3 The flap was harvested

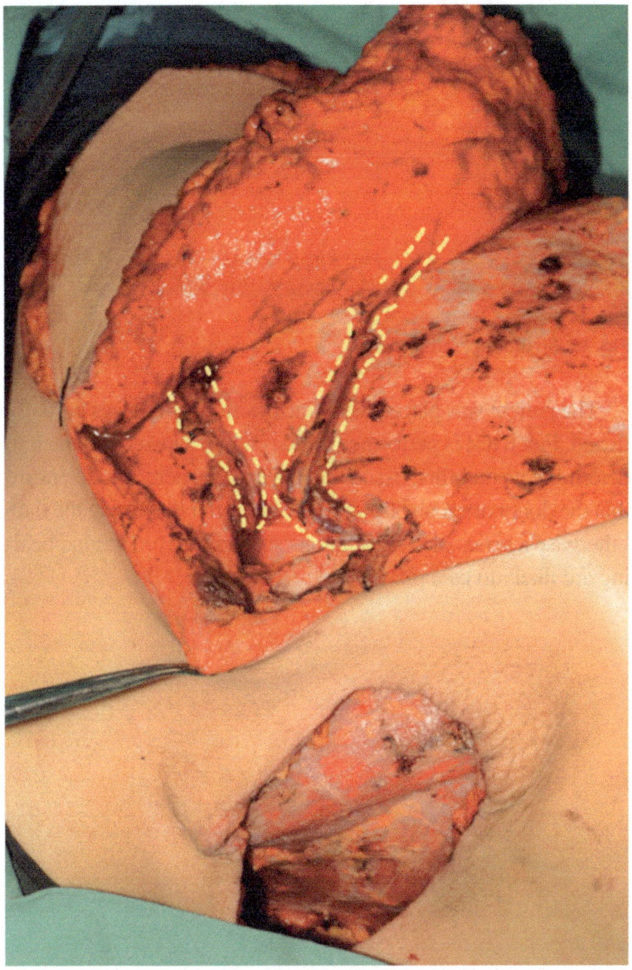

Fig. 12.4 End-to-end anastomosis (2A2V) between bilateral deep inferior epigastric vessels and proximal and distal ends of right internal thoracic vessels were made, respectively

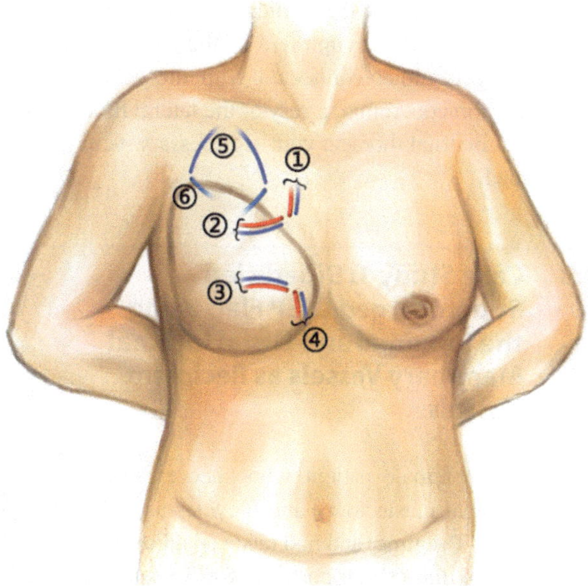

Fig. 12.5 Another vena comitan of the left DIEA and the left SIEV were anastomosed with two thoracoacromial veins, respectively. (1) Proximal IMA vessels; (2) Left deep inferior epigastric vessels; (3) Right deep inferior epigastric vessels; (4) Distal IMA vessels; (5) Concomitant veins of the thoracoacromial artery; (6) SIEV

Common recipient vessels used for anastomosis in breast reconstruction and chest wall reconstruction with bipedicled supercharged DIEP flaps are as follows:

1. Proximal + distal internal thoracic vessels.
2. Internal mammary vessels + lateral thoracic vessels.
3. Internal mammary vessels + transverse cervical vessels.
4. Internal mammary vessels + anterior serratus branch of thoracodorsal vessels.
5. Lateral thoracic vessels + thoracic acromial vessels.
6. Anterior serratus branch of thoracodorsal vessels + lateral thoracic vessels.
7. Proximal + distal lateral thoracic vessels.
8. Thoracoacromial vessels + lateral thoracic vessels.
9. Lateral thoracic vessels + thoracodorsal vessels.
10. Proximal + distal thoracic dorsal vessels.

We should be cautious about using free tissue flap for breast reconstruction in patients who once received chemotherapy on the ground that their vessels are commonly in poor condition and the perforators are degenerative and atrophic, making operation more difficult.

In many cases, the perforator flap of the deep inferior epigastric artery with bilateral vascular pedicles is reliable. The internal thoracic artery is generally accompanied by only one vein. In order to ensure the sufficient venous reflux of the flap, the other accompanying vein of the deep inferior epigastric artery is either connected with the accompanying vein of the thoracoacromial artery or the lateral thoracic vein or the distal internal thoracic vein, if necessary, vein grafting is performed.

12.3 Case Study 1: Bipedicled Supercharged DIEP Flap Using the Proximal and Distal Internal Mammary Vessels as Recipient Vessels

A 41-year-old female patient who once experienced right modified radical mastectomy and 6 cycles adjuvant chemotherapy (FEC-T regime) and had received adjuvant endocrine therapy (tamoxifen 60 mg per day) for 3 years was free of recurrence during follow-up. The pathological results at that time were histological grade III, ER70%, PR80%, HER2 –, ki67 level of 10% (pT2N1M0,IIb).

The patient received right breast reconstruction using a free bipedicled DIEP flap and laparoscopic left breast augmentation with prothesis via axillary incision.

The left deep inferior epigastric arteriovenous vessels carried by the flap were end-to-end anastomosed with the proximal ends of the internal thoracic artery and vein (1A1V), and the right deep inferior epigastric arteriovenous vessels were end-to-end anastomosed with the distal ends of the internal thoracic artery and vein (1A1V).

After operation, the patient recovered well, the incision healed well, and the appearance and function recovered satisfactorily (Figs. 12.6, 12.7, 12.8, 12.9, 12.10, 12.11, 12.12, and 12.13).

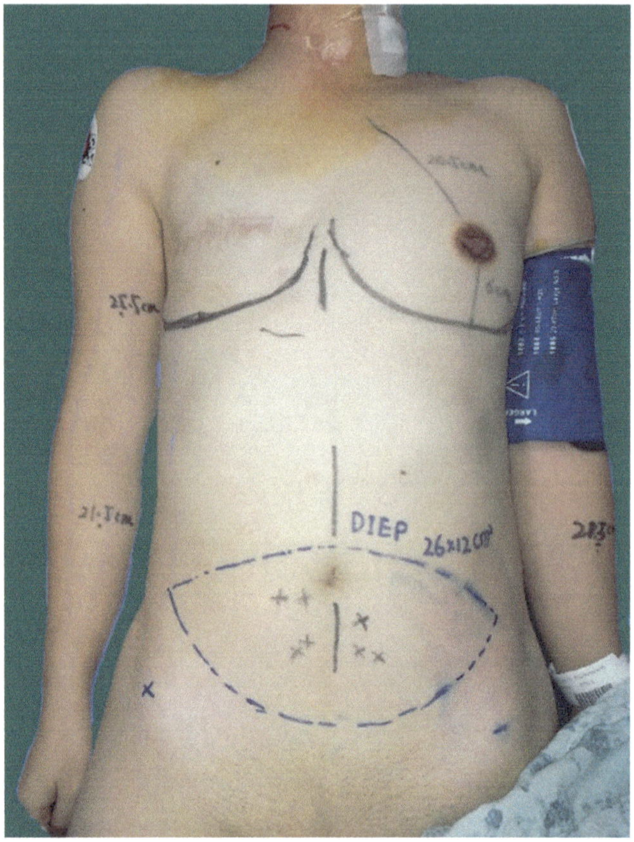

Fig. 12.6 Intraoperative design

The patient was placed in supine position with knees partially flexed. Pinch test is performed on the patient's lower abdomen to determine its mobility, tissue volume and elasticity and to ensure that the donor area can be closed directly after dissecting the flap, otherwise a series of complications such as delayed wound healing are likely to take place.

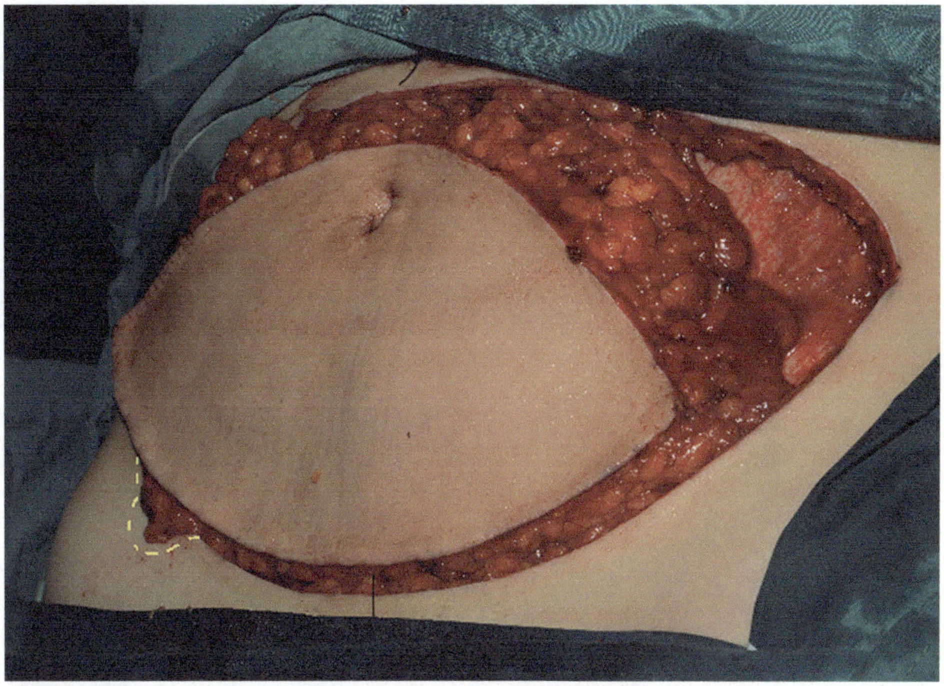

Fig. 12.7 The flap was raised and the right SIEV was carried in the flap

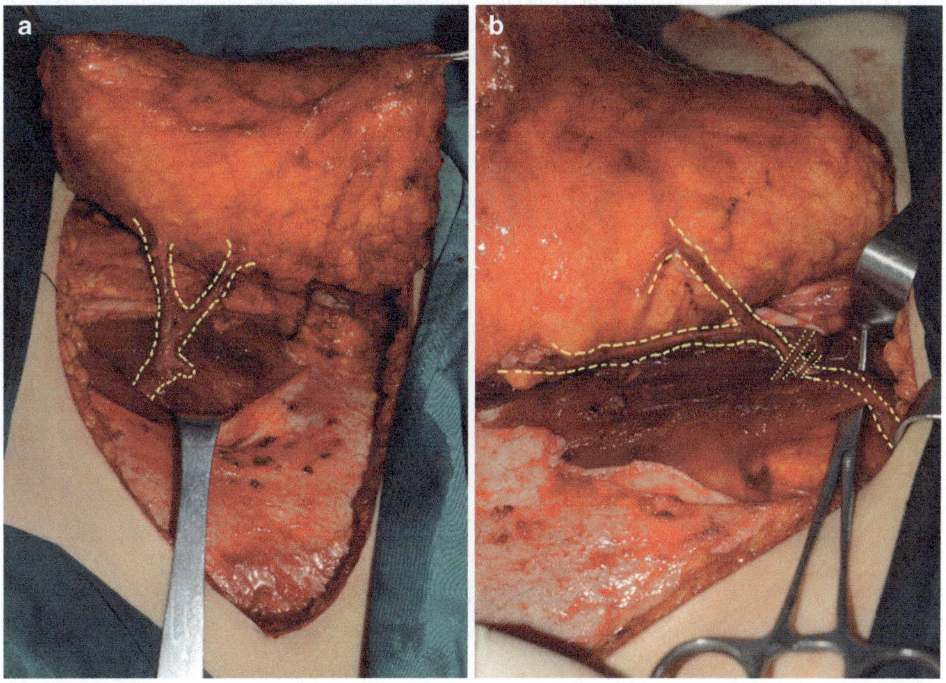

Fig. 12.8 (**a**, **b**) The perforators and vascular pedicles on both sides were separated in the muscle. The vascular pedicle was cut off from the origin

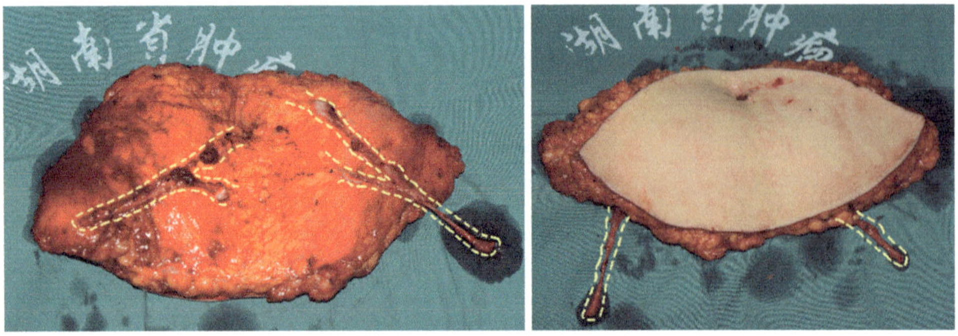

Fig. 12.9 The flap was harvested

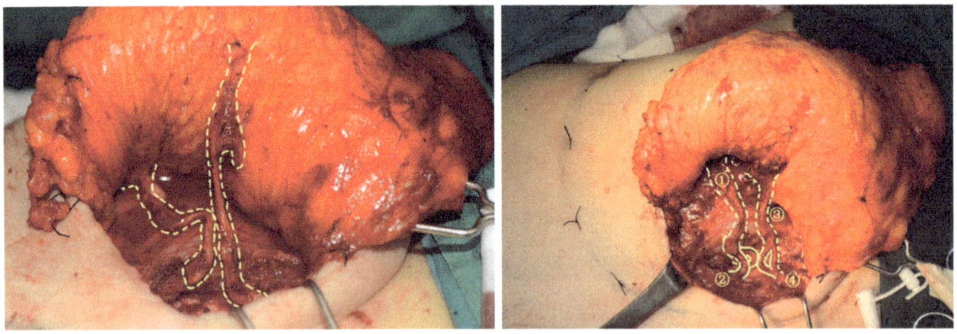

Fig. 12.10 The flap was transferred to the right chest, and the bilateral deep inferior epigastric vessels and the proximal and distal ends of the right IMA vessels were anastomosed, respectively (2A2V). (1) Right deep inferior epigastric vessels; (2) Proximal IMA vessels; (3) Left deep inferior epigastric vessels; (4) Distal IMA vessels

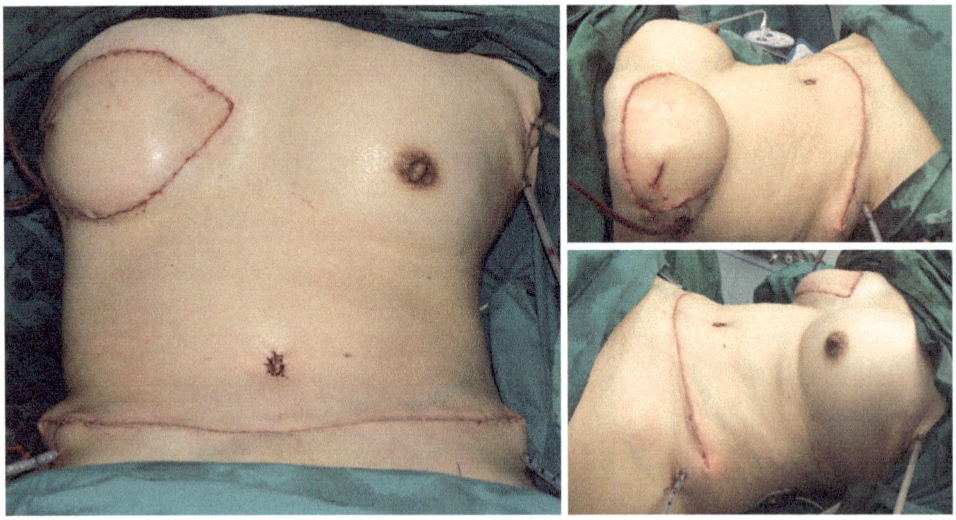

Fig. 12.11 Intraoperative view immediately after flap shaping. Laparoscopic left breast augmentation with prothesis via axillary incision was performed

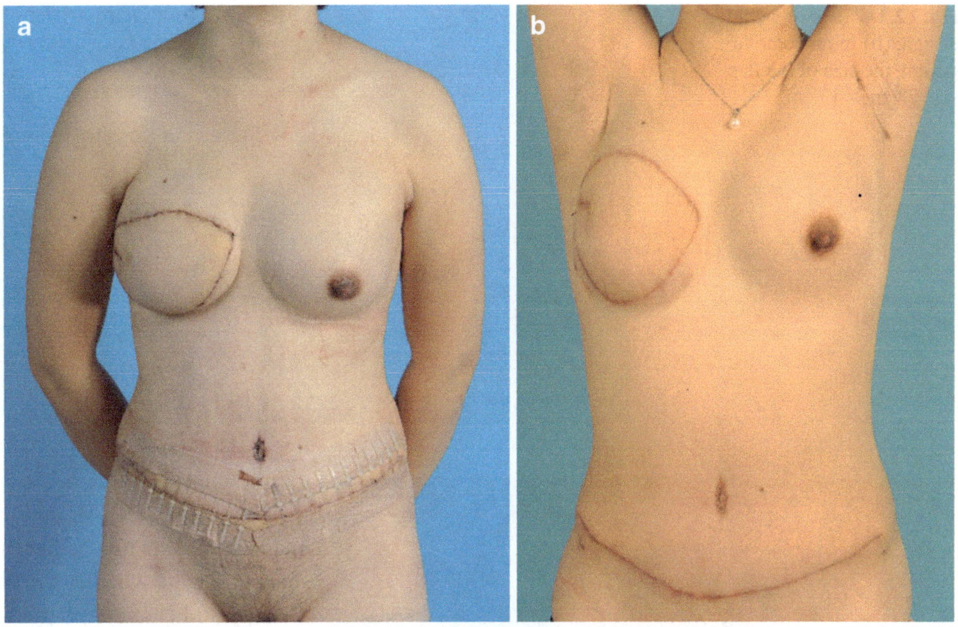

Fig. 12.12 (**a**) 2 weeks after operation. (**b**) The recovery of appearance and function was satisfactory at 3-month follow-up after operation

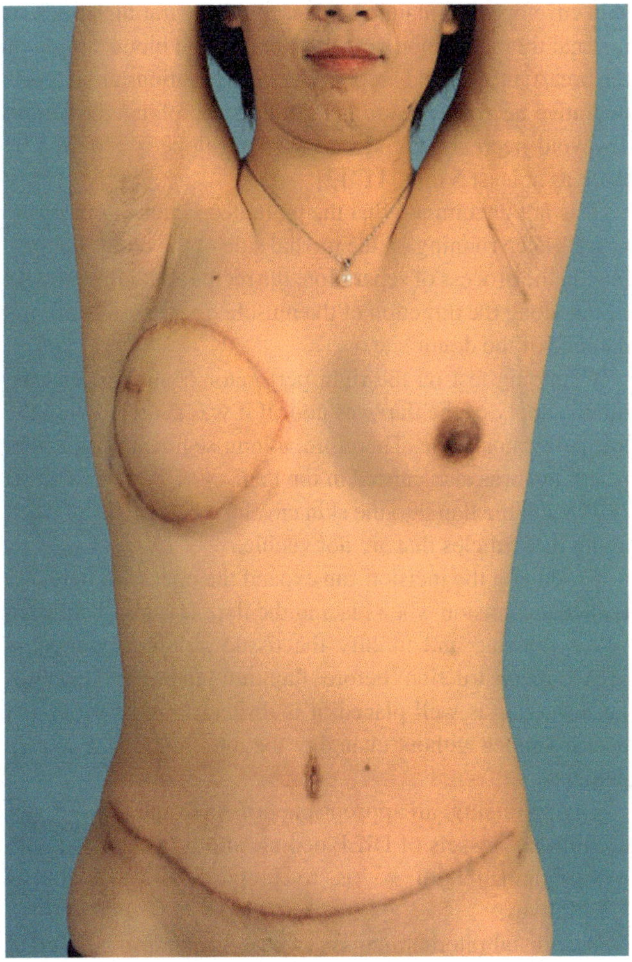

Fig. 12.13 12 months at follow-up, the appearance and function recovered satisfactorily

12.4 Case Study 2: Supercharged Vascular Anastomosis: The Anterior Serratus Branch of Thoracodorsal Vessel and the Proximal End of Internal Thoracic Vessels Were Used as Recipient Vessels

A 48-year-old female presented for left breast invasive ductal carcinoma (histology Grade III) diagnosed on lumpectomy 10 days ago.

At admission, left nipple-sparing mastectomy plus left sentinel lymph node biopsy plus breast reconstruction with DIEP flap were performed.

The size of the designed flap was about 28 cm × 13 cm, carrying the right SIEV of 7 cm in length. The right vascular pedicle about 11 cm long was connected with the anterior serratus branch of the left thoracodorsal vessel (1A1V) and the left deep inferior epigastric artery and vein were anastomosed end to end with the left internal thoracic vessels (1A1V).

Postoperative pathological examination showed that sentinel lymph nodes (0/4) and all margins were free of tumor (pT2N0M0, IIa). Immunohistochemical results were ER (−), PR(−), CerbB-2(−), ki67 index of 70%. The patient was subsequently transferred to the internal medicine department for comprehensive treatment.

The flap survived completely and the patients recovered satisfactorily during follow-up (Figs. 12.14, 12.15, 12.16, 12.17, 12.18, 12.19, 12.20, 12.21, 12.22, and 12.23).

Markings of the breasts and the abdomen were made when the patient standing before operation.

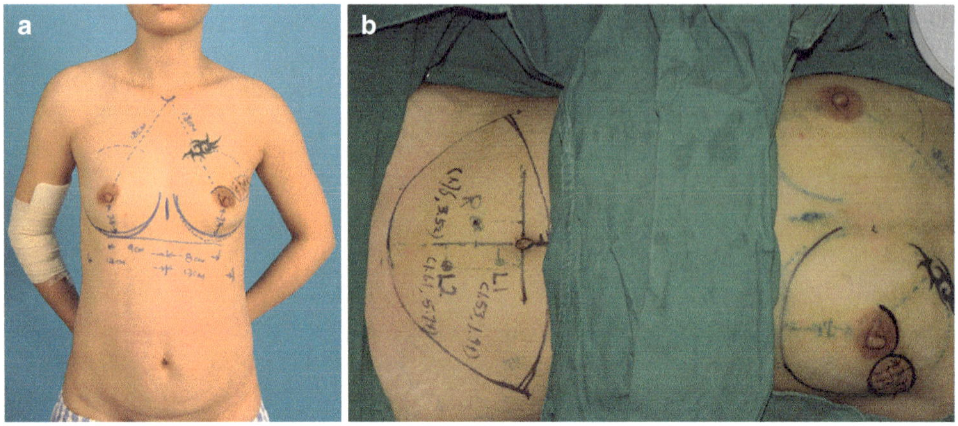

Fig. 12.14 (**a**) Preoperative design. (**b**) Intraoperative design, the size of the flap was 28 cm × 13 cm

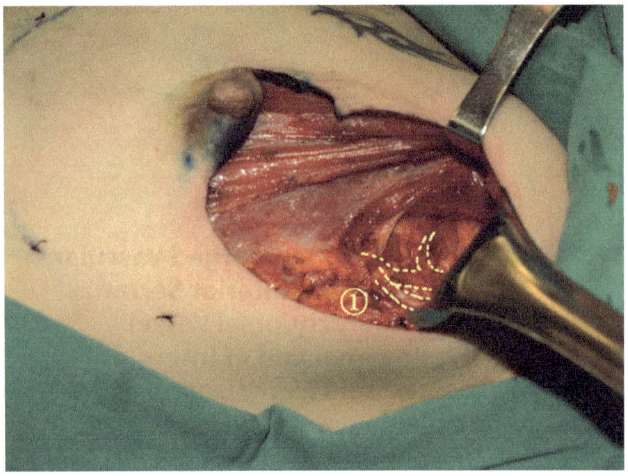

Fig. 12.15 Preparation of vessels in the receiving area. The anterior serratus branch of the left thoracodorsal vessels and the proximal end of the internal thoracic vessels were selected. (1) Anterior serratus branch of thoracodorsal vessels

On the chest wall, the boundary of the existing breast was marked. In the lower abdomen, the midline, peri-umbilicus, and the outline of oval flap in the lower abdomen were marked.

The patient lay on her back, and the position of major perforators were marked according to the results of CTA or MRA or by using an audible Doppler.

At the same time, we needed to move the tissue of the lower abdomen slightly upward to reduce the tension when closing the abdominal wall.

The abdominal wound can move down more than 7 cm.

Further, it is to determine whether to cut a single pedicle or double-pedicle flap according to the required tissue volume. If the patient received Cesarean section before, and the amount of tight abdominal tissue is less while more tissue needs to be cut, priority should be given to cutting bilateral vascular pedicle flaps. Whether turbocharged or supercharged vascular anastomosis is adopted is based on the actual perforator conditions. The decision as to using a flap with unilateral pedicled TRAM and contralateral FREE DIEP was made according to whether the patient can tolerate prolonged anesthesia and whether she once received preoperative radiotherapy and chemotherapy.

In immediate breast reconstruction, the natural inframammary fold should be conserved when separating the breast skin envelope; maintaining at least one penetrating branch of internal thoracic blood vessels to ensure the blood supply of the breast, nipple, and areola skin; being cautious about postoperative necrosis of skin margin due to prolonged traction. To avoid necrosis, the spared skin envelope is required as thick as at least 5 mm [11, 12].

It is not uncommon that the main deep inferior epigastric vessels keep running on the medial side of the rectus abdominis. In the process of separation, the rectus abdominis should be cut along the direction of the muscle fiber to minimize the damage of the donor site.

Clamping test on the right perforator confirmed that the blood supply of the flap was poor if it was pedicled with the left perforator alone. Therefore, a long segment of the right perforator was also carried in the flap.

Placing the flap into the skin envelope bears risks of damaging the pedicles that are not visible.

Extending the incision can expand the operation field and reduce the tension when placing the flap. It is also helpful to better evaluate and modify the tissue volume required in breast reconstruction before flap implantation. However, once the flap is well placed, it is difficult to take it out and trim it further without changing the direction of the double pedicles.

In flap raising, all appropriate branches and the superior continuous vessels of DIEP pedicle should be carried with a sufficient length so as to prepare for anastomosis alternatives.

The distal internal mammary vessels can also be used to anastomose a second pedicle after removal of partial costal cartilage; we usually assess which recipient vessel to be

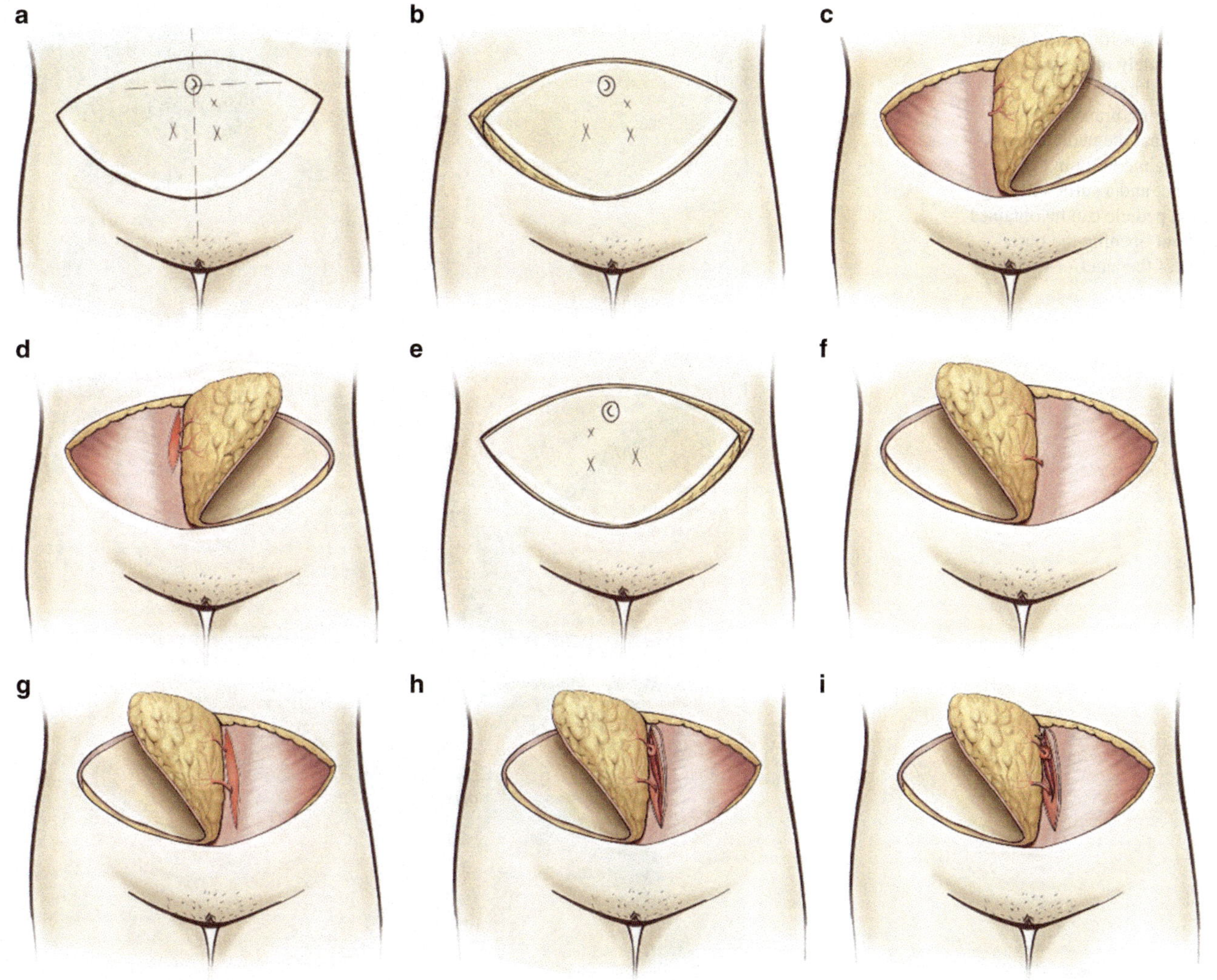

Fig. 12.16 Schematic diagram of flap design and cutting process. (**a**) Flap design; (**b**) Starting with cutting the subcutaneous tissue on one side; (**c**) Lifting the flap to expose the perforator of the right deep inferior epigastric artery; (**d**) The anterior sheath was cut longitudinally along the outer edge of the perforating branch to expose the deep part of the perforating branch. It was found that the right deep inferior epigastric perforating branches were thin; (**e**) The left flap was cut; (**f**) Lifting the left flap to expose two large perforating branches of deep inferior epigastric artery; (**g**) Cutting the anterior sheath and exposing the deep parts of the two perforating branches. It can be seen that the superior perforating branch was going through tendon inscriptions and the lower perforating branch was a musculocutaneous pattern; (**h**) It was difficult to completely remove the tendon inscriptions surrounding the perforator that was harvested to avoid vascular injury. Separation was continued at the level of the lower perforator in the muscle caudally toward the main trunk of deep inferior epigastric vessels and cephalically toward the superior perforator to avoid accidental injury; (**i**) The main artery of the deep inferior epigastric artery was ligated far from the superior perforating branch, and the vascular pedicle was separated retrogradely

connected with a second pedicle among all vascular candidates.

Rarely, the internal thoracic artery runs between the internal and external thoracic veins. The two venous pedicles can be revascularized with the proximal internal mammary veins. The proximal veins are preferred because the distal veins are likely to contain valves [13].

When there is only one internal thoracic vein, the distal end can be considered for anastomosis when blood regurgitation occurs after using heparinized saline for repeated rinse. The blood pressure is found to be higher in the proximal internal mammary artery than in the distal end, which is capable of providing the flap with sufficient blood perfusion.

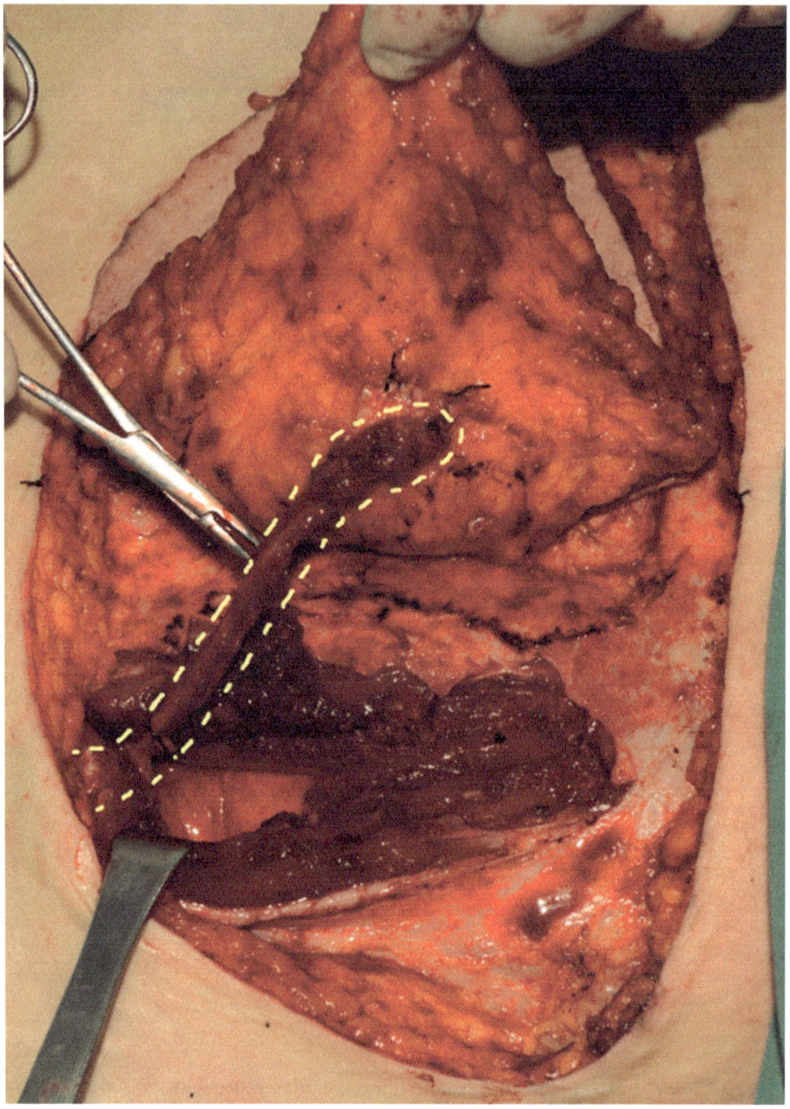

Fig. 12.17 The vascular pedicle was further separated retrogradely in the muscle proximal to the lower perforating branch. It was found that the pedicle kept running medially in the muscle, and a sufficient length of the pedicle can be obtained without opening the outer edge of the anterior sheath

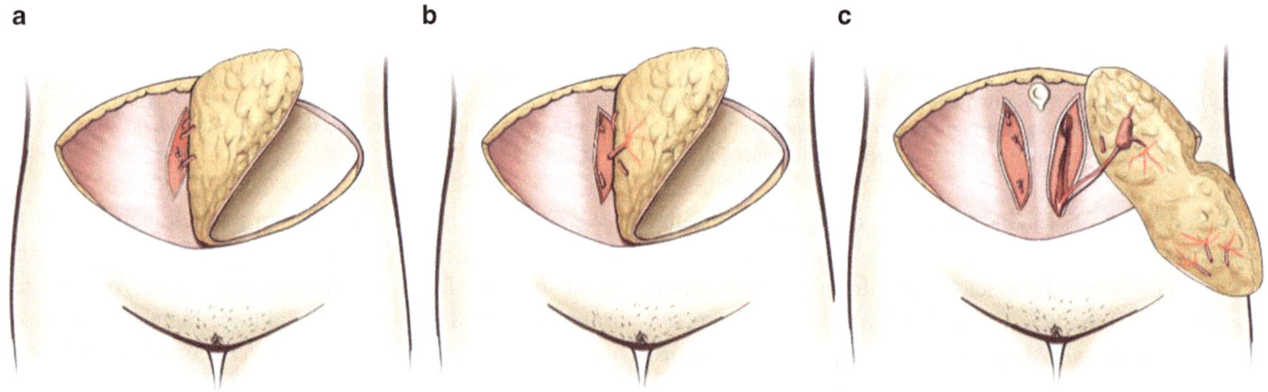

Fig. 12.18 Flap raising. (**a**) Cutting off two small perforating branches on the right side to further separate the flap; (**b**) Exposing another large DIEA musculocutaneous perforator close to the midline on the right side to complete flap harvest, and removing the umbilicus from the flap. Clamping test confirmed that the blood supply of the flap was unreliable, so the perforating branches were separated till a sufficient vascular length was obtained for turbocharge; (**c**) The flap was prepared and bilateral donor site damage was minimized

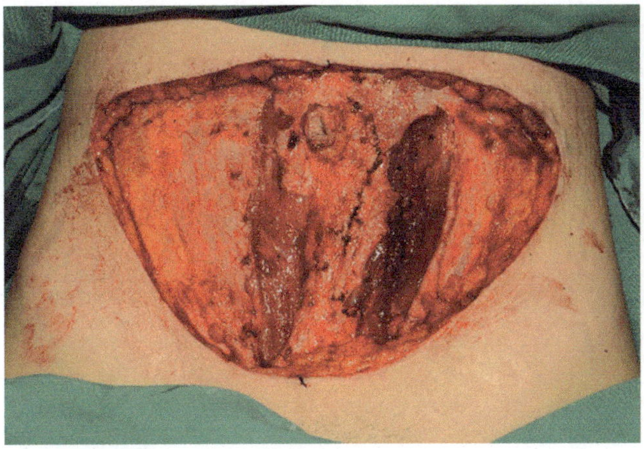

Fig. 12.19 Donor area view after flap removal. The integrity of rectus abdominis and its anterior sheath was preserved

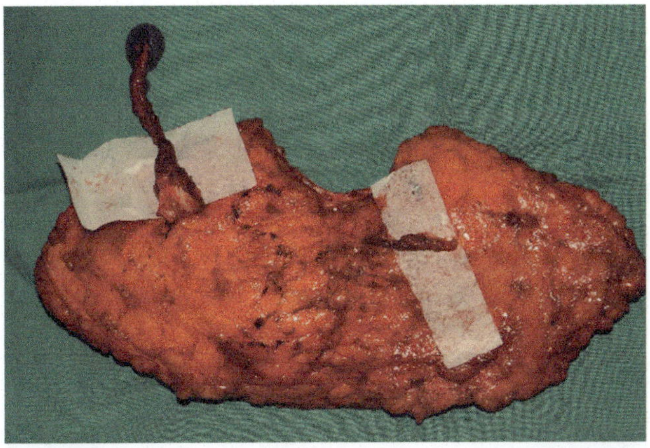

Fig. 12.20 The flap was harvested

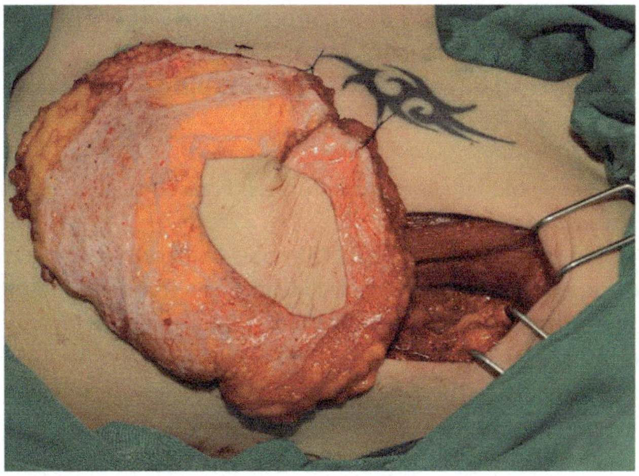

Fig. 12.21 The flap was transferred to the recipient area and de-epithelization was performed

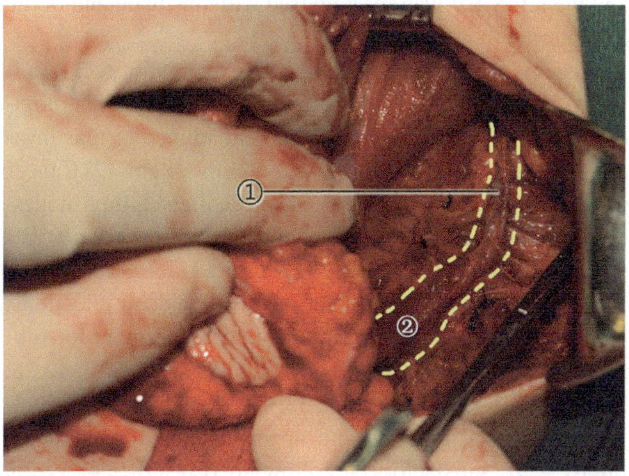

Fig. 12.22 The right DIEP was anastomosed with the anterior serratus branch of the left thoracodorsal vessel. The left DIEP was anastomosed with the left internal mammary vessel. (1) Anterior serratus branch of left thoracodorsal vessel; (2) Perforating branch of right deep inferior epigastric vessels

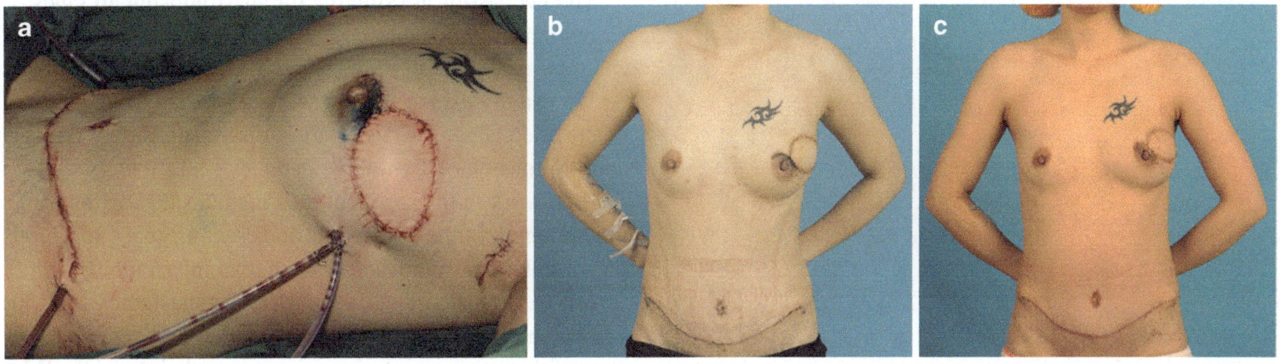

Fig. 12.23 (**a**) View immediately after operation; (**b**) Follow-up at 1 month after operation; (**c**) Follow-up at 9 months after operation

12.5 Case Study 3: Supercharged DIEP Flap Using Internal Mammary Vessels and Lateral Thoracic Vessels as Recipient

A 43-year-old female present for a left breast mass found for 1 week.

The patient received left NSM plus axillary lymph node dissection and breast reconstruction using a free DIEP flap.

The weight of the removed breast tissue and the bipedicled DIEP flap was 650 g and 980 g, respectively. Area IV and part of Area III of the flap were removed, and the remaining flap weighed 700 g.

The left internal thoracic vessels containing one artery (about 2 mm in caliber) and one vein (about 2 mm in caliber) communicated with the left deep inferior epigastric vessels. The right deep inferior epigastric artery and vein were anastomosed with the left lateral thoracic artery and vein (1A1V), and the left SIEV was anastomosed with the distal end of the left internal thoracic vein.

Results of routine pathological examination: (1) (left breast) Invasive ductal carcinoma (pT2N1M0,IIb), histological grade III, focal squamous differentiation, vascular invasion (+), mass size of about 2.5 cm × 2 cm × 1 cm; (2) Cancer metastasis was found in 1/15 of left axillary lymph nodes; (3) Margins were clear. Immunohistochemistry results: ER (−), PR (weak, < 1%), HER-2 (1 +), Ki-67 (1 +, about 30%).

The flap survived completely without any complications. The patient was transferred to oncology department for subsequent treatment (Figs. 12.24, 12.25, 12.26, 12.27, 12.28, 12.29, 12.30, 12.31, 12.32, 12.33, 12.34, and 12.35).

The sensory function and appearance of reconstructed breast were satisfactory at follow-up (Figs. 12.24, 12.25, 12.26, 12.27, 12.28, 12.29, 12.30, 12.31, 12.32, 12.33, 12.34, and 12.35).

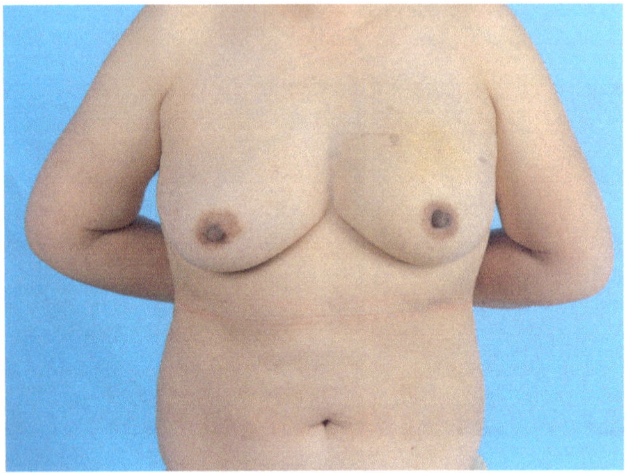

Fig. 12.24 Preoperative view

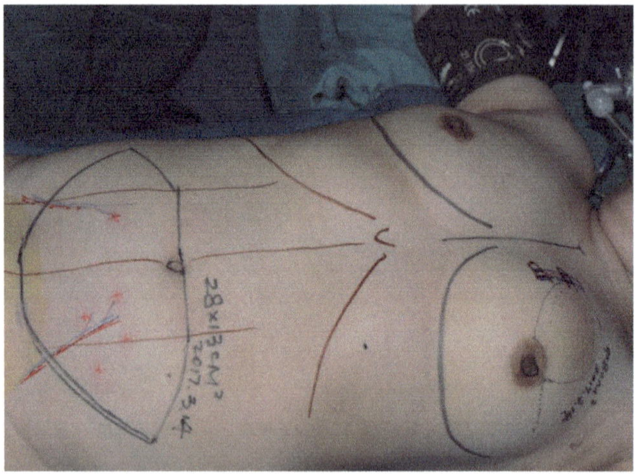

Fig. 12.25 Intraoperative design

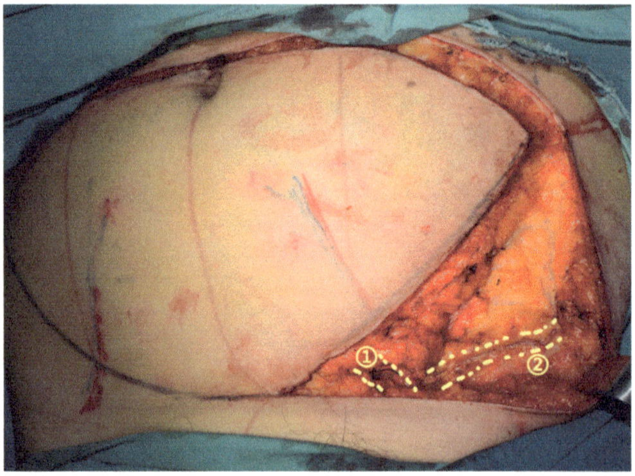

Fig. 12.26 Lifting the left flap, the SIEV was separated and carried in the flap. (1) SIEV; (2) Superficial circumflex iliac vein

Intramammary (IM) vessels are the most frequently used recipient vessels.

The thoracodorsal vessels and lateral thoracic vessels are also used.

The IM vessels are suitable for anastomosing all kinds of vascular pedicle because both the proximal and distal vessels can provide sufficient blood supply.

We usually excise costal cartilage at a length of 3 cm to create adequate space facilitating dissecting the IM vessels and the anastomosis with two pedicles.

Prep work in the recipient area includes harvesting a sufficient length of the IM vessels and creating space for multiple vascular anastomosis free of mutual interference.

It is very challenging to complete the anastomosis of four vessels in a narrow space, but the arterial and venous diameters of the two deep inferior epigastric pedicles and the IMA vessels in the thorax are highly matched, which is a favorable factor for anastomosis (Fig. 12.33).

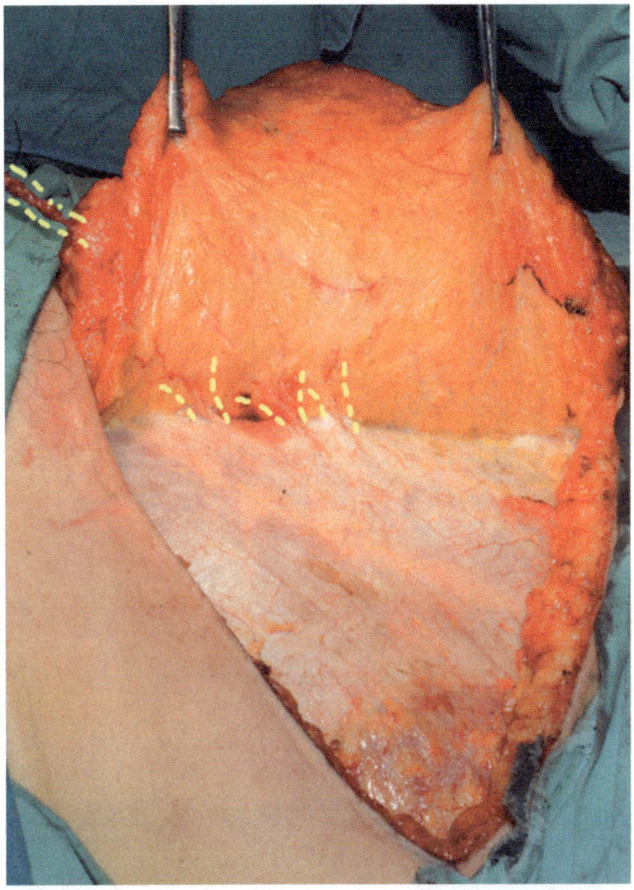

Fig. 12.27 The left perforators

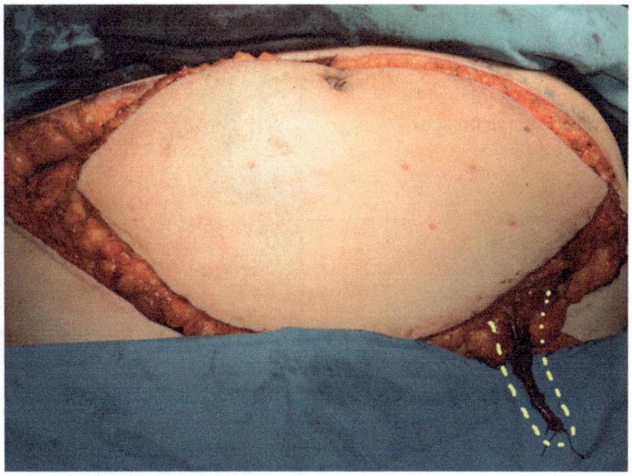

Fig. 12.28 The flap was attached to the abdominal wall only on the base and the SIEV was harvested

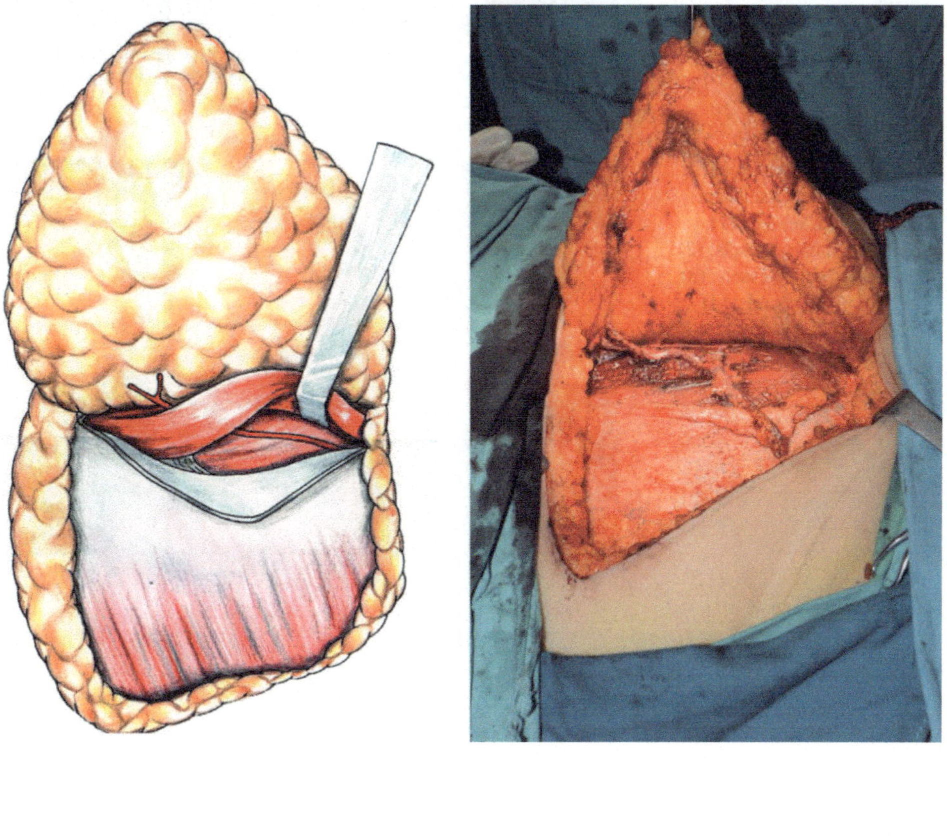

Fig. 12.29 The right deep inferior epigastric pedicle

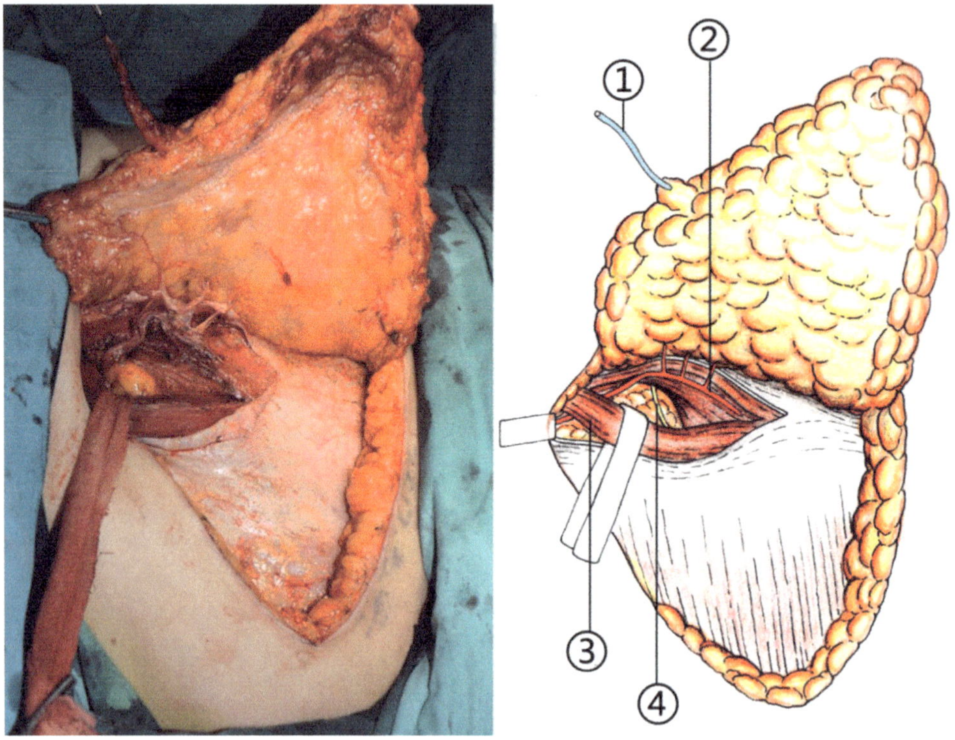

Fig. 12.30 The left deep inferior epigastric pedicle. (1) SIEV; (2) Perforating vessels; (3) Rectus abdominis; (4) Intercostal nerve branch

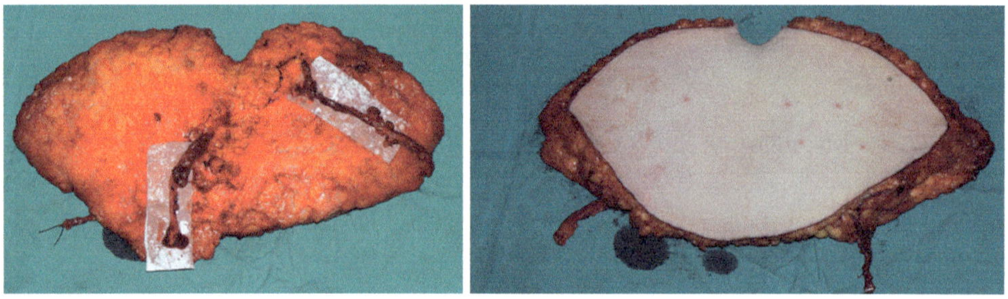

Fig. 12.31 A bilateral vascular pedicled skin flap was harvested

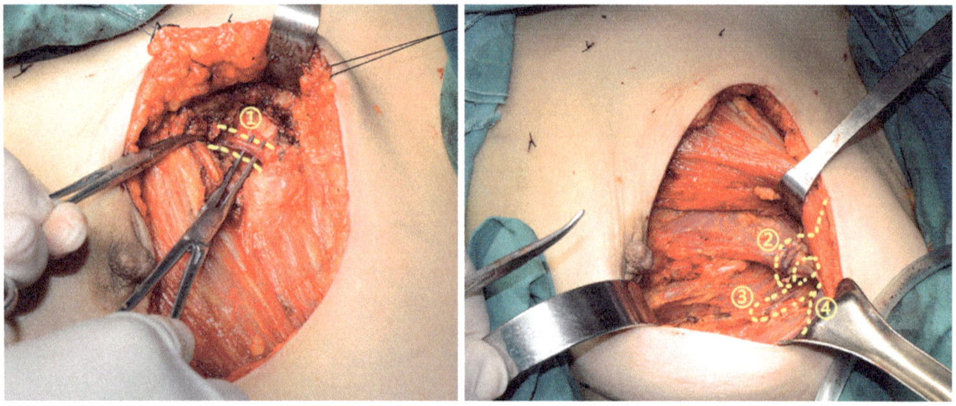

Fig. 12.32 Preparation of internal thoracic vessels and lateral thoracic vessels. (1) Internal mammary vessels; (2) Thoracic acromial vessels; (3) Lateral thoracic vessels; (4) Axillary vein

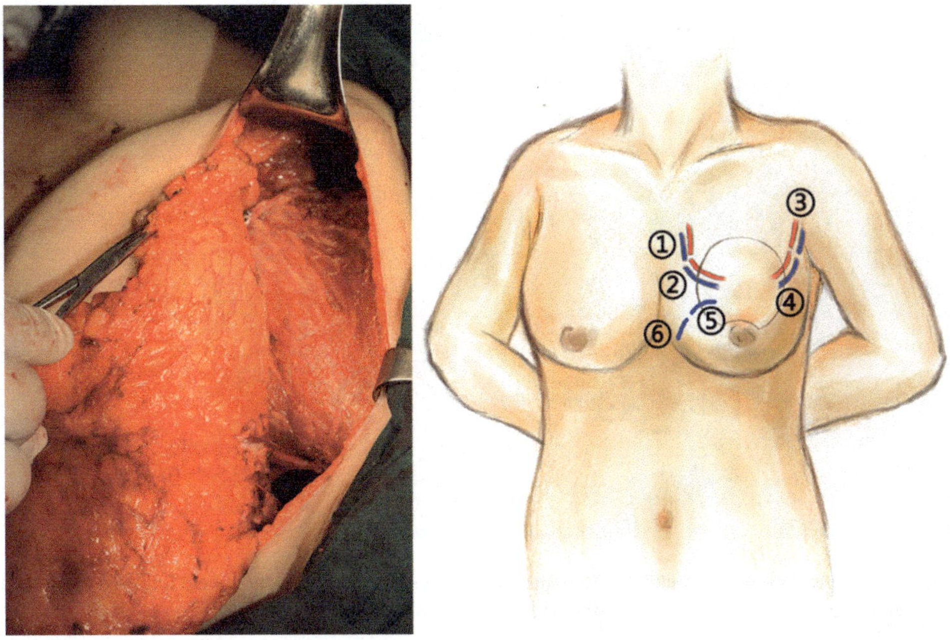

Fig. 12.33 Revascularization mode. The left internal thoracic artery and vein were prepared as recipient vessels. One arterial vessel with a diameter of about 2 mm and one venous vessel with a diameter of about 2 mm were anastomosed with the left deep inferior epigastric artery and vein, the right deep inferior epigastric artery and vein were anastomosed with the left lateral thoracic artery and vein (1A1V), and the left SIEV was anastomosed with the distal end of the left internal thoracic vein. (1) Internal mammary vessels; (2) Left deep inferior epigastric vessels; (3) Lateral thoracic vessels; (4) Right deep inferior epigastric vessels; (5) SIEV; (6) Distal internal thoracic vein

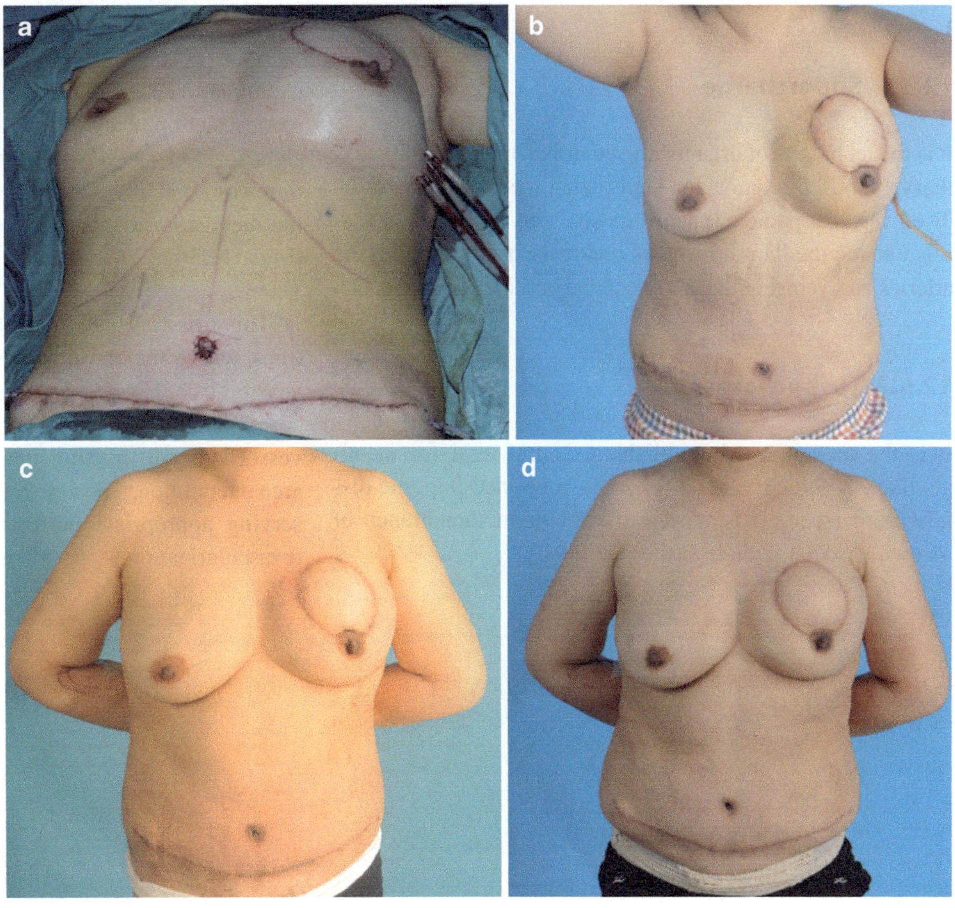

Fig. 12.34 (**a**) Appearance immediately after reconstruction; (**b**) One month at follow-up; (**c**) The patients were followed up at 3 months; (**d**) The patients were followed up at 12 months

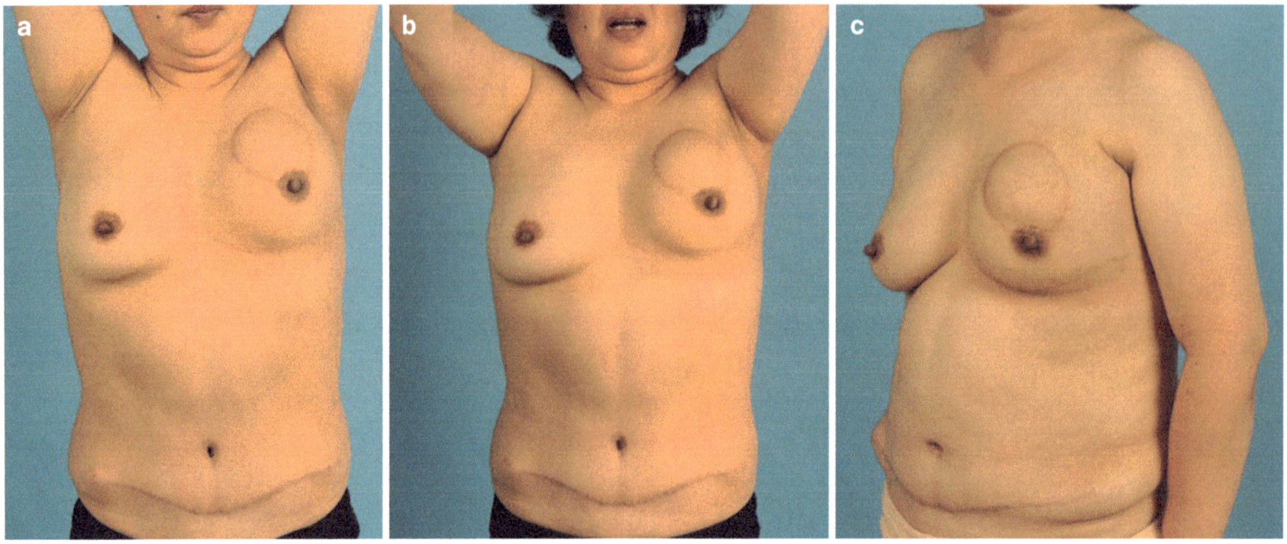

Fig. 12.35 (**a**) Function and appearance at 24 months of follow-up. (**b**) The appearance and function were followed up at 28 months after operation. (**c**) The appearance and function were followed up at 40 months after operation

Vascular coupler can reduce operation time and surgical complications [14].

During the long-term follow-up, the patient's body figure changed, but the reconstructed breast shape was still naturally satisfactory.

12.5.1 Supercharge

It is the technique of establishing contralateral (or distal) auxiliary blood circulation for super conjoined flap where the distal vascular pedicle is anastomosed with the recipient vessels outside the flap. It includes revascularization of both the arteries and veins, or the arteries alone or the veins alone, etc.

12.5.2 Turbocharge

It is the technique of establishing contralateral (or distal) auxiliary blood circulation for super conjoined flap, the distal vascular pedicle is anastomosed with another branch of its own vascular pedicle of the flap.

12.6 Case 4: Bipedicled DIEP Flap for Breast Reconstruction

The patient was a 42-year-old female who received left modified radical mastectomy and chemotherapy 6 years ago and had 5-year adjuvant endocrine therapy.

A mass on the left chest wall was found by self-examination. Left chest wall scar removal and left breast reconstruction using a free bilateral pedicled DIEP flap and right mastopexy were performed. The blood supply of the flap was good after operation, and the shape and function of the reconstructed breast were satisfactory during follow-up (Figs. 12.36, 12.37, 12.38, 12.39, 12.40, 12.41, 12.42, and 12.43).

This case was featured by a small internal thoracic venous trunk with a major venous perforator that was available for anastomosis. However, most of the patients with breast cancer experience chemotherapy before reconstruction that is vessel harmful, making major perforators in the recipient area uncommon. The case reminds us of identifying and conserving appropriate perforators in the receiving area for revascularization.

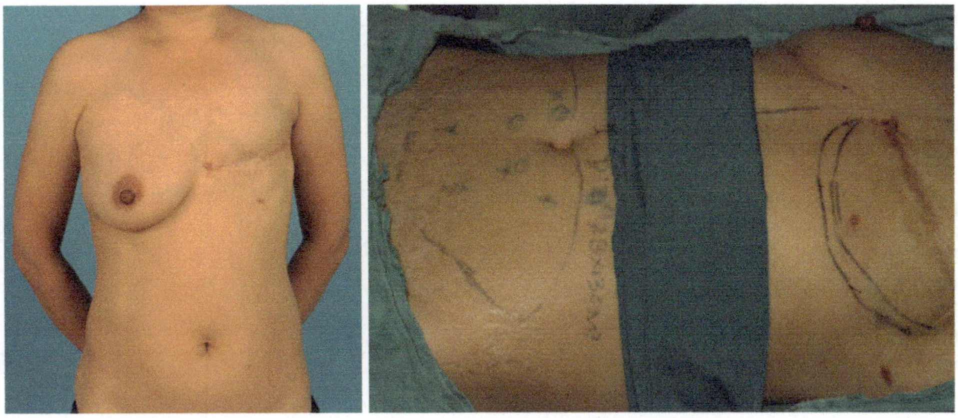

Fig. 12.36 Preoperative findings and intraoperative design

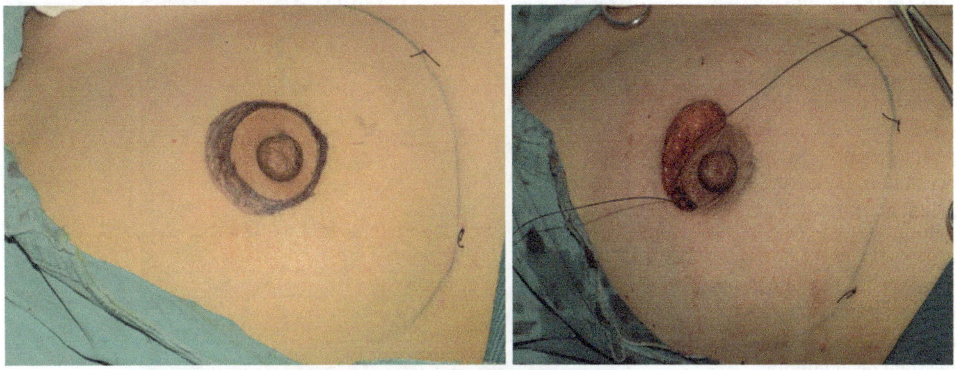

Fig. 12.37 The right breast sagged slightly. Removing part of the skin above the areola and folding the dermis posterior to the right nipple to improve projection

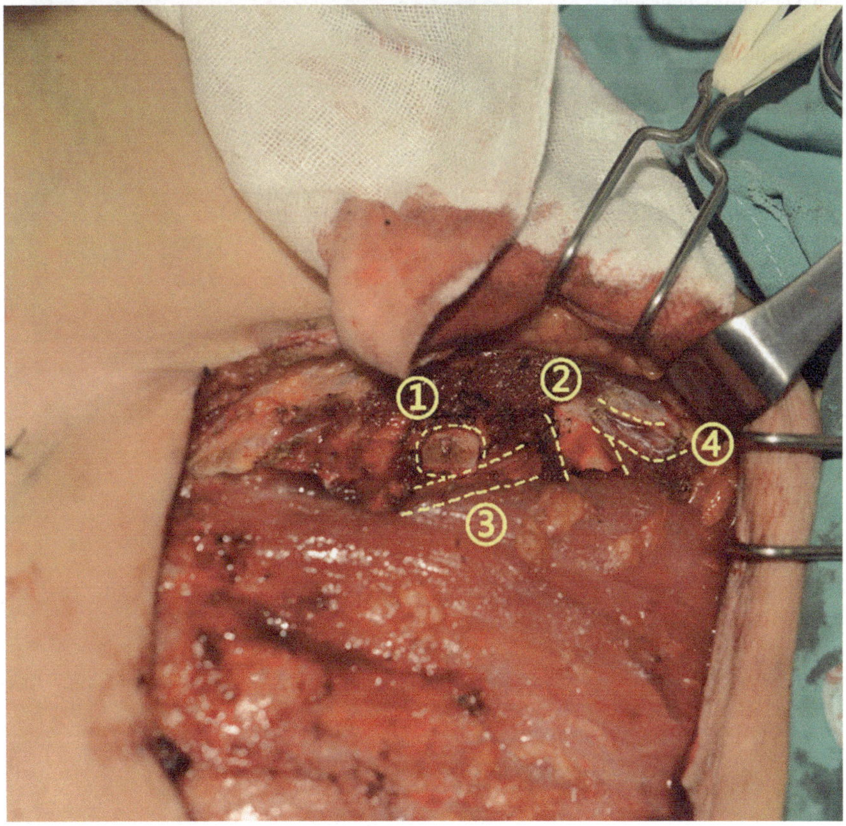

Fig. 12.38 The left chest skin bag was separated and the recipient vessels were prepared. We initially removed the third costal cartilage and found that the internal thoracic artery was large while the internal thoracic vein was small. We then found that the IM vascular perforator was in large caliber above the second rib cartilage that was hence cut off to prepare the venous perforator and the proximal end of the left internal thoracic vessels as recipient vessels

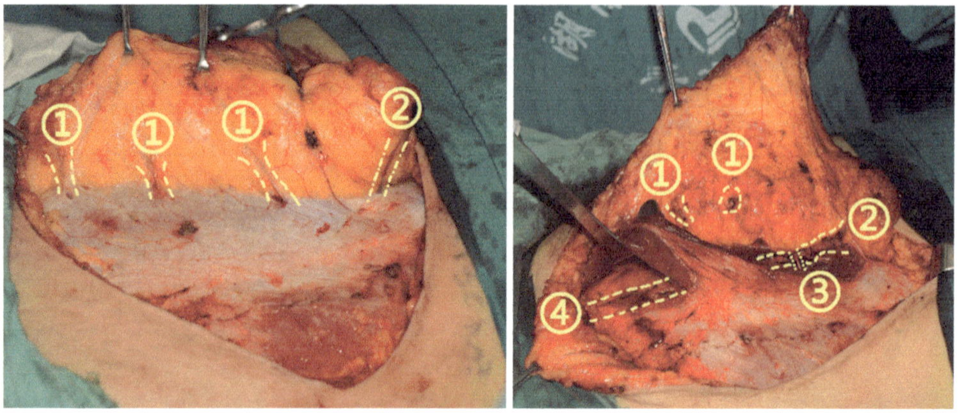

Fig. 12.39 Lifting the left DIEP flap, multiple sensory branches of intercostal nerve were found and included in the flap, the muscle nerve branches were preserved intact, and the flap was well prepared. (1) Sensory branch of intercostal nerve; (2) Perforating branch of deep inferior epigastric artery; (3) Muscular branches of intercostal nerve; (4) The main deep inferior epigastric vessels

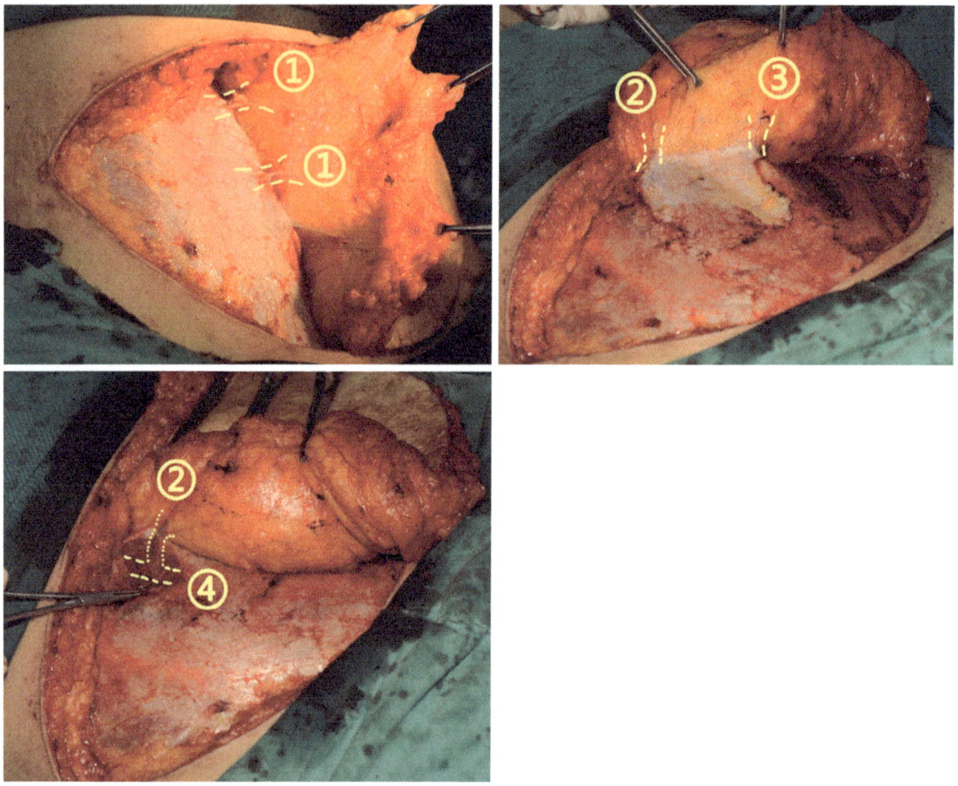

Fig. 12.40 Lifting the right DIEP flap, multiple intercostal nerve sensory branches were found and carried in the flap. Retrograde separation of the medial perforators revealed that the perforators came from the lateral branch of the deep inferior epigastric vessels that was dissected toward the vascular trunk till it was close to the emitting point, and completing the preparation of the right deep inferior epigastric artery perforator flap. (1) Sensory branch of intercostal nerve; (2) Paraumbilical perforator of deep inferior epigastric artery; (3) Septal perforator of deep inferior epigastric artery; (4) Lateral branch of deep inferior epigastric vessel

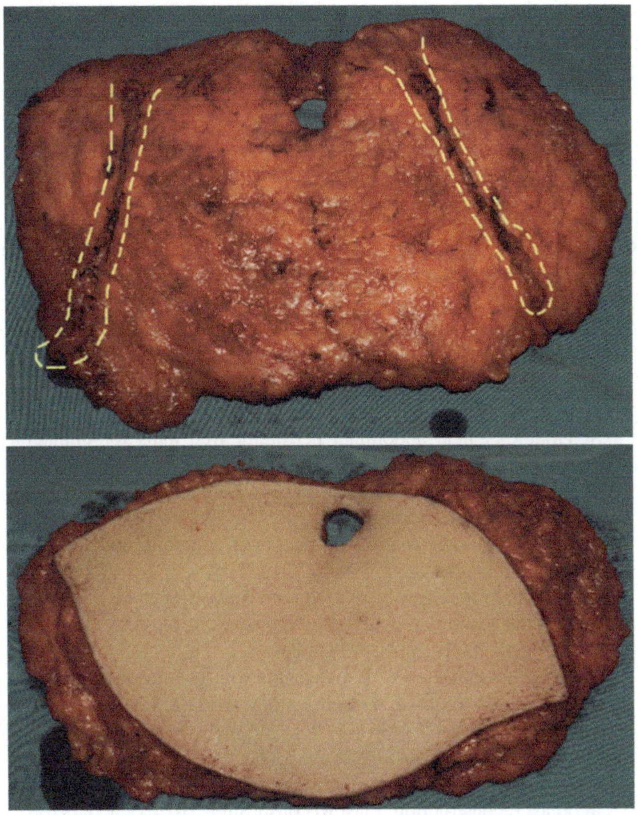

Fig. 12.41 Preparation of perforator flap of deep inferior epigastric artery with bilateral vascular pedicle

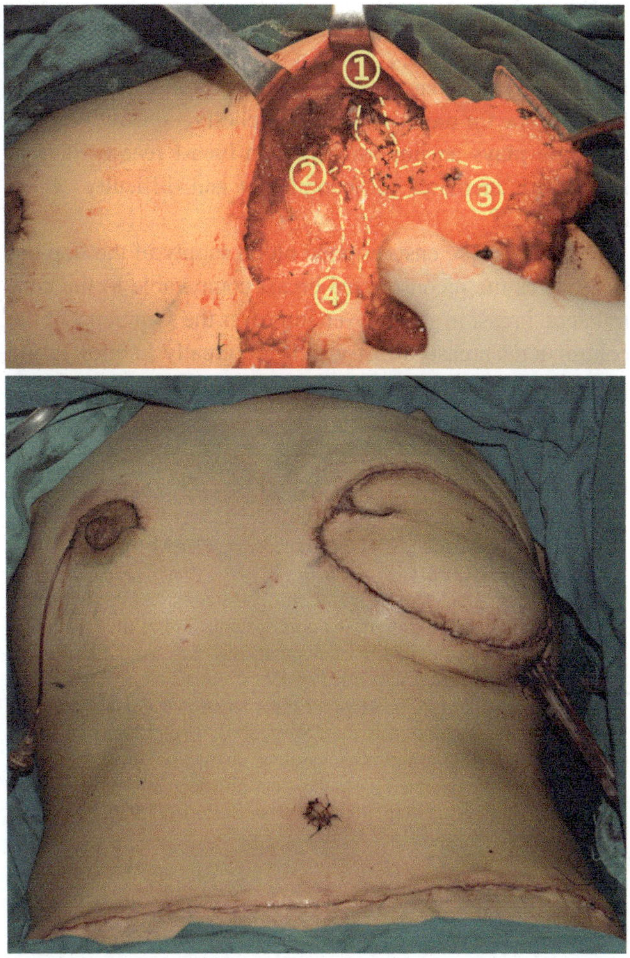

Fig. 12.42 Vascular anastomosis and breast reconstruction were finished. (1) The proximal end and perforating branches of internal thoracic artery and vein; (2) Distal internal thoracic artery and vein; (3) Left deep inferior epigastric vessel; (4) Right deep inferior epigastric vessel

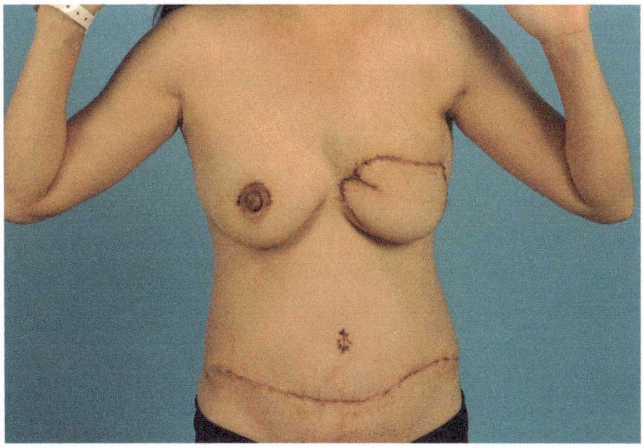

Fig. 12.43 The patient was discharged 6 days after operation

12.7 Summary

Bipedicled supercharged DIEP flap can reliably provide sufficient tissue for unilateral breast or chest reconstruction and therefore plays an important role in breast reconstruction, although it increases the complexity and difficulty of the operation.

This technique ensures good blood supply of the flap tissue, makes the reconstructed breast comparable to the contralateral breast in size or even improves the symmetry of the contralateral breast, all of which are greatly helpful to the psychological and physiological rehabilitation of patients.

References

1. Arnez ZM, Scamp T. The bipedicled free TRAM flap. Br J Plast Surg. 1992;45(3):214–8.
2. Pennington DG, Nettle WJ, Lam P. Microvascular augmentation of the blood supply of the contralateral side of the free transverse rectus abdominis musculocutaneous flap. Ann Plast Surg. 1993;31(2):123–6; discussion 126–7.
3. Lam TC, Sellars GD. Free perforator crossover TRAM flap for breast reconstruction. Ann Plast Surg. 2003;50(2):126–31.
4. Semple JL. Retrograde microvascular augmentation (turbocharging) of a single-pedicle TRAM flap through a deep inferior epigastric arterial and venous loop. Plast Reconstr Surg. 1994;93(1):109–17.
5. Keller A. Perfusion zones of the DIEP flap revisited: a clinical study. Plast Reconstr Surg. 2006;118(4):1076–7; author reply 1077.
6. Wong C, Saint-Cyr M, Mojallal A, et al. Perforasomes of the DIEP flap: vascular anatomy of the lateral versus medial row perforators and clinical implications. Plast Reconstr Surg. 2010;125(3):772–82.
7. DellaCroce FJ, Sullivan SK, Trahan C. Stacked deep inferior epigastric perforator flap breast reconstruction: a review of 110 flaps in 55 cases over 3 years. Plast Reconstr Surg. 2011;127(3):1093–9.
8. Agarwal JP, Gottlieb LJ. Double pedicle deep inferior epigastric perforator/muscle-sparing TRAM flaps for unilateral breast reconstruction. Ann Plast Surg. 2007;58(4):359–63.
9. Simon AM, Bouwense CL, McMillan S, Lamb S, Hammond DC. Comparison of unipedicled and bipedicled TRAM flap breast reconstructions: assessment of physical function and patient satisfaction. Plast Reconstr Surg. 2004;113(1):136–40.
10. Hamdi M, Khuthaila DK, Van Landuyt K, Roche N, Monstrey S. Double-pedicle abdominal perforator free flaps for unilateral breast reconstruction: new horizons in microsurgical tissue transfer to the breast. J Plast Reconstr Aesthet Surg. 2007;60(8):904–12; discussion 913–4.
11. Carlson GW. Skin sparing mastectomy: anatomic and technical considerations. Am Surg. 1996;62(2):151–5.
12. Torresan RZ, dos Santos CC, Okamura H, Alvarenga M. Evaluation of residual glandular tissue after skin-sparing mastectomies. Ann Surg Oncol. 2005;12(12):1037–44.
13. Mackey SP, Ramsey KW. Exploring the myth of the valveless internal mammary vein—a cadaveric study. J Plast Reconstr Aesthet Surg. 2011;64(9):1174–9.
14. Jandali S, Wu LC, Vega SJ, Kovach SJ, Serletti JM. 1000 consecutive venous anastomoses using the microvascular anastomotic coupler in breast reconstruction. Plast Reconstr Surg. 2010;125(3):792–8.

Bilateral Simultaneous Breast Reconstruction with Bilateral DIEP Flaps

13

Zan Li and Dequan Liu

Bilateral breast reconstruction is not simply repeating the operation of unilateral breast reconstruction [1–3]. It is much more complex, and it is more likely to reconstruct the symmetry of bilateral breasts [4, 5].

The complication rate of bilateral breast reconstruction with autologous tissue transplantation is about 30% worldwide [6–9].

A systematic review showed that the complication rate of breast reconstruction with bilateral DIEP flaps was 27.3–35.6%, bilateral gluteus maximus myocutaneous flaps was 15–36%, bilateral pedicled rectus abdominis flaps was 26.9%, and bilateral latissimus dorsi plus prosthesis was 29.7% [7, 8].

The rate of reoperation after free flap transplantation was 6.4–16.6%, and the rate of flap necrosis in different flap techniques was 2–20%.

According to Chun et al. [9], the satisfaction rate of patients after bilateral breast reconstruction with bilateral DIEP flaps was 92.6%.

The reported satisfaction rate by Drazan [6] was 96.2%.

The strength recovery of abdominal wall after breast reconstruction with bilateral DIEP flaps depends on the degree of injury to rectus abdominis muscle and nerves [10].

Other reports [11] further confirmed that bilateral breast reconstruction with bilateral DIEP flaps was associated with faster recovery, shortened hospitalization, and less complications compared with bilateral pedicled rectus abdominis flaps.

For bilateral breast reconstruction in obese patients and patients with large breasts, unilateral DIEP flap is often not enough [12–14]. The most satisfactory effect can be achieved by cutting two DIEP flaps based on independent vascular pedicle for reconstructing bilateral breasts [15–17].

Z. Li (✉)
Department of Oncology Plastic Surgery, Hunan Cancer Hospital, Changsha, Hunan, China

D. Liu
Department of Breast Surgery, Yunnan Cancer Hospital, Kunming, Yunnan, China

The condition, size, and location of perforator vessels are determined factors for the size of a DIEP flap. Nonetheless, the proportion of symmetrical distribution of perforator vessels on both sides of the abdominal wall is less than 50%, making operation adjustment necessary according to the actual anatomical characteristics in the actual clinical work [18–20].

Case Study 1: Bilateral Breast Reconstruction with Bilateral DIEP Flaps

The patient, a 20-year-old female, presented for recurrence after four breast lumpectomies previously because of multiple breast fibroadenomas on both side. She strongly requested for bilateral mastectomy. At admission, she underwent bilateral nipple-sparing mastectomies (NSMs) and breast reconstruction using free bilateral DIEP flaps.

The right breast was reconstructed with the DIEP flap based on the right deep inferior epigastric vessels that were anastomosed with the right internal thoracic artery and vein (1A2V). The left DIEP flap was used to reconstruct the left breast and the left deep inferior epigastric artery and vein were anastomosed with the left internal thoracic artery and vein (1A2V).

Postoperative pathological results diagnosed as multiple fibroadenomas of bilateral breasts.

Bilateral flaps survived well, no tumor recurrence was found after operation, and the appearance of reconstructed breast recovered satisfactorily during follow-up (Figs. 13.1, 13.2, 13.3, 13.4, 13.5, 13.6, 13.7, 13.8, 13.9, 13.10, 13.11, 13.12, and 13.13).

The patient once received four breast surgeries resulting in multiple scars. We performed NSMs through the superior medial incision scars and found multiple masses in the removed breast tissue.

Z. Li, D. Song (eds.), *Oncoplastic Flap Surgery*, https://doi.org/10.1007/978-981-19-8926-1_13

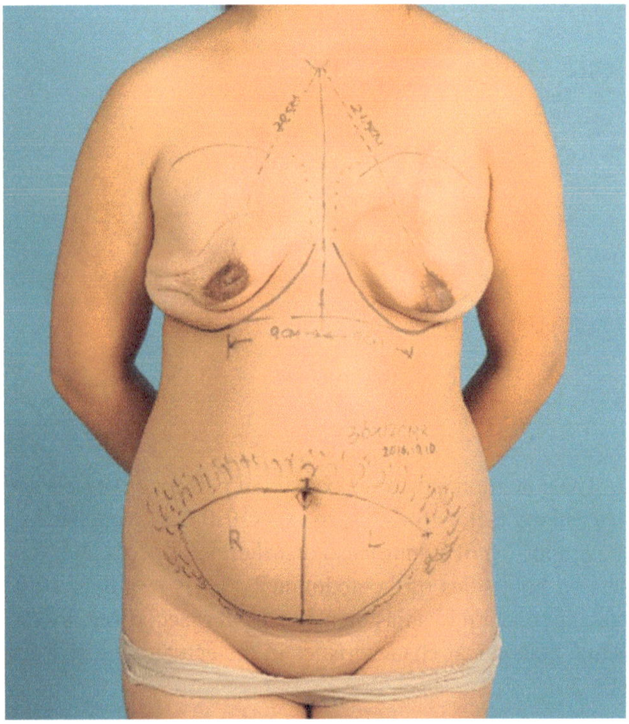

Fig. 13.1 Preoperative view

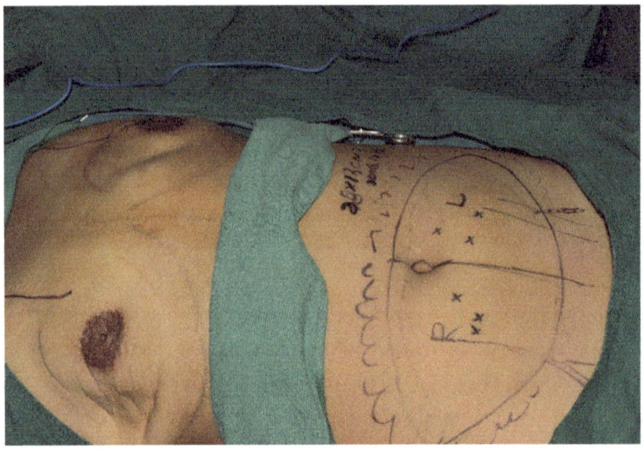

Fig. 13.2 Intraoperative design

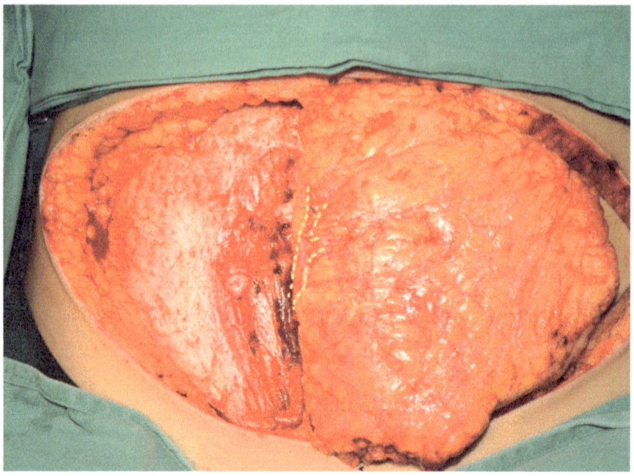

Fig. 13.3 Lifting the right flap to expose and separate the perforating vessels

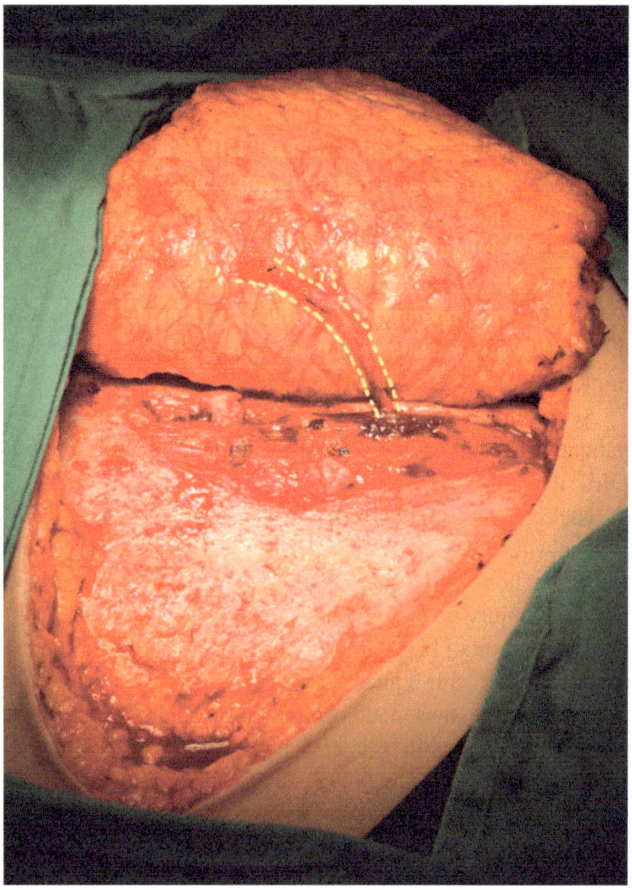

Fig. 13.4 The vascular pedicle of the perforating branch of the right deep inferior epigastric artery was separated

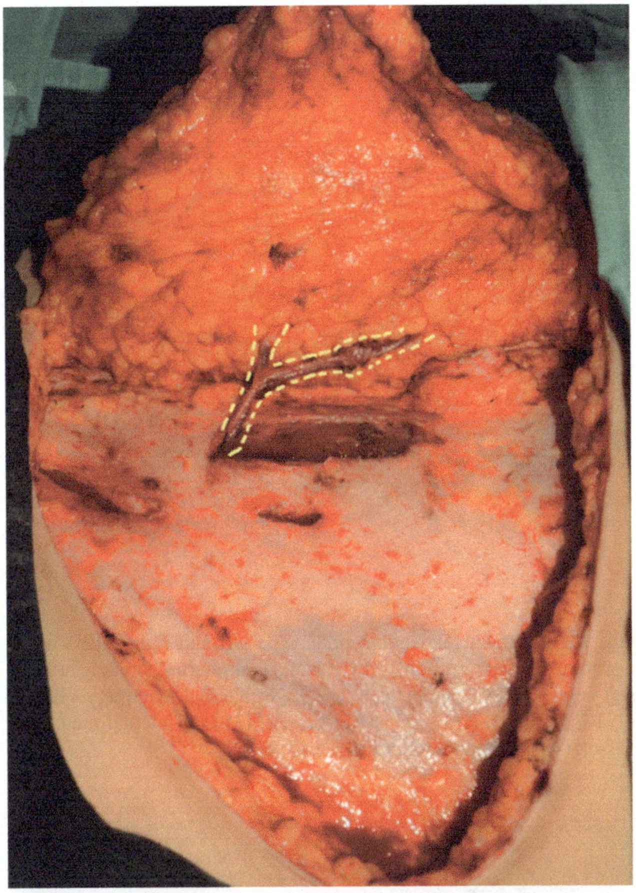

Fig. 13.5 The vascular pedicle of the perforating branch of the left deep inferior epigastric artery was separated

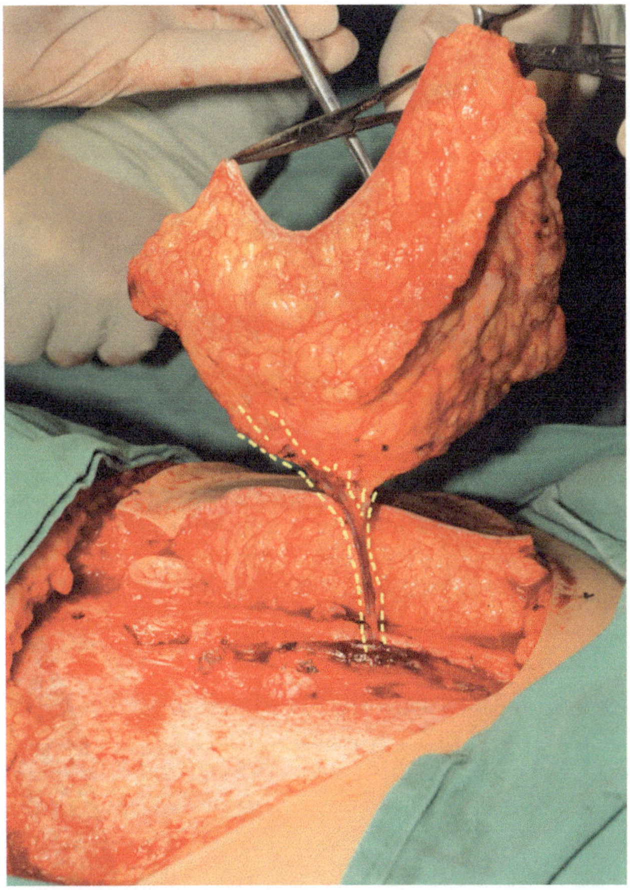

Fig. 13.7 The perforator flap of the right deep inferior epigastric artery was prepared

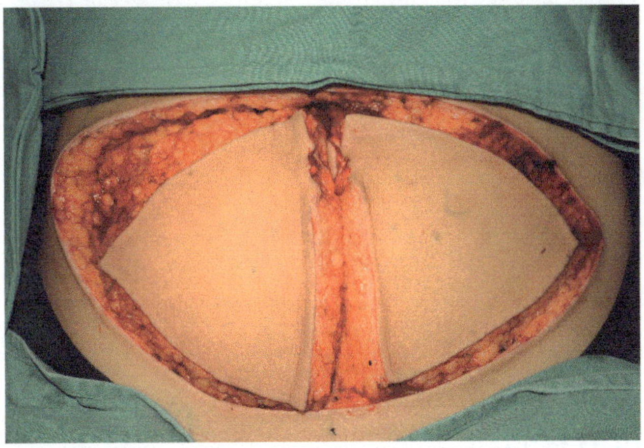

Fig. 13.6 The skin margins of bilateral DIEP flaps were cut open

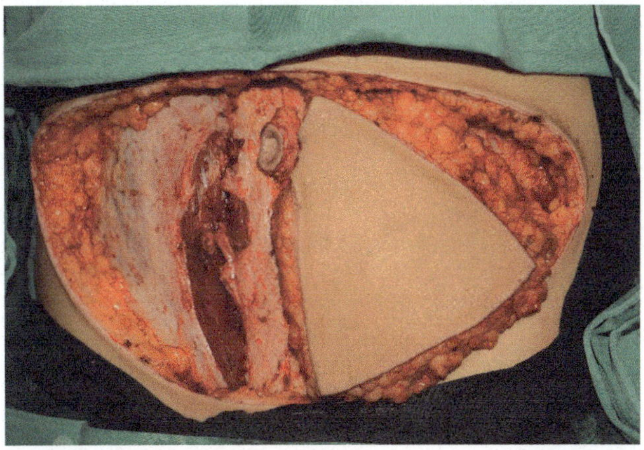

Fig. 13.8 The right flap was transferred to the right chest for vascular anastomosis, and raising the left flap followed

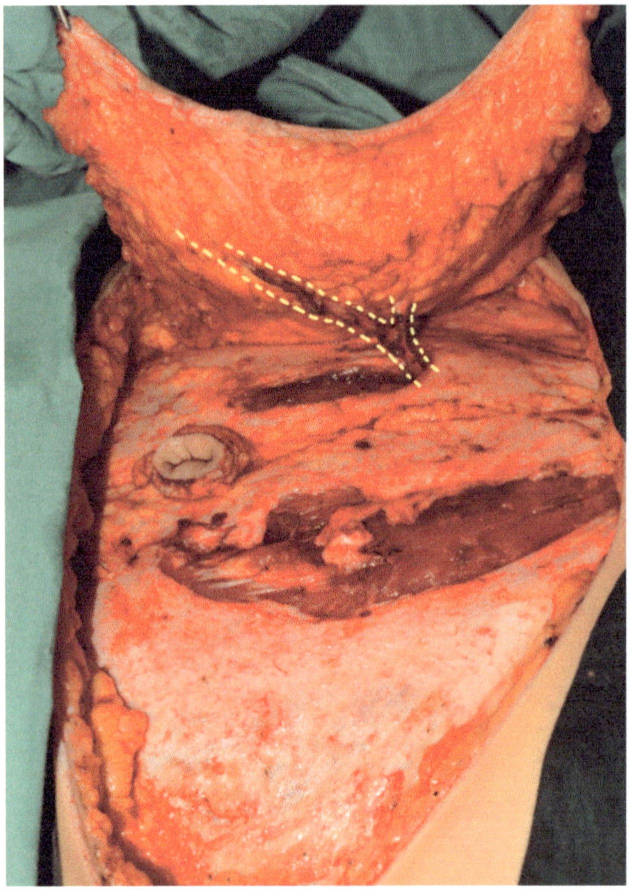

Fig. 13.9 The perforator flap of the left deep inferior epigastric artery was cut off

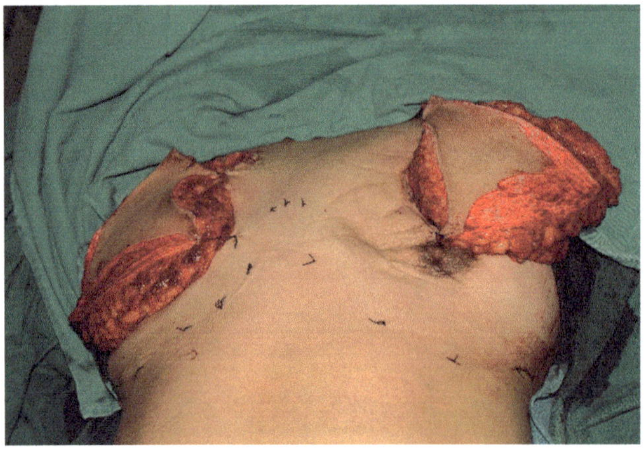

Fig. 13.10 Bilateral flap shaping

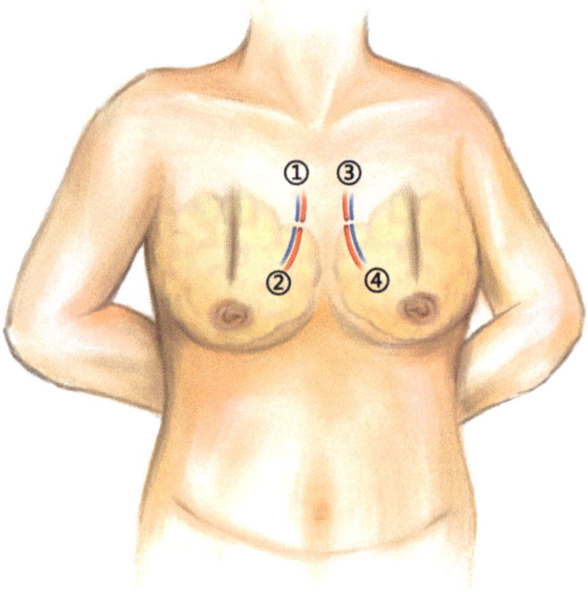

Fig. 13.11 Revascularization mode. The left and right DIEPs were anastomosed with the left and right bilateral internal thoracic arteries and veins (1A1V), respectively. (1) Right internal mammary vessels; (2) Right deep inferior epigastric vessels; (3) Left internal mammary vessel; (4) Left deep inferior epigastric vessel

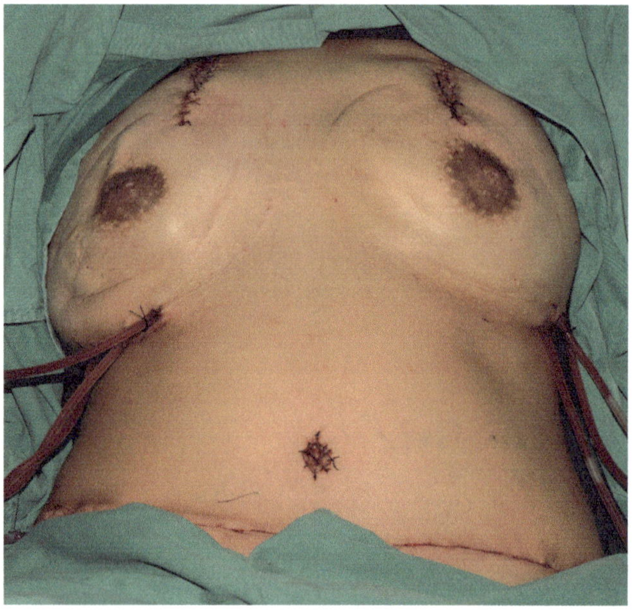

Fig. 13.12 Intraoperative view immediately after reconstruction

Case Study 2: Bilateral Breast Reconstruction with Bilateral DIEP Flaps

The patient, a 51-year-old female, who had found a right breast mass more than 1 month ago and once received modified radical mastectomy for left breast cancer 8 years ago.

A mass of about 3.5 cm × 3.0 cm in size was palpable 1 cm above the right areola on physical examination. The mass was hard with unclear boundary and poor mobility. No abnormality on physical examination was found on the left chest wall. In addition, an enlarged lymph node of 3.0 cm × 2.5 cm in size was palpated in the right armpit. It was hard with unclear boundary and poor mobility. Supra- and sub-clavicular lymph nodes were not palpable on either side.

Breast color Doppler ultrasound showed a solid mass in the upper quadrant of the right breast (BIRADS 5); enlarged lymph nodes were found in the right armpit with a high possibility of metastasis; no significantly enlarged lymph nodes were found in the left axillary or on bilateral supra- and subclavicular areas.

At admission, right modified radical mastectomy plus left chest wall scar removal and bilateral breast reconstruction using bilateral DIEP flaps were performed. The blood supply of the flap was good after operation. Comprehensive treatment was given subsequently. The shape and function of the reconstructed breast were satisfactory during follow-up (Figs. 13.14, 13.15, 13.16, 13.17, 13.18, 13.19, 13.20, and 13.21).

Although the flap pictures are put together here, in fact, the pedicle of the perforator flap of the left inferior abdominal artery is first transferred to the left breast defect area for vascular anastomosis. We first performed left breast reconstruction and revascularization of the left DIEP flap. Disconnection of the vascular pedicle of the right DIEP flap and right breast reconstruction followed, so as to avoid the occurrence of reperfusion injury caused by prolonged ischemia and shortened operation time.

The left internal thoracic artery was accompanied by one large vein and one small vein, which were comparable to the size of the left inferior abdominal vessels. The right lateral thoracic artery and vein and the anterior serratus branch of the right thoracodorsal artery were initially planned to be used as recipient vessels, the diameter of these vessels were later found to be only about 0.4 mm under the microscope, which was much smaller than that of the right deep inferior epigastric vessels (2.5 mm). Instead, the main trunk of the right thoracodorsal artery and vein was used. The reasons why we did not choose the right internal mammary vessels were as follows: (1) rib cartilage removal was required, and cutting off segments of bilateral costal cartilage may cause chest wall deformity and increase the risk of postoperative chest pain; (2) the right breast incision was extending laterally, which limited vision field on the medial side, and over-retraction of the incision was likely to damage the skin envelope; (3) the vascular pedicle of the right DIEP flap was cut off when the right lateral thoracic vessels were found to be inappropriate. Extra time would be required for preparing the right internal mammary vessels, which will increase the ischemia time of the flap and the possibility of ischemia-reperfusion injury of the flap.

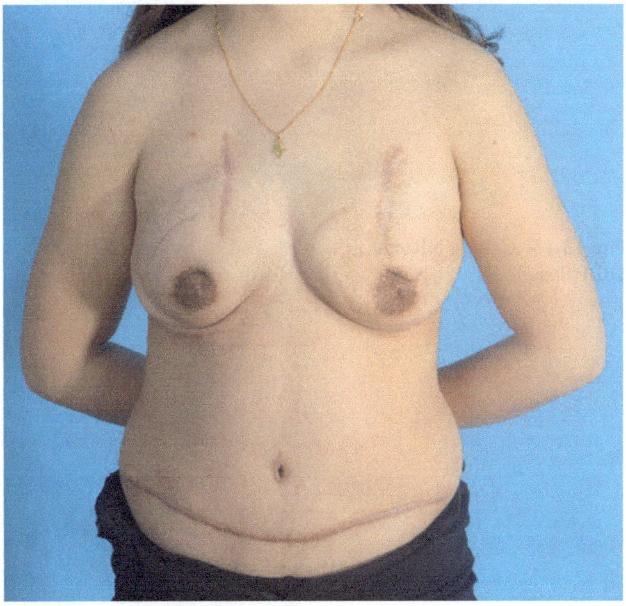

Fig. 13.13 6-month at follow-up after operation

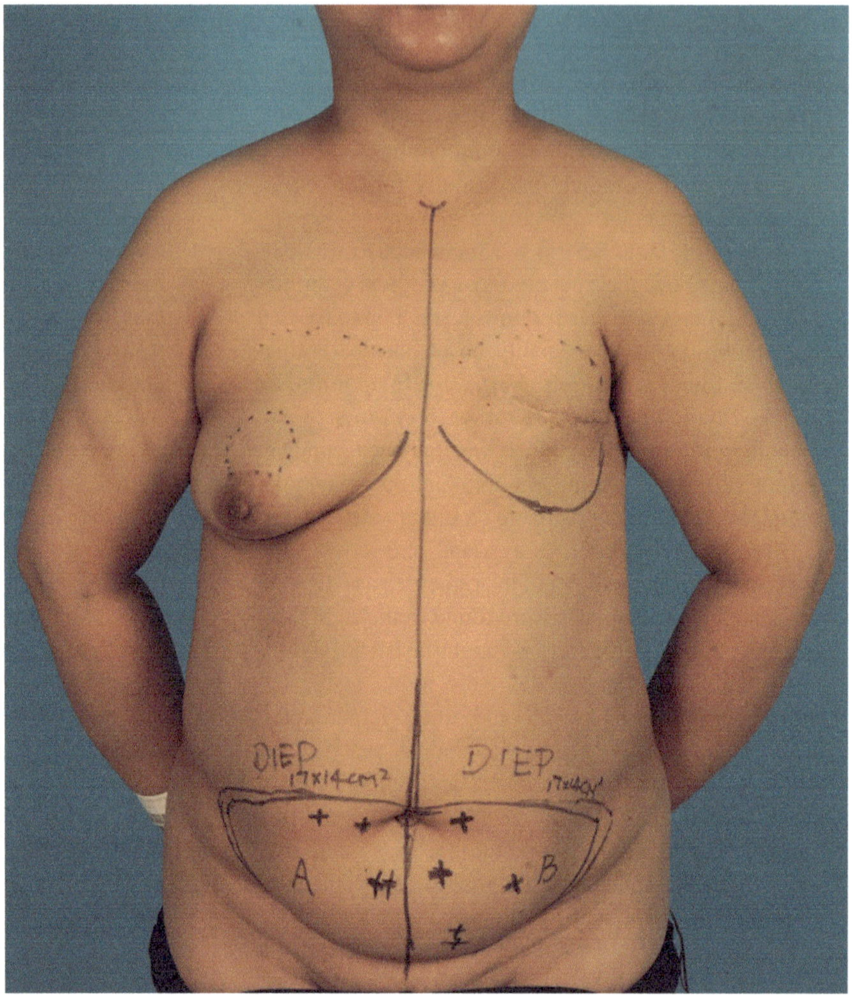

Fig. 13.14 Preoperative findings

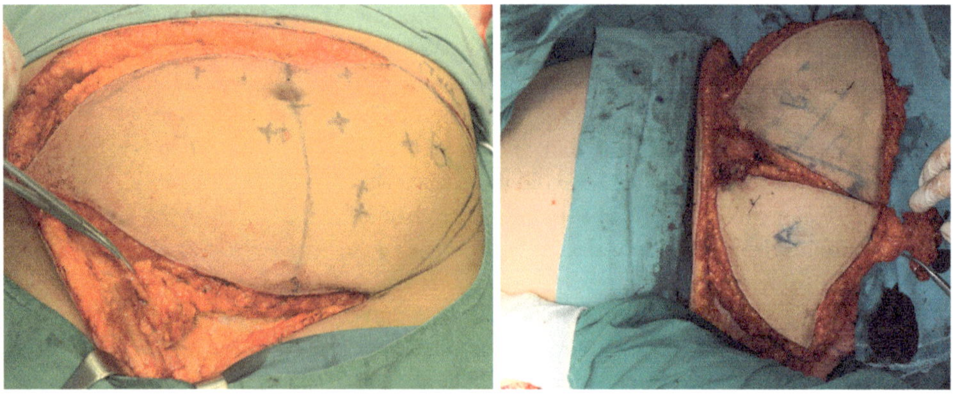

Fig. 13.15 Cutting bilateral DIEP flaps

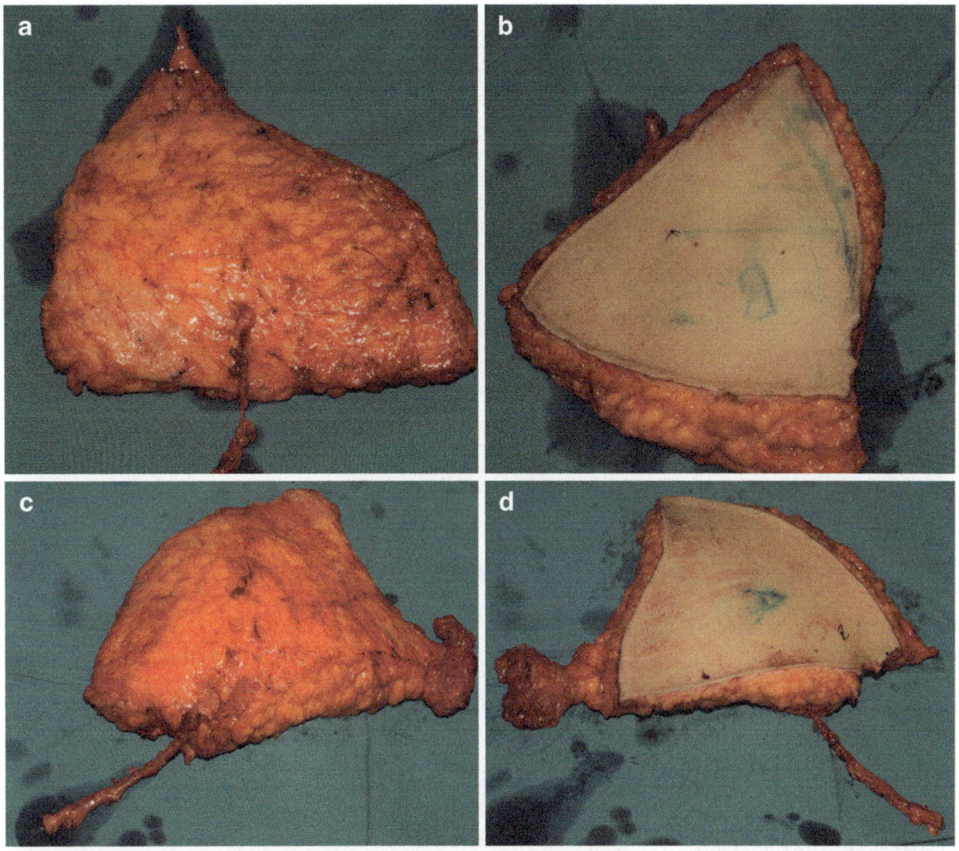

Fig. 13.16 The bilateral pedicled DIEP flap was split for transfer. (**a**, **b**) The left DIEP flap; (**c**, **d**) The right DIEP flap

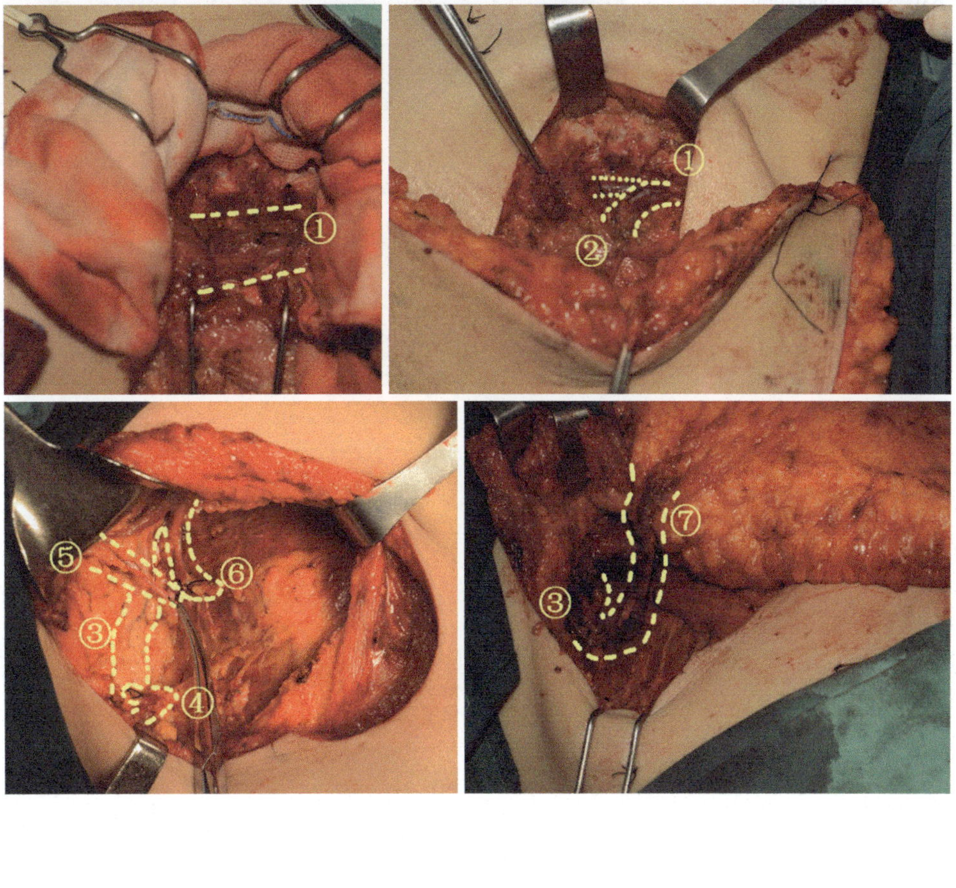

Fig. 13.17 Revascularization of bilateral flaps was completed. The left deep inferior epigastric vessels were anastomosed to the proximal ends of the left internal mammary vessels (A:*V* = 1:2), and the right deep inferior epigastric vessels were anastomosed to the right thoracodorsal vessels (A:*V* = 1:2). (1) Left internal mammary vessels; (2) Left deep inferior epigastric vessels; (3) Right thoracodorsal vessels; (4) Anterior serratus branch of right thoracodorsal vessel; (5) Right lateral thoracic vein; (6) Right lateral thoracic artery and vein; (7) Right deep inferior epigastric vessels

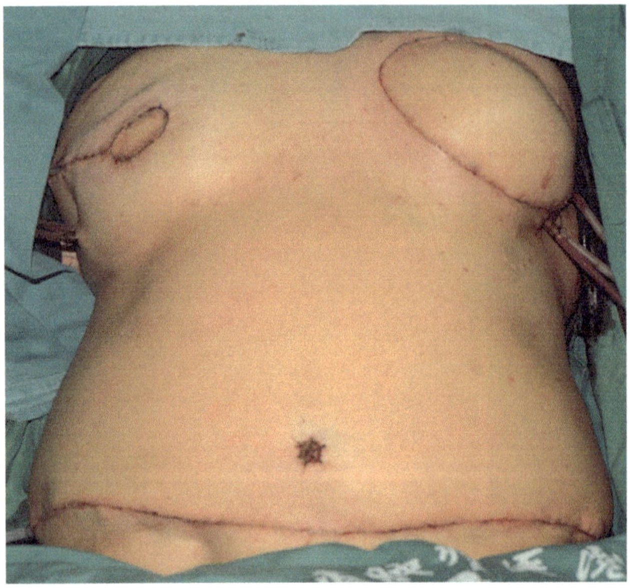

Fig. 13.18 Intraoperative view immediately after bilateral breast reconstruction

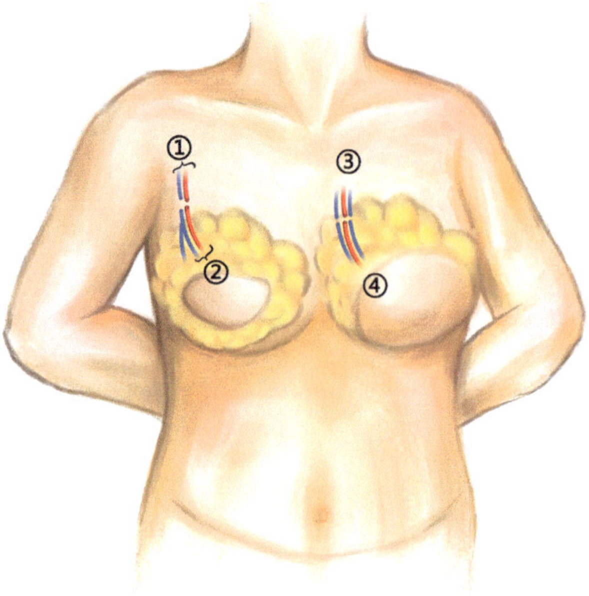

Fig. 13.19 Revascularization pattern of bilateral breast reconstruction

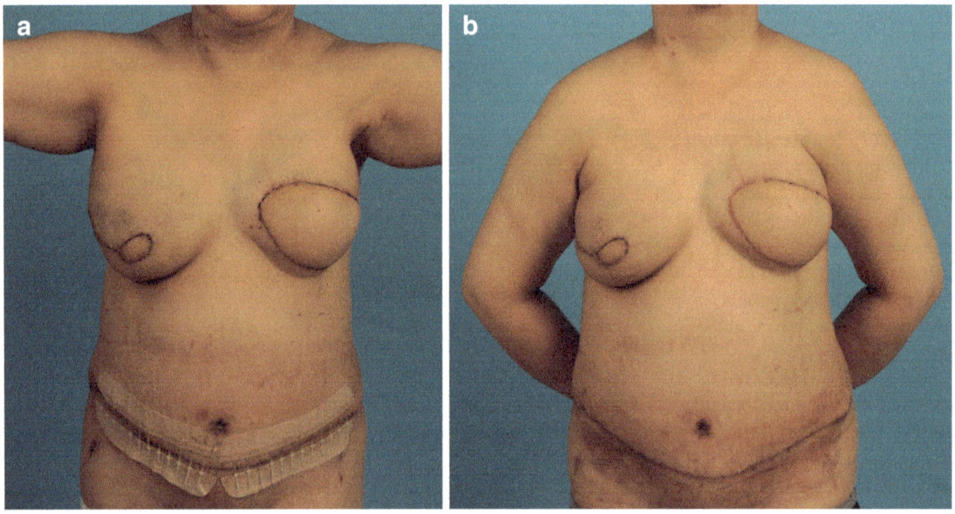

Fig. 13.20 (**a**) The patient was discharged 2 weeks after operation. (**b**) The appearance and function at follow-up of 28 days after operation

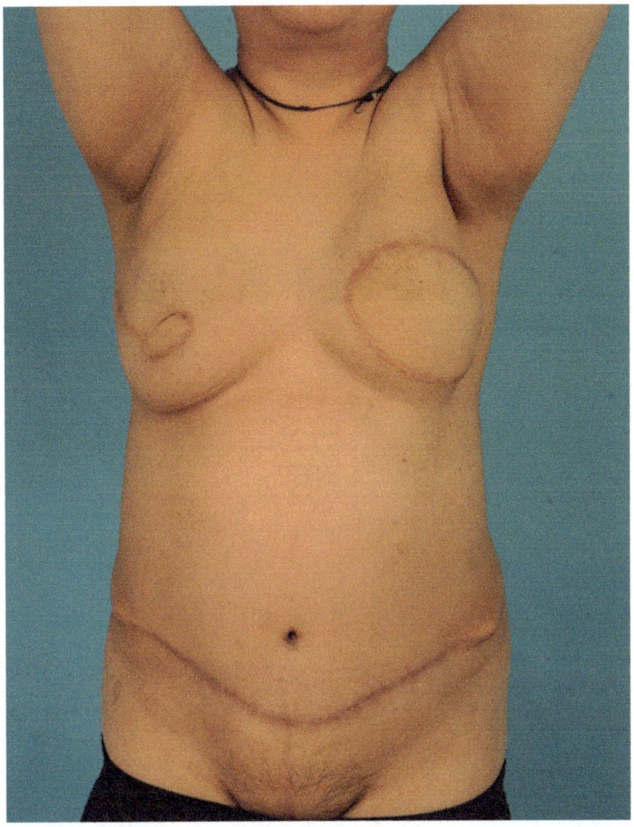

Fig. 13.21 Appearance and function at 12-month follow-up

References

1. Wormald JC, Wade RG, Figus A. The increased risk of adverse outcomes in bilateral deep inferior epigastric artery perforator flap breast reconstruction compared to unilateral reconstruction: a systematic review and meta-analysis. J Plast Reconstr Aesthet Surg. 2014;67(2):143–56.
2. Bodin F, Schohn T, Dissaux C, Baratte A, Fiquet C, Bruant-Rodier C. Bilateral simultaneous breast reconstruction with transverse musculocutaneous gracilis flaps. J Plast Reconstr Aesthet Surg. 2015;68(1):e1–6.
3. Ting J, Rozen WM, Le RCM, Ashton MW, Garcia-Tutor E. Predictors of blood transfusion in deep inferior epigastric artery perforator flap breast reconstruction. J Reconstr Microsurg. 2011;27(4):233–8.
4. Appleton SE, Ngan A, Kent B, Morris SF. Risk factors influencing transfusion rates in DIEP flap breast reconstruction. Plast Reconstr Surg. 2011;127(5):1773–82.
5. Tin SS, Wiwanitkit V. Patient satisfaction in bilateral and unilateral breast reconstruction. Plast Surg Nurs. 2014;34(4):164.
6. Drazan L, Vesely J, Hyza P, et al. Bilateral breast reconstruction with DIEP flaps: 4 years' experience. J Plast Reconstr Aesthet Surg. 2008;61(11):1309–15.
7. Paige KT, Bostwick J, Bried JT, Jones G. A comparison of morbidity from bilateral, unipedicled and unilateral, unipedicled TRAM flap breast reconstructions. Plast Reconstr Surg. 1998;101(7):1819–27.
8. Hankins CL, Friedman J. A 7-year experience in utilizing the latissimus dorsi myocutaneous flap for bilateral breast reconstruction. Ann Plast Surg. 2008;60(2):134–40.
9. Chun YS, Sinha I, Turko A, et al. Comparison of morbidity, functional outcome, and satisfaction following bilateral TRAM versus bilateral DIEP flap breast reconstruction. Plast Reconstr Surg. 2010;126(4):1133–41.
10. Selber JC, Fosnot J, Nelson J, et al. A prospective study comparing the functional impact of SIEA, DIEP, and muscle-sparing free TRAM flaps on the abdominal wall: part II. Bilateral reconstruction. Plast Reconstr Surg. 2010;126(5):1438–53.
11. Vega SJ, Bossert RP, Serletti JM. Improving outcomes in bilateral breast reconstruction using autogenous tissue. Ann Plast Surg. 2006;56(5):487–90; discussion 490–1.
12. Smith ML, Gandolfi BM, Dayan E, et al. Bilateral breast reconstruction from a single hemiabdomen using angiosome-based flap design. Plast Reconstr Surg. 2013;132(2):291–4.
13. Rozen WM, Ashton MW, Le RCM, Pan WR, Corlett RJ. The perforator angiosome: a new concept in the design of deep inferior epigastric artery perforator flaps for breast reconstruction. Microsurgery. 2010;30(1):1–7.
14. Holm C, Mayr M, Höfter E, Ninkovic M. Perfusion zones of the DIEP flap revisited: a clinical study. Plast Reconstr Surg. 2006;117(1):37–43.
15. Gilmour A, Mackay IR. Bilateral deep inferior epigastric perforator flaps based on unilateral perforators. J Plast Reconstr Aesthet Surg. 2013;66(6):848–50.
16. Saint-Cyr M, Schaverien MV, Rohrich RJ. Perforator flaps: history, controversies, physiology, anatomy, and use in reconstruction. Plast Reconstr Surg. 2009;123(4):132e–45e.
17. Taylor GI, Corlett RJ, Dhar SC, Ashton MW. The anatomical (angiosome) and clinical territories of cutaneous perforating arteries: development of the concept and designing safe flaps. Plast Reconstr Surg. 2011;127(4):1447–59.
18. Rozen WM, Ashton MW, Pan WR, Taylor GI. Raising perforator flaps for breast reconstruction: the intramuscular anatomy of the deep inferior epigastric artery. Plast Reconstr Surg. 2007;120(6):1443–9.
19. Rozen WM, Murray AC, Ashton MW, et al. The cutaneous course of deep inferior epigastric perforators: implications for flap thinning. J Plast Reconstr Aesthet Surg. 2009;62(8):986–90.
20. Rozen WM, Chubb D, Whitaker IS, Grinsell D, Ashton MW. Deep inferior epigastric perforators do not correlate between sides of the body: the role for preoperative imaging. J Plast Reconstr Aesthet Surg. 2010;63(12):e842–3.

14 Free DIEP Combined with SIEAP Flap for Unilateral Breast Reconstruction

Zan Li and Shu Liu

The human abdominal wall is the preferred flap donor area for autologous breast reconstruction, in which the deep inferior epigastric perforator (DIEP) flap and the superficial deep inferior epigastric artery perforator (SIEAP) flap are widely known [1]. However, the latter is not commonly used clinically due to its great anatomical variation.

In 1971, the first article on free SIEAP flap published by Antia and Buch [2] was about repairing facial soft tissue defects with SIEA flap.

Allen firstly used it for autologous breast reconstruction in 1989 [3].

In recent years, the technique of lower abdominal wall flap has been improved, and the injury of donor area is becoming smaller and smaller.

The first free flap from the abdominal wall is the transverse free rectus abdominis myocutaneous flap (TRAM), which requires partial or entire resection of the rectus abdominis muscle; then DIEP flap appeared, and the muscle and fascia are almost preserved.

Then, in 1989, it was reported that SIEAP flap can be used for breast reconstruction without damaging the abdominal wall.

This advantage is very important in the process of breast reconstruction, because the injury of rectus abdominis muscle or fascia will reduce the strength and integrity of abdominal wall barrier, which is bad for the surgical outcome.

Furthermore, studies have shown that SIEAP flaps have less damage to the donor site than DIEP flaps or free TRAM flaps [4, 5].

The DIEP flap proposed by Allen [1] in 1994 is better than SIEAP flap, for the former has longer vascular pedicle, larger anastomotic diameter, and larger amount of flap tissue. DIEP flap can also be prepared into different forms of tissue flaps, so it has been the most widely used [6].

Z. Li (✉)
Department of Oncology Plastic Surgery, Hunan Cancer Hospital, Changsha, Hunan, China

S. Liu
Department of Breast Surgery, Affiliated Hospital of Guizhou Medical University, Guiyang, Guizhou, China

14.1 Indications and Contraindications

The injury of abdominal donor site caused by SIEAP flap was lightest.

However, since its anatomy is extremely unstable, we prefer DIEP flap instead in clinical practice. In our clinical experience, SIEAP flap is more suitable for repairing limbs and the perineum, while breast reconstruction with free SIEAP flap alone is rarely implemented in Asian women, which may be related to the anatomical basis of Asian women. Therefore, SIEAP flap can only be regarded as a supplementary means in the flap selection of breast reconstruction [7].

14.1.1 Anatomy

In 1975, Taylor and Daniel published a study on the anatomy of the superficial deep inferior epigastric artery (SIEA) [8, 9].

This study found that SIEA was absent in 35% of the subjects, and its origin varied in the remaining subjects: 48% of SIEA shared a vascular trunk with the superficial circumflex iliac artery and 52% of SIEA directly came from the femoral artery.

In 2011, Piorkowski [10] used CT angiography (CTA) to evaluate if SIEA can be applied to SIEA flap. They found that 43% of the subjects had at least one SIEA, but only 21% of the patients had a SIEA with appropriate caliber for SIEA flap preparation.

Our clinical experience in dissecting the donor area of the lower abdominal wall to obtain free flap during breast reconstruction is basically consistent with the conclusions of those studies.

Of more than 300 patients in our study, 76% had a bilateral SIEA deficiency, and of the other 24% with SIEA, only 14% of patients had SIEA with appropriate caliber (no less than 1.5 mm).

Z. Li, D. Song (eds.), *Oncoplastic Flap Surgery*, https://doi.org/10.1007/978-981-19-8926-1_14

Based on the measurement of the following abdominal incision, only the minimum external diameter of SIEA larger than 1.5 mm is able to support a free flap.

In conclusion, only 14% of the patients in our study had SIEA suitable for free flap, which was significantly lower than that in the previous research conclusions, due to the anatomical difference between Chinese women and European and American women.

The root of SIEA from femoral artery can be found 2–5 cm below inguinal ligament.

It may originate independently or share the trunk with the superficial circumflex iliac artery.

Moreover, there are also variations in the origin of vascular pedicle, which may originate from profunda femoral artery or perineal artery.

SIEA and its adjacent accompanying veins usually run laterally to the deep inferior epigastric artery (DIEA).

SIEA originates from the deep surface of Scarpa fascia, but it will continue to move through the fascia and end into the superficial subcutaneous tissue.

The SIEA flap has two accompanying veins that run along the SIEA, flow into the great saphenous vein and superficial abdominal vein (SIEV), and finally flow into the femoral vein (Figs. 14.1 and 14.2).

The caliber of SIEV is usually large, namely, 2–3 mm, but it will gradually move away from SIEA to the inside, which may result in difficulty in vascular anastomosis and arterial torsion.

Therefore, the segment of the accompanying veins before confluence is usually used for pedicle.

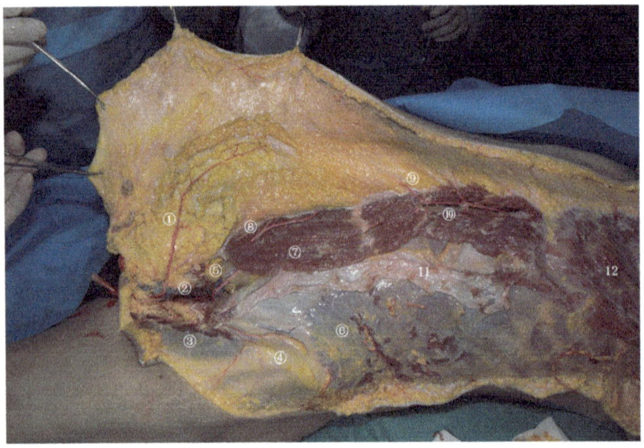

Fig. 14.1 Anatomy and location of superficial epigastric artery and deep inferior epigastric artery. (1) Superficial epigastric artery; (2) Femoral vein; (3) Sartorius muscle; (4) Anterior superior iliac spine; (5) Deep inferior epigastric vessels; (6) External oblique abdominal muscle; (7) Rectus abdominis; (8) Perforating branch of medial branch of deep inferior epigastric artery; (9) Perforating branch of superior epigastric artery; (10) Superior epigastric artery; (11) Anterior sheath of rectus abdominis; (12) Pectoralis major

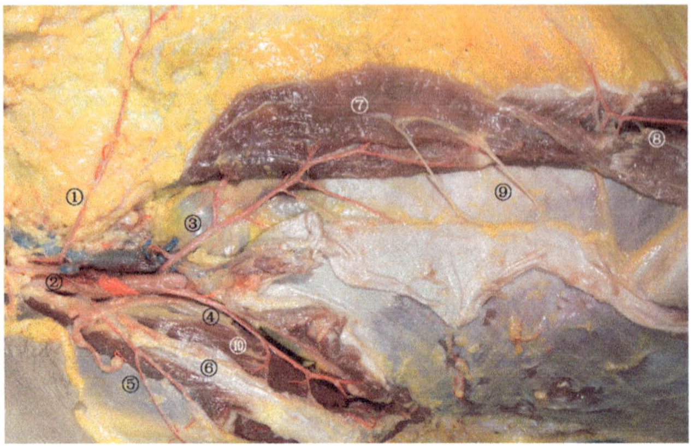

Fig. 14.2 The root of the superficial epigastric artery from the femoral artery can be found 2–5 cm below the inguinal ligament

The length of vascular pedicle in SIEAP flap is usually 5–8 cm, and the arterial diameter should be 1.1–1.9 mm throughout the whole process [11–14].

The SIEA flap consists of the lower abdominal wall area perfused by SIEA, but the lateral part of the flap coincides with the perforasome of the superficial circumflex iliac artery (SCIA) [6, 15–18].

The 10th to 12th intercostal nerves innervate the sensation in this area. If it is necessary to prepare sensory preserving flaps, they can also be carried in the flaps for flap sensory reconstruction [19, 20].

It may originate independently or share the trunk with the superficial iliac circumflex artery.

Whether one side of SIEA has an effect on tissue perfusion and venous reflux across the midline of the abdominal wall or not has been widely debated.

Some studies have concluded that it is quite difficult to predict venous return and blood perfusion across the midline.

However, other studies have found that it is possible to use tissues crossing the midline in areas III and IV [21, 22].

It is clinically observed that SIEA anatomical variation is great in Chinese female patients in terms of vascular existence, diameter, and length. Therefore, SIEAPF is only used as a supplement to deep inferior epigastric perforator flap (DIEPF) in daily clinical work.

Preoperative CTA can be used to judge whether SIEA exists and whether the caliber is appropriate. It can also be used to locate the route of relevant blood vessels in the flap [10].

Preoperative marks were made 8 h before operation.

The patient was placed in the supine position and both SIEAP flap and DIEP flap were marked on the abdomen at the same time.

During the operation, SIEAP or DIEP flap would be selected according to the standard approach.

Ipsilateral and contralateral flaps may be required during reconstruction, so all patients need to be marked bilaterally on the abdominal walls [7].

Firstly, the Doppler probe was used to determine how the SIEA and accompanying veins travel. The body surface location of the veins is often at the midpoint between the anterior superior iliac spine (ASIS) and pubic symphysis.

Next, SIEV was labeled. Compared with SIEA, it usually extends medially and runs among periumbilical arteriovenous perforations.

At this time, the perforator of the deep inferior epigastric artery was marked to provide anatomical reference for designing the shape and size of the flap.

When we mark the lower incision line, the incision needs to be designed low enough to dissect a SIEA with appropriate caliber.

According to the standard process, if the minimum diameter of the perforator is smaller than 1.5 mm, the DIEP flap should be cut instead for breast reconstruction.

The lower incision is started from above the midpoint of the pubic symphysis, extended to both sides with a slight upward arc, and ended at the anterior superior iliac spine (ASIS).

The incision is started from about 1.5–2 cm above the umbilicus with a shuttle-shaped flap.

The preparation of SIEAP flap should be started from the marked area of the lower abdominal wall on the same side of the breast to be reconstructed.

Carefully make an incision along the marked line and cut to the dermis.

Dissect the subcutaneous tissue carefully to avoid injury to SIEA, as it runs quite superficially in this area.

Before ligating the vascular pedicle of the disembodied SIEA flap, we should measure the diameter of the artery with the diameter measuring instrument of the vascular coupler.

If the blood vessels are as large as 1.5 mm in size with visible pulsation, dissection of the artery and its accompanying veins will be continued. It is important to continue dissecting only when the blood vessel is progressively thicker, usually without dissecting the blood vessel to its root.

A little subcutaneous tissue and fat are reserved around the vascular pedicle to protect the vascular pedicle. Only the anastomosis area at the end of the vascular pedicle needs to be thoroughly dissected for anastomosis.

Unilateral breast reconstruction is best achieved with the ipsilateral superficial epigastric artery perforator flap for the following three reasons:

1. The vascular pedicle of SIEA enters the abdominal wall tissue from the edge. When the ipsilateral flap is turned 180° to the chest wall, the vascular pedicle will get closer to the recipient vessel on the inner side of the chest wall.
2. When suturing the periumbilical incision to shape the ipsilateral flap, the flap will naturally become a cone on the inferolateral wall.
3. The implantation position of the ipsilateral flap makes the most unreliable part of the flap blood supply be placed in the marginal area rather than the main reconstruction area. On the contrary, the tissues at relatively high risk of necrosis are placed on the inner part of the contralateral flap, if necrosis appears, it would increase difficulty for further repair.

However, the SIEA on both sides needs to be evaluated before deciding which side of SIEA be used for vascular pedicle.

The evaluation mainly depends on the arterial diameter. If the diameter is smaller than 1.5 mm or the pulse is very weak, the contralateral SIEA will be the next assessment. If the contralateral SIEA is more satisfactory, the dissection is continued and reconstruction is performed with the contralateral flap.

If both SIEAs are unsatisfactory, we consider the deep perforator system to be more advantageous, and thus switch to DIEP flap.

Consistent with SIEAP flap, DIEP flap is also evaluated from the same side.

Similarly, evaluation starts from the lateral perforators to medial ones on the ipsilateral side. If none is available, evaluate the contralateral perforators.

During the operation, it is necessary to accurately compare the diameter of the recipient artery with that of SIEA. If the difference is >1 mm, it is strongly recommended to use DIEP flap instead.

Before the pedicle of the flap is broken, all the perforating vessels of the deep inferior epigastric artery should be blocked with a vascular clamp to determine the range of the flap that can be safely cut only by the blood supply of the superficial epigastric artery. If its blood supply is limited, the combined DIEPF + SIEAPF transplantation or the DIEP flap transplantation alone should be selected to reconstruct the breast.

In cases of mastectomy with skin or nipple preservation, the transplanted flap is simply used to fill the breast volume with little skin loss. Generally, a small skin island on the flap will be reserved for postoperative observation of blood supply, as well as for stage 2 nipple reconstruction and areola tattoo.

No matter what kind of mastectomy, the inframammary fold should be adjusted to the initially marked height, and the lateral edge of the skin envelope should be reconstructed if necessary.

When reconstructing the inframammary fold, the skin of the upper abdomen and chest will pull down the reconstructed inframammary fold, so it is necessary to raise the fold by 1–2 cm before closing the abdomen.

Some patients may need radiotherapy which is well tolerated by free flap autologous breast reconstruction, so we choose to carry out stage 2 breast reconstruction at least 6 months after radiotherapy.

The changes brought by radiotherapy and the choice of mastectomy method directly affect whether the chest wall skin can be retained or not during breast reconstruction. In patients with minimal skin changes after radiotherapy, flap shaping is similar to that in patient without radiotherapy.

If radiotherapy causes obvious changes to the skin of the chest wall, the scars and hardened, degenerative skin tissue left following mastectomy should be widely removed, a flap with preserved epidermis is able to achieve both volume filling and surface skin repair of the breast.

If planning to reconstruct the sensation of the flap, we usually choose the third anterior intercostal branch as recipient because it is anatomically constant and easy to obtain. It is usually found at the junction between the lower edge of the third rib and the sternum, where the nerve crosses the upper part of the intercostal vessel [23].

The nerve is carefully stripped from the blood vessel and cut down on the middle, after which the nerve is retrogradely separated to its maximum length in preparation for the nerve transplantation.

The sensory nerve carried by the flap is usually the sensory cutaneous branch of T11 or T12 [24]. We can usually find it near the lowest perforator when dissecting the abdominal wall.

The anastomosis of the vessels is difficult and technically demanding. In order to shorten the anastomotic distance and make the lumen more matched, we prefer to anastomose the accompanying vein of the superficial epigastric artery rather than the superficial epigastric vein with the recipient vein, because connecting the superficial epigastric vein will increase the risk of vascular pedicle torsion and flap complications.

If the accompanying veins are not enough, or additional veins need to be connected to improve the venous drainage of the flap, the anastomosis of the superficial epigastric vein should be considered.

When placing the flap, it is necessary to prevent the torsion of the vascular pedicle before entering the flap, or it will be destructive to the perfusion of the flap.

Another important point is that when the flap is implanted, the vascular pedicle of SIEA flap will make a big turn where it leaves the intercostal space and then enters the flap.

Vascular pedicle torsion and tortuosity are most likely to occur at this turning place.

If the patient has a history of radiotherapy on the reconstructed breast, it should be noted that poor skin elasticity will compress the skin flap and then the vascular pedicle with serious consequences.

After the flap is placed, observe for 3–5 min to determine the stability of the flap blood supply, and then adjust the patient to the semi sitting position in order to evaluate the symmetry of bilateral breasts. At the same time, placement of drainage tube of abdominal wound, reconstruction of umbilical position, and closure of abdominal donor area are performed.

14.2 Matters Needing Attention

14.2.1 Perfusion Evaluation

When the SIEAP flap with tissue volume across the midline is used, all tissues that may not survive, including any places with poor perfusion in area IV and area III, need to be removed.

The amount of tissue that can be used for reconstruction beyond the midline depends on the actual perfusion mode of each patient.

There are several methods to evaluate perfusion: (1) Leave the flap in situ, clamp its deep perforator and contralateral SIEA vascular pedicle, and there will be a boundary in the area of insufficient perfusion. (2) ICG fluoroscopy can help reflect the perfusion in practice and help determine how much of the flap requires removal.

14.2.2 Adjustment of Flap Placement

In the process of placing the flap into the chest envelope, the position of the flap needs to be carefully adjusted to prevent the tortuous compression of the vascular pedicle. Two points should be paid attention to:

1. Different from the vascular pedicle of DIEP flap, the superficial vascular pedicle enters from the lower edge of the flap.

   To facilitate anastomosis, the superficial vascular pedicle has to be introduced from superficial surface to deep surface of the flap and then turned 90° so as to approach the internal mammary vessels, which increases the risk of vascular pedicle torsion.
2. The vascular pedicle of SIEAP flap is also likely to get stuck where the pectoralis major muscle is opened.

Therefore, unlike the preparation of recipient blood vessels in cases of reconstruction using DIEP flap, the opening on the pectoralis major muscle should be as large as possible to prevent too much tension from compressing the vascular pedicle when SIEAP flap is used.

This is particularly important for patients with a history of radiotherapy. Radiotherapy would compromise the elastic and soft characteristics of chest skin and make adhesion worse. In order to avoid flap compression, it is recommended to expand the removal of the diseased skin.

14.2.3 Abdominal Drainage

The donor drainage tube of patients with SIEAP flap is usually placed longer than that of patients with DIEP flap, for which SIEA has a wider anatomical range in the groin and greater damage to the lymphatic system.

The drainage tube should be placed in situ until the daily drainage volume is less than 10 mL, which usually takes 1–2 weeks.

14.2.4 Postoperative Monitoring

The flap is observed every hour within the first 24 h after operation, and the posture test is carried out.

If there are no complications in the postural test, the patient can be transferred to the general ward as long as his vital signs are stable and his pain is well controlled.

As far as tolerable, patients are encouraged to get out of bed and walk 3–4 days after operation, so they can usually be discharged 5–7 days after operation.

14.3 Case 1: DIEP + SIEAP Breast Reconstruction

The patient, a 44-year-old female, recovered from right breast cancer after radical mastectomy 5 years ago. The original pathological results were: histological grade II of right breast invasive ductal carcinoma, cancer metastasis in 2/12 of right axillary lymph nodes, and immunohistochemistry: ER (−), PR (−), CerbB-2 (+), Ki-67 (20%).

The first operation after admission: free right DIEP flap and left SIEAP flap were transplanted to reconstruct the right breast.

After excision of the chest wall scar, the skin envelope was fully freed, and the right internal thoracic artery and vein and the right lateral thoracic artery and vein were prepared for revascularization.

The size of the designed flap was about 26 cm × 14 cm.

The superficial epigastric artery and vein were relatively thick and were retrogradely dissected along them to close to their emitting plane, with the vascular pedicle about 8 cm long. The DIEP flap pedicled with the right deep inferior epigastric artery and vein and the SIEAP flap pedicled with the left superficial epigastric artery and vein were harvested. The superficial epigastric artery and vein were anastomosed end to end with the right lateral thoracic vessels (1A1V), and the right deep inferior epigastric artery and vein were anastomosed end to end with the right internal thoracic artery and veins (1A2V).

The second operation: debridement + flap exploration.

Twelve hours after operation, cyanosis appeared on the outside of the flap and dark red blood was increasingly discharged in the drainage tube. Emergency surgical exploration: cyanosis was seen on the outside of the right chest flap, accounting for about 2/5 of the lateral flap. The lateral suture of the flap was disassembled, and the lateral flap was loosened. Obvious congestion and swelling on the outside of the flap was seen, so we remove 2/5 of the lateral flap until fresh blood flowed out at the cutting edge.

Rinse the wound. Two negative pressure drainage tubes were placed in the operation cavity for drainage. The wound was narrowed and sutured again, and the flap survived well (Figs. 14.3, 14.4, 14.5, 14.6, 14.7, 14.8, 14.9, 14.10, 14.11, 14.12, 14.13, 14.14, 14.15, 14.16, 14.17, and 14.18).

If removing a flap with superficial epigastric vessels, we should be careful to avoid the injury to ilioinguinal lymph nodes [11].

When we cut the flap with the superficial epigastric vessels as the pedicle, the vessel pedicle should be separated to its emitting plane as far as possible to obtain the maximum

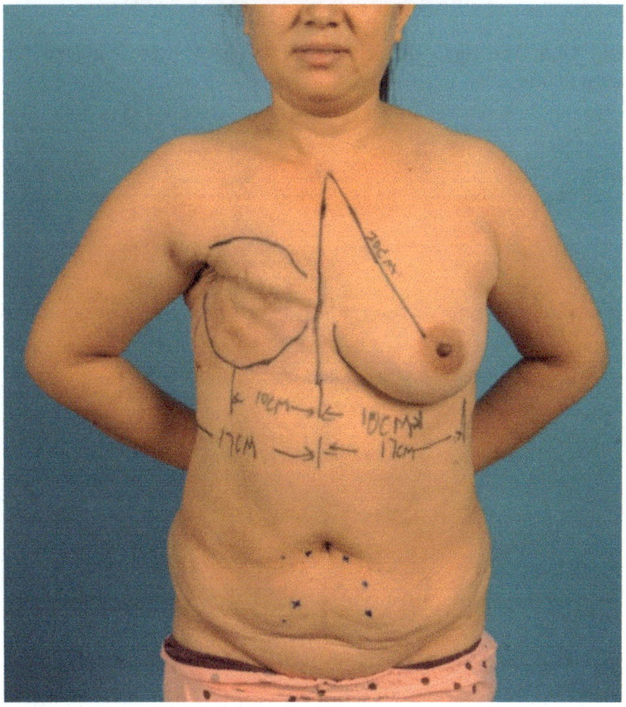

Fig. 14.3 Preoperative findings

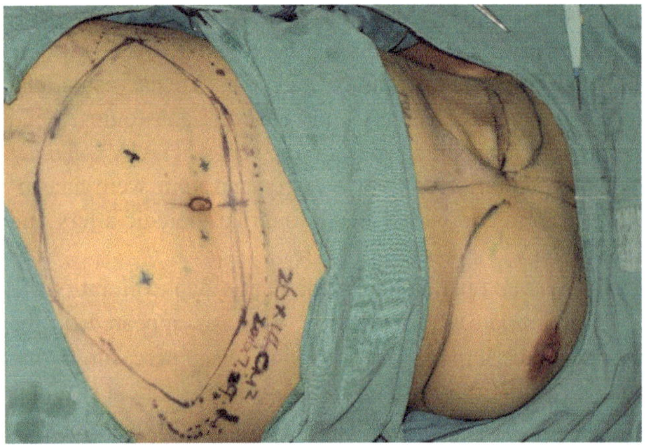

Fig. 14.4 Intraoperative design

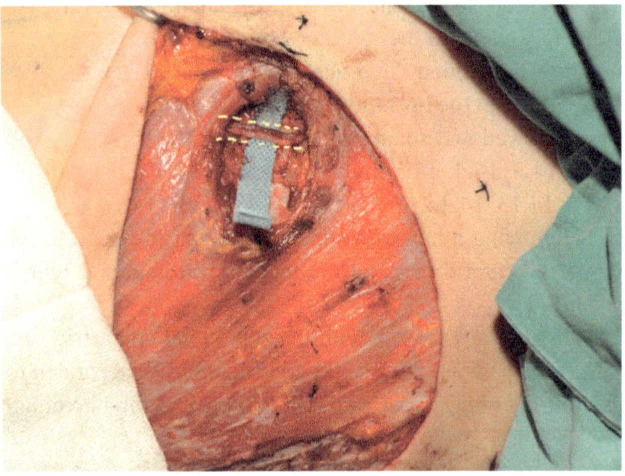

Fig. 14.5 The right internal mammary vessels were prepared for anastomosis

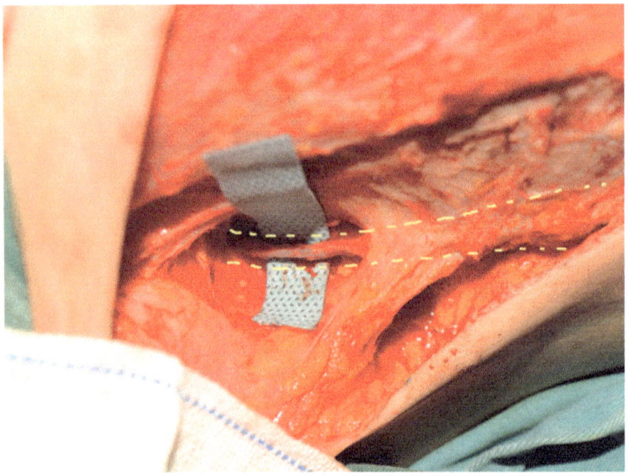

Fig. 14.6 The right lateral thoracic vessels were prepared for anastomosis

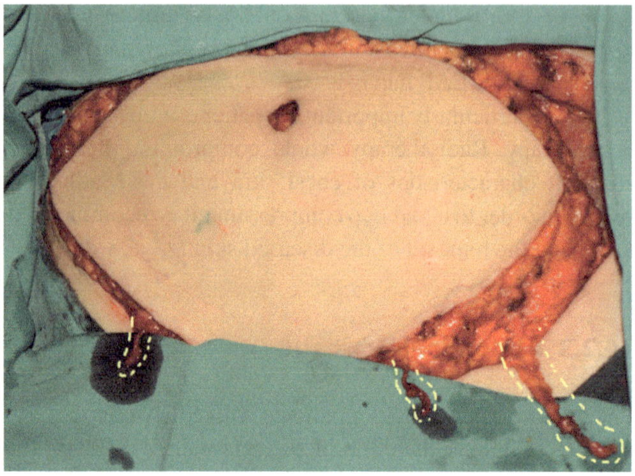

Fig. 14.7 The left superficial epigastric artery and vein and the right superficial epigastric vein were prepared

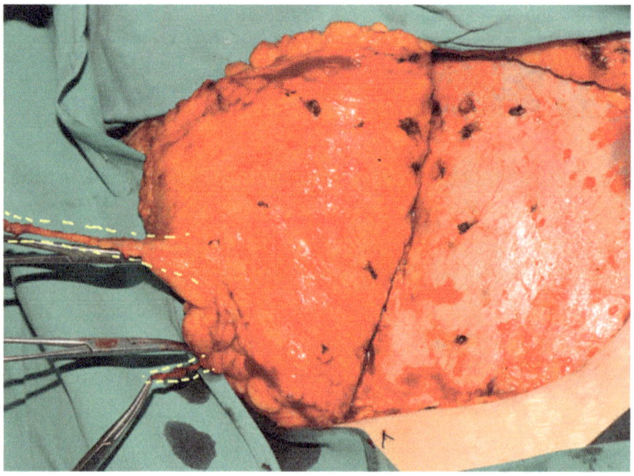

Fig. 14.8 No large perforating vessels were found in the left abdominal exploration

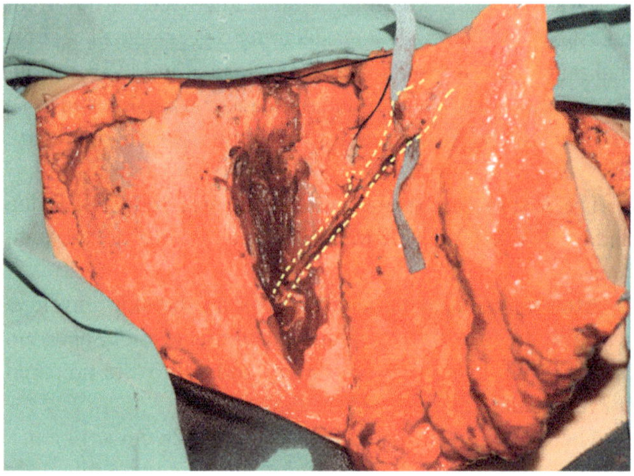

Fig. 14.9 The perforator and pedicle of the right deep inferior epigastric vessels were separated

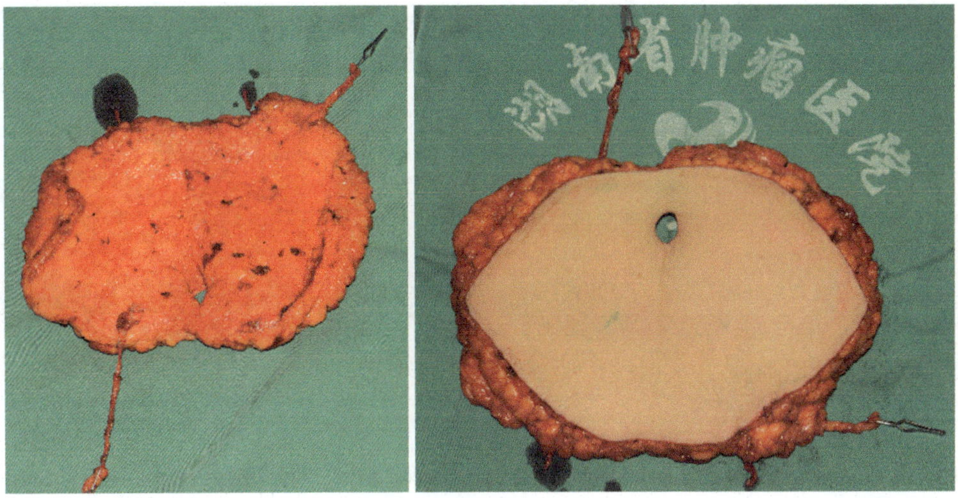

Fig. 14.10 Right DIEPF + left SIEAPF were ready

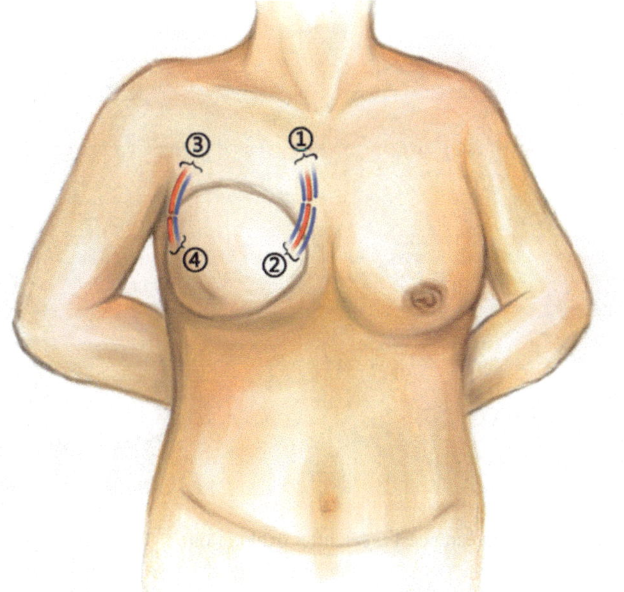

Fig. 14.11 Revascularization pattern: Left superficial epigastric vessels + right lateral thoracic vessels (1A1V); Right deep inferior epigastric artery and vein + right internal thoracic artery and vein (1A2V). (1) Right internal thoracic artery and vein; (2) Right deep inferior epigastric artery and vein; (3) Right lateral thoracic vessels; (4) Left superficial epigastric vessels

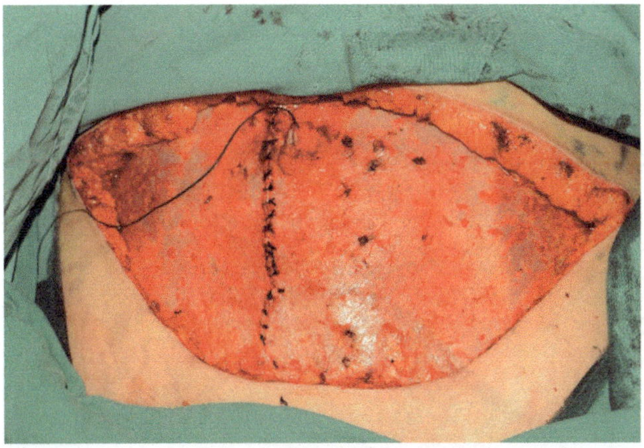

Fig. 14.12 Repair of anterior sheath of rectus abdominis muscle

length and diameter. As the superficial iliac circumflex vessels may be encountered while approaching the femoral artery area, they should be carefully separated.

However, the diameter of superficial epigastric vessels tends to vary a little, so there is no need to further separate when the appropriate diameter is reached in the clinical separation.

Once the flap is separated, the surface position of the vascular pedicle should be marked with a marker for subsequent anastomosis.

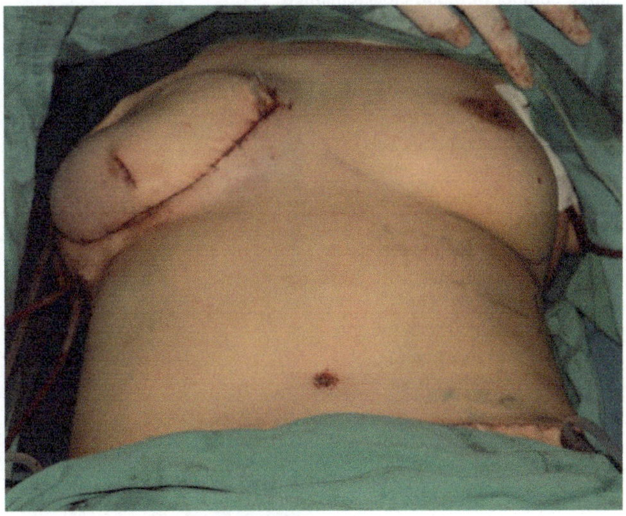

Fig. 14.13 An intraoperative view of immediate breast reconstruction

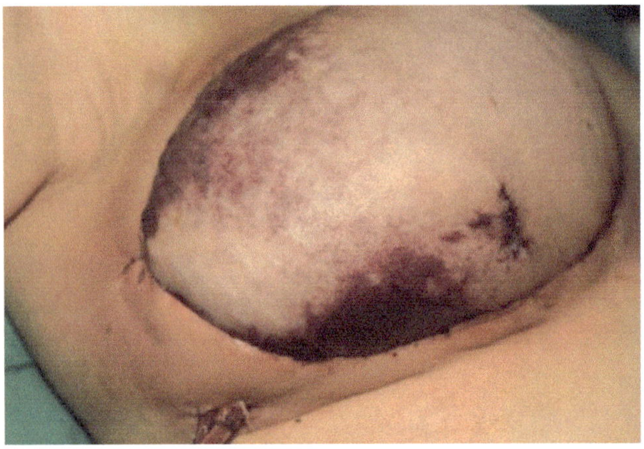

Fig. 14.14 Venous reflux obstruction in the flap area occurred 2 days after operation

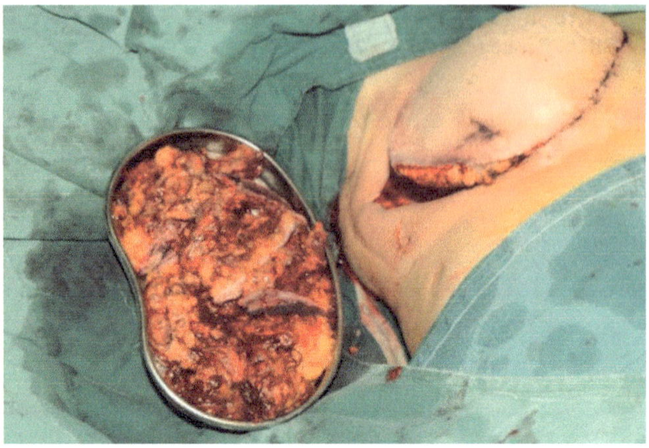

Fig. 14.16 Partial flap with congestion obstruction was removed, and the blood supply of the flap returned to normal

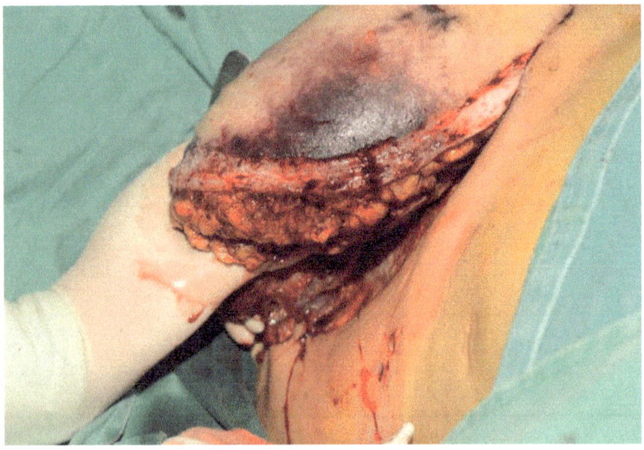

Fig. 14.15 Emergency exploration showed that bilateral anastomoses were unobstructed, congestion was obvious at the edge of the flap, and a large number of blood clots remained

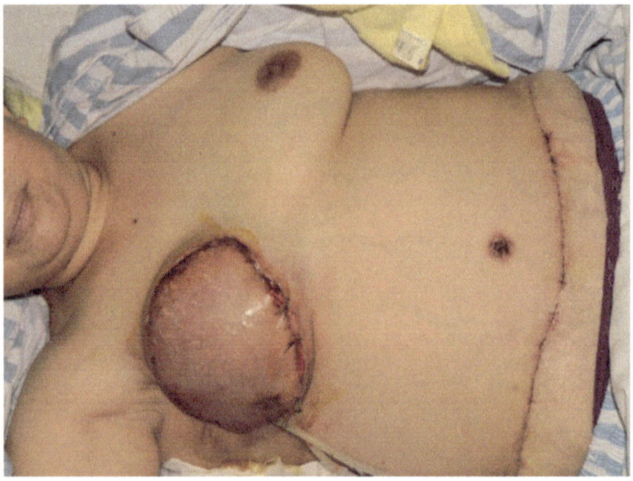

Fig. 14.17 Appearance 1 week after exploration

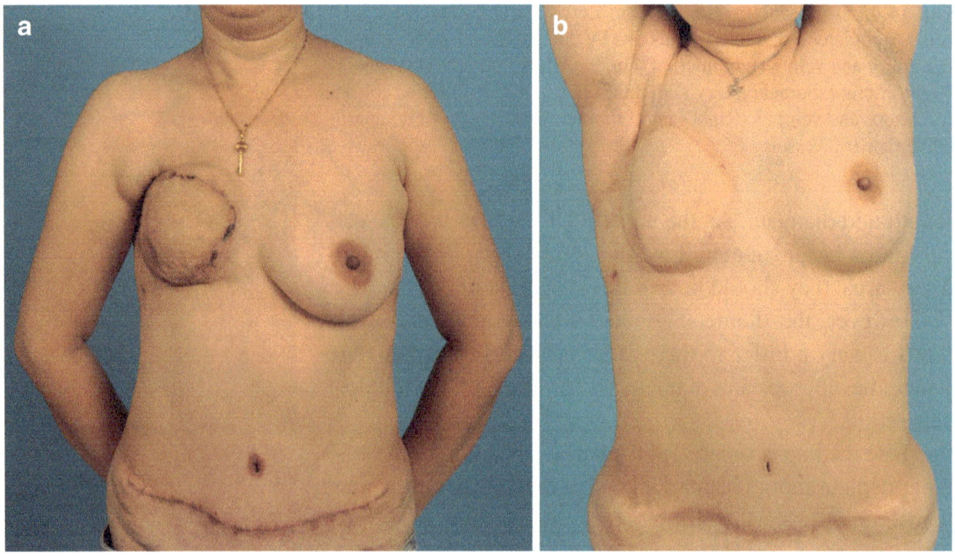

Fig. 14.18 (**a**) Postoperative follow-up in 2 months: the right reconstructed breast was significantly reduced due to the removal of some flap tissue. (**b**) Postoperative follow-up in 28 months: the right breast was slightly smaller than the left. The patient was satisfied with the appearance and function of the reconstructed breast and refused further fat transplantation

Put the flap edges back into the abdomen and fix them in the appropriate receiving area.

If bilateral reconstruction is planned, revascularization of the first flap should be performed before evaluating the feasibility of the contralateral superficial vessels for reconstruction use in terms of SIEA caliber and pulsation, otherwise the contralateral DIEP flap may be used instead.

The superficial epigastric vascular pedicle is difficult to place, because on the one hand, the vascular pedicle is short; on the other hand, the vascular pedicle is located at the edge of the flap, which makes it harder to adjust the flap and vascular pedicle.

14.3.1 Flap Adjustment

If the flap is too large for the residual chest skin envelope or the chest skin is removed extensively, excessive tension can also cause flap crisis.

For such a flap, we should trim it and implant it again in a tension-free manner.

The penumbra area of the flap can be evaluated clinically by fluorescence photography.

When the congestion is located in Area IV or the contralateral lateral area, the best solution is to remove it directly. If the congestion of the flap can be removed, it will reduce the venous load and improve the circulation of the whole flap.

14.4 Case 2: DIEP + SIEAP Breast Reconstruction 2

The patient, a 47-year-old female, was admitted after the diagnosis of right breast cancer. She underwent modified radical mastectomy for right breast cancer plus breast reconstruction using free right DIEP flap combined with right SIEAP flap.

The breast skin envelope was completely freed following radical mastectomy, and the right internal thoracic vessels and right lateral thoracic vessels were prepared for anastomosis.

The size of the lower abdominal flap was about 30 cm × 14 cm.

Lifting up the lower edge of the flap, we found that the superficial inferior epigastric arteries and veins on each side were relatively thick. We then dissected the vessels retrograde. The right vascular pedicle was about 10 cm long and the left was about 9 cm long. After adjusting the vascular body area of the flap, we adopted the right DIEP flap pedicled with the right deep inferior epigastric artery plus the right SIEAP pedicled with the right superficial epigastric vein. The right superficial epigastric artery and vein were anastomosed end to end with the distal end of the right internal thoracic artery and vein (1A1V), and the right deep inferior epigastric artery and vein were anastomosed end to end with the proximal end of the right internal thoracic artery and vein (1A2V).

The flap was viable after operation, with slight fat liquefaction at the flap edge that was solved after dressing change and the patient was then discharged from the hospital (Figs. 14.19, 14.20, 14.21, 14.22, and 14.23).

The superficial deep inferior epigastric artery originates from the femoral artery (57%) or the superficial circumflex iliac artery (43%), and runs deep into the Scarpa fascia below the inguinal ligament [25, 26].

After reaching above the inguinal ligament, it crosses Scarpa fascia and runs in the superficial subcutaneous tissue.

However, the superficial deep inferior epigastric artery was absent in 30% of patients. Even in patients with SIEA, the proportion of flap without sufficient blood supply still accounts for 50% [5].

SIEA flaps were used in only 35% of all patients [8].

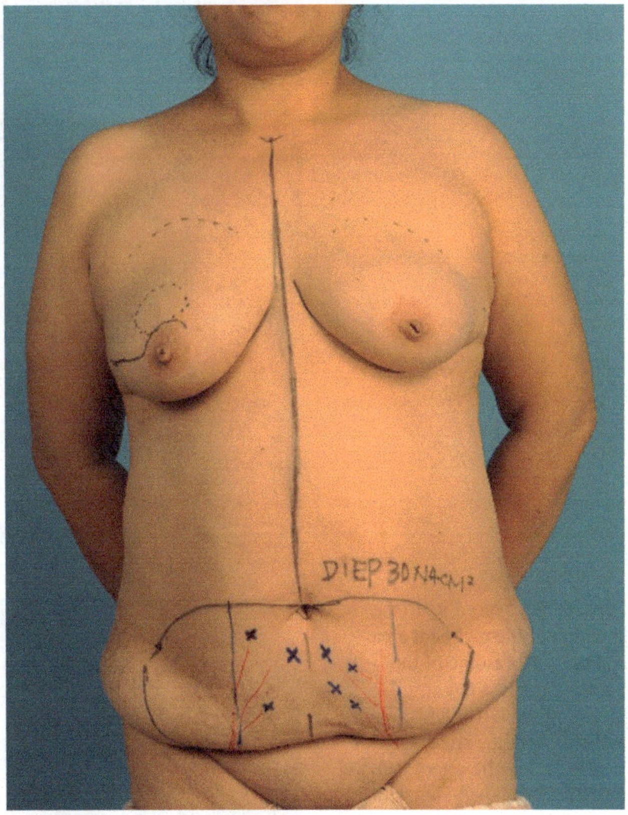

Fig. 14.19 A preoperative photo: abundant adipose tissue and skin tissue in the lower abdomen

Fig. 14.20 After modified radical mastectomy for right breast cancer, bilateral DIEP flaps and SIEAP flaps were cut off

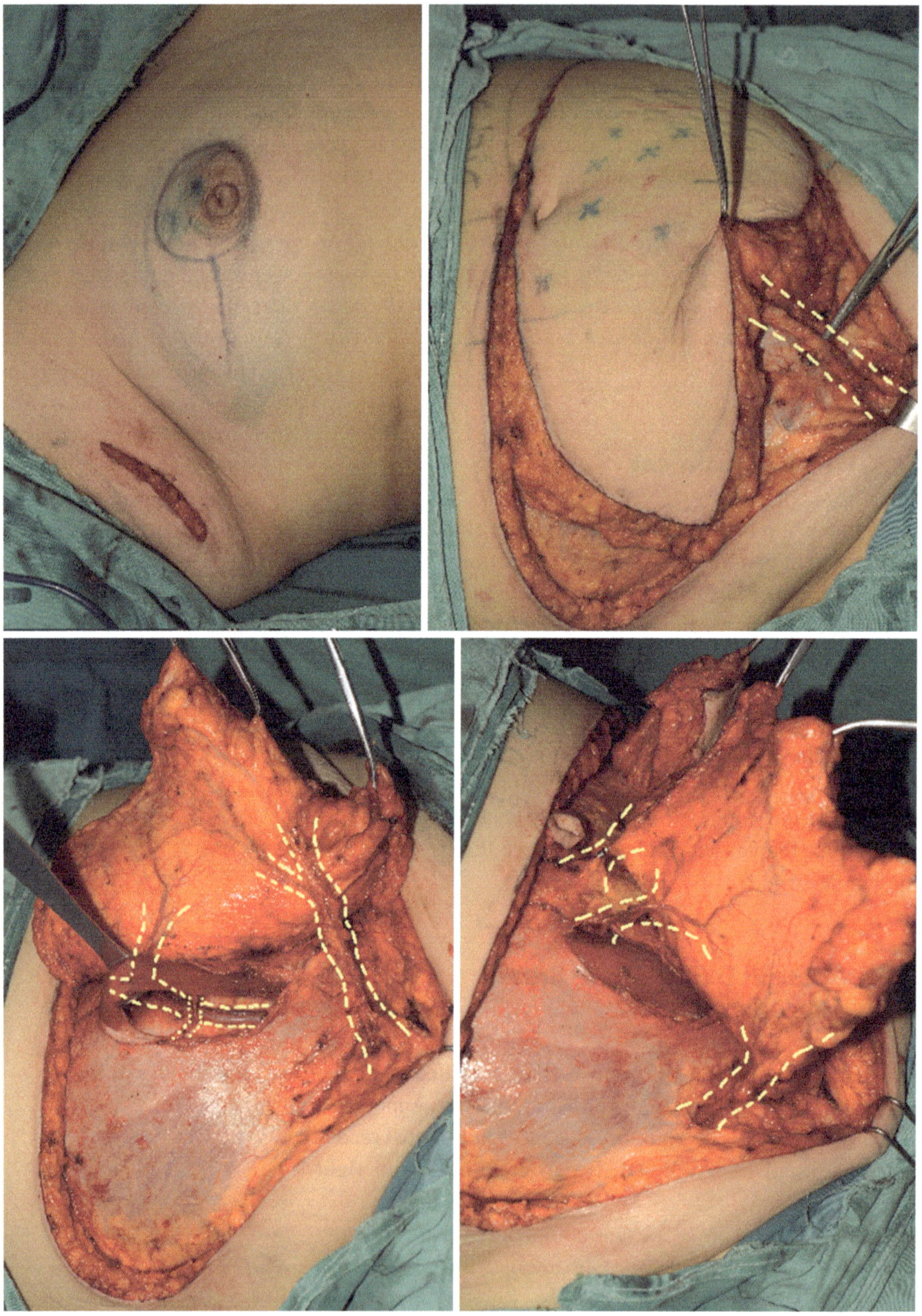

Fig. 14.21 According to the situation of the recipient area and the perforasome of the flap, a combined flap including the DIEP flap pedicled with the right inferior epigastric artery and the SIEAP flap pedicled with the right superficial epigastric artery and vein was adjusted too

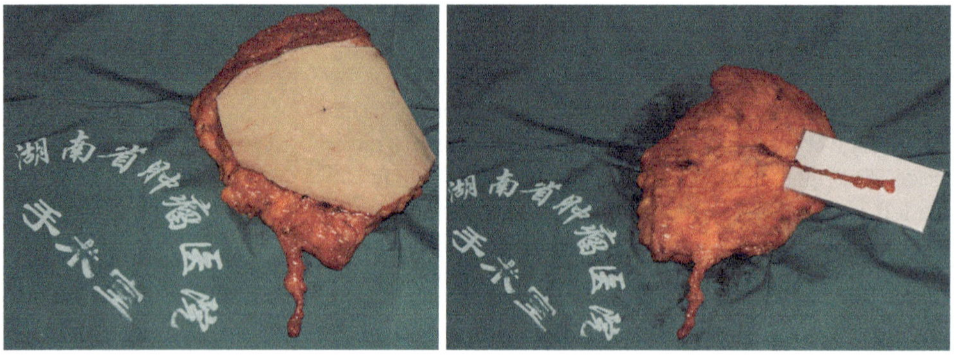

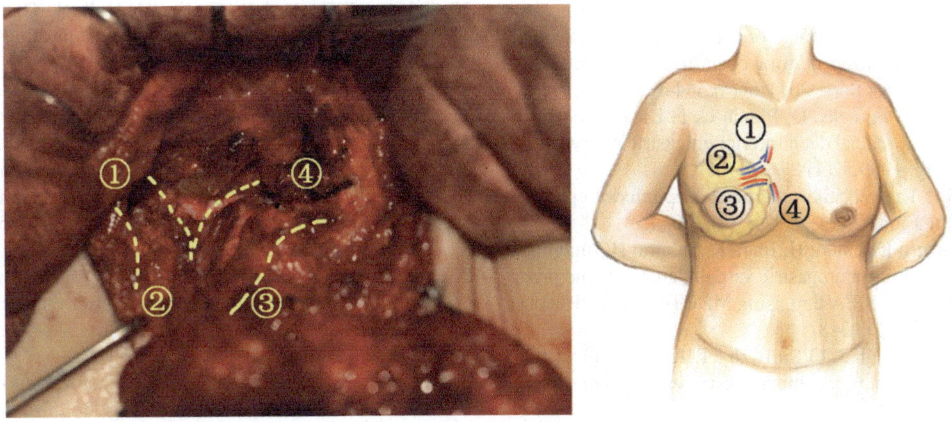

Fig. 14.22 The superficial epigastric artery and vein were anastomosed end to end with the distal end of the right internal thoracic artery and vein (1A1V), and the deep inferior epigastric artery and vein were anastomosed end to end with the proximal end of the right internal thoracic artery and vein (1A2V). (1) Proximal end of right internal thoracic artery and vein; (2) Right deep inferior epigastric artery and vein; (3) Right superficial epigastric artery and vein; (4) Distal end of right internal thoracic artery and vein

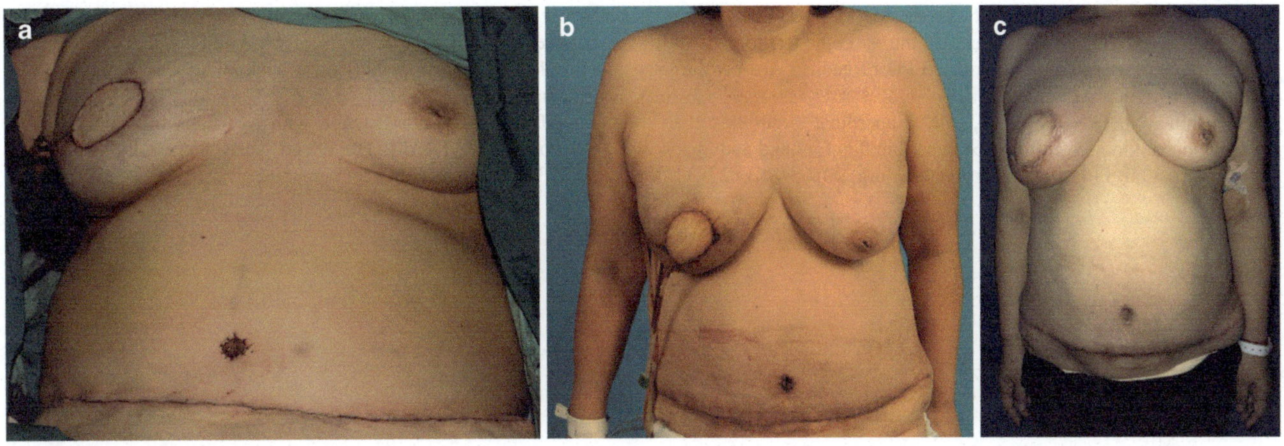

Fig. 14.23 (**a**) An intraoperative view of immediate breast reconstruction. (**b**) Hospital discharge in 2 weeks: the flap survived well and the effect of abdominal shaping was satisfactory. (**c**) Postoperative follow-up in 4 months: the patient was satisfied with the appearance of reconstructed breast and the effect of abdominal shaping

It is concluded that the superficial inferior epigastric artery flap is less reliable than DIEP flap in carrying the blood supply to Areas II and III [5, 27].

Overall, the thrombosis rate and total flap necrosis rate of SIEA flap are significantly higher than those of free TRAM or DIEP flap [27, 28].

References

1. Allen RJ, Treece P. Deep inferior epigastric perforator flap for breast reconstruction. Ann Plast Surg. 1994;32(1):32–8.
2. Antia NH, Buch VI. Transfer of an abdominal dermo-fat graft by direct anastomosis of blood vessels. Br J Plast Surg. 1971;24(1):15–9.
3. Healy C, Allen RJ. The evolution of perforator flap breast reconstruction: twenty years after the first DIEP flap. J Reconstr Microsurg. 2014;30(2):121–5.
4. Wu LC, Bajaj A, Chang DW, Chevray PM. Comparison of donor-site morbidity of SIEA, DIEP, and muscle-sparing TRAM flaps for breast reconstruction. Plast Reconstr Surg. 2008;122(3):702–9.
5. Chevray PM. Breast reconstruction with superficial deep inferior epigastric artery flaps: a prospective comparison with TRAM and DIEP flaps. Plast Reconstr Surg. 2004;114(5):1077–83; discussion 1084–5.
6. Schaverien M, Saint-Cyr M, Arbique G, Brown SA. Arterial and venous anatomies of the deep inferior epigastric perforator and superficial deep inferior epigastric artery flaps. Plast Reconstr Surg. 2008;121(6):1909–19.
7. Spiegel AJ, Khan FN. An intraoperative algorithm for use of the SIEA flap for breast reconstruction. Plast Reconstr Surg. 2007;120(6):1450–9.
8. Taylor GI, Daniel RK. The anatomy of several free flap donor sites. Plast Reconstr Surg. 1975;56(3):243–53.
9. Boyd JB, Taylor GI, Corlett R. The vascular territories of the superior epigastric and the deep inferior epigastric systems. Plast Reconstr Surg. 1984;73(1):1–16.

10. Piorkowski JR, DeRosier LC, Nickerson P, Fix RJ. Preoperative computed tomography angiogram to predict patients with favorable anatomy for superficial deep inferior epigastric artery flap breast reconstruction. Ann Plast Surg. 2011;66(5):534–6.
11. Arnez ZM, Khan U, Pogorelec D, Planinsek F. Breast reconstruction using the free superficial deep inferior epigastric artery (SIEA) flap. Br J Plast Surg. 1999;52(4):276–9.
12. Stern HS, Nahai F. The versatile superficial deep inferior epigastric artery free flap. Br J Plast Surg. 1992;45(4):270–4.
13. Fukaya E, Kuwatsuru R, Iimura H, Ihara K, Sakurai H. Imaging of the superficial deep inferior epigastric vascular anatomy and preoperative planning for the SIEA flap using MDCTA. J Plast Reconstr Aesthet Surg. 2011;64(1):63–8.
14. Reardon CM, O'Ceallaigh S, O'Sullivan ST. An anatomical study of the superficial deep inferior epigastric vessels in humans. Br J Plast Surg. 2004;57(6):515–9.
15. Nasir S, Aydin MA. Versatility of free SCIA/SIEA flaps in head and neck defects. Ann Plast Surg. 2010;65(1):32–7.
16. Aydin MA, Nasir S. Free SCIA/SIEA skin flap: a dual blood supply approach to groin region. Microsurgery. 2007;27(7):617–22.
17. Hester TR, Nahai F, Beegle PE, Bostwick J. Blood supply of the abdomen revisited, with emphasis on the superficial deep inferior epigastric artery. Plast Reconstr Surg. 1984;74(5):657–70.
18. Holm C, Mayr M, Höfter E, Ninkovic M. The versatility of the SIEA flap: a clinical assessment of the vascular territory of the superficial epigastric inferior artery. J Plast Reconstr Aesthet Surg. 2007;60(8):946–51.
19. Narushima M, Iida T, Kaji N, et al. Superficial circumflex iliac artery pure skin perforator-based superthin flap for hand and finger reconstruction. J Plast Reconstr Aesthet Surg. 2016;69(6):827–34.
20. Schlenz I, Kuzbari R, Gruber H, Holle J. The sensitivity of the nipple-areola complex: an anatomic study. Plast Reconstr Surg. 2000;105(3):905–9.
21. Granzow JW, Levine JL, Chiu ES, Allen RJ. Breast reconstruction using perforator flaps. J Surg Oncol. 2006;94(6):441–54.
22. Ulusal BG, Cheng MH, Wei FC, Ho-Asjoe M, Song D. Breast reconstruction using the entire transverse abdominal adipocutaneous flap based on unilateral superficial or deep inferior epigastric vessels. Plast Reconstr Surg. 2006;117(5):1395–403; discussion 1404–6.
23. Spiegel AJ, Salazar-Reyes H, Izaddoost S, Khan FN. A novel method for neurotization of deep inferior epigastric perforator and superficial deep inferior epigastric artery flaps. Plast Reconstr Surg. 2009;123(1):29e–30e.
24. Spiegel AJ, Menn ZK, Eldor L, Kaufman Y, Dellon AL. Breast reinnervation: DIEP neurotization using the third anterior intercostal nerve. Plast Reconstr Surg Glob Open. 2013;1(8):e72.
25. Fathi M, Hatamipour E, Fathi HR, Abbasi A. The anatomy of superficial deep inferior epigastric artery flap. Acta Cir Bras. 2008;23(5):429–34.
26. Kim BJ, Choi JH, Kim TH, Jin US, Minn KW, Chang H. The superficial deep inferior epigastric artery flap and its relevant vascular anatomy in Korean women. Arch Plast Surg. 2014;41(6):702–8.
27. Selber JC, Samra F, Bristol M, et al. A head-to-head comparison between the muscle-sparing free TRAM and the SIEA flaps: is the rate of flap loss worth the gain in abdominal wall function. Plast Reconstr Surg. 2008;122(2):348–55.
28. Lipa JE. Breast reconstruction with free flaps from the abdominal donor site: TRAM, DIEP, and SIEA flaps. Clin Plast Surg. 2007;34(1):105–21; abstract vii.

15 Simultaneous Contralateral Breast Reduction/Mastopexy with Unilateral Breast Reconstruction Using Free DIEP Flaps

Zan Li and Kun Wang

15.1 Background

In the past 60 years, development in medicine has greatly improved early diagnosis, precise staging, and comprehensive treatment of breast cancer, which contributed to the increasing survival rate of patients with breast cancer [1, 2].

In addition, technical advancement in breast surgery has remarkably enhanced the safety and effectiveness of sentinel lymph node biopsy, skin sparing radical mastectomy, and immediate breast reconstruction [3, 4].

The development of breast oncoplasty has raised the expectations of patients including extended survival time and tumor recurrence free interval as well as restoration of beautiful appearance and function of the breast [5–8].

Autologous breast reconstruction was commonly performed at delayed stage in the past, now it is well recognized that immediate reconstruction is better at constructing a natural and beautiful breast [9].

However, patients' cosmetic expectations frequently come true not simply by reconstructing the affected breast but also adjusting the shape, size, and symmetry of both breasts. Hakyal and Guay [1] reported that the proportion of breast adjustment subsequent to immediate breast reconstruction using autologous tissue (TRAM flap, muscle-sparing TRAM flap, and DIEP flap) for breast cancer was 11.3%.

Successful breast reconstruction they defined was that patients achieved satisfactory reconstructive outcome in only one anesthesia operation, otherwise failure was deemed.

At present, it is recognized that the criterion for successful and satisfactory breast reconstruction is not only to reconstruct a normal breast shape, but also to restore the symmetry of bilateral breasts to the greatest extent, which requires adjusting the contralateral breast such as contralateral breast augmentation, contralateral breast reduction, and contralateral mastopexy [1, 6–8, 10]. In Asian female patients, contralateral breast augmentation is the most frequently used breast adjustment [10].

In addition, it is worth noting that the rate of tumor tissue accidentally found in the contralateral breast tissue on pathological examination is 4.6% [11].

15.2 Timing of Operation

Stevenson and Goldstein [8] confirmed that unilateral autologous tissue breast reconstruction concurrent with contralateral breast adjustment was safe and cosmetically satisfactory.

Adjusting the contralateral breast simultaneously with reconstructing the affected breast using autologous tissue may provide with a better outcome [6].

The purpose of breast reconstruction is to reconstruct beautiful, symmetrical, and natural breasts. The most important measurement is the symmetry of bilateral breasts, which requires adjusting the contralateral breast, and often completed at a delayed timing [8, 12]. Delayed adjustment was thought to be better on the ground that the results of the reconstructed breast was time dependent [6].

Further studies have proved that the safety, cosmetic effect and satisfaction of immediate contralateral breast adjustment is as good as that of delayed surgery [10].

In addition, the coincidence of breast cancer can be investigated in dealing with the contralateral mammary glands [11].

At present, there is no final conclusion on when contralateral breast adjustment should be performed after breast reconstruction to achieve satisfactory results [6, 8, 11].

The timing of contralateral breast adjustment is still controversial [1].

Z. Li (✉)
Department of Oncology Plastic Surgery, Hunan Cancer Hospital, Changsha, Hunan, China

K. Wang
Breast-Conserving and Reconstructive Surgery, Multidisciplinary Cancer Treatment, Department of Breast Cancer, Cancer Center, Guangdong Provincial People's Hospital, Guangdong Academy of Medical Sciences, Guangzhou, Guangdong, China
e-mail: wangkun@gdph.org.cn

Z. Li, D. Song (eds.), *Oncoplastic Flap Surgery*, https://doi.org/10.1007/978-981-19-8926-1_15

Stevenson and Goldstein [8] first made a statistical comparison on the effect of delayed and immediate breast reconstruction with pedicled rectus abdominis flap transfer.

Losken [6] reported the recovery of 1394 patients who underwent contralateral breast adjustment without making a statistical comparison between the effects of immediate and delayed surgery.

Giacalone [7] reported 683 cases of breast reconstruction with autologous tissue and prosthesis to achieve bilateral breast symmetry, yet the timing of operation was not mentioned.

Some scholars evaluated the satisfaction after breast reconstruction using BREAST-Q questionnaire, which presented as a tool to measure the effect of breast reconstruction and contralateral breast adjustment. Their results proved that immediate reconstruction was associated with better effect and satisfaction [13].

Many scholars favor staged surgery [8, 14, 15], which has many advantages, such as shortened operation time, reduced blood loss, lowered possibility of breast asymmetry, and no interference with the implementation of comprehensive treatment.

When the patient's own conditions meet the requirements, autologous tissue transplantation should be first considered for breast reconstruction [5–8, 16, 17].

The indications of contralateral breast adjustment depend on the patient's breast condition, the operator's technical skills, the patient's expectations for breast shape, the surgical approach for breast cancer, and reconstruction methods [8, 18].

Indications for contralateral breast adjustment include:

1. The patient was not satisfied with contralateral breast ptosis or hypertrophy.
2. The volume and shape of the reconstructed breast were not matched with that of the contralateral breast.
3. Breast ptosis is graded II or III level and significant vacancy is observed on the superior breast.

The occurrence of contralateral breast cancer can also be investigated in contralateral breast adjustment [11].

15.3 Preoperative Design and Donor Site Preparation

The new inframammary fold (IMF) and the upper margin of the breast as well as the new nipple position on the contralateral breast are marked when the patient is standing. The distance from the nipple to the sternum in Asian women is generally 19–21 cm.

Surgery was underwent by three teams at the same time. One team prepares breast skin envelope and recipient vessels. The second team completes free flap harvest and vascular anastomosis, and the third group performs adjustment of the contralateral breast.

Hidalgo et al. [19, 20] reported the details of contralateral breast surgery including inverted "T" incision and vertical incision, which can be flexibly selected.

The method of mastopexy depends on the degree of breast ptosis. Benelli method is applied for a moderately ptotic breast, an inverted "T" incision and vertical incision are used for the correction of severe breast ptosis.

Breast reduction can be completed by an inverted "T" incision introduced by Hidalgo, where the second to third and fourth to sixth internal thoracic perforating vessels were preserved to provide sufficient blood supply for the nipple areola complex and the upper chest wall skin [21].

Some scholars simultaneously performed immediate breast reconstruction and contralateral breast augmentation endoscopically. The symmetry of bilateral breasts was satisfactory, the appearance was beautiful, and the patient satisfaction was high [10, 22].

Shaping of the reconstructed breast with autologous tissue should be done according to the size and shape of the modified breast on the other side.

Case Study 1: Unilateral Breast Reconstruction with DIEP Flap Plus Contralateral Breast Augmentation with Prothesis: The Internal Thoracic Vessels and Lateral Thoracic Vessels Used as Recipient

The patient was a 51-year-old female, who once received right radical mastectomy for breast cancer plus left mastectomy plus left breast reconstruction with prosthesis. She was given 4 cycles of chemotherapy after operation. After comprehensive treatment, the patient recovered. Subsequently, prosthesis displacement and capsule contracture occurred. She underwent right chest scar resection, right breast reconstruction with free DIEP flap, capsulectomy, and prothesis replacement. Bilateral deep inferior epigastric arteries and veins were end-to-end anastomosed with the proximal and distal ends of the right internal thoracic arteries and veins, respectively. The new prosthesis placed into the left breast was 215 cc in size.

The flap survived completely, bilateral breasts were symmetrical, and the function and appearance recovered satisfactorily. Tumor recurrence was negative on pathological examination (Figs. 15.1, 15.2, 15.3, 15.4, 15.5, 15.6, 15.7, and 15.8).

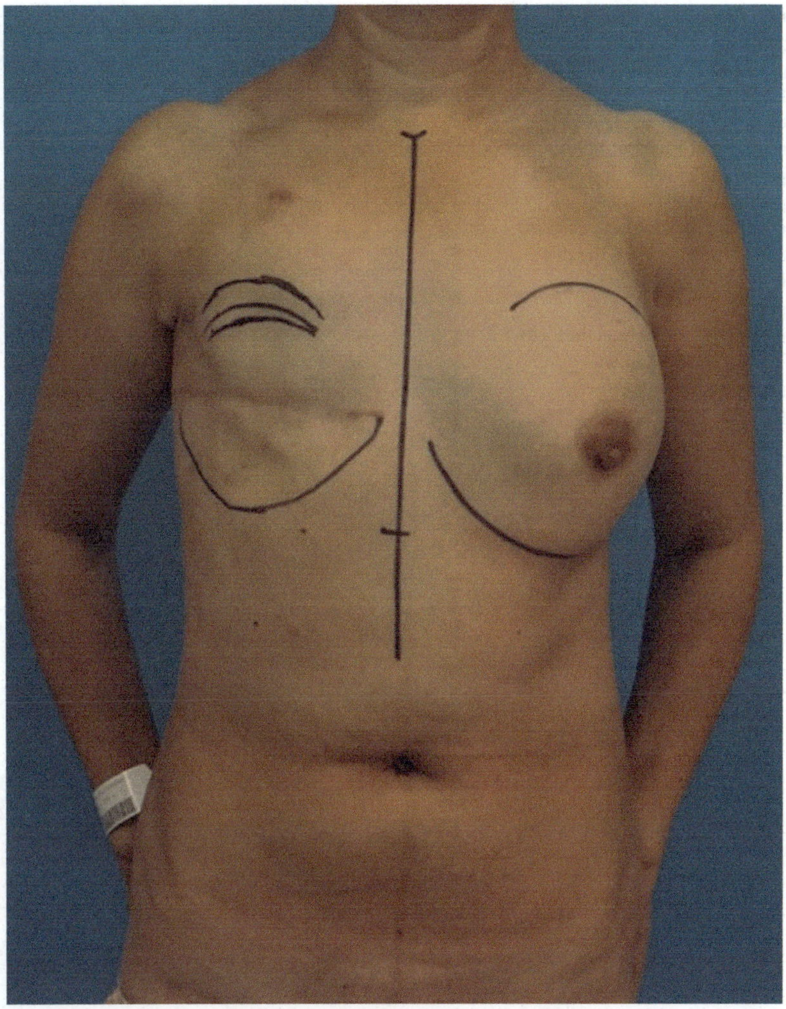

Fig. 15.1 Preoperative findings and design

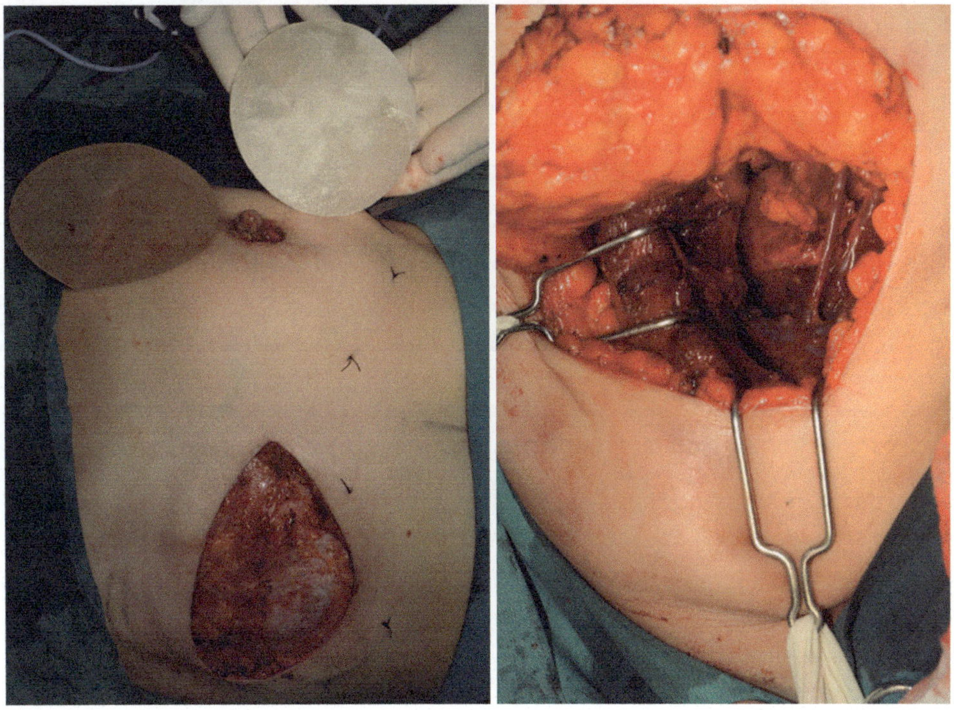

Fig. 15.2 Prosthesis replacement was performed on the left breast through the original areola incision, and the skin envelope was prepared after scar resection of the right chest wall. The vessels in the receiving area were lateral thoracic vessels and internal thoracic vessels

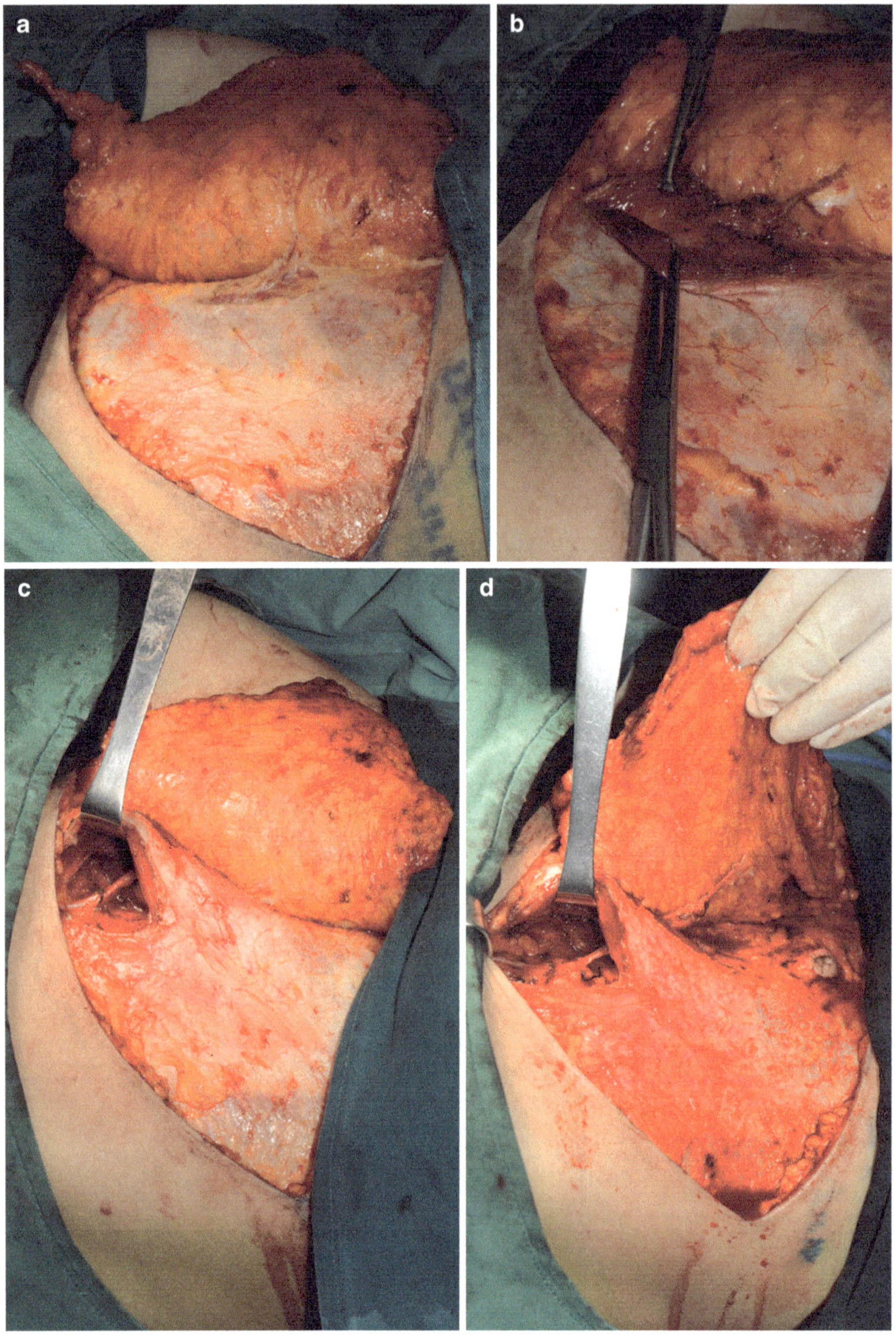

Fig. 15.3 Flap cutting process. (**a**) Exposing the perforating vessels of the left lower abdomen. (**b**) Opening the anterior sheath and retrogradely separating the perforating vessels toward the posterior sheath. (**c**) A modified incision was used to expose and separate the deep inferior epigastric vascular pedicle and the adjacent intercostal nerve branches. (**d**) The left DIEP flap was prepared in rendezvous method

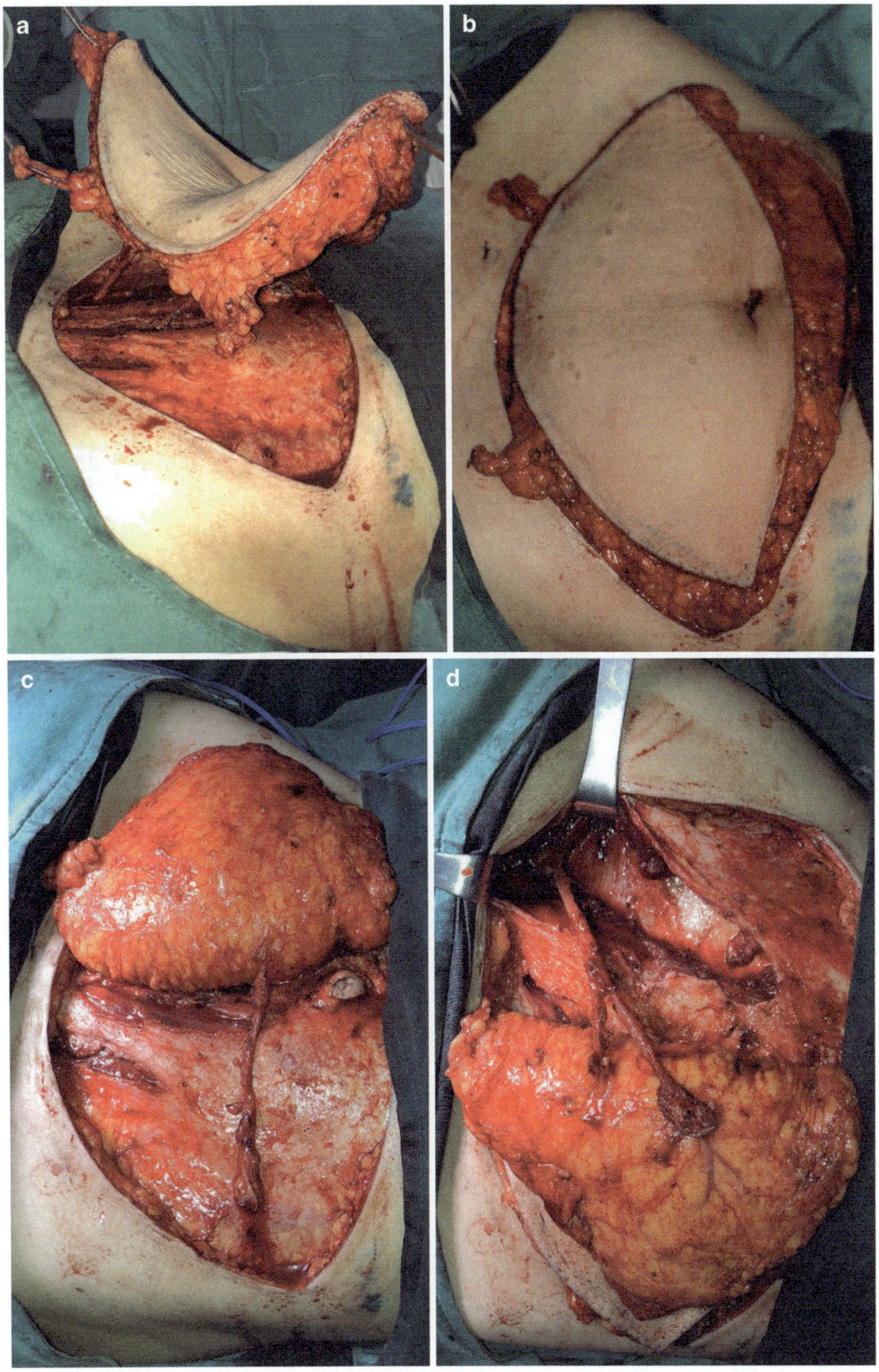

Fig. 15.4 The vascular pedicle of the flap was separated. (**a**) Preparing a DIEP flap with bilateral vascular pedicles, both of which continued with the medial perforators on each side. (**b**) The reserved SIEVs on both sides were overfilled. (**c**) Retrograde extraction of the left vascular pedicle from the intramuscular tunnel. (**d**) The right vascular pedicle was separated retrogradely till where it was close to the emitting plane

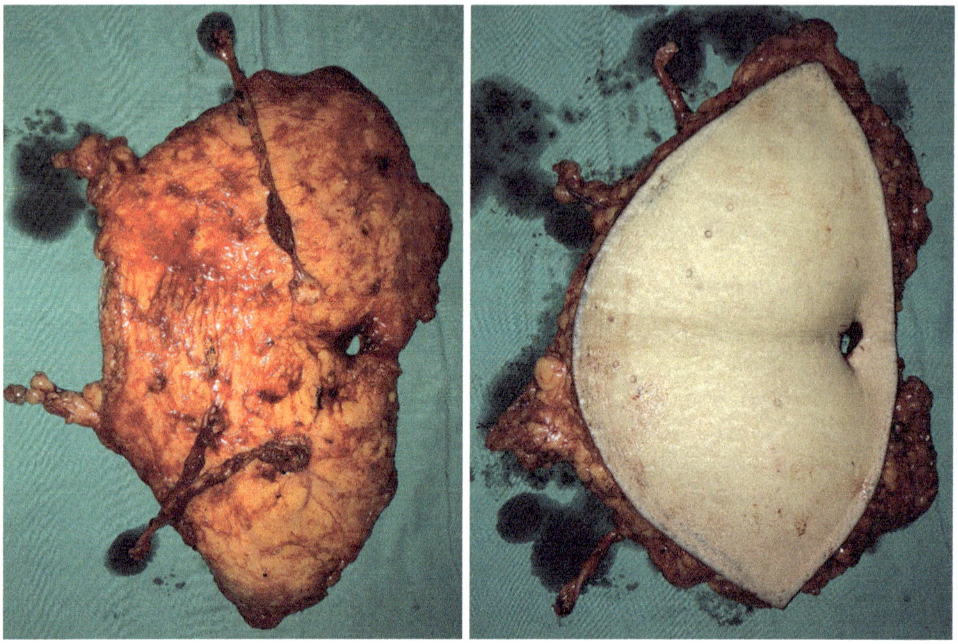

Fig. 15.5 The front and back of the flap

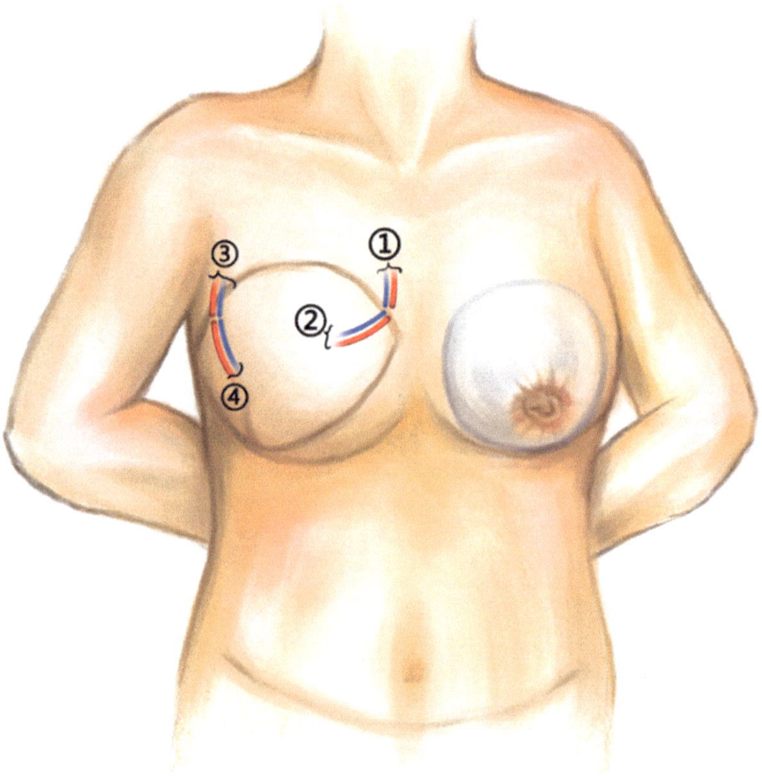

Fig. 15.6 Revascularization mode. (1) Internal mammary vessels; (2) Right deep inferior epigastric vessels; (3) Lateral thoracic vessels; (4) Left deep inferior epigastric vessel

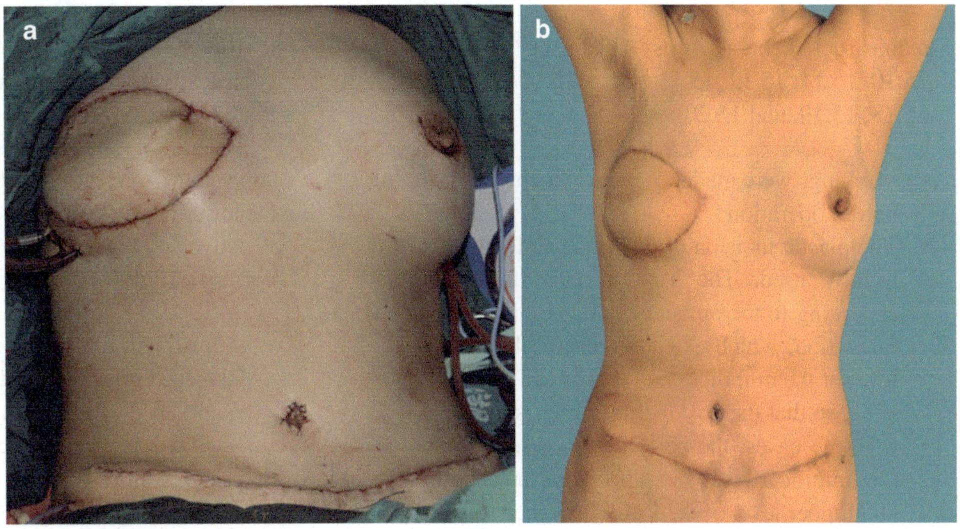

Fig. 15.7 (**a**) Intraoperative view immediately after reconstruction; (**b**) 3 months at follow-up

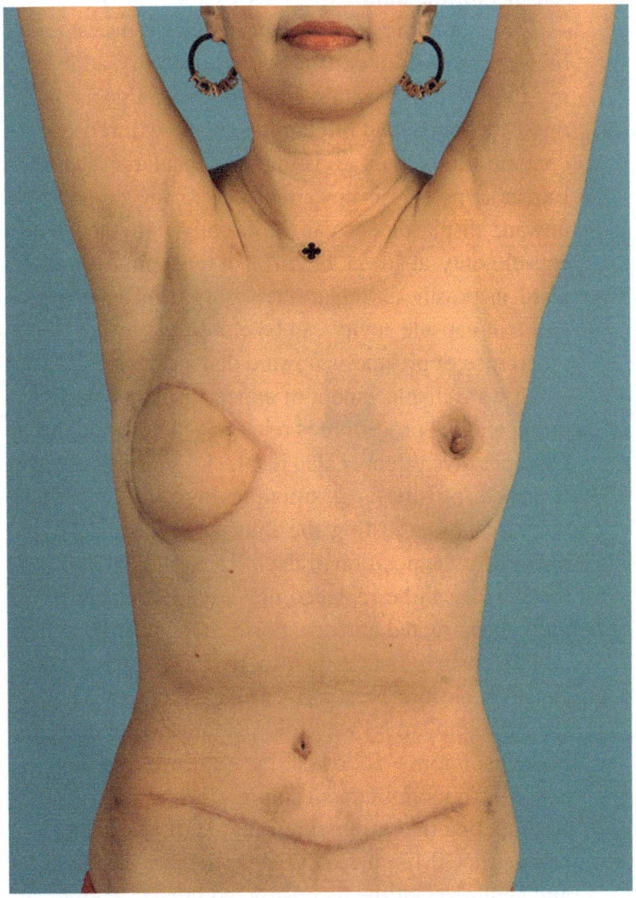

Fig. 15.8 10 months at follow-up after operation

Case Study 2: Unilateral Breast Reconstruction with DIEP Flap After Removal of Displaced Tissue Expander Plus Contralateral Mastopexy

A 31-year-old woman underwent right modified radical mastectomy plus immediate dilator implantation after 6 cycles of neoadjuvant chemotherapy in a local hospital.

Postoperative radiotherapy was given and tissue expansion was continued after radiotherapy.

The expander had been moving upward for 2 years before the patient received capsulectomy, expander removal, and free DIEP flap transplantation for right breast reconstruction plus left mastopexy through double peri-areola incision.

After the scar on the right chest wall and expander were removed, the right internal thoracic artery and its accompanying veins were separated for anastomosis. The size of the designed flap was about 26 cm × 12 cm. A DIEP flap based on bilateral vascular pedicles was prepared.

The right and left deep inferior epigastric artery and vein were anastomosed with the proximal and distal ends of the right internal thoracic artery and vein, respectively.

The left mastopexy was performed using double peri-areola incision. The flaps survived well, bilateral breasts were symmetrical, and the functional feeling of reconstructed breast was satisfactory (Figs. 15.9, 15.10, 15.11, 15.12, 15.13, 15.14, 15.15, 15.16, 15.17, 15.18, 15.19, and 15.20).

- Markings were made when the patient was standing before operation.
- The plastic incision of the lower abdominal wall is usually used. The harvest range is determined according to the amount of abdominal fat and skin relaxation, which extends upward above or to the level of the umbilicus and downward as low as possible, so that the postoperative scar is hidden.
- In some cases, the perforating vessels lie beyond the umbilical level and adipose tissue accumulates at a higher level of the lower abdomen, resulting in harvesting a flap from a higher level of the lower abdomen. Patients should be informed.
- Expander displacement: where the expander is placed is responsible for the postoperative effect of two-stage prothesis-based reconstruction. Subpectoral expander is commonly displaced by the inferior pectoralis major muscle that has not been interrupted.
- The displacement often occurs with the lower part of tissue expander, frequently resulting in extremely high or low level expander. In immediate breast reconstruction, the expander is often placed behind the pectoralis major muscle. Where the pectoralis major muscle ends inferiorly is higher than the level of the inframammary fold, as a result, the position of the subpectoral expander is often too high.
- If it is a slight asymmetry, we can usually correct it by adjusting the capsule cavity during prosthesis replacement. In cases with significant expander displacement or asymmetrical inframammary folds, we need to surgically adjust the position of the expander as soon as possible. Expander displacement would lead to tissue over-expansion at where expansion is not required. This is commonly seen when the expander shifts upward and dilates the superior chest skin, ending up with thin soft tissue on the upper breast and insufficient expansion on the lower breast. This can be solved by adjusting early the expander position and good long-term outcome can be often accomplished.
- The most important goal of one-stage implantation of expander is to level the inframammary fold close to that of the opposite side.

The asymmetry of bilateral inframammary folds will become obvious during expansion.

In patients with high reconstructed IMF, it can be corrected by removing the lower capsule and separating downward in the process of prosthesis replacement.

If the tissue covering the prosthesis is too thin to be completely removed, capsulotomy can be made in parallel or crisscross pattern.

Prothesis implant follows. The symmetry of the reconstructed IMF and the naturality of the semi-circle shape of the lower breast is determined in upright position.

Adverse events of prothesis/expander implant and corresponding solutions:

1. Adjustment of capsule space: Patients with prothesis-based breast reconstruction may have asymmetric breasts, which often needs reoperation.

   Expander or prosthesis misplacement, inappropriate volume or size of breast prosthesis, mismatched size of tissue expander, insufficient expansion, and unsatisfactory position are leading reasons for the failure of cavity establishment.

   Corresponding approaches include removal of breast prosthesis or expander, capsulectomy, adjusting IMF, renewing a tissue expander as large as the opposite breast, and implanting a new textured silicone prothesis after adjusting the capsular space.
2. Expander/prosthesis upward displacement: expander upward displacement can be usually corrected by capsulotomy at lower breast and separating downward in prosthesis replacement surgery. The upper space of capsule cavity can be closed to prevent the recurrence of prosthesis upward displacement.

   Upward displacement of expander can be easily corrected, the procedure is relatively simple and the postoperative effect is also ideal.
3. Expander/prosthesis positioning low: this can be corrected by adjusting the inferior capsule cavity upward. If the position of the inframammary fold is too low, it can be replaced upward simultaneously and reconstructed at a new position.

   It is usually necessary to perform intracavity capsular closure to adjust the capsular space and raise the implant by wall folding suture or horizontal capsulotomy followed by suture using non-absorbable monofilament suture.
4. Remodeling the inframammary fold: it is crucial to reconstruct IMF since it directly affects the shape and symmetry of the reconstructed breast.

   In cases of downward displacement of the expander or prosthesis, evaluation of the reconstructed IMF should be conducted when the patient is upright. The descending IMF is raised following implant replacement.

   Before operation, when the patient is standing, the descended IMF is evaluated and where the new IMF should be is determined.

The IMF is lifted by folding and sewing the redundant capsule on the lower breast.

If the IMF position is quite low, we can also remove some capsular tissue horizontally, and then close the gap by intracavity approximating the lateral sides with 3-0 Prolene suture. If the IMF is still lower than expected, repeat the above procedure.

For patients with obesity and thick subcutaneous adipose tissue, the IMF of the reconstructed breast is not so remarkable as that on the opposite side and a larger breast prosthesis is needed.

The symmetry of bilateral IMFs is very important to breast cosmetology. To achieve symmetry in patients with remarkable IMF line of the healthy breast, the reconstructed IMF should be further lowered by removing focal subcutaneous tissue and interrupted suturing the superficial fascia and the opened inferior capsule.

Do not resect the entire capsule, otherwise the prosthesis is likely to shift downward when a large-sized prothesis is implanted.

5. Lateral or medial displacement of dilator/prosthesis: Naturally, the breast tissue distributes between the para-sternum and the anterior axillary line with fullness on the medial breast.

   Many reconstructed breasts based on implant incline laterally, resulting in reduced fullness on the upper part of the breast and rubbing between the medial arm and the lateral breast. Lateral displacement is probably caused by excessive lateral dissection, or accidental entry of the implant into the previously separated subaxillary cavity, or attraction by lateral tissue and gravity when the patient is in supine position.

   Lateral displacement of the implant can be corrected by suturing the lateral capsule or splitting and reconnecting the lateral capsule to increase the capsular thickness. Two or three rows of capsular suture using non-absorbable suture are commonly used to provide sufficient repair strength and ensure the lasting effect.

   Preoperative markings are made when the patient is standing. The breast prosthesis is manually mobilized to a normal position to outline the range of capsular separation and where capsular suture internally would be.

   Medial displacement of breast prothesis is the most difficult to be dealt with and commonly requires multiple methods including release of the lateral capsule, replacement of prosthesis, and suture of the capsule parallel to the lateral edge of the sternum.

   In almost all cases, capsulectomy is required and the anterior and posterior sides of the capsule are lifted to form capsule valves, subsequently pushing the prothesis laterally to evaluate the adjustment result of medial displacement and making marks on the skin.

6. Poor projection of the reconstructed breast: it is commonly improved by replacing with a prothesis of better projection. Focal poor projection is frequently found on the inferior-medial or inferior breast, which can be solved by capsulotomy (a radial or cross-shaped incision at horizontal level), focal capsulectomy, or subtotal capsulectomy.

   The main purpose of these surgical methods is to minimize the pressure and restraint exerted by the capsule on the prosthesis surface.

   However, the tissue covering the prosthesis in patients undergoing breast reconstruction is generally weak and should be taken good care of.

7. Skin wrinkles:these often appear in patients with immediate breast reconstruction based on implant and greatly affect the aesthetic effect of the surgery.

   The main reason for skin wrinkle is filling insufficiency by prothesis or tissue. Other reasons include vacancy above the upper pole of the prosthesis, tissue used for cover or filling is insufficient, wrinkles under tension on textured prosthesis, mismatch between breast prosthesis and capsule cavity, etc.

   The breast reconstruction–related skin wrinkles are hardly radically eliminated and are likely to reoccur due to tissue attraction, which should be well informed to patients.

   Wrinkles that are caused by insufficient tissue for cover or filling can be removed by autologous fat grafting.

   We suggest that focal wrinkles together with significant breast deformity or pain due to capsular contracture (Baker IV capsular contracture) are resolved by capsulotomy or capsulectomy and filling with autologous tissue (latissimus dorsi flap, rectus abdominis flap, perforator flap of deep inferior epigastric artery, etc.).

   If skin wrinkles are caused by the mismatch between the size and volume of the prosthesis and the capsule cavity, treatment needs to focus on the mismatched problem.

   It is difficult to repair the wrinkles after breast reconstruction. Treatment usually includes tightening the capsule to slightly change the capsule space, adjustment of the size or the volume or the surface characteristics or all of them of the prosthesis, or increasing the covering tissue with autologous fat grafting.

8. Implant leakage and capsular contracture: if implant leakage is not treated in time, the capsular contracture around the implant will occur.

   If capsular contracture occurs, the size and volume of the capsular cavity must be restored by capsular resection.

   These additional procedures also increase the possibility of bilateral breast asymmetry. Therefore, once implant leakage is found, it needs to be treated as soon as possible.

   If silicone gel prosthesis rupture is considered, magnetic resonance imaging is required for evaluation and prosthetic replacement or autologous tissue breast reconstruction is optional. In our center, we prefer rectus abdominis flap or perforator flap of deep inferior epigastric artery or latissimus dorsi myocutaneous flap when reconstruction based on implant fails.

   Capsular contracture is more common and serious in breast reconstruction with prosthesis implantation than in breast augmentation, which may be related to the quality and quantity of the covering tissue. In many patients with breast reconstruction with prosthesis implantation, the covering tissue often gets hard after operation.

   For the treatment of capsular contracture, it is necessary to change the local tissue conditions through capsular resection to provide fresh tissue and a suitable space for the new prosthesis.

   For breast cancer patients undergoing breast reconstruction, we should be cautious with performing capsulectomy because the tissue covering the prosthesis is thin.

9. Insufficient tissue for filling or coverage: deficient subcutaneous adipose tissue is often seen in patients receiving breast reconstruction with prosthesis implantation.

   A common situation is that the amount of tissue in the upper part of the breast after prosthesis implantation is insufficient, resulting in a local hollow between above the prosthesis and the surrounding tissue.

   Another situation is that the tissue covering the prosthesis is insufficient leading to poor feeling of the reconstructed breast.

   To solve the above issues, we often perform autologous fat grafting. After stewing and purification, we inject the extracted fat on multiple levels and directions with a blunt needle with a diameter of 1.5–2.0 mm into the depressed area. According to the degree of depression, multiple injections may be required.

At present, satisfaction survey of breast cancer treatment shows that patients are no longer satisfied with long-term survival and are even hoping to restore the aesthetics of the breast with minimal damage, cost, and hospital stay.

Contralateral breast adjustment concurrent with unilateral breast reconstruction will not increase surgical complications, however, Asian women are not likely to accept additional surgery simply for aesthetic purposes. Instead, they care greatly about how the surgical outcome can minimize the impact on future work and life. Communication between doctors and patients is very important, and operators should also accurately grasp the surgical indications to obtain satisfactory clinical results.

We prefer to perform surgical adjustment of the opposite breast simultaneously with unilateral breast reconstruction. Adjustments include breast augmentation, mastopexy, and breast reduction.

To achieve the symmetrical effect of bilateral breasts, re-operation may be required where adjustment of both the reconstructed breasts and the opposite breast can be performed simultaneously. If cosmetic surgery of the opposite breast is done when the reconstructed breast is well shaped, asymmetry may happen and require one more correction operation.

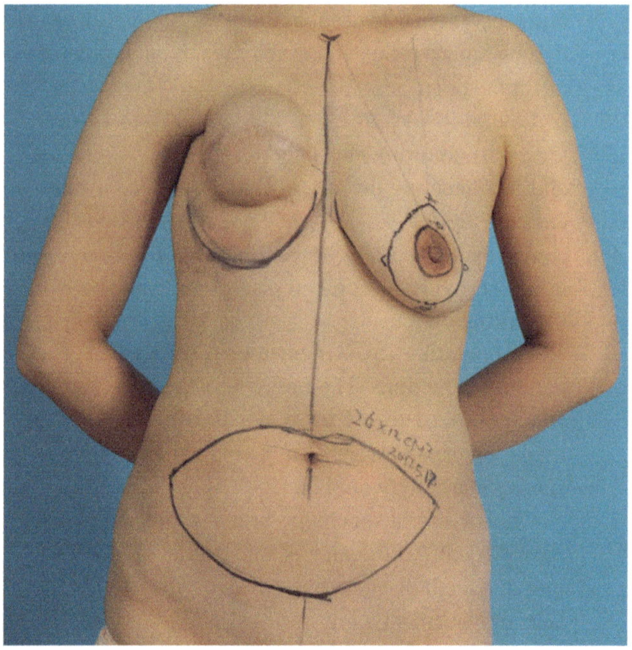

Fig. 15.9 Preoperative design

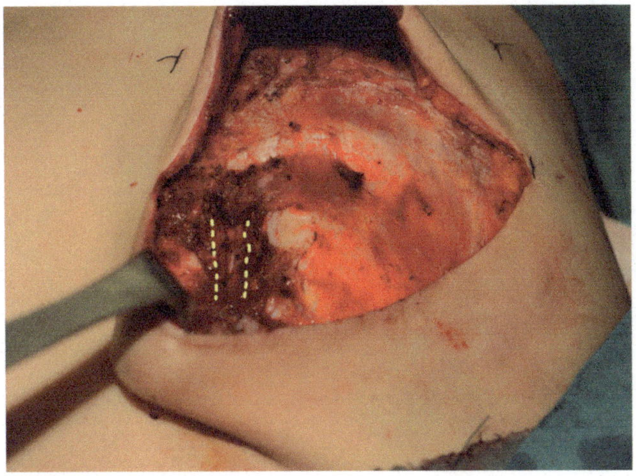

Fig. 15.10 The expander and the capsule were removed and the internal mammary vessels were prepared

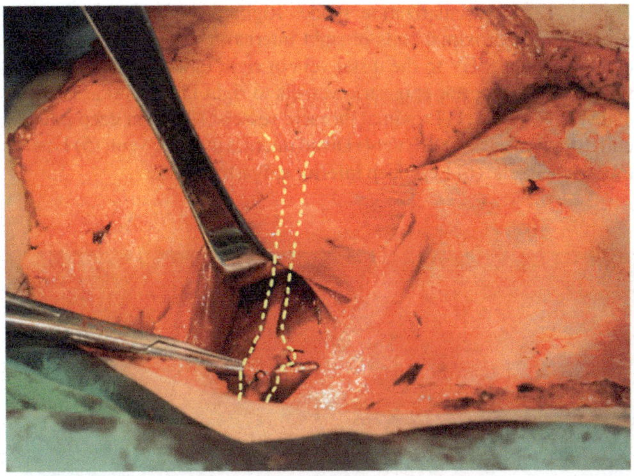

Fig. 15.11 Separating the left deep inferior epigastric perforator and vascular pedicle

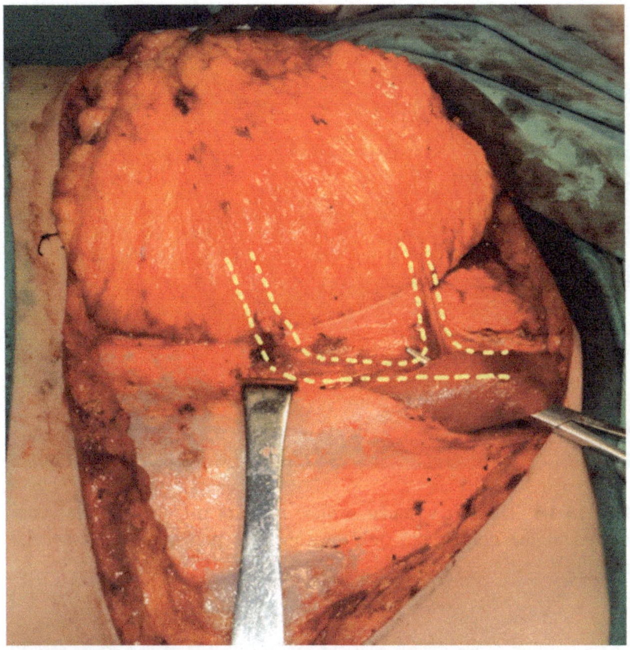

Fig. 15.12 Separating the right deep inferior epigastric perforator and vascular pedicle

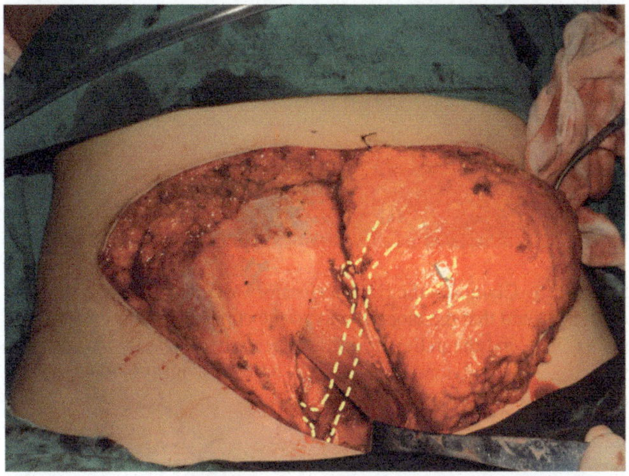

Fig. 15.13 Separation of right vascular pedicle was completed

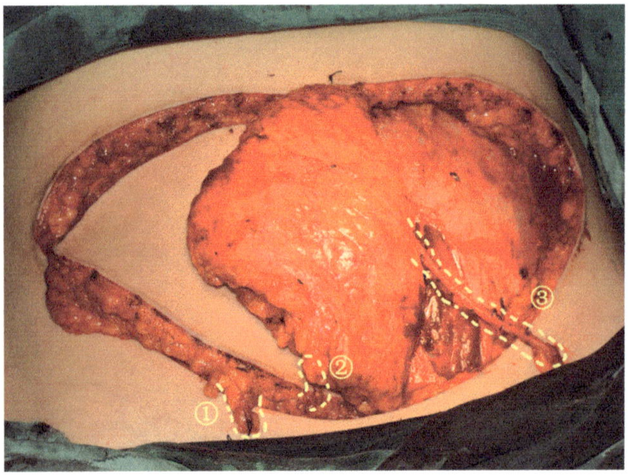

Fig. 15.14 The left vascular pedicle was cut off, the flap was connected to the donor area only by the right perforator and vascular pedicle

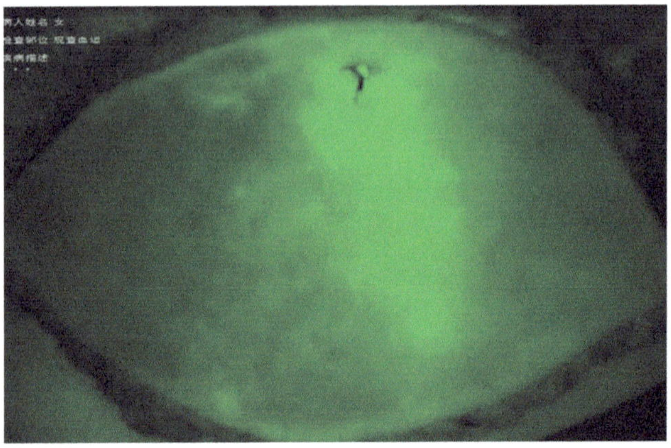

Fig. 15.15 Clamping the right perforator vascular pedicle, ICG angiography found that the blood supply to the opposite side of the flap was insufficient, and the patient had insufficient abdominal fat. As a result, the whole lower abdominal tissue was needed, requiring bilateral vascular pedicles for blood supply

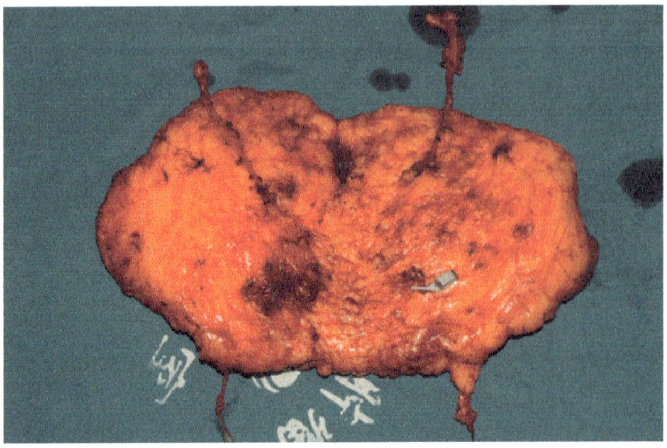

Fig. 15.16 A double DIEP flap carrying bilateral SIEVs

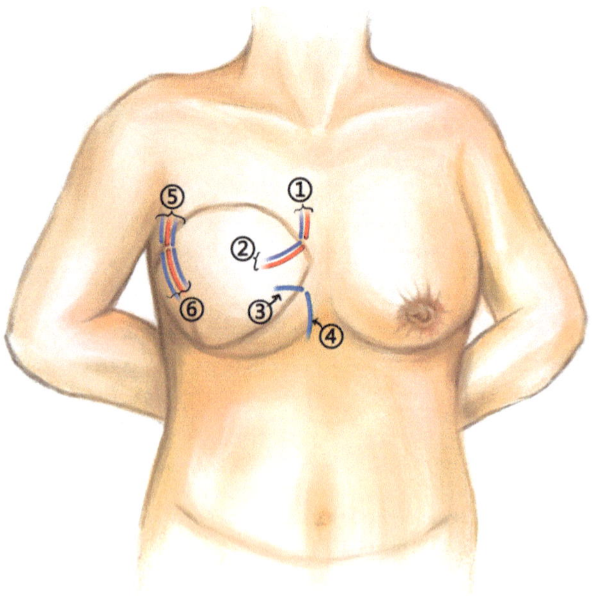

Fig. 15.17 Revascularization mode. Right deep inferior epigastric vessels to the proximal ends of right internal thoracic artery and vein (1A1V). Right SIEV to the distal vein of right internal mammary vessel. Left deep inferior epigastric vessels to right lateral thoracic artery and vein (1A2V). (1) Proximal thoracic vessels; (2) Right deep inferior epigastric vessels; (3) SIEV; (4) Distal internal thoracic vein; (5) Lateral thoracic vessels; (6) Left deep inferior epigastric vessel

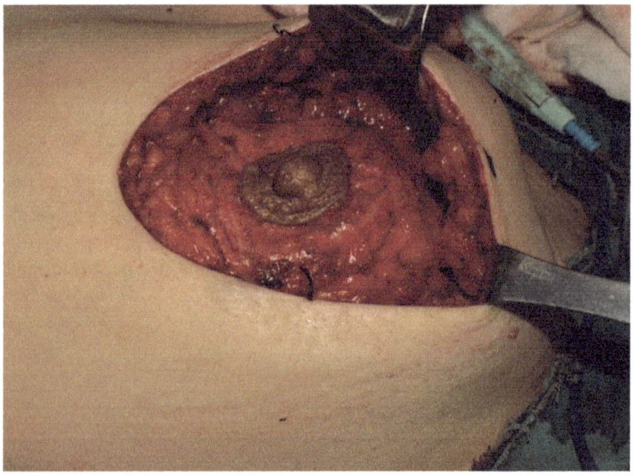

Fig. 15.18 Left mastopexy using round-block method

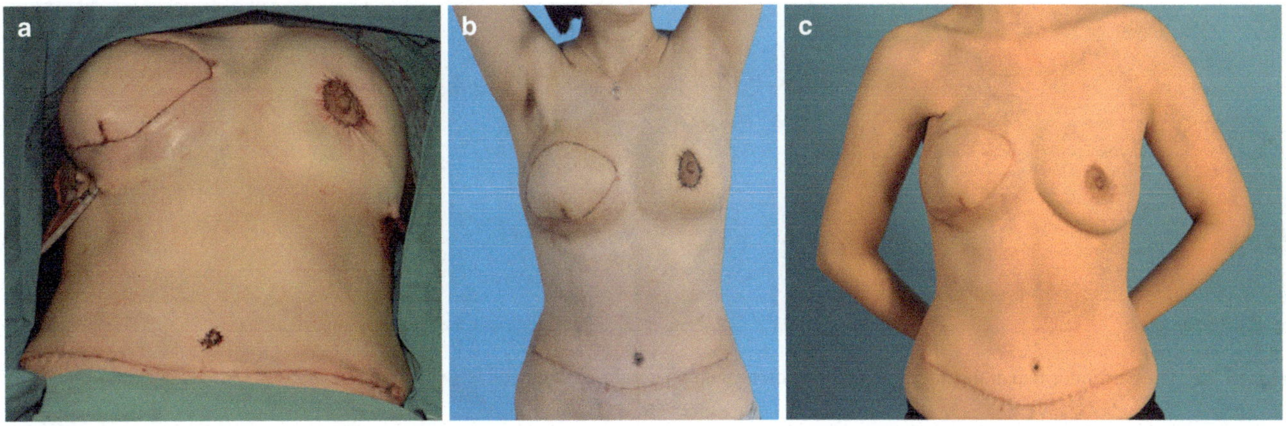

Fig. 15.19 (**a**) Intraoperative view immediately after reconstruction. (**b**) Follow-up at 6 months after operation. (**c**) Follow-up at 10 months after operation

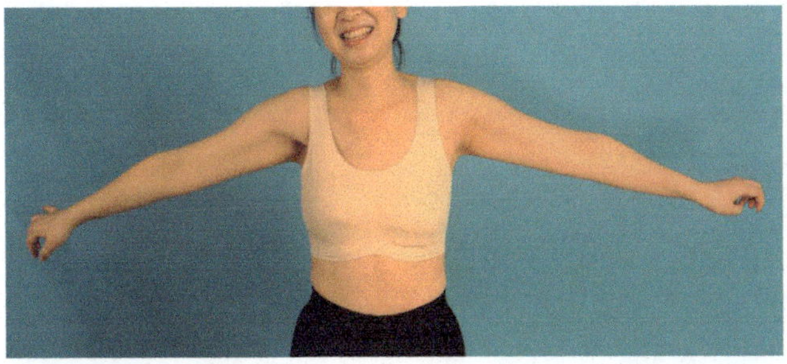

Fig. 15.20 The patient's function and appearance recovered satisfactorily

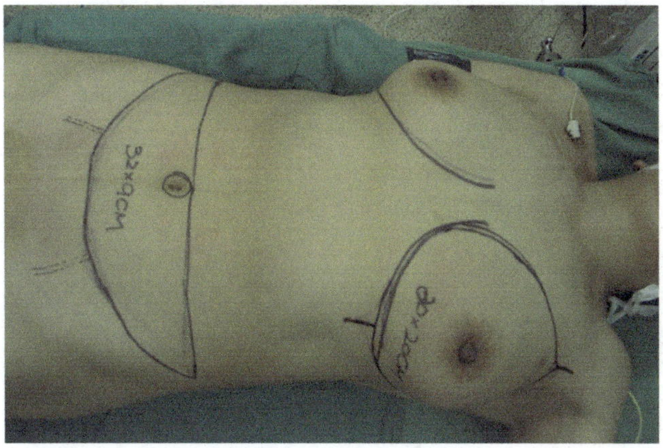

Fig. 15.21 Preoperative view

Case Study 3: Unilateral Breast Reconstruction and Contralateral Mastopexy

The patient, 46 years old, received left modified radical mastectomy plus breast reconstruction with free DIEP flap and adjuvant chemotherapy 10 years ago. In recent years, the bilateral breast asymmetry was increasingly significant featured by the reconstructed breast shrinking. The patient was admitted for left chest wall scar plasty and left nipple reconstruction and left breast fat filling as well as right breast reduction (Figs. 15.21, 15.22, 15.23, 15.24, and 15.25).

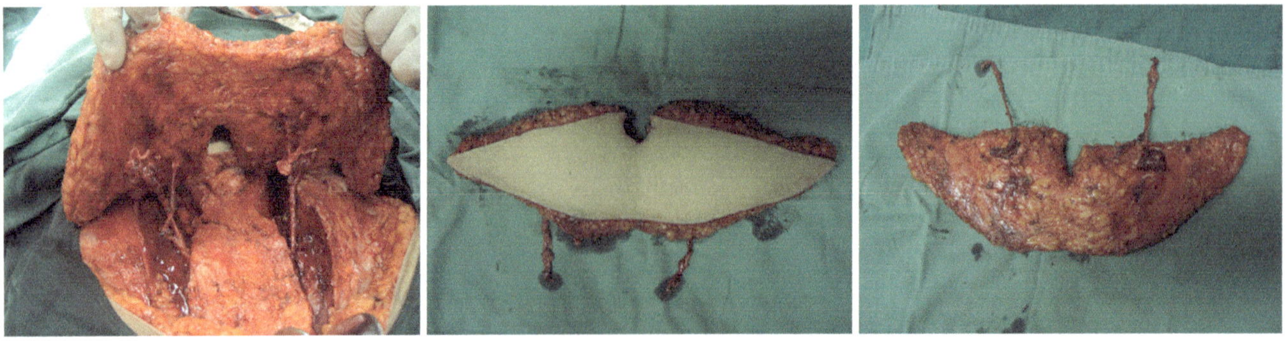

Fig. 15.22 The perforator flap of the inferior epigastric artery with bilateral vascular pedicles was cut off

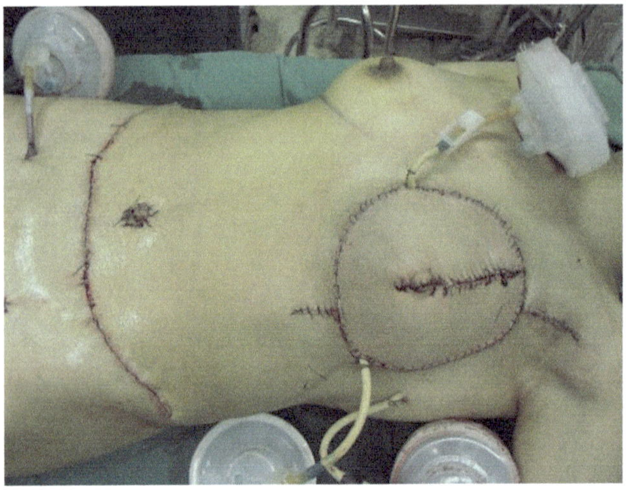

Fig. 15.23 Intraoperative view immediately after reconstruction

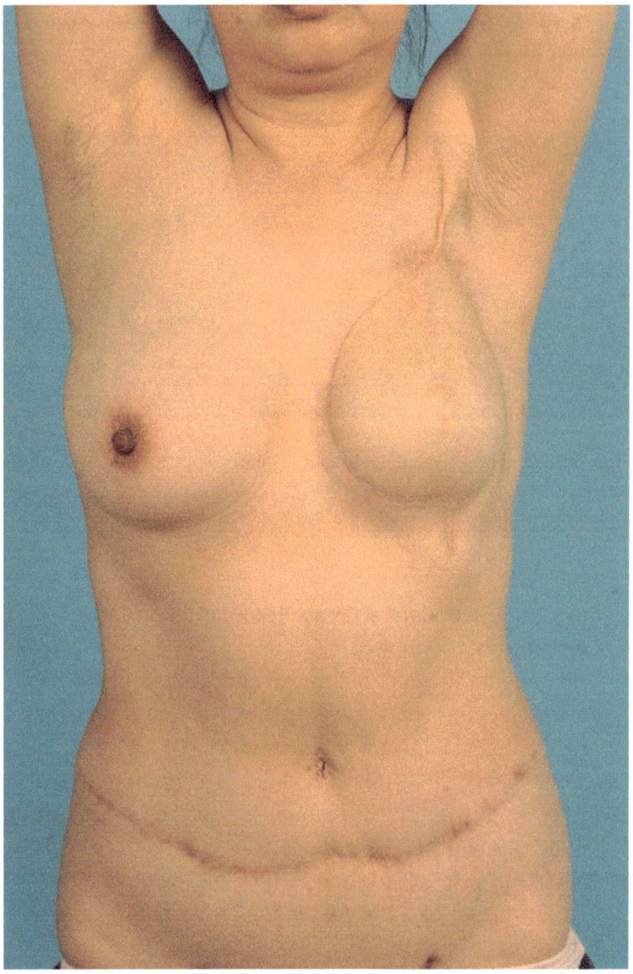

Fig. 15.24 10 years at follow-up after operation

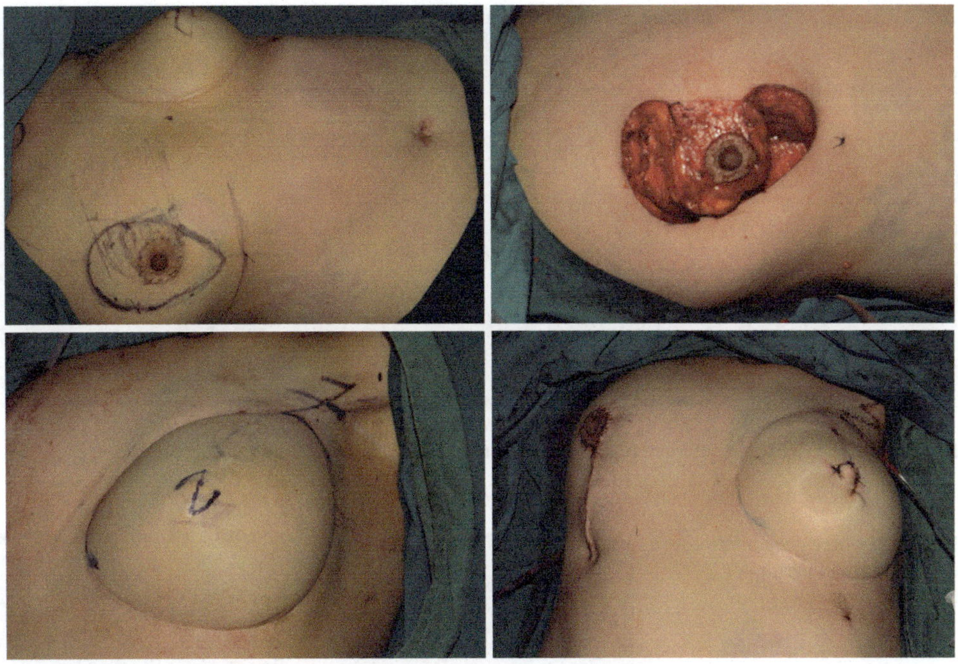

Fig. 15.25 Right mastopexy, left nipple reconstruction, and axillary scar plasty using Z-shaped incision were performed

> **Case Study 4: Unilateral Breast Reconstruction and Contralateral Mastopexy**
>
> A 46 year-old patient received left modified radical mastectomy plus breast reconstruction with free DIEP flap and adjuvant chemotherapy 10 years ago. In recent years, the bilateral breast asymmetry was increasingly significant featured by the reconstructed breast shrinking. The patient was admitted for scar adjustment and left nipple reconstruction and left breast fat filling as well as right breast reduction (Figs. 15.26, 15.27, 15.28, 15.29, and 15.30).

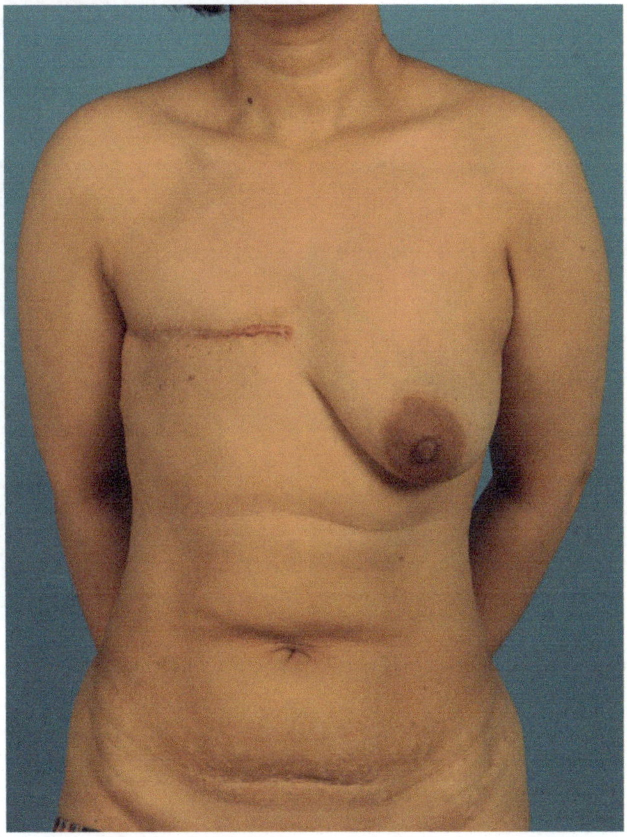

Fig. 15.26 Preoperative view

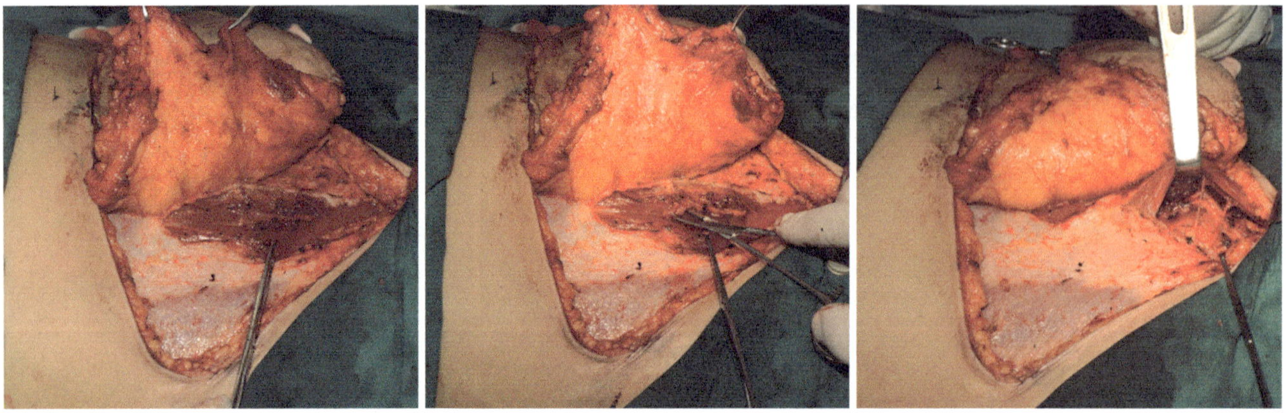

Fig. 15.27 The right deep inferior epigastric artery and the perforating vessels were separated

Fig. 15.28 Free deep inferior epigastric artery perforator flap was prepared

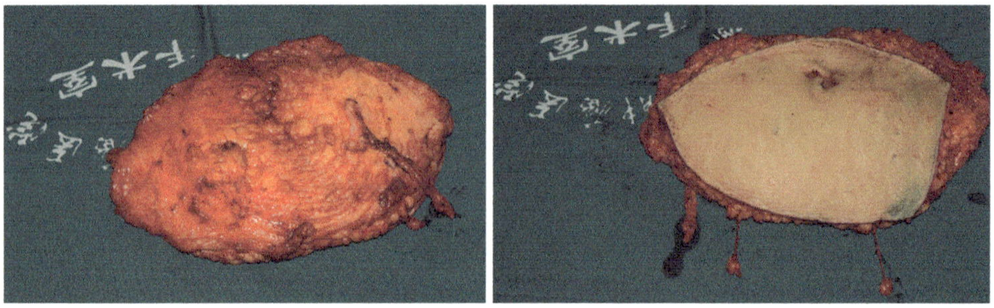

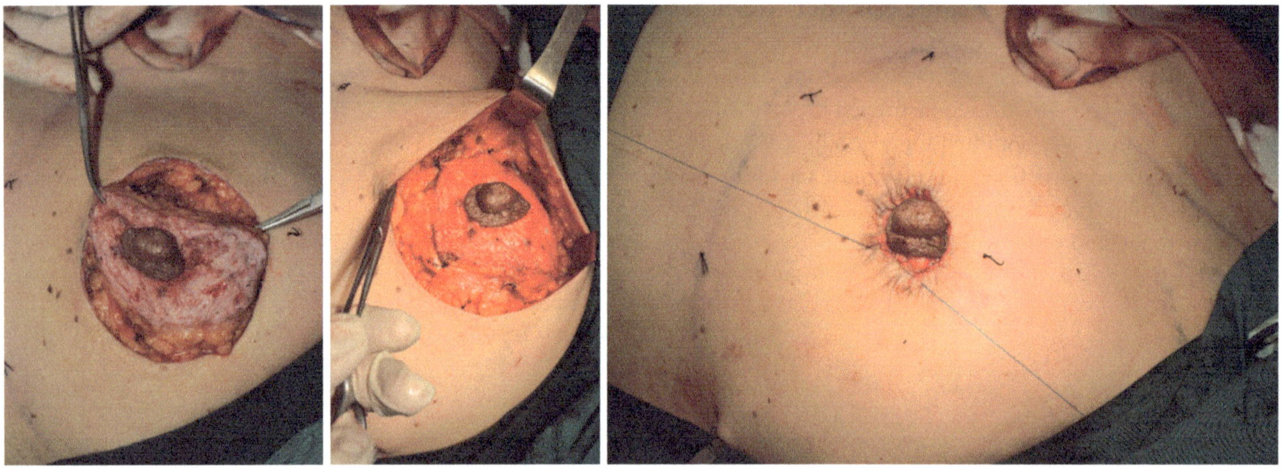

Fig. 15.29 Left mastopexy was done by round-block method

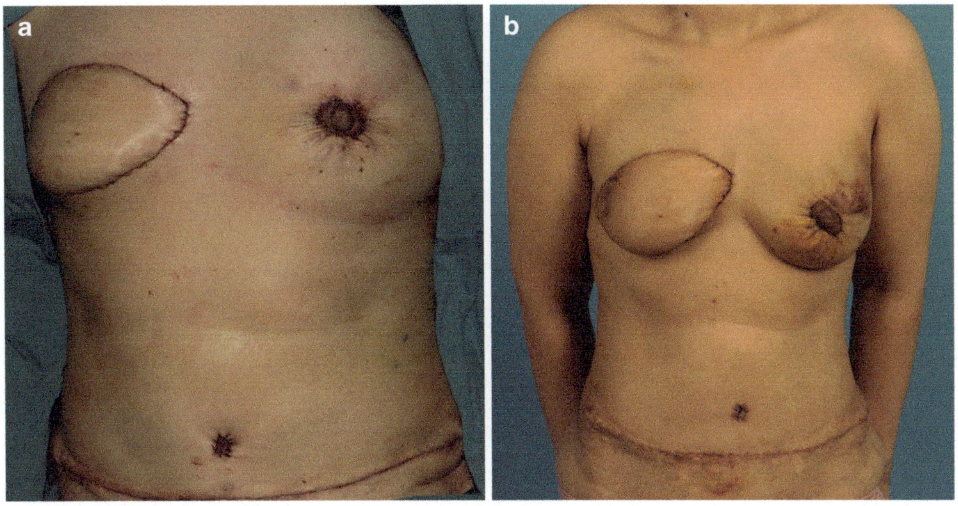

Fig. 15.30 (**a**) The blood supply of the flap was good during the operation; (**b**) 10 days after operation, the patient was discharged with good symmetry and satisfactory appearance of bilateral breasts

References

1. Haykal S, Guay N. One hundred forty-one consecutive attempts at autologous tissue single-stage breast cancer reconstruction. Ann Plast Surg. 2009;63(1):21–7.
2. Kroll SS, Schusterman MA, Tadjalli HE, Singletary SE, Ames FC. Risk of recurrence after treatment of early breast cancer with skin-sparing mastectomy. Ann Surg Oncol. 1997;4(3):193–7.
3. Kronowitz SJ, Chang DW, Robb GL, et al. Implications of axillary sentinel lymph node biopsy in immediate autologous breast reconstruction. Plast Reconstr Surg. 2002;109(6):1888–96.
4. Omranipour R, Bobin JY, Esouyeh M. Skin Sparing Mastectomy and Immediate Breast Reconstruction (SSMIR) for early breast cancer: eight years single institution experience. World J Surg Oncol. 2008;6:43.
5. Nahabedian MY. Symmetrical breast reconstruction: analysis of secondary procedures after reconstruction with implants and autologous tissue. Plast Reconstr Surg. 2005;115(1):257–60.
6. Losken A, Carlson GW, Bostwick J, Jones GE, Culbertson JH, Schoemann M. Trends in unilateral breast reconstruction and management of the contralateral breast: the Emory experience. Plast Reconstr Surg. 2002;110(1):89–97.
7. Giacalone PL, Bricout N, Dantas MJ, Daurés JP, Laffargue F. Achieving symmetry in unilateral breast reconstruction: 17 years experience with 683 patients. Aesthet Plast Surg. 2002;26(4):299–302.
8. Stevenson TR, Goldstein JA. TRAM flap breast reconstruction and contralateral reduction or mastopexy. Plast Reconstr Surg. 1993;92(2):228–33.
9. Saint-Cyr M, Schaverien MV, Rohrich RJ. Perforator flaps: history, controversies, physiology, anatomy, and use in reconstruction. Plast Reconstr Surg. 2009;123(4):132e–45e.
10. Ulusal BG, Cheng MH, Wei FC. Simultaneous endoscope-assisted contralateral breast augmentation with implants in patients undergoing postmastectomy breast reconstruction with abdominal flaps. Plast Reconstr Surg. 2006;118(6):1293–302.
11. Petit JY, Rietjens M, Contesso G, Bertin F, Gilles R. Contralateral mastoplasty for breast reconstruction: a good opportunity for glandular exploration and occult carcinomas diagnosis. Ann Surg Oncol. 1997;4(6):511–5.
12. Granzow JW, Levine JL, Chiu ES, Allen RJ. Breast reconstruction with the deep inferior epigastric perforator flap: history and an update on current technique. J Plast Reconstr Aesthet Surg. 2006;59(6):571–9.
13. Pusic AL, Klassen AF, Scott AM, Klok JA, Cordeiro PG, Cano SJ. Development of a new patient-reported outcome measure for breast surgery: the BREAST-Q. Plast Reconstr Surg. 2009;124(2):345–53.
14. Chang DW, Kroll SS, Dackiw A, Singletary SE, Robb GL. Reconstructive management of contralateral breast cancer in patients who previously underwent unilateral breast reconstruction. Plast Reconstr Surg. 2001;108(2):352–8; discussion 359–60.
15. Labandter HP, Dowden RV. Surgical considerations in managing the remaining breast during postmastectomy breast reconstruction. Clin Plast Surg. 1984;11(2):365–8.
16. Nahabedian MY, Galdino G. Symmetrical breast reconstruction: is there a role for three-dimensional digital photography. Plast Reconstr Surg. 2003;112(6):1582–90.
17. Hartrampf CR. The transverse abdominal Island flap for breast reconstruction. A 7-year experience. Clin Plast Surg. 1988;15(4):703–16.
18. Gill PS, Hunt JP, Guerra AB, et al. A 10-year retrospective review of 758 DIEP flaps for breast reconstruction. Plast Reconstr Surg. 2004;113(4):1153–60.
19. Hidalgo DA. Improving safety and aesthetic results in inverted T scar breast reduction. Plast Reconstr Surg. 1999;103(3):874–86; discussion 887–9.
20. Linderman R. Current trends in breast reduction. Plast Reconstr Surg. 2000;106(2):512.
21. Hidalgo DA, Elliot LF, Palumbo S, Casas L, Hammond D. Current trends in breast reduction. Plast Reconstr Surg. 1999;104(3):806–15; quiz 816; discussion 817–8.
22. Huang JJ, Wu CW, Leon LW, Lin CY, Nguyen DH, Cheng MH. Simultaneous contralateral breast reduction/mastopexy with unilateral breast reconstruction using free abdominal flaps. Ann Plast Surg. 2011;67(4):336–42.

Sensory Reconstruction for the Reconstructed Breast

16

Zan Li and Pengcheng Su

The breast reconstruction with free autologous tissue transplantation contributes to natural appearance and long-lasting effect, avoiding various surgical risks and complications of prosthesis implants. With the continuous improvement of surgical technique, patients' expectations for breast reconstruction are rising, including reconstruction of nipple areola complex, sensory restoration of the reconstructed breast, and good recovery of the donor site without affecting future life.

Female patients undergoing breast reconstruction are eager to obtain a breast with normal sensation. Hence, the deep inferior epigastric artery perforator flap with sensory nerve is the most promising means to improve the odds of sensory recovery of the flap. However, the surgical outcome is still uncertain, and it is discrepant among the reports [1].

The sensory nerves of the breast come from the lateral and anterior branches of the second–sixth intercostal nerves, and the sensation of the nipple areola complex is dominated by the fourth or fifth intercostal nerves.

The nerves are commonly cut off during modified radical mastectomy resulting in the decline of postoperative sensory function. It is reported that the sensation of the reconstructed breast may resume naturally, yet differences in reports are great.

At present, sensory nerves from T10 to T12 are carried in the perforator flap of the deep inferior epigastric artery and anastomosed with the fourth or fifth intercostal nerve in order to restore the sensation of the flap.

Measurement results of the sensory recovery of the reconstructed breast flap varied greatly. Some reports found no effect at all, while others reported that the sensory recovery of the flap with sensory nerve was significantly improved.

Z. Li (✉)
Department of Oncology Plastic Surgery, Hunan Cancer Hospital, Changsha, Hunan, China

P. Su
Department of Breast and Thyroid Surgery, People's Hospital of XinJiang Uygur Autonomous Region, Urumqi, Xinjiang, P. R. China

Many scholars have reported that rectus abdominis skin flaps and deep inferior epigastric artery perforator skin flaps without nerve anastomosis show symptoms of spontaneous sensory recovery [2–7].

It was advocated that the proportion of good or satisfactory sensory recovery of autologous tissue transplantation for breast reconstruction at 2–5 years of follow-up was 6–31% [3, 5–7].

Although sensory reconstruction has become the second criterion of successful breast reconstruction, many scholars do not recommend sensory nerve reconstruction. The reasons include the following [5, 8]: (1) the flap has the function of spontaneous sensory recovery; (2) it is difficult to find the nerve in the receiving area; (3) it increases the damage of donor and recipient areas; and (4) it increases the complexity of the operation and operation time.

However, in cases with spontaneous sensation recovery of the flap, the recovery of pressure sensation is usually unsatisfactory and varies greatly. The sensory threshold of a reconstructed breast is ten times higher than that of a normal breast [2, 4–6].

Slezak [4] firstly reported that in three cases undergoing breast reconstruction, sensory innervation was completed by anastomosing the sensory nerve of the flap to the fourth intercostal nerve.

It was described that to innervate the flap, the sensory anterior branch of the fourth intercostal nerve alone was connected to the segmental nerve of the rectus abdominis, which mainly contains motor fibers.

The application of DIEP flap in breast reconstruction is not only better at reducing donor site injury [9] but also helps better understand the three-dimensional anatomy of movement and sensory nerves of the rectus abdominis muscle, preparing the surgeon the technical ability to separate and dissect the sensory branches entering the segmental nerves of the rectus abdominis, so as to complete the pure sensory nerve suture at the level of the third and fourth intercostal nerves in the chest receiving area (as shown in Fig. 16.1) [10].

Z. Li, D. Song (eds.), *Oncoplastic Flap Surgery*, https://doi.org/10.1007/978-981-19-8926-1_16

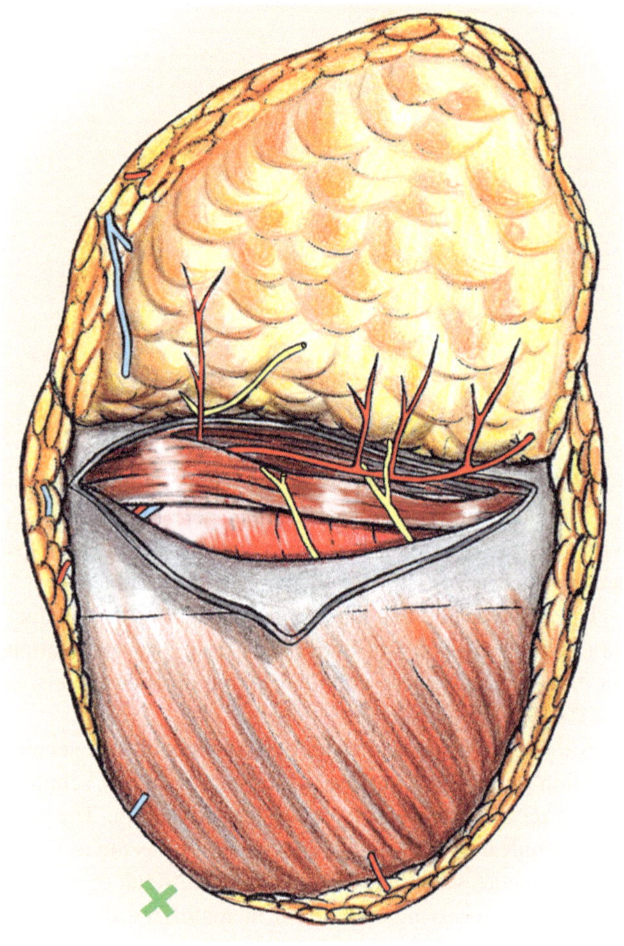

Fig. 16.1 Schematic diagram of the motor and sensory branches of the intercostal nerves and their anatomical relationship with the deep inferior epigastric vessels and their perforating branches

Many studies have found that 60–80% of the flaps in patients with breast reconstruction using DIEP flap resume sensation even without rebuilding the continuity of sensory nerves, questioning the necessity of reconstructing the sensation of the flap [1, 11]. It is further found that the sensory recovery usually starts from the periphery than from the deep surface to the center of the flap, and the resulting outcome is satisfactory [12]. However, neither the mechanism of flap spontaneous sensory recovery has not been fully studied nor the associated factors are reported [1].

More studies have shown that flap innervation can greatly improve the effect of breast reconstruction and patient satisfaction as well as reduce trauma to the reconstructed breast. The sense of pressure and temperature is better in a sensation-reconstructed flap than that with spontaneous sensory recovery [5, 13–15].

Santanelli [16] believed that the time of sensory recovery of an innervated DIEP flap was not significant as that with spontaneous sensory recovery.

Blondeel [15] reported about a modified DIEP flap for breast reconstruction where the sensory nerves were carried on the flap and anastomosed with the fourth intercostal nerve to reconstruct the sensory function of the flap.

Spiegel [17] also completed a similar operation, using the third intercostal nerve as the recipient nerve. Further studies have proved that sensory nerve anastomosis can improve the sensory recovery of the flap. Although the procedure will prolong the operation time, it is of great importance especially in delayed breast reconstruction [15].

16.1 Selecting Nerves

There are multiple sensory nerve candidates that are carried on the flap. The third and fourth intercostal nerves are commonly used, yet the fourth intercostal nerve is at a lower position, which increases the difficulty of anastomosis and flap placement. These nerves are often cut off during radical mastectomy, making it difficult to be exposed in delayed breast reconstruction.

We prefer the sensory branch close to the perforator vessel pedicle for innervation of the flap (as shown in Figs. 16.2 and 16.3). Moreover, the third intercostal nerve is preferred as the receiving nerve because it is constant in anatomy and convenient for anastomosis. Also, there are two outstanding advantages of using this nerve (as shown in Fig. 16.4) [17]:

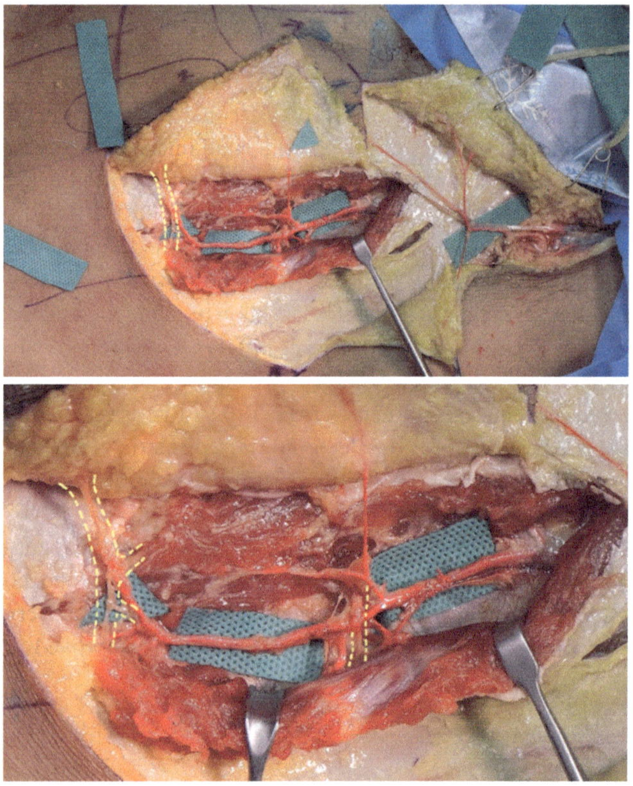

Fig. 16.2 The anatomical relationship between the deep inferior epigastric vessels and their perforating branches and the intercostal nerves was investigated on a cadaver to determine the positional relationship between the sensory branches of the intercostal nerve and the vascular pedicle

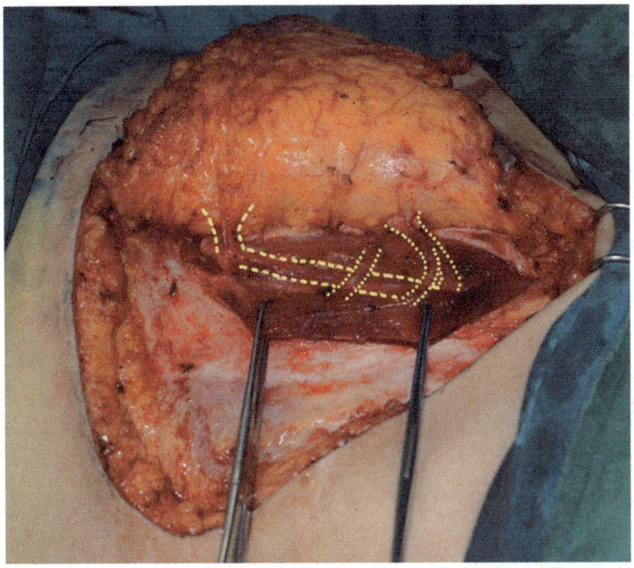

Fig. 16.3 The relationships of the deep inferior epigastric vascular pedicle and its perforating branch and the intercostal nerve and its sensory branch were examined during the operation

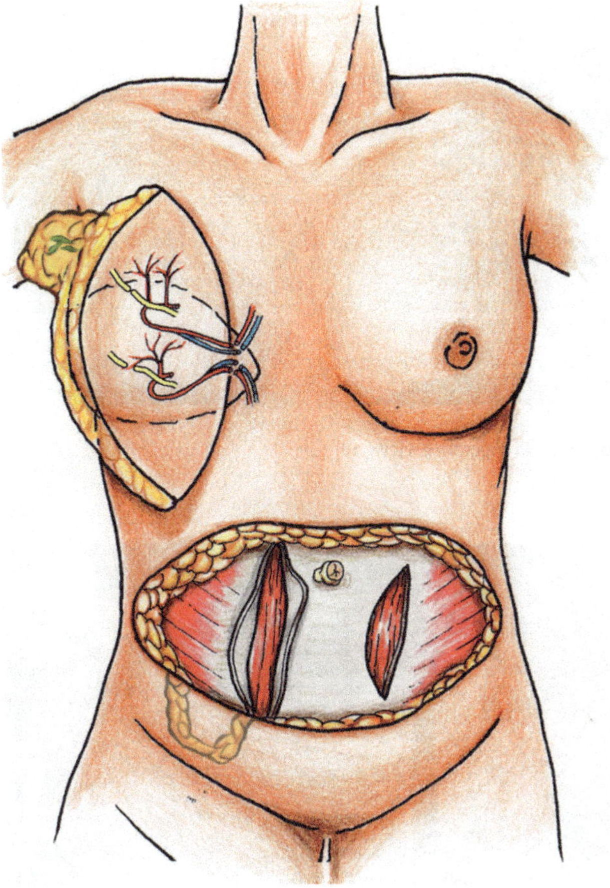

Fig. 16.4 Breast reconstruction with innervated free DIEP flap

1. In order to prolong the length of the sensory nerve of the flap for anastomosis and placement of the flap, we usually retrogradely separate the sensory nerve to the deep surface of the rectus abdominis. Separating the sensory branch and motor branch of the intercostal nerve entirely will increase the damage to the donor area. To minimize additional injuries to the rectus abdominis, we select the intercostal nerve close to the perforator vascular pedicle. If the position of the motor branch and vascular pedicle is too complex to be separated, the intercostal nerve will be directly disconnected to reduce the difficulty of operation.
2. To minimize the injury of donor site, extra opening on the rectus abdominis and anterior sheath of the rectus abdominis is not recommended.

It was proved that reconstructing the flap sensation improved both patient satisfaction and quality of life. Although the procedure prolongs the operation time and increases the complexity of the operation, it will pay off [5].

Outcome measurement of flap sensation reconstruction includes the blood supply of the flap tissue, postoperative radiotherapy, smoking history, diabetes concomitance, and other related situations.

Before surgery, we should understand whether the sensory recovery of the reconstructed breast is expected except breast shape restoration [18].

Case Study 1: Sensory Innervation in Breast Reconstruction

A 31-year-old female patient presented for left breast invasive carcinoma on biopsy (cT2NM0, stage IIb) and underwent modified radical mastectomy for left breast cancer and breast reconstruction using a free DIEP flap carrying sensory nerve. The postoperative flap was in good viability, and the patient was transferred to internal medicine department for further comprehensive treatment. No major complications occurred during follow-up, and the patient's functional feeling and appearance recovered satisfactorily (Figs. 16.5, 16.6, 16.7, 16.8, 16.9, 16.10, 16.11, 16.12, 16.13, and 16.14).

Notes

- This patient's concomitant vein of the deep inferior epigastric artery was small, which significantly increased the difficulty of operation.
- The actual clinical effect of immediate breast reconstruction using free DIEP flap carrying intercostal

sensory nerve branch for sensory reconstruction warrants further clinical evaluation.
- To facilitate flap shaping and vascular anastomosis, how is the incision modified?
- Two sensory nerves on the left were carried. One nerve was accompanied by a perforator, and the other was accompanied by its nutrient vessels instead of perforator.
- Is it likely that a nerve obtains better blood supply by the concomitant perforator, contributing to better sensory recovery?
- Adjacent to the first perforator, the nerve accompanied by the second perforator was included in the flap. However, how to balance flap shaping and nerve placement before operation or during flap raising is yet to be determined.
- Multiple sensory nerves had been carried in the flap, yet it was difficult to use them all for sensory reconstruction.
- The recipient nerve was the third intercostal nerve, and its accompanying intercostal artery was large which can be used for vascular anastomosis.
- A few vessels in the receiving area can be used for re-vasculization, including the lateral thoracic artery and vein, the thoracodorsal artery and its anterior serratus muscle branch, a large branch of the anterior serratus muscle branch, and a large muscle branch artery and vein in the pectoralis major muscle.
- Additional venous reflux was established by using a large muscular venous branch of the pectoralis major muscle and the lateral thoracic vein.
- Dissection of the intramammary area can be obviated if the lateral thoracic vessels or other axillary vessels are suitable for re-vasculizing the flap. Nonetheless, vascular placement is a tricky point under such circumstance, and how the operating table and the ipsilateral arm should be posed may be considered.
- The issue as to using a long length of the thoracodorsal vessels for anastomosis needs to be further analyzed.

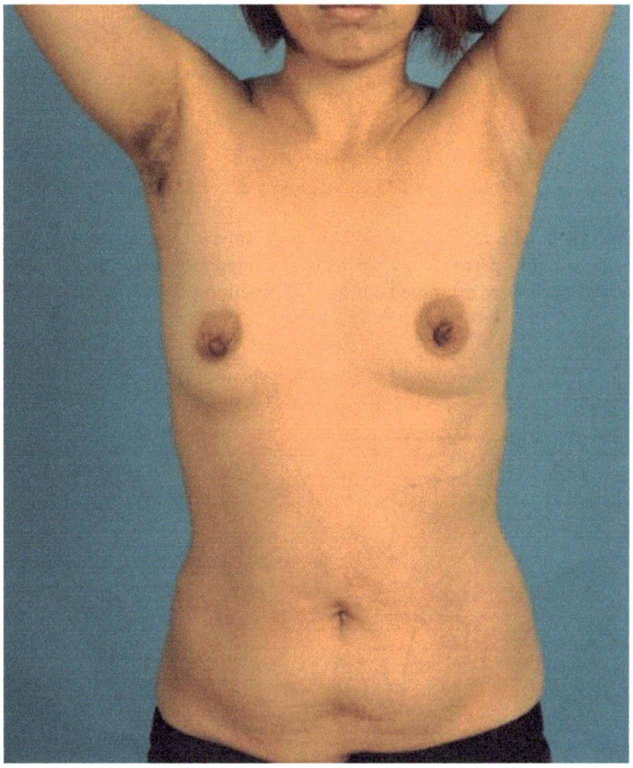

Fig. 16.5 Preoperative view

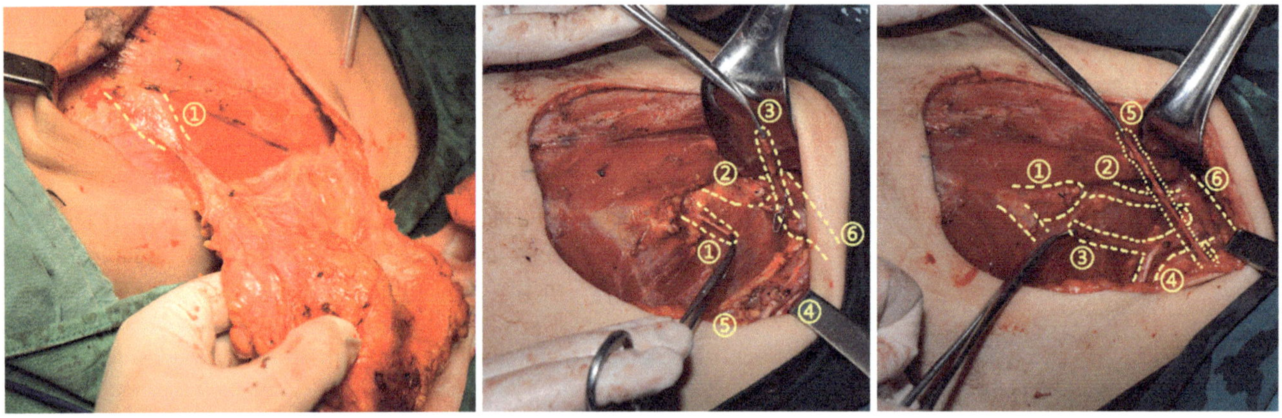

Fig. 16.6 Preparing recipient vessels after modified radical mastectomy. (1) Intercostal vascular nerve bundle. (2) Lateral thoracic artery and vein. (3) Lateral thoracic vein. (4) Thoracodorsal vascular nerve bundle. (5) Intercostal brachial nerve. (6) Axillary vein

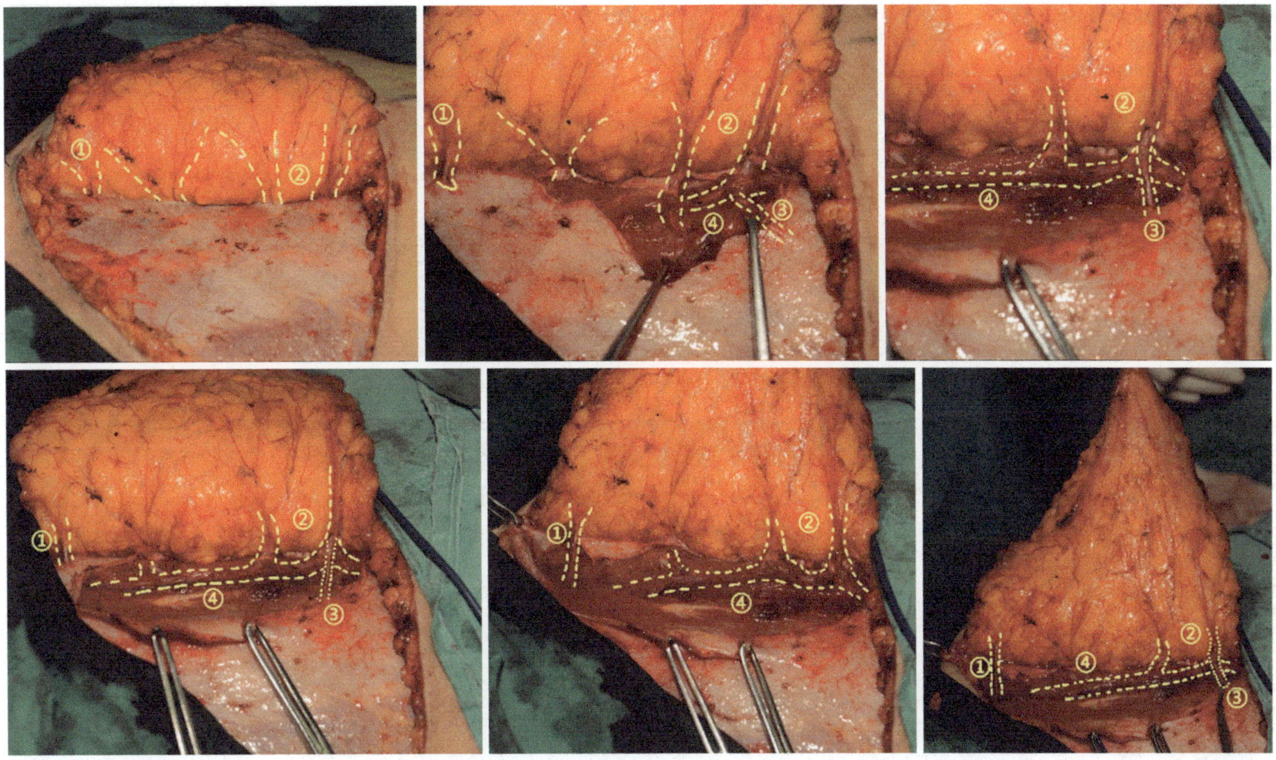

Fig. 16.7 Separation of the perforator and flap sensory nerve. (1) Sensory branch of the intercostal nerve 1; (2) perforating vessels; (3) sensory branches of the intercostal nerve; and (4) deep inferior epigastric vascular pedicle

Fig. 16.8 Clamping the right perforator suggested that the flap was in good blood supply based on the left vascular pedicle alone

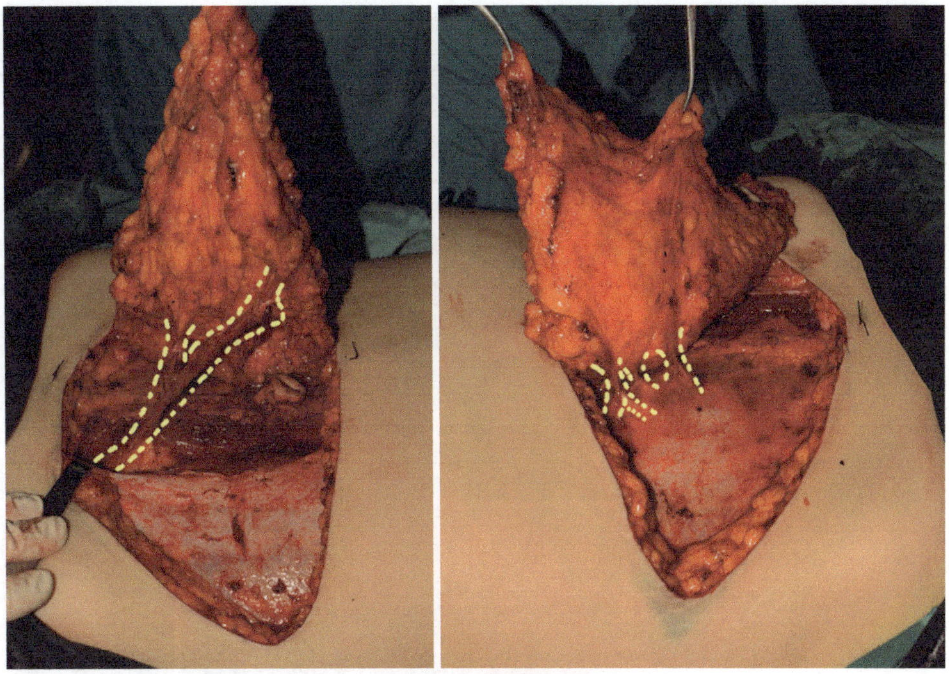

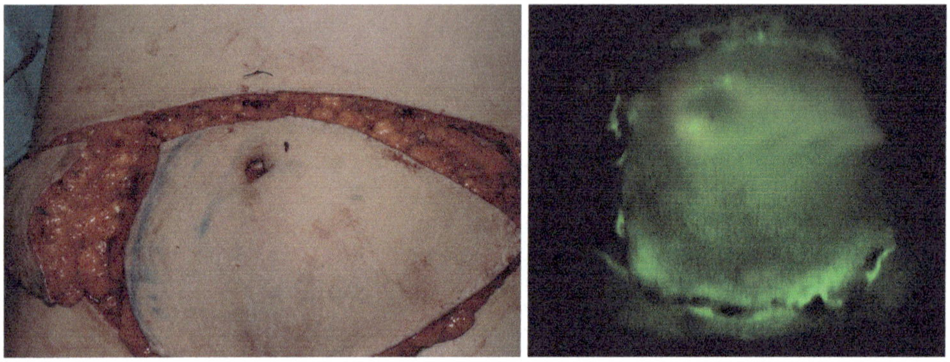

Fig. 16.9 Intraoperative ICG angiography was used to determine the blood supply of the flap, and the AREA IV was removed because of poor perfusion

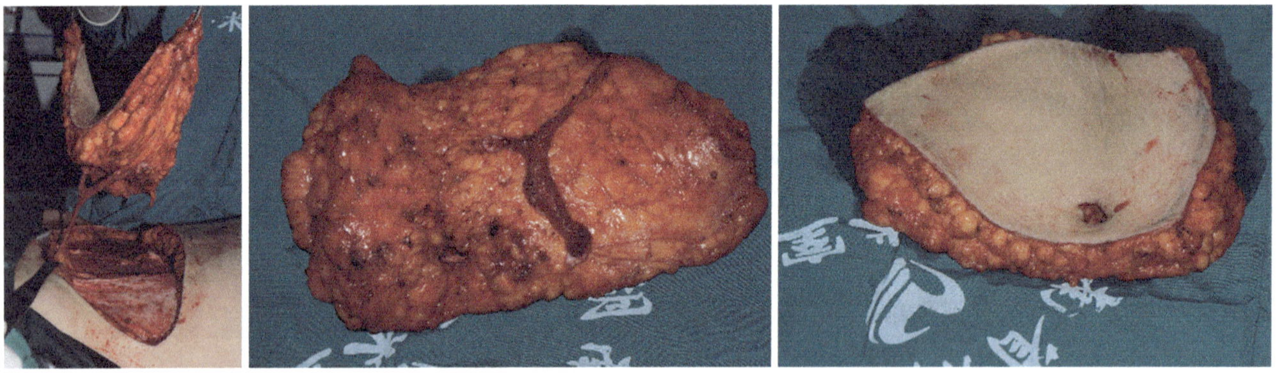

Fig. 16.10 The perforator flap of the deep inferior epigastric artery with the sensory branch of the intercostal nerve was cut

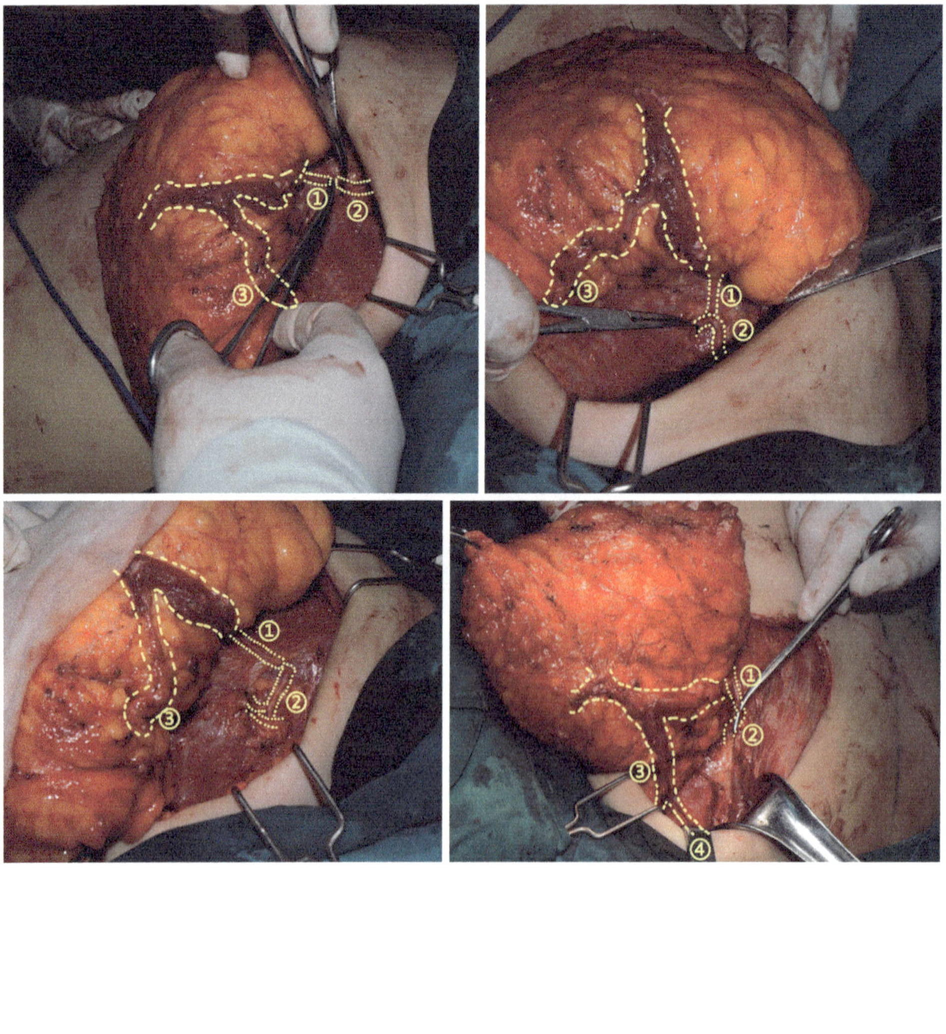

Fig. 16.11 Flap vascular anastomosis and sensory nerve reconstruction were completed. (1) Sensory branches of the intercostal nerve of the flap; (2) third intercostal nerve; (3) deep inferior epigastric vascular pedicle; and (4) lateral thoracic artery and vein and pectoralis major muscle branch vein

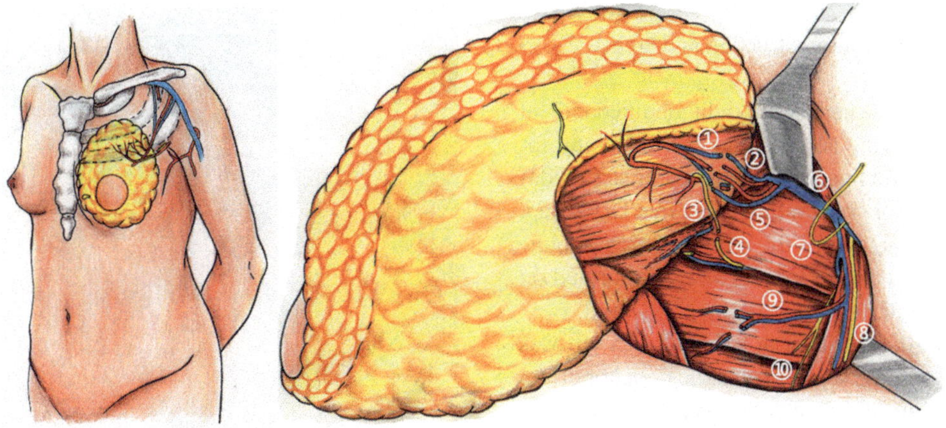

Fig. 16.12 Vascular and sensory reconstruction model of breast reconstruction. (1) Deep inferior epigastric artery and vein; (2) pectoralis major muscle branch artery and vein; (3) sensory branches of the intercostal nerve of the flap; (4) third intercostal nerve; (5) lateral thoracic artery and vein; (6) axillary vein; (7) intercostal brachial nerve; (8) thoracodorsal vascular nerve bundle; (9) anterior serratus branch of the thoracodorsal vessels; and (10) long thoracic nerve

Fig. 16.13 Intraoperative view immediately after reconstruction

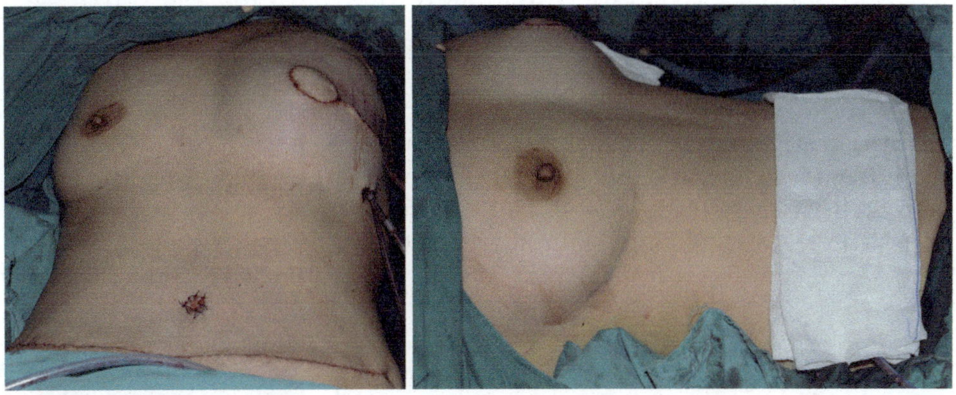

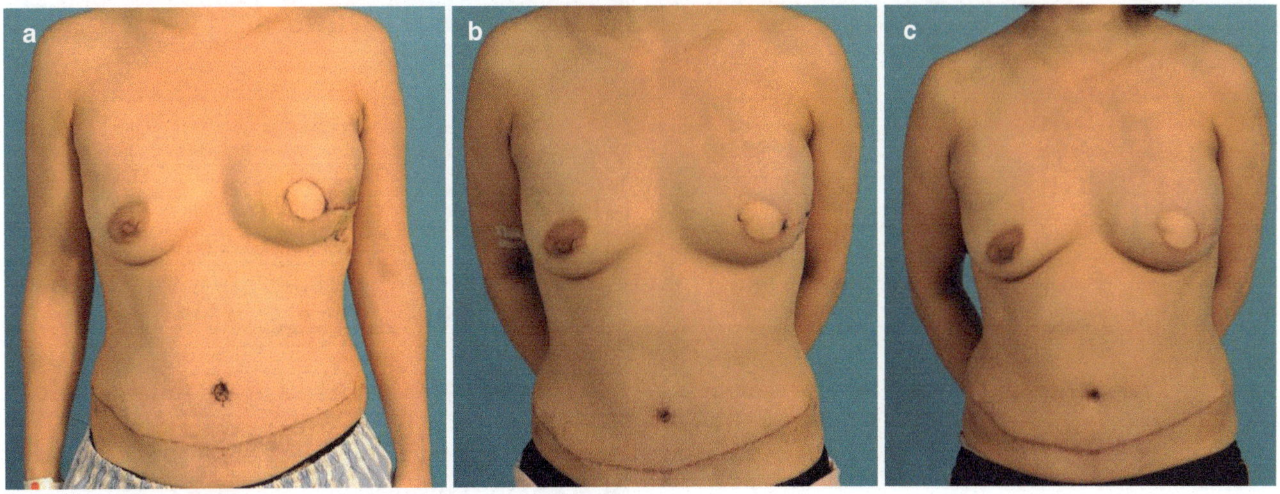

Fig. 16.14 (**a**) The appearance of reconstructed breast at 2 weeks after operation. (**b**) The appearance of reconstructed breast at 4 weeks after operation. (**c**) The appearance of reconstructed breast was satisfactory 6 months after operation

Case Study 2: Sensory Reconstruction and Breast Reconstruction

A 39-year-old female underwent right modified radical mastectomy following neoadjuvant chemotherapy for breast cancer 3 years ago. She received breast reconstruction and sensory restoration using free DIEP flap.

After the preparation of the receiving area, a huge defect of about 20 cm × 11 cm in size was formed on the right chest wall.

The third costal cartilage at a length of 3 cm was resected near the right sternum, and the perichondrium and intercostal muscle were cut to prepare the internal thoracic artery and its accompanying veins.

The size of the designed flap was about 28 cm × 14 cm in size.

The vascular pedicle was about 11 cm long. The bilateral deep inferior epigastric arteries and veins were end-to-end anastomosed with the internal thoracic arteries and veins (1A2V), and the SIEV was end-to-end anastomosed with the distal end of an internal thoracic vein. The blood supply of the flap was good after re-vasculization.

The patient recovered well after operation (Figs. 16.15, 16.16, 16.17, 16.18, 16.19, 16.20, 16.21, 16.22, 16.23, 16.24, 16.25, 16.26, 16.27, 16.28, 16.29, 16.30, 16.31, 16.32, 16.33, 16.34, 16.35, and 16.36).

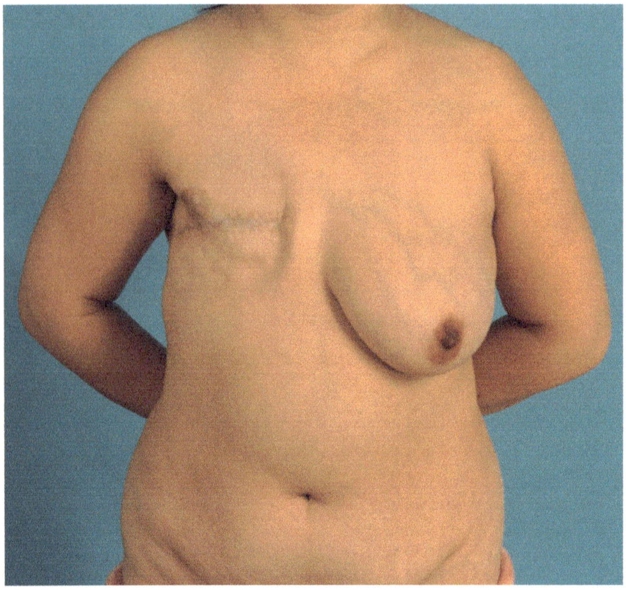

Fig. 16.15 Preoperative view

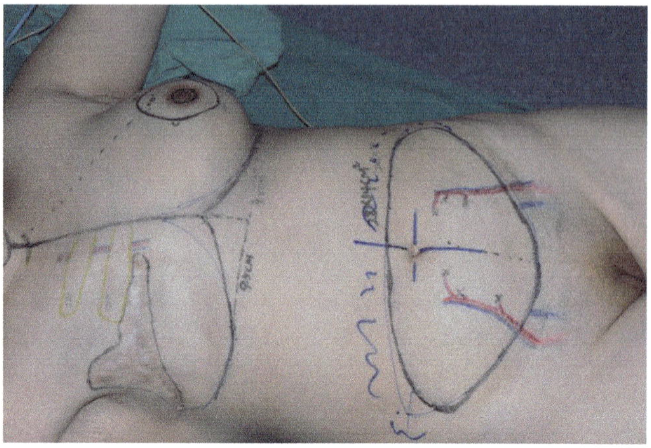

Fig. 16.16 Markings

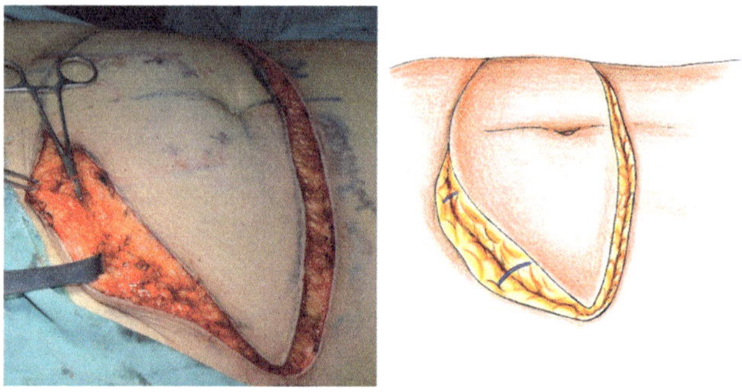

Fig. 16.17 The left SIEV was carried in the flap

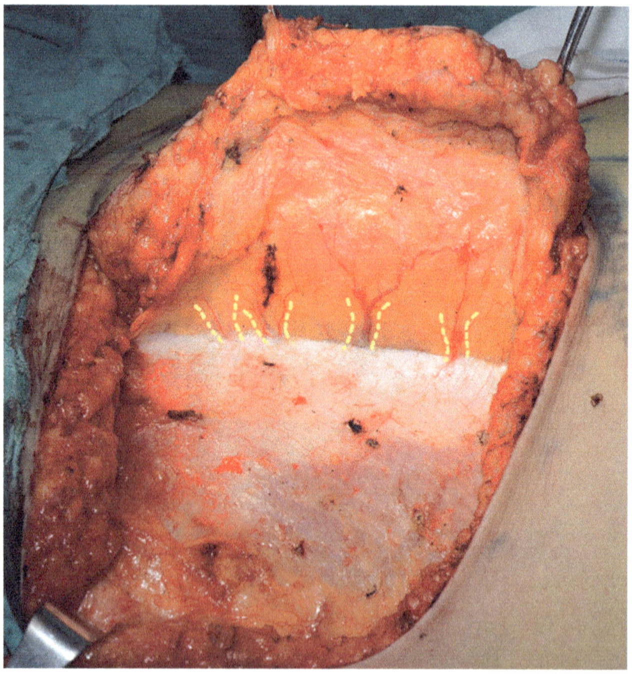

Fig. 16.18 Perforators

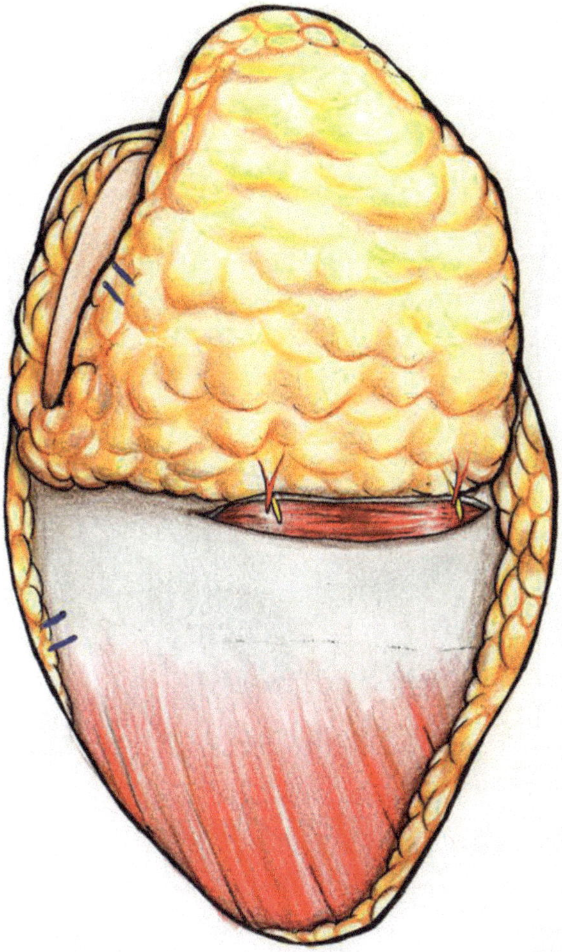

Fig. 16.19 Cutting the anterior sheath longitudinally along the lateral edge of the right perforator to expose the deep vessel. Multiple sensory branches of intercostal nerves accompanying the perforators were found

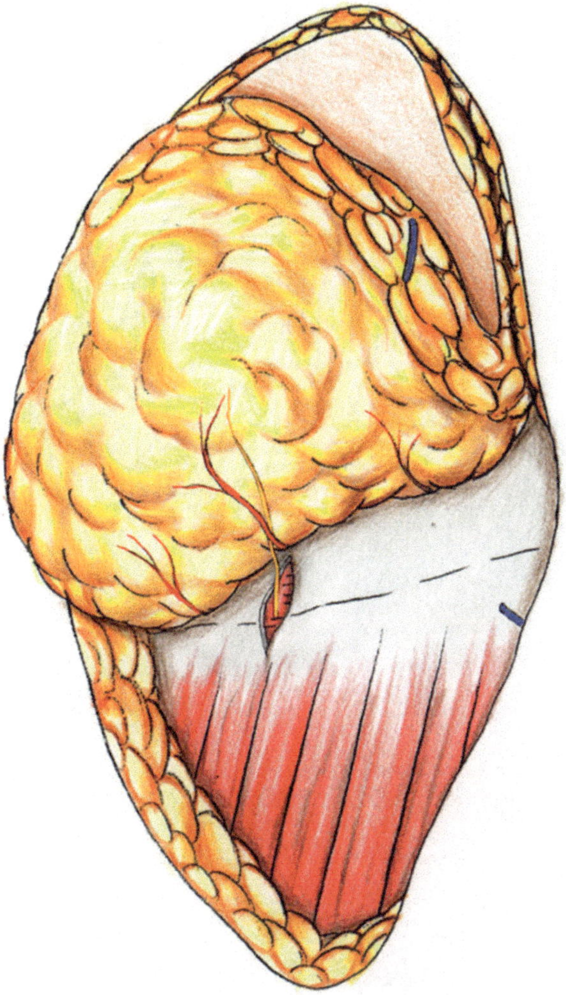

Fig. 16.20 Further incising the anterior sheath to reveal more perforating vessels and how the nerves traveled

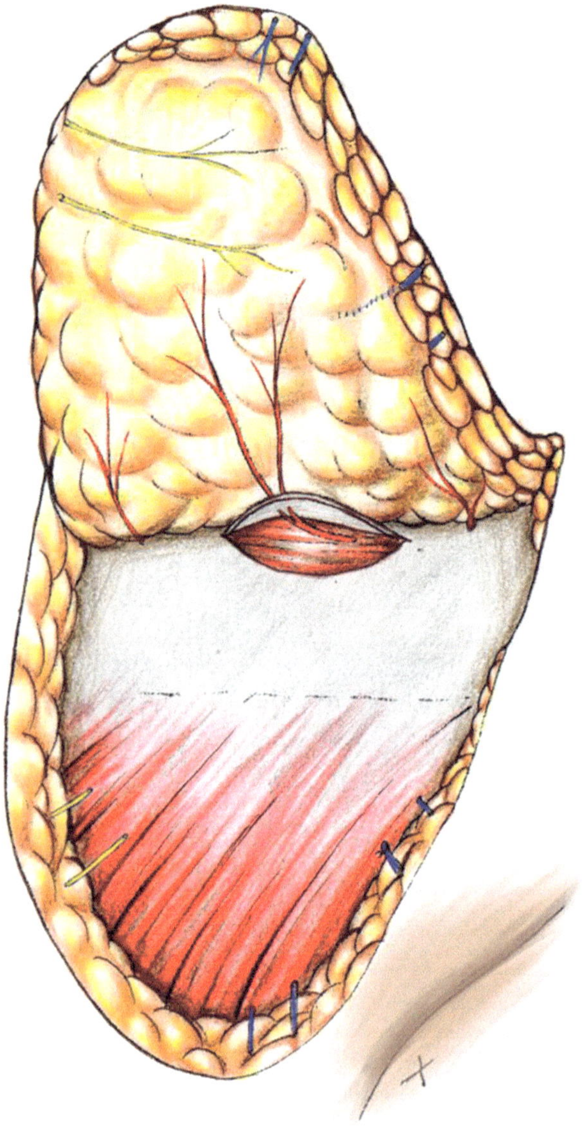

Fig. 16.21 Dissecting the right deep inferior epigastric perforator

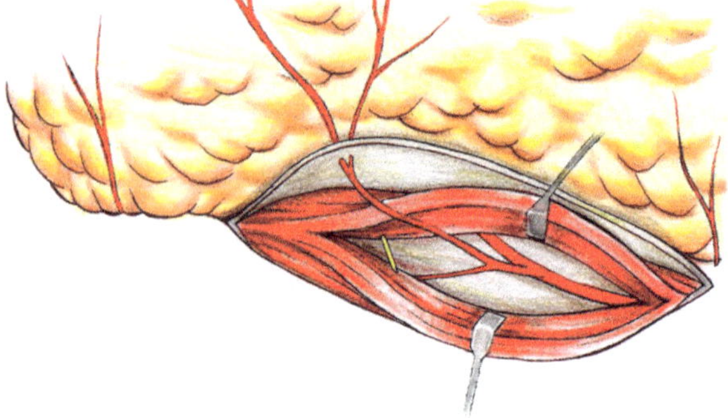

Fig. 16.22 Retrograde separation of the right perforator and the vascular trunk in the muscle toward the posterior sheath

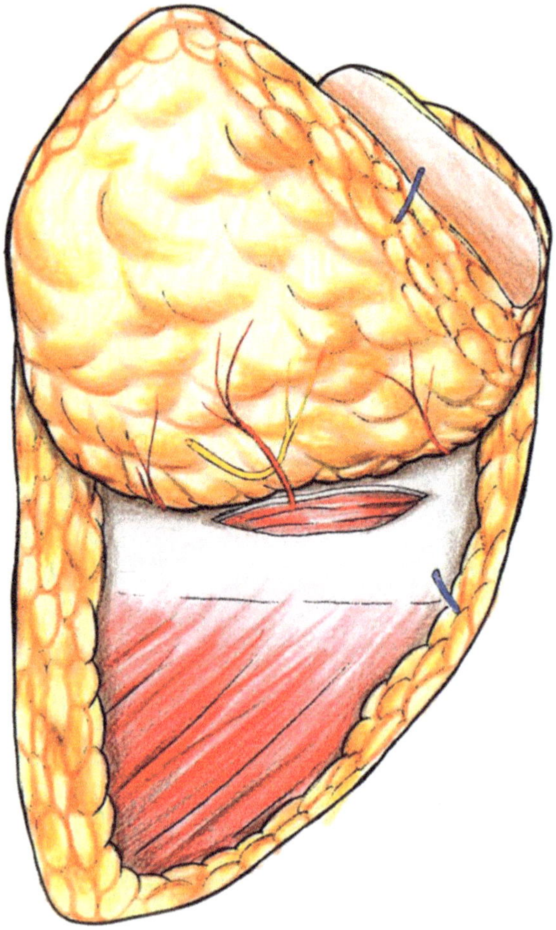

Fig. 16.23 A long segment of the sensory branch of the intercostal nerve was carried in the flap

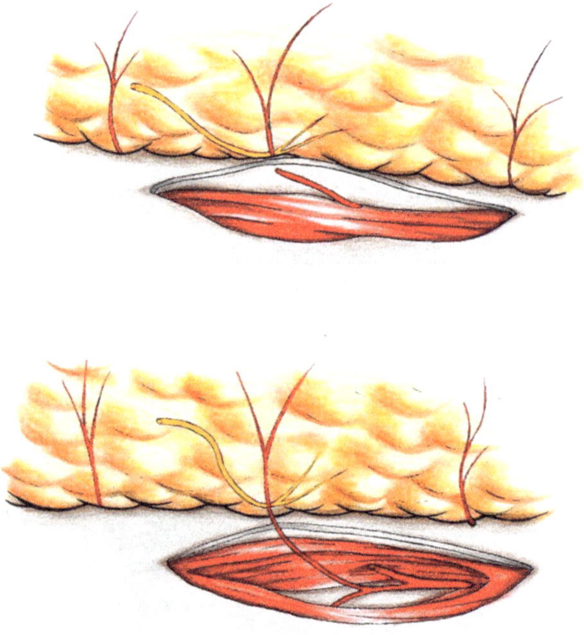

Fig. 16.24 Carefully protecting where the perforating vessels and the sensory branches of the intercostal nerve entered the flap

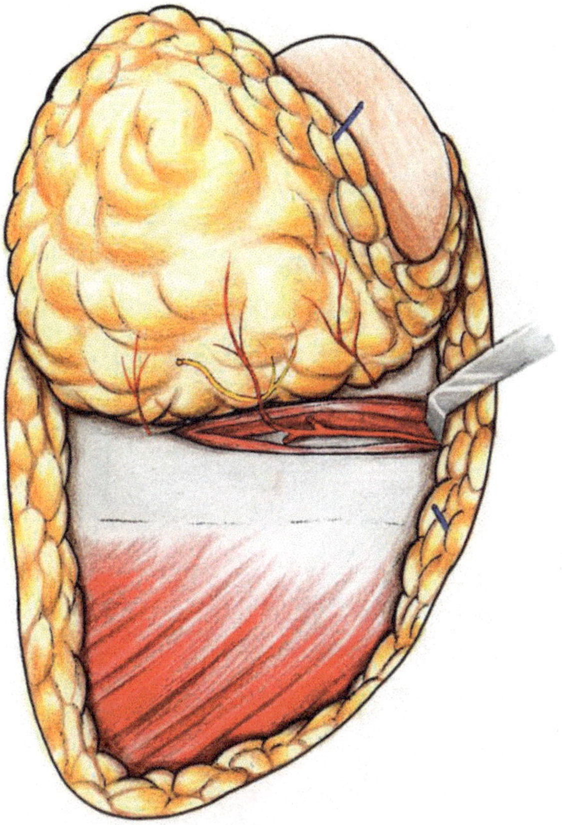

Fig. 16.25 The right vascular pedicle ran a long way inside the rectus abdominis muscle

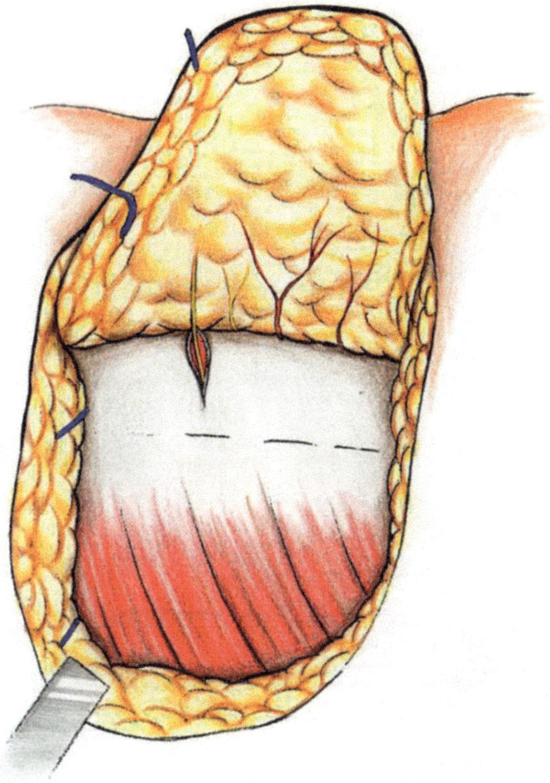

Fig. 16.26 The left perforating vessels

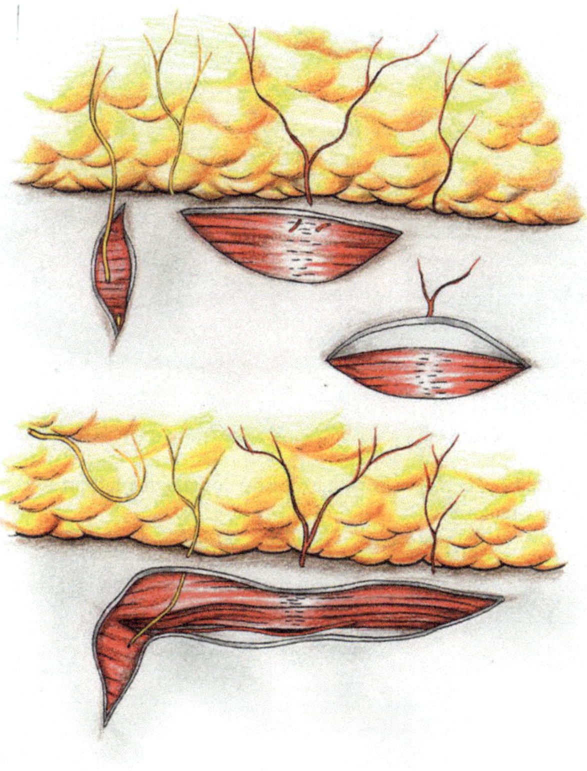

Fig. 16.27 Opening the anterior sheath and retrogradely separating the perforator vessel and vascular pedicle in the rectus abdominis muscle

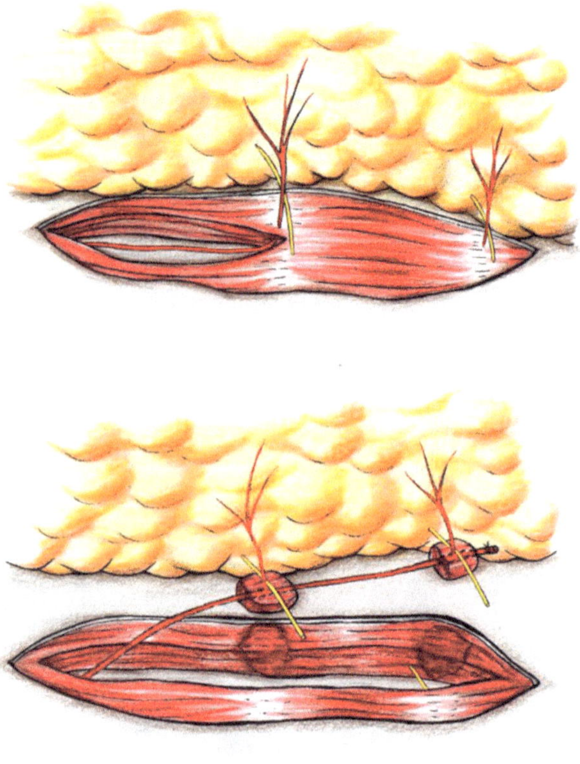

Fig. 16.28 It was difficult to skeletonize a perforator going through the tendinous inscriptions. A small amount of tendinous inscriptions surrounding the perforating branch was carried

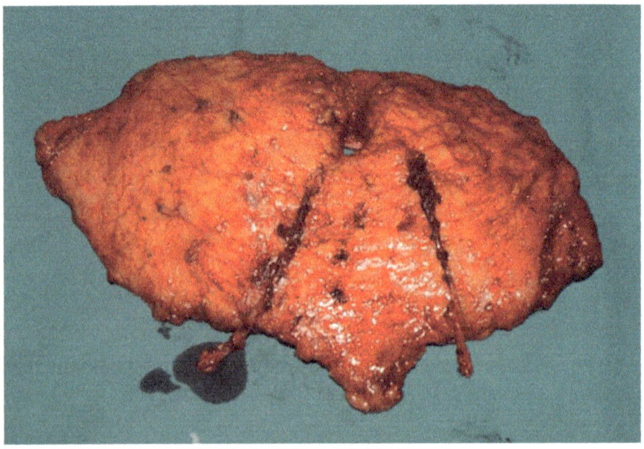

Fig. 16.29 The flap was with excessive volume; the left area IV was partially removed

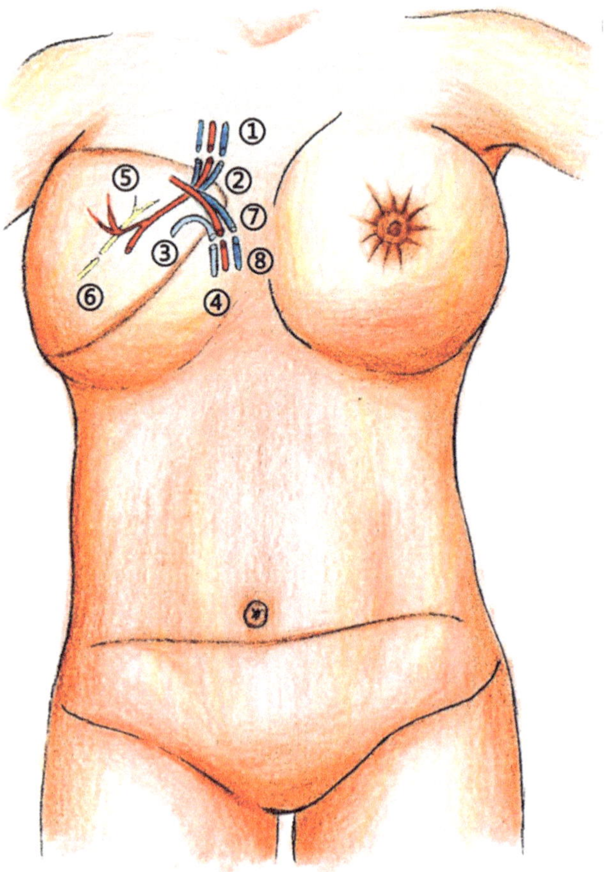

Fig. 16.30 Pattern of revascularization: the right deep inferior epigastric vessels were anastomosed to the proximal ends of the right internal thoracic vessels, the left deep inferior epigastric vessels were anastomosed to the distal ends of the right internal thoracic vessels, the right SIEV was anastomosed to the distal end of the right internal thoracic vein, and the sensory branch of the intercostal nerve carried on the flap was anastomosed to the third intercostal nerve. (1) Proximal end of the right internal mammary vessels; (2) right deep inferior epigastric vessels; (3) right SIEV; (4) distal end of the right internal thoracic vein; (5) the sensory branch of the intercostal nerve; (6) third intercostal nerve; (7) left deep inferior epigastric vessels; (8) distal end of the right internal mammary vessels

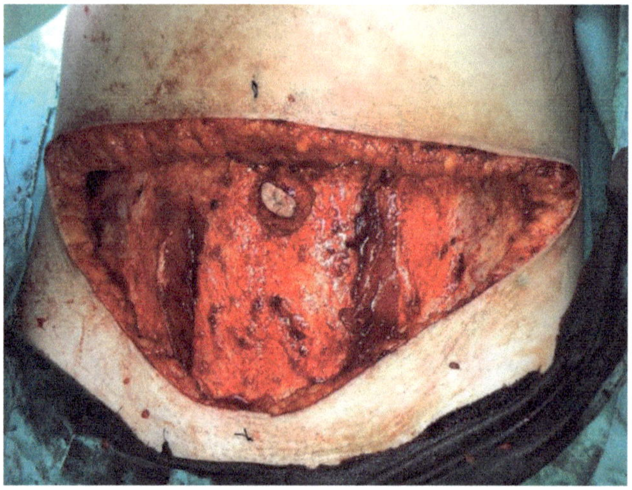

Fig. 16.31 Donor site after flap raising

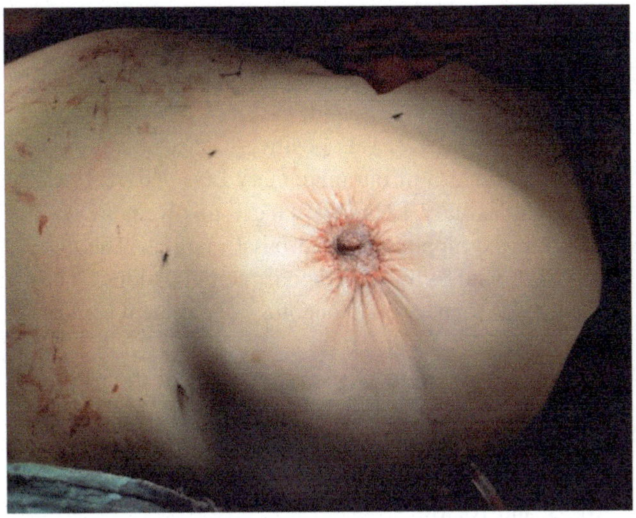

Fig. 16.32 Left mastopexy by round-block method

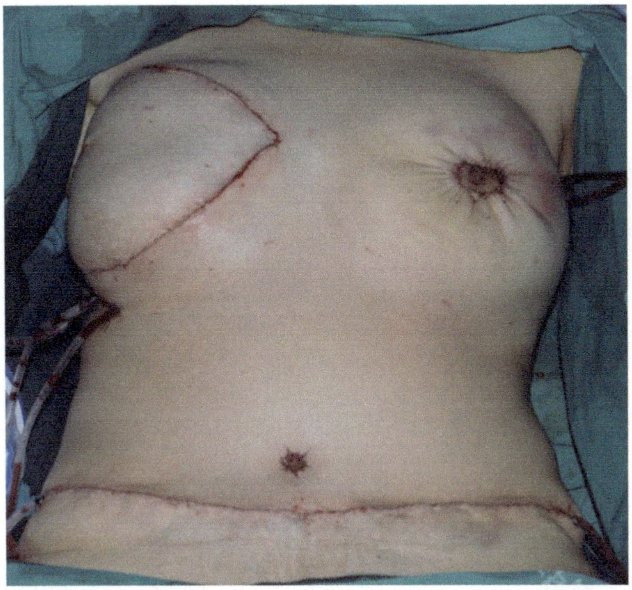

Fig. 16.33 Intraoperative view immediately after reconstruction

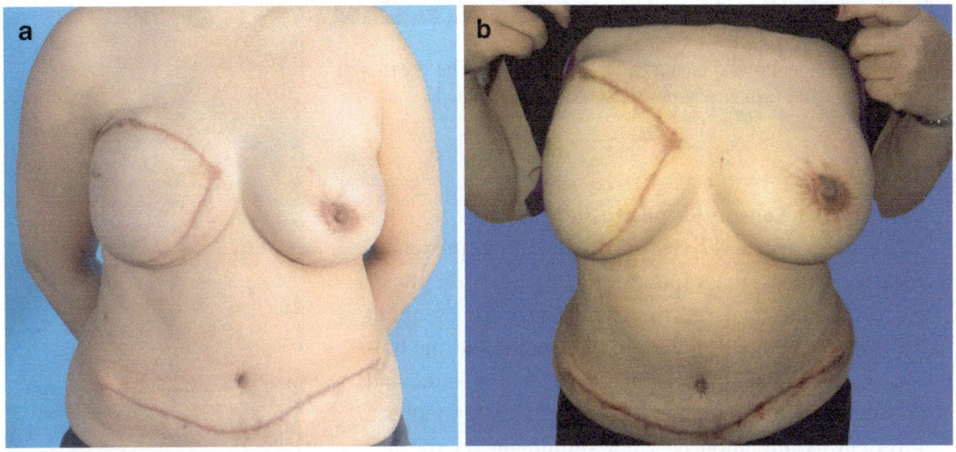

Fig. 16.34 Satisfactory breast shape and function during postoperative follow-up. (**a**) The patients were followed up at 12 months after operation. (**b**) The patients were followed up at 16 months after operation

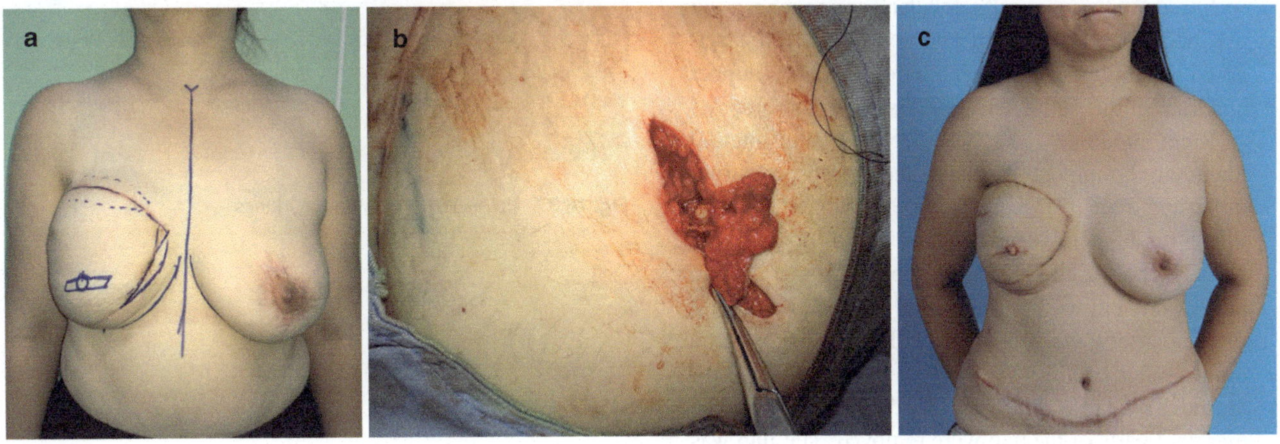

Fig. 16.35 (**a**) Nipple reconstruction 28 months after operation. (**b**) Using the costal cartilage cut off in the previous operation as a pad, a trilobal flap was designed to reconstruct the nipple. (**c**) The appearance of reconstructed nipple was satisfactory

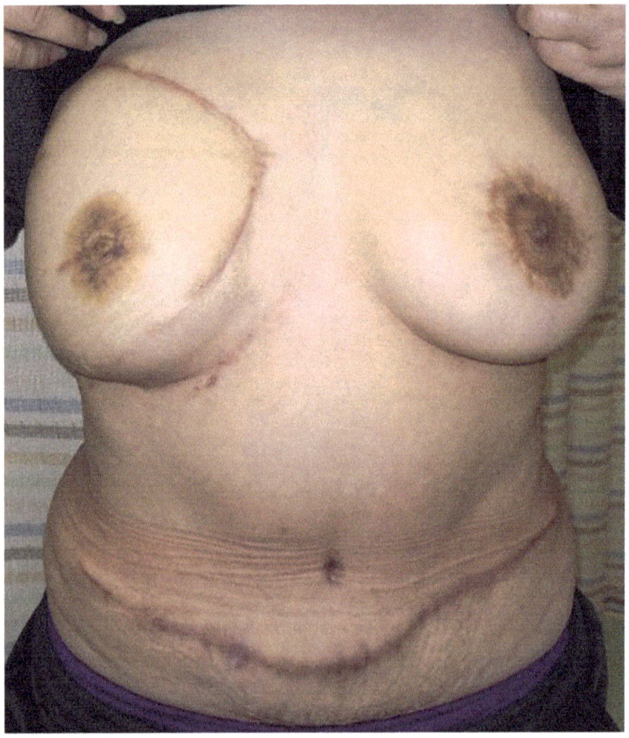

Fig. 16.36 Follow-up at 6 months after areola tattoo. The breast scar was significant and further scar plastic surgery was planned

Case Study 3: Sensory Reconstruction

The patient was a 47-year-old female who presented for a right breast mass found for half a year. On physical examination, tissue thickening as wide as about 5.0 cm × 6.0 cm was found on the lateral- and medial-upper quadrants of the right breast. It was hard and bumpy without definite boundary or tenderness. Physical examination was not significant on the left breast and regional lymph nodes.

Intraductal cancer with lobular carcinogenesis on the medial-upper quadrant and invasive ductal carcinoma with intraductal carcinoma on the lateral-upper quadrant of the right breast was diagnosed on biopsy.

Right modified radical mastectomy plus internal mammary lymph node excision and breast reconstruction using free DIEP skin flap were performed. A DIEP flap with bilateral deep inferior epigastric vascular pedicles was used. The left deep inferior epigastric artery and vein were anastomosed with the left lateral thoracic artery and vein (1A2V). The left SIEV and a branch of the axillary vein were end-to-end anastomosed. The flap was in good blood circulation and the marginal parts of the flap were removed. The flap was in good viability after operation. The results of postoperative pathological examination showed that right breast invasive ductal carcinoma was histological grade II, intraductal carcinoma and lobular and fat tissue involvement were found; the size of the mass was 6.5 cm × 3 cm; LVI was positive. Cancer metastasis was found in 3/3 of intramammary LNs and 15/19 of the right axillary LNs. No cancer involvement was found in the nipple, skin and basal margins. The flap survived well without obvious complications. The patient was transferred to oncology department for further treatment.

The functional and sensory recovery of the reconstructed breast were satisfactory (Figs. 16.37, 16.38, 16.39, 16.40, 16.41, 16.42, 16.43, 16.44, 16.45, 16.46, 16.47, 16.48, 16.49, 16.50, 16.51, 16.52, 16.53, 16.54, 16.55, and 16.56).

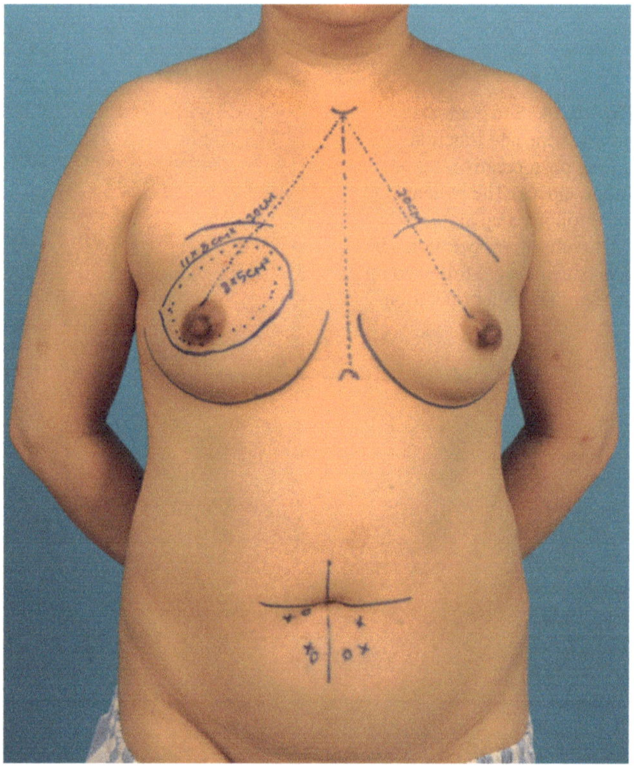

Fig. 16.37 Preoperative view and markings

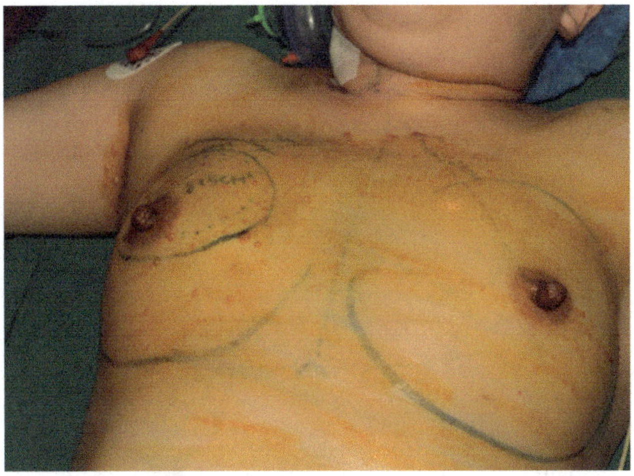

Fig. 16.38 Markings

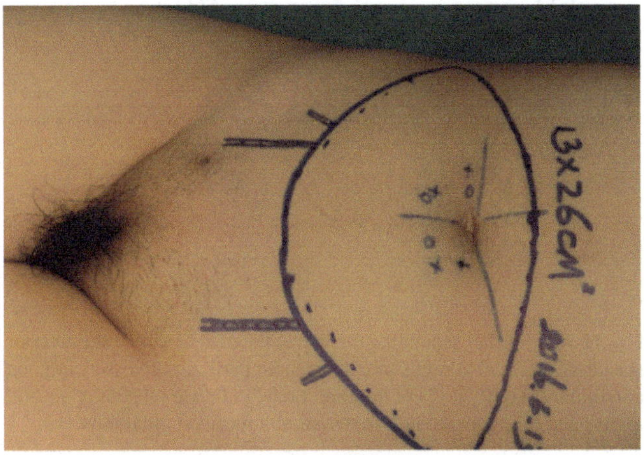

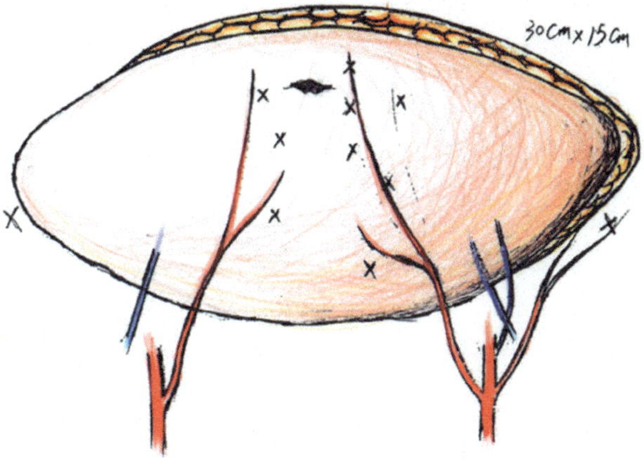

Fig. 16.39 Design of DIEP flap. Pencil Doppler was used to determine the position of perforating vessels. Flap raising started from the proximal part and the left margin

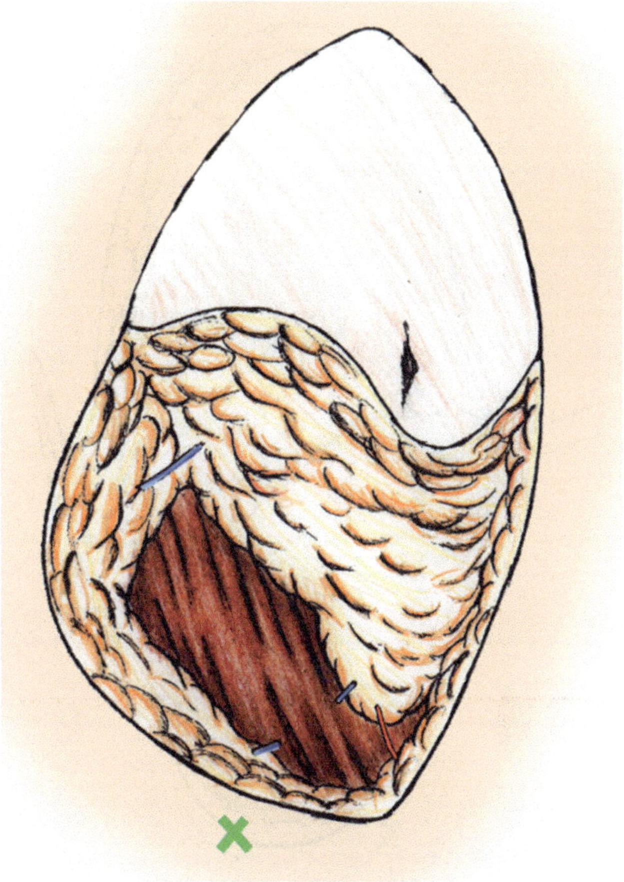

Fig. 16.40 Lifting the flap from outside to inside on the aponeurosis surface of the external oblique muscle, ligating the branches of the superficial iliac circumflex vessels and intercostal vessels

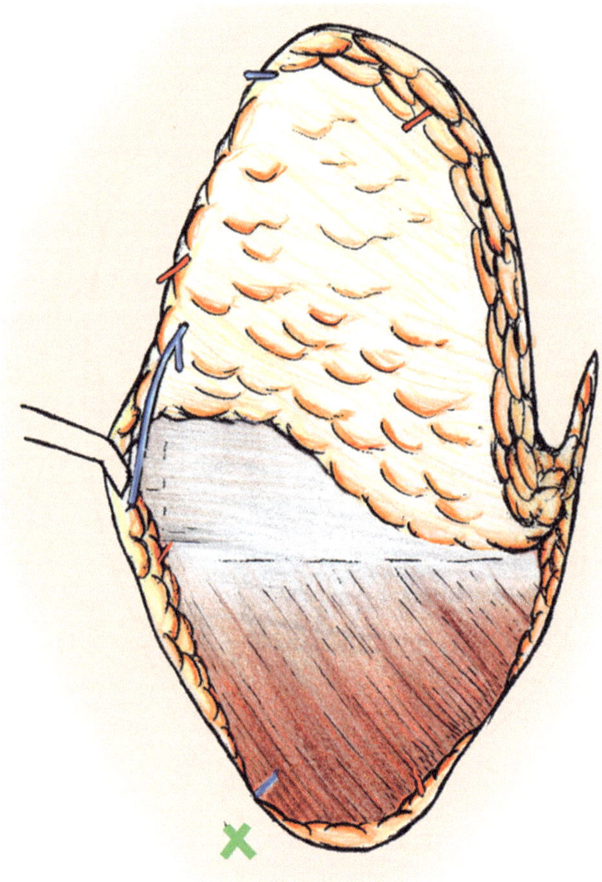

Fig. 16.41 Further lifting the distal end of the flap and preserving the SEIV as long as 7 cm. In this case, the SIEV was slightly medial and retrogradely separated till the aponeurosis surface of the external oblique muscle. The tributaries of the SEIV were ligated

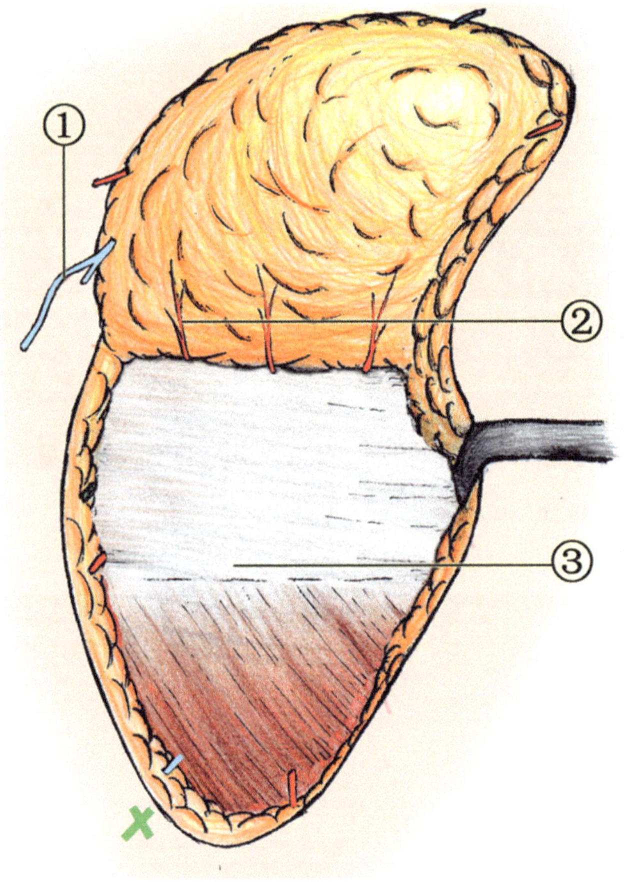

Fig. 16.42 Further separating the flap to the medial side of the anterior sheath of rectus abdominis to expose three perforating vessels in good conditions. (1) SIEV; (2) perforating branch of deep inferior epigastric artery; and (3) aponeurosis of external oblique abdominal muscle

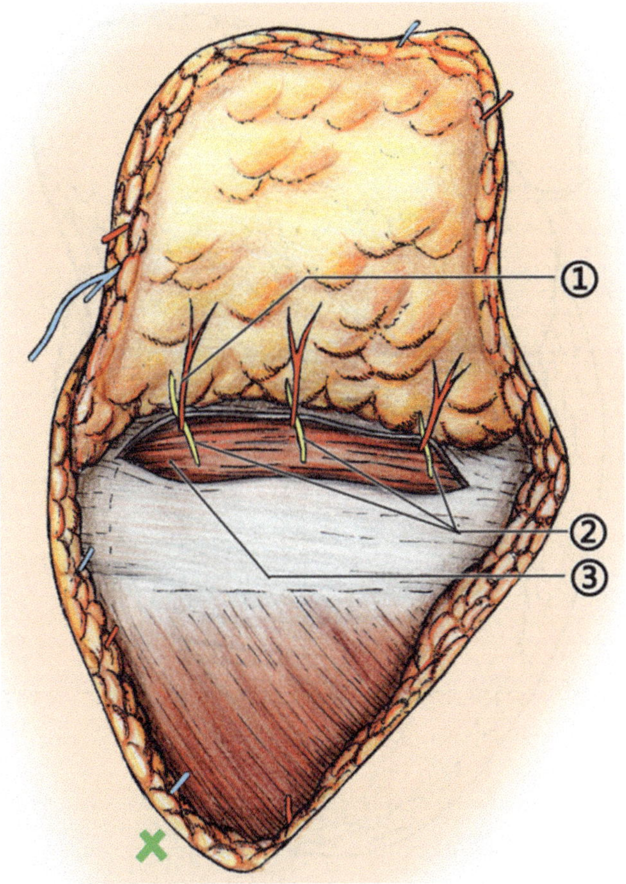

Fig. 16.43 Cutting the anterior sheath longitudinally along the outer edge of the three perforating branches and retrogradely intramuscular separating the perforating branches toward the vascular trunk. It can be seen that the perforating branches intersected with the sensory branch of the intercostal nerve which should be carefully preserved. (1) Perforating branch of the deep inferior epigastric artery. (2) Sensory branch of the intercostal nerve. (3) Rectus abdominis

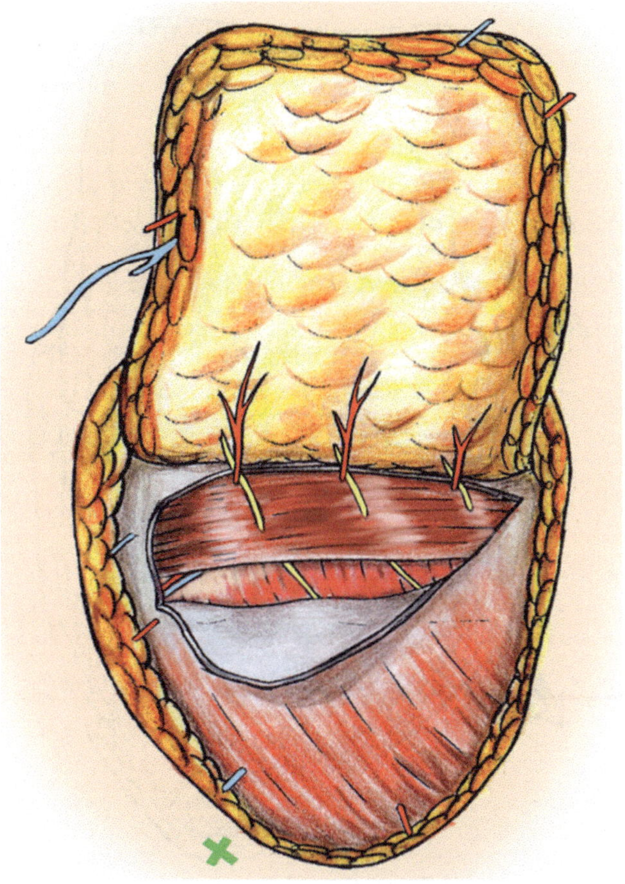

Fig. 16.44 Extending the opening of the anterior sheath laterally to fully expose the outer edge of the rectus abdominis, the trunk of the deep inferior epigastric vessels, and the intercostal nerve

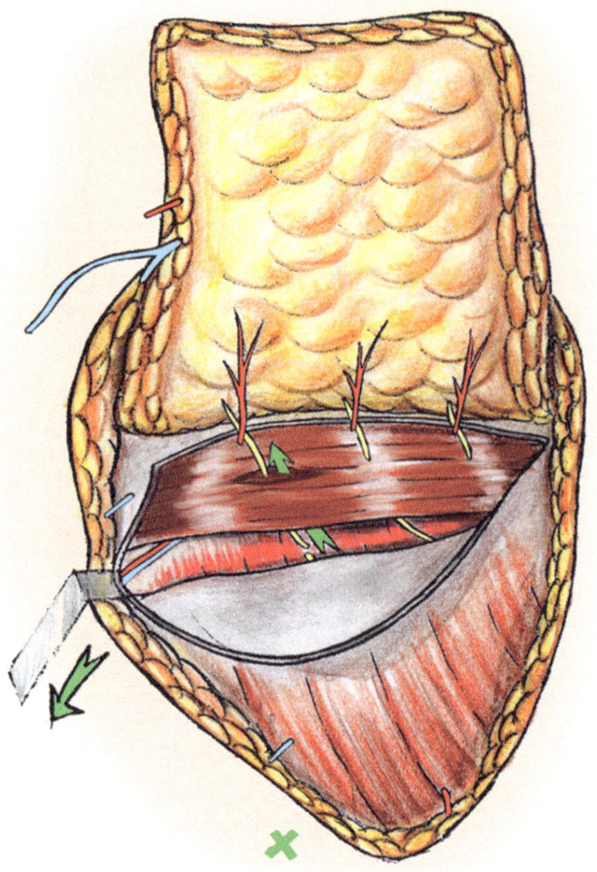

Fig. 16.45 The sensory branch of the intercostal nerve was separated in the muscle using rendezvous method and cut off at the outer edge of the anterior sheath and extracted retrogradely. Further separating the deep inferior epigastric blood vessels anterogradely

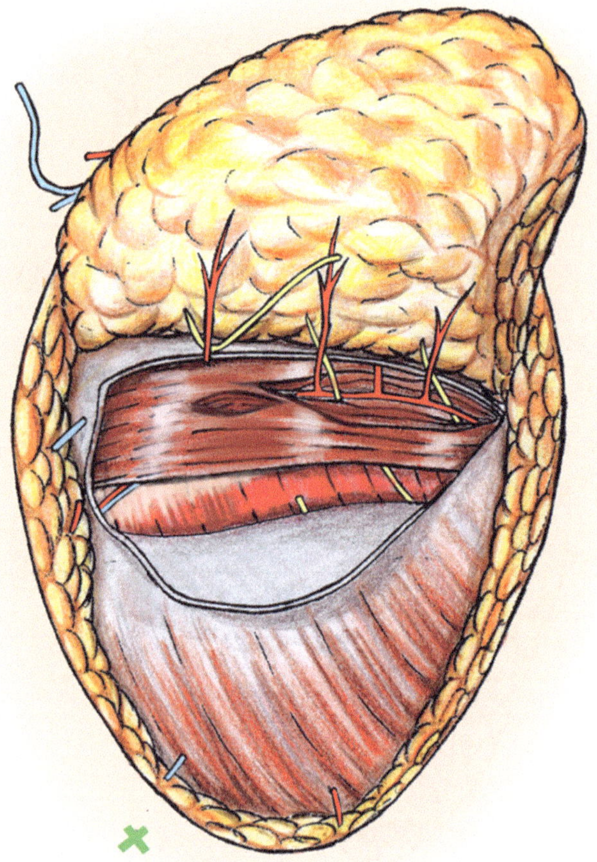

Fig. 16.46 Three perforators and the crisscrossing sensory branches of intercostal nerves that entered the flap were separated using rendezvous method. The vascular trunk bifurcated a large medial perforator and then traveled beneath the anterior sheath, along the surface of the rectus abdominis between the first and second perforators

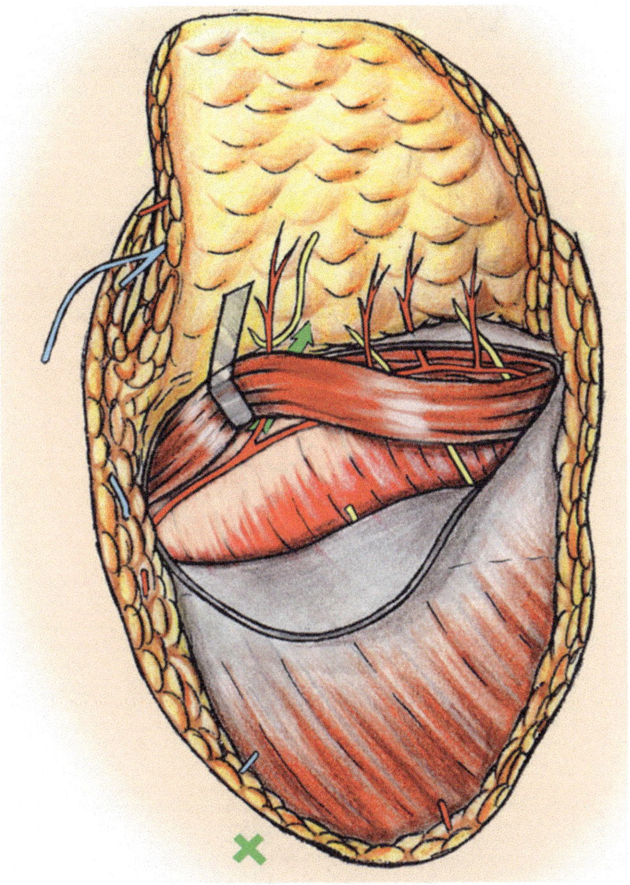

Fig. 16.47 Dissection medially along the surface of the anterior sheath to reveal a large perforator. The deep inferior epigastric vessels that were separated anterogradely beneath the rectus abdominis sent out a major perforator medially. Preserving the integrity of a large intercostal nerve

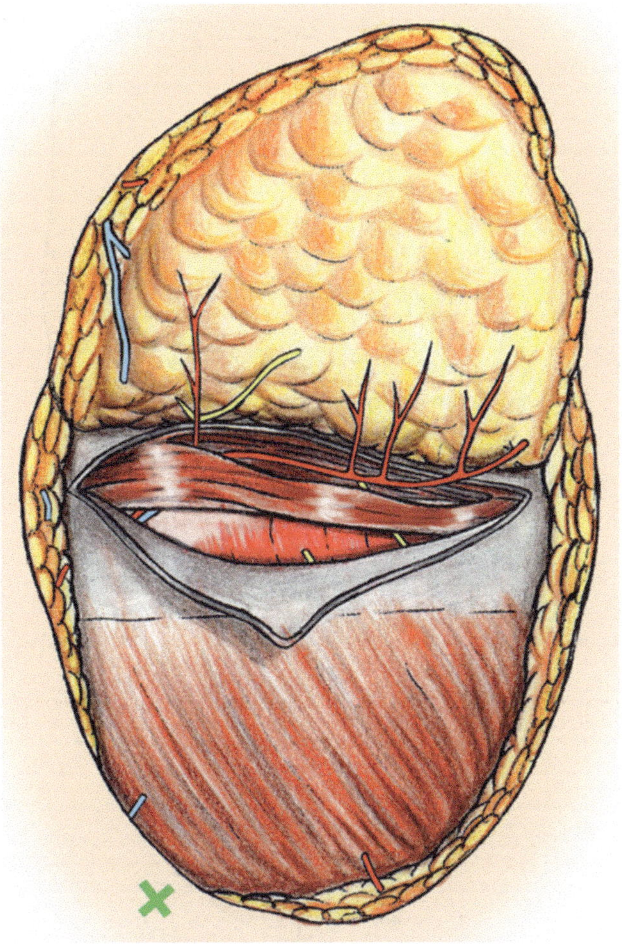

Fig. 16.48 Separating the deep inferior epigastric vessels as long as possible caudally for re-vasculization

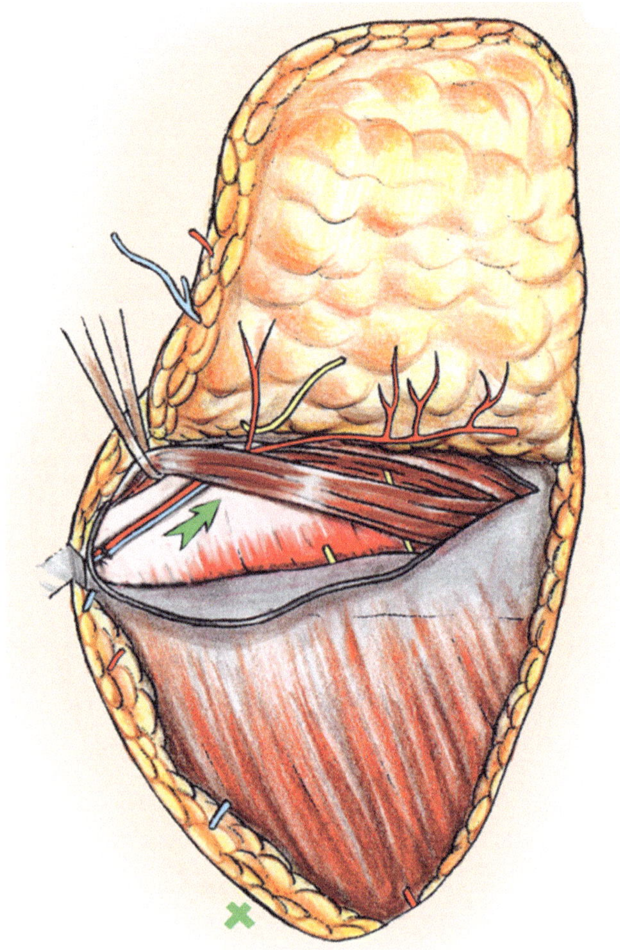

Fig. 16.49 The flap was freed; the deep inferior epigastric vessels were disconnected where it originated from and extracted retrogradely through the rectus abdominis to avoid damaging the muscle. The intercostal nerves innervated the upper rectus abdominis were maintained

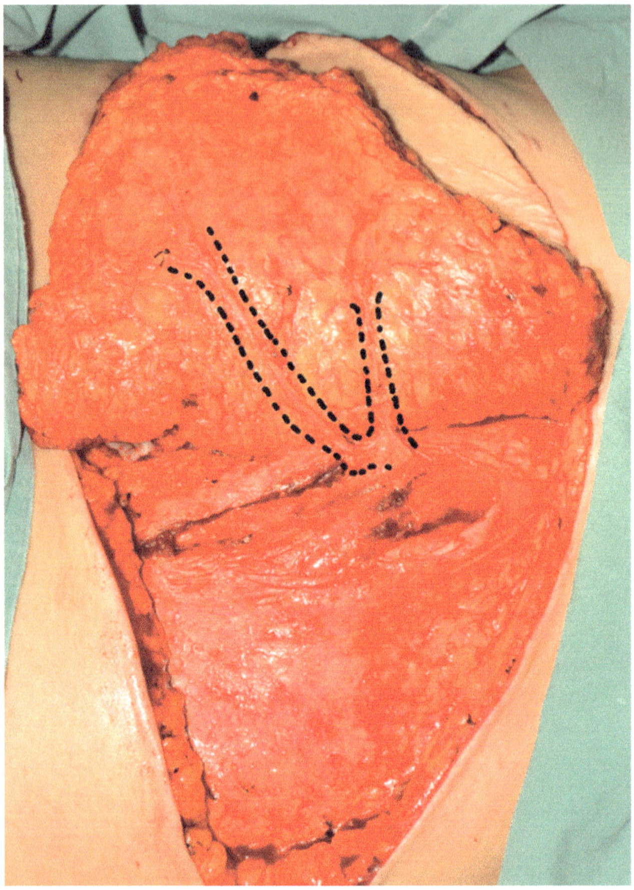

Fig. 16.50 Separation of right perforator vessels

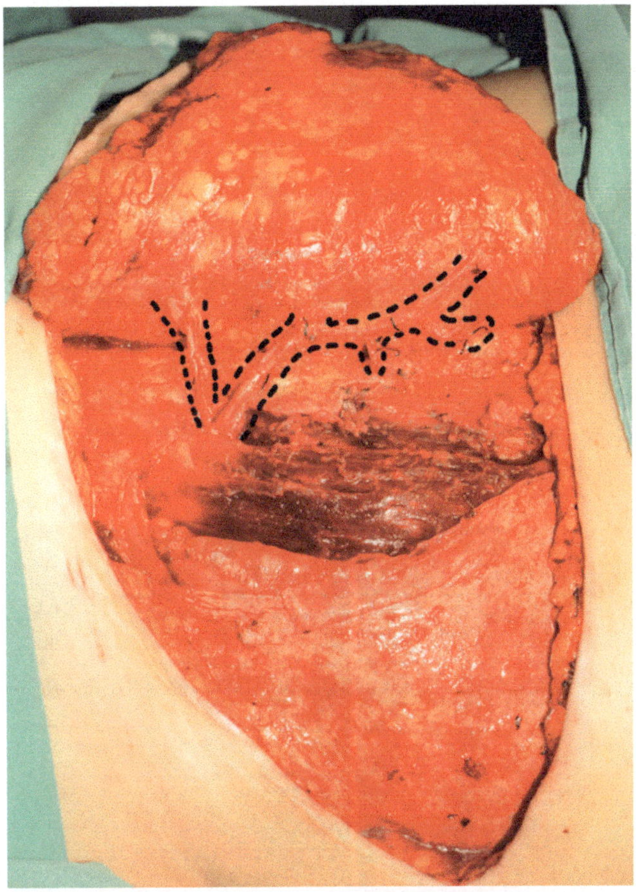

Fig. 16.51 Separation of left perforator vessels

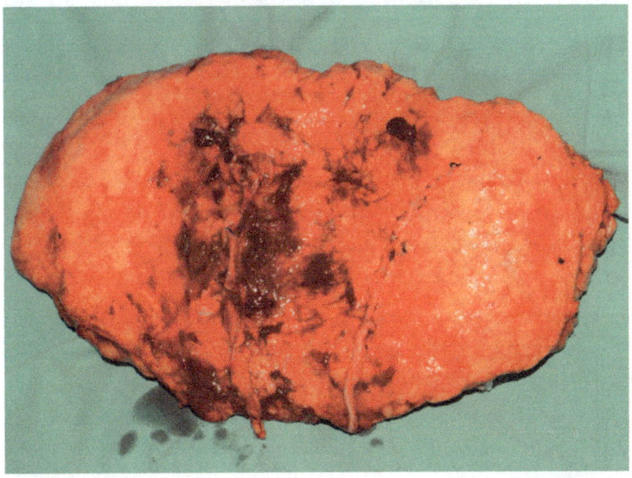

Fig. 16.52 A bilateral pedicled DIEP flap was prepared

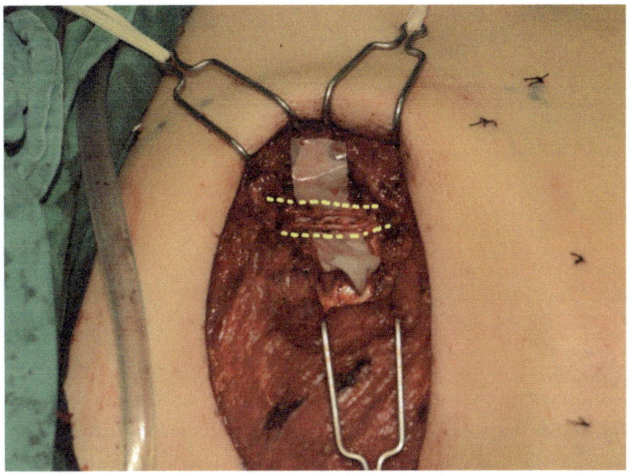

Fig. 16.53 Preparation of the right intramammary blood vessels

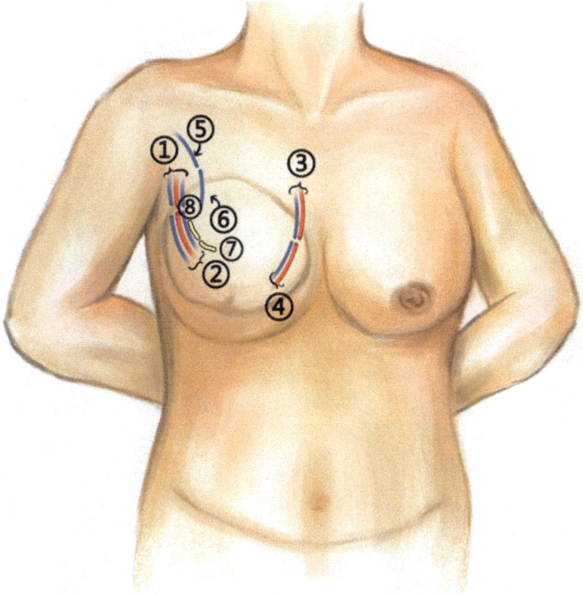

Fig. 16.54 Pattern of revascularization and sensory reconstruction: left deep inferior epigastric vessels to right lateral thoracic vessels (A: $V = 1:2$); left SIEV to right lateral thoracic vein; and right deep inferior epigastric vessels to right internal mammary vessels (A: $V = 1:1$). (1) Lateral thoracic vessels. (2) Left deep inferior epigastric vessels. (3) Internal mammary vessels. (4) Right deep inferior epigastric vessels. (5) Lateral thoracic vein. (6) SIEV. (7) The sensory branch of the intercostal nerve carried in the flap. (8) Sensory branch of the intercostal nerve in the receiving area

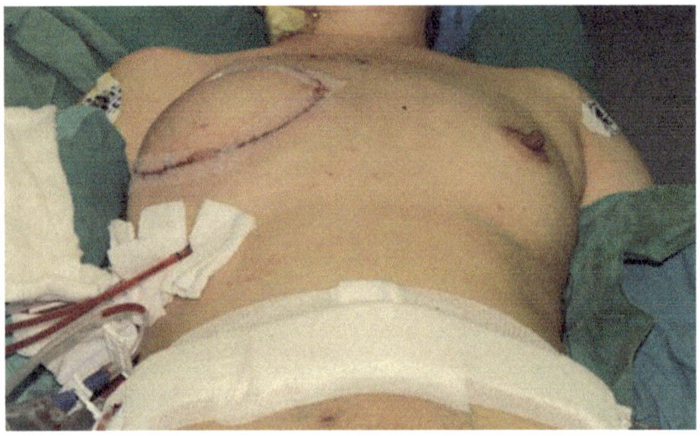

Fig. 16.55 Intraoperative view immediately after reconstruction

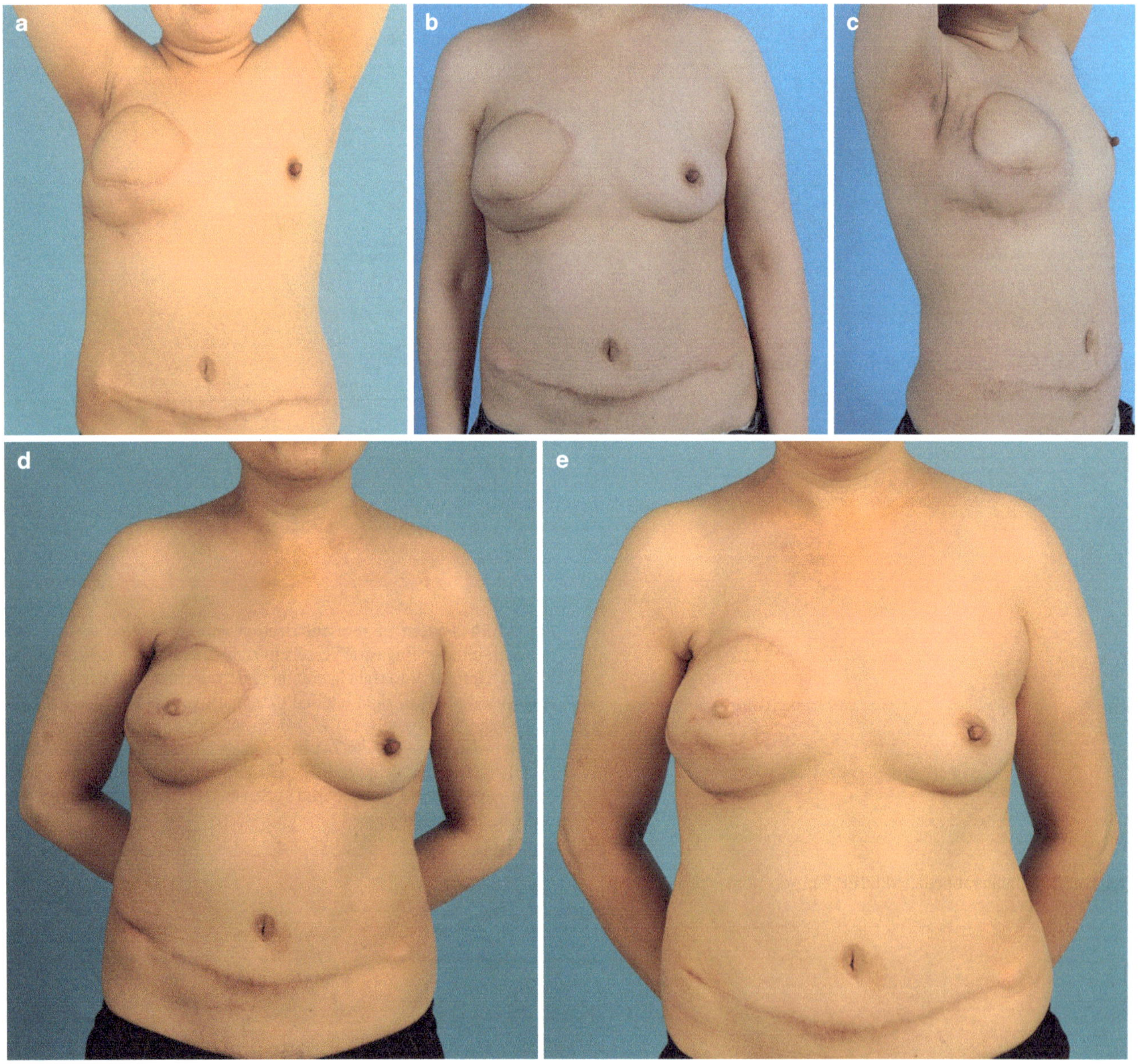

Fig. 16.56 (**a**) 12 months at follow-up; (**b**, **c**) 18 months at follow-up; (**d**) follow-up at 3 months after nipple reconstruction; (**e**) follow up at 8 months after nipple reconstruction

References

1. Shridharani SM, Magarakis M, Stapleton SM, Basdag B, Seal SM, Rosson GD. Breast sensation after breast reconstruction: a systematic review. J Reconstr Microsurg. 2010;26(5):303–10.
2. Lapatto O, Asko-Seljavaara S, Tukiainen E, Suominen E. Return of sensibility and final outcome of breast reconstructions using free transverse rectus abdominis musculocutaneous flaps. Scand J Plast Reconstr Surg Hand Surg. 1995;29(1):33–8.
3. Shaw WW, Orringer JS, Ko CY, Ratto LL, Mersmann CA. The spontaneous return of sensibility in breasts reconstructed with autologous tissues. Plast Reconstr Surg. 1997;99(2):394–9.
4. Slezak S, McGibbon B, Dellon AL. The sensational transverse rectus abdominis musculocutaneous (TRAM) flap: return of sensibility after TRAM breast reconstruction. Ann Plast Surg. 1992;28(3):210–7.
5. Temple CL, Tse R, Bettger-Hahn M, MacDermid J, Gan BS, Ross DC. Sensibility following innervated free TRAM flap for breast reconstruction. Plast Reconstr Surg. 2006;117(7):2119–27; discussion 2128–30.
6. Liew S, Hunt J, Pennington D. Sensory recovery following free TRAM flap breast reconstruction. Br J Plast Surg. 1996;49(4):210–3.
7. Place MJ, Song T, Hardesty RA, Hendricks DL. Sensory reinnervation of autologous tissue TRAM flaps after breast reconstruction. Ann Plast Surg. 1997;38(1):19–22.
8. Temple CL, Ross DC, Kim S, et al. Sensibility following innervated free TRAM flap for breast reconstruction: part II. Innervation improves patient-rated quality of life. Plast Reconstr Surg. 2009;124(5):1419–25.
9. Blondeel N, Vanderstraeten GG, Monstrey SJ, et al. The donor site morbidity of free DIEP flaps and free TRAM flaps for breast reconstruction. Br J Plast Surg. 1997;50(5):322–30.
10. Blondeel PN, Boeckx WD. Refinements in free flap breast reconstruction: the free bilateral deep inferior epigastric perforator flap anastomosed to the internal mammary artery. Br J Plast Surg. 1994;47(7):495–501.
11. Blondeel PN. One hundred free DIEP flap breast reconstructions: a personal experience. Br J Plast Surg. 1999;52(2):104–11.
12. Stromps JP, Bozkurt A, Grieb G, Kim BS, Wiezik M, Pallua N. Spontaneous reinnervation of deep inferior epigastric perforator flaps after delayed breast reconstruction. J Reconstr Microsurg. 2016;32(3):169–77.
13. Yap LH, Whiten SC, Forster A, Stevenson HJ. Sensory recovery in the sensate free transverse rectus abdominis myocutaneous flap. Plast Reconstr Surg. 2005;115(5):1280–8.
14. Yano K, Hosokawa K, Takagi S, Nakai K, Kubo T. Breast reconstruction using the sensate latissimus dorsi musculocutaneous flap. Plast Reconstr Surg. 2002;109(6):1897–902; discussion 1903.
15. Blondeel PN, Demuynck M, Mete D, et al. Sensory nerve repair in perforator flaps for autologous breast reconstruction: sensational or senseless. Br J Plast Surg. 1999;52(1):37–44.
16. Santanelli F, Longo B, Angelini M, Laporta R, Paolini G. Prospective computerized analyses of sensibility in breast reconstruction with non-reinnervated DIEP flap. Plast Reconstr Surg. 2011;127(5):1790–5.
17. Spiegel AJ, Menn ZK, Eldor L, Kaufman Y, Dellon AL. Breast reinnervation: DIEP neurotization using the third anterior intercostal nerve. Plast Reconstr Surg Glob Open. 2013;1(8):e72.
18. Spiegel AJ, Salazar-Reyes H, Izaddoost S, Khan FN. A novel method for neurotization of deep inferior epigastric perforator and superficial deep inferior epigastric artery flaps. Plast Reconstr Surg. 2009;123(1):29e–30e.

17 Free DIEP Flap with Ilioinguinal Lymphoid Tissue for Breast Reconstruction and Treatment of Upper Limb Lymphedema

Zan Li, Jie Ma, Xiaomin Yang, Jianghua Ou, Dequan Liu, Yiyin Tang, and Shu Liu

17.1 Summary

Radical mastectomy not only leads to permanent breast missing but also constitutes an independent risk factor for lymphedema after breast cancer surgery. Upper limb lymphedema is most commonly seen after breast cancer treatment.

With the development of society and the improvement of people's living standards, more and more patients with upper limb lymphedema ask for treating lymphedema and reconstruction of breast shape and function [1, 2].

Axillary sentinel lymph node biopsy, lymph node dissection, and radiotherapy can lead to upper limb lymphedema in breast cancer patients.

According to the latest literature, the probability of upper limb lymphedema after breast cancer patients undergoing axillary lymph node dissection is 19.9% [3].

The cause of lymphedema is the damage of lymphatic system, manifesting pathologically as tissue fibrosis, impaired immune function, and subcutaneous fat hypertrophy.

Z. Li (✉)
Department of Oncology Plastic Surgery, Hunan Cancer Hospital, Changsha, Hunan, China

J. Ma
Department of Breast Surgery, Tangshan People's Hospital, Tangshan, HeBei, China

X. Yang
Department of Breast Surgery, Tumor Hospital of Shaanxi Province, Xi'an, Shaanxi, China

J. Ou
Department of Breast Surgery, Plastic and Reconstructive Surgery, The Affiliated Tumor Hospital of Xinjiang Medical University, Urumqi, Xinjiang, China

D. Liu · Y. Tang
Department of Breast Surgery, Yunnan Cancer Hospital, Kunming, Yunnan, China

S. Liu
Department of Breast Surgery, Affiliated Hospital of Guizhou Medical University, Guiyang, Guizhou, China

Due to lymph and protein extravasation and damage to local immune response, patients with lymphedema are prone to soft tissue infection, which seriously affects the quality of life and even endangers the life of patients.

Current studies have shown that the transplantation of lymphoid tissue flap can promote the regeneration of axillary lymphatic system, the anti-inflammatory response, and anti-fibrosis response in axillary region and alleviate the progress of limb lymphedema [3–5].

Lower abdominal tissue is not only the best donor area for autologous breast reconstruction but also a common donor area for lymphoid tissue flap [6].

The most commonly used lower abdominal flaps include the perforator flap of the deep inferior epigastric artery, muscle-sparing rectus abdominis flap, and the perforator flap of the superficial epigastric artery [7].

The free DIEP flap with iliac inguinal lymphatic tissue can reconstruct the breast shape and the axillary lymphatic system altogether.

17.2 Surgical Methods

17.2.1 Flap Design

The flap is designed based on the perforator positions fixed by preoperative CTA and Doppler imaging. The flap is 1–2 cm above the umbilical level on the upper edge, as wide as up to 14 cm reaching above the anterior superior iliac spine on both sides, carrying the iliac inguinal lymphoid tissue flap on one side.

17.2.2 Receiving Area Preparation

The patients were placed in supine position. The operation was performed by two groups. One group removed the chest wall scar and prepared the skin envelope and recipient blood vessels. If the thoracodorsal vessels were chosen, the

Z. Li, D. Song (eds.), *Oncoplastic Flap Surgery*, https://doi.org/10.1007/978-981-19-8926-1_17

latissimus dorsi muscle was separated toward the midline from the lateral side, and the vascular pedicle was prepared with a sufficient length. The anterior serratus branches were cut off.

If the internal mammary vessels were chosen, the third or second rib cartilage at a length of about 2–3 cm was removed to expose the vessels.

17.2.3 Flap Raising

Another group harvested the DIEP flap with iliac inguinal lymphoid tissue. Flap raising started from the lower edge of the flap; large SIEVs that were encountered would be prepared as long as possible and carried in the flap. The iliac inguinal lymphoid tissue flap was raised in the superficial subcutaneous layer and separated from the aponeurosis surface of the external oblique muscle. The flap was then lifted from the outside to the inside toward the anterior sheath of the rectus abdominis where the perforators of the deep inferior epigastric vessels were unveiled. Cutting the anterior sheath of the rectus abdominis longitudinally lateral to the selected perforator which was retrogradely separated in the muscle till the vascular trunk was seen. The rectus abdominis was pulled medially, and the separation of the vascular pedicle was completed using rendezvous method. Now, the flap was fed by the pedicles only, when the flap was determined in good blood supply, disconnecting the vascular pedicle and transferring the flap to the chest defect (Fig. 17.1).

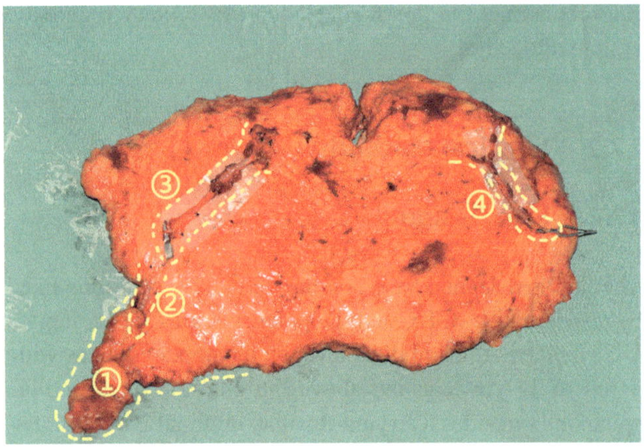

Fig. 17.1 Preparation of the perforator flap of the deep inferior epigastric artery with ilioinguinal lymphoid tissue flap was completed. (1) Ilioinguinal lymphoid tissue flap. (2) Superficial circumflex iliac vessels. (3) Left deep inferior epigastric vessels. (4) Right deep inferior epigastric vessels

17.2.4 Breast Reconstruction and Vascular Anastomosis

The flap was placed obliquely or longitudinally in the breast defect with the right side facing upward and temporarily fixed on the chest wall using 4-0 absorbable suture, placing the vascular pedicle at an appropriate position, and completing the vascular anastomosis under microscope. The deep inferior epigastric perforator vessels were anastomosed with the internal thoracic vessels or thoracodorsal vessels (Fig. 17.2). After confirming that the distal flap and the lymphatic tissue flap were in good blood supply, place the lymphatic tissue flap to cover the axillary blood vessels. De-epithelization boundary of the flap was dependent on the actual range of skin defects in the recipient area (Fig. 17.3). It should be reassured that the vascular pedicle was well placed as soon as shaping completed. Several vacuum-drainage tubes were dwelled, and the incision was closed after double checking on wound bleeding.

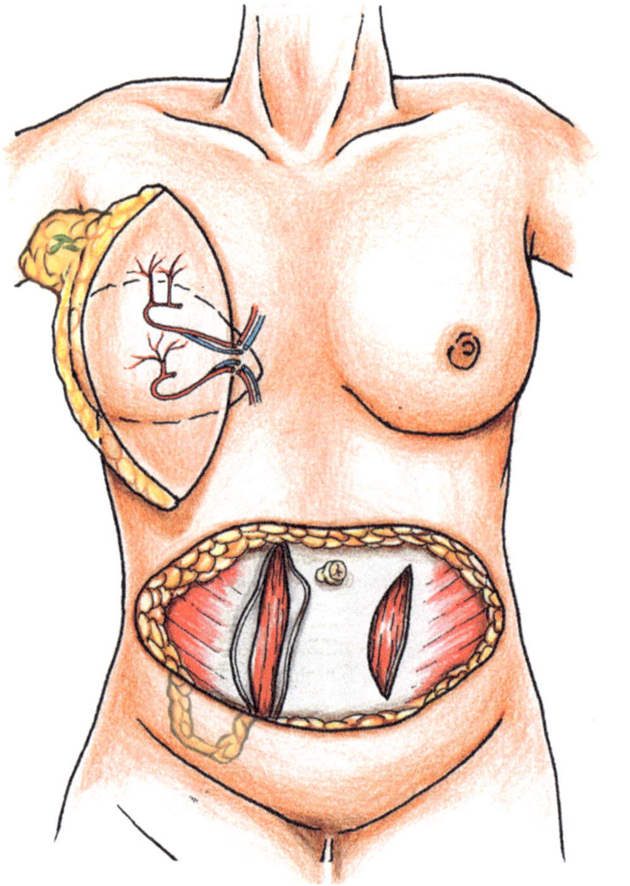

Fig. 17.2 Schematic diagram of revascularization and axillary lymphatic system reconstruction using a DIEP flap with ilioinguinal lymphoid tissue flap

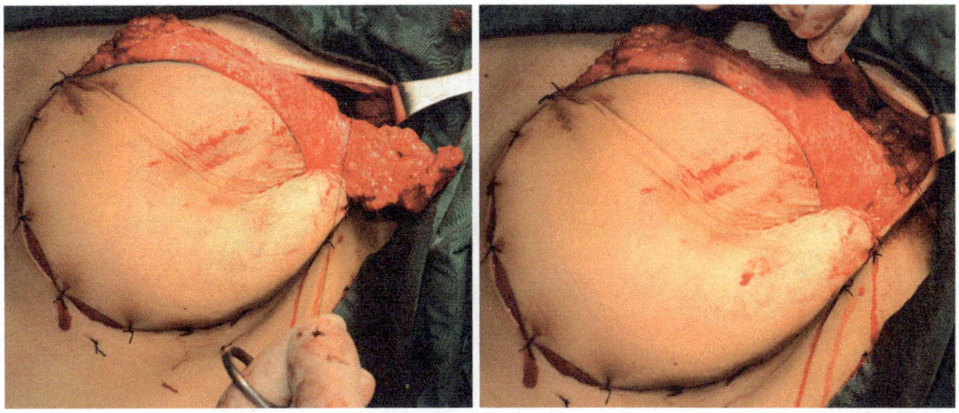

Fig. 17.3 After revascularization of the flap, the lymphoid tissue flap was placed around the axillary vascular brachial plexus

17.2.5 Postoperative Treatment

The abdomen was bandaged immediately after operation to reduce the tension of wound.

The flap was kept warm using baking lamp if necessary. The patients maintained an upright position of the upper body, and both hip joints were flexed, treated with volume expansion, analgesia, anticoagulation, antispasmodic, anti-infection, and so on.

The blood supply of the flap was observed once per hour in the initial 3 days after operation and once every 4 h from the fourth day after operation. In the case of congestion and swelling of the flap, vascular crisis was assessed and treated in time.

Patients were encouraged to carry out leg lifting and knee-ankle flexion and extension activities in bed on the third day after operation to prevent thrombosis. Patients were guided to be ambulatory 3–6 days after operation.

The color and amount of draining discharge determine the timing of tube withdrawal. Previous experimental studies proved that lymphatic tissue regeneration became mature 2–6 months after operation [8].

The patient actively exercised the affected shoulder under the guidance of physical rehabilitation therapist after operation. Compression stocking on the affected upper limb was in persistent use within 6 months after operation; afterwards, the duration of compression stocking use depends.

Case Study 1

A 50-year-old female presented for right upper limb lymphedema and neuralgia following right modified radical mastectomy for breast cancer 2 years before.

At admission, the circumferential diameter of the affected limb was measured, which was 3.5 cm and 8 cm larger than the opposite at 10 cm above and below the elbow. A DIEP flap carrying an ilioinguinal lymphatic tissue flap was used to reconstruct the breast shape and right axillary lymphatic system (Fig. 17.4).

The operation was performed by two groups. One group removed the chest wall scar and separated the skin envelope, cutting the third costal cartilage at a length of 2.5 cm near the right sternum the perichondrium and intercostal muscle and preparing the internal thoracic vessels.

A bipedicled DIEP flap carrying the right ilioinguinal lymphatic tissue flap was harvested. The flap was 28.0 cm × 13.0 cm in size and 3.8 cm in thickness. The length of left and right vascular pedicles were 9.8 cm and 10.2 cm, and the vessel diameters on each side were 2.1 mm and 2.2 mm, respectively.

The weight of the flap was 395 g. When it was determined that the blood supply of the flap and lymphatic tissue flap was good, the flap was transferred to repair the breast defect. The two vascular pedicles of the flap were anastomosed with the proximal and distal ends of the right internal mammary vessels (A: $V = 1:1$). The blood supply of the flap was good. The lymphatic tissue flap was placed around the axillary vessels and sutured for immobilization. Three vacuum-drainage tubes were dwelled, and the flap donor area was closed without tension.

The patient recovered uneventfully. At 9 months of follow-up, the appearance and function of the abdominal donor area were good; only linear scar was found. The reconstructed breast shape was satisfactory. After 6 months of postoperative rehabilitation treatment, the circumferential diameter of the affected limb was measured, which was equal to that at 10 cm above the elbow and 1 cm smaller at 10 cm below the elbow than the opposite upper limb (Figs. 17.4, 17.5, 17.6, 17.7, 17.8, 17.9, 17.10, 17.11, 17.12, 17.13, 17.14, and 17.15).

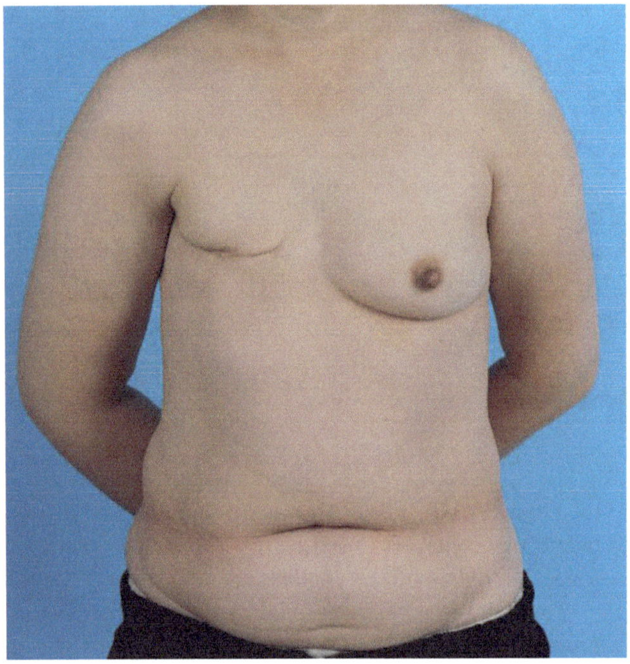

Fig. 17.4 Preoperative findings

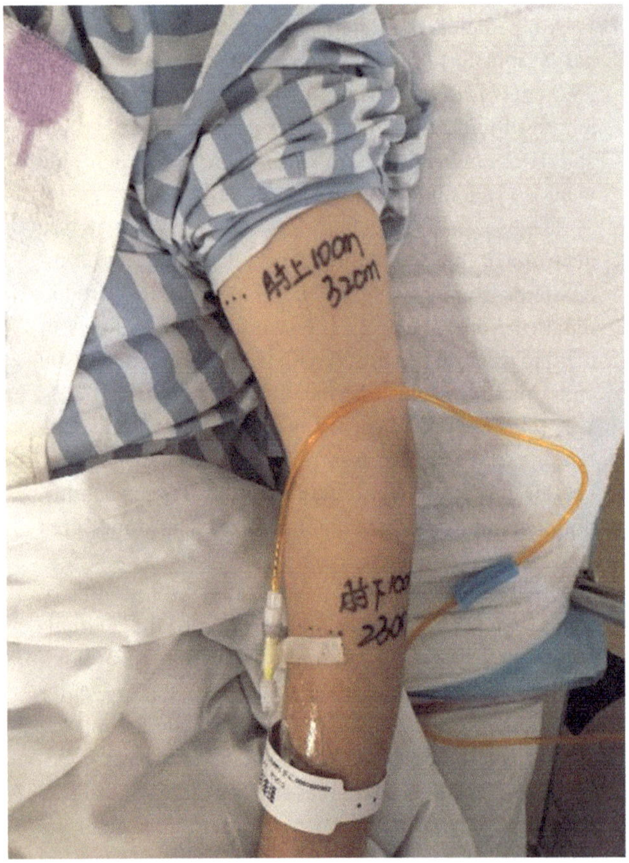

Fig. 17.5 Preoperative measurement of the circumference of the unaffected upper limb

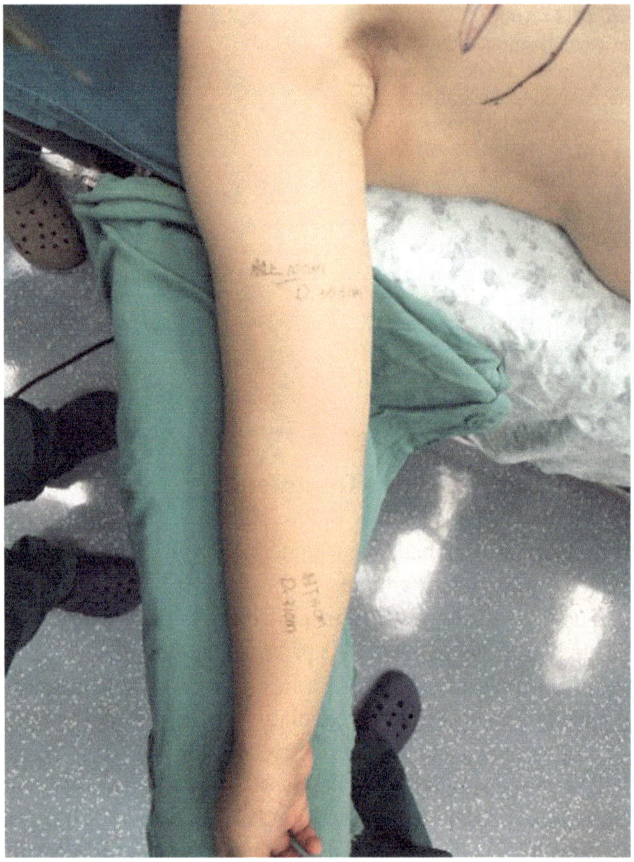

Fig. 17.6 Measuring the circumferential diameter of the affected upper limb before operation

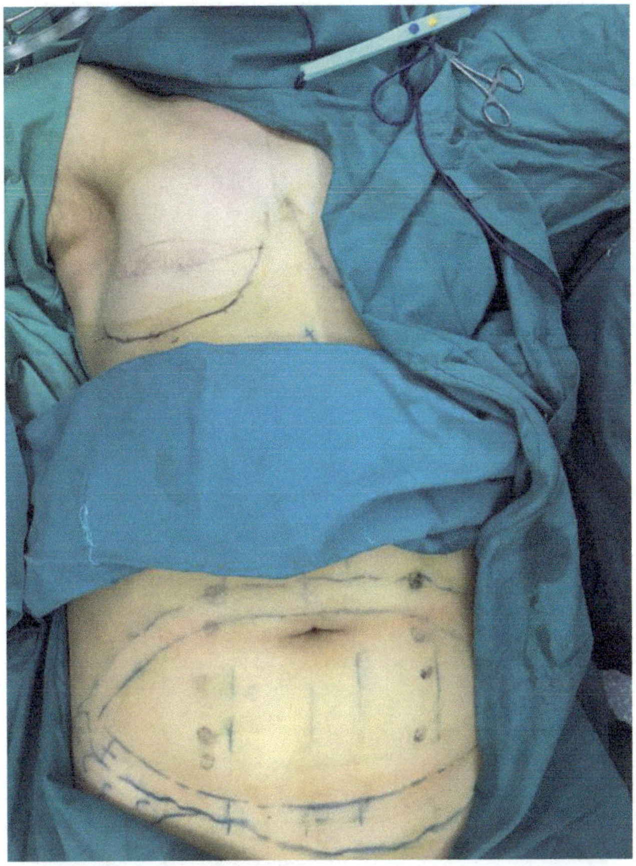

Fig. 17.7 Intraoperative design

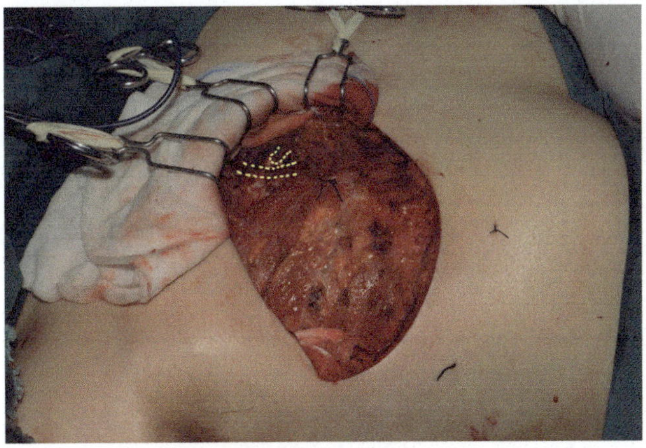

Fig. 17.8 Preparation of the right internal mammary vessels

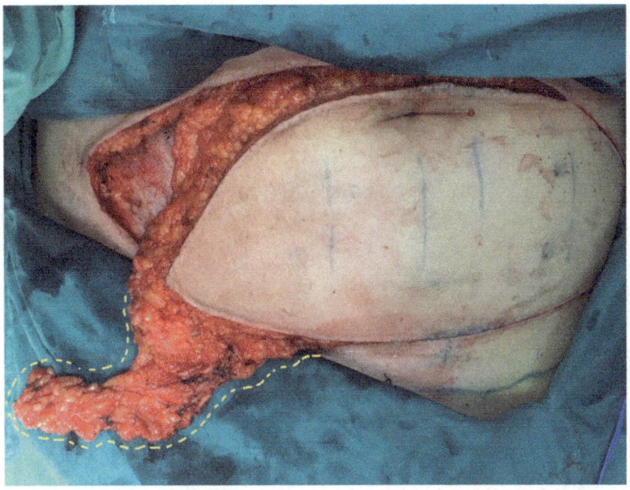

Fig. 17.9 Harvesting the right ilioinguinal lymphatic tissue flap

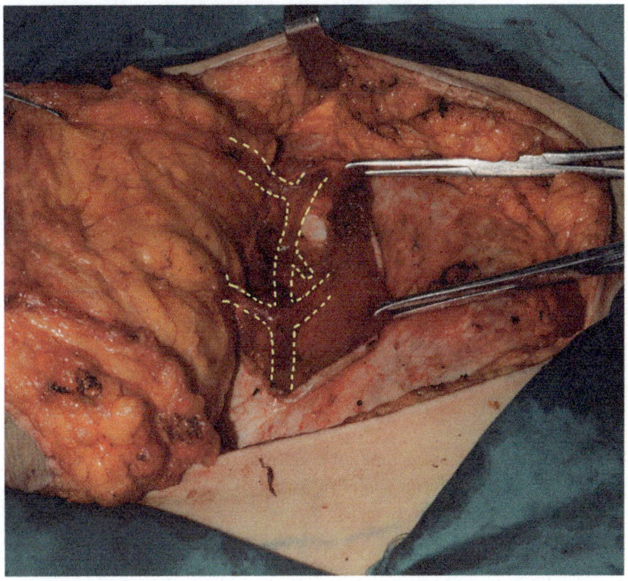

Fig. 17.10 Separating the left deep inferior epigastric vascular pedicle and perforator

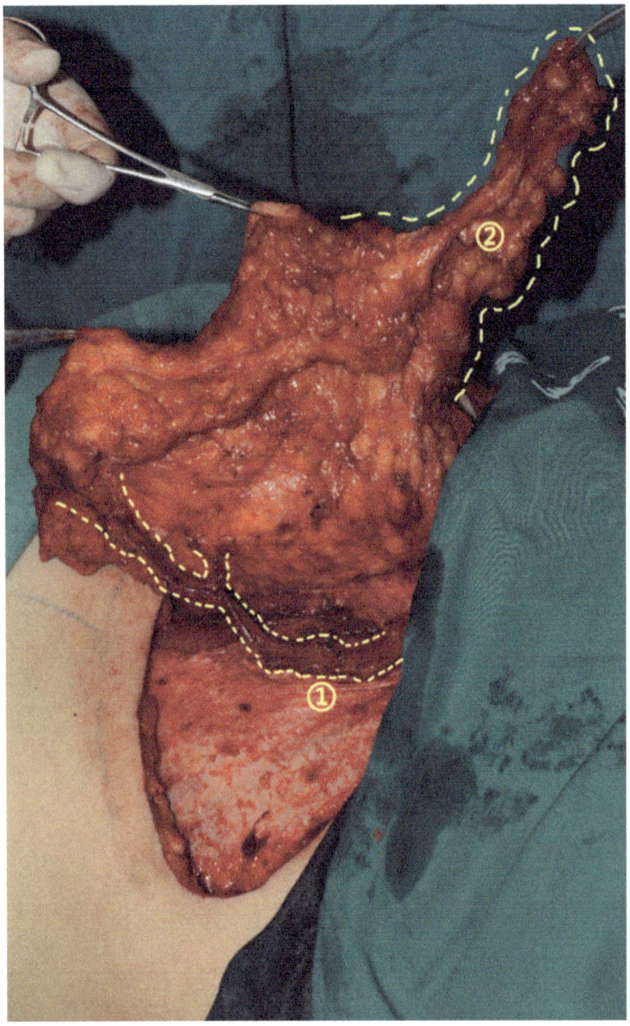

Fig. 17.11 The right deep inferior epigastric vessels and perforator were prepared. (1) Deep inferior epigastric vessels. (2) Lymphatic tissue flap

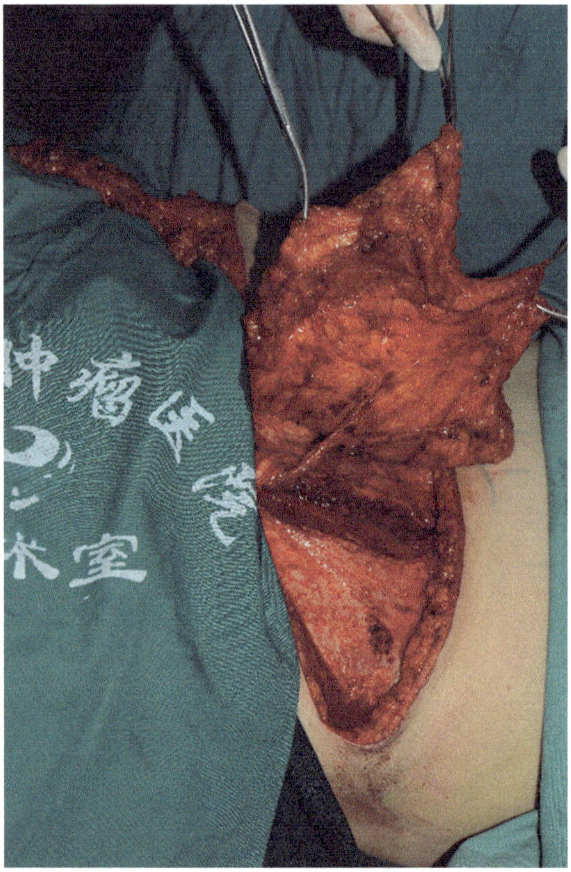

Fig. 17.12 A bipedicled DIEP flap with right ilioinguinal lymphatic tissue flap was harvested

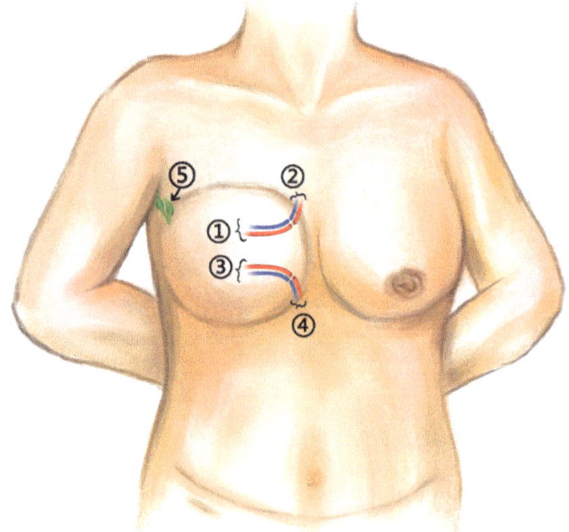

Fig. 17.13 Placement of the lymphatic tissue flap and revascularization pattern. The right deep inferior epigastric artery and vein were anastomosed with the proximal ends of the right internal thoracic artery and vein (1A1V), the left deep inferior epigastric artery and vein were anastomosed with the distal ends of the right internal thoracic artery and vein (1A1V), and the right lymphatic tissue flap was transplanted into the right axilla. (1) Right deep inferior epigastric vessels. (2) Proximal internal mammary vessels. (3) Left deep inferior epigastric vessels. (4) Distal internal mammary vessels. (5) Lymphatic tissue flap

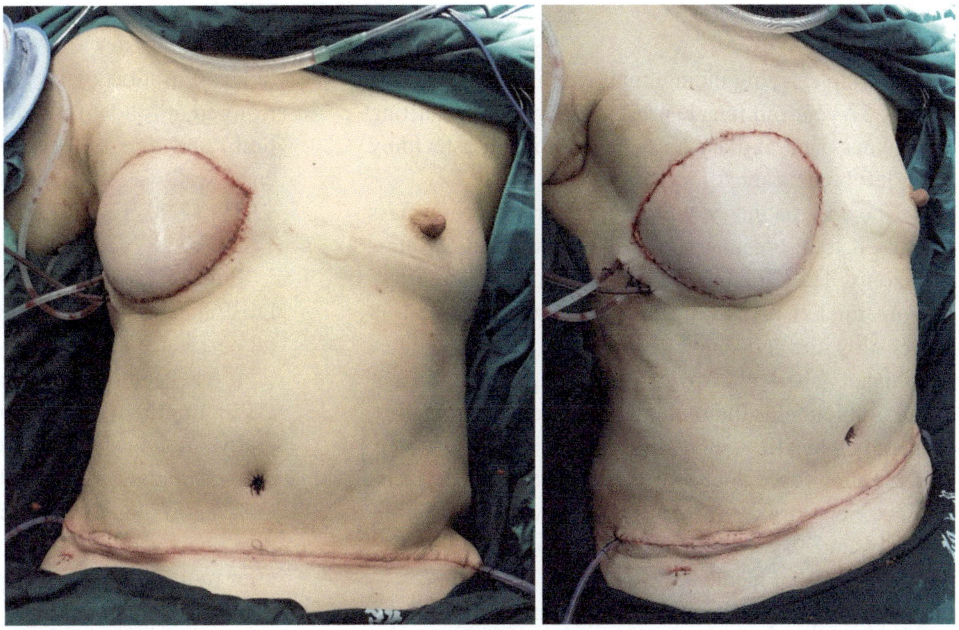

Fig. 17.14 Intraoperative view immediately after reconstruction

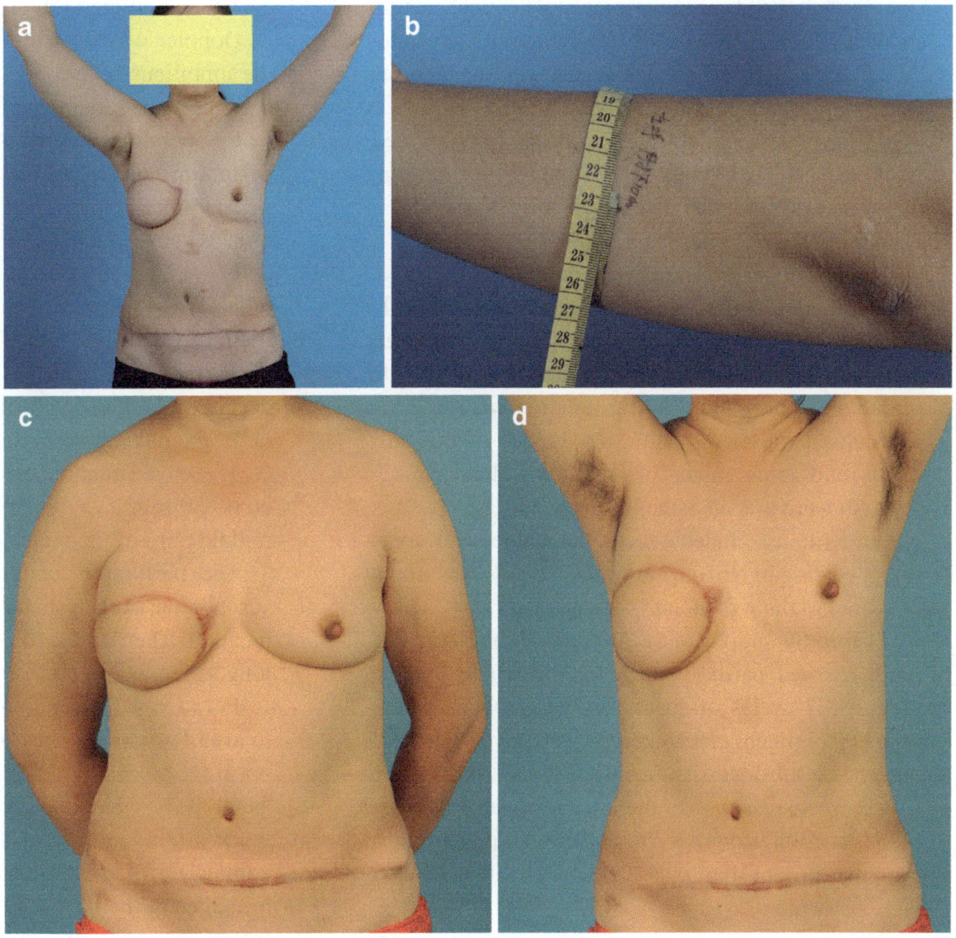

Fig. 17.15 (**a**) The reconstructed breast appearance and upper limb function at follow-up of 3 months after operation. (**b**) The arm circumference of the affected limb decreased significantly 6 months after operation. (**c**, **d**) At follow-up of 12 months, the function of the affected limb was significantly improved, and the bilateral arm circumference was almost the same

Case Study 2

DIEP flap carrying ilioinguinal lymphatic tissue flap.

A 57-year-old female presented for shoulder lifting weakness and axillary ulcer after radical mastectomy for left breast cancer 13 years before.

She was diagnosed with left axillary ulcerous mass and left total brachial plexus injury after radical mastectomy. The patient received modified radical mastectomy for left breast cancer in 2002 and weakness in elevating the left shoulder followed. She was given adjuvant chemotherapy with cyclophosphamide + doxorubicin plus fluorouracil (CAF) regime and radiotherapy when the axillary ulcer occurred and persisted. The patient once applied herbal medicine on the ulcer. Since February 2014, the ulcer has worsened significantly and exacerbated after external application of Chinese herbal medicine.

Pathological examination on tumor excision biopsy diagnosed as high-grade spindle cell malignant tumor of the left chest wall, i.e., squamous cell metaplasia carcinoma, based on immunohistochemical results showed ER (−), PR (−), HER-2 (−), and Ki67 index (about 45%). On physical examination, an ulcerous and bumpy mass in size of about 5 cm × 4 cm was found in the left axilla; it was hard and immobilized. As wide as about 15 cm × 10 cm, redness surrounding the mass was also seen. No significance was found in examining the right breast and armpit.

The left upper limb was with pitting edema (grade 3), and the left shoulder was too weak to elevate. The elbow wrist joint was active, extension of each finger joint was limited, finger flexion function was OK, the thumb abduction and palming function were OK, the left deltoid muscle strength was graded 4, the teres major and teres minor of latissimus dorsi muscle strength were graded 5, the biceps brachii triceps muscle strength was graded 4+, and the whole hand sensation decreased. No obvious abnormality was found proximal to the wrist joint.

Electromyography of the left upper limb (local hospital) showed partial damage of the whole brachial plexus. Six cycles of docetaxel and carboplatin regimen (TP regimen) chemotherapy were given. The axillary tumor subsided significantly.

Complete resection of the left chest wall lesion and reconstruction using free DIEP flap with iliac inguinal lymphatic tissue flap plus brachial plexus neurolysis were performed.

The patient recovered well after operation. The shoulder joint continued to adduct and compress the flap, resulting in local necrosis which was repaired by local flap transfer with satisfactory outcome. The functional sensation of the left upper limb was partially restored at follow-up. Edema receded in the left upper limb, and the sensory function of the reconstructed chest wall was satisfactory (Figs. 17.16, 17.17, 17.18, 17.19, 17.20, 17.21, 17.22, 17.23, 17.24, 17.25, 17.26, 17.27, 17.28, 17.29, 17.30, and 17.31).

Preoperative imaging was used in the design of DIEP flap similar to designing the anterolateral femoral perforator flap.

It has been reported that results based on practical CT angiography have a good correlation with intraoperative findings [9]. Blondeel et al. preferred the use of color Doppler scanning [10]. We usually utilize both CTA and color Doppler in patients undergoing complex chest wall defect repair and breast reconstruction after multiple chemotherapy to reduce the risk of surgery and complications.

The patient was in supine position, and the whole abdomen was disinfected including the bilateral low costal arch, bilateral thighs, and the perineum.

Doppler was used to locate the perforators around the umbilicus before operation, which was helpful to determine the reliable perforators.

Preoperative imaging is important to ensure that the perforators are in the center of the flap particularly when a small flap is raised. It is not necessary to determine whether the deep inferior epigastric artery exists before operation because its anatomical existence is relatively constant.

Because the position of the flap completely depends on the position of the selected perforators, the final design of the flap can be determined only after finding large and pulsing perforators.

The most suitable perforators can usually be found at 10–30 mm away from the umbilicus medial to the middle third of the rectus abdominis.

The perforators support the dense subcutaneous vascular network systems which are mutually communicating. The flap can be designed in any direction as long as it contains a large periumbilical perforator.

For safety, the range of the flap should not extend to area IV which is beyond the contralateral semilunar line. A unilateral flap can be oblique and reaches as far as the rib edge. The subcutaneous vascular network orients mainly at an angle of 45° to the horizontal level. Densely distributing perforating branches of the deep inferior epigastric artery can be found around the umbilicus. Therefore, the oblique design of the flap around the umbilicus is the most reliable.

The skin of the flap was cut till the anterior sheath of rectus abdominis and at least one perforator were included in the flap according to the results of preoperative Doppler detection.

The medial edge of the flap is located in the midline, and the lateral end of the flap can reach the costal arch.

Starting from the lateral edge, the flap was raised from the fascia and separated toward the semilunar line.

The first perforator can be found within a few centimeters from the semilunar line and assessed by its diameter and pulsation.

The second large perforator near the umbilicus was found as flap raising continued. The flap was designed based on these two perforators.

Experience summary: (1) Anatomical essentials of the brachial plexus. (2) The lesion resection was very complex requiring multidisciplinary cooperation (thoracic surgery, orthopedics, oncoplastic surgery, microsurgery).

The application of skin grafting highlighted the importance of supporting structures. The reason for partial necrosis of the flap above the axilla was that the flap was compressed due to the absence of supporting structure on the shoulder.

Herein the injury of abdominal donor area was minimized, that is, retracting the rectus abdominis fibers to both sides through the incision on the surface of the perforating vessels, and retrogradely separating the vascular pedicle till obtaining a sufficient length instead of widely cutting of the lateral rectus abdominis, so as to preserve the integrity of the anterior sheath of the rectus abdominis to the greatest extent.

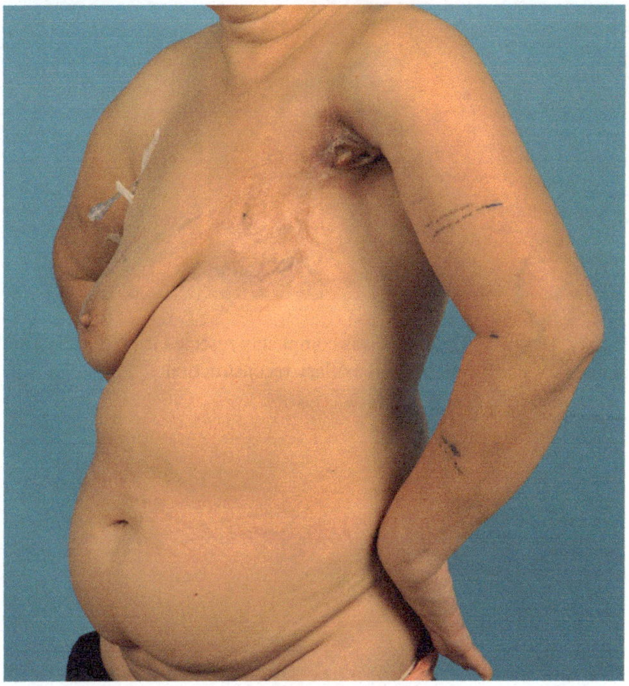

Fig. 17.16 Preoperative findings

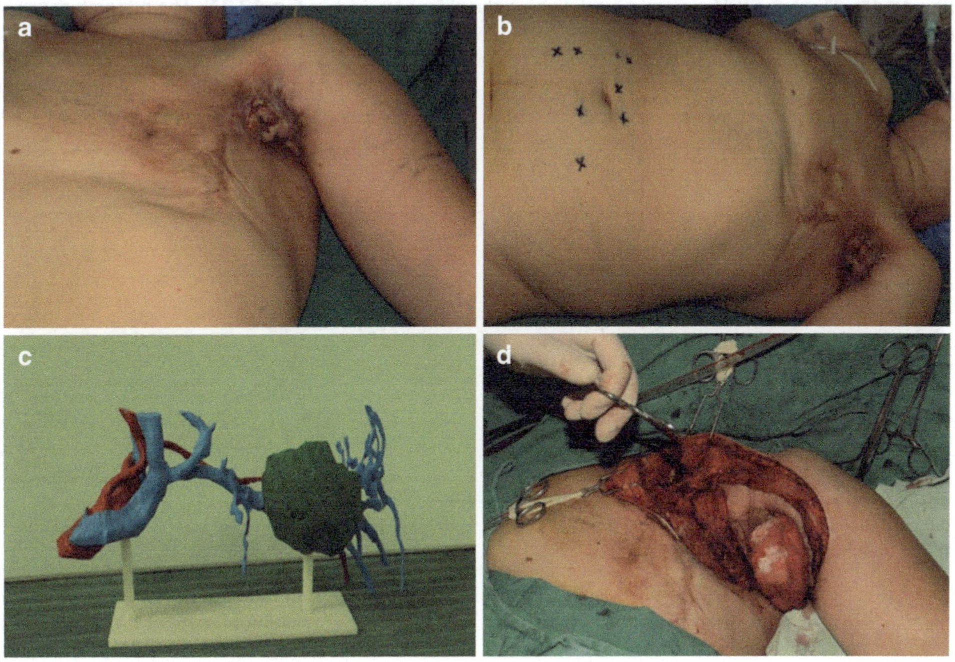

Fig. 17.17 (**a**) Patient positioning. (**b**) Perforator location based on CTA. (**c**) Three-dimensional printing model based on CTA on the left upper limb. (**d**) Complete resection of the tumor, releasing the brachial plexus and axillary artery and vein

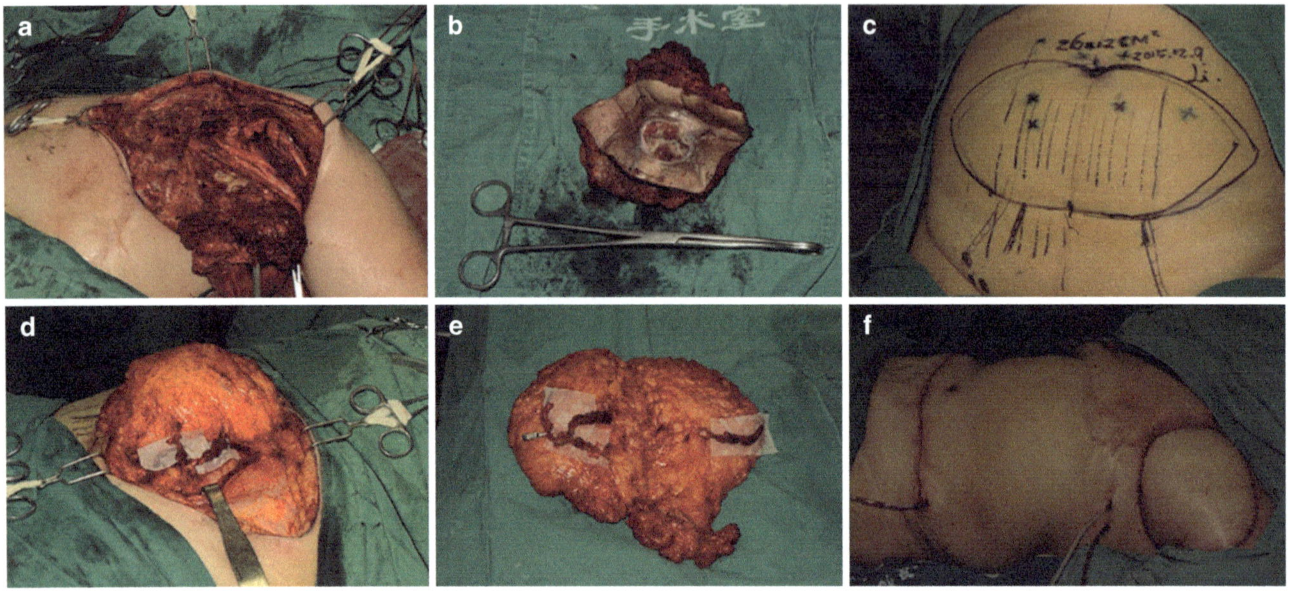

Fig. 17.18 (a–f) The lesion was completely resected from the chest wall. A free DIEP flap with the right inguinal lymphatic tissue flap was transplanted for chest wall and left axillary reconstruction

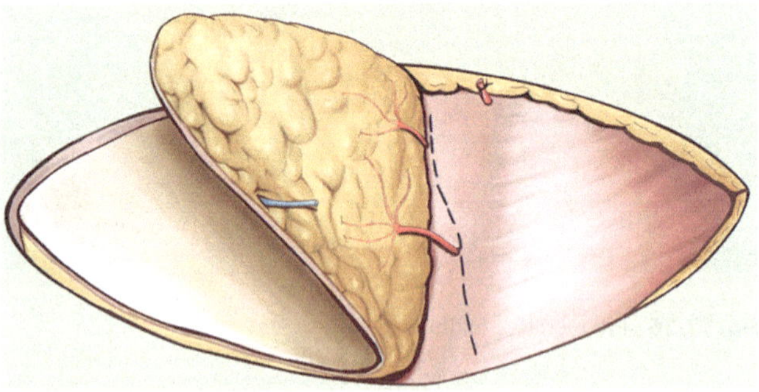

Fig. 17.19 The left SIEV was preserved, cutting the skin edge in a circular way and revealing two perforators on the left, of which the superior one was marginal and hence given up

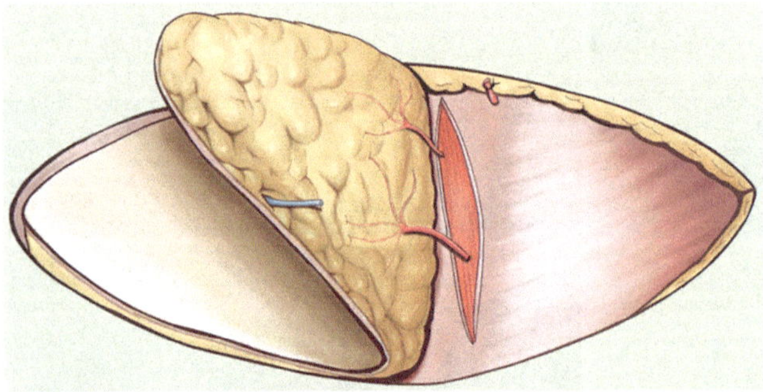

Fig. 17.20 Longitudinally incising the anterior sheath at the outer edge of the perforators and displaying the relationship of the two perforators and the muscle

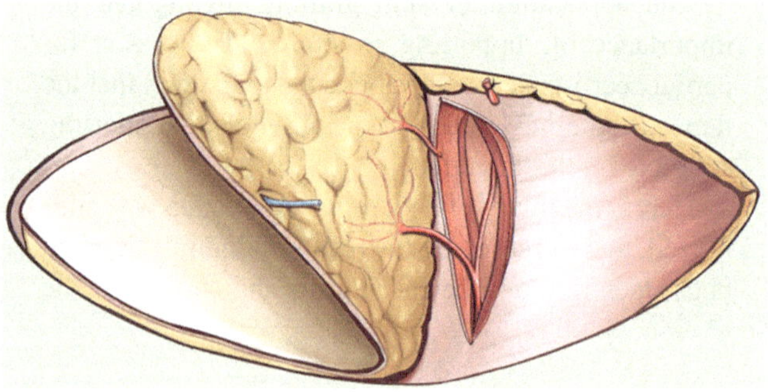

Fig. 17.21 The perforators were separated toward the vascular trunk, and the muscle was longitudinally opened, carefully lifting the flap to fully expose the anterior sheath of rectus abdominis for further dissection of blood vessels. In slim patients, the deep inferior epigastric blood vessels are faintly visible when the flap is slightly lifted upward

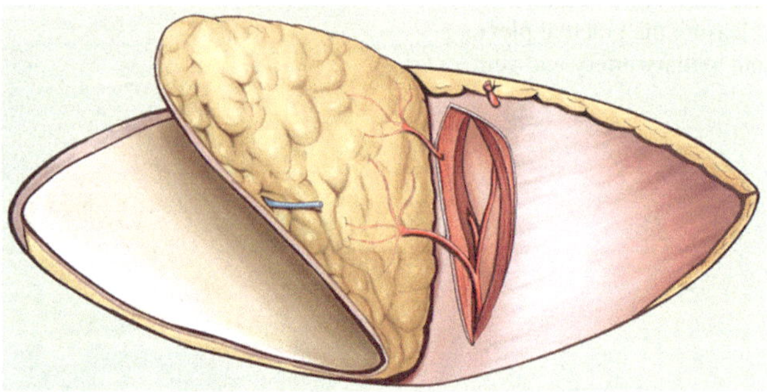

Fig. 17.22 The vascular pedicle was found to run outward on antero-grade separation and not to continue with the perforators in retrograde muscle separation along the perforating branch. Carefully dissect the anterior sheath of the rectus abdominis around the first perforator, cutting off the accompanying sensory nerve

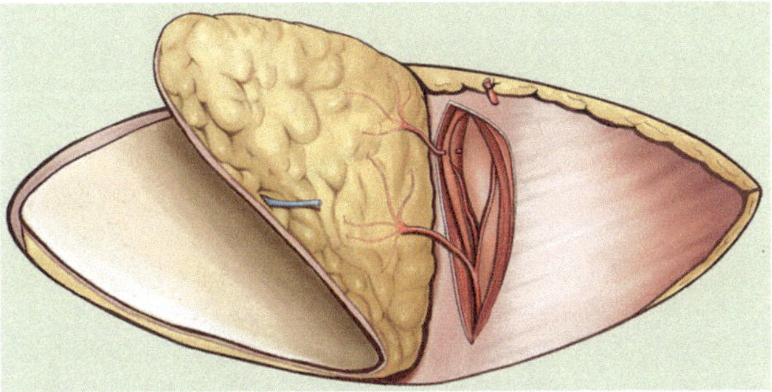

Fig. 17.23 The vascular pedicle was explored in the muscle far from the lower perforating branch and found to bifurcate a large medial perforator to the medial side of the muscle. Open the fascia around the second perforating branch, bluntly separating muscle fibers and exposing the deep inferior epigastric vessels

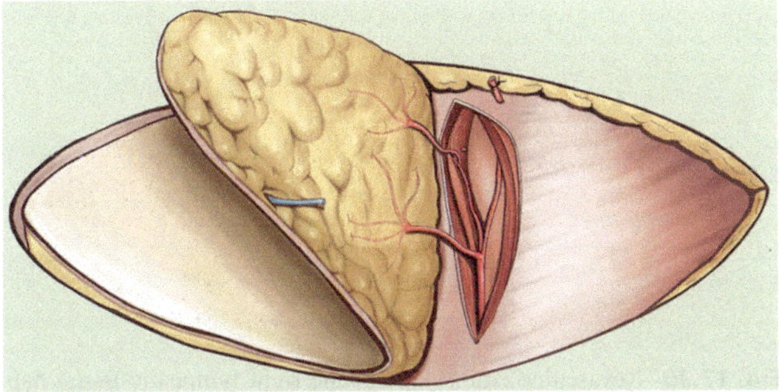

Fig. 17.24 It was determined that the middle perforator and the lower perforator shared a common vascular trunk, yet they were far from each other horizontally resulting in cutting off the muscle fibers in between. Dissection of the deep inferior epigastric blood vessels in a circle pattern and a suspending ring was placed around the vascular pedicle. The collateral vessels of rectus abdominis were ligated and severed. The deep inferior epigastric vessels were dissected caudally by blunt separation of the muscle. The posterior sheath of the rectus abdominis was not damaged

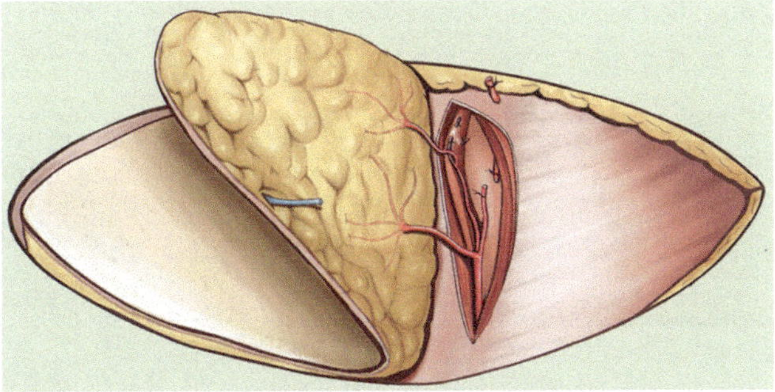

Fig. 17.25 The medial branch was separated till the level of the middle perforator, where they were found to not be continuous

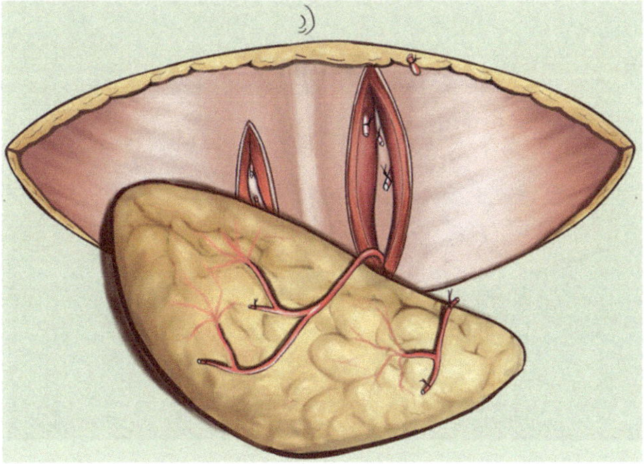

Fig. 17.26 Further separating the medial perforator. It was initially thought that its intramuscular segment of the middle perforator was straight which was later found to be the intercostal nerve branch and its nutrient vessels crossing with the perforator. The nerve and its feeding vessels were cut off, and the intramuscular segment of the perforator was determined to travel toward the midline and converge into the medial branch

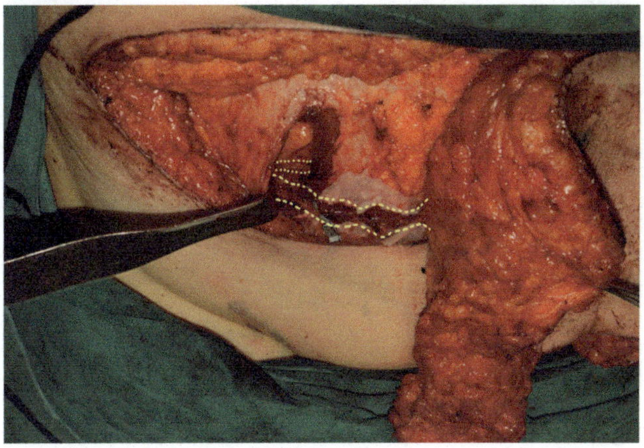

Fig. 17.27 Depending on the desired pedicle length, the deep inferior epigastric vessels were separated retrogradely where they originated from the external iliac artery without further incision of the abdominal skin

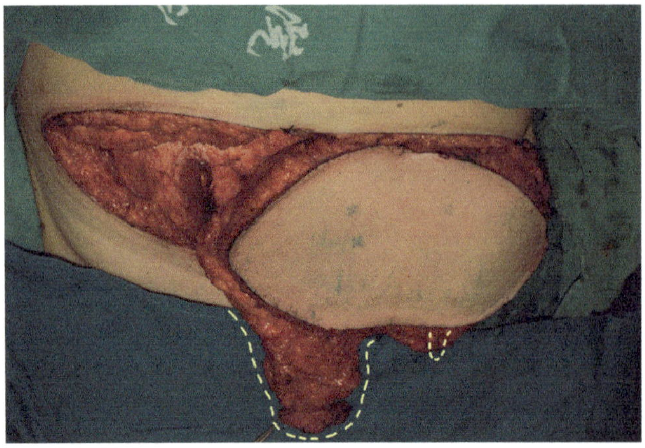

Fig. 17.28 Ligating the deep inferior epigastric vascular pedicle proximal to the perforator and providing blood supply to the flap by the distal end of the pedicle

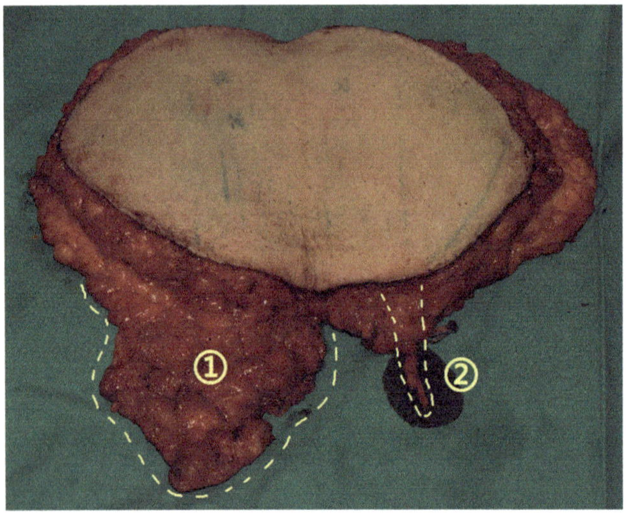

Fig. 17.29 The DIEP flap was prepared. If necessary, the flap can be thinned by removing excess adipose tissue, leaving only the tissue around the subcutaneous vascular plexus and perforating branches. The distal part of the right flap carried some inguinal lymph nodes in order to further reduce the edema of the left upper limb. Suture the rectus abdominis, indwelling drainage tubes, and closing anterior sheath of rectus abdominis. Finally, close the skin. (1) Lymphatic tissue flap; (2) SIEV

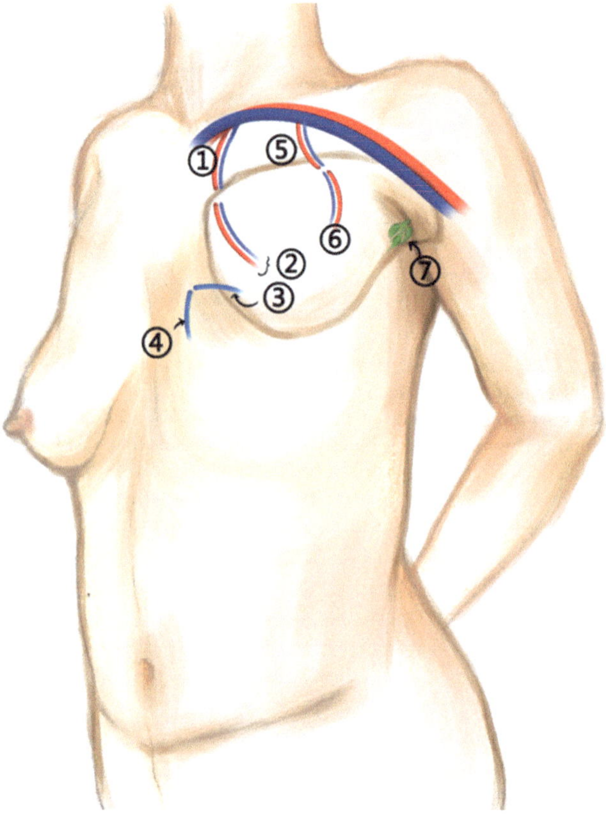

Fig. 17.30 Revascularization pattern: the right lymphatic tissue flap was placed in the left armpit, the right deep inferior epigastric vessels were anastomosed with the left thoracoacromial blood vessels, the left deep inferior epigastric vessels were anastomosed with the proximal ends of the left internal mammary blood vessels, and the left SIEV was anastomosed with the distal end of the left internal mammary vein. (1) Internal mammary vessels. (2) Left deep inferior epigastric vessels. (3) SIEV. (4) Distal internal thoracic vein. (5) Thoracic acromial vessels. (6) Right deep inferior epigastric vessels. (7) Lymphatic tissue flap

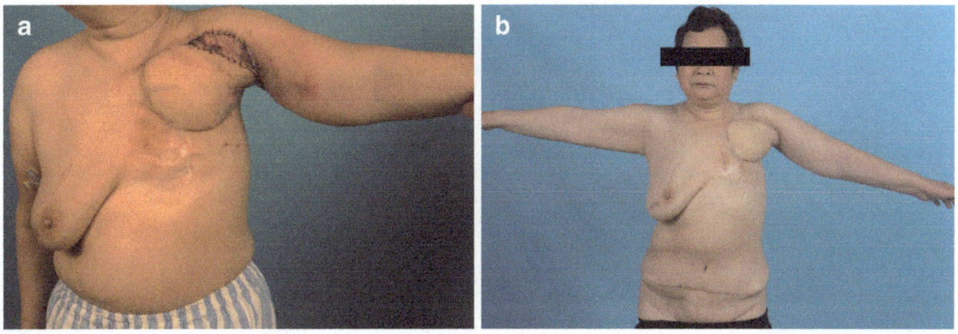

Fig. 17.31 (**a**) Half a month after operation. (**b**) Two years at follow-up. There was no recurrence of tumor and no obvious edema of upper limb, and the function was significantly improved

Case Study 3

DIEP flap with ilio-inguinal lymphatic tissue flap.

A 39-year-old female presented for local recurrence with the right breast skin extensively invaded after breast-conserving surgery, adjuvant chemotherapy, and radiotherapy 7 years ago. Right radical mastectomy plus reconstruction using free bipedicled DIEP flap was performed after admission.

The internal mammary vessels at a length of 1 cm between the second and third ribs, one set of the lateral thoracic vessels at a length of 2 cm, and a lateral thoracic venous branch of the axillary vein at a length of 2 cm were reserved.

A perforator flap pedicled with bilateral deep inferior epigastric arteries was prepared.

The right deep inferior epigastric artery and vein were anastomosed with the right lateral thoracic artery and vein (1A2V), and the left deep inferior epigastric artery and vein were anastomosed with the right internal thoracic artery and vein (1A1V).

Postoperative pathological examination: (1) (Right breast) fibrous tissue hyperplasia and degenerative cancerous nests were observed which was induced by chemotherapy (pathology remission grade 1a). (2) Cancer invasion was found in the papillary stroma, adipose tissue, and dermis; margins were clear of tumor. (3) (Right axillary) no cancer metastasis was found in lymph nodes 0/1.

Immunohistochemistry: ER (about 70%, medium, strong), PR (about 1%, strong), CerbB-2 (2 +), and Ki-67 about 20%.

The patient recovered well after operation, and the flap survived completely. The functional and sensory recovery of the right upper limb was satisfactory at follow-up, there was no obvious edema of the right upper limb, and the sensory function of the reconstructed chest wall was satisfactory (Figs. 17.32, 17.33, 17.34, 17.35, 17.36, 17.37, 17.38, 17.39, 17.40, 17.41, and 17.42).

Key points of operation: flap harvest methods minimizing abdominal donor site injury to the greatest extent have been previously described. Briefly, when revealing and separating the vascular pedicle, the rectus abdominis fibers should retracted to each side instead of being widely disconnected, so as to preserve the integrity of the anterior sheath of the rectus abdominis to the greatest extent.

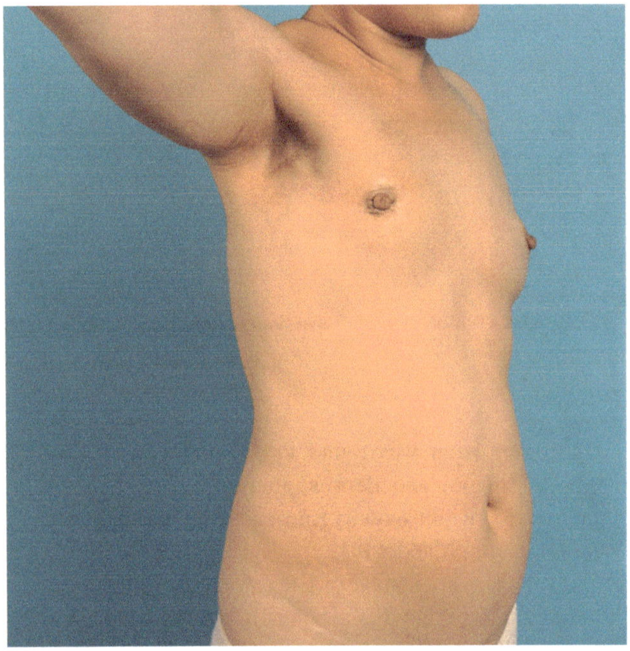

Fig. 17.32 Preoperative findings

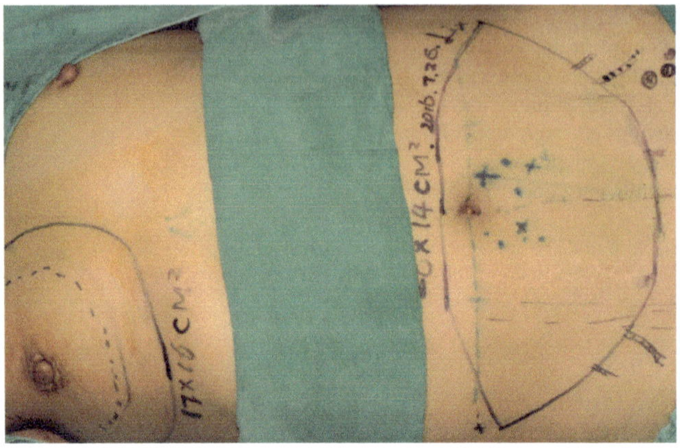

Fig. 17.33 Intraoperative design

Fig. 17.34 The tumor was removed according to "no touch" principle

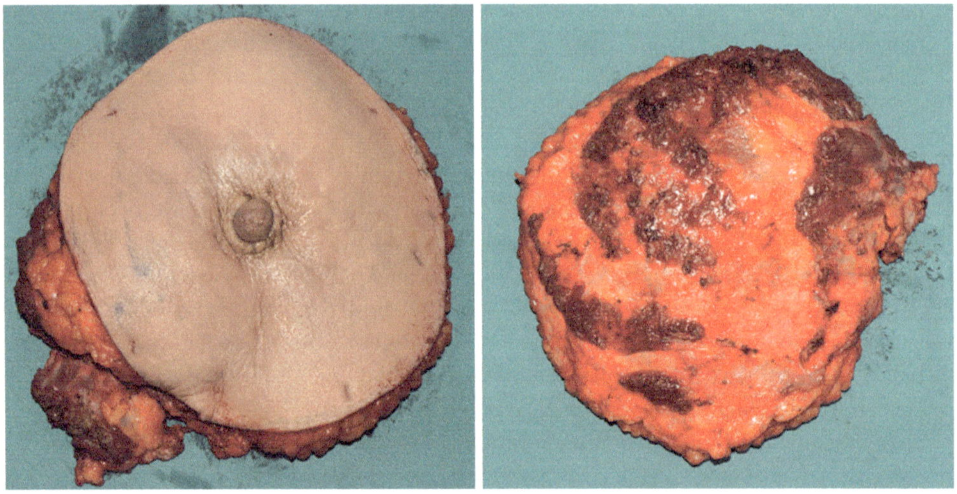

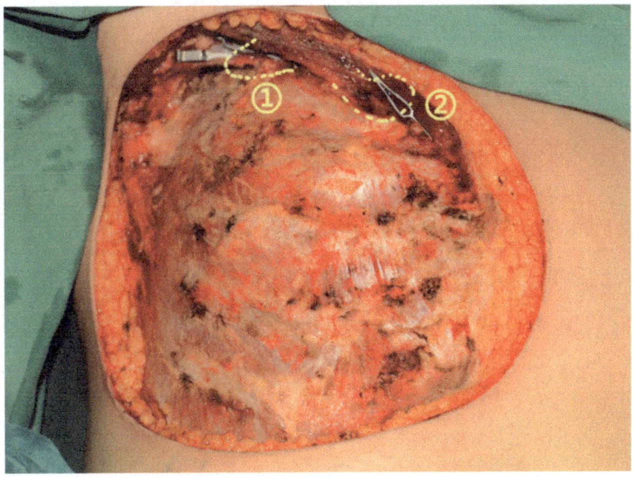

Fig. 17.35 Extensive skin and soft tissue defects were left on the chest wall, and the thoracoacromial vessels, internal mammary vessels, and lateral thoracic vessels were retained as the recipient vessels

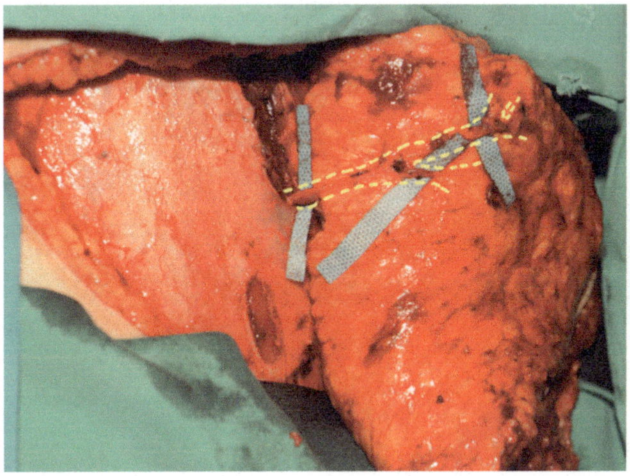

Fig. 17.37 The perforating vessels were retrogradely separated till the vascular trunk using a modified method

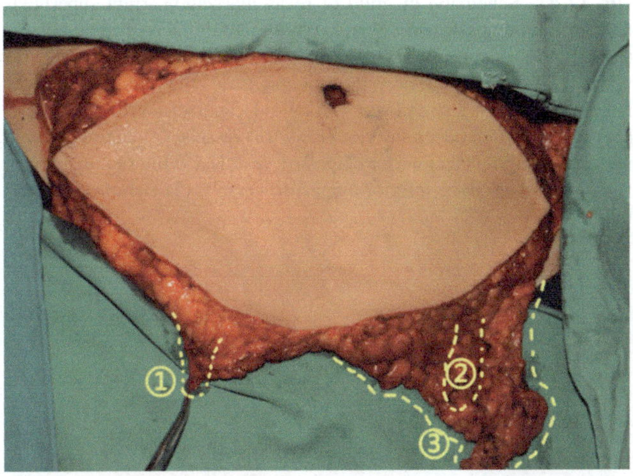

Fig. 17.36 The margins of the flap were completely cut, carrying the left SIEV and the right inferior superficial epigastric artery and vein. The left iliac inguinal lymphatic tissue flap was also harvested. (1) Superficial deep inferior epigastric artery and vein; (2) left SIEV; (3) left ilioinguinal lymphatic tissue flap

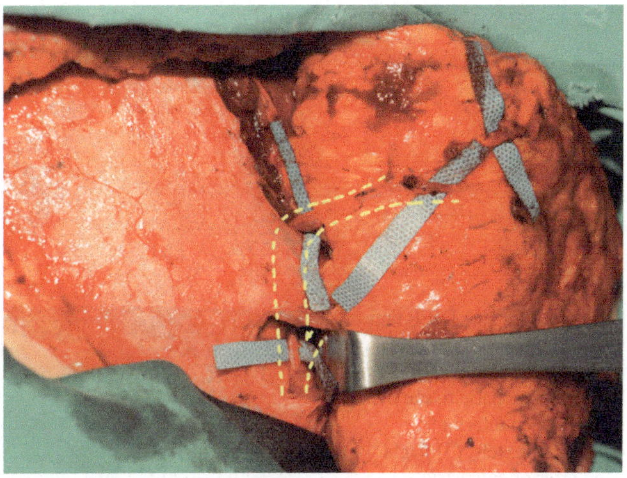

Fig. 17.38 Making an auxiliary incision on the lateral edge of the anterior sheath, retracting the rectus abdominis to expose the proximal end of the vascular trunk. Separation of the vascular pedicle was completed beneath the rectus abdominis using rendezvous method

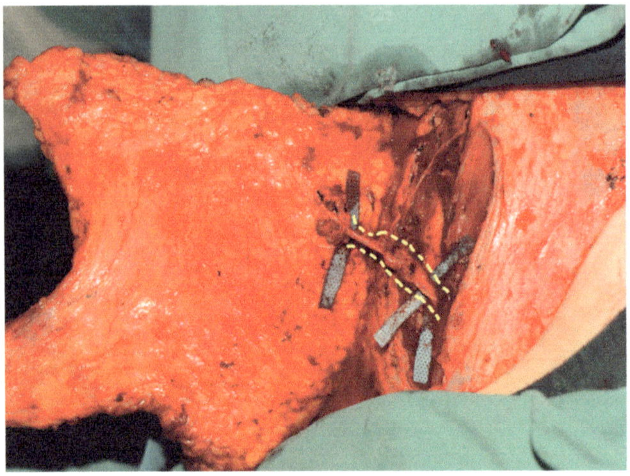

Fig. 17.39 The perforating branch and vascular pedicle were exposed and separated by the modified method to preserve the integrity of the rectus abdominis and anterior sheath to the greatest extent. The perforating branch and vascular pedicle of the left deep inferior epigastric artery were separated retrogradely in the muscle

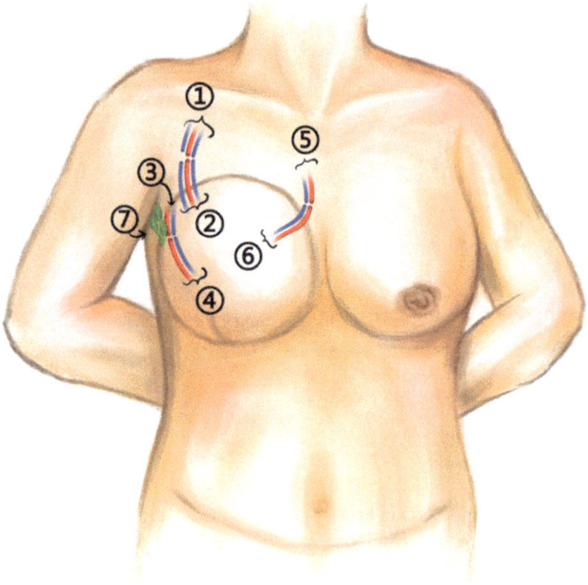

Fig. 17.41 Schematic diagram of revascularization: right superficial deep inferior epigastric artery and vein to right thoracoacromial vessels (1A2V); right deep inferior epigastric vessels + right lateral thoracic vessels (1A1V), and left deep inferior epigastric artery and vein to right internal thoracic artery and vein (1A1V). (1) Thoracic acromial vessels. (2) right superficial deep inferior epigastric vessels. (3) lateral thoracic vessels. (4) right deep inferior epigastric vessels. (5) Internal mammary vessels. (6) Left deep inferior epigastric vessels. (7) Lymphatic tissue flap

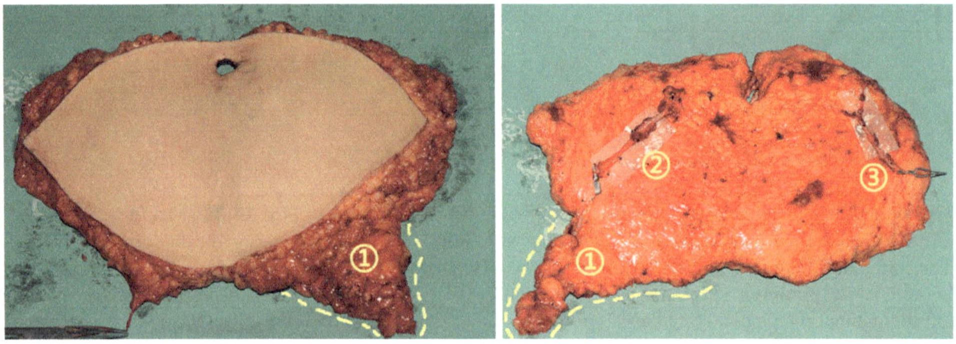

Fig. 17.40 A free DIEP flap with left inguinal lymphatic tissue flap was prepared. (1) Inguinal lymphatic tissue flap. (2) Left deep inferior epigastric vessels. (3) Right deep inferior epigastric vessels

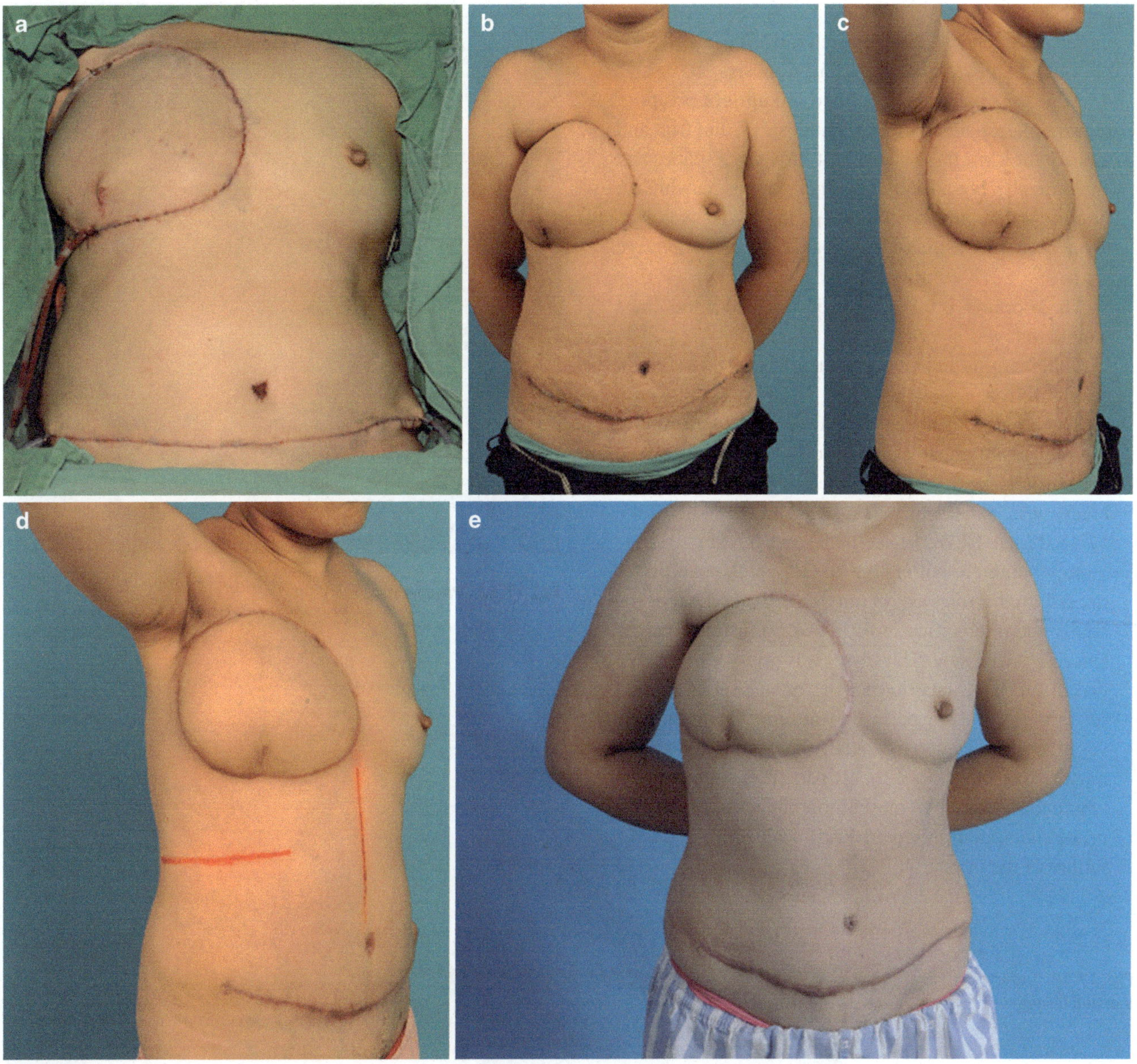

Fig. 17.42 (**a**) Intraoperative view immediately after operation. (**b**) Appearance 2 months after operation. (**c**) Follow up at 6 months after operation. (**d**) 12 months of follow-up. (**e**) 18 months of follow-up

Case Study 4

Breast reconstruction with free DIEP flap with iliac inguinal lymphatic tissue flap using the distal end of internal thoracic vessels and lateral thoracic vessels as recipient vessels.

The patient was a 37-year-old female admitted for left breast cancer (cT2N2M0, stage IIIA), Immunohistochemistry results were ER (−), PR (−), CerbB-2 (1+), and Ki-67 40%. The tumor was downstaged to cT1N0M0, stage I after neoadjuvant chemotherapy using EC followed by T regime.

Left modified radical mastectomy plus free bilateral pedicled DIEP flap transplantation for breast reconstruction was then performed. The left second and third ribs were partially removed; the left internal thoracic vessels and lateral thoracic vessels were prepared.

The removed breast tissue weighed 710 g. The free bipedicled DIEP flap with inguinal lymphatic tissue flap was 30 cm × 12 cm in size and weighed 770 g.

The two deep inferior epigastric vessels were end-to-end anastomosed with the proximal ends of the left internal thoracic artery and vein (1A1V) and the lateral thoracic vessels (1A1V), respectively. The blood supply of the flap was good after anastomosis.

Adjust the patient's upper body to upright position; remove marginal flap tissue on both sides; and trim and modify the skin flap according to the size, shape, and anatomical boundary of the opposite breast. Intermittent fixation of the deep flap tissue was performed to reconstruct the subaxillary and cleavage shape.

Three drainage tubes were placed under the chest wound that was closed layer by layer.

Skin margins and the subareolar tissue were clear of tumor on frozen section.

The breast and axillary adipose tissue were sent to routine pathological examination. The flap survived uneventfully, and the appearance of the reconstructed breast was satisfactory (Figs. 17.43, 17.44, 17.45, 17.46, 17.47, 17.48, 17.49, 17.50, and 17.51).

Key points for cutting the DIEP flap: the two perforators initially traveled obliquely on the surface of the rectus abdominis muscle for a certain distance before entering the muscle. The vessel was pretty thin when it was distal to the superior perforator, and the main vessel ran a long distance in the muscle. Separating the vascular pedicle deep beneath the rectus abdominis muscle was the most difficult part in raising the flap, where there were two muscular branches and inappropriate manipulation would lead to bleeding and even failure of the operation.

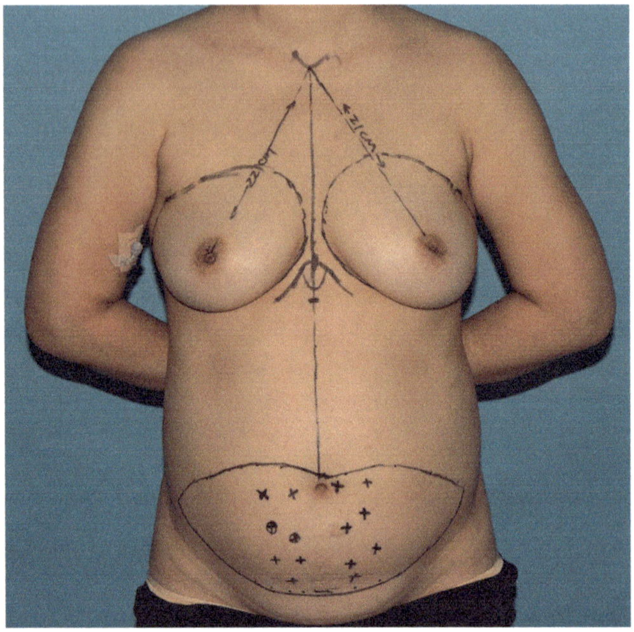

Fig. 17.43 Preoperative marking

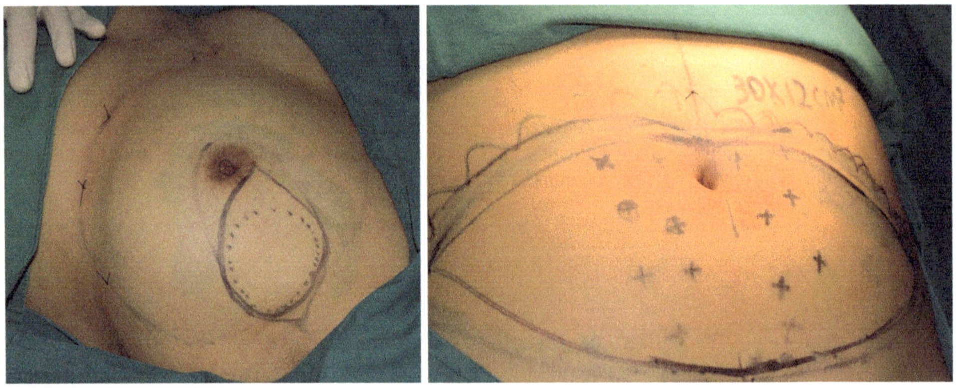

Fig. 17.44 Intraoperative incision design

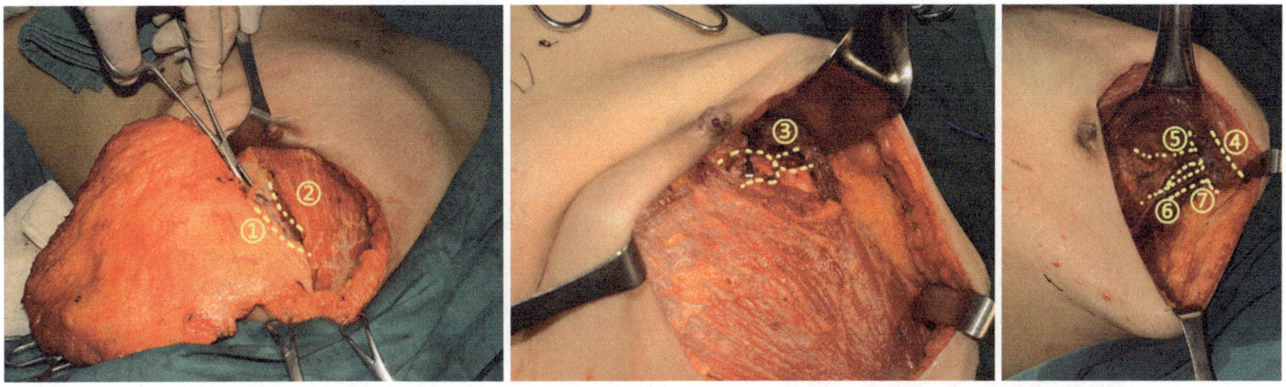

Fig. 17.45 Preparation of vessels in the receiving area. (1) Where the lateral thoracic artery entered the anterior serratus muscle. (2) Pectoralis major. (3) Proximal and distal ends of the internal mammary vessels. (4) Axillary vein. (5) Injured lateral thoracic artery and vein. (6) Another intact lateral thoracic vein. (7) Long thoracic nerve

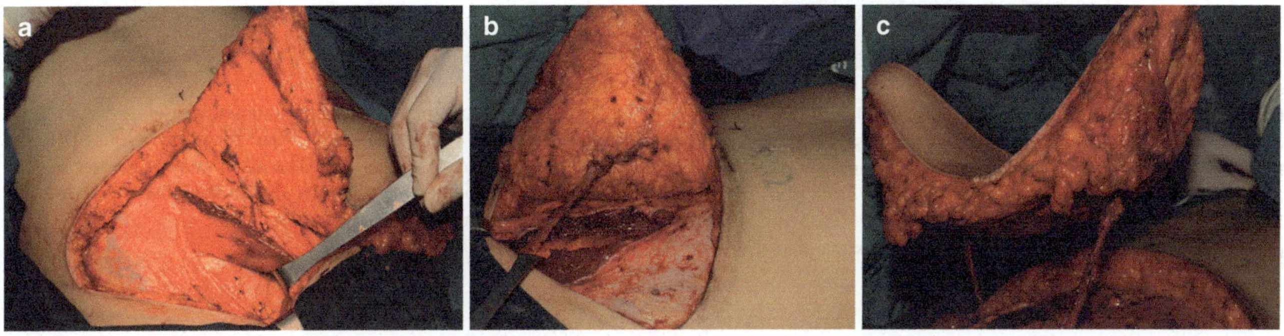

Fig. 17.46 (**a**) The right vascular pedicle was separated. (**b**) The left vascular pedicle was separated. (**c**) Clamping test determined that the flap was in good blood supply only when bilateral vascular pedicles were included; therefore, a bipedicled DIEP flap was prepared

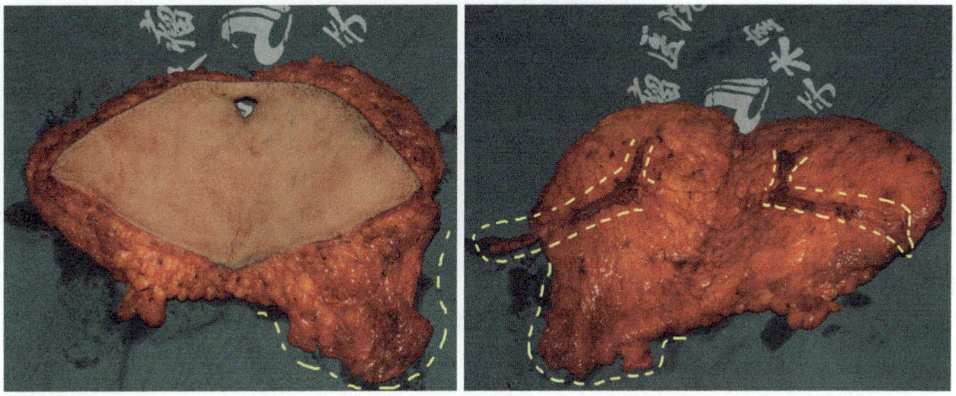

Fig. 17.47 The left ilioinguinal lymphatic tissue flap was carried to prevent upper limb lymphedema

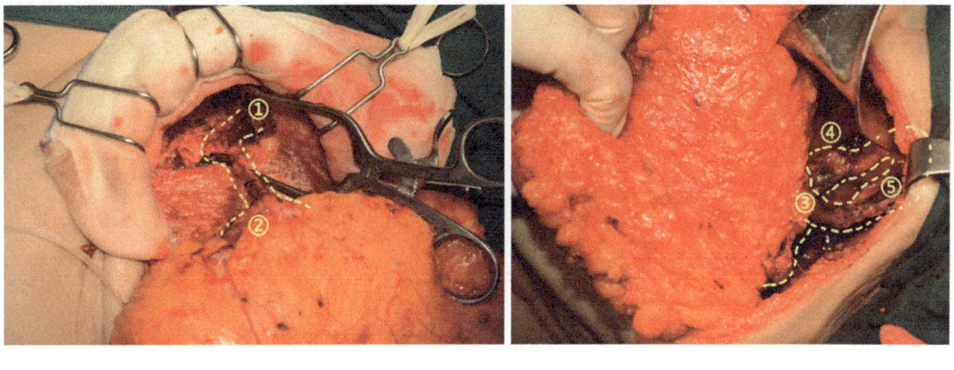

Fig. 17.48 Bilateral vascular pedicles re-vasculization was completed, and the blood circulation of the flap was satisfactory. (1) Proximal thoracic vessels. (2) Left deep inferior epigastric vessels. (3) Right deep inferior epigastric vessels. (4) Distal ends of lateral thoracic artery and vein. (5) Proximal end of another lateral thoracic vein

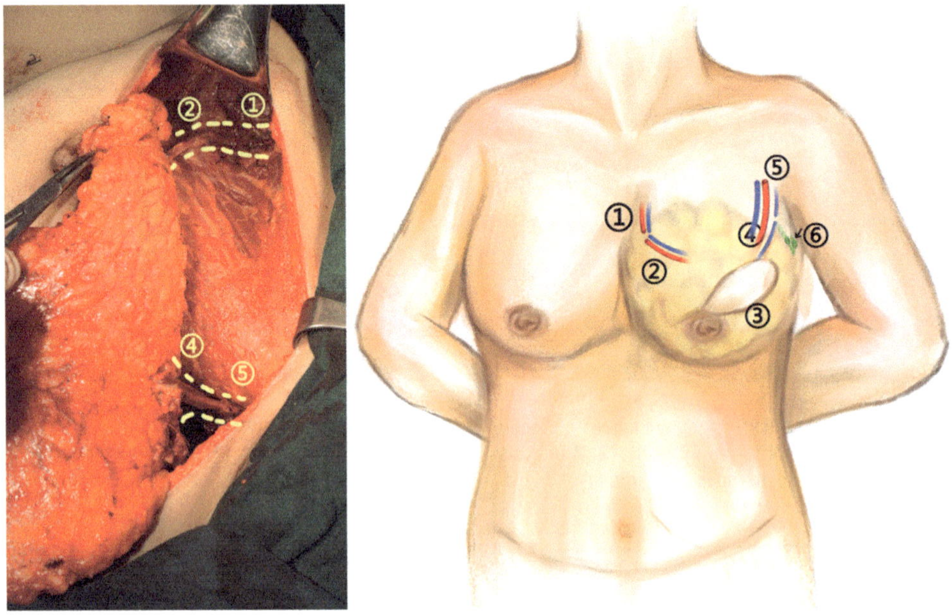

Fig. 17.49 Revascularization of flap was completed. Vascular anastomosis mode: the left deep inferior epigastric vessels were anastomosed with the proximal ends of the left internal mammary vessels (1A1V), the right deep inferior epigastric vessels to the distal ends of the left lateral thoracic vessels (1A1V), and the other accompanying vein of the right deep inferior epigastric vessels to the proximal end of the other left lateral thoracic vein. (1) Proximal thoracic vessels. (2) Left deep inferior epigastric vessels. (3) Skin island for observation. (4) Right deep inferior epigastric vessels. (5) The distal ends of the lateral thoracic artery and vein and the proximal ends of the other lateral thoracic vein. (6) Left ilioinguinal lymphatic tissue flap

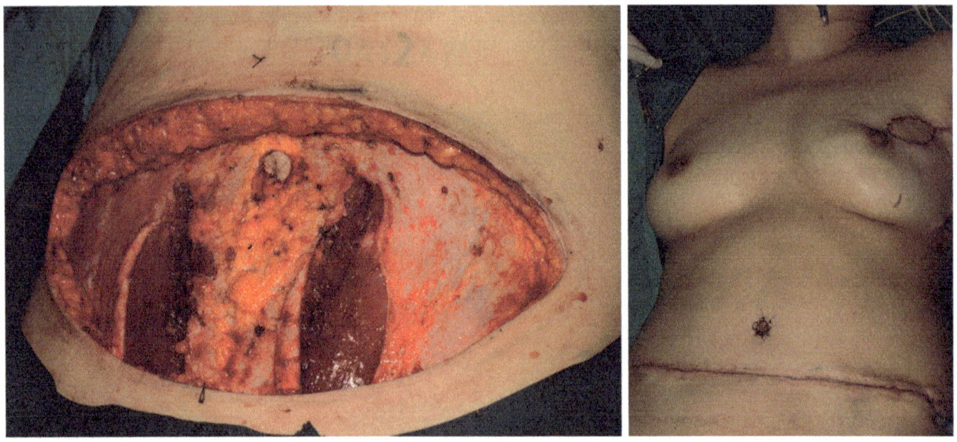

Fig. 17.50 The rectus abdominis and anterior sheath of the donor area were completely preserved. Intraoperative view immediately after breast reconstruction

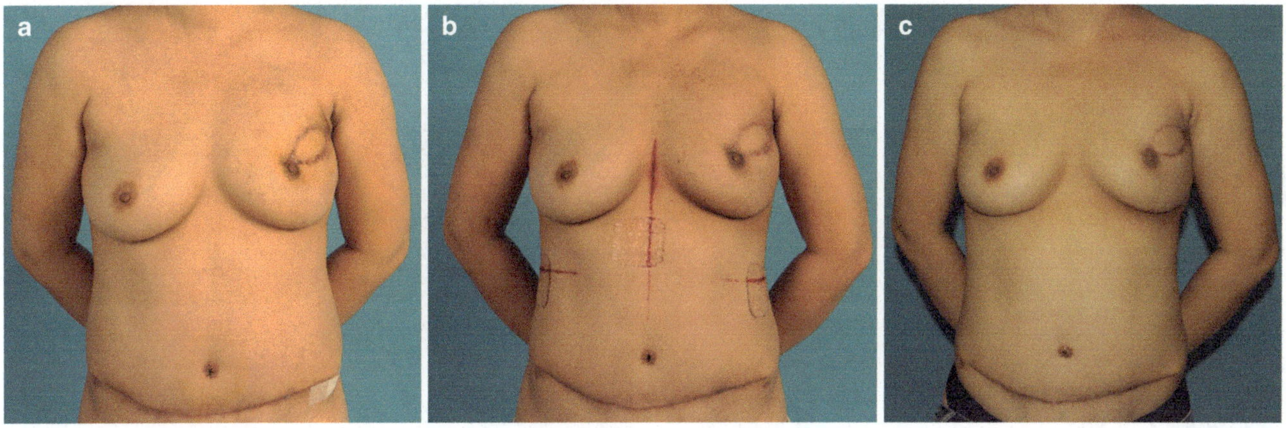

Fig. 17.51 (**a**) 3-month follow-up after operation. (**b**) The patients were followed up at 6 months after operation. (**c**) The patients were followed up at 15 months after operation

Case Study 5

Chest wall reconstruction using unilateral DIEP flap containing ipsilateral iliac inguinal lymphatic tissue flap based on superficial deep inferior epigastric artery and contralateral pedicled TRAM flap: the distal ends of thoracic acromial vessels and lateral thoracic vessels were used as recipient vessels.

After neoadjuvant chemotherapy with AC-T regime for left breast cancer, a 41-year-old female received right extended radical mastectomy and reconstruction using unilateral DIEP flap containing ipsilateral iliac inguinal lymphatic tissue flap based on superficial deep inferior epigastric artery and contralateral pedicled TRAM flap. After completing radical mastectomy, the right thoracoacromial vessels and lateral thoracic vessels were prepared.

The size of the flap was 28 cm × 14 cm. The deep inferior epigastric vessels in the vascular pedicle of the DIEP flap were end-to-end anastomosed with the proximal ends of the right thoracoacromial artery and vein (1A1V) and the superficial deep inferior epigastric artery and vein end-to-end with the lateral thoracic vessels (1A1V). After anastomosis, the blood supply of the flap was good. The reconstruction of the chest wall was completed, and three chest wound drainage tubes were placed. The flap survived uneventfully. Further comprehensive treatment was carried out, and the appearance and function of the reconstructed chest wall were satisfactory (Figs. 17.52, 17.53, 17.54, 17.55, 17.56, 17.57, 17.58, 17.59, 17.60, 17.61, and 17.62).

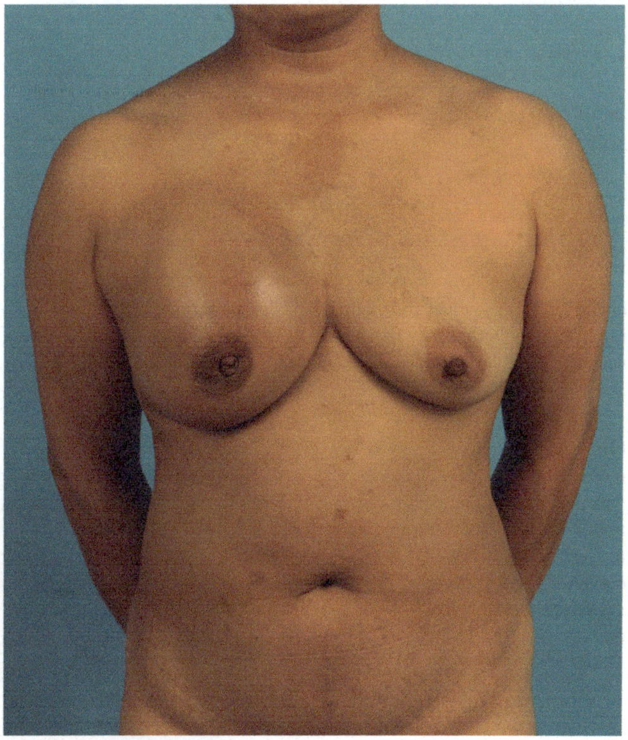

Fig. 17.52 Preoperative findings

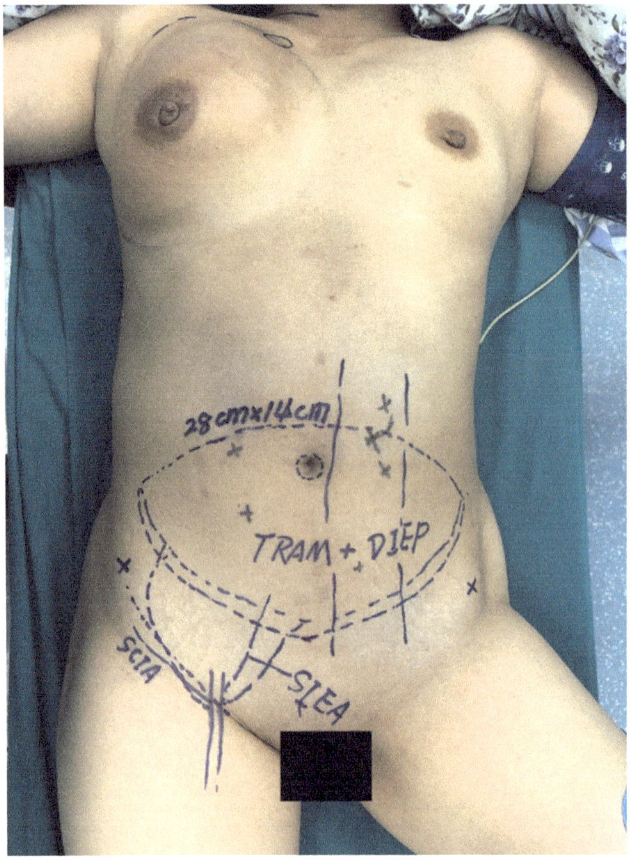

Fig. 17.53 Design of the right DIEP flap containing ipsilateral iliac inguinal lymphatic tissue flap based on superficial deep inferior epigastric artery and left pedicled TRAM flap

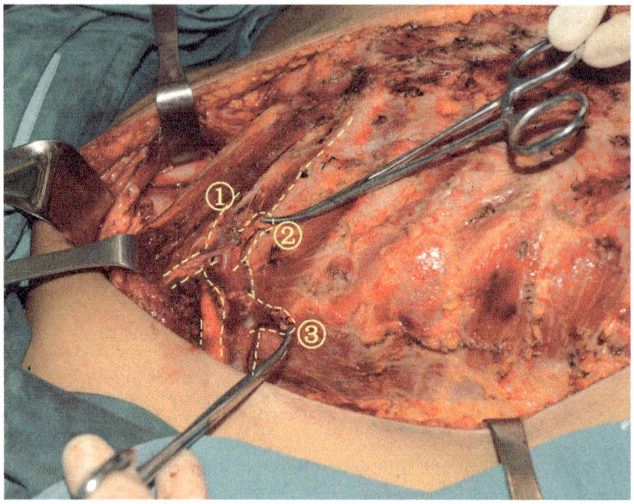

Fig. 17.55 Preparation of thoraco-acromial vessels and lateral thoracic arteries and veins in the receiving area

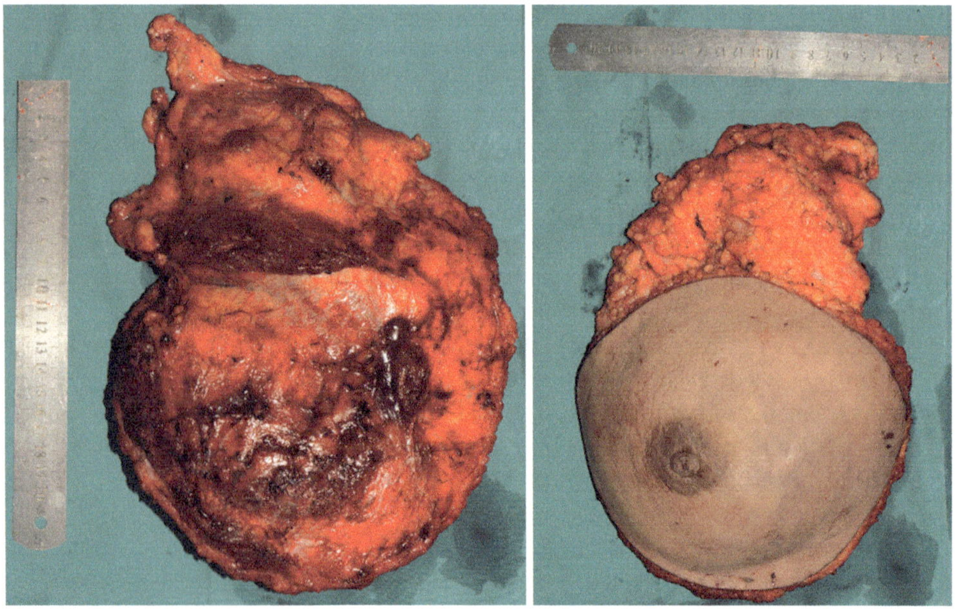

Fig. 17.54 Radical mastectomy for breast cancer was performed. The pectoralis major and pectoralis minor muscles were removed; the clavicular end of pectoralis major and nerve were preserved

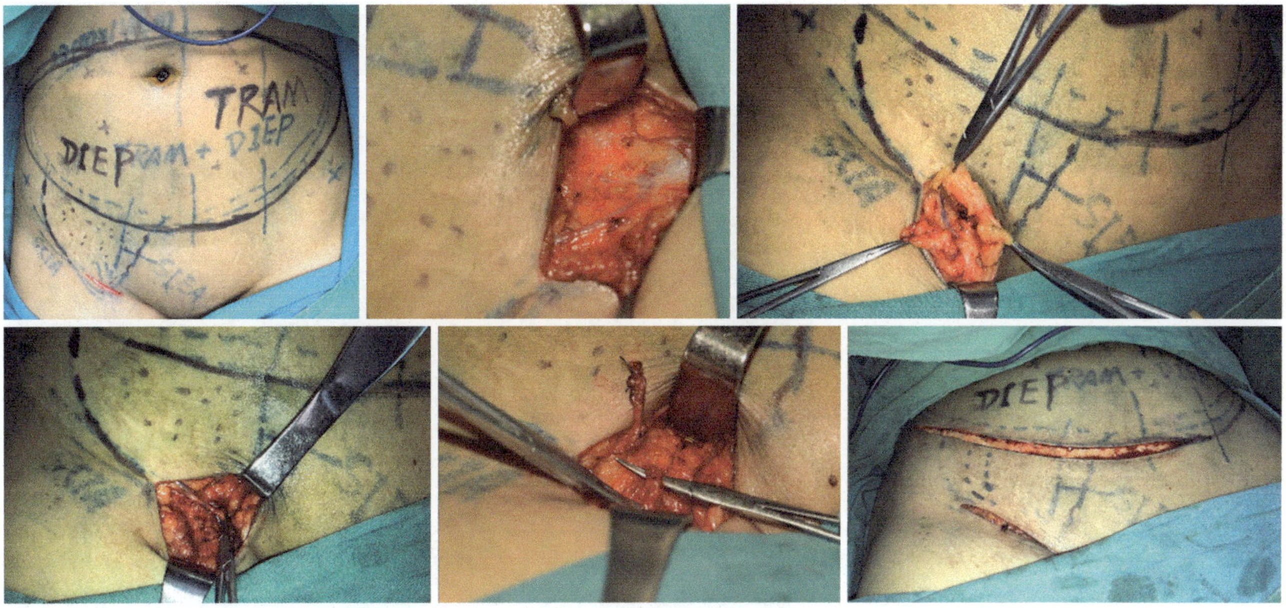

Fig. 17.56 The iliac inguinal lymphatic tissue flap pedicled with the right superficial deep inferior epigastric abdominal artery was harvested through an auxiliary incision

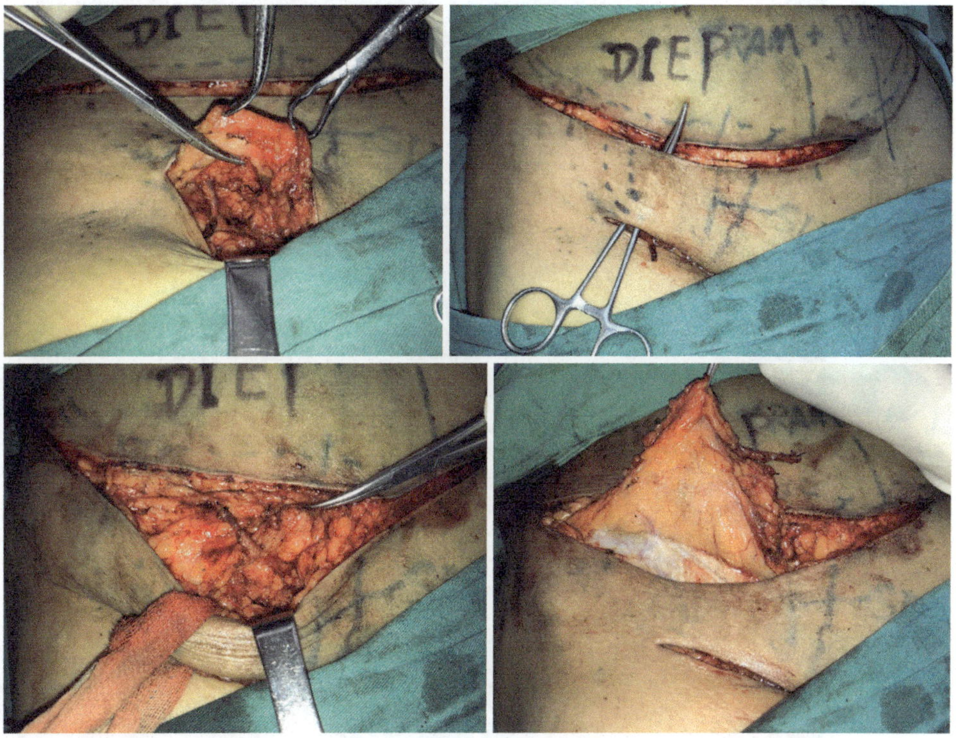

Fig. 17.57 The iliac inguinal lymphatic tissue flap pedicled with the right superficial deep inferior epigastric abdominal artery was raised using rendezvous method

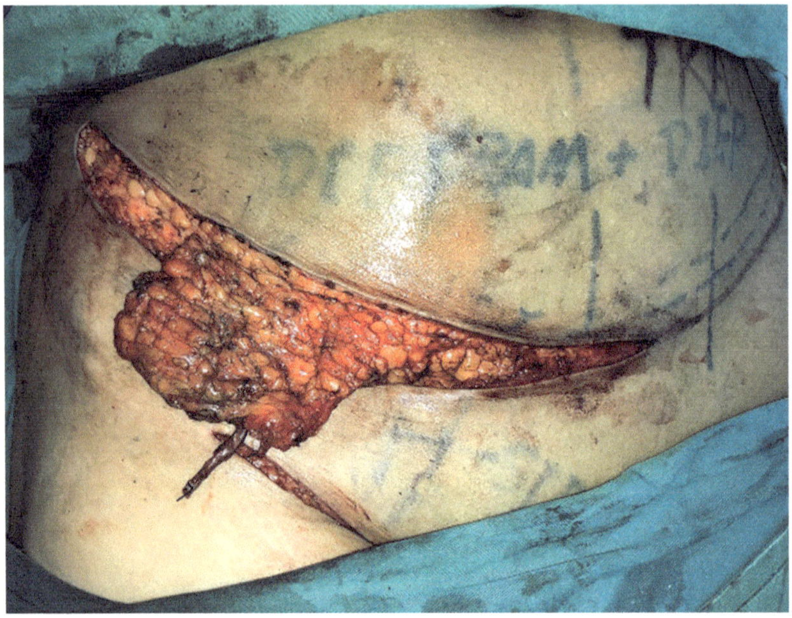

Fig. 17.58 The iliac inguinal lymphatic tissue flap pedicled with the right superficial deep inferior epigastric abdominal artery was prepared

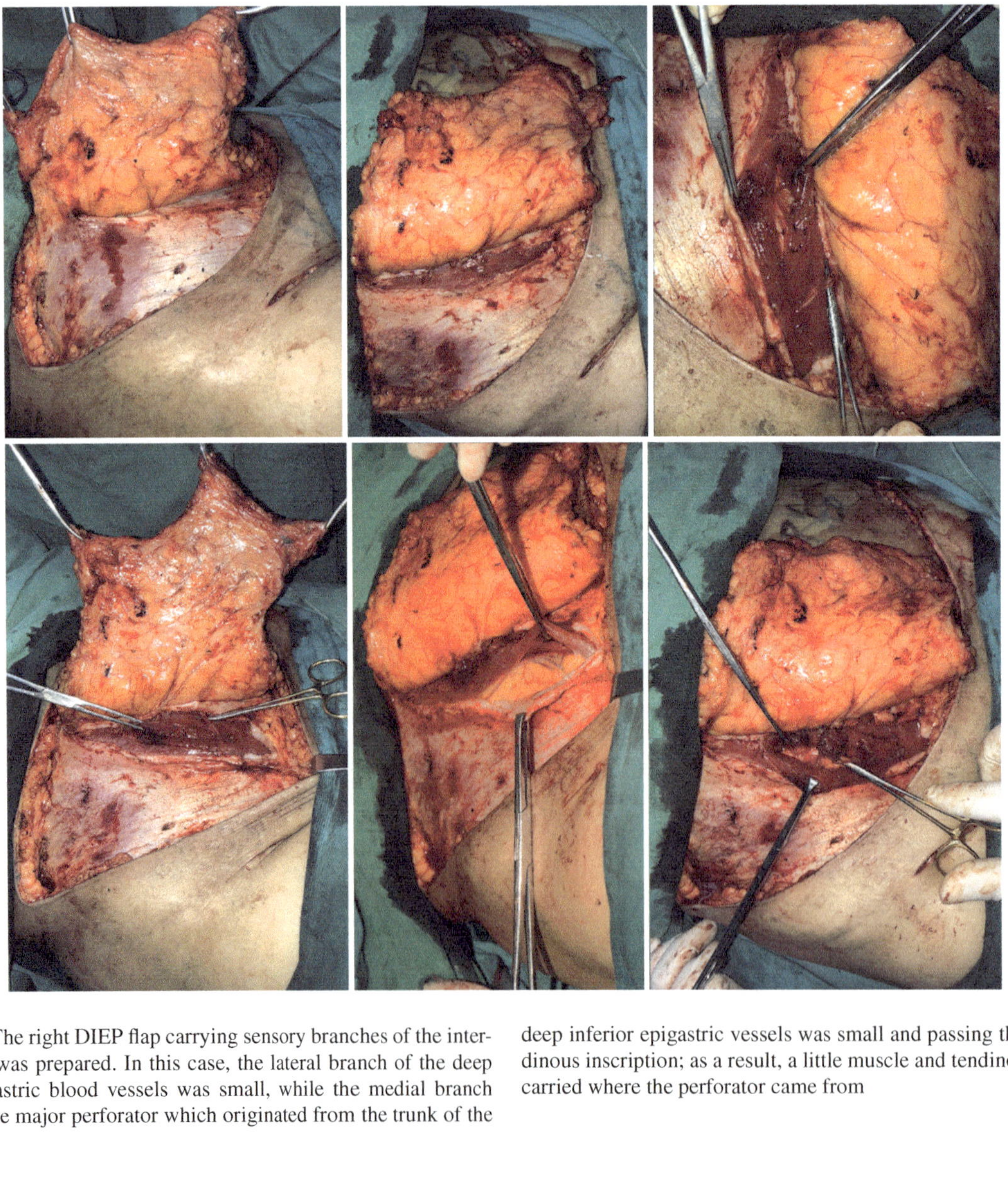

Fig. 17.59 The right DIEP flap carrying sensory branches of the intercostal nerve was prepared. In this case, the lateral branch of the deep inferior epigastric blood vessels was small, while the medial branch was large. The major perforator which originated from the trunk of the deep inferior epigastric vessels was small and passing through the tendinous inscription; as a result, a little muscle and tendinous tissue were carried where the perforator came from

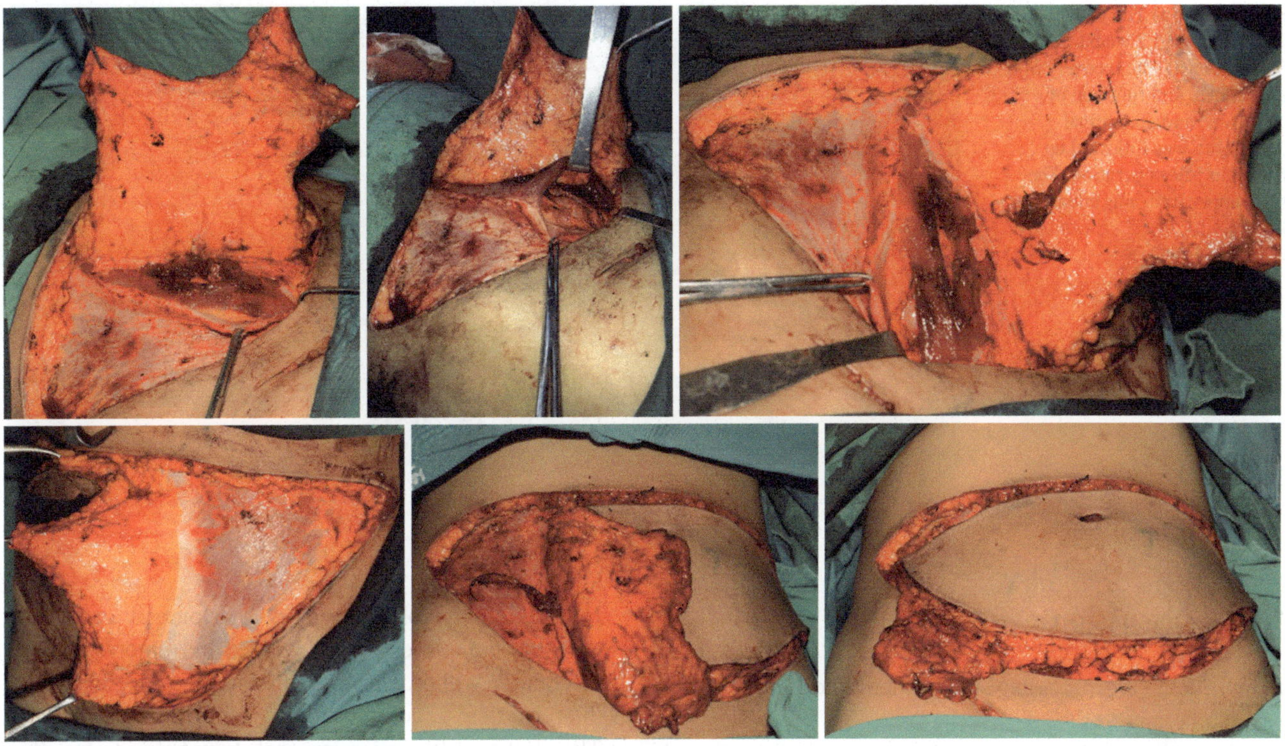

Fig. 17.60 The right DIEP flap and ipsilateral ilioinguinal lymphatic tissue flap pedicled with the right superficial deep inferior epigastric artery were raised

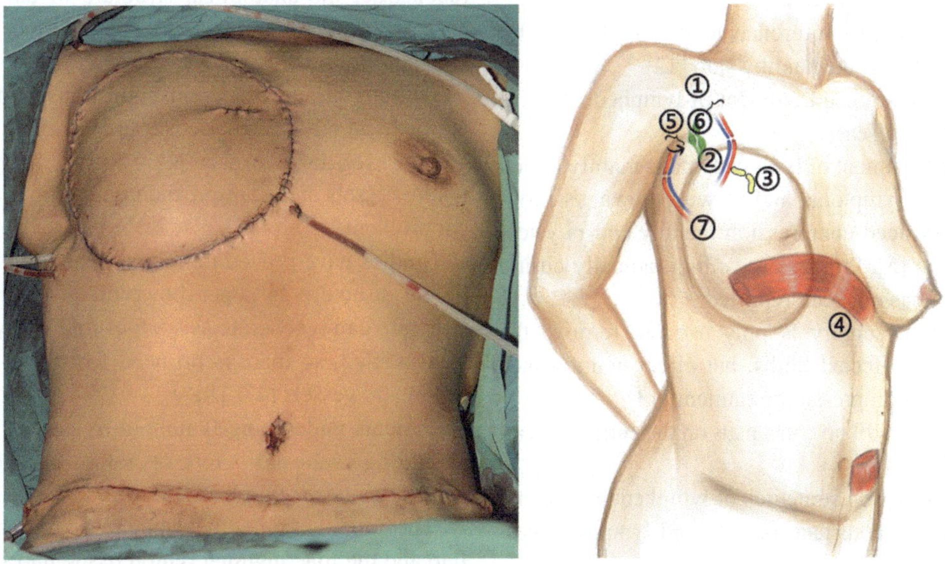

Fig. 17.61 Transferring the combined flap to the right chest wall through the subcutaneous tunnel on the upper abdomen, anastomosing the artery and vein of the DIEP flap with the right thoracoacromial artery and vein (1A1V), and anastomosing the sensory branch of the intercostal nerve with the third intercostal nerve in the receiving area. The blood supply of the flap was satisfactory after further anastomosis of the right superficial deep inferior epigastric artery and vein with the right lateral thoracic artery and vein (1A1V). The lymphatic tissue flap covered the axillary vessels and brachial plexus nerve. Indwelling drainage tube and suturing the subcutaneous tissue and skin. (1) Right thoracoacromial artery and vein. (2) Deep inferior epigastric artery and vein. (3) The sensory branch of intercostal nerve was anastomosed with the third intercostal nerve in the receiving area. (4) Rectus abdominis pedicle. (5) Right lateral thoracic artery and vein. (6) Ilioinguinal lymphatic tissue flap. (7) Right superficial deep inferior epigastric artery and vein

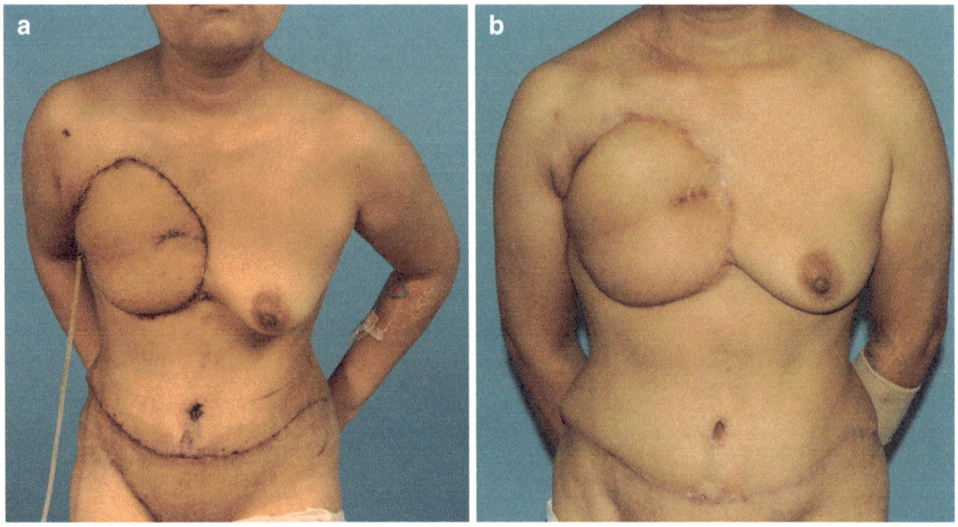

Fig. 17.62 (**a**) The patient was discharged 2 weeks after operation. (**b**) The recovery of appearance and function of chest wall and abdominal donor area was followed up 6 months after operation. The right upper limb was edema free

17.3 Discussion

Lymphedema is progressing slowly after radical mastectomy or radiotherapy.

The diagnosis of lymphedema is mainly based on clinical manifestations. In the early stage, it is mainly characterized by accumulation of interstitial fluid. As the disease progresses, subcutaneous fat and fibrous tissue continue to increase [11].

The affected limb circumference tends to increase by 10% or more than that of the healthy side [12].

The best time for surgical treatment of lymphedema is at the early stage of the disease.

At present, the treatment of lymphedema is mainly aimed at reducing clinical symptoms and slowing down its progress. Patients often need compression therapy and physical therapy for lifetime [5]. Progress regarding radically curing limb lymphedema has not been reported.

Volume reduction surgery is only used to remove the excess tissue of the affected limbs, but effect maintenance requires continuous compression treatment [13].

Up to now, there is still no consensus on the surgical treatment of lymphedema.

Surgical reconstruction strategies of lymphedema mainly include lymphangiovenous anastomosis and lymphatic vessel transplantation [5].

Different from lymph node or lymphatic tissue transplantation, lymphangiovenous anastomosis does not increase the risk of lymphedema in the donor area.

It should be noted that there is not enough data to confirm the long-term patency after anastomosis.

The main challenge is to prevent the reflux of the venous system, which is also the main reason for the blockage of lymphatic venous anastomosis [14].

In addition, lymphatic venous anastomosis cannot be used in the limbs previously involved by tumors, because this technique will provide a channel for tumor cells to enter the blood system directly from the lymphatic vessels.

The cutting-edge microsurgical lymphatic tissue flap transplantation is expected to improve lymphatic function in patients with lymphedema after breast cancer surgery.

The purpose of lymphatic tissue flap transplantation is to reconstruct the anatomical structure of axillary lymphatic vessels and further reconstruct the lymphatic function of swollen limbs [15].

Autologous micro-lymph node transplantation was first applied and reported by Becker [16] in 2006.

However, how to accurately locate the functional lymphatic vessels in the armpit and upper limb is a difficult clinical problem.

Studies have proved that the regeneration ability of lymphatic structure is super powerful. The lymphatic tissue structure can regenerate as soon as that the lymph nodes are transplanted, so there is no need for micro-anastomosis of lymphatic vessels [17, 18].

Patients undergoing lymphoid tissue flap transplantation should be evaluated before operation to determine that the cancer has been completely removed.

The combination of the deep inferior epigastric perforator flap and the iliac inguinal lymph tissue flap share the advantages of each flap, which is particularly suitable for breast reconstruction in breast cancer patients with upper limb lymphedema following breast surgery [19].

So far, 4 studies including 64 patients have investigated the effect of lymph node transplantation to the armpit [16, 19–21].

Although the actual therapeutic effect of lymph node transplantation warrants further clarification in large sample randomized controlled studies [20], the previously reported surgical effect is relatively satisfactory, and more than half of the patients have reduced circumferential diameter of the upper arm [22–24].

These reports suggest that lymph node transplantation may be effective in patients with lymphedema, especially in patients with limb erysipelas or neuralgia.

The lymphatic micro-anastomosis between the recipient area and the donor area is only theoretically feasible. In practice, it is very difficult to find functional lymphatic vessels in the axillary recipient area. We use the lymphatic tissue flap to cover and wrap the brachial plexus and axillary blood vessels to reconstruct the axillary lymphatic system relying on the immediate lymphatic regeneration ability of the flap.

The results of experimental animal studies showed that the maturation of lymphatic vessels after lymph node transplantation was slow. It took at least 6 months for the establishment and maturation of new lymphatic systems to evolve into real collecting lymphatic vessels [8, 25].

Therefore, the effect of deep inferior epigastric artery perforator flap with iliac inguinal lymphatic tissue flap in the treatment of upper limb lymphedema can be objectively evaluated at least 6–12 months when the patient can reduce the frequency of pressure bandage.

There were few reports on the injury of the donor area caused by the cutting of the DIEP flap with the iliac inguinal lymphatic tissue flap [23, 26].

In 2013, the occurrence of lymphedema in donor area was first reported internationally [27, 28].

However, this represents only a small proportion of the total number of patients receiving lymph node transplantation.

None of these reports can determine the long-term impact of lymph node transplantation on lymphedema limbs.

During follow-up in our serial cases, no functional impairment such as swelling and pain of the lower limbs on the side of the donor area was found.

In practice, we modified the design of lymphatic tissue flap to minimize the injury of donor area, which was more conservative than that in previous reports.

According to anatomical studies, the lymphatic vessels and lymph nodes that were mainly responsible for lower limb lymphatic drainage located in the central and medial regions of the groin should be avoided in raising the lymphatic tissue flap.

Recent studies demonstrated that breast cancer patients with recurrent skin and soft tissue infection and neuralgia of the lymphedema upper limb after radical breast surgery and axillary lymph node dissection were the best candidates for lymphatic tissue flap transplantation [29].

Which side of ilioinguinal lymphatic tissue flap is harvested is dependent on the blood supply of the flap. Re-vasculization of bilateral deep inferior epigastric vascular pedicles or of unilateral pedicle on the same side of the lymphatic tissue flap can ensure sufficient blood supply of the flap. At present, there is no consensus on the reconstruction scheme for patients with lymphedema, and none of the existing techniques is applicable to all patients with lymphedema.

Future studies need to classify all reconstruction techniques and determine their specific indications. We also need to evaluate the impact of lymph node transplantation on recipient and donor areas, so as to further determine the indications of lymph tissue flap transplantation.

The significance of preventive resection of ilioinguinal lymphatic tissue flap for the prevention of upper limb lymphedema warrants further clinical statistical research.

References

1. Chang DW, Kim S. Breast reconstruction and lymphedema. Plast Reconstr Surg. 2010;125(1):19–23.
2. Xiao Zhou, Bo Zhou, Zan Li. The history and current situation of oncoplastic surgery in China—oncology surgeons have the responsibility to cure tumors, and also have the obligation to give patients a healthy and beautiful life. Chin J Otorhinolaryngol Skull Base Surg2016. (02): 85–90.
3. DiSipio T, Rye S, Newman B, Hayes S. Incidence of unilateral arm lymphoedema after breast cancer: a systematic review and meta-analysis. Lancet Oncol. 2013;14(6):500–15.
4. Viitanen TP, Visuri MT, Sulo E, Saarikko AM, Hartiala P. Anti-inflammatory effects of flap and lymph node transfer. J Surg Res. 2015;199(2):718–25.
5. Suami H, Chang DW. Overview of surgical treatments for breast cancer-related lymphedema. Plast Reconstr Surg. 2010;126(6):1853–63.
6. Healy C, Allen RJ. The evolution of perforator flap breast reconstruction: twenty years after the first DIEP flap. J Reconstr Microsurg. 2014;30(2):121–5.
7. Xiao Zhou, Dajiang Song, Zan Li. The development of perforator flap and its application in oncoplastic surgery. Chin J Aesthet Plast Surg 2017. 28(2): 69–72.
8. Tammela T, Saaristo A, Holopainen T, et al. Therapeutic differentiation and maturation of lymphatic vessels after lymph node dissection and transplantation. Nat Med. 2007;13(12):1458–66.
9. Al-Dhamin A, Berry R, Prasad V, Martin A, Morris SF. Coding system for computed tomographic angiography of deep inferior epigastric artery perforators in DIEP flaps. Plast Reconstr Surg. 2012;129(2):387e–8e.
10. Sönmez TT, Al-Sawaf O, Brandacher G, et al. A novel laser-Doppler flowmetry assisted murine model of acute hindlimb ischemia-reperfusion for free flap research. PLoS One. 2013;8(6):e66498.
11. Brorson H. Adipose tissue in lymphedema: the ignorance of adipose tissue in lymphedema. Lymphology. 2004;37(4):175–7.
12. Armer JM, Stewart BR. A comparison of four diagnostic criteria for lymphedema in a post-breast cancer population. Lymphat Res Biol. 2005;3(4):208–17.
13. Warren AG, Brorson H, Borud LJ, Slavin SA. Lymphedema: a comprehensive review. Ann Plast Surg. 2007;59(4):464–72.
14. Uhrin P, Zaujec J, Breuss JM, et al. Novel function for blood platelets and podoplanin in developmental separation of blood and lymphatic circulation. Blood. 2010;115(19):3997–4005.

15. Slavin SA, Upton J, Kaplan WD, Van den Abbeele AD. An investigation of lymphatic function following free-tissue transfer. Plast Reconstr Surg. 1997;99(3):730–41; discussion 742–3.
16. Becker C, Assouad J, Riquet M, Hidden G. Postmastectomy lymphedema: long-term results following microsurgical lymph node transplantation. Ann Surg. 2006;243(3):313–5.
17. Slavin SA, Van den Abbeele AD, Losken A, Swartz MA, Jain RK. Return of lymphatic function after flap transfer for acute lymphedema. Ann Surg. 1999;229(3):421–7.
18. Tobbia D, Semple J, Baker A, Dumont D, Johnston M. Experimental assessment of autologous lymph node transplantation as treatment of postsurgical lymphedema. Plast Reconstr Surg. 2009;124(3):777–86.
19. Saaristo AM, Niemi TS, Viitanen TP, Tervala TV, Hartiala P, Suominen EA. Microvascular breast reconstruction and lymph node transfer for postmastectomy lymphedema patients. Ann Surg. 2012;255(3):468–73.
20. Viitanen TP, Visuri MT, Hartiala P, et al. Lymphatic vessel function and lymphatic growth factor secretion after microvascular lymph node transfer in lymphedema patients. Plast Reconstr Surg Glob Open. 2013;1(2):1–9.
21. Dancey A, Nassimizadeh A, Nassimizadeh M, Warner RM, Waters R. A chimeric vascularised groin lymph node flap and DIEP flap for the management of lymphoedema secondary to breast cancer. J Plast Reconstr Aesthet Surg. 2013;66(5):735–7.
22. Cheng MH, Chen SC, Henry SL, Tan BK, Lin MC, Huang JJ. Vascularized groin lymph node flap transfer for postmastectomy upper limb lymphedema: flap anatomy, recipient sites, and outcomes. Plast Reconstr Surg. 2013;131(6):1286–98.
23. Poon Y, Wei CY. Vascularized groin lymph node flap transfer for postmastectomy upper limb lymphedema: flap anatomy, recipient sites, and outcomes. Plast Reconstr Surg. 2014;133(3):428e.
24. Zeltzer AA, Hamdi M. Operative treatment of peripheral lymphedema: a systematic meta-analysis of the efficacy and safety of lymphovenous microsurgery and tissue transplant. Plast Reconstr Surg. 2014;134(3):491e–2e.
25. Lähteenvuo M, Honkonen K, Tervala T, et al. Growth factor therapy and autologous lymph node transfer in lymphedema. Circulation. 2011;123(6):613–20.
26. Azuma S, Yamamoto T, Koshima I. Donor-site lymphatic function after microvascular lymph node transfer should be followed using indocyanine green lymphography. Plast Reconstr Surg. 2013;131(3):443e–4e.
27. Pons G, Masia J, Loschi P, Nardulli ML, Duch J. A case of donor-site lymphoedema after lymph node-superficial circumflex iliac artery perforator flap transfer. J Plast Reconstr Aesthet Surg. 2014;67(1):119–23.
28. Vignes S, Blanchard M, Yannoutsos A, Arrault M. Complications of autologous lymph-node transplantation for limb lymphoedema. Eur J Vasc Endovasc Surg. 2013;45(5):516–20.
29. Nahabedian MY. Microvascular breast reconstruction and lymph node transfer for postmastectomy lymphedema patients. Gland Surg. 2012;1(1):1–2.

Experience Sharing in Handling Difficult Cases of Breast Reconstruction with DIEP Flap

18

Zan Li, Zhuangqing Yang, Huaihua Qi, Kun Wang, Wuping Zheng, Pengcheng Su, and Haiyan Gao

In the past 15 years, breast reconstruction using microsurgical technique has become popular.

Due to reduced abdominal complications and good long-term cosmetic effect, patient reported outcome is generally great [1–3].

Deep inferior epigastric perforator flap (DIEP) transplantation for breast reconstruction is the most widely used autologous breast reconstruction. However, a recent survey among oncoplastic surgeons showed that microsurgical technique was used in less than one fifth of breast reconstruction cases with flap transplantation [4].

In clinical practice, breast reconstruction with autologous free flap transplantation is a surgical field that requires cooperation of multidisciplinary teams and bears high surgical risk and many clinical variations. It is experience and technically demanding. Every perioperative detail should be taken seriously.

Some studies have shown the formulation and adjustment of reconstruction scheme are more likely to be affected by its feasibility, the operator's preference, and the hospital platform than by the anatomy and reconstructive outcome and function [5, 6].

Plastic microsurgical reconstruction plan of free flap transplantation is more complex than that of implant prosthesis or pedicled flap. It requires operators to receive more professional training and patients to tolerate longer operation time and hospitalization time.

Therefore, many breast cancer treatment centers have not yet carried out perforator flap surgery which are normally carried out in medical-university-affiliated hospitals, teaching hospitals, and large tertiary hospitals [7].

The US National College of Surgery established the national certification program for breast centers, which provides a comprehensive guideline for breast cancer treatment and emphasizes the indications for plastic surgeons to use perforator flaps for breast reconstruction.

If patients are diagnosed with breast cancer in centers without microsurgery and treated with oncological medicine and want to undergo perforator flap reconstruction surgery, they have to be referred to centers with microsurgical department, which may interrupt the comprehensive tumor treatment [8, 9].

For a long time, the work related to repair and reconstruction has been completed by plastic surgeons. Oncoplastic surgery regarding the tumor of body surface is independently described in various versions of plastic surgery monographs, while the contents related to postoperative repair and reconstruction of tumors in eyelids, scalp, mouth, breast, external genitalia, and other parts are discussed separately in various relevant monographs, accounting for only a small proportion.

Under the current specialist training system in China, oncological surgeons hardly receive formal and systematic

Z. Li (✉)
Department of Oncology Plastic Surgery, Hunan Cancer Hospital, Changsha, Hunan, China

Z. Yang
Department of Mammary Surgery, The Third Affiliated Hospital of Kunming Medical University (Yunnan Cancer Hospital, Yunnan Cancer Center), Kunming, Yunnan, China

H. Qi
Department of Breast Surgery, Tangshan People's Hospital, Tangshan, Hebei, China

K. Wang
Breast-Conserving and Reconstructive Surgery, Multidisciplinary Cancer Treatment, Department of Breast Cancer, Cancer Center, Guangdong Provincial People's Hospital, Guangdong Academy of Medical Sciences, Guangzhou, Guangdong, China
e-mail: wangkun@gdph.org.cn

W. Zheng
Department of Breast and Thyroid Surgery at the Second Affiliated Hospital of Hainan Medical College, Haikou, Hainan Province, China

P. Su
Department of Breast and Thyroid Surgery, People's Hospital of XinJiang Uygur Autonomous Region, Urumqi, Xinjiang, P. R. China

H. Gao
Department of Breast Surgery, Changzhou Tumor Hospital, Changzhou, P. R. China

Z. Li, D. Song (eds.), *Oncoplastic Flap Surgery*, https://doi.org/10.1007/978-981-19-8926-1_18

training of flap surgery, which hampers the technical development of tissue repair and reconstruction in oncosurgical treatment.

Some patients are forced to give up radical surgery because of lacking effective means of repair. Some radical operations such as facial surface tumor radical correction and modified radical mastectomy of breast cancer resulted in serious body deformities and dysfunction.

Some doctors began to explore the application of plastic surgery technique in oncological surgery, and some radical tumor surgeries also achieved good therapeutic results due to the introduction of plastic surgery technique.

Tumor plastic surgery combines the theories and techniques of tumor surgery, plastic surgery, microsurgery, and flap surgery. On the basis of multidisciplinary comprehensive treatment (MDT), it is a cross surgical and marginal department characterized by planned radical tumor resection and one-stage repair and reconstruction [10, 11].

The formal name of tumor plastic surgery at home and abroad appeared for the first time in the article Talking About The Necessity of Tumor Plastic Surgery on pages 694–695, Volume 10, issue 12, *China Tumor Magazine*, 2001. The article formally put forward the concept of tumor plastic surgery and briefly described the historical background, name, nature, scope, treatment principle, and problems to be studied of tumor plastic surgery [12, 13].

In February 2013, Zhou Xiao, Cao Yilin, and Hu Bingqiang, together with experts in relevant fields at home and abroad, published a monograph on tumor plastic surgery, which was the first professional treatise at home and abroad to systematically elaborate the theoretical system of tumor plastic surgery. The monograph systematically expounds the preparation skills and clinical application of skin flaps commonly used in tumor plastic surgery.

In August 2017, the monograph *Oncoplastic Surgery* was collected by Springer press and translated into English version *Oncoplastic Surgery*, which was published and distributed all over the world.

We are committed to the development of perforator flap program to meet the requirements of routine implementation of this kind of complex surgery.

It is very important to gain microsurgical experience by performing a large number of operations. The curative effect of patients after reconstruction is related to the amount of autologous microsurgeries performed by the institution [14].

Compared with plastic surgeons with sufficient microsurgical reconstruction experience, inexperienced doctors encounter more obstacles [15].

After implementation of the specialty training program, improvement of postoperative outcome has been continuously reported in other surgical and tumor fields [16].

Establishment of perforator flap reconstruction program enables the existing breast cancer treatment center to receive patients referred from other local and regional hospitals. Building a comprehensive breast treatment program in neglected areas can increase patient satisfaction and help select reconstruction plans with high success rate [17].

Standardized reconstruction microsurgery can make efficient use of personnel and resources, improve medical quality and patient safety, and reduce the cost of treatment [8].

At the initial stage of the project, we need to consider designing and modifying the perioperative clinical path and the reconstruction sequence of postoperative perforator flap, predict disease progress in patients undergoing microsurgery, and assist them to participate in other disciplines or medical services.

Measures for postoperative monitoring and initial recovery may vary according to institutions. Similarly, the time spent in ICU may also be different.

Due to the differences in surgeons' preferred postoperative analgesia methods, the combination of anesthesia and analgesic drugs may be valuable.

Cooperation between breast cancer treatment projects in clinical institutions can simplify the referral process and reduce the unnecessary time cost of reconstruction consultation.

At the same time, the coordination of pre-anesthesia assessment should also be taken into account.

Some studies have improved efficiency and reduced complications by describing the incidence of perforator flap complications and typical microsurgical learning curve [18–22].

Excellent know-how and sound perioperative management will certainly help patients obtain the best recovery effect.

The experience gained from patient selection, flap design, and intraoperative decision-making is very important for the long-term success of plastic surgeons and perforator flaps.

Flap viability is crucial, which requires careful planning throughout the whole process.

Methods and techniques of preoperative vascular selection include color Doppler ultrasound, CTA, and MRA.

Postoperative flap monitoring methods include (1) clinical experience for observation; (2) finger pulse oxygen monitoring; (3) near-infrared spectroscopy; (4) photoelectric volume diagram; (5) body surface temperature measurement; (6) fluorescence measurement; (7) microdialysis; (8) ultrasound; (9) Doppler; (10) impedance plethysmography; (11) confocal microscope; (12) nuclear medicine; (13) subcutaneous pH meter; (14) hydrogen removal method; (15) monitoring flap; and (16) white light spectral analyzer.

In few clinical cases, the blood vessels are well filled, and the flap is in good blood supply after intraoperative vascular anastomosis in flap transplantation. However, regional venous congestion occurs in the early stage after operation, which manifests as a well-defined area instead of the entire flap with venous reflux obstruction. Emergency exploration will be given in cases with gradually expanded congested areas, where the anastomotic patency is evaluated and the congested tissue is removed to improve venous drainage.

Case Study 1: Flap Venous Congestion Intervened by Emergency Exploration

A 32-year-old female presented for a right breast mass found for more than 1 month. It was diagnosed on biopsy as invasive carcinoma of the right breast (cT2N1M0, stage IIb). Modified radical mastectomy and free deep inferior epigastric perforator flap for one-stage breast reconstruction were performed. The right deep inferior epigastric artery and vein were anastomosed end-to-end with the lateral thoracic artery and vein branch (1A1V). The other accompanying vein of the deep inferior epigastric artery was anastomosed with the distal end of the lateral thoracic vein. The blood supply of the flap was satisfactory. Signs of venous congestion on the lateral margins of the flap occurred 6 h after breast reconstruction without worsening or remission symptomatic treatment. The flap exploration was performed 24 h after operation and found that the vascular anastomosis was unobstructed, yet about 100 mL of blood clot was collected under the flap. Venous congestion was dominant in the subcutaneous layer at the edge of the flap. The blood clot and the congested tissues were removed until fresh red blood flowed out at the edge of the flap. Hemostasis and wound lavage was conducted, two vacuum-suction drainage tubes were placed, and then the wound was closed. The amount of intraoperative bleeding was about 100 mL. After operation, the flap survived and the reconstructed breast was slightly smaller than the opposite side. It was going to be corrected by fat transplantation later (Figs. 18.1, 18.2, 18.3, 18.4, 18.5, 18.6, 18.7, 18.8, 18.9, 18.10, 18.11, 18.12, 18.13, and 18.14).

Flap trimming needs to be flexibly adjusted because excessive tension can also cause flap crisis.

For congested flap that was salvaged, we should trim it accordingly and re-put it into the skin envelope in a tension-free manner.

In order to ensure blood supply, ICG angiography can be used to evaluate where the flap was in poor perfusion.

If the congestion part of the flap can be removed, especially when it is located in area IV or contralateral lateral area, the best solution is to remove it directly, which will reduce the venous load and improve the circulation of the whole flap.

Hematoma and seroma are one of the common complications after flap transplantation. Based on clinical observation, we found that over-perfusion of the flap was more common. The reason is that the flap blood cannot be simply drained by the anastomosed vein, and excessive static blood in the flap tissue is likely to form hematoma, which can be coped with by the following methods: (1) additional anastomosis of the contralateral vascular pedicle; (2) anastomosing ipsilateral or contralateral SIEV; and (3) removing the tissue with serious venous reflux obstruction.

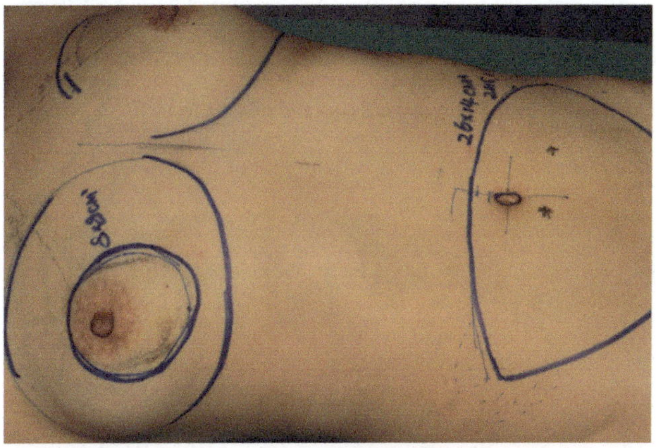

Fig. 18.1 Intraoperative design

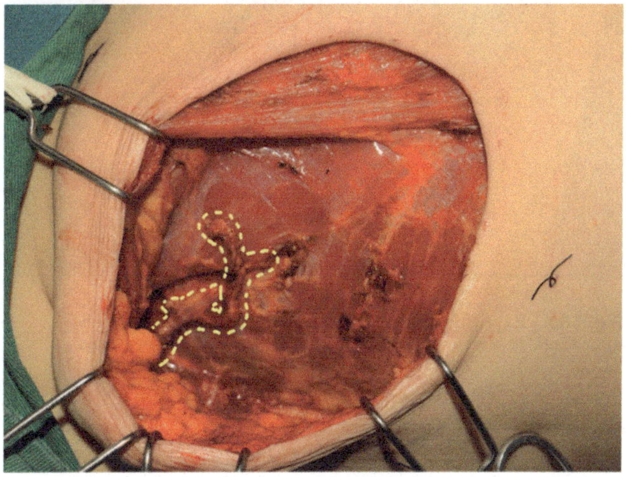

Fig. 18.2 Preparation of lateral thoracic vessels in the receiving area was completed

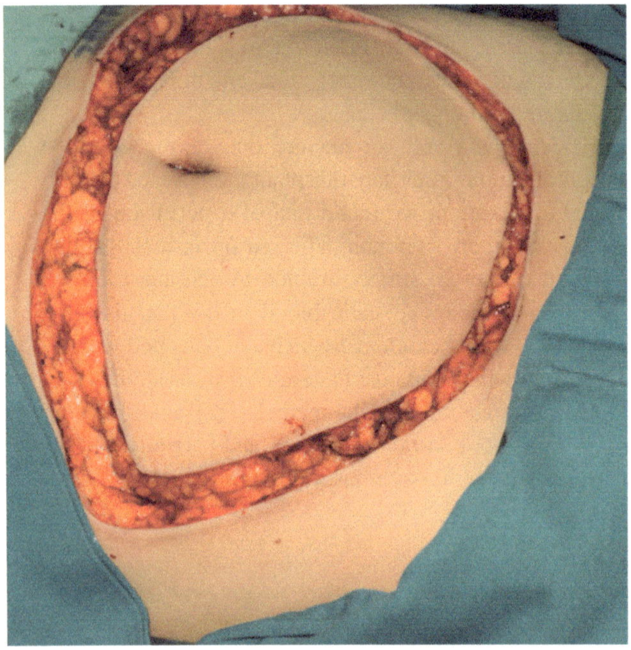

Fig. 18.3 Incising skin flap margins and subcutaneous tissue

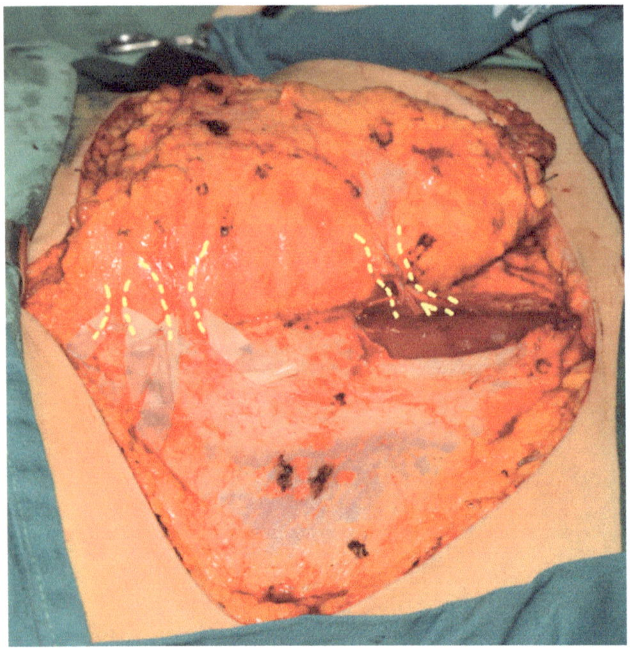

Fig. 18.4 Exposing and separating the right perforator

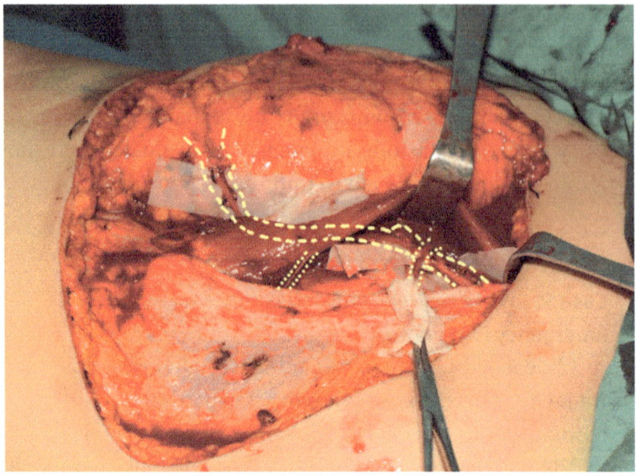

Fig. 18.5 Dissecting the entire vascular pedicle

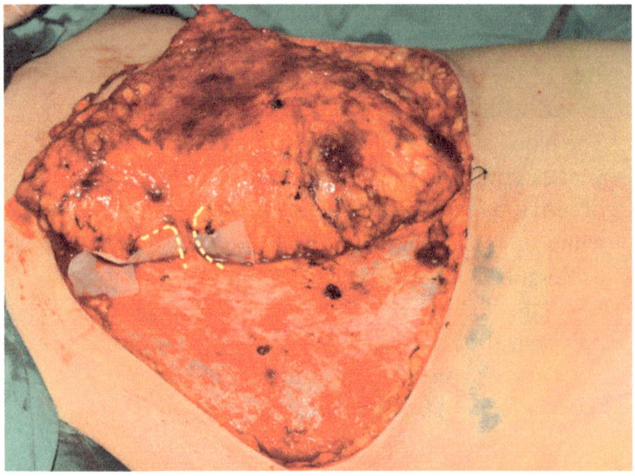

Fig. 18.6 Revealing the left perforator

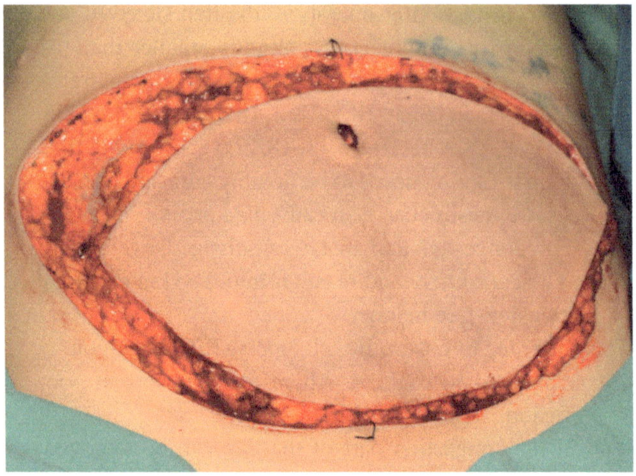

Fig. 18.7 After the flap was cut, obvious obstruction of venous reflux was seen

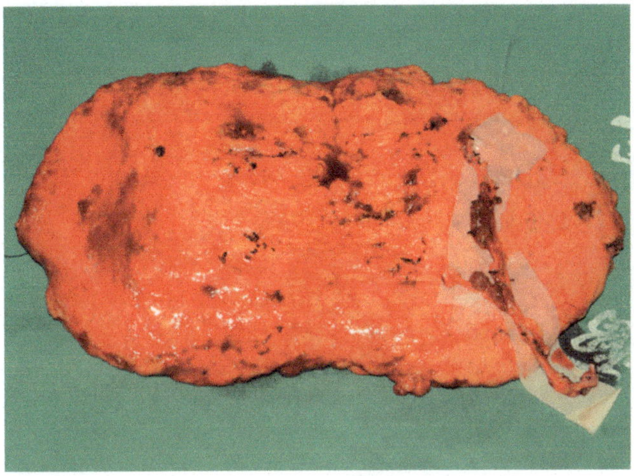

Fig. 18.8 The flap was cut off

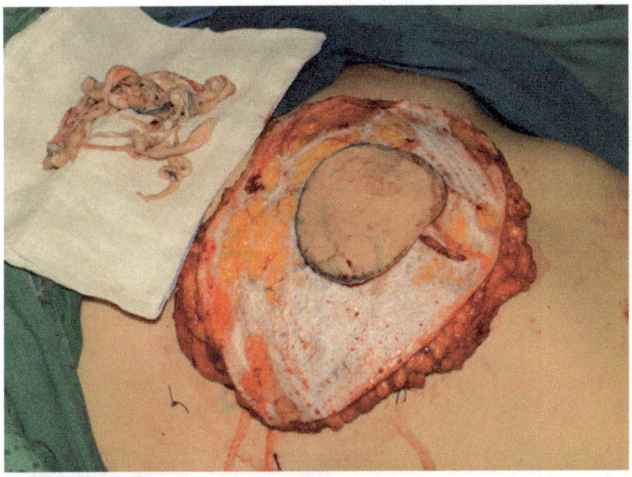

Fig. 18.9 Removing the tissue of area IV of the flap and the epidermis of the flap to complete breast shaping

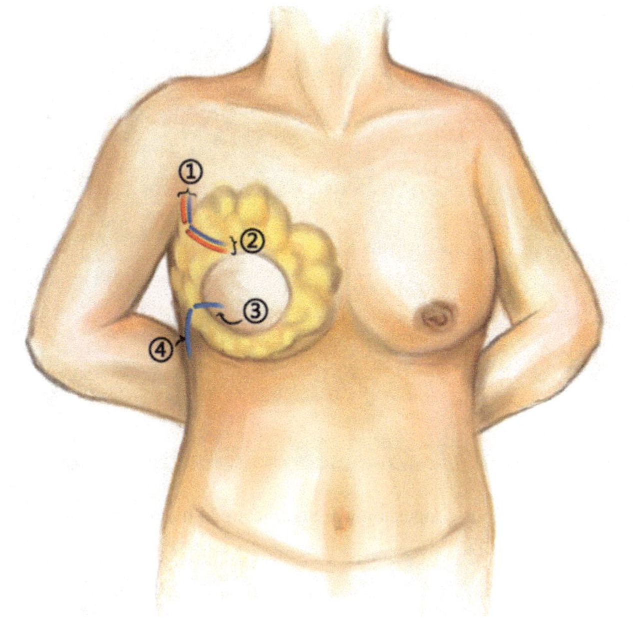

Fig. 18.10 Revascularization mode: right deep inferior epigastric vessels to right lateral thoracic artery and vein (A: v = 1:1). Right SIEV to right lateral thoracic vein. (1) Lateral thoracic vessels. (2) Right deep inferior epigastric vessels. (3) Right SIEV. (4) Distal lateral thoracic vein

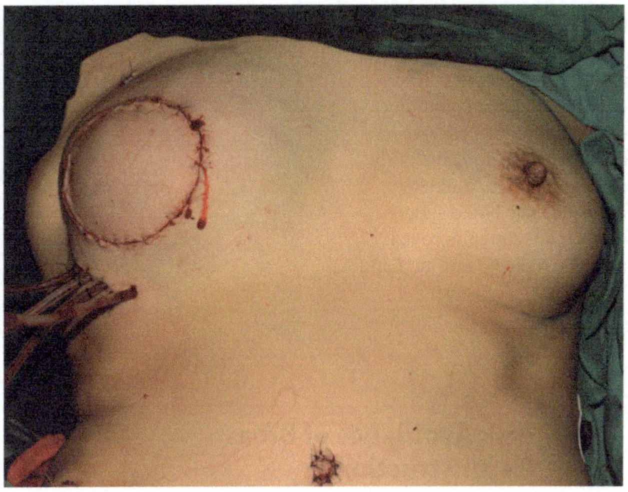

Fig. 18.11 Intraoperative view immediately after reconstruction. Mild over-perfusion of the flap was found

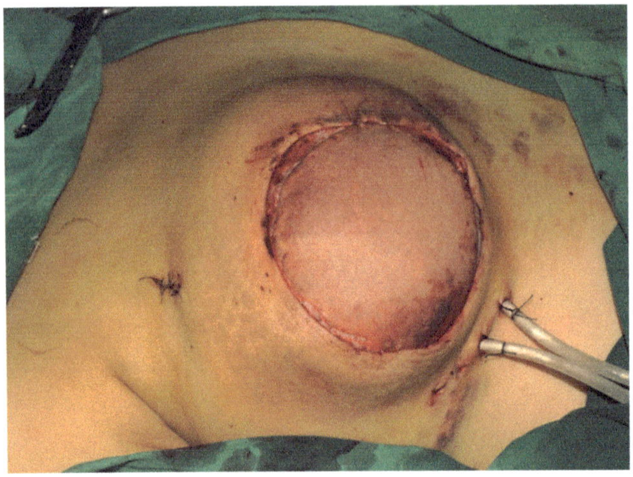

Fig. 18.12 Venous congestion was significant 24 h after operation

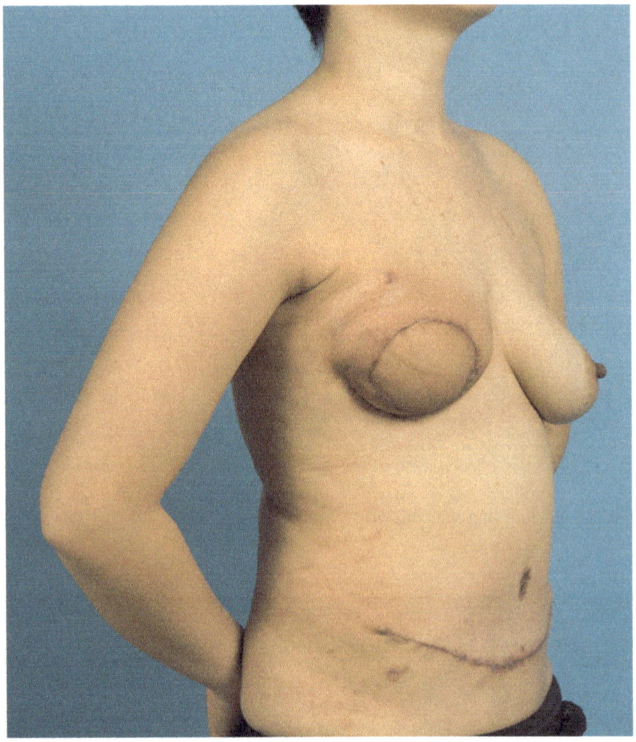

Fig. 18.14 Two months after operation

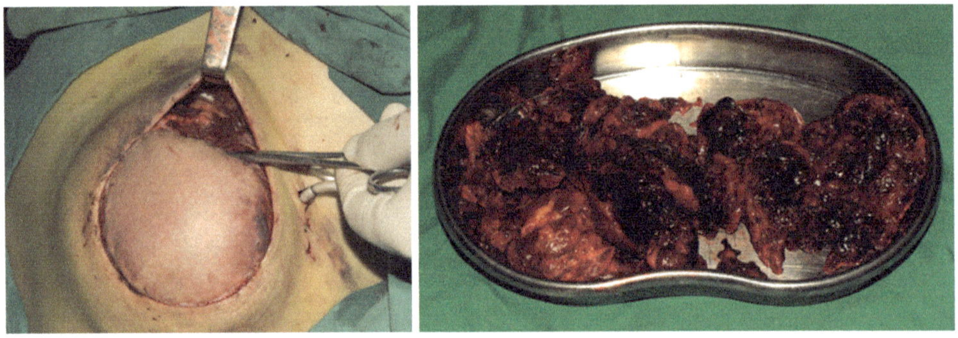

Fig. 18.13 Emergency exploration found that the anastomoses were unobstructed, a large number of hematoma was removed, and the congestion area of the flap was further completely removed. The blood supply was significantly improved after the reduction of the flap

18.1 Risk Avoidance of Breast Reconstruction

The main causes of complications and failure of breast reconstruction with autologous tissue transplantation include the following:

1. Improper choice of operation mode.
2. Failure to optimize the operation mode.
3. Inadequate preoperative planning.
4. The treatment of intraoperative problems is not in place.
5. 5 Postoperative complications are not treated in time.

Patient selection indicators included body mass index, history of smoking and diabetes, risk factors for vascular events, autoimmune condition, and general health [23, 24].

Case Study 2: Anatomical Variations of the Flap Vascular Pedicle

The patient was a 43-year-old female presented for left breast mass found for 1.5 years.

Left breast-invasive carcinoma of histological grade II (cT4N1M0) was diagnosed based on biopsy and preoperative imaging. Left radical mastectomy + left pedicled rectus abdominis flap (TRAM) for chest wall reconstruction were performed under general anesthesia after chemotherapy.

Postoperative pathology results were as follows: (1) Left breast-invasive lobular carcinoma, vascular, and nerve invasion (+), the size of the mass was about 3 cm × 2.5 cm × 2.5 cm; (2) 2/15 of left axillary lymph nodes were found with cancer metastasis; (3) the nipple was involved; and (4) no cancer involvement was found in the skin and basal margin. ER (80%+), PR (90%+), HER-2(0), and KI-67(20–30%+) (pT4N1M0). The flap survived uneventfully and the patient was transferred to oncology department for subsequent treatment. The function and appearance of chest wall recovered satisfactorily during follow-up (Figs. 18.15, 18.16, 18.17, 18.18, 18.19, 18.20, 18.21, 18.22, 18.23, 18.24, 18.25, 18.26, and 18.27).

The decision-making of the rectus abdominis flap or deep inferior epigastric artery perforator flap is based on multiple factors, including the operator's experience and expertise and previous history abdominal liposuction. In addition, if unilateral DIEP dysplasia is found during operation, contralateral TRAM flap should be considered.

The middle and lower perforating branches were retrogradely divided to the upper edge of the pubic symphysis and entered the posterior sheath.

How to deal with the lateral perforating branch?

What are the key points of muscle separation? Key points for judging the direction of perforating branches?

Under such circumstance, the possibility of operation failure increases. Due to anatomical variation, emphasis on skeletonizing the vascular pedicle to prepare a free perforator flap will cause extensive injury to rectus abdominis in the donor area, seriously affecting muscle function and strength. Considering operation time, operation difficulty, and risk, pedicled TRAM flap or muscle-sparing TRAM flap was also a good candidate.

Failure summary: It was anatomical variation rarely seen. The vascular pedicle was retrogradely separated in the muscle along the perforator. The pedicle was found to come from an unknown muscle branch medial to the rectus abdominis muscle. The vascular trunk actually traveled from the outside to the inside to the deep surface of the rectus abdominis muscle, and sent out multiple large muscle branches which zigzagged and further bifurcated the middle and lower perforators. To avoid failure, we should pay attention to the change of diameter and running direction when separating the vascular pedicle retrogradely and do not ligate the distal end. When the pedicle was found to become smaller and run medially, the optimal solution was to immediately expose the proximal end of the vascular trunk to confirm its diameter and travelling direction and then to make adjustment.

Consider that the patient had received 12 cycles of systemic chemotherapy before, and the perforator vessels were in poor condition. In order to ensure the safety of the operation, the left pedicled TRAM flap was harvested. Since the right perforators were not available, they were not re-vascularized. We removed the area IV and anastomosed the right SIEV with the left SIEV; the flap was in good blood supply and viable.

Summary of experience: In the process of cutting the DIEP flap, we should be aware of the anatomical variations of blood vessel. It is best to expose the proximal deep inferior epigastric vessels and then separate it in rendezvous manner. During retrograde separation of perforating branches, do not easily ligate any large branches, especially when the main trunk is not determined, the operation field must be fully exposed before accurate judgment can be made.

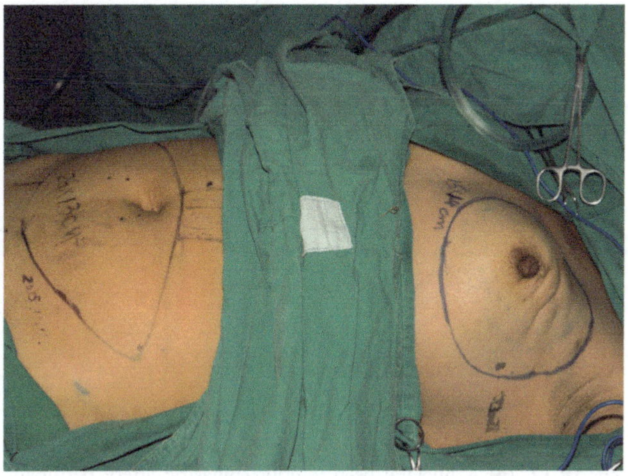

Fig. 18.15 Designed resection range during operation. The designed size of the flap was 26 cm × 13 cm

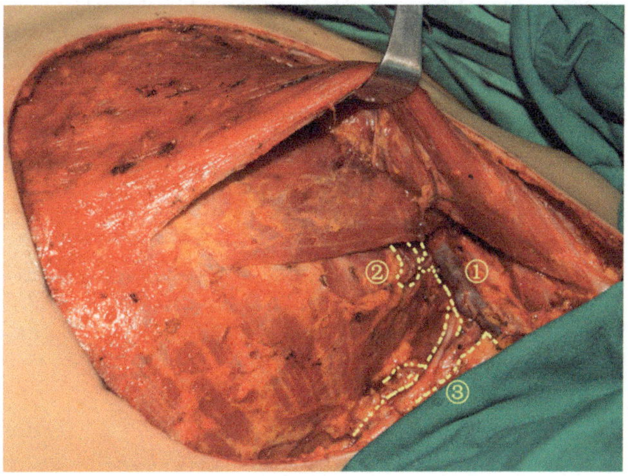

Fig. 18.16 The lesion was completely removed and the vascular pedicle in the recipient area was prepared. (1) Axillary vein. (2) Lateral thoracic vessels. (3) Thoracodorsal vessels and nerves

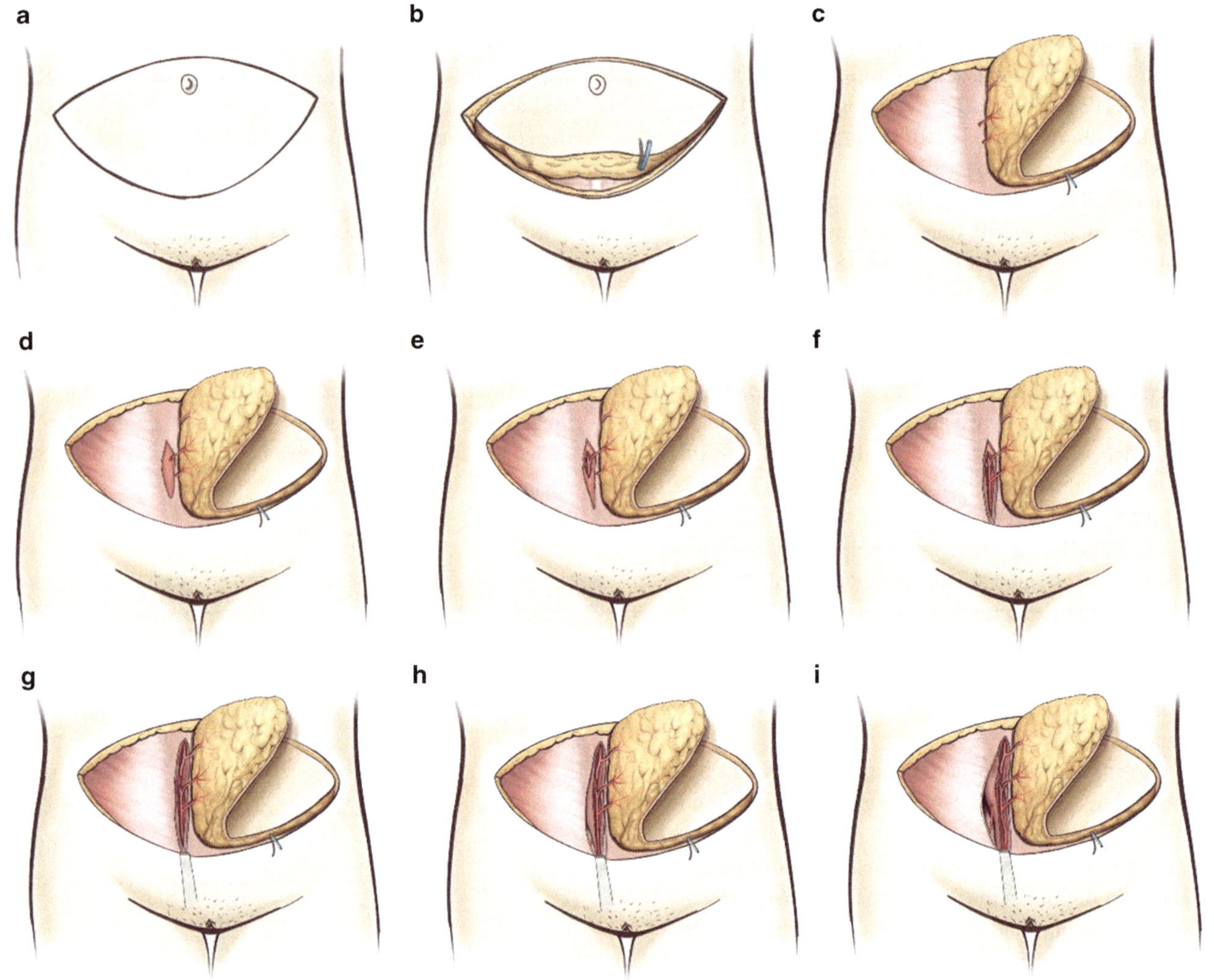

Fig. 18.17 (**a**) A bilateral deep inferior epigastric artery perforator flaps was planned before operation, and the rectus abdominis myocutaneous flap transfer for repair was actually completed. (**b**) The SIEV (V) was isolated. Lifting the flap on the surface of the anterior sheath of rectus abdominis and carrying the left SIEV (V). (**c**) The flap was separated from right to left to expose three perforating branches, which were located at paraumbilical, middle, and inferior-medial level, respectively. (**d**) The anterior sheath was cut along the outside of the middle perforator, and it was found that the perforator ran caudally beneath the anterior sheath. (**e**) The muscle separation was difficult, and the inferior and middle perforators were separated instead. (**f**) The middle and lower perforating branches shared a common trunk and went deep into the muscle. (**g**) Turn to lift the lateral anterior sheath, expose the main trunk of the deep inferior epigastric artery, and evaluate the lower two perforating branches. (**h**) Instead, the para-umbilical perforator was separated and found to be vertically descending in the superficial layer of the muscle, which had been broken earlier as the muscular perforator. (**i**) Intramuscular exploration along the trunk showed that the trunk sent out the paraumbilical perforator which was broken by mistake

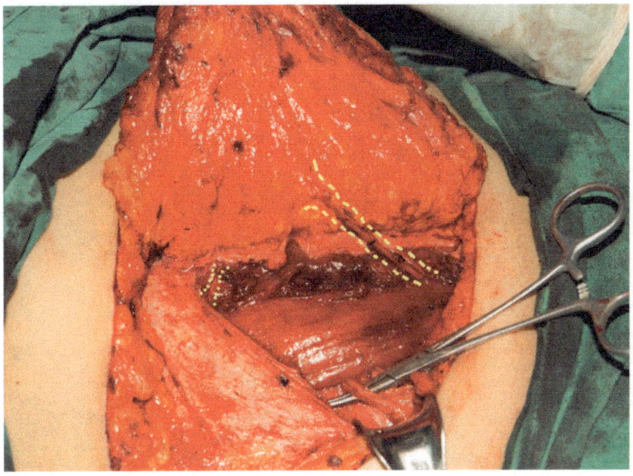

Fig. 18.18 Exposing the main deep inferior epigastric blood vessels at the lateral edge of the rectus abdominis

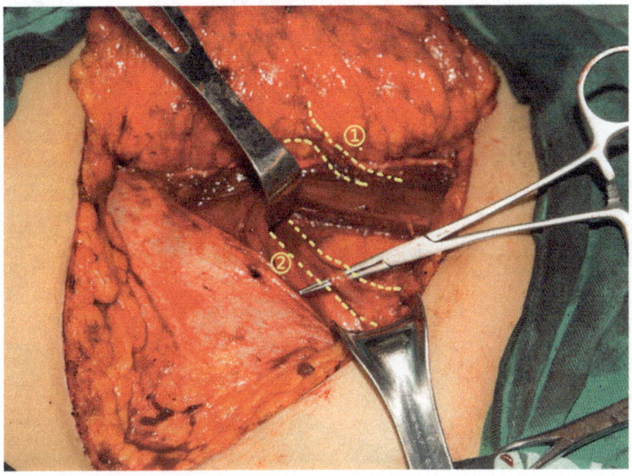

Fig. 18.19 Further separation found that the vascular pedicle of the flap was not the main deep inferior epigastric vessels. (1) Flap vascular pedicle. (2) The main deep inferior epigastric vessels

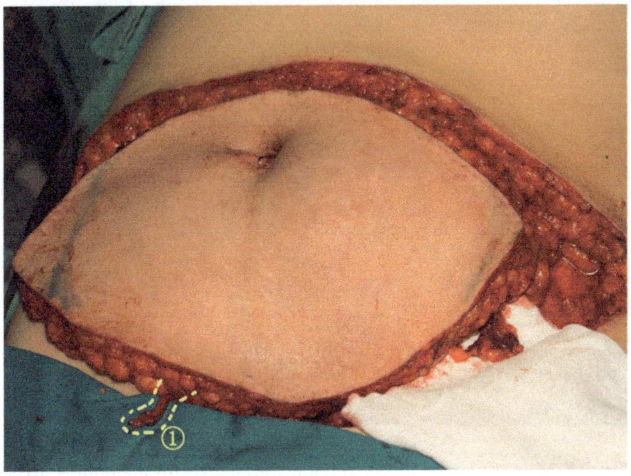

Fig. 18.20 Operation plan adjustment: the left rectus abdominis flap with pedicle was cut off. (1) Vascular pedicle of the right flap

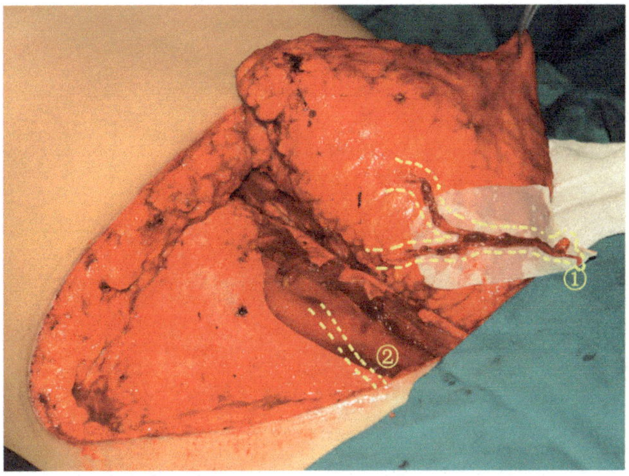

Fig. 18.21 The vascular pedicle of the right flap was examined and found to be unfilled and useless. (1) Flap vascular pedicle; (2) deep inferior epigastric vessels

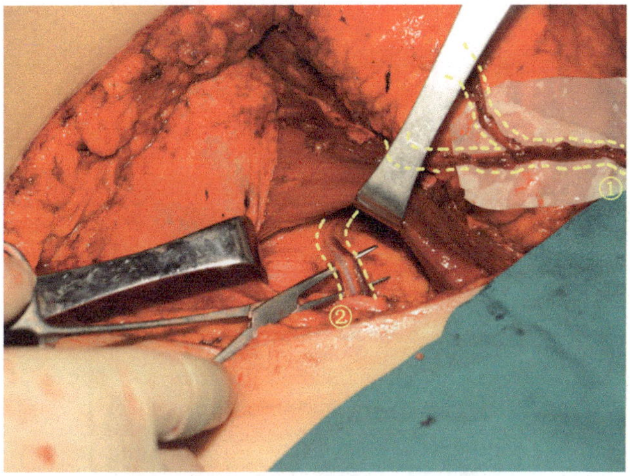

Fig. 18.22 Why the vascular trunk was missed were discussed later. (1) Flap vascular pedicle; (2) deep inferior epigastric vessels

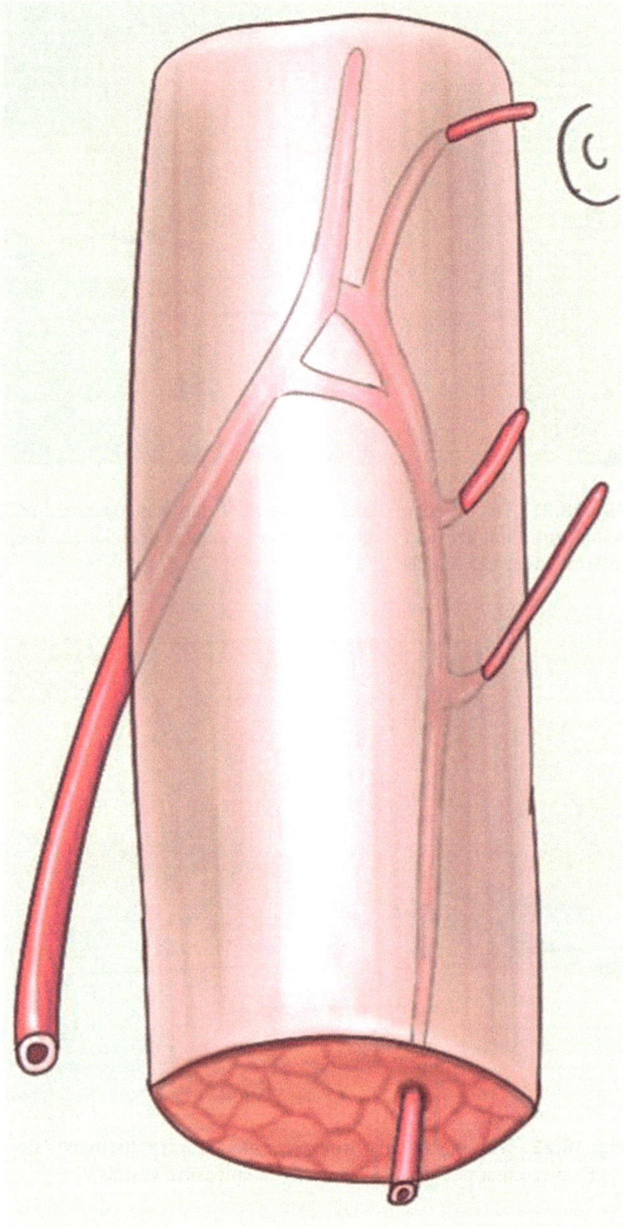

Fig. 18.23 The anatomy of three perforators

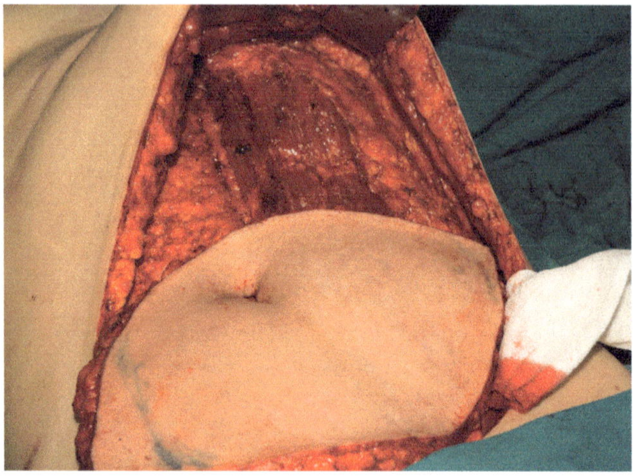

Fig. 18.24 Completing the preparation of the left pedicled rectus abdominis flap

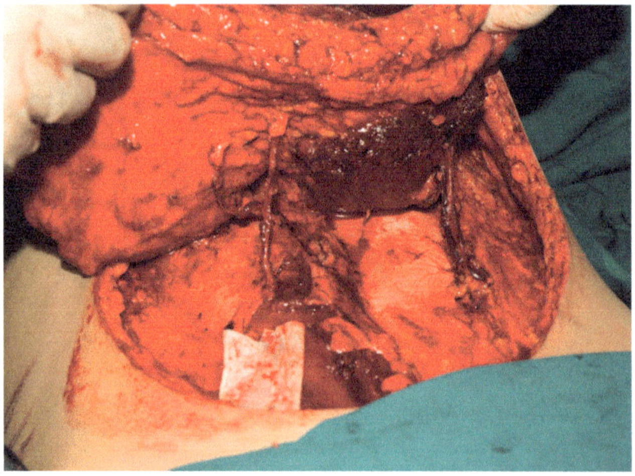

Fig. 18.25 The rectus abdominis flap was prepared

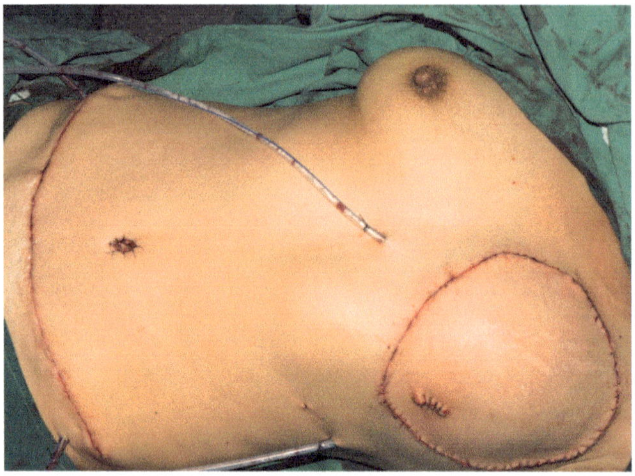

Fig. 18.26 Left breast reconstruction with left rectus abdominis myocutaneous flap was finished

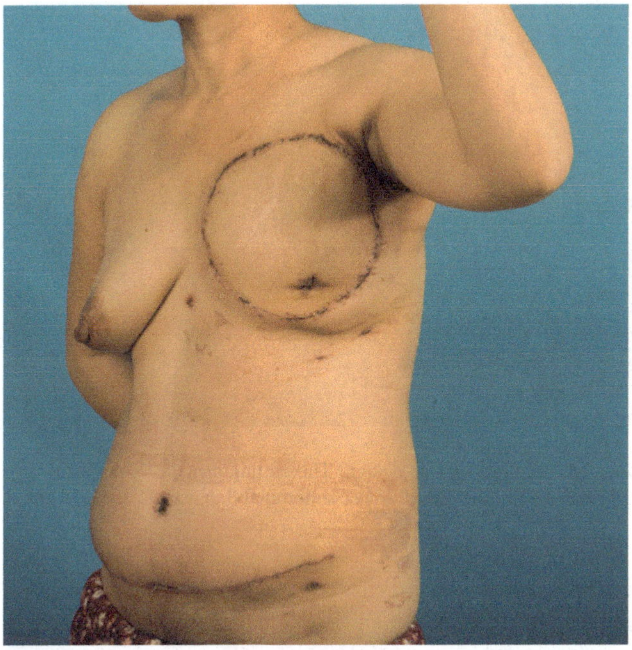

Fig. 18.27 One month after operation

Case Study 3: Repairing Chest Wall Defect with Anterolateral Femoral Flap

The patient was a 64-year-old male presented for chest wall recurrence for 6 months after comprehensive treatment for left breast cancer 28 years before. Left chest wall mucinous carcinoma was diagnosed. The patient received 19 cycles of chemotherapy before admission to our hospital where extended resection of left chest wall mass + the entire left chest wall removal + chest wall repair with pedicled rectus abdominis myocutaneous flap combined with free deep inferior epigastric artery perforator flap + mesh + bone cement were performed.

The third, fourth, fifth, and sixth ribs and most of the corresponding sternum were removed; only the right sternum with a width of about 5–7 mm was retained, and the left chest wall was completely removed.

The proximal ends of the internal thoracic artery and vein as well as the left lateral thoracic vessels were reserved.

Skin margins were clear of tumor by frozen section. The mesh was firmly sutured with the defect edge of the left chest wall, and the bone cement formed two artificial ribs to strengthen the ribs and sternum.

The right pedicled TRAM flap and left DIEP flap were harvested and transferred to the chest defect through the subcutaneous tunnel. Anastomosing the vascular pedicle of the left DIEP flap with the left lateral thoracic artery and vein (1A2V) under the microscope, and connecting the reserved SIEV with a branch of thoracodorsal vein.

The results of routine pathological examination were as follows: (1) (chest wall mass) diagnosed as metastatic breast mucinous carcinoma involving ribs; (2) no cancer invasion was found at the cutting edge; and (3) pericardial surface was clear of cancer invasion.

After operation, the chest wall tissue and flap edges were partially necrotic, resulting in exposure of the bone cement and mesh. After multiple debridement and vacuum-assisted suction, a free anterolateral femoral flap was transplanted to repair the secondary defect. The flap survived smoothly. At 2-year follow-up, the patient's chest wall function and appearance recovered satisfactorily, and there were no obvious complications in the flap donor area. The patient died of heart attack 28 months after operation (Figs. 18.28, 18.29, 18.30, 18.31, 18.32, 18.33, 18.34, 18.35, 18.36, 18.37, 18.38, 18.39, 18.40, 18.41, 18.42, 18.43, 18.44, 18.45, 18.46, 18.47, 18.48, 18.49, 18.50, 18.51, 18.52, 18.53, 18.54, 18.55, 18.56, 18.57, and 18.58).

Keep as many available recipient vessels as possible.

The preserved vascular pedicle included the pectoralis major branch of thoracoacromial vessels, two sets of lateral thoracic arteries and veins, and one set of internal thoracic artery and vein. The distal internal mammary vessels were deficient.

Initially, a large concomitant vein was found above the anterior sheath and vanished beneath the anterior sheath, because it was damaged accidentally. We later found that it did not come from the trunk of the deep inferior epigastric vessels; instead it was a vein unrelated to the perforator on the ground of which both perforators and their accompanying veins were intact after flap harvest.

In practice, it is not uncommon to find the pure venous perforator in the process of flap cutting. We should pay attention to distinguish it from the perforator. The most reliable way is to observe its pulsation, or gently pinch it with your fingers to determine the arterial pulsation. Large vein perforator together with small deep inferior epigastric perforator that go through the anterior sheath of the rectus abdominis is a rare case.

All perforating vessels in the half epigastric wall should be evaluated as comprehensively as possible before the perforating vessels of the flap are fully determined.

The deep inferior epigastric blood vessels were retrogradely separated to obtain a sufficient length, and an intramuscular branch was ligated and disconnected.

During the operation, this branch was mistaken as a simple muscle branch instead of the proximal source of the medial perforator.

Confusion and difficulty in judging perforator condition: neither the nutrient vessels of intercostal nerve nor the nutrient vessels of deep vein (V) can be used as the vascular pedicle of flap.

The anterior sheath of the rectus abdominis and the rectus abdominis between two parallel incisions did not need to be cut off. In this case, the anterior sheath was cut off; the integrity of rectus abdominis was preserved.

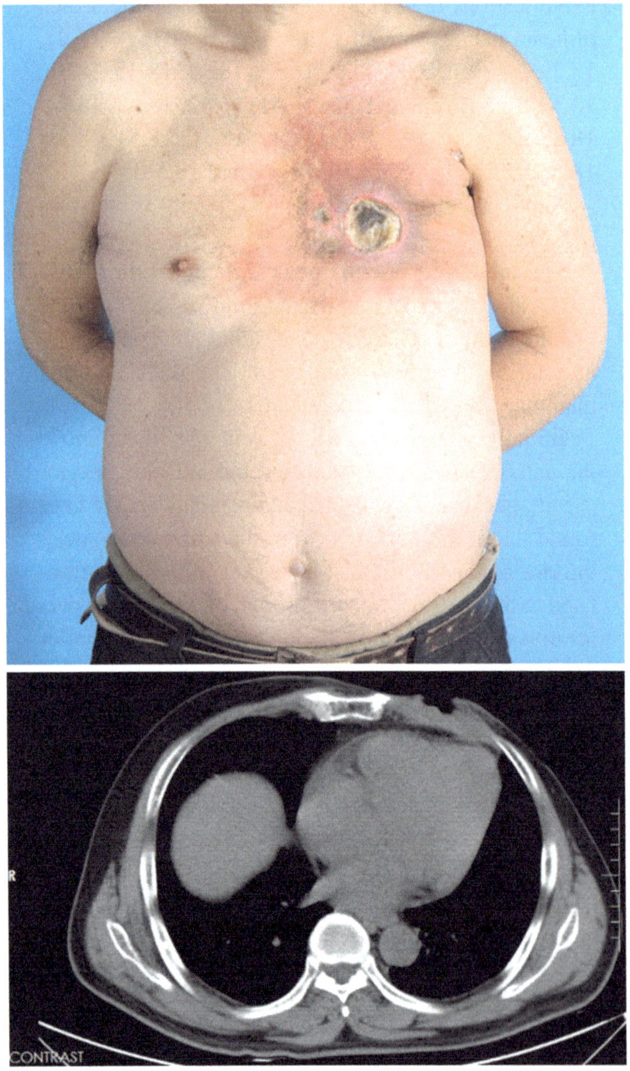

Fig. 18.28 Preoperative view and CT imaging

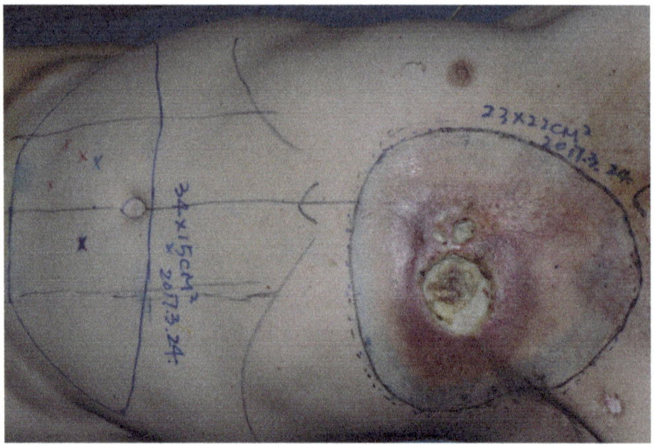

Fig. 18.29 Preoperative design. The cutting range of chest wall was 23 cm × 22 cm; the size of lower abdominal flap was 34 cm × 15 cm

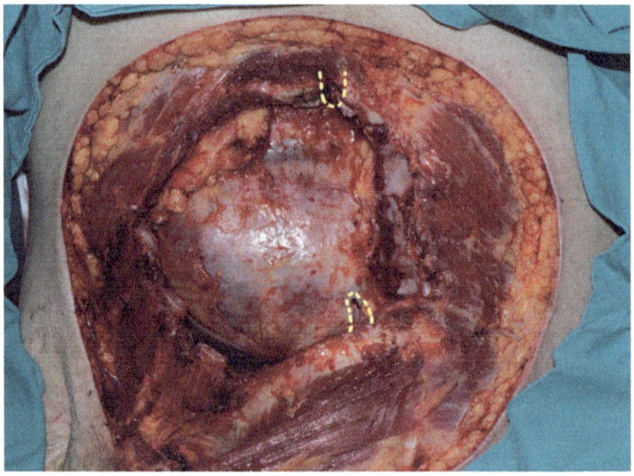

Fig. 18.30 Extended tumor resection

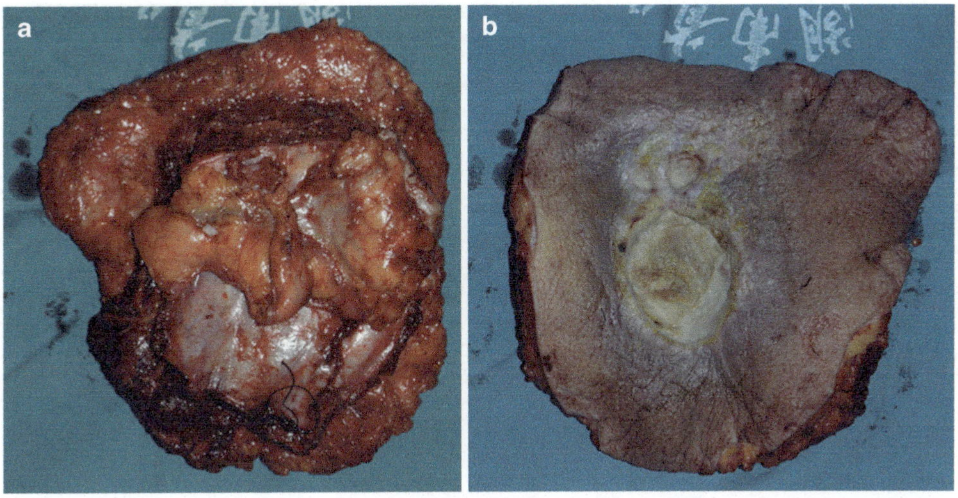

Fig. 18.31 (**a**) Depth of tumor resection. (**b**) The size of tumor resection range

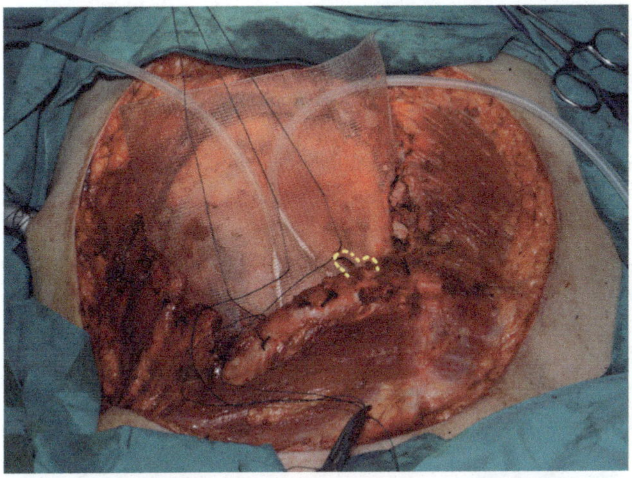

Fig. 18.32 Repair of chest wall defect with mesh

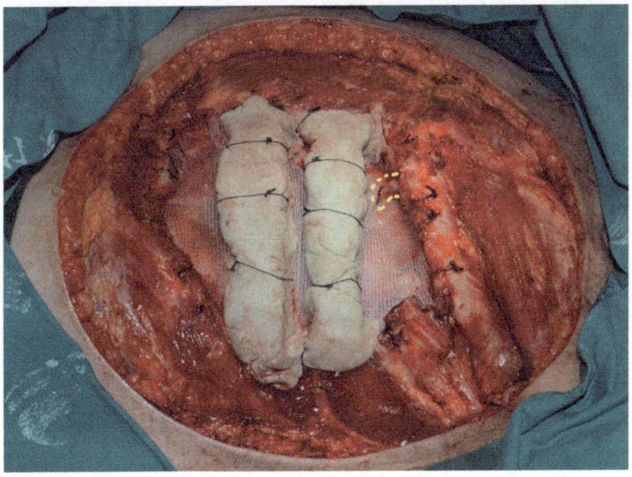

Fig. 18.33 Reconstruction of chest wall structure with bone cement. The vascular pedicle was separated during the operation. It was found that the vascular condition of this patient was very poor after chemotherapy and radiotherapy

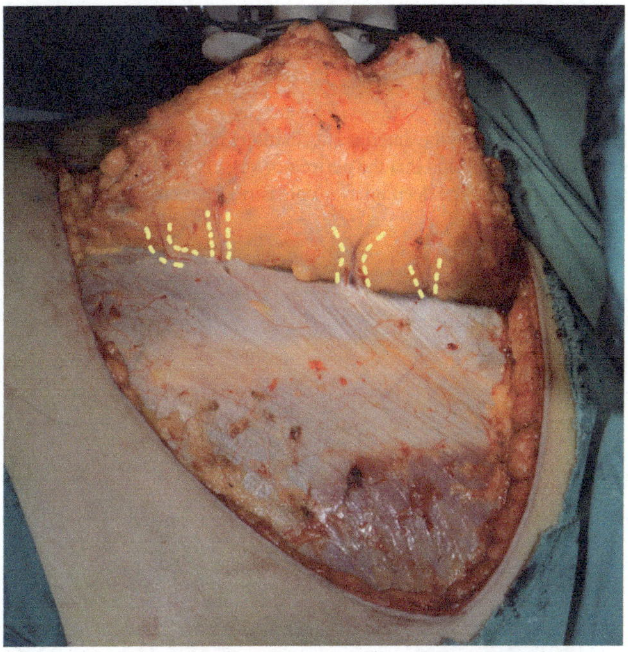

Fig. 18.34 Preoperative CTA was not given due to iodine allergy. According to the Doppler imaging, lifting the left flap to expose multiple perforator vessels

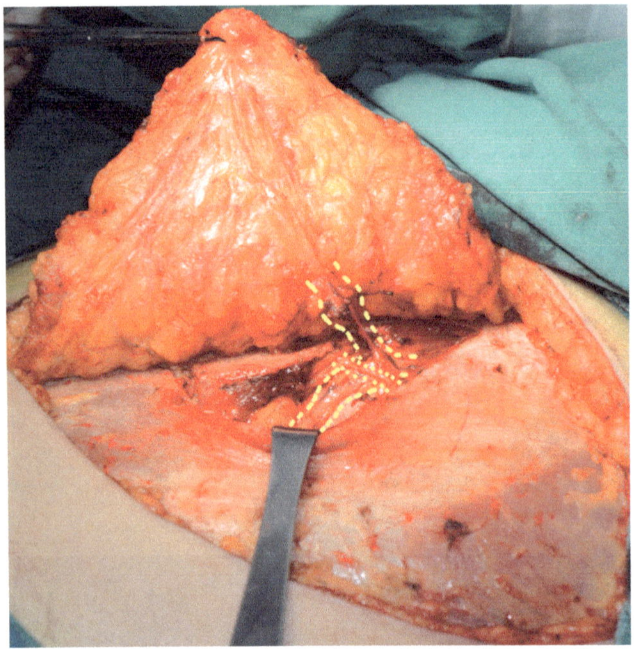

Fig. 18.35 Cutting the anterior sheath along the perforator, and retrograde separation found that the perforator vessels were small, exposing a long segment of the deep inferior epigastric vascular pedicle

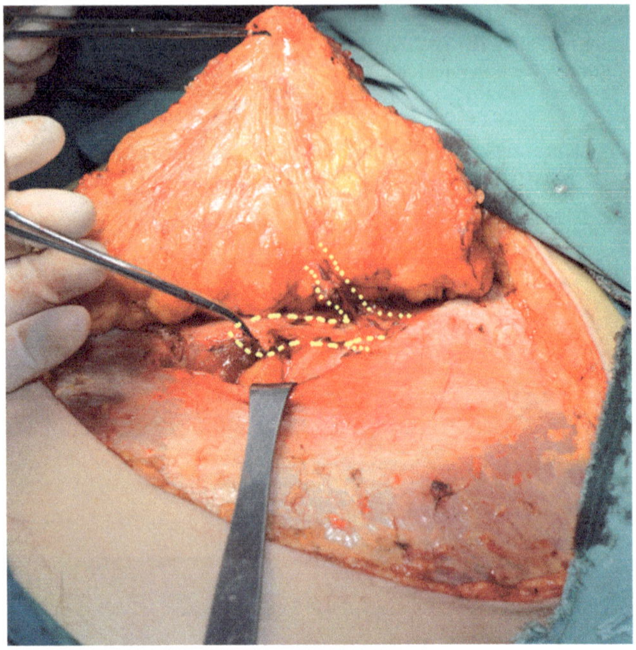

Fig. 18.37 Both perforators were desired; to avoid damaging too much rectus abdominis, we decided to cut off blood vessels to preserve rectus abdominis

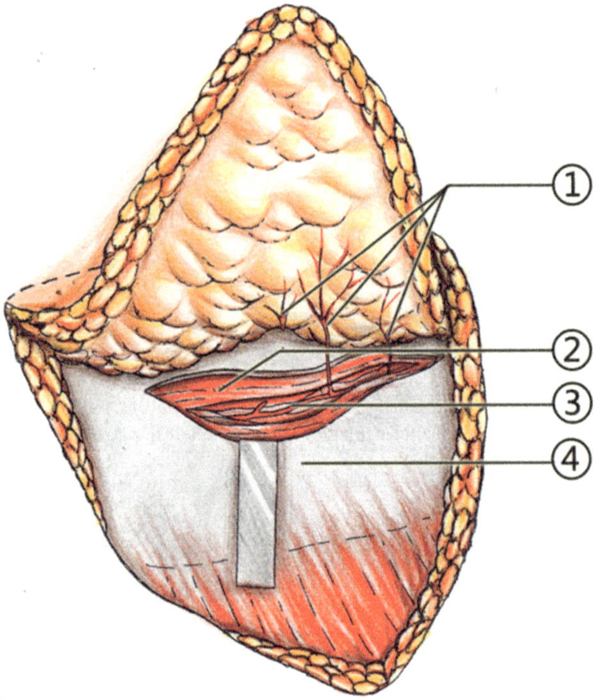

Fig. 18.36 It was suspected that this perforating branch was not the major left perforator; to avoid increasing injury, further exploration from caudal side to cephalic side showed that there was another large perforator near the midline. (1) Perforating vessels. (2) Rectus abdominis. (3) Deep inferior epigastric vessels. (4) Aponeurosis of external oblique abdominal muscle

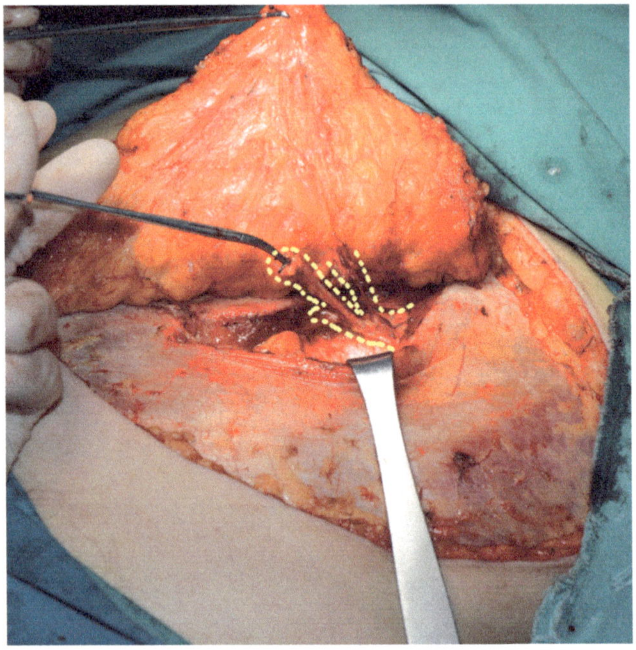

Fig. 18.38 Vascular pedicle separation was completed

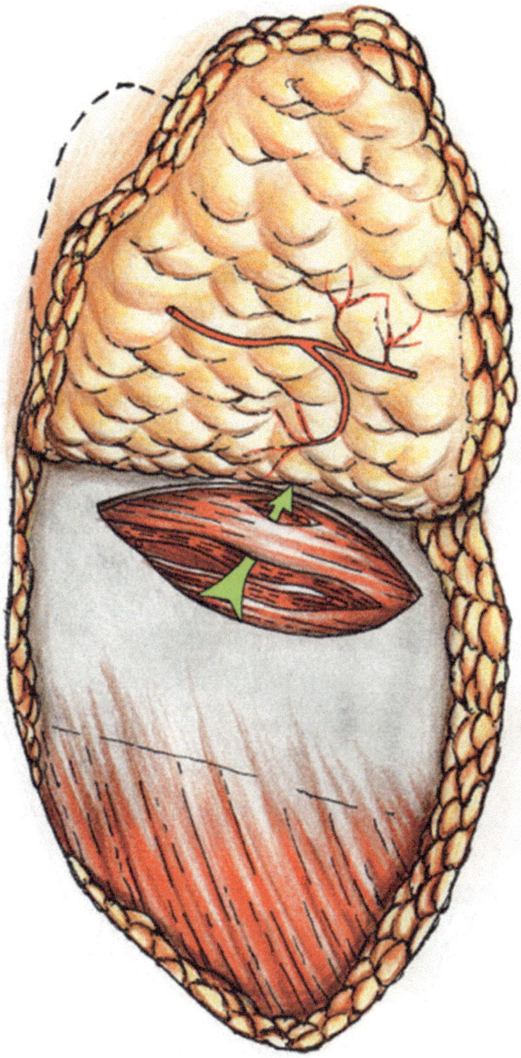

Fig. 18.39 After ligation and disconnection of the vascular pedicle, it was led out from the distal end and passed through the rectus abdominis tunnel on the deep surface of the large branch of the intercostal nerve, which retained the integrity of the rectus abdominis muscle to the greatest extent and the vegetative nerve

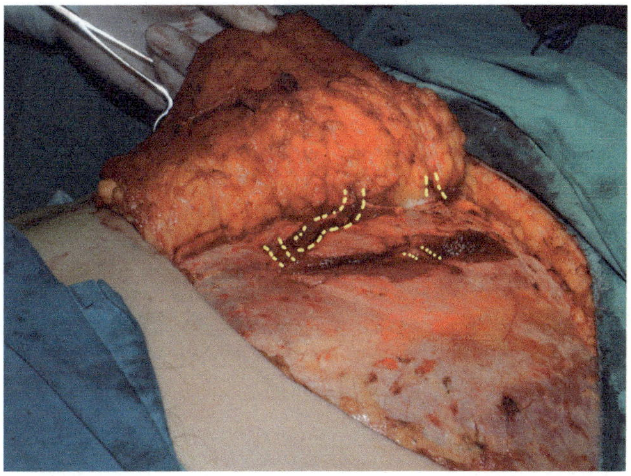

Fig. 18.40 Further separating flap toward the inside, exposing the real large perforating vessels of the left abdomen, cutting the anterior sheath longitudinally to reveal the underneath blood vessels, and determining that the main trunk was the medial branch previously exposed and ligated on the outside

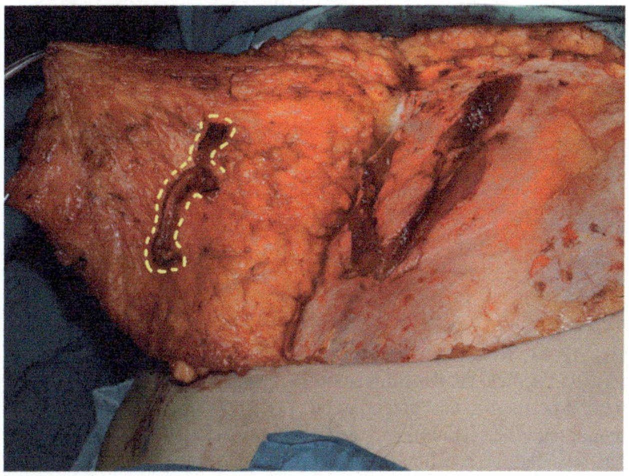

Fig. 18.41 The medial perforator vessel was separated through intramuscular tunnel, and the left DIEP flap was cut off

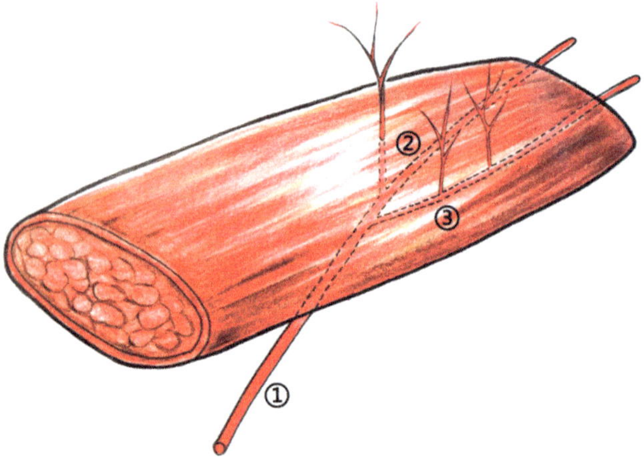

Fig. 18.42 Actual anatomical vascular form of DIEP flap. (1) The main deep inferior epigastric vessels. (2) Medial branch. (3) Lateral branch

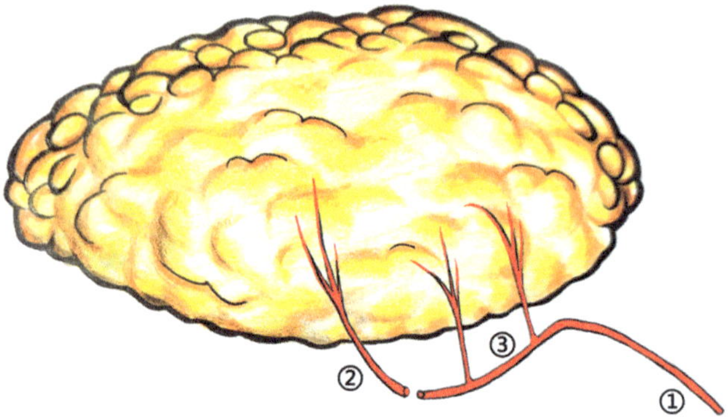

Fig. 18.45 Anastomosing the medial branch with the distal end of the lateral vascular pedicle of the flap, extending the effective length of the vascular pedicle. (1) The main deep inferior epigastric vessels. (2) Medial branch. (3) Lateral branch

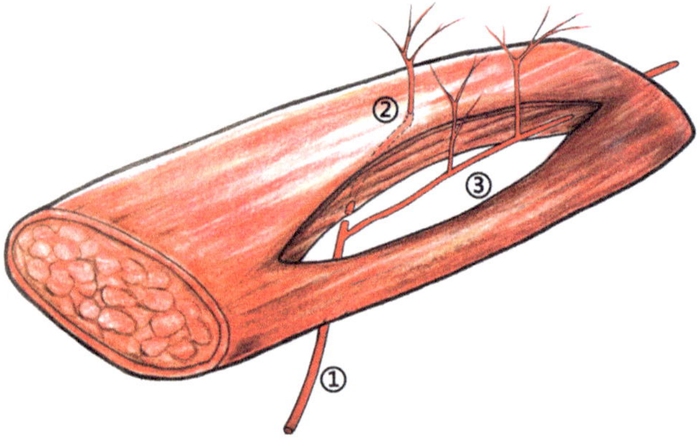

Fig. 18.43 Retrogradely separating of the lateral perforator and its vascular pedicle to the bifurcation facing inside, further ligating the medial perforator, and preparing the vascular pedicle with a sufficient length, and then ligation and disconnection were performed. This step has revealed the position of the medial perforator. (1) The main deep inferior epigastric vessels. (2) Medial branch. (3) Lateral branch

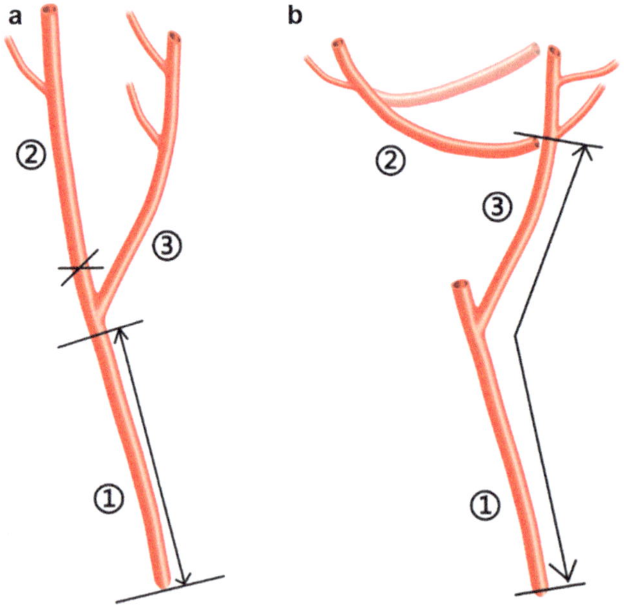

Fig. 18.46 (**a**, **b**) Schematic diagram of vascular pedicle extension. Vascular anastomosis reconstruction mode: turbocharge—anastomosing the medial perforator vessel with the distal end of the deep inferior epigastric vessels. The advantages are as follows: (1) The rectus abdominis muscle is preserved to the greatest extent; the medial perforator is repositioned to effectively prolong the length of vascular pedicle. (1) The main deep inferior epigastric vessels. (2) Medial branch. (3) Lateral branch

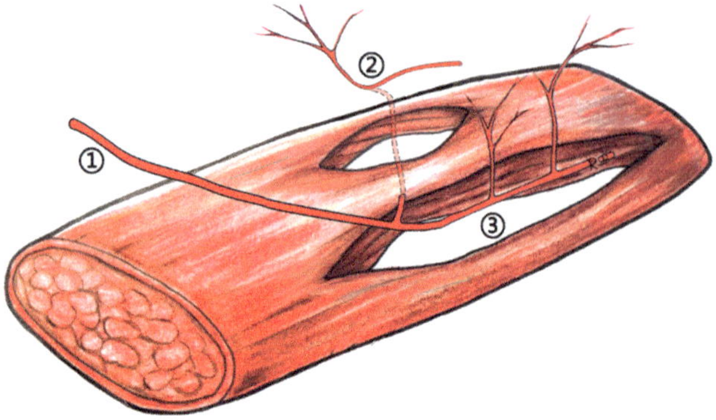

Fig. 18.44 Pulling away the lateral vascular pedicle, further separating the medial perforator medially and freeing the medial perforator vascular pedicle in the muscle in rendezvous manner

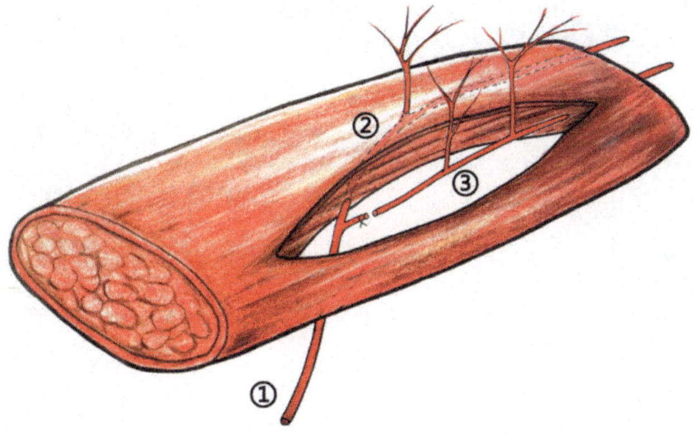

Fig. 18.47 Lifting the flap, directly ligating and disconnecting the lateral perforator, exposing the large medial perforator, and retrogradely separating the perforator in the muscle toward outside. The adjustment of vascular pedicle position is more flexible, and the placement of flap is more flexible. Reasonable design can further prolong the effective vascular length for repair. (1) The main deep inferior epigastric vessels. (2) Medial branch. (3) Lateral branch

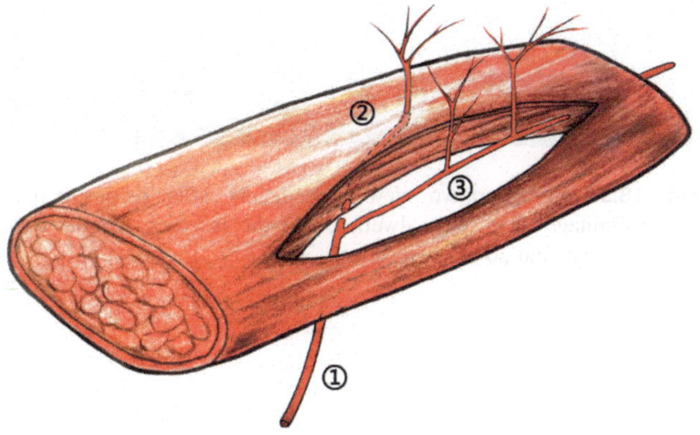

Fig. 18.48 After exposing the lateral perforating branch, retrograde separation continues to the trunk and its medial bifurcation. Ligating and disconnecting it far from the bifurcation. (1) The main deep inferior epigastric vessels. (2) Medial branch. (3) Lateral branch

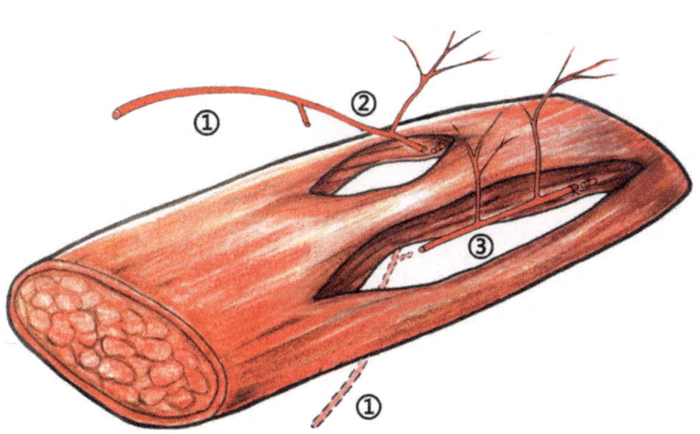

Fig. 18.49 Further separating the flap to the medial side, completely exposing the medial perforator vessels, and separating the medial perforator and the main vascular pedicle in rendezvous manner. (1) The main deep inferior epigastric vessels. (2) Medial branch. (3) Lateral branch

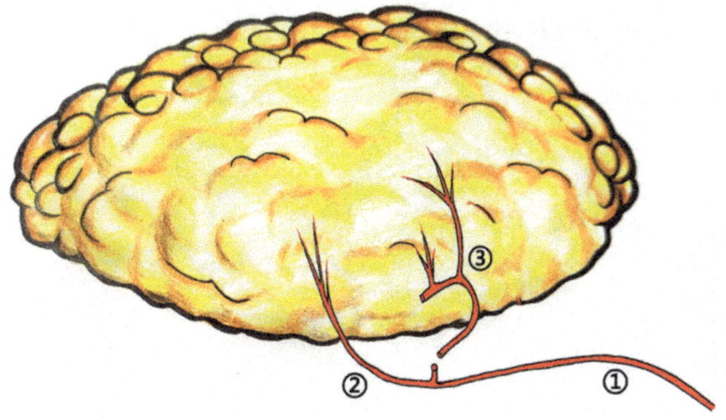

Fig. 18.50 Ligating and disconnecting the vascular pedicle from the point close to the origin, retrogradely extracting it from the intramuscular tunnel, and anastomosing the distal end of the lateral perforator vascular pedicle with the medial perforator vascular pedicle for turbocharge. (1) The main deep inferior epigastric vessels. (2) Medial branch. (3) Lateral branch

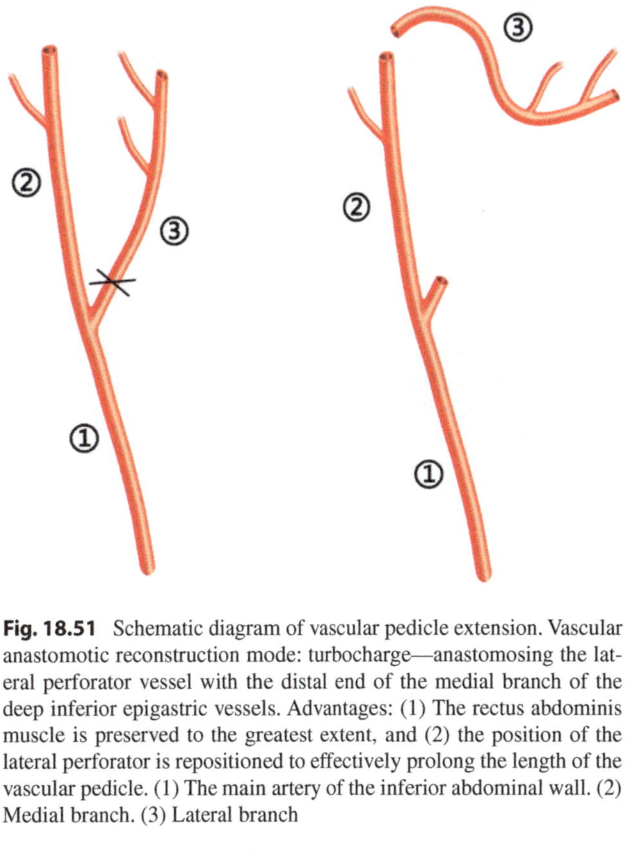

Fig. 18.51 Schematic diagram of vascular pedicle extension. Vascular anastomotic reconstruction mode: turbocharge—anastomosing the lateral perforator vessel with the distal end of the medial branch of the deep inferior epigastric vessels. Advantages: (1) The rectus abdominis muscle is preserved to the greatest extent, and (2) the position of the lateral perforator is repositioned to effectively prolong the length of the vascular pedicle. (1) The main artery of the inferior abdominal wall. (2) Medial branch. (3) Lateral branch

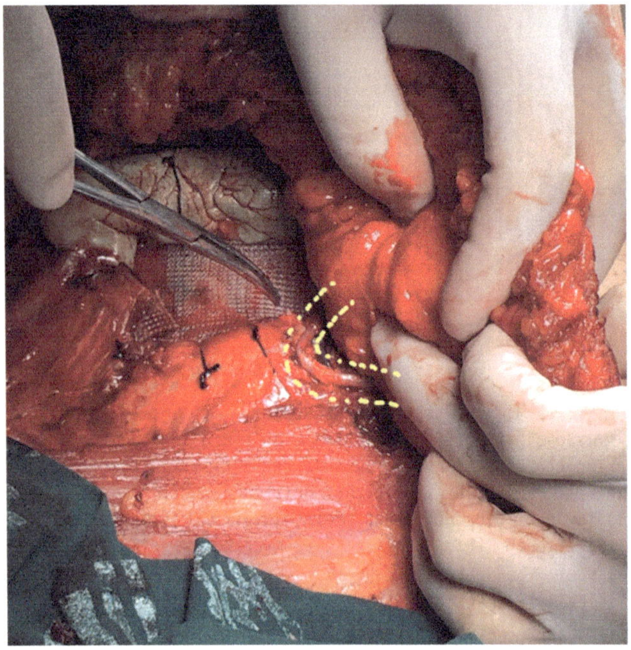

Fig. 18.52 Vascular anastomosis: pay attention to the protection of surrounding soft tissue, which can effectively avoid vasospasm

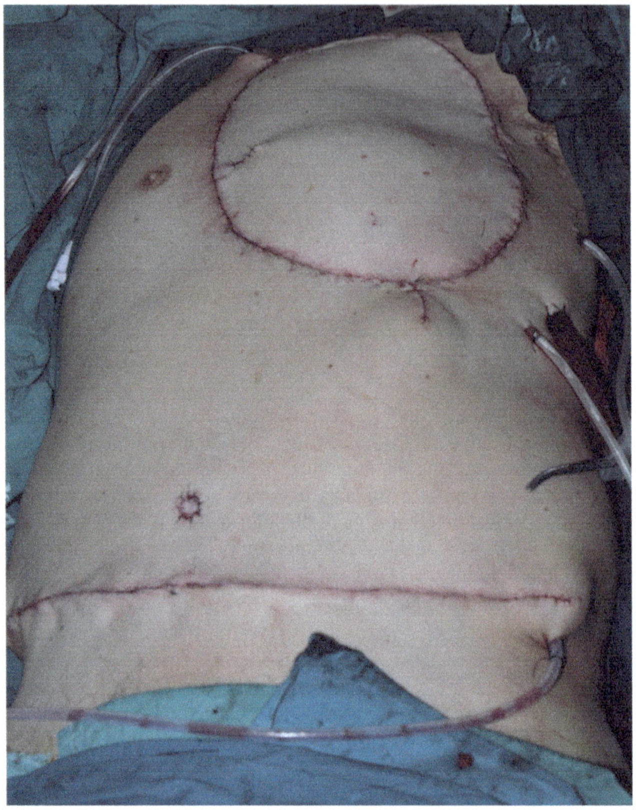

Fig. 18.54 Intraoperative view immediately after reconstruction. Three drainage tubes were dwelled, and the insertion lengths were 15 cm, 20 cm, and 20 cm, respectively

Fig. 18.53 Placement of the vascular pedicle after the placement of the skin flap with and without costal cartilage removal

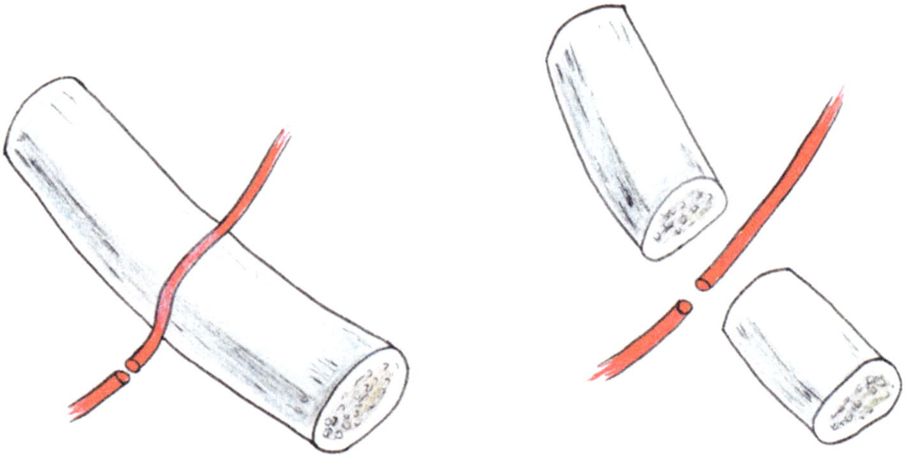

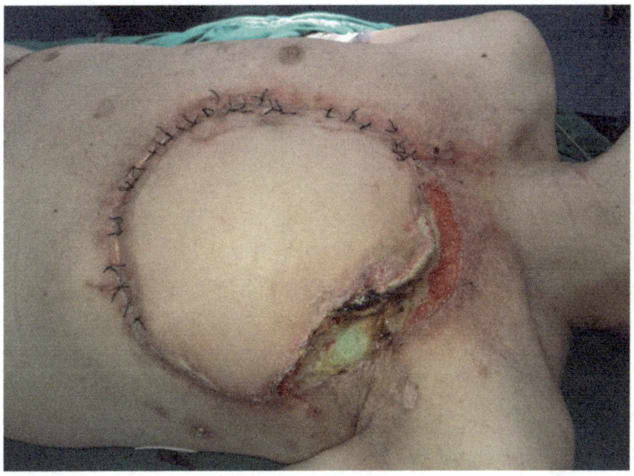

Fig. 18.55 Most of the flaps survived after operation, while the surrounding tissues manifest progressive necrosis, resulting in exposure of bone cement and mesh

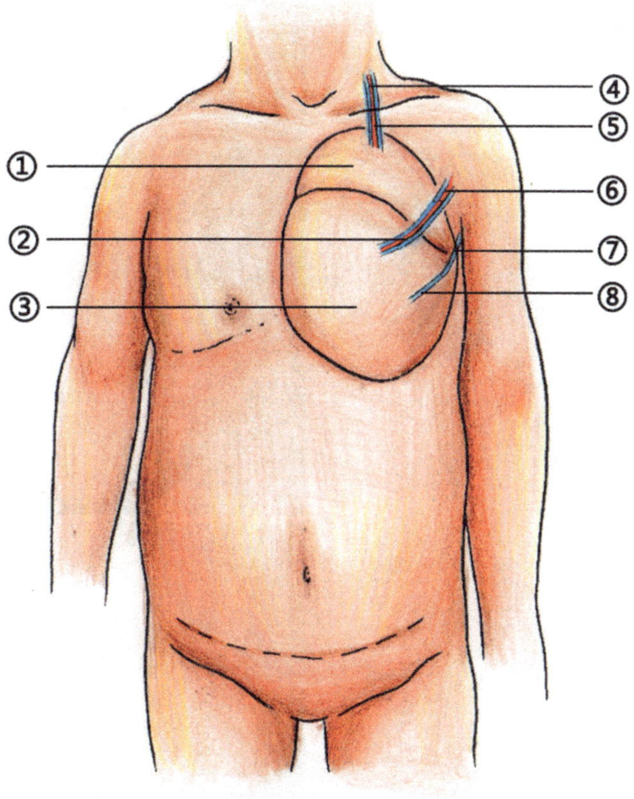

Fig. 18.57 Revascularization pattern: left deep inferior epigastric vessels + left lateral thoracic vessels (1A2V); right SIEV + anterior serratus branch of left thoracodorsal vein. (1) Anterolateral femoral perforator flap. (2) Left deep inferior epigastric vessel. (3) Perforator flap of the deep inferior epigastric artery. (4) Transverse cervical vessels. (5) Descending branch of the lateral femoral circumflex vessel. (6) Lateral thoracic vessels. (7) Anterior serratus branch of the thoracodorsal vein. (8) SIEV

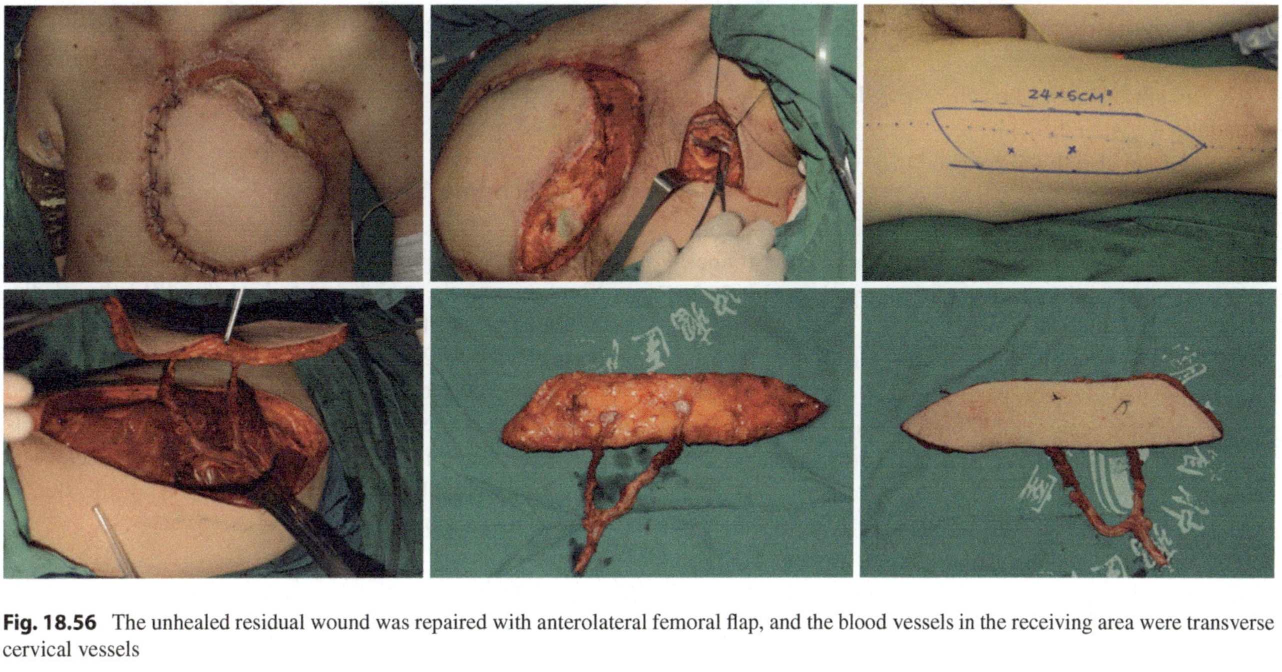

Fig. 18.56 The unhealed residual wound was repaired with anterolateral femoral flap, and the blood vessels in the receiving area were transverse cervical vessels

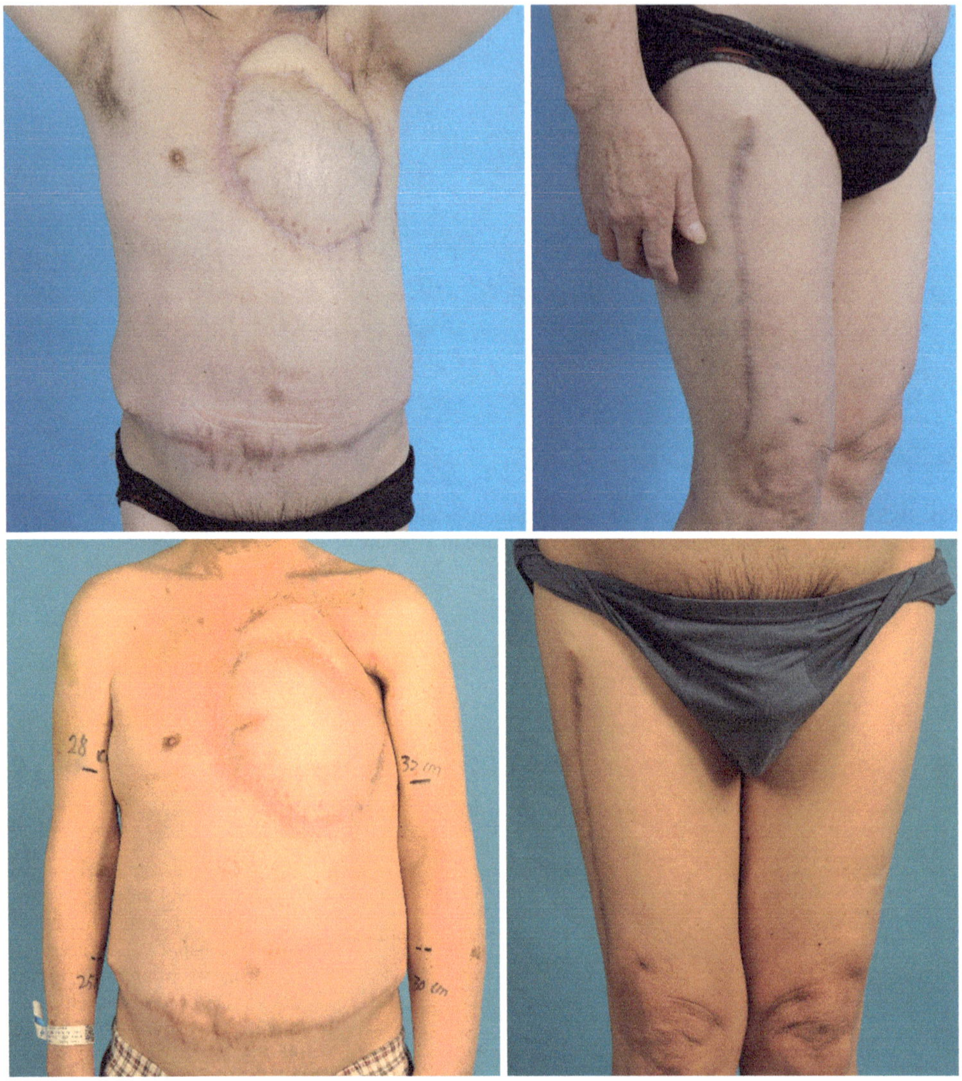

Fig. 18.58 16-month follow-up after operation

18.1.1 Downsides of Flap Raising in This Case

1. The length of lateral branch reserved was not sufficient making decision difficult.
2. The anterior sheath did not need to be cut completely; the solution diagram is shown below.
3. The lateral perforator can be sacrificed, and the perforator can be separated directly into the intramuscular tunnel.
4. What is the significance of supercharged repair? Reflect on what should be done.
5. Issues as to vascular anastomosis: insufficient length of vascular pedicle, complete removal of costal cartilage and complete separation of blood vessels should be done, and soft tissue protection at base was required.

During the operation, we mistaken the large subcutaneous vein accompanied by the small perforator as the pedicle; otherwise it would be cut off and flap separation continued medially, raising the left DIEP flap pedicled with the large medial perforator. See the following scheme.

18.1.2 Scheme 1 Summary

It is very important to understand and master the anatomy of perforating vessels, which can reduce the difficulty of dissection. There are three anatomical forms of deep inferior epigastric vessels [25].

The most common is that the main blood vessel is divided into medial and lateral branches, and the perforating vessels originate beneath or inside the rectus abdominis muscle. The area of blood supply by the perforator entering the skin is called the perforasome.

Generally speaking, the lateral perforators run vertically and a short distance in the muscle, while the medial perforators travel obliquely and a long distance in the muscle, making separation difficult.

The other two vascular anatomical forms include single vascular pedicle and three vascular pedicle types [26].

When the vascular pedicle is divided into internal and external branches in rectus abdominis, in some cases, the position of internal and external perforating vessels is outward, which should be noted (Figs. 18.42, 18.43, 18.44, 18.45, and 18.46).

18.1.3 Redesign Scheme 2 (Fig. 18.47)

The flap was cut only with the large medial perforator as the pedicle.

Parallel auxiliary incision was made from the outside of the anterior sheath.

Lifting the rectus abdominis muscle from outside to inside to expose the main deep inferior epigastric vessels.

The main deep inferior epigastric vessels and perforating branches were separated in rendezvous manner. See scheme 3 (Figs. 18.48, 18.49, 18.50, 18.51, and 18.52).

Option 3:

The vascular conditions of patients with chemotherapy and radiotherapy were very poor.

The preserved vascular pedicle included two sets of lateral thoracic arteries and veins and one set of internal thoracic artery and vein. Vascular anastomosis mode: The internal thoracic artery and vein were anastomosed with the deep inferior epigastric artery and vein.

Note: The placement of vascular pedicle is very important. It is necessary to remove the part of the second costal cartilage when the length of vascular pedicle is insufficient, the space of anastomotic vessels is insufficient, and the tension is large.

In order to place the vascular pedicle without torsion, the possible compression of the vascular pedicle after flap suture should be considered.

There are two anastomosis patterns. The second can prolong the length of vascular pedicle, but the diameter of the first one is more matched (Fig. 18.53).

There are three most important points in vascular anastomosis: (1) anastomotic tension, (2) matching of anastomotic diameter, and (3) enough space for anastomosis.

18.1.4 Vascular Pedicle Repair and Repositioning

Although the free vascular pedicle is very fragile, it usually becomes the most stable part after vascular anastomosis, especially when coupler is used.

Therefore, venous reflux disorder is mostly due to vascular pedicle injury or distortion, which has nothing to do with vascular anastomosis.

However, when anastomosing with the internal mammary blood vessels, whether the ribs are removed or not, the blood vessels may be distorted at the junction between the pectoralis major muscle and the ribs.

When exploring the distortion of vascular pedicle, we should focus on checking whether there is torsion of vascular pedicle, because blindly repeating anastomosis will not improve the undetected distortion or vascular pedicle injury. Such useless efforts will only lead to further ischemia, failure to solve the actual problem, and shortening the rescue time window.

Long vascular pedicle is best preserved in stage II chest wall reconstruction and breast reconstruction, and short pedicle is more likely to be used in stage I. The position of the combined flap can be slightly adjusted and transferred clockwise or counterclockwise to improve the tension.

Multiple small auxiliary covert free retraction can make the wound converge to the center and reduce the tension of the flap.

It is not uncommon for breast cancer patients to receive chest wall radiotherapy and systemic chemotherapy for a long time. The operator must master remedial measures; otherwise it will lead to more serious and acute complications.

Conclusion: There are two most difficult points in cutting the DIEP flap: (1) location, exposure, and selection of perforators; (2) separation of perforating branches penetrating tendinous inscriptions; and (3) combined utilization of different perforators and their vascular pedicles.

For the breast cancer patients, there are many risks that cannot be completely anticipated before the completion of the breast reconstruction with DIEP flap transplantation. The most common and tricky difficulty is the poor vascular characteristics caused by radiotherapy and chemotherapy, which is manifested by the separation of the vascular pedicle and the separation of vessels in the recipient area. This requires the operator's excellent vascular anastomosis technique to avoid the risk. Pedicled rectus abdominis myocutaneous flap combined with the free deep inferior epigastric artery perforator flap to reconstruct the breast can be the first choice in patients with poor general conditions or vascular conditions due to multiple cycles of chemotherapy and radiotherapy [27].

Case Study 4: Patients with Poor General Conditions and Poor Vascular Conditions of the Flap

The patient was a 34-year-old female presented for left breast cancer (cT4N2M0 phase III A, ER (−), PR (−), HER-2 (−)) previously treated with chemotherapy (TEC regime) and which responded partially.

The patients were treated with radical mastectomy of left breast cancer + pedicled rectus abdominis myocutaneous flap combined with perforator flap of deep inferior epigastric artery for reconstruction. Dissecting the left internal thoracic artery and vein and the lateral thoracic artery and vein which were anastomosed with the deep inferior epigastric artery and vein (1A2V).

Postoperative pathological examination showed that the histology of left breast-invasive ductal carcinoma was grade III, cancer metastasis was found in 1/18 of left axillary lymph nodes' cancer involvement (not involving epidermis) was found in nipple, vascular invasion (+); and no cancer involvement was found in skin and basal margins (pT3N1M0, stage IIIa). Immunohistochemistry showed ER (−), PR (−), CerbB-2 (1 +), and Ki-67 about 60%.

The flap was still partially liquefied and necrotic and healed after debridement and suture, and the patient was transferred to internal medicine department for further systematic treatment.

The appearance and function of the chest wall recovered well during follow-up (Figs. 18.59, 18.60, 18.61, 18.62, 18.63, 18.64, 18.65, 18.66, 18.67, 18.68, 18.69, 18.70, 18.71, 18.72, 18.73, 18.74, 18.75, and 18.76).

Difficult points: This case represents the actual clinical situation that it is difficult to achieve perfect anatomy. It was very difficult to complete micromanipulation and flap resection. Long-term chemotherapy had led to disappearance or waning of perforating vessels.

It is still a difficult clinical problem to retain the perforating branch of the lateral or medial row.

It was difficult to obtain satisfactory perforators in this case: No suitable perforators of the lateral branch whose large medial perforator was located in the muscle, making separation very difficult. Moreover, the main large perforator passing through the anterior sheath was basically directly below the navel. In order to explore the blood vessels, the flap will not be separated to this range. We must rely entirely on preoperative CTA and operator experience.

Necrosis appeared in area three of the right rectus abdominis flap. It was reconstruction with transplantation of the right pedicled rectus abdominis flap combined with the left free DIEP flap. We assumed that the main reason was the systemic skin and soft tissue injury caused by chemotherapy, the skin flap blood supply of this patient was significantly worse than that of normal people, and the secondary reason should be the blood supply zoning characteristics of the rectus abdominis flap.

Breast reconstruction surgery is difficult and requires multidisciplinary team cooperation, as well as full communication and cooperation between doctors and patients. For a very small number of patients who are difficult to communicate, hesitant, and distrusting medical staff, breast reconstruction surgery should not be implemented [28].

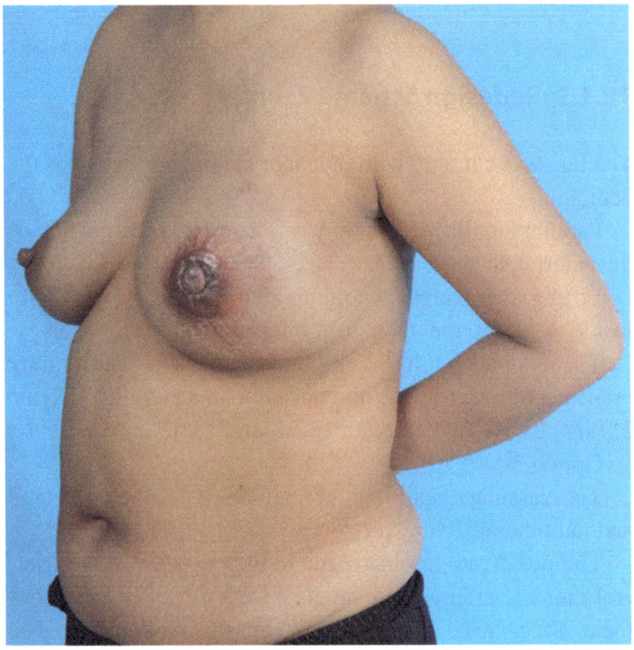

Fig. 18.59 Preoperative findings

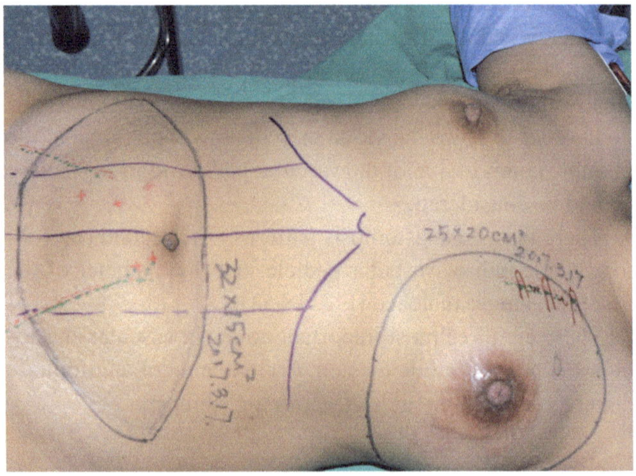

Fig. 18.60 Intraoperative design

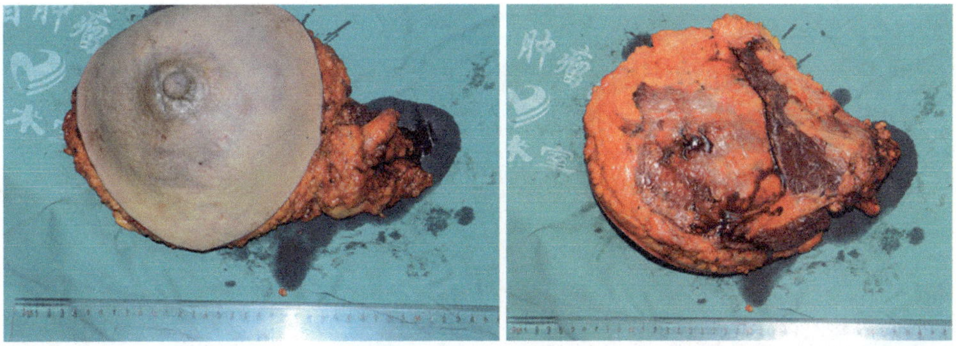

Fig. 18.61 Resection of lesion tissue completed

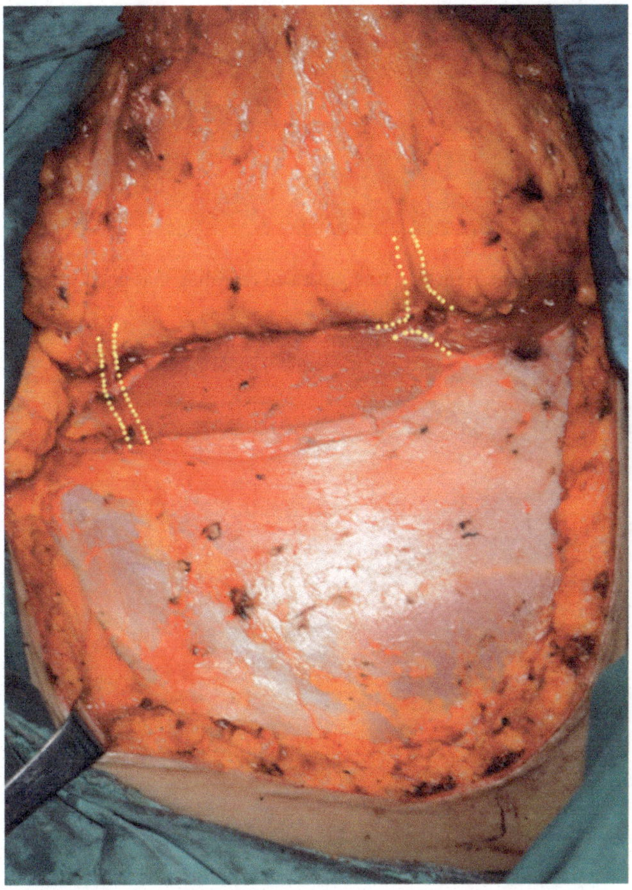

Fig. 18.62 Preserving bilateral SIEVs

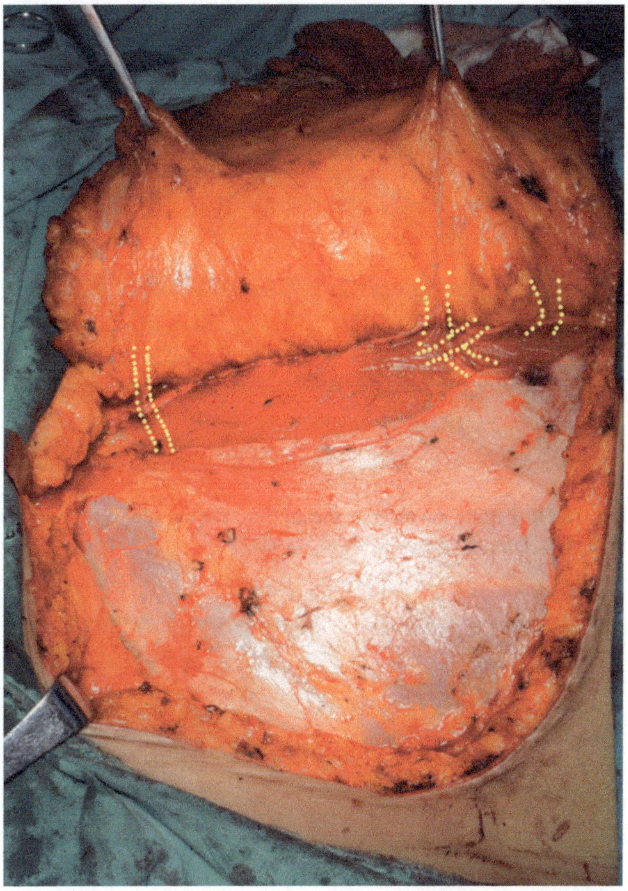

Fig. 18.63 Lifting the left flap to expose four small perforators, and the perforator above the umbilicus was slightly large; the anterior sheath was cut to expose the small perforating branches and the deep inferior epigastric vascular pedicle

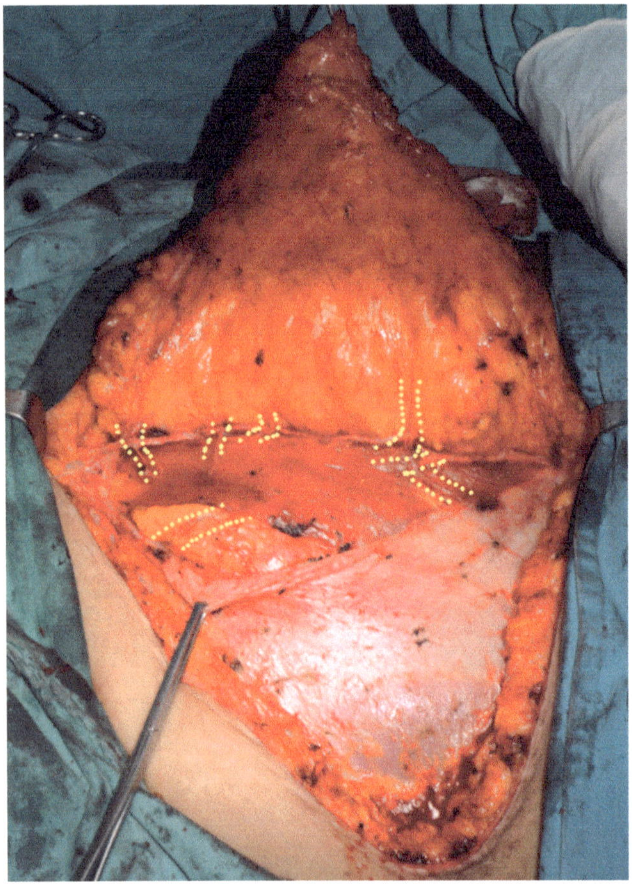

Fig. 18.64 Lifting the anterior sheath from the outside to expose the main deep inferior epigastric blood vessels

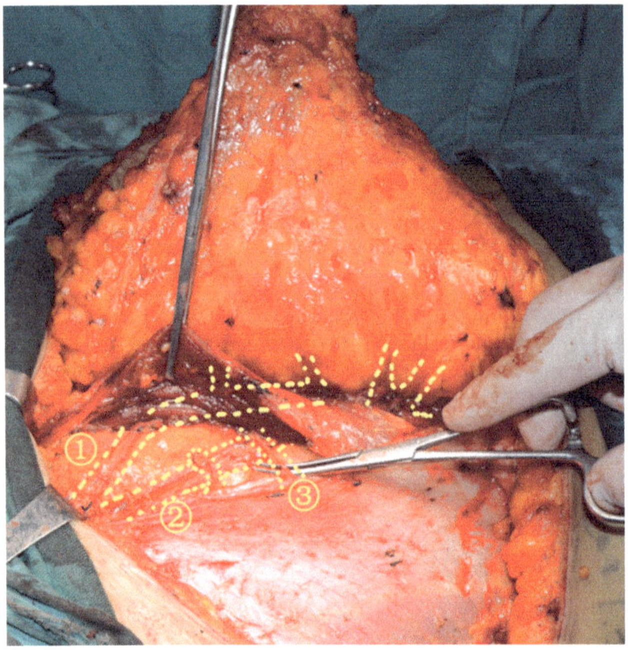

Fig. 18.65 It was found that the two main branches did not share a common vascular trunk. (1) Medial branch. (2) Lateral branch. (3) Intercostal nerve

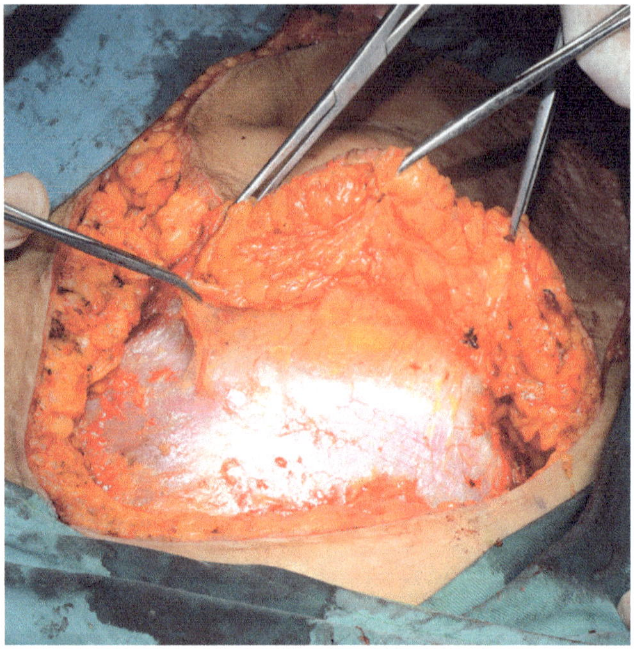

Fig. 18.66 The right flap was separated revealing that good perforators were absent near the umbilicus

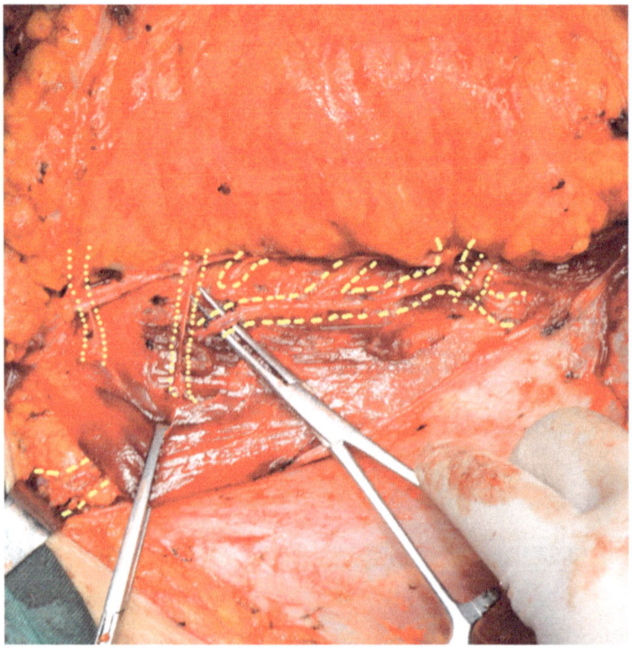

Fig. 18.67 The vascular pedicle was separated retrogradely in the muscle along the left perforator. It can be seen that it was the medial branch sharing the vascular trunk with the lateral branch, albeit lying low

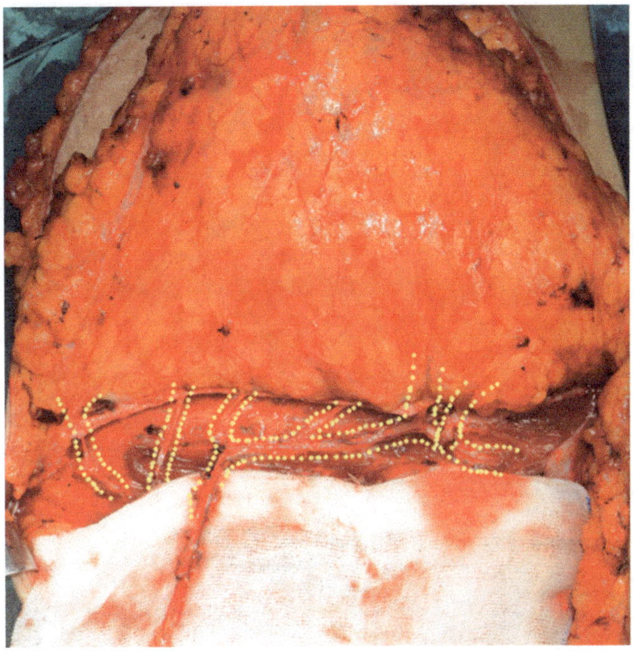

Fig. 18.68 Ligating the deep inferior epigastric blood vessels at the origin level and the lateral branch, the perforators were all from the medial branch. The medial branch and its trunk were conserved intact. The two perforating vessels in the lower abdomen came from the main deep inferior epigastric vessels. They were too low to be used because the length of the effective vascular pedicle was insufficient

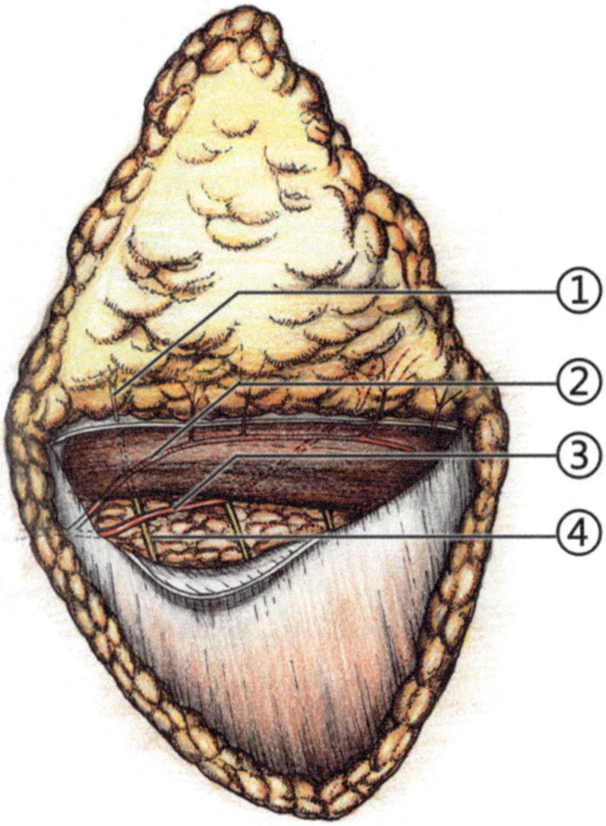

Fig. 18.70 When the flap was further separated to the inside, the major perforator was found, which was very large and came from the large medial branch far from the lateral branch. (1) Intercostal nerve; sensory nerve. (2) Medial branch of deep inferior epigastric vessel. (3) Lateral branch of deep inferior epigastric vessel. (4) Intercostal nerve

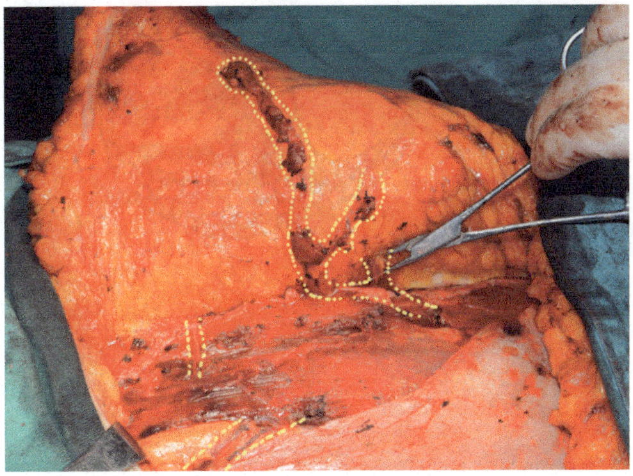

Fig. 18.69 Separation of the medial branch was performed in rendezvous manner

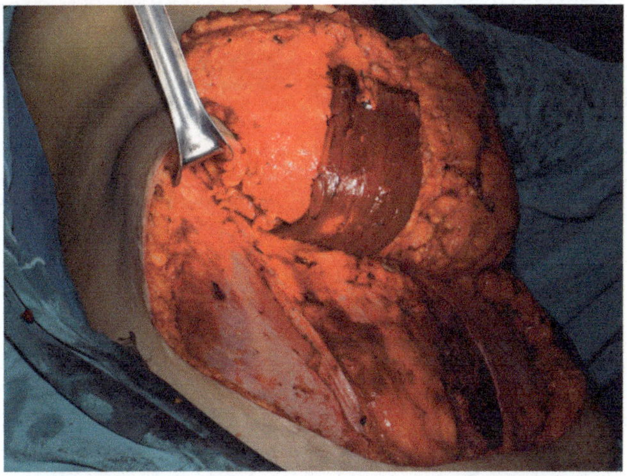

Fig. 18.71 No suitable right DIEPs were found; the pedicled rectus abdominis myocutaneous flap was raised

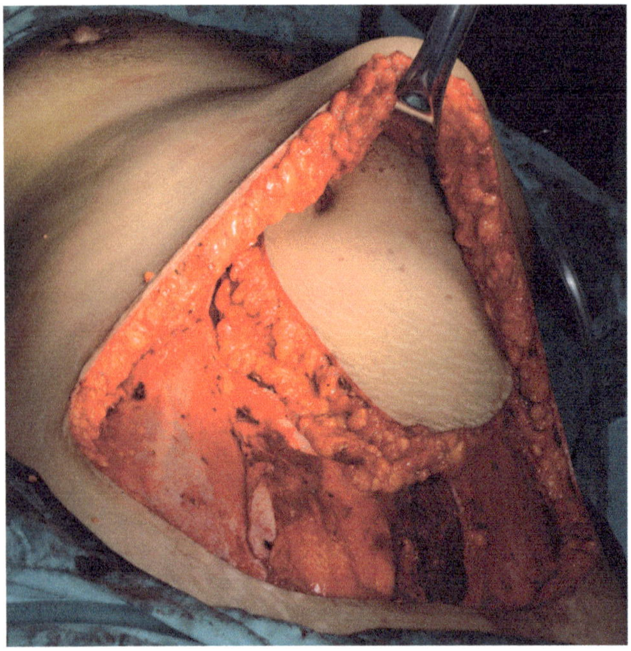

Fig. 18.72 Retrogradely extracting the medial branch of the left vascular pedicle through the rectus femoris tunnel

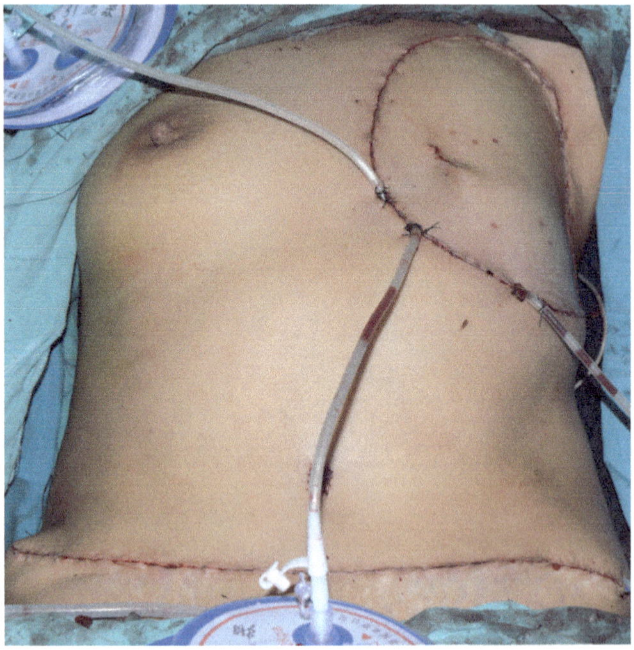

Fig. 18.74 Intraoperative view immediately after reconstruction

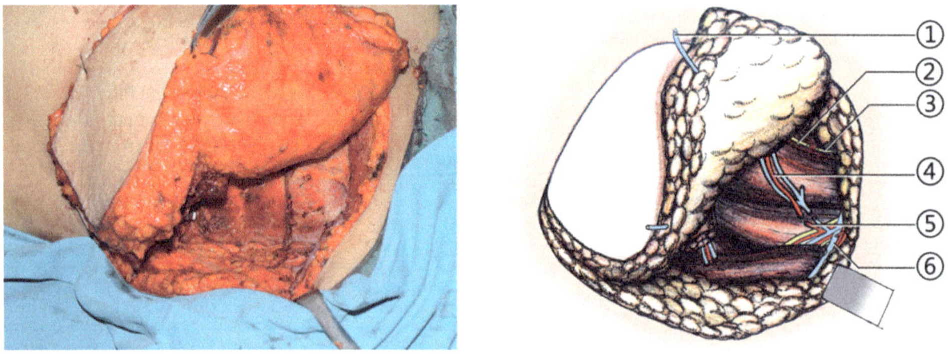

Fig. 18.73 Pattern of flap revascularization. (1) SIEV; (2) sensory branch of intercostal nerve; (3) sensory branch of intercostal nerve in the receiving area; (4) left deep inferior epigastric vessel; (5) anterior serratus branch of thoracodorsal vessels; and (6) thoracodorsal vessels

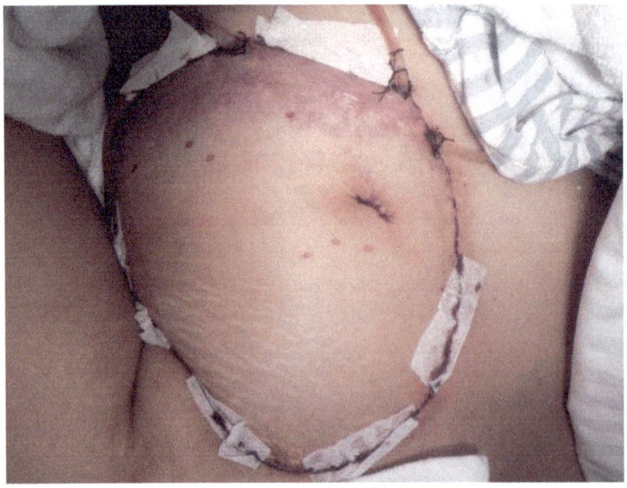

Fig. 18.75 Partial liquefaction and necrosis of the flap occurred 3 days after operation, and no obvious signs of infection were found

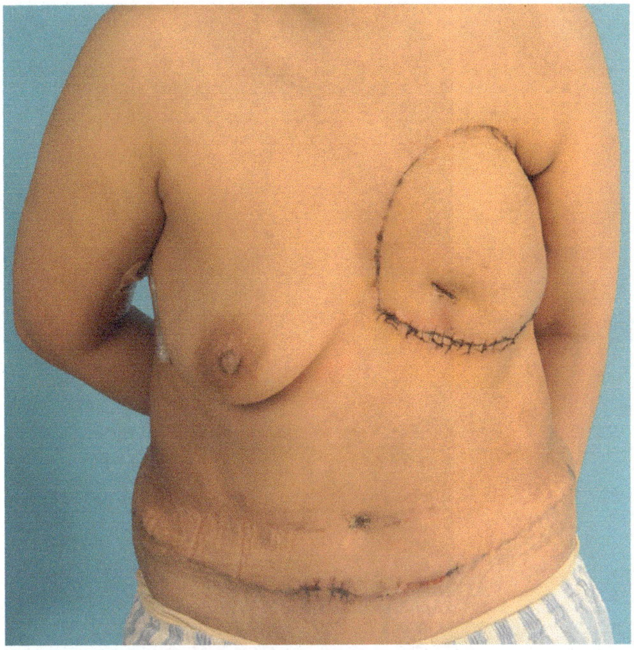

Fig. 18.76 Partial fat liquefaction and necrosis of the flap after operation which was solved by debridement. The patient was discharged 15 days after operation

Case Study 5: Failure of Breast Reconstruction Due to Patient Incooperation

A 55-year-old female patient underwent modified radical mastectomy for right breast cancer in the external hospital. She experienced repeated wound unhealing after operation, resulting in extensive scar healing, affecting the limb function and chest wall appearance. Bilateral pedicled DIEP flaps for staged II right breast reconstruction was performed.

The proximal and distal ends of the internal thoracic vessels were prepared as recipient. The blood supply of the flap was good during the operation. Seventy-two hours after the operation, the patient refused flap monitoring by medical staff and put on clothes inversely and slept with the back collar just pressing on the vascular pedicle of the flap. The blood supply of the flap turned poor, and the surgical exploration was refused, resulting in complete necrosis of the flap and failure of the operation (Figs. 18.77, 18.78, 18.79, 18.80, 18.81, 18.82, 18.83, 18.84, 18.85, 18.86, and 18.87).

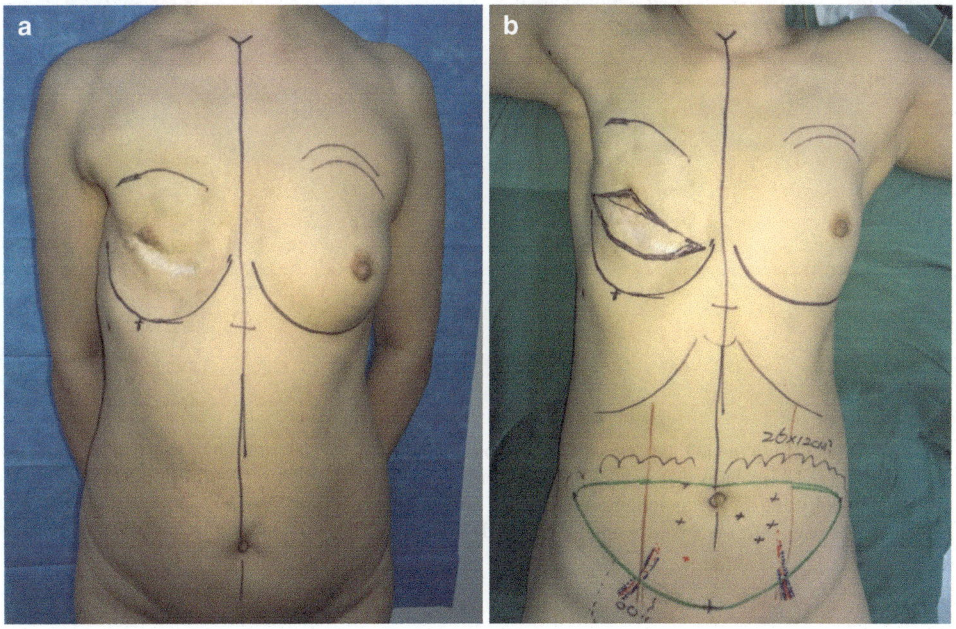

Fig. 18.77 (**a**) Preoperative view. (**b**) Intraoperative design

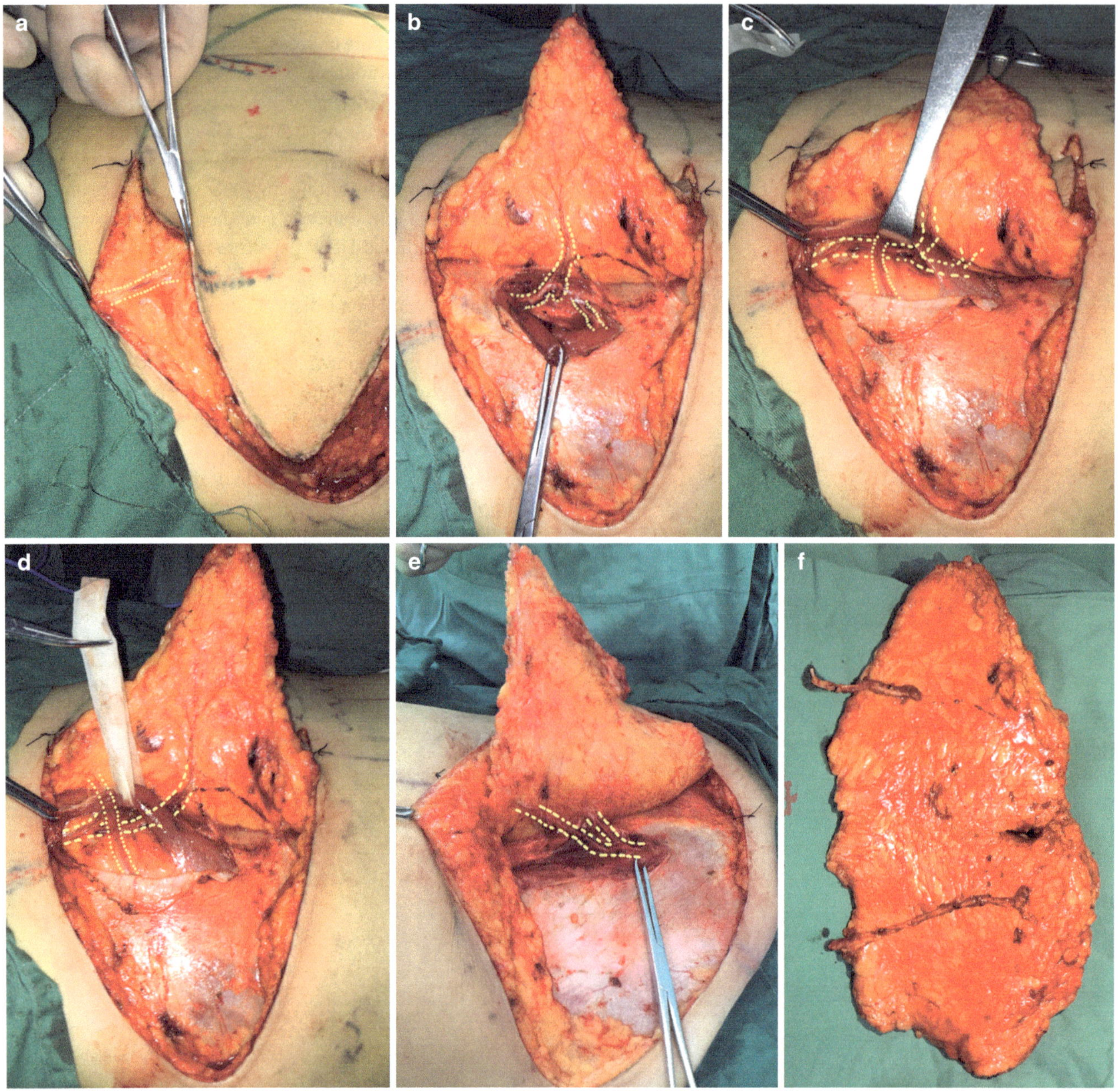

Fig. 18.78 (**a**) Lifting the left flap, exposing and separating the SIEV. (**b**) Perforator and vascular pedicle were separated from rectus abdominis muscle. (**c**) Lifting the rectus abdominis muscle to expose the proximal end of the deep inferior epigastric blood vessel. (**d**) Completing the separation of the right deep inferior epigastric blood vessel and perforator. (**e**) The anatomical separation of the left vascular pedicle and perforator was completed. (**f**) The perforator flap of the bilateral pedicled deep inferior epigastric blood vessel was cut off

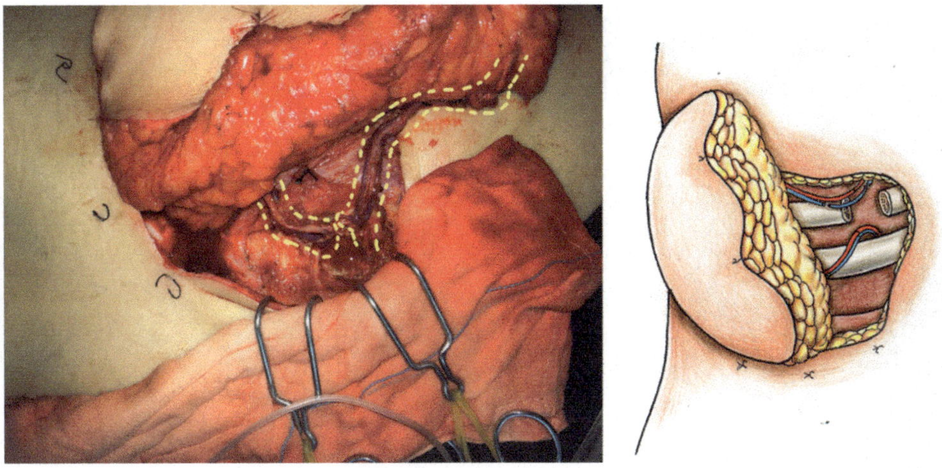

Fig. 18.79 Bilateral deep inferior epigastric vascular pedicle anastomosed with proximal and distal thoracic vessels, respectively

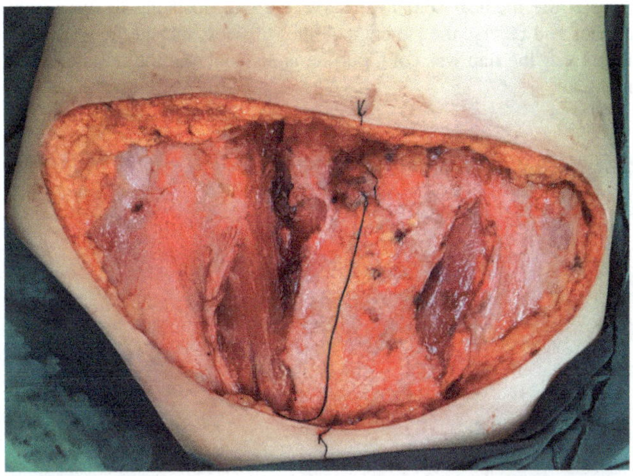

Fig. 18.80 The integrity of rectus abdominis and anterior sheath in the flap donor area was preserved and repaired in situ

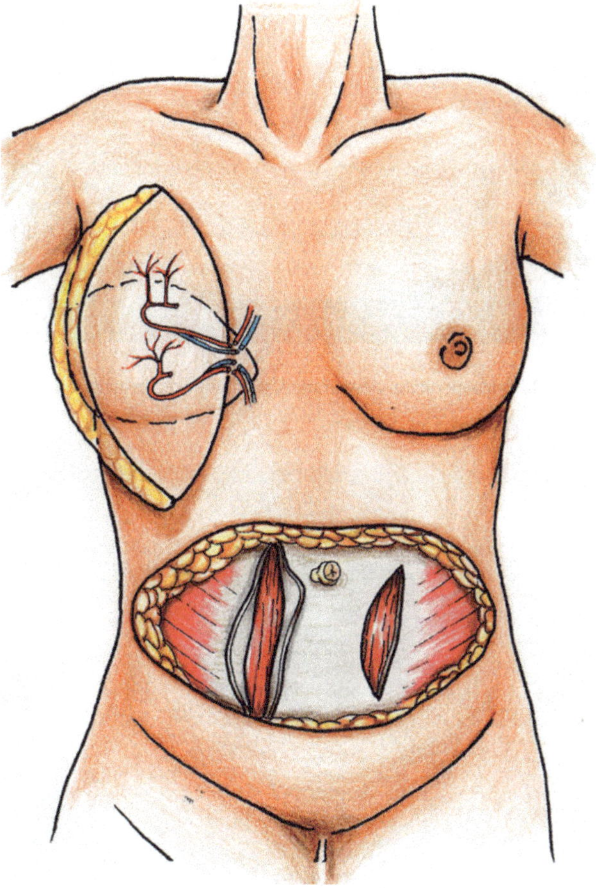

Fig. 18.81 Further shaping after revascularization of flap

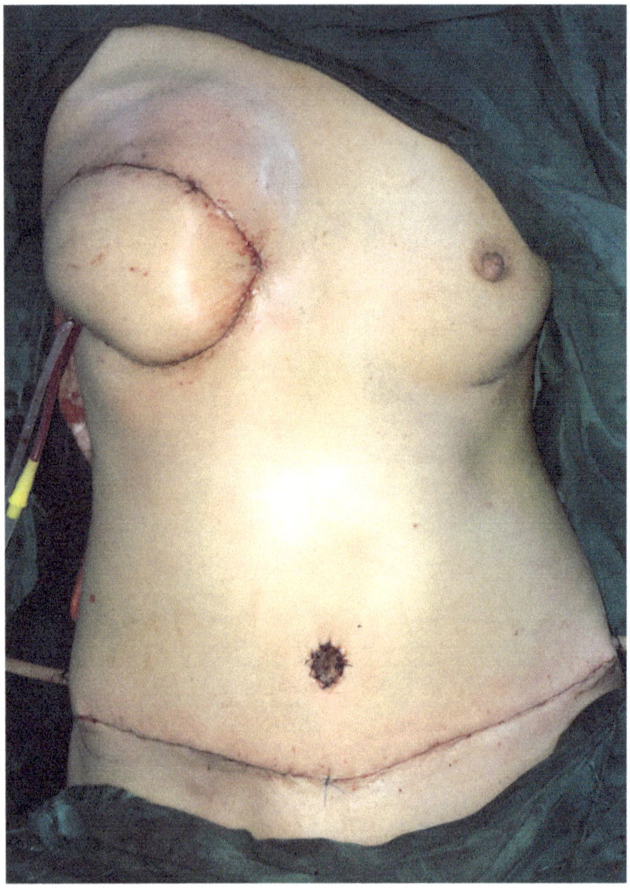

Fig. 18.82 Intraoperative view immediately after reconstruction

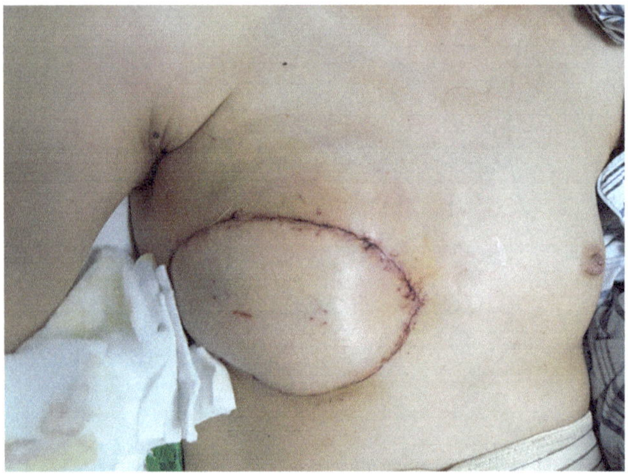

Fig. 18.83 The blood supply of the flap was good 3 days after operation

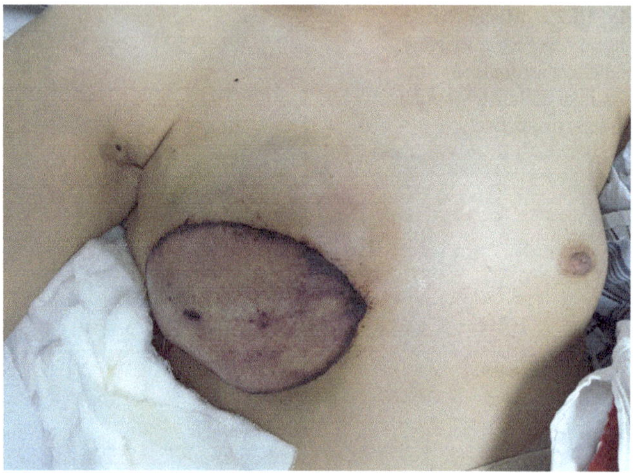

Fig. 18.84 On the evening of the third day after operation, the patient refused the medical staff to observe the flap, insisting to wear tight clothes and reverse the patient's clothes to sleep, locked the ward, and found that the flap was cold, purple, and swollen in the middle of the night

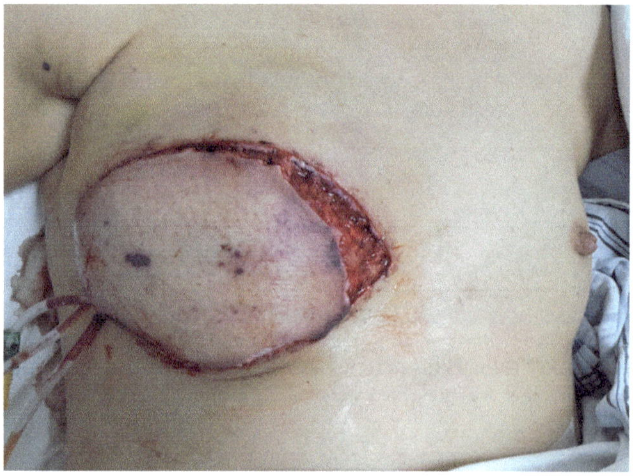

Fig. 18.85 The medical staff found that the collar of the reverse patient's suit was just stuck on the vascular pedicle of the flap, resulting in obvious dents. The flap was bruised and the skin temperature was low. They immediately loosened the patient's suit. The doctor asked for emergency vascular exploration for the patient. The patient was impatient, agitated, and refused. Four hours later, part of the suture of the flap was removed; the blood circulation improved and the bruise was reduced. After that, the patient still refused the doctor's suggestion of emergency vascular exploration

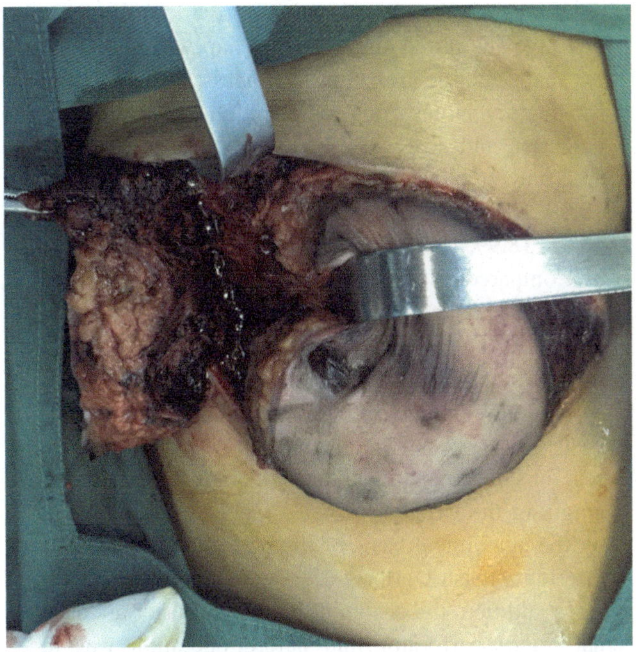

Fig. 18.86 Skin flap blackening and necrosis 7 days after operation

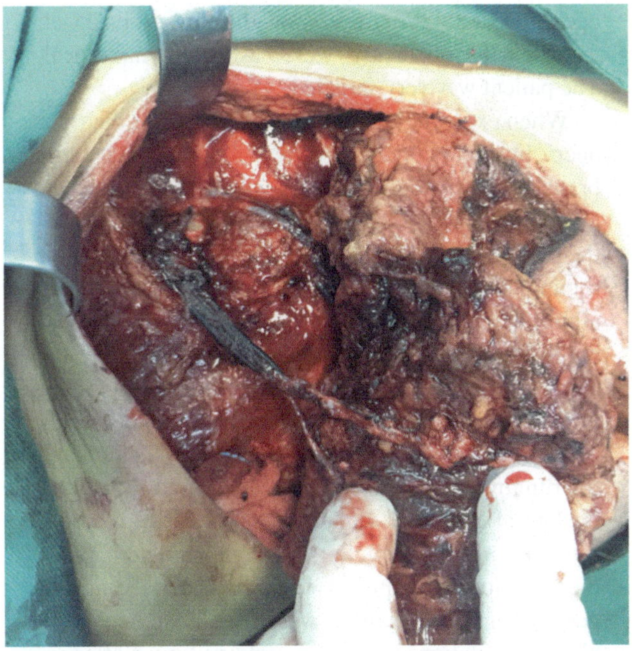

Fig. 18.87 Taking out the necrotic flap, separating the wound edge, and closing it directly

18.1.5 Experience and Lessons of Surgical Failure

1. Improvement of Surgical Technique
   (a) Pay attention to the angle of vascular pedicle to avoid torsion and vascular transplantation.
   (b) If the blood vessels in the thorax have been planned to be anastomosed at both ends, the cutting plane should not be too proximal or distal, and midline is appropriate.
   (c) The DIEP flap should be separated carefully, and the vascular pedicle should not be damaged.
   (d) When the diameter of the anastomotic vessel is less than 1.5 mm, the use of vascular coupler shall be avoided because the use of vascular coupler will further reduce the lumen and increase the risk of vascular embolism.
2. Lesson Summary

   After the operation, the patient was extremely uncooperative. On the third night, he wore tight underwear and reversed the patient's clothes, resulting in the collar jamming and pressing the flap. The ward was tightly locked and refused the hourly flap observation by doctors and nurses. At 1 a.m., the flap became cold and spotted. The suture removal was refused, and purple spots appeared on the edge of the flap. All the sutures of the breast were removed at 9 a.m. on the fourth day after operation. The color of the flap improved, the skin temperature increased, and progressive ecchymosis appeared 2 days later, and finally the flap was necrotic.

   Analysis of causes: After external force compression for more than 5 h, the skin temperature decreased. It was determined that external force compression was the main cause of skin flap necrosis: The skin flap was anastomosed with 2A2V. If there was a problem with venous anastomotic bridging, the skin flap should show venous crisis, the skin flap should be swollen obviously, the skin temperature remained warm, the skin flap became obviously purple, and ecchymosis occurred in the whole region. In this patient, only ecchymosis occurred at the edge of the flap, the skin temperature decreased, there was no obvious purple swelling, there was no large-area blood stasis of the whole flap, and there was no obstruction of venous reflux on the surface. However, the decrease of skin temperature of the flap was consistent with the lack of arterial blood supply, and the obstruction of venous reflux would not lead to the decrease of skin temperature. Moreover, the flap was re-vascularized with 2a2v after operation, and the slight perfusion was greater than the flow. Arterial blood supply is absolutely safe. The flap was stable in the first 3 days after operation, which basically eliminates the possibility of problems in vascular anastomosis. The actual situation of this flap was that the anastomotic arteries and veins were blocked at the same time, so there was obvious lack of arterial blood supply without poor venous reflux. The only explanation is that the local pressure of the collar was stuck on the arteriovenous anastomosis, especially when the anastomotic stoma of bilateral arteries were clamped at the same time, it can be seen that the pressure of collar clamp was great.

Case Study 6: Salvaging a DIEP Flap Deprived of Blood Supply After Harvest

The patient was a 46-year-old female. Modified radical mastectomy for bilateral breast cancer + FREE DIEP flap transplantation for breast reconstruction were performed under general anesthesia. Before operation, the bilateral DIEP flap was designed to be cut and transplanted for bilateral breast reconstruction immediately. During the operation, it was actually found that the left perforator was too small to offer sufficient blood supply, and the right perforator and vascular pedicle were relatively small. The blood vessels and rectus abdominis were closely connected, and the blood vessels were brittle. A small amount of rectus abdominis muscle were carried around the perforator and vascular pedicle. The size of the right DIEP flap was 14 cm × 12 cm, and the vascular pedicle was anastomosed with the internal vessels of the left thorax (A: v = 1:2). It was found that the left perforating branch was tortuous resulting in poor blood supply of the flap. Instead, the right perforator flap based on the profunda femoral artery was designed and transferred to the left breast defect, and the vascular pedicle was anastomosed with the right thoracodorsal vessels (A: v = 1:2). After confirming that the blood supply of bilateral flaps was satisfactory, further shaping was carried out. After indwelling the drainage tube, the wound margin was sutured in layers, and the flap donor area was closed directly. The blood supply of the flap was good, and the shape and function of the reconstructed breast were satisfactory. No obvious complications such as fat liquefaction and necrosis were found in the flap donor area, and only linear scars were left (Figs. 18.88, 18.89, 18.90, 18.91, 18.92, 18.93, 18.94, 18.95, 18.96, 18.97, 18.98, 18.99, 18.100, and 18.101).

Compared with the right reconstructed breast, the left breast was relatively flat. The main reason was that the length of vascular pedicle was limited, so it was impossible to fully shape the right DIEP flap.

Although the length of the right deep inferior epigastric artery was long, it carried two perforator vessels for safety, resulting in the reduction of the effective length of the vascular pedicle, which was determined by the anatomical basis of the perforator of the deep inferior epigastric artery.

In addition, the design of bilateral inferior abdominal artery perforator flap before operation was to ensure that the reconstructed bilateral breasts were similar in size and texture. The actual situation can be flexibly adjusted during operation. First, ensure the operation safety. After operation, the flap survived well and the bilateral breasts were basically symmetrical. The patient was very satisfied.

When exposing the perforating branch of the right deep inferior epigastric artery, although a large branch of the vascular network was seen in the subcutaneous fascia layer, it was found that the diameter of the perforating branch was significantly reduced after tracing back to the deep inferior epigastric artery along the perforating branch, indicating that the real major perforating branch was hidden behind the small perforating branch, and both perforating branches were tendinous perforating branches. Therefore, it was difficult to completely understand the running course of the perforator. After separating the lateral perforator vessel, it was considered that the separation of the pedicle had been completed. When the tendinous inscriptions was further cut, the medial perforator vessel pedicle was cut off, and then the blood circulation of the flap remained poor after re-anastomosing the internal perforator vessels under the microscope which was attributed to prolonged ischemia of the flap.

Fig. 18.88 Preoperative view

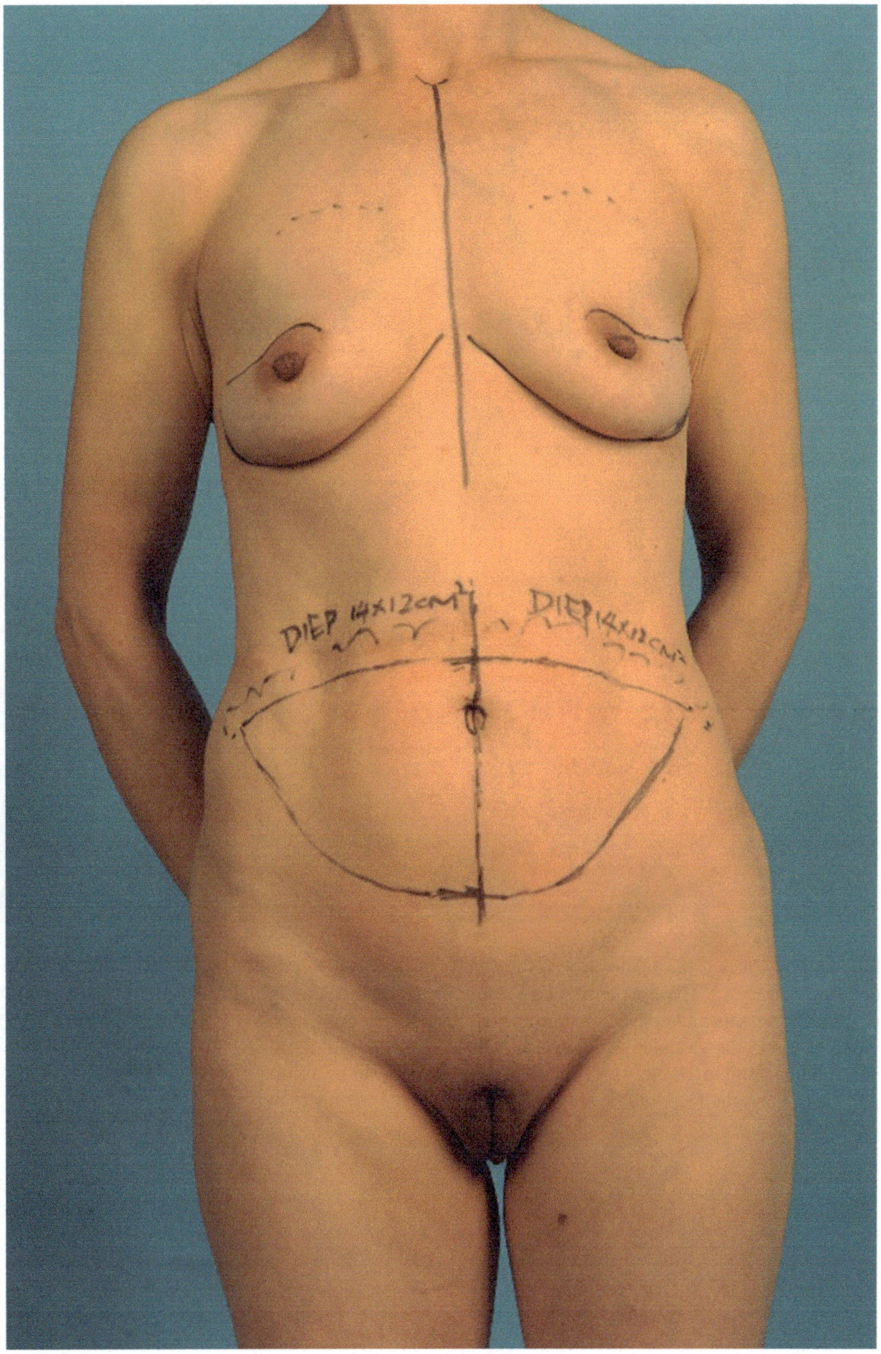

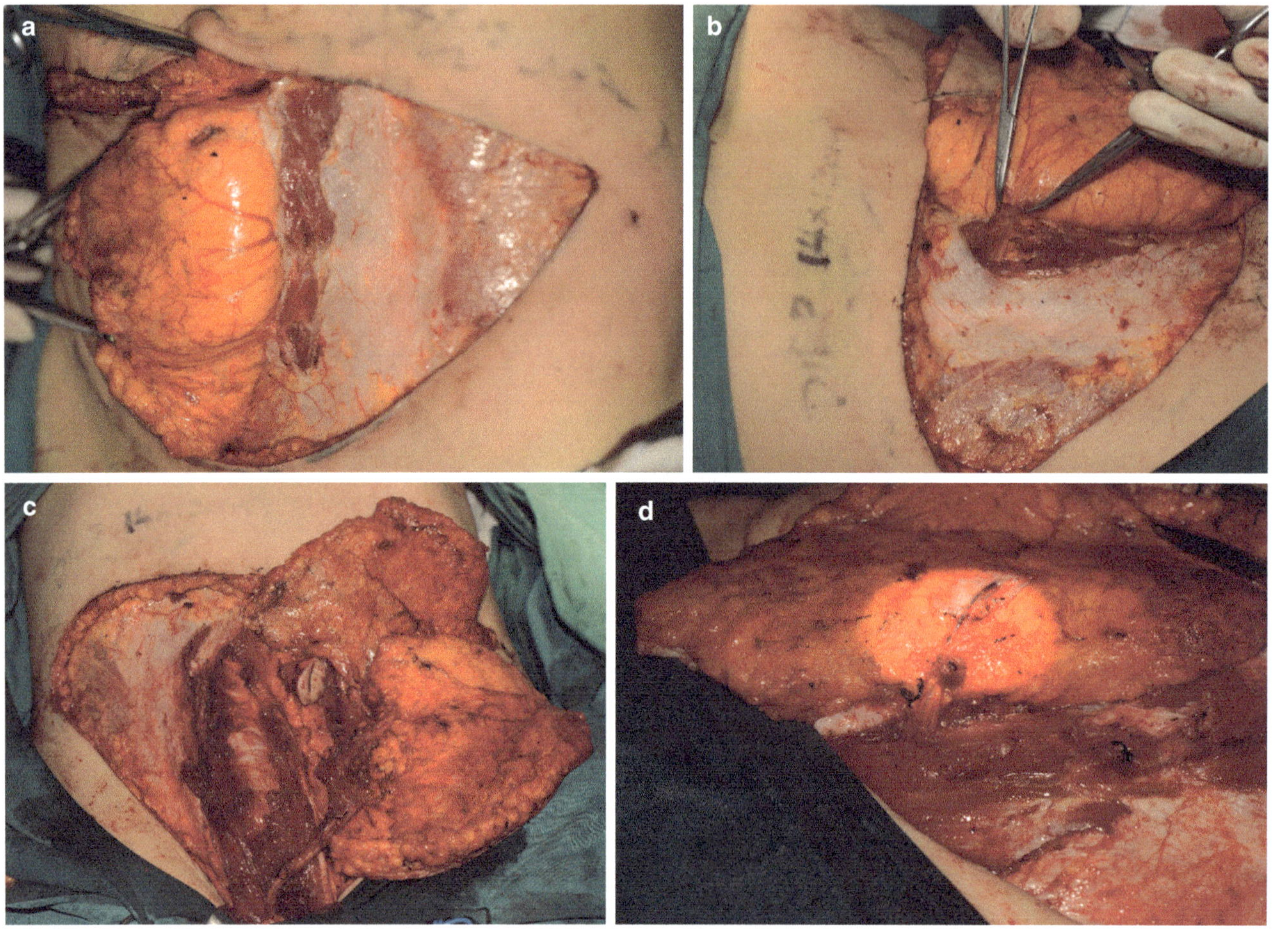

Fig. 18.89 Cutting the bilateral perforator flaps of the deep inferior epigastric artery. (**a**) Expose perforating vessels. (**b**) After exposing the perforating vessels and converging into the left deep inferior epigastric vascular trunk, the vascular pedicle was cut and separated with a little surrounding tendon tissue. (**c**) The perforating branch and vascular pedicle of the right deep inferior epigastric artery adhered closely to the rectus abdominis muscle. The muscle bundle carrying the medial part of the right rectus abdominis muscle was cut and retained around the vascular pedicle for safety. (**d**) The filling of the perforating branch of the left inferior abdominal wall became worse, and there was no significant improvement after exploration, so it was abandoned

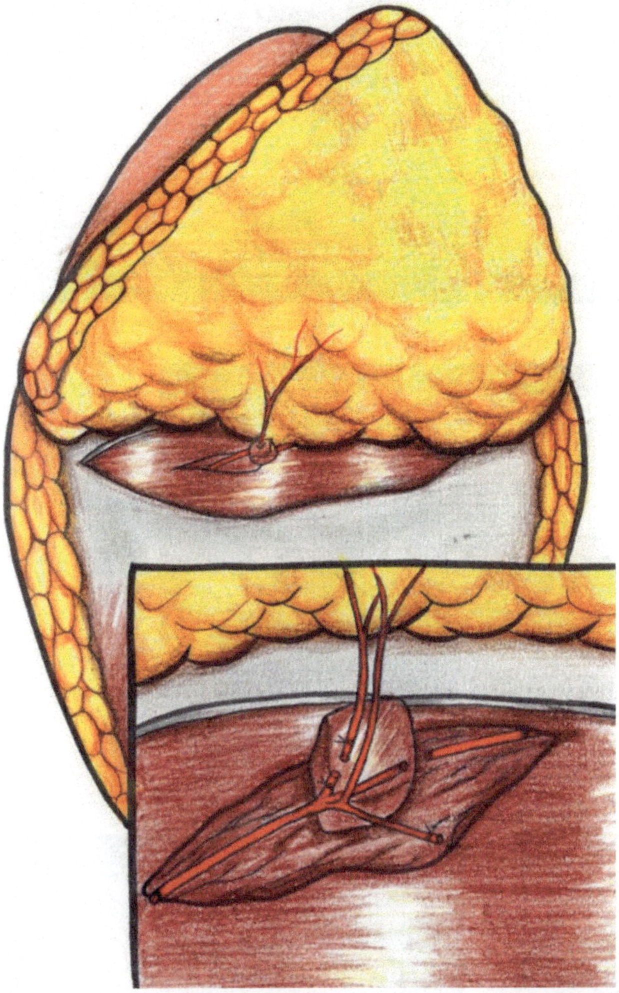

Fig. 18.90 Schematic diagram of the actual situation of accidental injury of the perforating branch of the left deep inferior epigastric artery

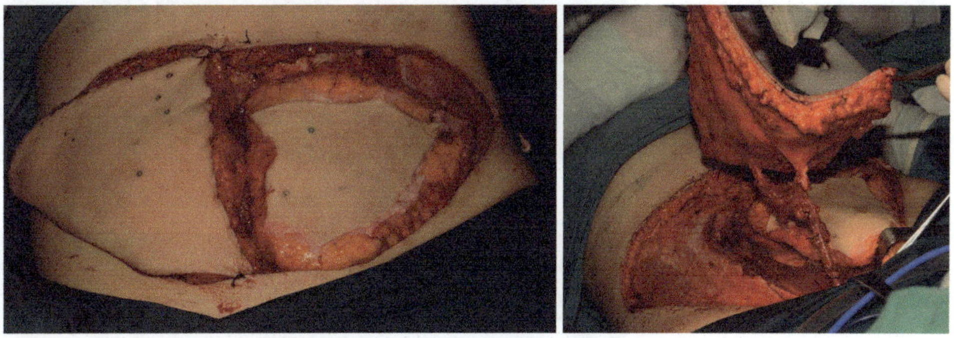

Fig. 18.91 Preparation of perforator flap of deep inferior epigastric artery with partial rectus abdominis muscle on the right side

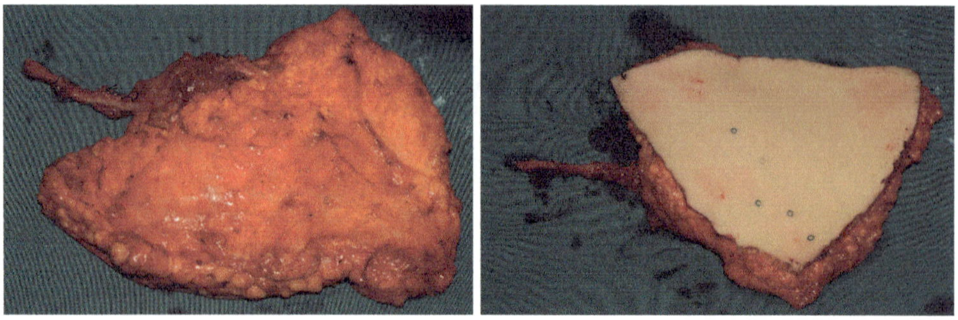

Fig. 18.92 The perforator flap of the right deep inferior epigastric artery was cut off

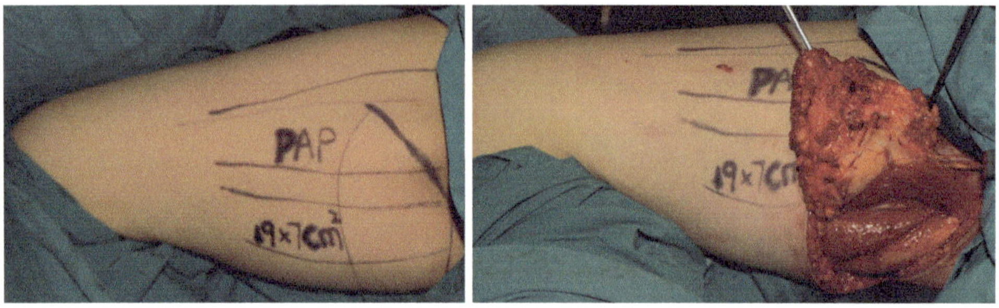

Fig. 18.93 The perforator flap of the posterior medial femoral artery of the right thigh was designed and cut. The flap size was 19 cm × 7 cm; the approach of exploring the perforating vessels from the rear to the front was used to expose the larger perforating vessels on the surface of the adductor major

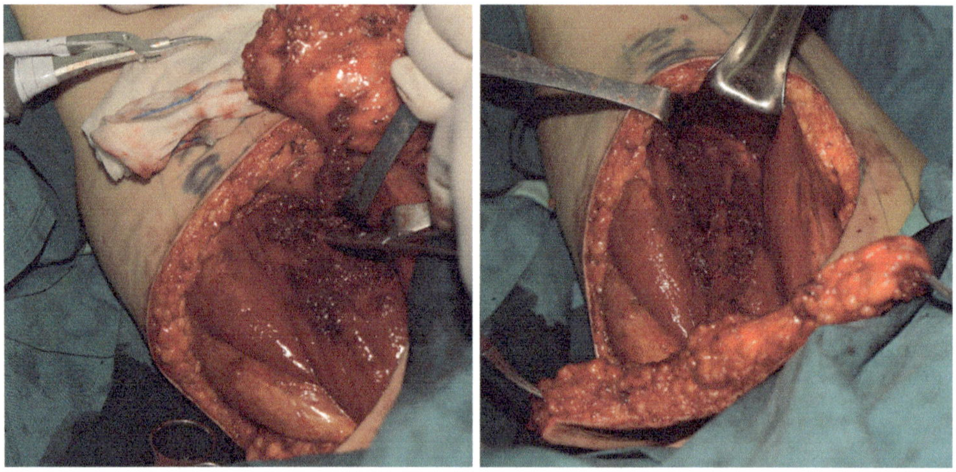

Fig. 18.94 Retrograde separation of perforating vessels of adductor major to the plane from profunda femoral vessels

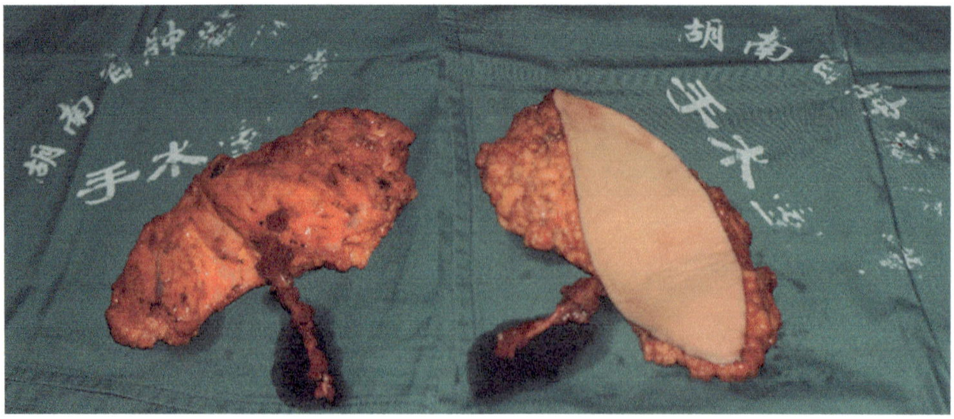

Fig. 18.95 The profunda femoral artery perforator flap was cut off

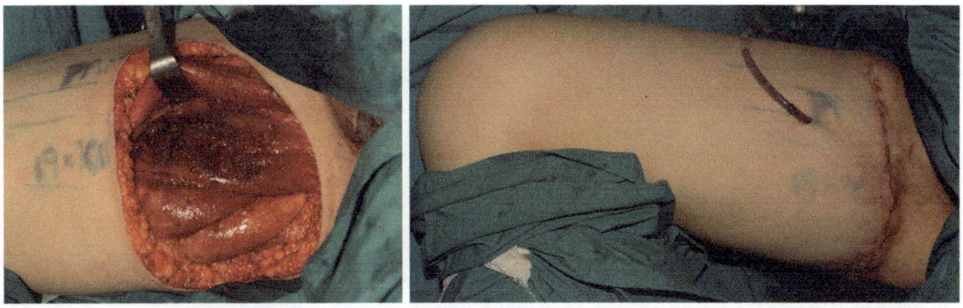

Fig. 18.96 The donor area of the perforator flap of the profunda femoral artery was slightly damaged and closed directly, leaving only linear scars

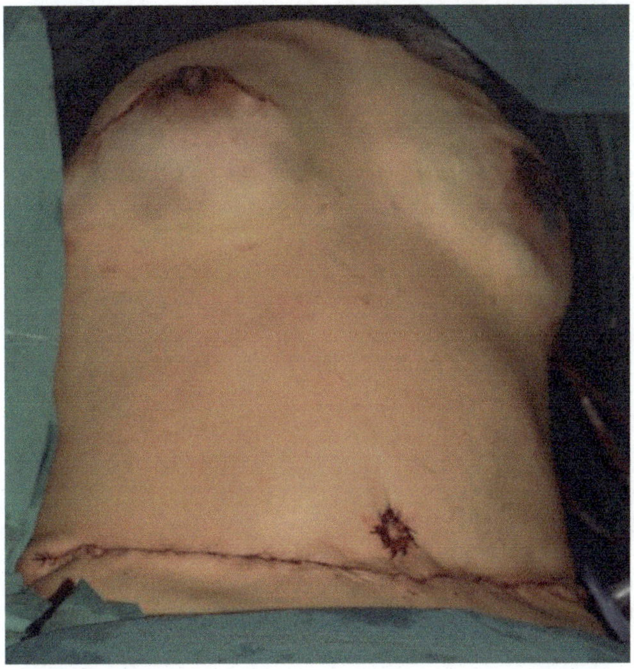

Fig. 18.97 Intraoperative view immediately after bilateral breast reconstruction

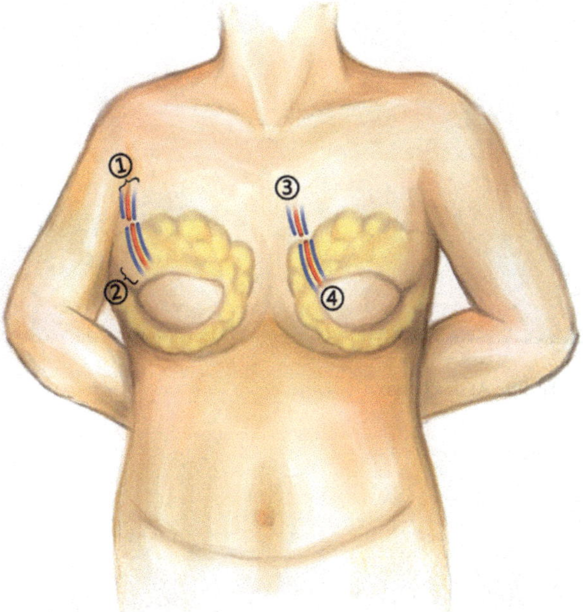

Fig. 18.98 Schematic diagram of revascularization mode. The vascular pedicle of the perforator flap of the right deep inferior epigastric artery was anastomosed with the left internal thoracic vessels (A: V = 1:2), and the perforator vascular pedicle of the profunda femoral artery at the inner and posterior side of the right thigh was anastomosed with the right thoracodorsal vessels (A: V = 1:2). (1) Right thoracodorsal vessels. (2) Right profunda femoral artery perforator pedicle. (3) Proximal ends of left internal mammary vessel. (4) Right deep inferior epigastric vessels

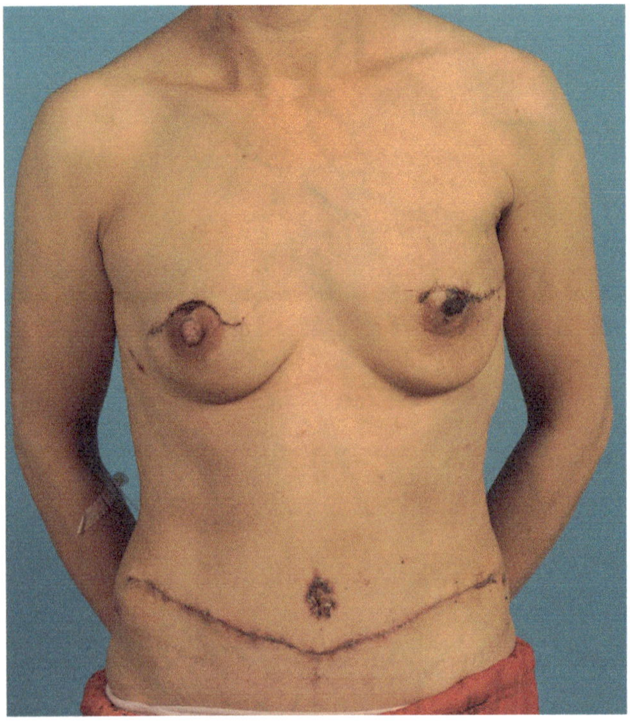

Fig. 18.99 At discharge

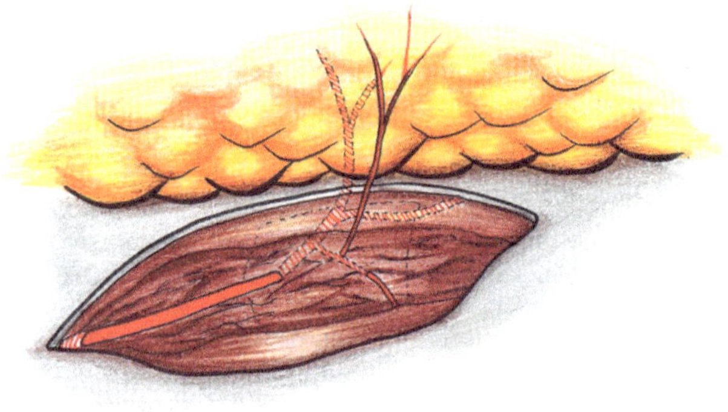

Fig. 18.100 Summary of the failure of the perforator flap of the left deep inferior epigastric artery

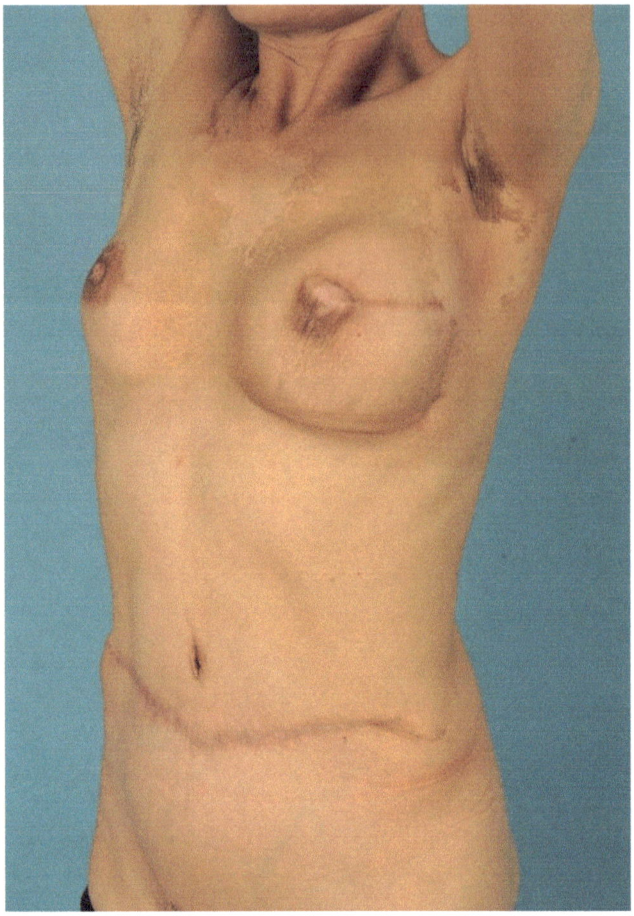

Fig. 18.101 Follow-up at 8 months after operation and 1 month after radiotherapy

18.2 Summary of the Perioperative Precautions of Breast Reconstruction and Chest Wall Reconstruction

18.2.1 Preoperative Preparation

1. Ward: Perform abdominal vascular color Doppler ultrasound and Doppler vascular positioning. If possible, CTA is feasible to determine abdominal vascular positioning. The history of menstruation and ongoing infection should be known. Patients should have a clear understanding of the operation and surgical indications and strongly desire breast reconstruction. Electrolyte disorder, hypoproteinemia, anemia, and other general conditions should be dealt with in advance. Abdominal belt is prepared.

2. Operating room: A foldable, side-lying, adjustable operating table is required. It is suggested to prepare a spacious operating room, two sets of operating lights, two scrub nurses, three sets of instruments, and replacing the instruments after the resection of the primary focus. Operating microscope, micro-instrument, vascular clamp, 9-10, 10-0 micro suture, heparin saline, methylene blue solution, two sets of manual unipolar electric knives, one set of foot controlled bipolar electrocoagulation, two sets of negative pressure aspirators, and sharp knife blades are prepared.
3. Intraoperative: For infected wounds, preoperative bacteria culture and antibiotic sensitivity test are required. Antibiotics; is needed Fluid infusion or even blood transfusion is a must; pressor drugs such as ephedrine, epinephrine, norepinephrine and dopamine and anticoagulant drugs should be avoided; the patient is placed in a semi-recumbent position before suturing the abdominal donor area.

18.2.2 Postoperative Treatment Plan

1. Anti-infection
2. Antispasmodic
3. Anticoagulation
4. Correcting hypoproteinemia
5. Correcting anemia
6. Edema palliation: maizhilin tablets (sodium aescinate tablets), albumin

Close observation and guidance after operation include the following:

1. The color and quantity of wound drainage.
2. Blood supply and exudation of displaced umbilicus.
3. Skin flap color, skin temperature, and blood stasis.
4. Check whether the clothes are jammed.

- The dressing shall be replaced in time, the indoor temperature shall be appropriate, and the baking lamp shall not be used as possible.
- The patient is kept in a semi-sitting position with hip flexion and knee flexion.
- Three days after the operation, the patient begins to be ambulatory. While stuck on bed, the patient should keep massaging the hands and feet to prevent thrombosis. If the flap is found to be swelling significantly, sutures should be removed in time, and smoking should be strictly prohibited indoors.
- Blood cell analysis, liver and kidney function, and electrolyte are checked on the first, third, and seventh day after operation.

References

1. Damen TH, Timman R, Kunst EH, et al. High satisfaction rates in women after DIEP flap breast reconstruction. J Plast Reconstr Aesthet Surg. 2010;63(1):93–100.
2. Momoh AO, Colakoglu S, Westvik TS, et al. Analysis of complications and patient satisfaction in pedicled transverse rectus abdominis myocutaneous and deep inferior epigastric perforator flap breast reconstruction. Ann Plast Surg. 2012;69(1):19–23.
3. Tønseth KA, Hokland BM, Tindholdt TT, Abyholm FE, Stavem K. Quality of life, patient satisfaction and cosmetic outcome after breast reconstruction using DIEP flap or expandable breast implant. J Plast Reconstr Aesthet Surg. 2008;61(10):1188–94.
4. Davis GB, Lang JE, Peric M, et al. Breast reconstruction satisfaction rates at a large county hospital. Ann Plast Surg. 2014;72(Suppl 1):S61–5.
5. Kruper L, Holt A, Xu XX, et al. Disparities in reconstruction rates after mastectomy: patterns of care and factors associated with the use of breast reconstruction in Southern California. Ann Surg Oncol. 2011;18(8):2158–65.
6. Albornoz CR, Bach PB, Pusic AL, et al. The influence of sociodemographic factors and hospital characteristics on the method of breast reconstruction, including microsurgery: a U.S. population-based study. Plast Reconstr Surg. 2012;129(5):1071–9.
7. Panchal H, Matros E. Current trends in postmastectomy breast reconstruction. Plast Reconstr Surg. 2017;140(5S Advances in Breast Reconstruction):7S–13S.
8. Lee BT, Yueh JH, Chen C, Lin SJ, Tobias AM, Slavin SA. Establishment of perforator flap programs for breast reconstruction: the New England program experience. Plast Reconstr Surg. 2009;124(5):1410–8.
9. Matros E, Yueh JH, Bar-Meir ED, Slavin SA, Tobias AM, Lee BT. Sociodemographics, referral patterns, and Internet use for decision-making in microsurgical breast reconstruction. Plast Reconstr Surg. 2010;125(4):1087–94.
10. Xiao Zhou, Dajiang Song, Zan Li. The development of perforator flap and its application in oncoplastic surgery Chin J Aesthet Plast Surg2017. 28(2): 69–72.
11. Zhang S, Song D. The discovery, development history and clinical implications of perforator flaps. Chin J Reparat Reconstr Surg. 2017;07:769–72.
12. Zhou X, Hu B, Luo Y. Talking about the necessity of the formation of oncoplastic surgery. Chin Cancer. 2001;12:14–5.
13. Zhou X, Zhou B, Li Z. The history and current situation of oncoplastic surgery in China—oncology surgeons have the responsibility to cure tumors, and also have the obligation to give patients a healthy and beautiful life. Chin J Otorhinolaryngol Skull Base Surg. 2016;02:85–90.
14. Albornoz CR, Cordeiro PG, Hishon L, et al. A nationwide analysis of the relationship between hospital volume and outcome for autologous breast reconstruction. Plast Reconstr Surg. 2013;132(2):192e–200e.
15. Kulkarni AR, Sears ED, Atisha DM, Alderman AK. Use of autologous and microsurgical breast reconstruction by U.S. plastic surgeons. Plast Reconstr Surg. 2013;132(3):534–41.
16. Dumon KR, Edelson PK, Raper SE, Foster-Kilgarriff K, Williams NN. Implementation of designated bariatric surgery program leads to improved clinical outcomes. Surg Obes Relat Dis. 2011;7(3):271–6.
17. Bible KC, Smallridge RC, Morris JC, et al. Development of a multidisciplinary, multicampus subspecialty practice in endocrine cancers. J Oncol Pract. 2012;8(3 Suppl):e1s–5s.
18. Ali SR, Chetwynd-Stapylton R, Holmes WJM, Vermaak L, Wilson SM. Time to re-group and save: do we routinely need to perform group-and-save in patients undergoing free deep inferior epigas-

tric perforator (DIEP) flap breast reconstruction. J Plast Reconstr Aesthet Surg. 2018;71:780.
19. Demir A, Kucuker I, Keles MK, Demirtas Y. The effect of learning curve on flap selection, re-exploration, and salvage rates in free flaps; a retrospective analysis of 155 cases. Microsurgery. 2013;33(7):519–26.
20. Hallock GG. Is there a "learning curve" for muscle perforator flaps. Ann Plast Surg. 2008;60(2):146–9.
21. Busic V, Das-Gupta R, Mesic H, Begic A. The deep inferior epigastric perforator flap for breast reconstruction, the learning curve explored. J Plast Reconstr Aesthet Surg. 2006;59(6):580–4.
22. Damen TH, Morritt AN, Zhong T, Ahmad J, Hofer SO. Improving outcomes in microsurgical breast reconstruction: lessons learnt from 406 consecutive DIEP/TRAM flaps performed by a single surgeon. J Plast Reconstr Aesthet Surg. 2013;66(8):1032–8.
23. Seidenstuecker K, Munder B, Mahajan AL, Richrath P, Behrendt P, Andree C. Morbidity of microsurgical breast reconstruction in patients with comorbid conditions. Plast Reconstr Surg. 2011;127(3):1086–92.
24. Tosun Z, Karabekmez FE, Duymaz A, Ozkan A, Keskin M, Avunduk MC. Preventing negative effects of smoking on microarterial anastomosis. Ann Plast Surg. 2010;65(1):91–5.
25. Mathes DW, Neligan PC. Preoperative imaging techniques for perforator selection in abdomen-based microsurgical breast reconstruction. Clin Plast Surg. 2010;37(4):581–91, xi.
26. Moon HK, Taylor GI. The vascular anatomy of rectus abdominis musculocutaneous flaps based on the deep superior epigastric system. Plast Reconstr Surg. 1988;82(5):815–32.
27. Patel AJK, Razzano S, Sassoon EM, Figus A. Split pedicle for bilateral free deep inferior epigastric perforator flap breast reconstruction: use of contralateral recipient vessels with radiotherapy damage. Microsurgery. 2017;37(7):837–8.
28. Thorarinsson A, Fröjd V, Kölby L, Lidén M, Elander A, Mark H. Patient determinants as independent risk factors for postoperative complications of breast reconstruction. Gland Surg. 2017;6(4):355–67.

Evolution, Anatomy, Advantages and Disadvantages, and Harvest Techniques of Profunda Artery Perforator Flap

19

Dajiang Song and Narushima Mitsunaga

19.1 History

In 1987, Taylor and Palmer introduced the concept of vascular territories (angiosomes) [1], and then koshima and SOEDA reported the perforator flap technology [2]. Various forms of free flaps have been applied to many parts of the human body and different fields of surgery and have become important technical means in plastic reconstruction surgery [3].

Despite many types of free flaps have already been used for breast reconstruction and chest wall reconstruction, there are still great demands to find new and better flaps to meet different needs [4–6].

Since the first report by Allen in 1992, the deep inferior epigastric artery perforator flap (DIEP) has gradually become the gold standard for breast reconstruction [5].

However, in clinical practice, we found that 25% of women are not suitable for breast reconstruction by the lower abdominal wall as the donor area.

The relative contraindications of breast reconstruction with DIEP include previous history of abdominal wall plastic surgery, previous history of fat aspiration, certain special abdominal surgery, history of abdominal cesarean section with obvious scar, young infertility, lack of abdominal subcutaneous fat, and patients who refused to use abdomen as the flap donor area.

In these cases, we prefer profunda artery perforator (PAP). For breast reconstruction, the profunda artery perforator flap is a good alternative to abdominal flap.

PAP flap is a flap designed and harvested based on the gracilis muscle and its posterior thigh tissue [7], which has become a new alternative in breast reconstruction [8–10].

According to the literatures, the concept of PAP flap refers to the medial posterior thigh flap [11] and can be transformed into different fashions, such as advanced flap [12], transposition flap [13], pedicled flap, and free flap [14, 15].

Allen et al. used this perforator flap in 27 patients for breast reconstruction, and the cosmetic effect is satisfactory [16, 17].

Satake et al. reported that the flap, as the posteromedial thigh flap, was successful in 70 cases of breast reconstruction [18].

Haddock et al. reported the application of 101 PAP flap in breast reconstruction [19].

It was generally believed that the inner thigh cannot provide enough amount of flap tissue than the lower abdomen, but this limitation can also be overcome with improved modifications.

It has been reported that by using bilateral PAP flaps, more tissue could be obtained in breast reconstruction cases of female with fuller shape [20].

Based on the clinical experience in our center, free or pedicled PAP flap transplantation has been routinely used in the reconstruction of breast, head, and neck defects and perineum repair after tumor resection [9, 14, 15, 21, 22].

19.2 Vascular Anatomy

The lower edge of the gluteal sulcus is regarded as the upper boundary and the iliotibial tract the outer boundary, the adductor longus the inner boundary, and the popliteal fossa the lower boundary.

The major muscles in the posterior inner side of the thigh are the posterior thigh muscles (biceps femoris, semitendinosus, and semimembranosus muscles) supplied by the deep artery.

The posterior inner thigh flap is supplied by the fasciocutaneous vascular network formed by the descending branch of the inferior gluteal artery and the perforating branches of the profunda femoral artery [23].

D. Song (✉)
Department of Oncology Plastic Surgery, Hunan Cancer Hospital, Changsha, Hunan, China

N. Mitsunaga
Mie University Graduate School of Medicine Plastic and Reconstructive Surgery, Tsu, Mie, Japan
e-mail: sancho-ps@umin.ac.jp

Z. Li, D. Song (eds.), *Oncoplastic Flap Surgery*, https://doi.org/10.1007/978-981-19-8926-1_19

However, although the profunda femoral artery is the main supplying artery of the posteromedial thigh region, the following arteries also contribute to the regional blood supply: medial femoral circumflex artery, pudendal artery, and inferior gluteal artery [18].

The first medial perforating branch of the profunda femoral artery enters the adductor muscle and sends out perforating branches to nourish the posteromedial skin of the thigh.

Some anatomical and imaging studies have confirmed the reliability and consistent distribution of medial perforating branches.

Anatomical studies show that the first and second perforating branches of the profunda femoral artery supply blood to most areas of posterior thigh, and the supply range of the inferior gluteal artery is determined as the skin of the inferior gluteal sulcus area (Fig. 19.1) [7, 23].

However, the main disadvantage of the posteromedial thigh perforator flap is the necessary change of body position due to the harvest of the flap.

Therefore, the early clinical application of this flap is the reconstruction of pressure ulcer [13].

The profunda femoral artery is stemmed from the femoral artery 3.5 cm below the inguinal ligament. It first courses on

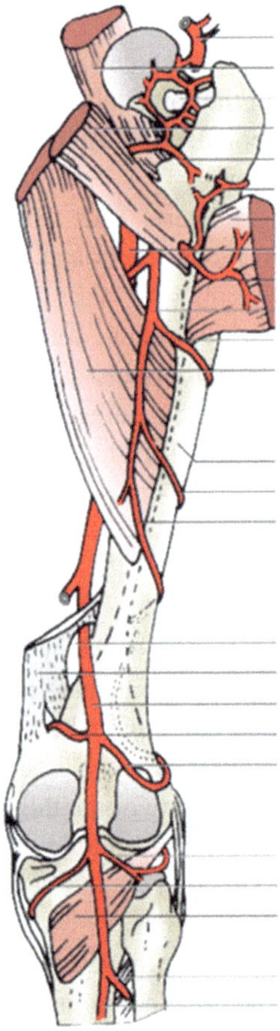

Fig. 19.1 Applied anatomy of the profunda femoral artery

the lateral side of the femoral artery and then spirals backward behind the inguinal ligament and descends alongside the medial femur.

After travelling through the posterior thigh, the profunda femoral artery sends out three main perforating branches.

In reconstruction surgery, because of a more medial location and a more ideal perfusion mode, we often prefer the first or second perforator as the vascular pedicle of the PAP flap (Fig. 19.1) [16].

Haddock et al. reported that according to CT angiography and magnetic resonance angiography, the first medial perforator of profunda femoral artery is the most common perforator (85.6% in the thigh), which is 3.8 cm away from the midline and 5 cm below the gluteal sulcus, and often passes through the adductor [24].

Saad et al. found that the average length of perforating branches was 10.6 cm and the average diameters of arteries and veins were 2.3 mm and 2.8 mm, respectively [8].

The profunda femoral artery has four perforating branches between the medial and lateral femoral circumflex arteries [25]. The first perforator originates from the proximal part of the adductor brevis or the space between adductor brevis and the pubic muscle, which provides branches to the adductor magnus and gracilis. The second perforator courses in front of the adductor brevis. The third branch travels under the adductor brevis. The second and third perforators supply the semimembranosus, biceps femoris, and lateral femoral muscles. The fourth perforator is the most variable in anatomy and is considered as the terminal branch of the profunda femoral artery. The fourth perforator pierces the muscular septum or becomes a musculocutaneous perforator like the other three perforators.

All these perforators locate deep to the skin and supply the flap with perforators of musculocutaneous or muscular septum [24].

Among them, the first and second perforating branches usually have skin branches passing through the posterior inner side of the thigh.

These perforators arise either from the musculocutaneous perforators of the adductor magnus or sometimes between the gracilis and adductor magnus or between the adductor magnus and semimembranosus muscle (Fig. 19.2) [8, 26].

There are three modes of vascular anatomical variation of the posteromedial perforating branches of the profunda femoral artery: the perforating branch of the muscular septum artery between the gracilis muscle and the adductor major, the perforating branch of the muscular skin of the adductor major, and the perforating branch of the muscular septum between the adductor major and the semimembranosus muscle (Fig. 19.3) [25].

In addition to the great adductor perforator vessels from the profunda femoral artery, medial femoral perforator vessels including the direct perforator of the femoral artery and

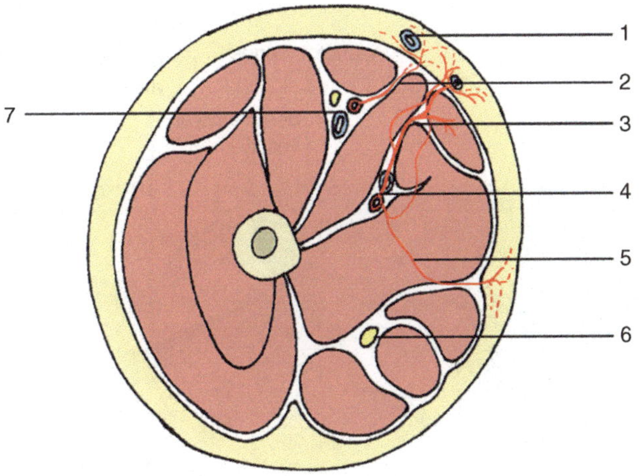

Fig. 19.2 The type and cross-sectional diagram of posterior medial femoral perforator. (1) Great saphenous vein. (2) Direct cutaneous branch of femoral artery. (3) The musculocutaneous perforators of gracilis and adductor longus from the profunda femoral artery. (4) Profunda femoral vessels. (5) Musculocutaneous perforator of adductor major. (6) Sciatic nerve. (7) Femoral artery, vein, and saphenous nerve

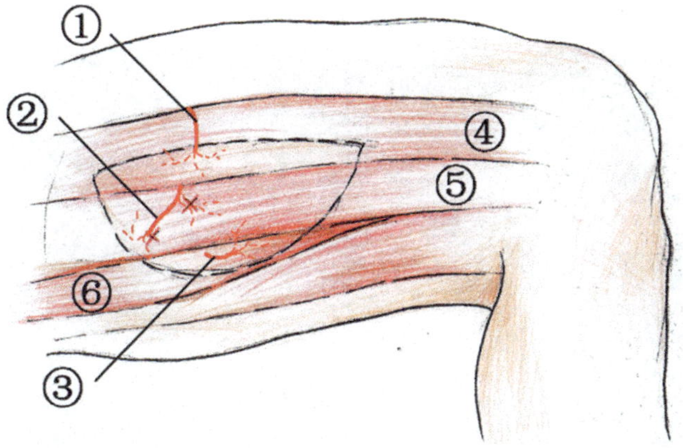

Fig. 19.3 Main vascular source and medial surface of the medial femoral perforator flap. (1) Perforating branch of the deep femoral artery. (2) Perforating branch of the gracilis muscle. (3) Perforating branch of the adductor major. (4) Adductor longus. (5) Gracilis muscle. (6) Adductor major

the gracilis perforator vessels from the profunda femoral artery are also common clinical findings (Figs. 19.4, 19.5, and 19.6) [27].

In clinical practice, we found that the femoral artery perforator flap can be consistently and reliably obtained, which was in line with other reports. In most cases, a direct femoral artery perforator can be found at the medial and lateral edges of the sartorius muscle, mostly in the area 10 cm below and 4 cm beside the anterior superior iliac spine. The diameter of the perforator artery is usually about 1.0–1.2 mm, and the diameter of the vein is usually about 1.5–2.0 mm [28].

According to the "GENT" consensus on the terminology for perforator flap [29], we believe that the naming of flap

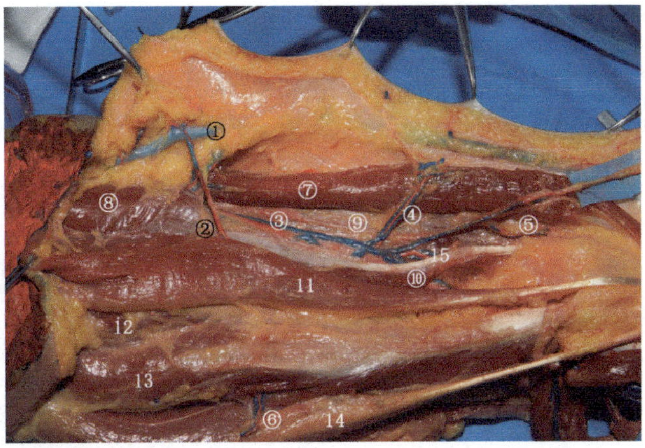

Fig. 19.4 Clinical anatomy of direct cutaneous perforator of the femoral artery and perforator of the profunda femoral artery. (1) Great saphenous vein. (2) Perforating branch of the profunda femoral artery in front of the gracilis muscle. (3) Femoral artery and vein. (4) Direct cutaneous branch of the descending genicular artery. (5) Saphenous artery. (6) Perforating branch of the profunda femoral artery from the surface of the semimembranosus muscle. (7) Sartorius muscle. (8) Adductor longus. (9) Saphenous nerve. (10) Adductor major. (11) Gracilis muscle. (12) Adductor major. (13) Semimembranosus muscle. (14) Semitendinosus muscle. (15) Articular branch of the descending knee artery

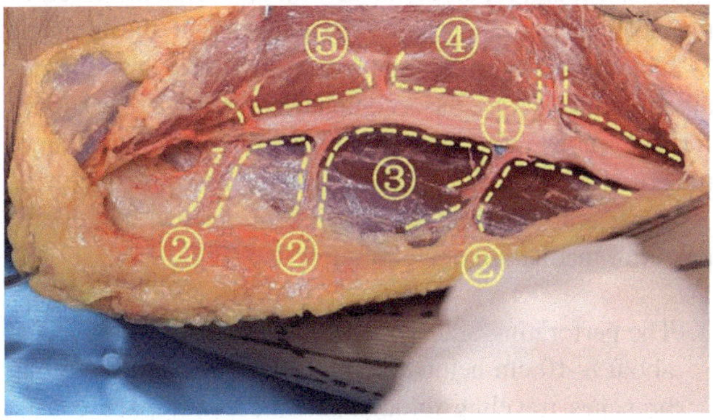

Fig. 19.5 Exposure and separation of medial femoral direct cutaneous perforator pedicled with femoral artery

should be based on the anatomical skin area. Therefore, it is more appropriate to call it posterior-medial thigh perforator flap, because not all perforators arise from the profunda femoral artery [30].

However, in clinical practice, the femoral artery perforator flap often has a small vascular diameter and short vascular pedicle, which is not suitable for breast reconstruction. Therefore, in international literatures, PAP flap is still used to indicate the posterior medial femoral perforator flap as a common practice. Similar to the half-moon-like transverse upper gracilis flap (TUG) or gracilis myocutaneous flap, the posterior medial femoral perforator flap has perforator vessels with larger diameter, longer vascular pedicle, and less complex flap anatomy. The vascular pedicle length of the pro-

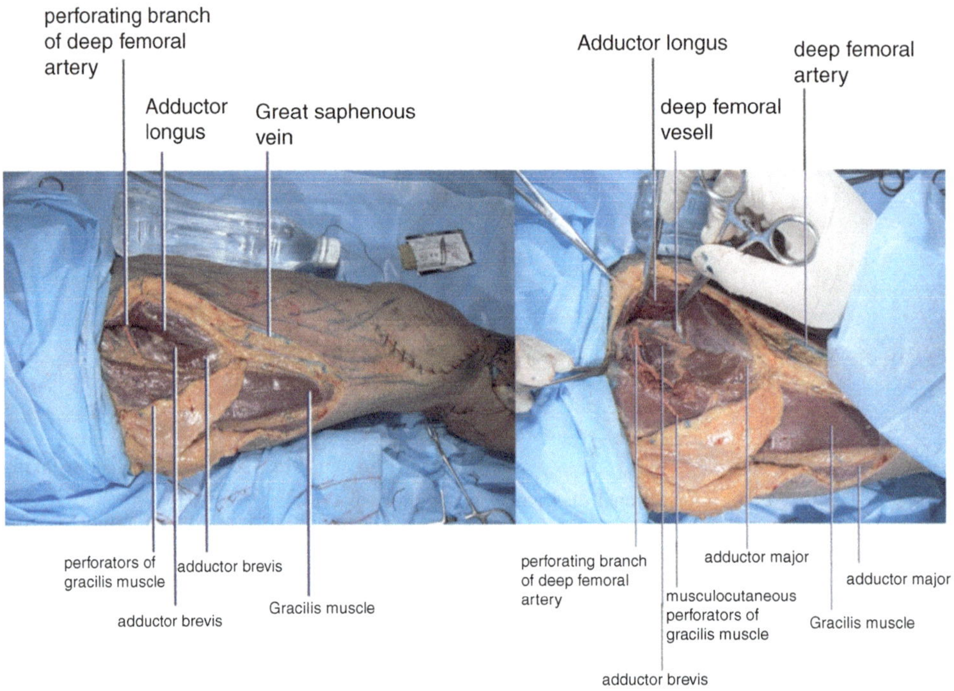

Fig. 19.6 Anatomical structure exposure and separation of the gracilis perforator flap pedicled with the profunda femoral artery

funda femoral artery perforator flap ranges from 8 to 13 cm, which is enough for anastomosis with the recipient vessels of the neck, limbs, and chest. The diameter of the artery is 2–2.5 mm, and there are usually two accompanying veins. In all our clinical cases, the accompanying veins were sufficient for the venous reflux of the flap when the perforator flap of the posterior medial femoral artery was cut and reconnected.

There are three reasons why it is simpler to harvest the posterior medial femoral perforator flap (Fig. 19.7):

1. The perforating branch of PAP flap is commonly located about 8–10 cm below the inguinal fold. The perforating branches traveling through intermuscular space can be often found in PAP flap, which makes the anatomy of the flap simpler [25, 26].
2. In addition, the vascular pedicle of the posteromedial femoral deep artery perforator flap usually has a straighter course than the anterolateral femoral perforator flap, so the anatomy for the perforators is simpler and less tortuous.
3. The musculocutaneous perforators in the vascular pedicle of free DIEP or ALT flap may be tortuous. The operation can be complex and require higher anatomical technology. In comparison, the vascular pedicle anatomy of PAP flap is simpler.

It has been reported that the number of perforator vessels in the profunda femoral artery perforator flap group is more than that in the anterolateral femoral perforator flap (2.0:1.5) [31].

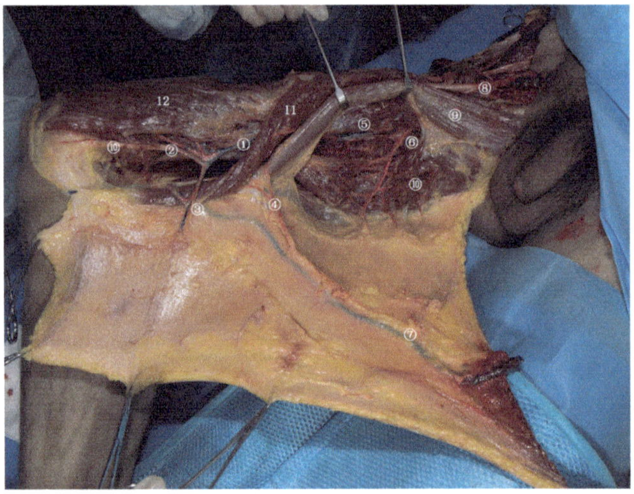

Fig. 19.7 The anatomy of the profunda femoral artery, femoral artery, and their medial femoral perforating vessels is simpler and less tortuous, and the anatomical separation is relatively easy. (1) Descending genicular artery. (2) Articular and muscular branches of the descending knee artery. (3) Saphenous artery. (4) Direct cutaneous branch of the femoral artery. (5) Profunda femoral artery. (6) The cutaneous perforator of adductor major from the profunda femoral artery. (7) Great saphenous vein. (8) Femoral artery. (9) Gracilis muscle. (10) Adductor major. (11) Sartorius muscle. (12) Medial femoral muscle

According to our experience, more perforators with appropriate size can be found in the posteromedial thigh (adductor region) than in the anterolateral thigh.

In our case, at least four perforating branches of appropriate size can be detected in the whole adductor major region and seven perforating branches to the maximum. There were

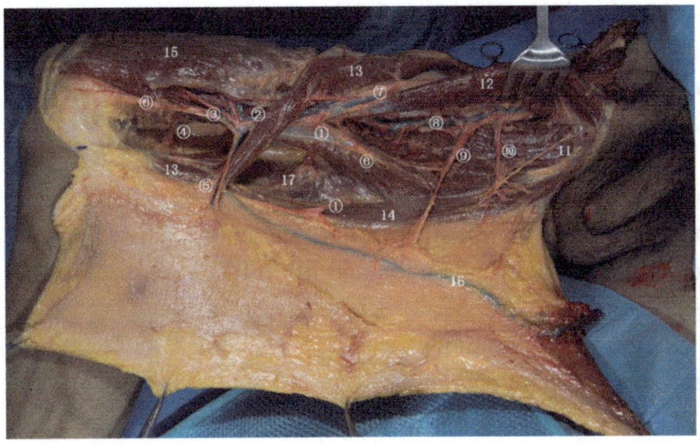

Fig. 19.8 The profunda femoral artery, the femoral artery, and their medial femoral perforating vessels commonly have multiple branches. The design size, position, and form of the flap are relatively flexible and unrestricted. (1) The perforating branch of the medial femoral muscle skin from the femoral artery. (2) Descending genicular artery. (3) Articular branch of the descending knee artery. (4) Medial superior genicular artery. (5) Saphenous artery. (6) Adductor major. (7) Femoral artery and vein. (8) Profunda femoral artery. (9) The anterior perforating branch of the adductor magnus from the profunda femoral artery. (10) Gracilis muscle branch. (11) Anterior branch of the obturator nerve. (12) Adductor longus. (13) Sartorius muscle. (14) Gracilis muscle. (15) Medial femoral muscle. (16) Great saphenous vein. (17) Semimembranosus muscle

only 1–3 perforating branches of appropriate size in the anterolateral femoral skin area. Therefore, several perforating branches of appropriate size can be obtained. According to this anatomical basis, the profunda femoral artery perforating branch flap can be designed as a chimeric flap or double flaps which can be harvested at one donor area at the same time (Fig. 19.8).

The perforating branches of the profunda femoral artery in the adductor magnus region are usually divided into 3–4 groups. In the posteromedial femoral artery perforating flap, the perforating branches of each group are usually adjacent to each other and share a common trunk, making it more likely to contain ≥2 perforating branches. In contrast, in the anterolateral thigh perforator flap, the perforators in the anterolateral thigh skin area are usually at least 5 cm apart, so it takes more time to separate the perforators, with higher technical requirements and increased surgical risk (Fig. 19.9).

According to our anatomy and clinical findings, there are three common patterns of adductor major perforator vessels (Figs. 19.10 and 19.11).

The second mode is that the adductor major branch from the profunda femoral artery sends out two perforator vessels in the adductor major into the subcutaneous tissue.

The third mode is that the adductor major branches of the profunda femoral artery at different segments send out perforating vessels into the subcutaneous tissue.

We found that most of the perforators of the profunda femoral artery are musculocutaneous perforators (40/32 (80%)) and 8/40 (20%) are musculoseptal perforators, which is consistent with that reported by Angrigiani et al. [11]. Despite the increased anatomical difficulty of the musculocutaneous perforator, muscle damage in the donor area, and

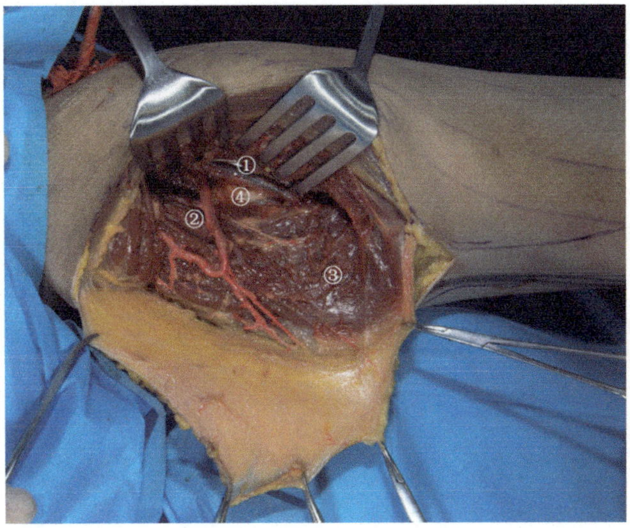

Fig. 19.9 In the adductor major region, the course of perforating branches from the profunda femoral artery in the muscle are usually straight and can directly dissected with ease. (1) Profunda femoral artery and vein. (2) Great adductor branch. (3) Adductor major. (4) Adductor brevis

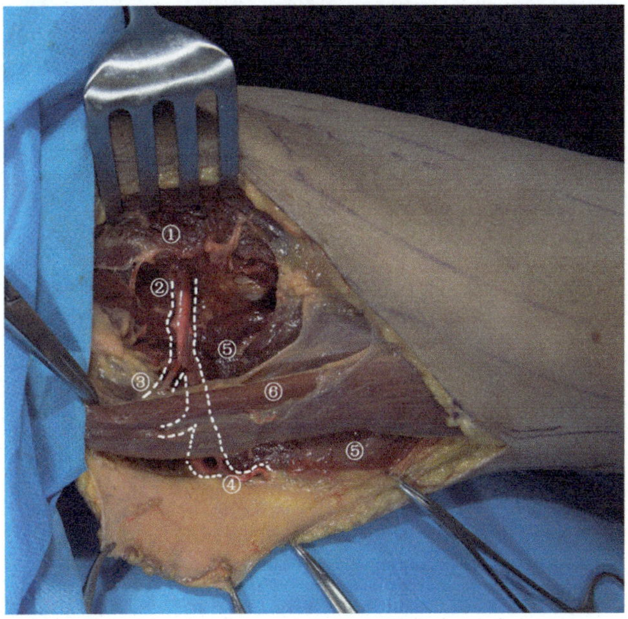

Fig. 19.10 The first mode of the great adductor perforator vessel: the great adductor vessel from the profunda femoral artery sends out the perforator vessel from the front and rear of the gracilis muscle into the subcutaneous tissue, respectively. (1) Adductor longus. (2) Adductor major branch of the profunda femoral artery. (3) Gracilis muscle branch from the great adductor branch. (4) The cutaneous branch from the great adductor branch. (5) Adductor major. (6) Gracilis muscle

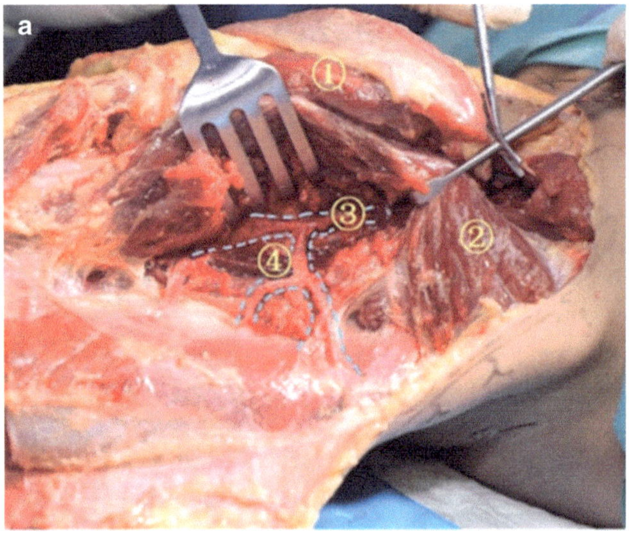

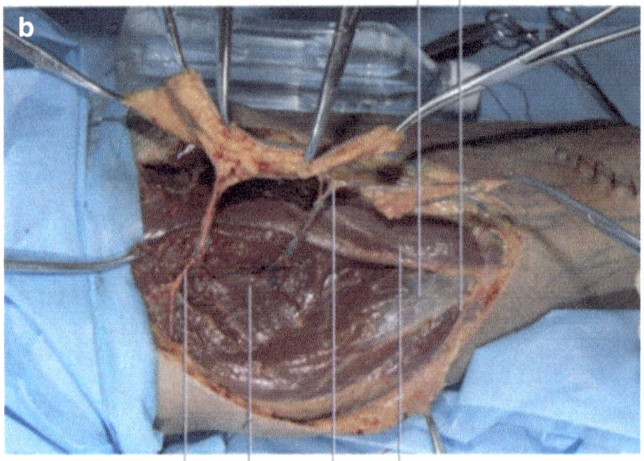

Fig. 19.11 (**a** and **b**) Show the surgical anatomy and the other two common perforator location patterns of the posterior medial thigh deep artery perforator flap

the anatomical difficulty of the posterior medial perforator flap of the thigh, the additional anatomical separation within the muscle is conducive to harvest a longer vascular pedicle. Also, the muscle flap can be more easily dissected [32].

Similar to the anterolateral femoral perforator flap, the posteromedial femoral deep artery perforator flap of the thigh can also be transformed into the chimeric myocutaneous flap to repair the wound and fill in the dead space at the same time (Figs. 19.12, 19.13, and 19.14).

Simulated operation procedures of medial femoral chimeric perforator myocutaneous flap are shown in Figs. 19.15, 19.16, 19.17, 19.18, 19.19, and 19.20.

The chimeric medial femoral perforator myocutaneous flap pedicled with profunda femoral artery has the following advantages:

1. The skin flap has pale color, soft texture, no hair growth, appropriate thickness, and is easy for shaping.
2. There are many perforating branches in the medial femoral area, and the vascular body area is large. The vascular anatomy is consistent. Compared with the anterolateral perforating branch flap, the medial femoral perforating branch flap can provide tissue with similar volume.
3. The profunda femoral artery perforator flap can carry the muscle flap at the same time and become a chimeric muscle flap, which is enough to close the dead space, facilitate the shaping, improve the surgical outcomes, and reduce the incidence of postoperative complications.
4. The perforating vessels mostly run along the gap between the adductor longus and gracilis femoris. The perforating muscles are not deep tissues, and therefore the incision and separation of the flap is relatively simple.
5. The medial femoral vascular body area of five profunda femoral arteries is large, the blood supply of the flap is reliable, and the anti-infectivity is potent.
6. The medial femoral perforator flap with a width of about 8 cm can easily and directly close the donor area and avoid skin-grafting in the donor area.
7. The supply area is normally concealed and the appearance is satisfactory.

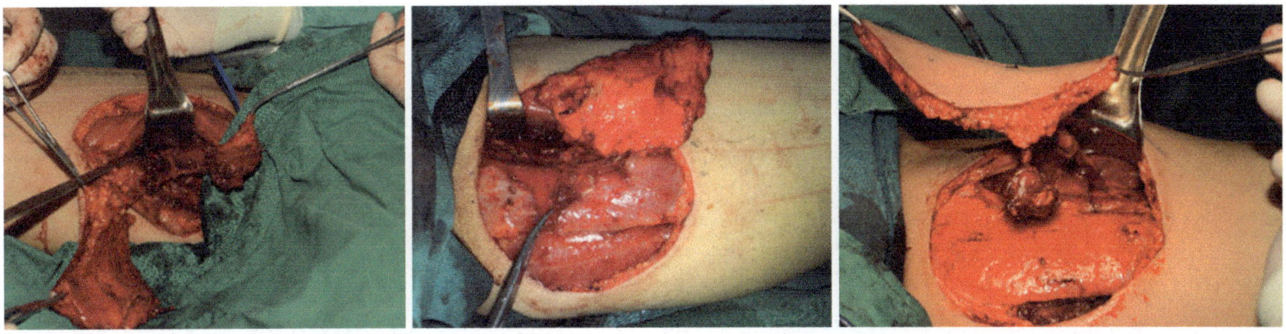

Fig. 19.12 For different forms of posteromedial femoral flap, the muscle flap cannot be cut with the direct cutaneous branch of the femoral artery. (1) Medial femoral chimeric myocutaneous flap of the adductor major branch. (2) Medial femoral chimeric myocutaneous flap with gracilis branch. (3) Medial femoral perforator flap pedicled with direct cutaneous branch of the femoral artery

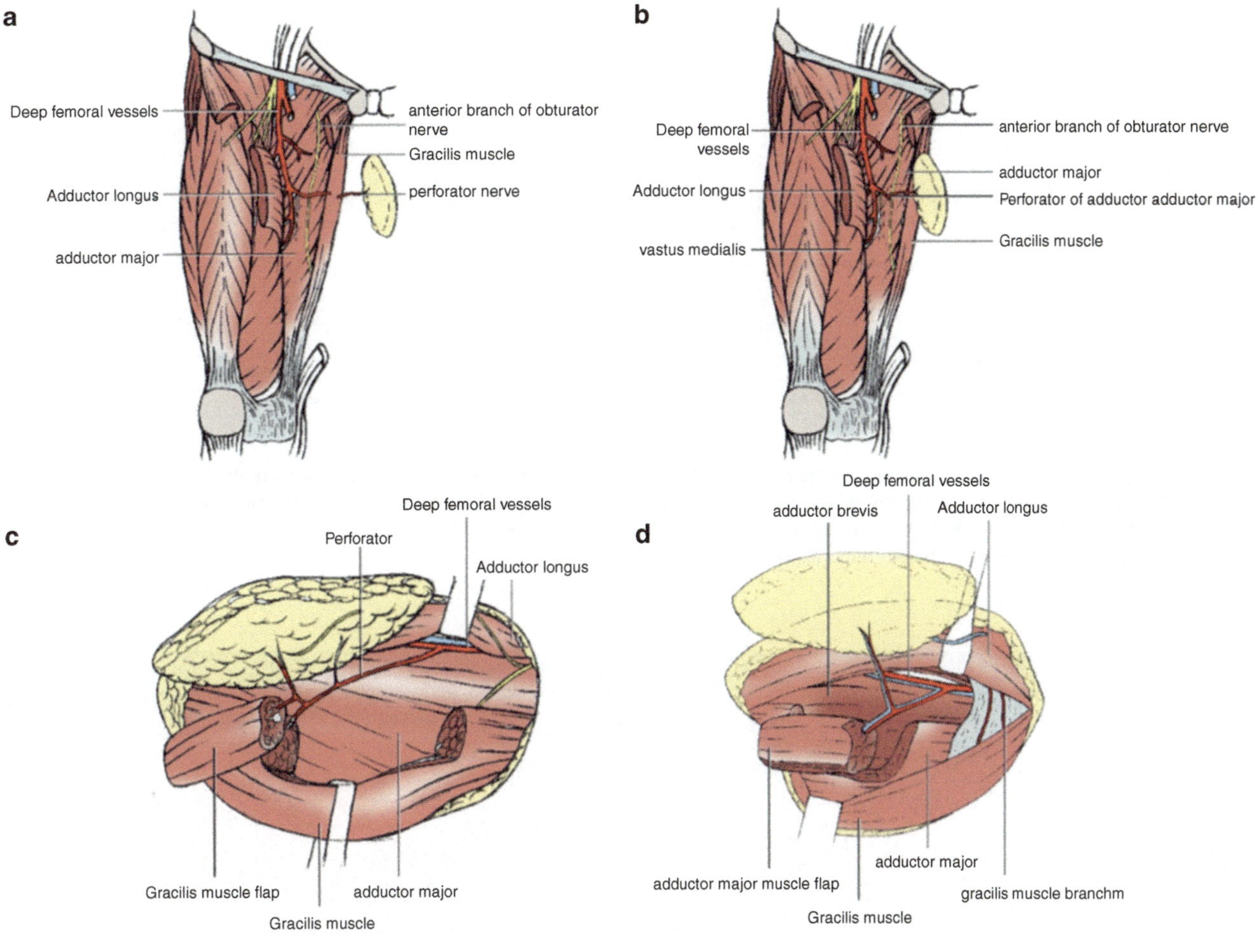

Fig. 19.13 Schematic diagram of two commonly used profunda femoral artery pedicled chimeric myocutaneous flaps. (**a**) Schematic diagram of the gracilis muscle branch embedded with medial femoral myocutaneous flap (front view). (**b**) Schematic diagram of the medial femoral myocutaneous flap embedded with adductor major muscle branch (front view). (**c**) Schematic diagram of the gracilis muscle branch embedded with medial femoral myocutaneous flap (local view). (**d**) Schematic diagram of the adductor major muscle branch embedded with medial femoral myocutaneous flap (local view)

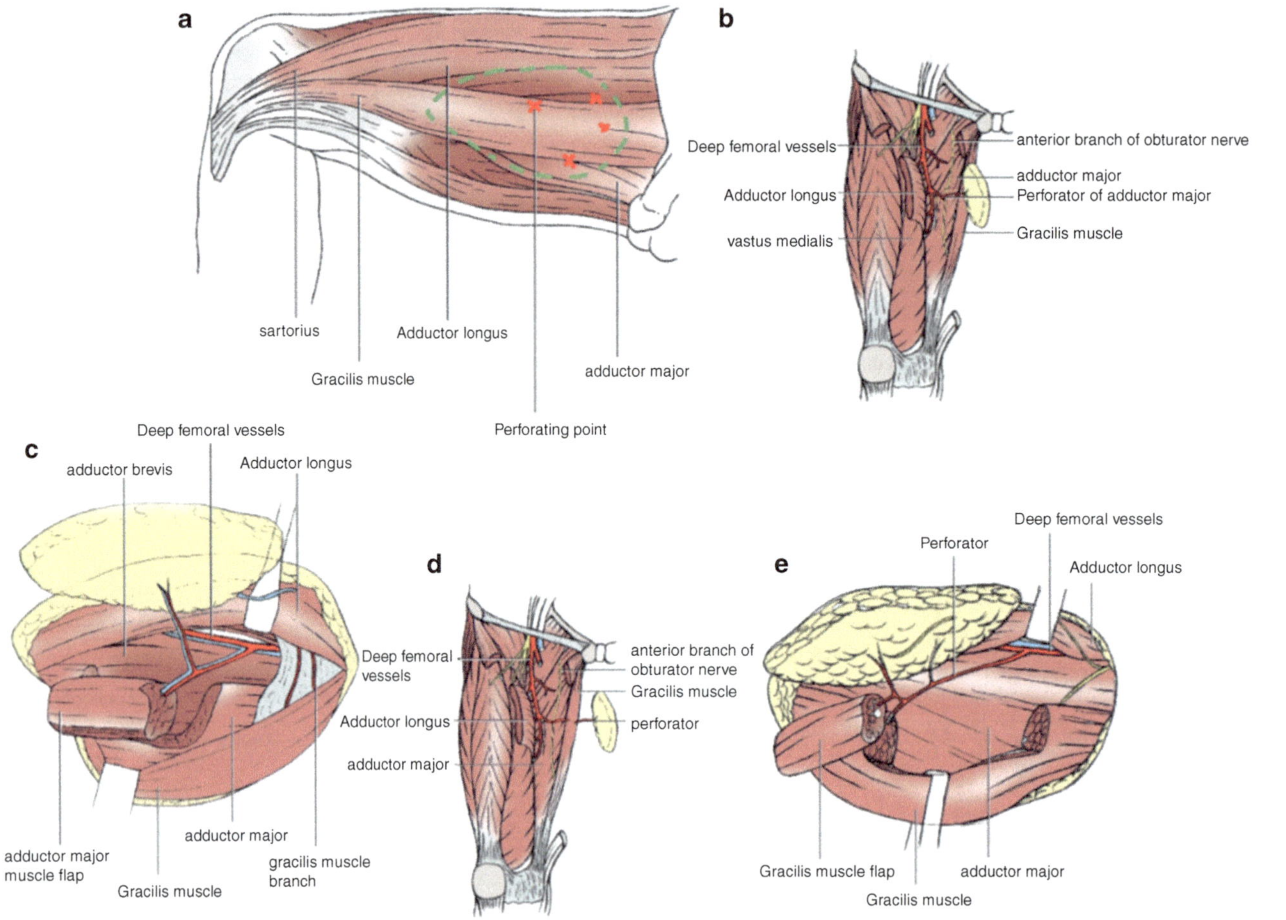

Fig. 19.14 Schematic diagram of design and cutting of free profunda femoral artery pedicled chimeric perforator myocutaneous flap. (**a**) Flap design and applied anatomy. (**b**, **c**) Applied anatomy and excision of the free profunda femoral artery pedicled chimeric perforator adductor magnus myocutaneous flap. (**d**, **e**) Applied anatomy and cutting of free profunda femoral artery pedicled chimeric perforator the gracilis myocutaneous flap

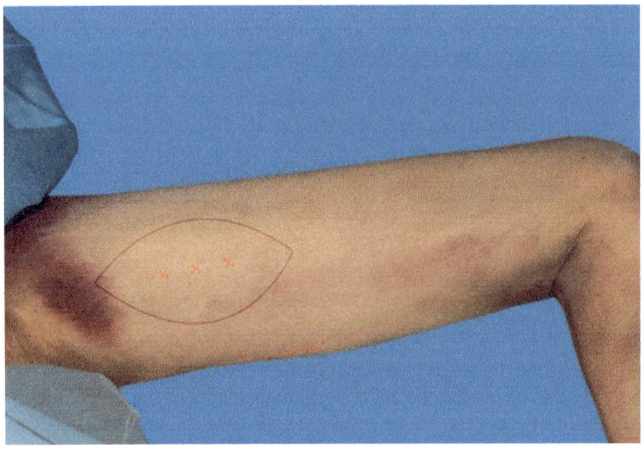

Fig. 19.15 Design of the medial femoral perforator myocutaneous flap

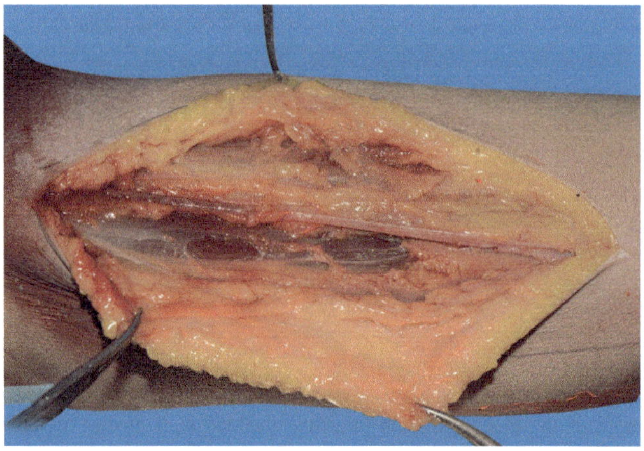

Fig. 19.16 Lift the flap from front to back to preserve the integrity of the great saphenous vein and expose the adductor longus muscle

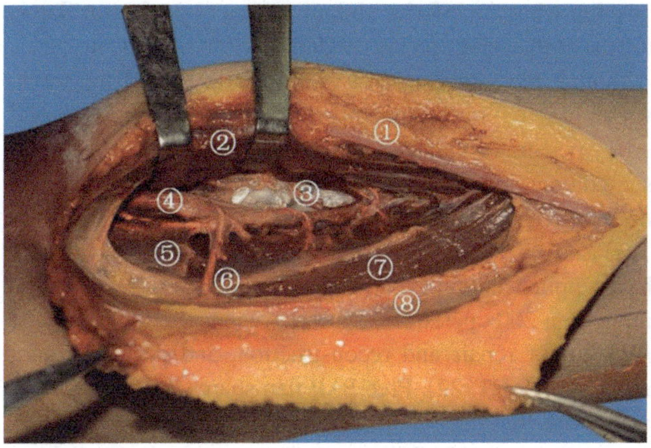

Fig. 19.17 Plane of separating perforating vessels to profunda femoral vessels. (1) Great saphenous vein. (2) Adductor longus. (3) Muscular septum. (4) Profunda femoral vessels. (5) Adductor brevis. (6) Vascular pedicle of the gracilis muscle. (7) Adductor major. (8) Gracilis muscle

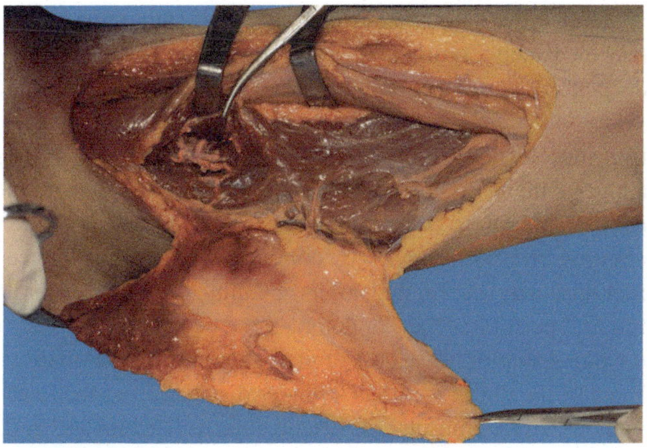

Fig. 19.18 Lift the flap further back to expose the adductor major and its profunda femoral vascular perforator on the surface

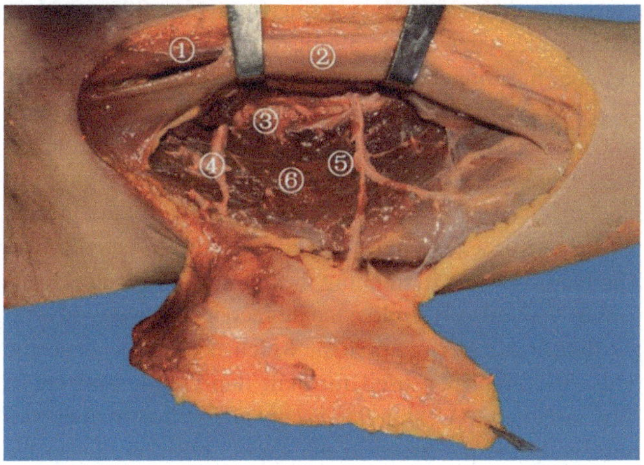

Fig. 19.19 Retrograde separation of adductor major perforator vessels to the plane of profunda femoral vessels. (1) Adductor longus. (2) Gracilis muscle. (3) Profunda femoral vessels. (4) Adductor major perforator 1. (5) Adductor major perforator vessel 2. (6) Adductor major

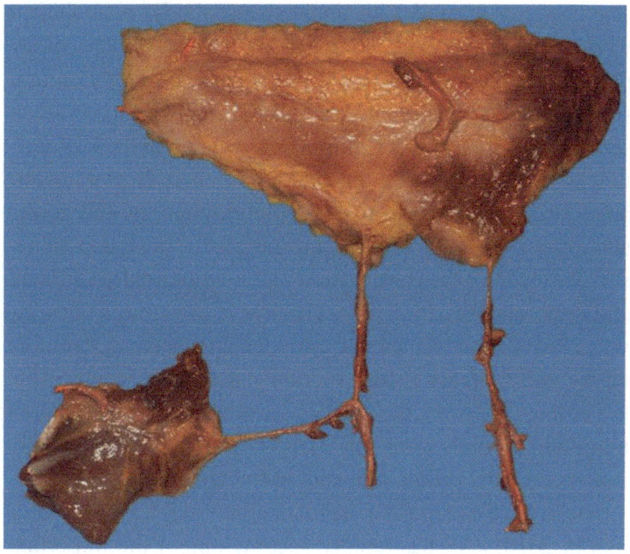

Fig. 19.20 The excision of the chimeric adductor major perforator myocutaneous flap is completed

8. There is little anatomical variation in chimeric myocutaneous posterior medial thigh perforator flap, and the flap can always be obtained.
9. There is less hair in the medial than anterolateral areas of the thigh.

Disadvantages

1. The location of perforator vessels is not fixed. Sometimes a single thin perforator is insufficient to supply a large flap. It is necessary to carry an additional perforator, which therefore increases the operation time and donor site injury.
2. The diameter of perforator vessels is often small. If a large area of flap is required, carrying double perforator vessels is necessary as a safe procedure.
3. The length of vascular pedicle is mostly about 7 cm, which is difficult to be extended further. When the recipient area repair needs a longer vascular pedicle, vascular transplantation for bridging or other flap donor areas should be selected. The specific surgical methods will be described in detail in the following chapters.

19.3 Indication

As the technology developed, all patients undergo magnetic resonance angiography (MRA) and CT angiography (CTA) to help locate and dissect the perforators during operation in order to shorten the operation time [24, 33]. The ideal group of patients for breast reconstruction using profunda femoral artery perforator (PAP) flap are those with small- to medium-sized breasts and not suitable for lower abdominal flap.

Therefore, compared with apple-shaped body, pear-shaped women are more suitable for PAP flap. However, many patients receiving PAP flap have had previous abdominal surgery, such as abdominal wall plastic surgery and cesarean section, and the problem of most patients is the lack of sufficient abdominal fat. At the same time, there is more available fat stored in the posterior thigh than in the lower abdomen [34]. PAP flap is conventionally designed transversely for breast reconstruction and longitudinally for head and neck reconstruction [35]. The scar of donor area of transverse PAP flap is located in the hidden area and is acceptable to the most breast reconstruction patients. However, if a larger flap is needed, the flap design should be converted to a longitudinal mode to obtain a larger width and flap volume, followed by the primary closing of the wound [36].

Since the first report of profunda femoral artery perforator flap in 2010, PAP has rapidly become one of the important alternatives for autologous breast reconstruction in patients who are not suitable for inferior abdominal artery perforator flap. The perforator flap of profunda femoral artery has many advantages. It has a long vascular pedicle and appropriate vascular caliber. It can cut a large amount of tissue. It can be designed into a perfect cone while retaining the muscle function. At the same time, the scar position of the donor area is hidden, and the aesthetic effect is satisfactory. The perforator flap of profunda femoral artery has many advantages. The diameter of perforator artery and vein of profunda femoral artery is perfectly matched with that of internal thoracic artery and vein, and the length of vascular pedicle can reach 10 cm, which makes the operation of vascular anastomosis, flap implantation, and breast shaping convenient [37, 38]. Moreover, a flap of crescent, transverse, and longitudinal design is sufficient to form good three-dimensional shape for the reconstructed breast [39].

Unlike the gluteal artery perforator flap, the harvest of the profunda femoral artery perforator flap does not affect the shape of hip postoperatively. Better still, the posteromedial femoral region can often provide flap with enough volume to resemble the amount of mastectomy tissue despite patients of different sizes. In addition, the profunda femoral artery perforator flap requires no dissection of the inguinal lymphatic vessels, so there is little lower extremity lymphedema after operation. Besides, based on the distribution of the posterior thigh cutaneous plexus in the deeper surface of the flap, the flap can also be used as a sensory flap for transplantation.

Another advantage is that the contour of the inner thigh can be modified after the flap dissection, and the profunda femoral artery perforator flap can be obtained in the lithotomy position, so no position change is needed in the process of breast reconstruction.

In the field of breast reconstruction, the profunda femoral artery perforator flap is to the transverse gracilis myocutaneous flap what the inferior abdominal artery perforator flap is to the transverse rectus abdominis myocutaneous flap. Although the sampling area is similar to that of the transverse gracilis myocutaneous flap, the profunda femoral artery perforator flap has more advantages, such as large tissue volume, longer vascular pedicle, hidden donor scar, and no sacrifice of muscle and function.

Based on the above researches, in the past 7 years, we have applied the profunda femoral artery perforator flap in more than 200 operations of breast reconstruction, head and neck tumor repair and reconstruction, and perineal tumor repair [9, 15, 21, 22]. Free PAP flap shares common advantages with free DIEP flap and free ALT flap, which expands the application of PAP flap in various reconstruction fields.

In contrast, the donor scar of profunda femoral artery perforator flap is located in the medial and posterior medial thigh and is hard to be noticed. The scar is still hidden from the rear observation. In addition, the change of the inner thigh shape is small, and the integrity of the gluteal fold is unaffected. As for donor site complications, although temporary myasthenia symptoms were reported in two cases in the deep artery perforator flap group, no permanent myasthenia symptoms were reported. Because the adductor group has five muscles, the functional damage after dissecting the adductor major can be easily compensated by the remaining adductor major and other adductor groups. According to literatures and our study, we found that the range of knee mobility may be limited after obtaining the anterolateral femoral perforator flap. In contrast, the deep artery perforator flap group did not have limited knee movement, mainly because the donor area has a longer distance from the knee without dissecting any important muscles, ligaments, and fascia structures that affect knee movement. In the PAP flap, the skin hair of the posterior medial thigh is less, and the scar of the donor area can be well covered. In our cases, the thickness of the perforator flap of the posterior medial femoral artery varied significantly, ranging from 15 to 30 mm. Most patients receiving tumor plastic repair and reconstruction had poor nutritional status with subsequent subcutaneous fat loss. The posteromedial thigh perforator flap tends to be of moderate thickness, which is ideal for breast reconstruction and head and neck reconstruction. When a thicker posteromedial femoral profunda femoral artery perforator flap is used to repair a superficial defect, the flap can be modified. The method refers to thinning the anterolateral femoral perforator flap [40–43]. Unlike the thoracodorsal artery perforator flap or hip perforator flap, which needs to change the body position when used for skin flap cutting and breast reconstruction, PAP skin flap is applied to breast reconstruction while the patient is in the supine position during the entire operation. PAP flap provides a longer vascular pedicle without sacrificing the appearance of the donor area, which happens in the hip perforator flap. Also, In PAP flap, there is little chance of sciatic nerve complications which may occur when dissecting the hip perforator flap. In the relatively thin patients, the posterior thigh tissue has stronger plasticity and more tissue volume than the abdominal and hip tissue. PAP flap can be used as a good donor alternative for patients with small breast and abdomen who are not suitable for breast reconstruction. According to our clinical cases, the application of PAP flap in carefully selected patients can provide an appropriate amount of tissue to cover the breast defect. The width of the flap is based on the pinch test and the closure of the donor site, usually about 7 cm. The scar of the flap donor area can be hidden in the hip femoral fold.

19.4 Preoperative Design

We usually take out preoperative marking lines for patients the day before operation. With the patient in standing position, the inferior gluteal fold as the upper boundary of the surgical incision is marked, and the second marking line 6–7 cm below the upper boundary is marked as the lower boundary of the flap. Also, the lateral boundary marking is set at the end point of the inferior gluteal fold or the area slightly lateral to the end point, and then the patient is transferred to the supine position with thigh abduction. The medial boundary is marked from the groin posterior with abundant lymphatic vessels to the rear of the adductor longus (Fig. 19.21).

According to the aforementioned markings, the typical PAP flap defined is a transverse crescent flap or a longitudinal flap of spindle shape, which can also be designed into a multi-leaf shape. The scar after donor area closure is in "T" shape, in order to obtain a larger amount of tissue. Then, the patient is transferred into the lithotomy position, and the main puncture fulcrum was marked according to the preoperative imaging results [44, 45].

The main perforating branch is commonly located 3–6 cm below the gluteal fold and 4 cm within the posterior boundary of gracilis muscle. After markings, the perforator location is confirmed again by handheld Doppler on the operating table. Mostly, patients have a sufficient number of perforators passing through the adductor major and distributed in the profunda femoral artery perforator flap, but in some cases, the most suitable perforators may also travel in the further posterior area. In these case, we can choose the perforator from the descending branch of the inferior gluteal artery (femoral gluteal artery flap) or replace it with the perforator of the profunda femoral artery closer to the posterior area. If the size and location of the perforator are not satisfactory, we can also use the gracilis myocutaneous flap as a bailout option. In addition, pressing the skin pattern into a "boomerang" shape to retain the main perforating branches is another choice to deal with the advantageous perforating branches walking in the rear.

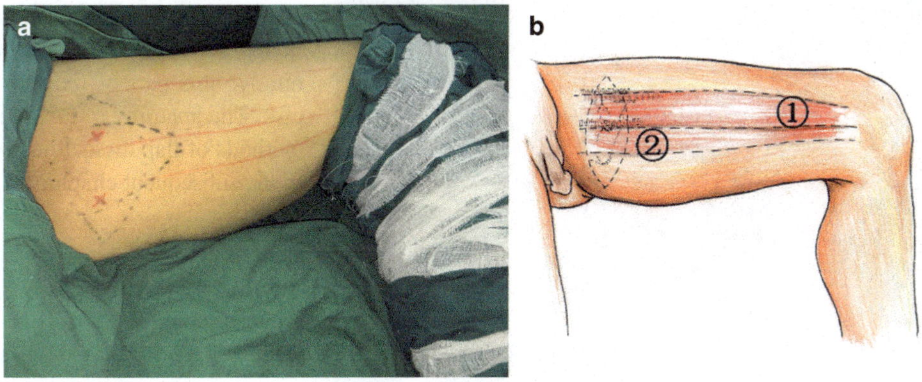

Fig. 19.21 Preoperative design of PAP flap. (**a**) preoperative markings; (**b**) illustration by drawing

19.5 Operation Process

In order to facilitate the localization and anatomy of perforating branches, so as to shorten the operation time, it is recommended that all patients undergo magnetic resonance angiography (MRA) and CT angiography (CTA) (Fig. 19.22) [8, 46].

The perforating branch is located 2 cm behind the gracilis muscle and 6 cm below the gluteal fold.

There are three perforating vessels passing through the adductor major on the inner side of the right thigh. Before operation, it was decided to choose the left thigh as the flap donor area.

The patient takes the supine position, followed by preoperative preparations for both lower limbs, disinfection, and draping. Usually, there are two groups of surgeons during the operation. Most incisions for flap perforator exploration require a position with thigh abduction. The thigh needs to be fixed in the retraction position only when the incision is taken in outmost area. During the operation, we should avoid oblique upward incision throughout the whole process, especially when close to the sciatic fat pad which bears the weight of the body, so as to avoid accidental injury of the important tissue structures. The location of the lower incision line depends on the amount of tissue required and the location of the main perforating branches. After the markings of four sides are confirmed, we lift the flap from front to back, vertically incise the gracilis fascia at the posterior edge of the gracilis muscle, and pull the muscle forward. Then, the gracilis fascia is vertically opened near the posterior edge of the gracilis and the front edge of the adductor, and the fascia behind the gracilis and the fascia on the surface of the adductor major are incised. The fascia of the adductor major is subsequently opened to confirm the main perforating branch, track it to the deep surface of the muscle, and find the origin of the perforating branch from the profunda femoral artery. At this very moment, it is important to further separate the perforating vessel of adductor major into the yellow adipose tissue space on the deep surface of adductor major. The length of vascular pedicle ranges from 8 to 12 cm. The average diameter of artery reaches 2.2 mm, and the average diameter of vein reaches 2.7 mm. Once the flap is removed, the wound drainage tube is placed and the donor area is sutured in layers. The drainage tube is retained for at least 1 week. We usually select the internal mammary vessels in the recipient area as the recipient anastomotic vessels. Similarly, the thoracodorsal vessels, lateral thoracic vessels, and thoracic acromial vessels can also be used as the recipient vessels for donor-recipient area vascular anastomosis (refer to the chapter on recipient area vascular selection). Generally, the perforator flap of the profunda femoral artery is often in conical shape in order to facilitate implantation and shaping. We reserve a part of the skin island for observation to monitor the blood supply of the flap postoperatively. In the secondary reconstruction of nipple areola, we will remove this part of the skin island that has completed the task. The anatomy of PAP flap varies, and there are multiple methods of flap dissection, which will be described in detail in the subsequent chapters of operation introduction.

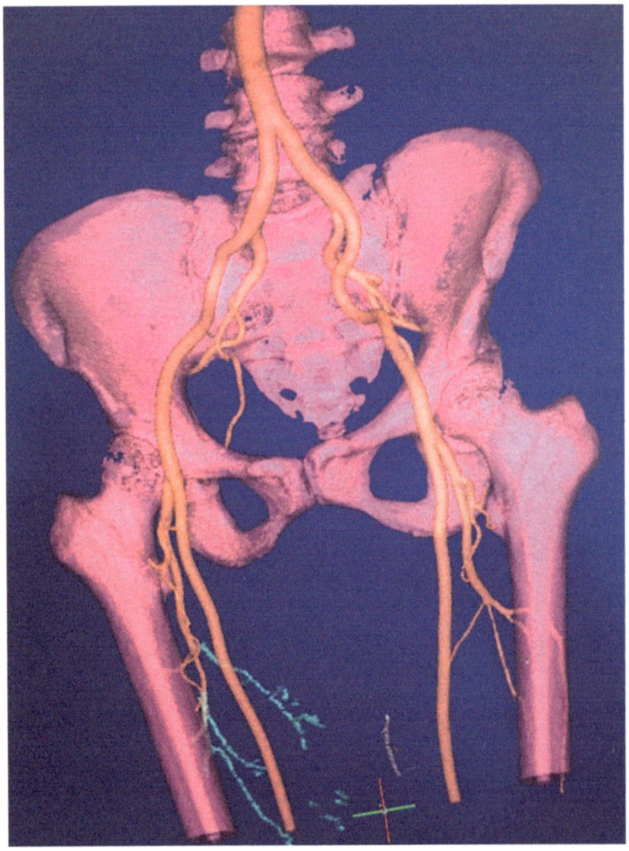

Fig. 19.22 CTA shows that there is a large perforator vessel passing through the adductor magnus on the inner side of the left thigh

19.6 Postoperative Care

After 1–2 h of observation in the recovery room, the patient can be transferred to the general ward. During this period, we should observe the blood supply of the flap every 1 h and focus on the condition of skin island. In clinical practice, we found that photographic evaluation is a very accurate method to evaluate the blood supply of the skin island. In terms of postoperative analgesia, we mainly use nonsteroidal anti-inflammatory drugs. In addition, in the morning of the first day after operation, the urethral catheter can be removed, and the patient can have regular meals and be encouraged to take early exercise. The patient can be discharged 4–7 days after operation.

19.7 Discussion

Based on our experience from more than 100 cases of profunda femoral artery perforator flap transplantation, less than 10% of the patients with small-scale fat liquefaction necrosis after one-stage operation can be solved during the two-stage reconstruction. Similarly, the postoperative donor site hematoma in the 10% of cases can also be solved by further drainage, surgical exploration, and removal of hematoma. Lymphatic leakage in the donor area can also be avoided by fine design and operation. The diameter of the perforating vessels of the profunda femoral artery is perfectly matched with that of the vessels in the chest recipient area. There is less hair on the posteromedial femoral skin and more perforating vessels in the posteromedial femoral area. The length of the vascular pedicle is sufficient. The vascular pedicle of the posteromedial femoral artery perforating branch usually runs in a straighter course than that of the anterolateral femoral perforating branch flap, so the dissection of the perforating branch is more simple and direct. The thickness of the flap can be flexibly adjusted, and the tissue is soft and easy to shape. The ideal group of patients for breast reconstruction with PAP flap are those with small- to medium-sized breasts and sufficient fat on the inner thigh. Because of its advantages, the inner and posterior thigh area as a donor area for breast reconstruction is gradually accepted by patients and medical community.

19.8 Conclusions

The profunda femoral artery perforator flap is a reliable flap with consistent perforator anatomy. In various reconstruction fields, there are many perforating branches in the posteromedial region of the thigh, and the length and diameter of the vascular pedicle are matched with the recipient vessels. The donor scar is hidden and the risks of complications are rather low. The profunda femoral artery perforator flap can be used as a main flap in different reconstruction fields and can be used as a desired donor alternative for two-stage breast reconstruction.

References

1. Taylor GI, Palmer JH. The vascular territories (angiosomes) of the body: experimental study and clinical applications. Br J Plast Surg. 1987;40(2):113–41.
2. Koshima I, Soeda S. Deep inferior epigastric artery skin flaps without rectus abdominis muscle. Br J Plast Surg. 1989;42(6):645–8.
3. Saint-Cyr M, Schaverien MV, Rohrich RJ. Perforator flaps: history, controversies, physiology, anatomy, and use in reconstruction. Plast Reconstr Surg. 2009;123(4):132e–45e.
4. Patel NG, Ramakrishnan V. Microsurgical tissue transfer in breast reconstruction. Clin Plast Surg. 2017;44(2):345–59.
5. Healy C, Allen RJ. The evolution of perforator flap breast reconstruction: twenty years after the first DIEP flap. J Reconstr Microsurg. 2014;30(2):121–5.
6. Zhang S, Song D. The discovery, development history and clinical implications of perforator flaps. Chin J Reparat Reconstr Surg. 2017;07:769–72.
7. Ahmadzadeh R, Bergeron L, Tang M, Geddes CR, Morris SF. The posterior thigh perforator flap or profunda femoris artery perforator flap. Plast Reconstr Surg. 2007;119(1):194–200; discussion 201–2.
8. Saad A, Sadeghi A, Allen RJ. The anatomic basis of the profunda femoris artery perforator flap: a new option for autologous breast reconstruction—a cadaveric and computer tomography angiogram study. J Reconstr Microsurg. 2012;28(6):381–6.
9. Dajiang Song, Zan Li, Xiao Zhou. Application of profunda femoral artery perforator flap in breast reconstruction. Chin J Plast Surg2017. (6): 412–416.
10. Fosseprez P, Gerdom A, Servaes M, Deconinck C, Pirson G, Berners A. [Profunda artery perforator flap: reliable secondary option for breast reconstruction?]. Ann Chir Plast Esthet. 2017;62(6):637–45.
11. Angrigiani C, Grilli D, Thorne CH. The adductor flap: a new method for transferring posterior and medial thigh skin. Plast Reconstr Surg. 2001;107(7):1725–31.
12. Fujii M, Terashi H, Hashikawa K, Tahara S. Functional reconstruction of large anogenital defects with bilateral V-Y advancement posterior thigh fasciocutaneous flaps. J Plast Reconstr Aesthet Surg. 2007;60(11):1208–13.
13. Unal C, Ozdemir J, Yirmibesoglu O, Yucel E, Agir H. Use of inferior gluteal artery and posterior thigh perforators in management of ischial pressure sores with limited donor sites for flap coverage. Ann Plast Surg. 2012;69(1):67–72.
14. Dajiang Song, Zan Li, Xiao Zhou. Free profunda femoral artery pedicled gracilis chimeric musculocutaneous perforator flap for repair of defects after oral and buccal cancer surgery Chin J Plast Surg2017. 33(4): 242–247.
15. Dajiang Song, Zan Li, Xiao Zhou. Clinical application of free medial femoral chimeric perforator myocutaneous flap in the repair of defects after tongue cancer surgery. Chin J Otorhinolaryngol Head Neck Surg2017. 52(4): 278–282.
16. Allen RJ, Haddock NT, Ahn CY, Sadeghi A. Breast reconstruction with the profunda artery perforator flap. Plast Reconstr Surg. 2012;129(1):16e–23e.
17. Allen RJ, Lee ZH, Mayo JL, Levine J, Ahn C, Allen RJ. The profunda artery perforator flap experience for breast reconstruction. Plast Reconstr Surg. 2016;138(5):968–75.
18. Satake T, Muto M, Ko S, Yasumura K, Ishikawa T, Maegawa J. Breast reconstruction using free posterior medial thigh perforator flaps: intraoperative anatomical study and clinical results. Plast Reconstr Surg. 2014;134(5):880–91.
19. Haddock NT, Gassman A, Cho MJ, Teotia SS. 101 consecutive profunda artery perforator flaps in breast reconstruction: lessons learned with our early experience. Plast Reconstr Surg. 2017;140(2):229–39.
20. Blechman KM, Broer PN, Tanna N, Ireton JE, Ahn CY, Allen RJ. Stacked profunda artery perforator flaps for unilateral breast reconstruction: a case report. J Reconstr Microsurg. 2013;29(9):631–4.
21. Zhou X, Song D, Li Z. The development of perforator flap and its application in oncoplastic surgery. Chin J Aesthet Plast Surg. 2017;28(2):69–72.
22. Dajiang Song, Zan Li, Xiao Zhou. Observation of curative effect of different forms of free profunda femoral artery pedicle chimeric perforator myocutaneous flap in the repair of defects after

tongue cancer surgery. Chin J Reparat Reconstr Surg2017. 31(06): 696–701.
23. Hupkens P, Ozturk E, Wittens S, Hoevenaren IA, Kooloos JG, Ulrich DJ. Posterior thigh perforator flaps: an anatomical study to localize and classify posterior thigh perforators. Microsurgery. 2013;33(5):376–82.
24. Haddock NT, Greaney P, Otterburn D, Levine S, Allen RJ. Predicting perforator location on preoperative imaging for the profunda artery perforator flap. Microsurgery. 2012;32(7):507–11.
25. DeLong MR, Hughes DB, Bond JE, Thomas SM, Boll DT, Zenn MR. A detailed evaluation of the anatomical variations of the profunda artery perforator flap using computed tomographic angiograms. Plast Reconstr Surg. 2014;134(2):186e–92e.
26. Scaglioni MF, Kuo YR, Yang JC, Chen YC. The posteromedial thigh flap for head and neck reconstruction: anatomical basis, surgical technique, and clinical applications. Plast Reconstr Surg. 2015;136(2):363–75.
27. Haddock N, Nagarkar P, Teotia SS. Versatility of the profunda artery perforator flap: creative uses in breast reconstruction. Plast Reconstr Surg. 2017;139(3):606e–12e.
28. Ratanshi I, McInnes CW, Islur A. The proximal superficial femoral artery perforator flap: anatomic study and clinical cases. Microsurgery. 2017;37(6):581–8.
29. Blondeel PN, Van Landuyt KH, Monstrey SJ, et al. The "Gent" consensus on perforator flap terminology: preliminary definitions. Plast Reconstr Surg. 2003;112(5):1378–83; quiz 1383, 1516; discussion 1384–7.
30. Sinna R, Boloorchi A, Mahajan AL, Qassemyar Q, Robbe M. What should define a "perforator flap". Plast Reconstr Surg. 2010;126(6):2258–63.
31. Shieh SJ, Chiu HY, Yu JC, Pan SC, Tsai ST, Shen CL. Free anterolateral thigh flap for reconstruction of head and neck defects following cancer ablation. Plast Reconstr Surg. 2000;105(7):2349–57; discussion 2358–60.
32. Hurwitz ZM, Montilla R, Dunn RM, Patel NV, Akyurek M. Adductor magnus perforator flap revisited: an anatomical review and clinical applications. Ann Plast Surg. 2011;66(5):438–43.
33. Agrawal MD, Thimmappa ND, Vasile JV, et al. Autologous breast reconstruction: preoperative magnetic resonance angiography for perforator flap vessel mapping. J Reconstr Microsurg. 2015;31(1):1–11.
34. Buescher TM, Andry D, Brown T, Vargo J, Nazir N, Andrews BT. Inset of unilateral dual microvascular breast reconstruction using nonabdominal free tissue transfer. Plast Reconstr Surg. 2016;138(1):42–8.
35. Ito R, Huang JJ, Wu JC, Lin MC, Cheng MH. The versatility of profunda femoral artery perforator flap for oncological reconstruction after cancer resection—clinical cases and review of literature. J Surg Oncol. 2016;114(2):193–201.
36. Scaglioni MF, Chen YC, Lindenblatt N, Giovanoli P. The vertical posteromedial thigh (vPMT) flap for autologous breast reconstruction: a novel flap design. Microsurgery. 2017;37(5):371–6.
37. Stalder MW, Lam J, Allen RJ, Sadeghi A. Using the retrograde internal mammary system for stacked perforator flap breast reconstruction: 71 breast reconstructions in 53 consecutive patients. Plast Reconstr Surg. 2016;137(2):265e–77e.
38. Buescher T, Przylecki WH, Holding J, et al. Evaluation of complications associated with flap/pedicle inset techniques for unilateral breast reconstruction utilizing dual transverse upper gracilis (TUG) or profunda artery perforator (PAP) flaps. Plast Reconstr Surg. 2015;136(4 Suppl):90–1.
39. Hupkens P, Hameeteman M, Westland PB, Slater NJ, Vasilic D, Ulrich DJ. Breast reconstruction using the geometrically modified profunda artery perforator flap from the posteromedial thigh region: combining the benefits of its predecessors. Ann Plast Surg. 2016;77(4):438–44.
40. Song D, Li Z, Zhou X. Observation of curative effect of free sensory ultra-thin anterolateral thigh perforator flap in repairing wounds at donor site. Chin J Reparat Reconstr Surg. 2017;31(08):987–91.
41. Xie S, Deng X, Chen Y, et al. Reconstruction of foot and ankle defects with a superthin innervated anterolateral thigh perforator flap. J Plast Surg Hand Surg. 2016;50:1–8.
42. Kimura N. A microdissected thin tensor fasciae latae perforator flap. Plast Reconstr Surg. 2002;109(1):69–77; discussion 78–80.
43. Koshima I, Fukuda H, Yamamoto H, Moriguchi T, Soeda S, Ohta S. Free anterolateral thigh flaps for reconstruction of head and neck defects. Plast Reconstr Surg. 1993;92(3):421–8; discussion 429–30.
44. Scaglioni MF, Eder M, Giovanoli P. The use of inverted-L posteromedial thigh (L-PMT) flap for autologous breast reconstruction: a case report. Microsurgery. 2018;38(5):558–62.
45. Date S, Ciudad P, Maruccia M, Chen HC. Breast reconstruction using the geometrically modified profunda artery perforator flap from the posteromedial thigh region: combining the benefits of its predecessors. Ann Plast Surg. 2017;79(1):124.
46. Wong C, Nagarkar P, Teotia S, Haddock NT. The profunda artery perforator flap: investigating the perforasome using three-dimensional computed tomographic angiography. Plast Reconstr Surg. 2015;136(5):915–9.

Vascular Variations and Approaches of PAP Flap

20

Dajiang Song and Narushima Mitsunaga

The posteromedial femoral perforator flap is regarded as a reliable choice for reconstructing defects in various parts of the body [1]. By understanding the anatomical study of the perforating branch of the profunda femoral artery, the vascular area of the perforating branch of the profunda femoral artery includes the whole medial and posterior thigh area [2]. After obtaining the vertically designed medial femoral perforator flap, the laser-assisted indocyanine green angiography system further confirmed the size of the vascular body area of the perforator of the profunda femoral artery.

20.1 Anatomy

The branch from the profunda femoral artery on the outside of the femoral artery courses deep into the posterior thigh septum and then separates into the internal and external branches before sending out the perforating artery. In the adductor septum, the medial branch sends out the first perforating branch to supply the gracilis and adductor major, and most of traveling course is located in the muscular septum [2]. Previous cadaver study found that the perforating branch was the thickest where the perforator was passing through the adductor muscle at 8 cm from the distal groin and 2 cm from the posterior edge of the gracilis muscle (Fig. 20.1) [3]. The average length of vascular pedicle is about 10 cm. In the study of cadaver and computed tomography angiography, the average arterial diameter is 2.3 mm and 2.7 mm, respectively [4, 5]. In CT study, the total number of perforating branches on the posterior medial side of each thigh ranged from two to five, and at least three perforating branches were found in more than 80% cases. Among 37.5% of male patients and 18.2% of female patients, the perforating branches came from the same vessel [5].

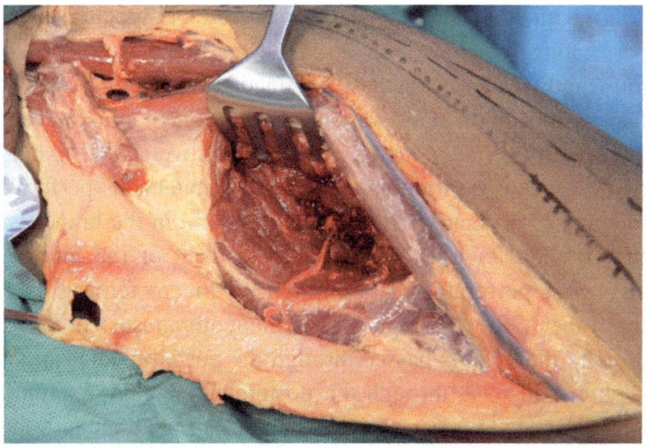

Fig. 20.1 The largest posteromedial femoral perforator often passes through the adductor major and enters the subcutaneous tissue

On average, there were 2 perforators (range, 1–3 perforators) in the posteromedial profunda femoral artery perforator flap group and 1.5 perforators (range, 1–3 perforators) in the anterolateral femoral perforator flap group. The difference between the two groups was statistically significant ($P = 0.0176$). Therefore, the design of posteromedial femoral flap is more flexible than anterolateral femoral flap [6].

According to anatomical research, the average distance from the posteromedial femoral puncture fulcrum to the fold is 3.5 cm. The distance from the fulcrum to the central line is 6.2 cm. All perforating branches are located between the adductor major and semitendinosus muscles. All perforating branches travel in short distance between the muscles so that an anatomical cavity can be easily dissected within the thigh muscles. From this area, the vessels can easily be traced to the origin of the profunda femoral artery through the loose space. The average length of vascular pedicle was 10.6 cm [4]. However, according to our clinical findings, it is still a complex procedure to separate the vascular perforators in the muscle before there is access into the loose tissue, which is

D. Song (✉)
Department of Oncology Plastic Surgery, Hunan Cancer Hospital, Changsha, Hunan, China

N. Mitsunaga
Mie University Graduate School of Medicine Plastic and Reconstructive Surgery, Tsu, Mie, Japan
e-mail: sancho-ps@umin.ac.jp

Z. Li, D. Song (eds.), *Oncoplastic Flap Surgery*, https://doi.org/10.1007/978-981-19-8926-1_20

hindered by limited visual field and a great number of vascular branches. It is reported that the average diameter of perforating artery is 2.3 mm, and the average diameter of vein is 2.8 mm among foreign population, but that of the Chinese population is obviously far from this level.

Foreign clinical anatomy reports have found the following three main perforator patterns [7]: (1) septal perforator between gracilis and adductor magnus (2/40 (5%)); (2) musculocutaneous perforator of adductor major (32/40 (80%)); and (3) septal perforators of adductor major and semimembranosus muscles (6/40 (15%)). We found that most of the perforating branches of 40/32 (80%) are muscle perforating branches, and 8/40 (20%) are muscle septal perforating branches, which were consistent with that reported by Angrigiani et al. Although the damage rate of myocutaneous perforating branches is high, which may increase the anatomical difficulty of the posterior medial perforating branch flap of the thigh, the additional separation of muscle can obtain a longer flap vascular pedicle. An average of five ± two cutaneous perforators, 35% musculocutaneous perforators and 65% septal perforators were found in the branches of profunda femoral artery. Eighty percent of the muscle cutaneous perforators pass through the biceps femoris and the other 20% through the semimembranosus muscle. Among them, 31% passed through the posteromedial thigh septum and 69% through the posterolateral thigh septum. The average diameter of the perforating branch was 0.8 ± 0.3 mm. The average length of vascular pedicle from deep fascia was 29 ± 14 mm, and that from femoral artery was 68 ± 33 mm. The average area of cutaneous vessels of profunda femoral artery was 229 ± 72 cm^2, and each perforator was 46 ± 13 cm^2. In the previous research, the average perforator length was 10.3 cm (range 8–13 cm), which was enough to connect the recipient vessels reconstructed in the head and neck [2].

The first perforating branch of profunda femoral artery mainly provides the blood supply for adductor and gracilis. The second and third perforators supply the semimembranosus, biceps femoris, and lateral femoral muscles. All these perforating arteries include myocutaneous and/or septal perforating arteries. We found more anatomical patterns of perforating branches based on clinical experience, including direct perforating branch flap of femoral artery, perforating branch flap of adductor longus muscle, and perforating branch flap of gracilis muscle. Except for the direct perforating branch of the femoral artery, all other perforating vessels originate from the profunda femoral artery, which will be introduced in detail in this section.

20.1.1 Preoperative Planning/Flap Design

The suitable perforating branch of profunda femoral artery is detected by thigh CTA, MRA, or handheld Doppler device, and a marking of a shape of vertical ellipse is taken along the inner thigh. If the perforating branch is located too far posterior, attention needs to be paid not to set the front edge of the flap too far interior, because the flap with increased width must contain additional perforating branches.

20.2 Discussion of Clinical Experience

In this chapter, we will systematically introduce in detail the clinical cases of reconstruction of breast, head and neck, trunk, and lower limb defects using posteromedial femoral perforator flap with different design methods, including transverse, longitudinal, oblique, and chimeric designs [7–9].

In the attempt to expand the application of the profunda femoral artery perforator flap, Song et al. first described a larger tissue volume of anterior femoral flap and the characteristics of multifunctional flap such as sensory reconstruction, chimeric transplantation, composite repair, and blood flow bridging. It is important to note that anterolateral femoral flap is still one of the most diversified flaps in the field of repair and reconstruction [10–12]. Although the complex anatomical structure of the anterolateral thigh does have great potential in complex tissue reconstruction, the anatomy of the posteromedial thigh flap pedicles with the perforating branch of the vertical profunda femoral artery varies considerably, and the dissecting methods are various and diverse [13, 14].

Compared with the transversely designed PAP and TUG flaps, the vertically designed medial femoral perforator flap can dissect a larger amount of tissue [14], and the largest flap in our case is 30 cm × 3 cm × 10 cm, which is enough for medium-sized breast reconstruction. The flap donor area can also be closed primarily, and the cosmetic results can be desirable.

Compared with the conventional free flap (TUG, PAP) from the medial thigh, the advantages of the vertically designed medial femoral perforator flap include the following:

1. The length of the vascular pedicle is up to 10 cm and even exceeds 10 cm [15]. In comparison, the length of the vascular pedicle of TUG flap is shorter (6–8 cm) [16].
2. As for the diameter of vascular pedicle, the diameter of TUG, VUG, PAP, and PMT flaps is about 2 mm, which are suitable for microvascular anastomosis [15, 16].
3. In the transverse design of PAP and TUG flaps, the donor scar can be well hidden [15, 16]. However, influenced by the gravity, the scar will move down seriously, and the subsequent rupture of the labia majora may be a serious complication [16]. The vertical scar of the donor area of the vertically designed posteromedial femoral perforator flap and VUG attenuates the tension that surround the

thigh, which prevent the sagging of the scar or the aggravation of the cleft labia majora [16].

4. Compared with TUG and VUG flaps, the vertically designed posteromedial femoral perforator flap does not damage the lymphatic structure due to its posterior position in the inner thigh.
5. TUG and VUG are myocutaneous flaps compared with the vertically designed posteromedial perforator flap, and the volume loss caused by muscle atrophy after denervation should be considered [16].

In our experience, the vertical profunda femoral artery perforator free flap provides an additional option for a variety of reconstruction. Although the perforator of the profunda femoral artery has been widely described through cadaveric and radiographic studies, the clinical application of using this flap as a free flap is rare. Angrigiani et al. first described this flap by autopsy and the application of this free flap in burn scar contracture and lower limb reconstruction [17]. Allen et al. described the anatomical characteristics of deep artery perforator flap through autopsy and angiography and summarized the clinical experience of breast reconstruction with deep artery perforator flap [4, 15, 18]. This flap has a crescent design on the inner upper side of the thigh, which is conducive to create a conical shape for breast reconstruction, but it is more diversified and suitable for reconstruction in other body areas [17]. In non-breast reconstruction, we usually prefer vertical or upright design, which provides a wide range of applications, minimizes incision tension, and provides more perforator selections.

There is less injury in the donor site of vertical profunda femoral artery perforator flap than that of anterolateral femoral flap. The donor scar of anterolateral femoral flap is located in the front of the thigh, and the corresponding perforator of profunda femoral artery is located in the posteromedial thigh. In addition, in male patients, the vertical profunda femoral artery perforator flap area often has less body hair than the anterolateral femoral area. Sensory abnormalities in the lateral thigh occurred in up to 24% of the patients due to the dissection of the anterolateral femoral flap. Although there were few reports on sensory evaluation in the posteromedial femoral region, sensory abnormalities in patients after the operation of vertical profunda femoral artery perforator flap were fairly rare [19].

Combined with the clinical experience, we adjusted the specific dissecting method of the flap based on the perforating vessels on different muscle surfaces from the anterior, medial, and posterior sides of the thigh and systematically introduced the dissecting approaches and operation key points of different forms of medial femoral perforating flap. In the process of clinical application of PAP flap in the repair and reconstruction of various defects, we found that the sources of perforating vessels of medial thigh and posterior medial thigh were diverse, and their positions varied dramatically. Next, we will introduce them one by one following the order from front to back in the medial thigh.

20.3 Typical Case 1: Medial Femoral Flap Pedicled with Direct Perforating Branch of the Femoral Artery

The perforating vessels from the femoral artery can often be separated and exposed on the surface of the adductor longus. According to our experience, the advantage is that more than one perforating vessel is commonly found in the muscular septum, which is easy to separate and offers multiple choices. The disadvantage is that the vascular pedicle is short and the vascular diameter is small, so it is difficult to place and anastomose the vascular pedicle. However, when a suitable perforating vessel cannot be found in the posteromedial thigh, it can still be served as an alternative (Figs. 20.2, 20.3, 20.4, 20.5, 20.6, 20.7, and 20.8) [20].

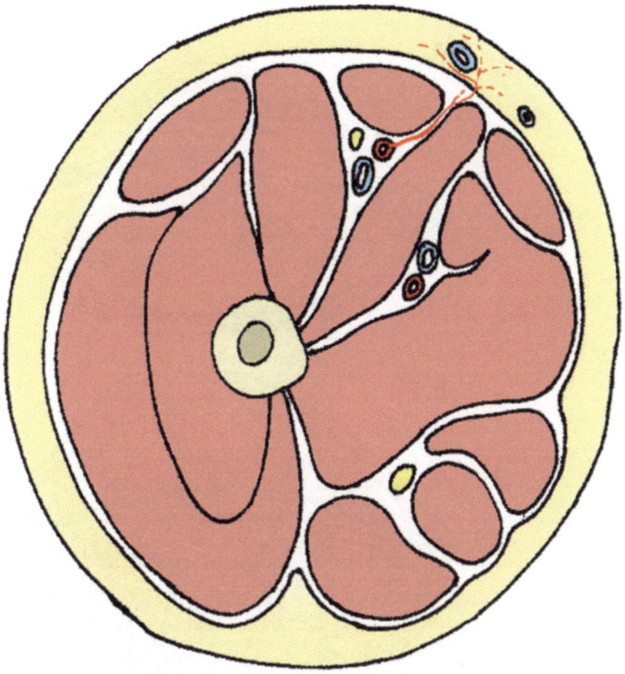

Fig. 20.2 Cross-sectional anatomy of direct perforating branch of the femoral artery

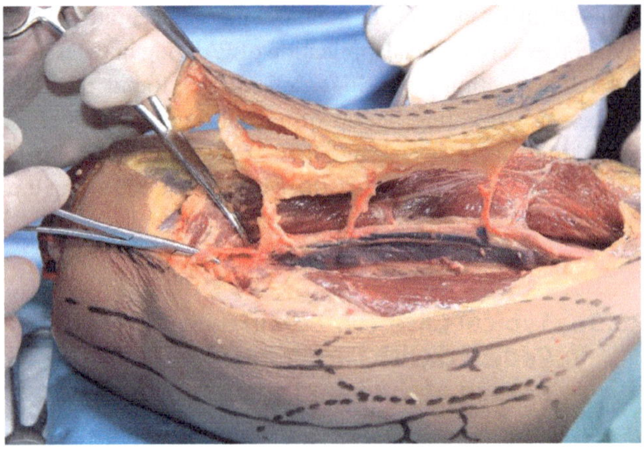

Fig. 20.3 Multiple direct cutaneous perforating branches from the femoral artery enter the skin between the adductor longus muscle and the medial femoral muscle

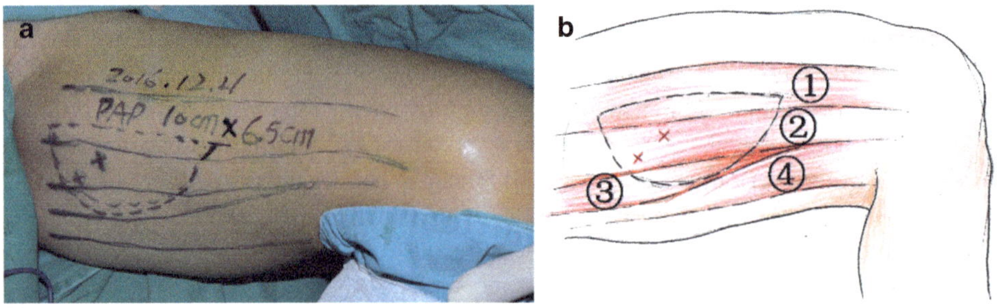

Fig. 20.4 The medial femoral flap pedicled with the direct perforating branch of the femoral artery should still use the adductor longus gracilis as the vascular body area. (1) Adductor longus. (2) Gracilis muscle. (3) Adductor major. (4) Semimembranosus muscle

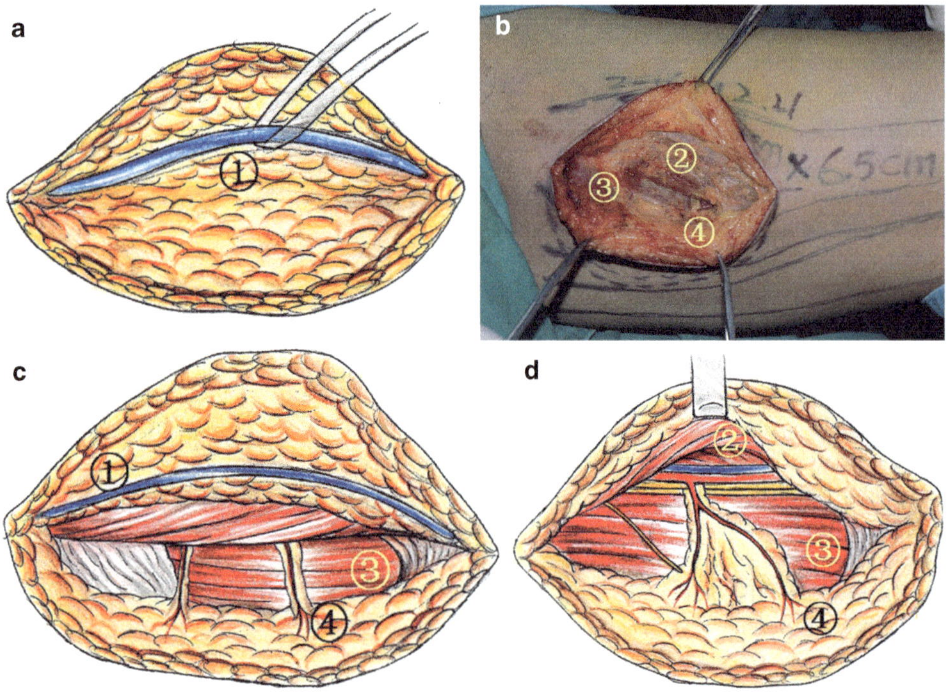

Fig. 20.5 Lift the front edge of the incision flap to directly expose the great saphenous vein and turn the great saphenous vein forward. Further lift the flap backward, the layer is the surface of deep fascia, and two perforators are exposed. The deep fascia was cut longitudinally along the front edge of the two perforating branches. It was found that the two perforating branches shared a common trunk within the muscle septum and came from the femoral artery and vein. In addition, a thick branch of the saphenous nerve was sent into the flap. The position of passing through and out of the skin was the muscle septum between the medial femoral muscle and the adductor longus muscle. (1) Great saphenous vein. (2) Medial femoral muscle. (3) Adductor longus. (4) Perforating vessels

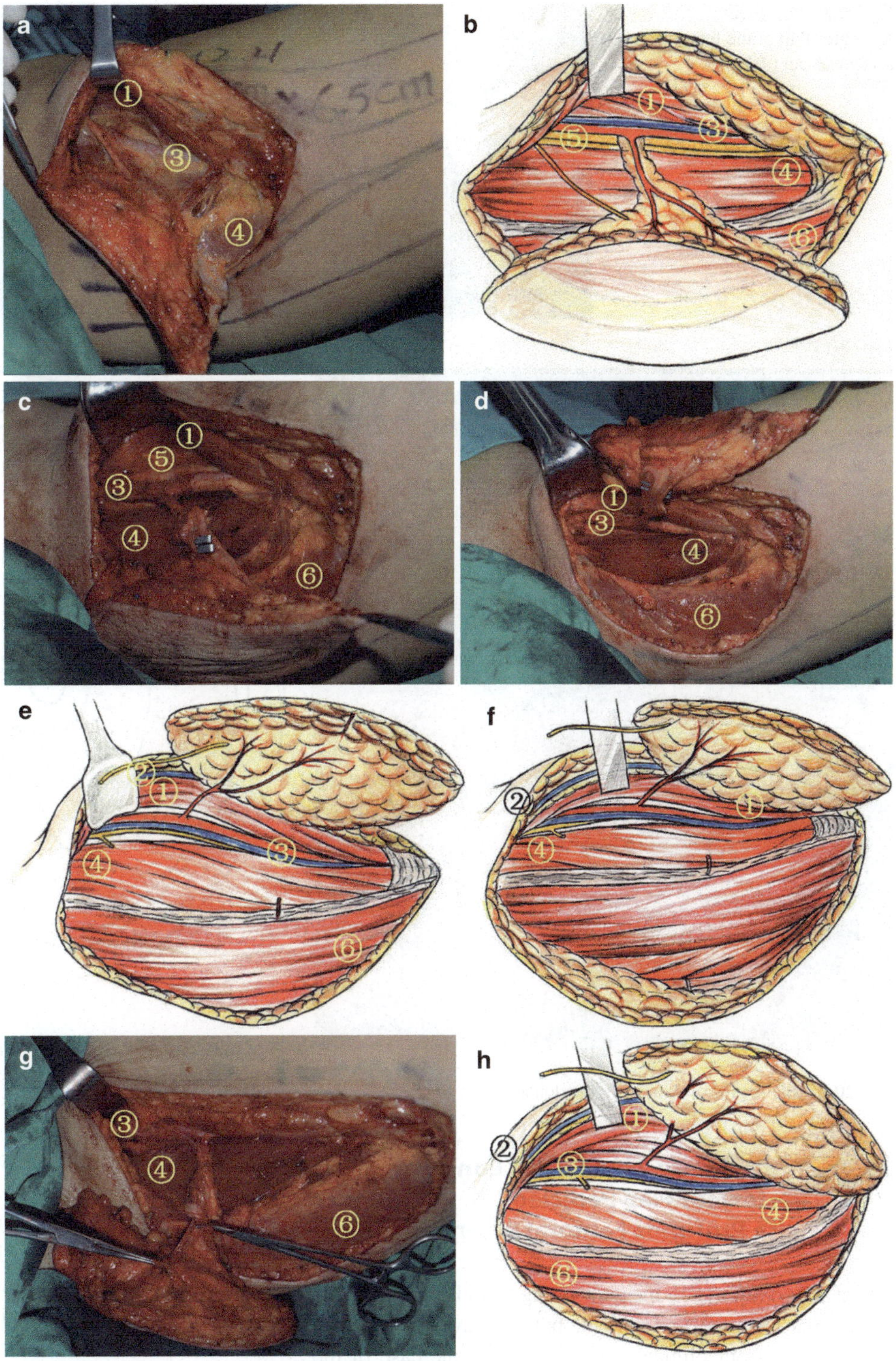

Fig. 20.6 Retrograde separation of perforator vessels from femoral vessels, circular incision of other skin edges of the flap, and complete lifting of the flap. A non-thick perforator vessel was found at the posterior edge of the flap between gracilis and adductor major. The flap was lifted completely. Only the perforator of the femoral artery with two branches was used as the pedicle. The long segment of the sensory branch of the free femoral nerve was left in the flap and separated from the posterior edge of the flap donor area. It was revealed that there was a thick perforator vessel between the adductor major and the semimembranosus muscle, which was reserved for use. Trace the perforating branch of femoral artery to its issuing plane, and ligate the proximal perforating branch to prolong the vascular pedicle. (1) Medial femoral muscle. (2) Great saphenous vein. (3) Femoral vessels. (4) Adductor longus. (5) Saphenous nerve. (6) Gracilis muscle

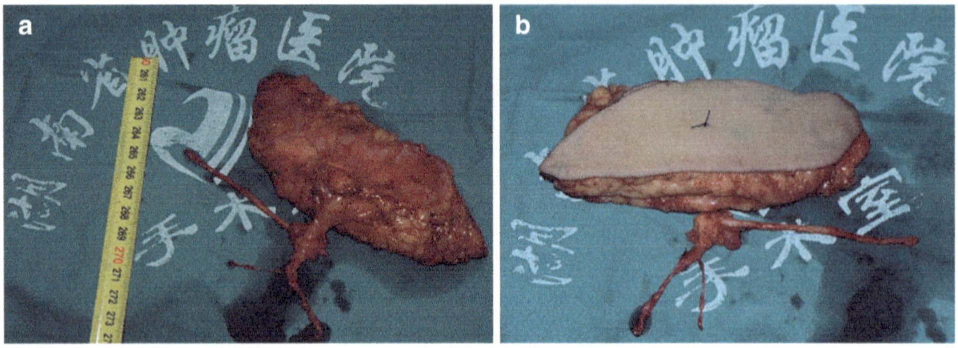

Fig. 20.7 The direct perforator flap of the femoral artery was cut off

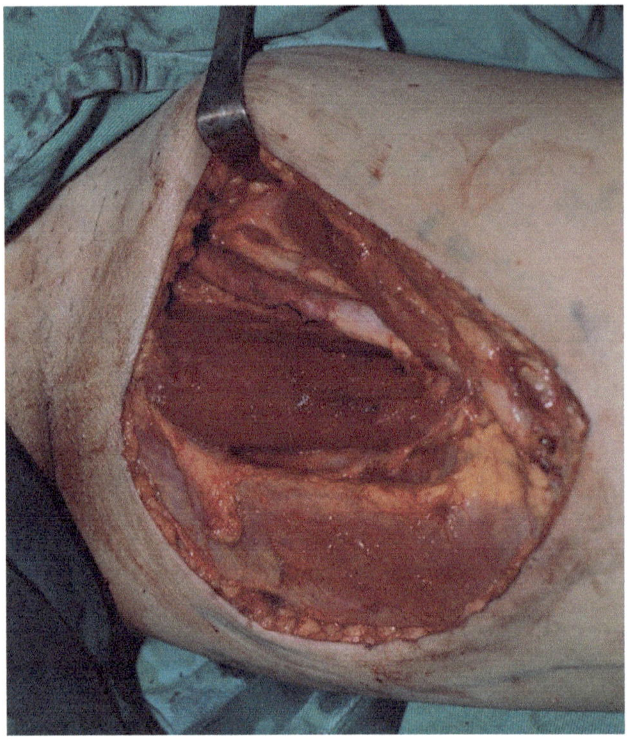

Fig. 20.8 The degree of damage in the donor area is small

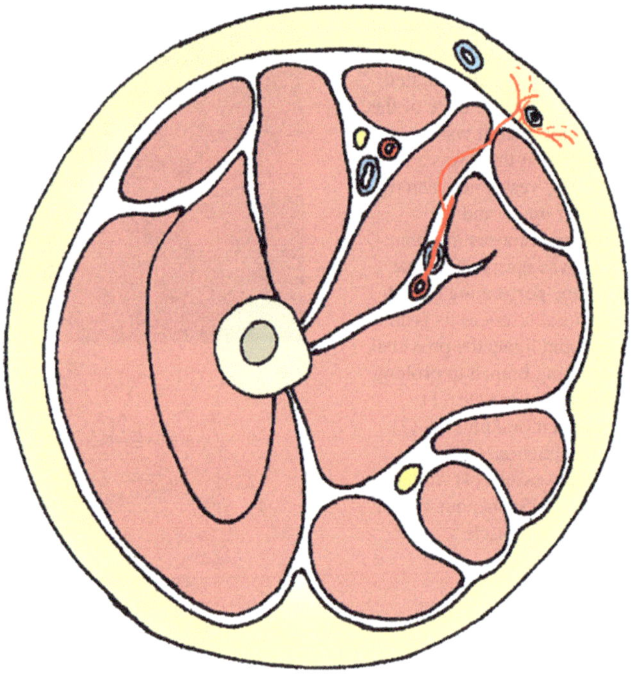

Fig. 20.9 Schematic cross-section of anatomical type 1 of perforating branch of adductor longus muscle. Anatomical type: adductor longus perforator flap (profunda femoral artery pedicle)

20.4 Typical Case 2: Adductor Longus Perforator Flap Pedicled with Profunda Femoral Artery

There are no reports on the perforating vessels of the adductor longus at home and abroad, but we have encountered three cases in our clinical work, including one case of the perforating vessels of the adductor longus directly from the profunda femoral artery and two cases from the main branches of the gracilis muscle. The dissecting methods are not remotely different. The perforating vessels commonly pass through the adductor longus, but the separation field is often limited, so the difficulty of procedures does not reduce.

In this typical case, there was no large cutaneous perforator in the gracilis muscle branch and no large perforator vessel in the adductor major. The only large perforator in the inner thigh came from the adductor longus muscle. Retrograde separation confirmed that the cutaneous perforator does not arise from the gracilis muscle branch. The long segment of the adductor longus muscle separated the perforator to the plane of profunda femoral vessels. The vascular pedicle was 8.2 cm long and the vessel diameter is 1.0 mm (Figs. 20.9, 20.10, and 20.11).

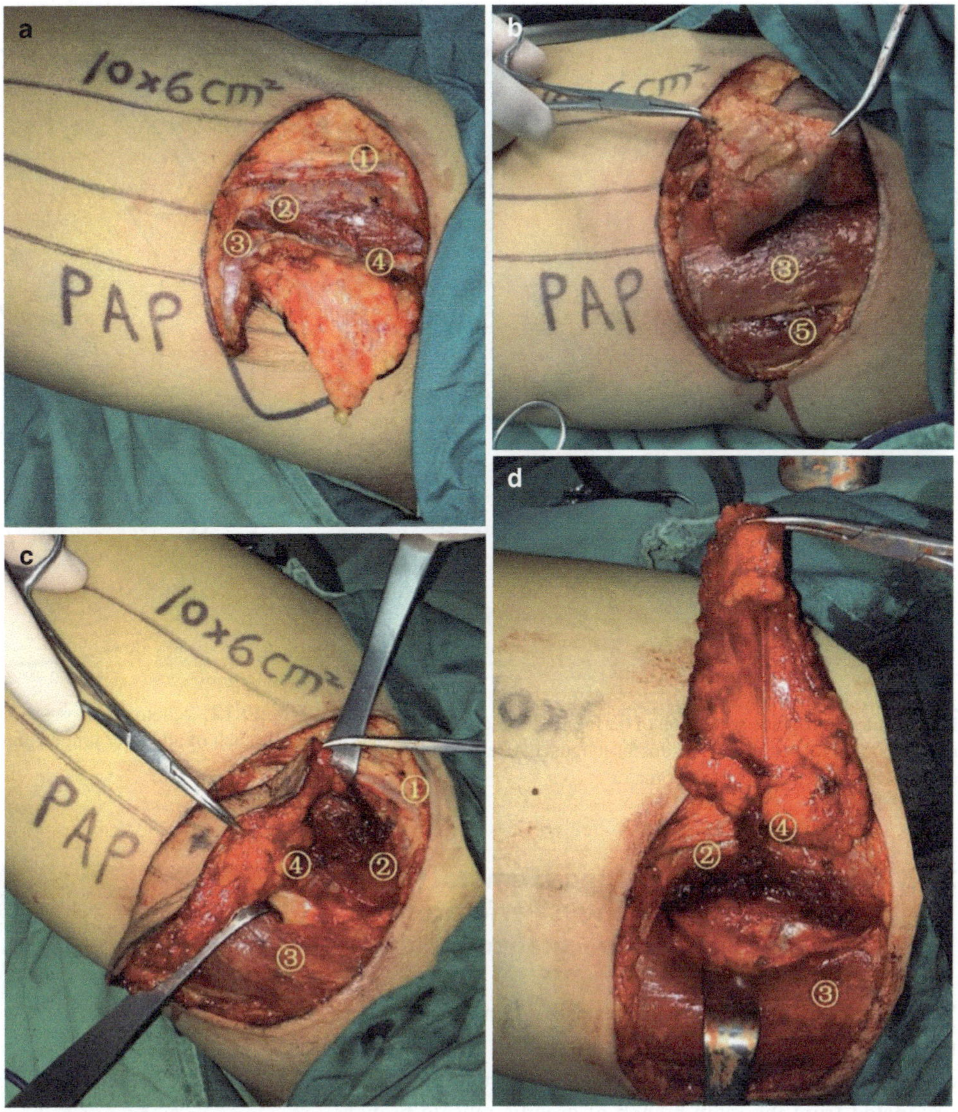

Fig. 20.10 Lift the flap to separate the perforator vessels, and it can be seen that the perforator vessel originates from the surface of the long adductor muscle. No other suitable perforator vessels are found on the surface of the gracilis muscle, which turns retrograde to separate the perforator vessels in the long adductor muscle. (1) Great saphenous vein. (2) Adductor longus. (3) Gracilis muscle. (4) Musculus adductor longus. (5) Adductor major

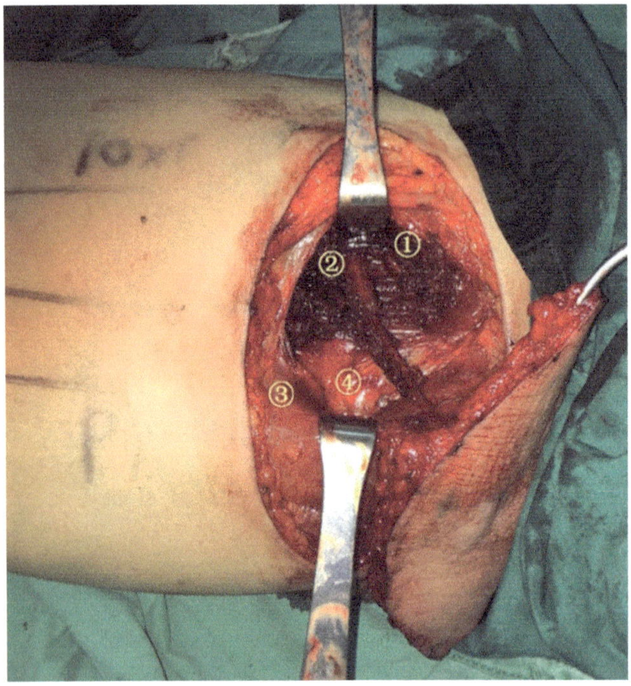

Fig. 20.11 Retrograde separation of perforating vessels to the plane of profunda femoral vessels. (1) Adductor longus. (2) Perforating vessels. (3) Gracilis muscle. (4) Adductor major

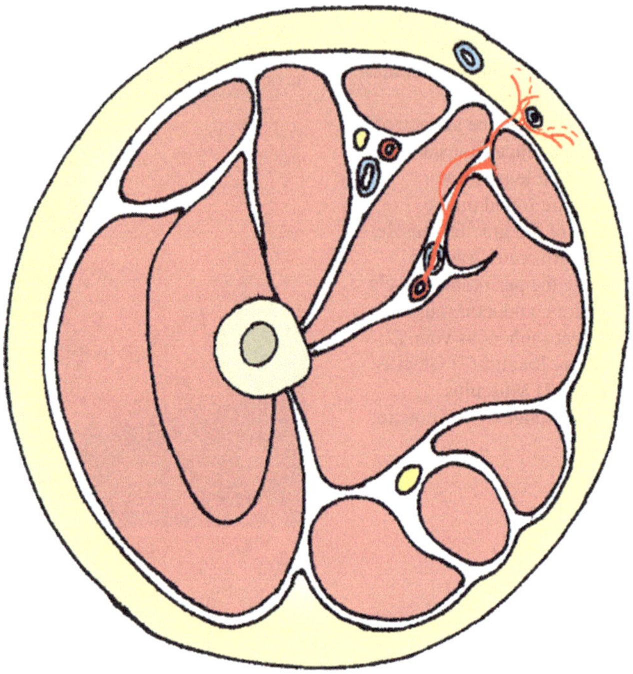

Fig. 20.12 Schematic cross-section of anatomical type 2 of perforating branch of adductor longus muscle

20.5 Typical Case 3: Profunda Femoral Artery Adductor Longus Perforator Gracilis Chimeric Myocutaneous Flap

When repair by different tissues is needed clinically, the chimeric myocutaneous flap is the best choice. In this typical case, the perforating branch of adductor longus muscle skin originated from the main branch of gracilis muscle branch. The design of chimeric myocutaneous flap has multiple choices, including adductor longus muscle flap and gracilis muscle flap (Figs. 20.12, 20.13, 20.14, 20.15, 20.16, 20.17, and 20.18).

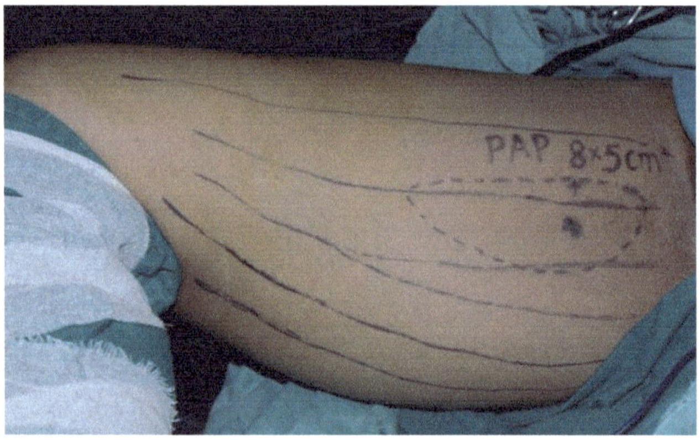

Fig. 20.13 Design of longitudinal flap and exploratory incision according to preoperative Doppler detection of perforating vessels, and the anterior edge was incised for exploration

Fig. 20.14 Expose the trunk of the great saphenous vein and the branch entering the flap, and ligate the long segment of the branch and leave it in the flap

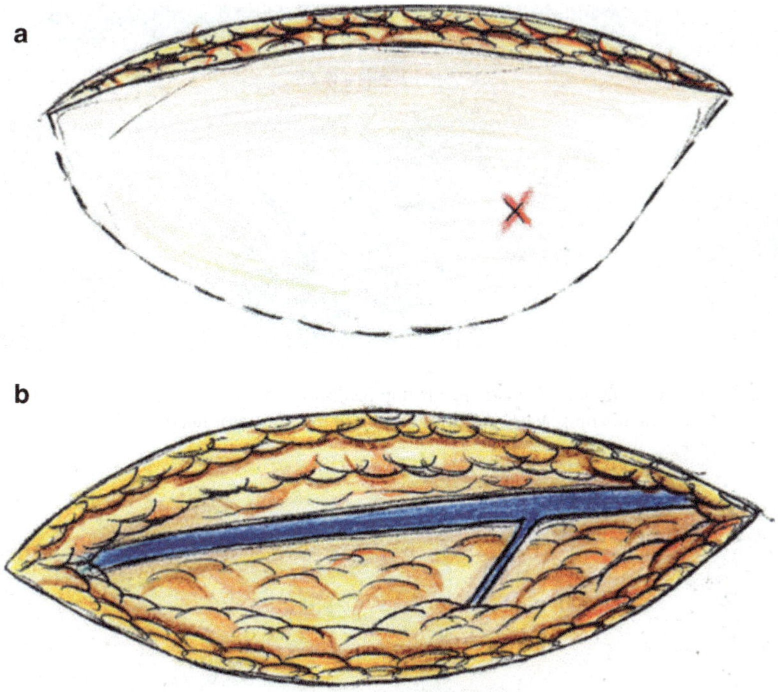

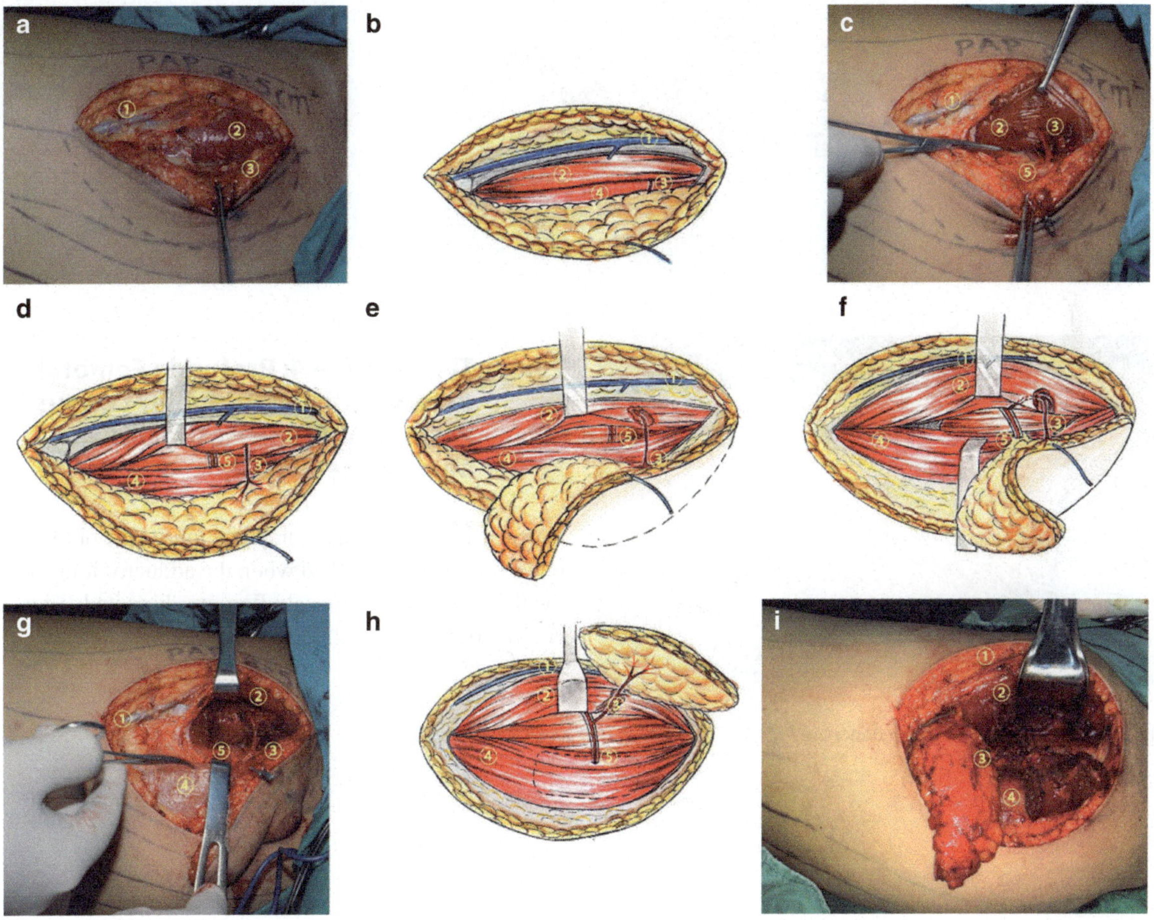

Fig. 20.15 Dissect the deep fascia lengthwise on the surface of the adductor longus, lift the flap from front to back, expose a perforating branch on the surface of the adductor longus, and retrograde separation found that it came from the vascular pedicle of the gracilis muscle branch. Cut the flap with it as the pedicle, and cut the gracilis muscle flap with the gracilis muscle branch as the pedicle. (1) Great saphenous vein. (2) Adductor longus. (3) Perforating vessels of the adductor longus. (4) Gracilis muscle. (5) Vascular pedicle of the gracilis muscle branch

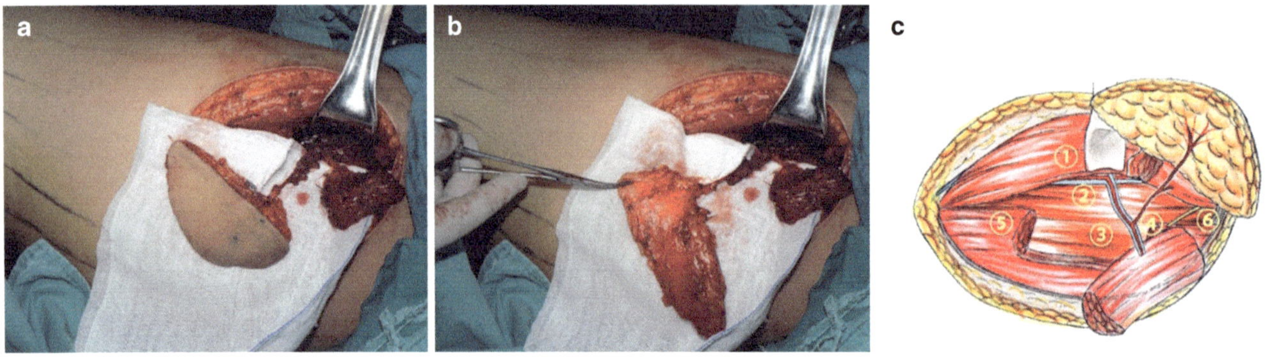

Fig. 20.16 The chimeric myocutaneous flap has been cut. (1) Adductor longus. (2) Profunda femoral vessels. (3) Adductor major. (4) Vascular pedicle. (5) Gracilis muscle. (6) Anterior branch of the obturator nerve

Fig. 20.17 The chimeric myocutaneous flap has been cut

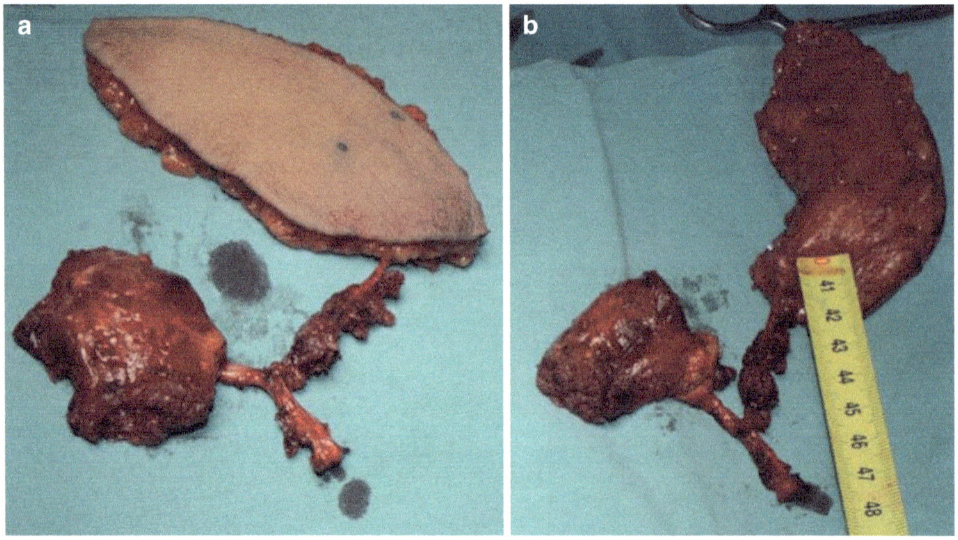

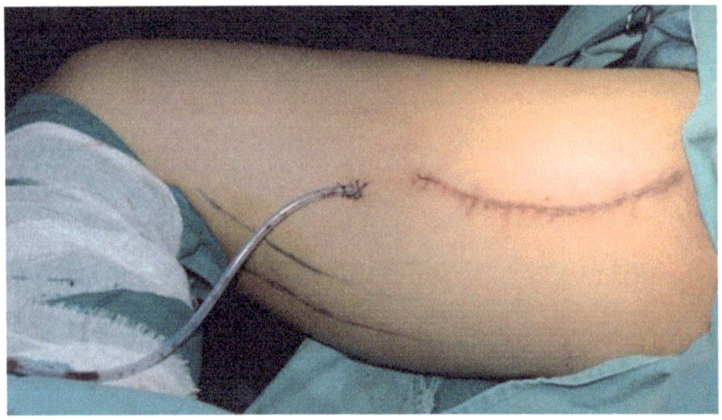

Fig. 20.18 Direct closure of the flap donor area

20.6 Typical Case 4: Profunda Femoral Artery Pedicled Adductor Longus Perforator Chimeric Gracilis Myocutaneous Flap

In order to minimize the donor site injury, the obturator nerve integrity can be preserved when the adductor longus perforator flap and gracilis muscle flap are dissected (Figs. 20.19, 20.20, 20.21, and 20.22).

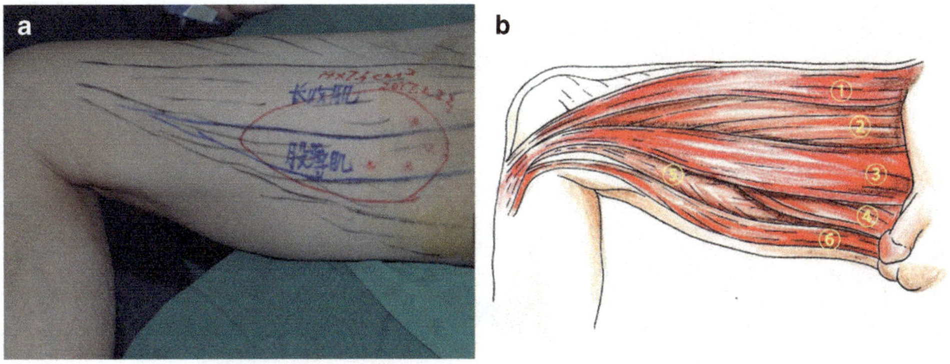

Fig. 20.19 Design of chimeric myocutaneous flap pedicled with profunda femoral artery. (1) Sartorius muscle. (2) Adductor longus. (3) Gracilis muscle. (4) Adductor major. (5) Semimembranosus muscle. (6) Semitendinosus

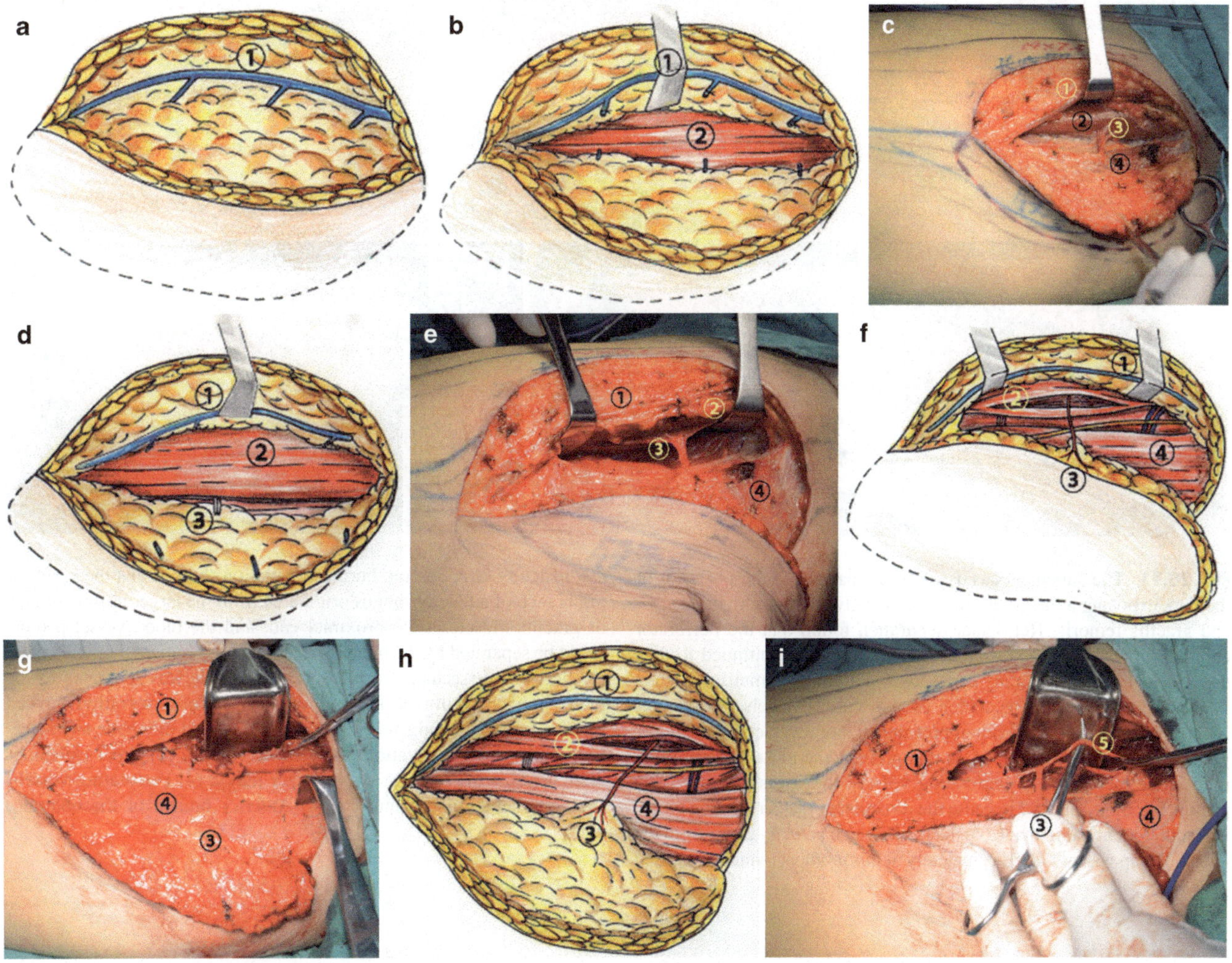

Fig. 20.20 First cut the anterior edge to expose the great saphenous vein. The continuity of great saphenous vein was preserved, and multiple branches of the flap were ligated. Then, lift the flap from front to back, and dissect the layer: the surface of the deep fascia. The adductor longus muscle and gracilis muscle were separated to expose a large perforator vessel The perforator vessel was retrogradely separated into the adductor longus muscle. The proximal end of the posterior edge of the flap was incised, and the flap was lifted from proximal to distal from the deep surface of the deep fascia, without exposing other perforating vessels on the surface of the gracilis muscle. (1) Great saphenous vein. (2) Adductor longus. (3) Perforating vessels. (4) Gracilis muscle. (5) Anterior branch of the obturator nerve

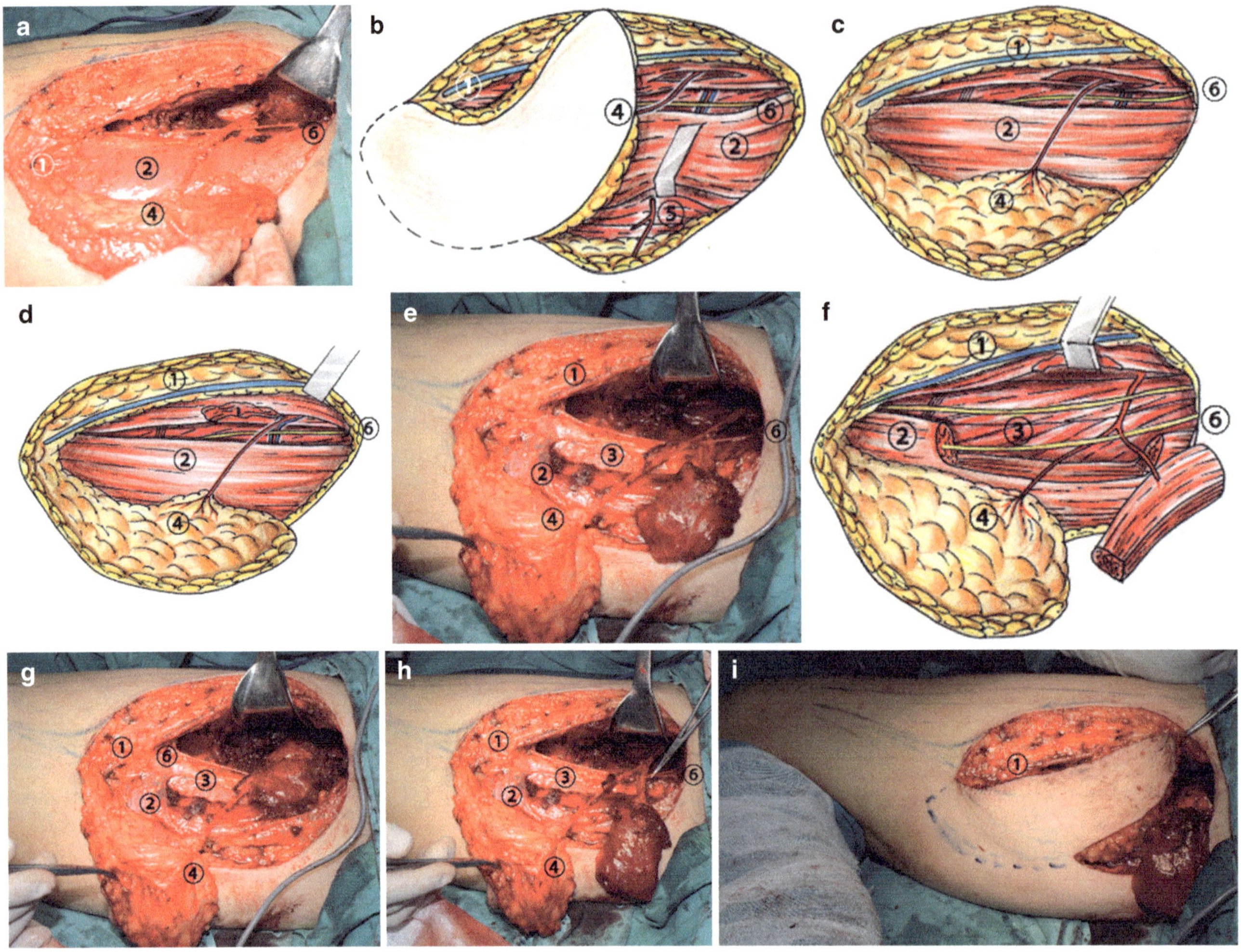

Fig. 20.21 The subcutaneous tissue was separated to the posterior of the flap, exposing a thick perforator vessel between the adductor major and gracilis femoris. Retrograde separation found that the perforator entered the deep surface of the adductor major and continued to dive deeply, and the perforator vessel was commonly small. We then switched to the further separation of perforating vessels of adductor longus, and two long branches of profunda femoral vessels entering the gracilis muscles were retained. In this process, the most difficult thing is to judge the source of perforating vessels: the femoral artery? The profunda femoral artery? Because the direction of the perforating vessel was rather identical to that from the front, which actually came from the rear. The flap was not lifted completely at this moment, which increased the difficulty of operation. Further separation showed that the perforating branch of adductor longus originated from the larger muscle branch of gracilis muscle at the proximal end, and the blood vessel pedicle could be separated by the bilateral method. The segmental gracilis muscle flap was dissected, and the vascular pedicle was separated to the plane from the profunda femoral vessel. Careful observation showed that two accompanying veins joined into one, and the mode and selection of flap revascularization changed accordingly. (1) Great saphenous vein. (2) Gracilis muscle. (3) Adductor major. (4) Perforating vessels. (5) Semimembranosus muscle. (6) Anterior branch of the obturator nerve

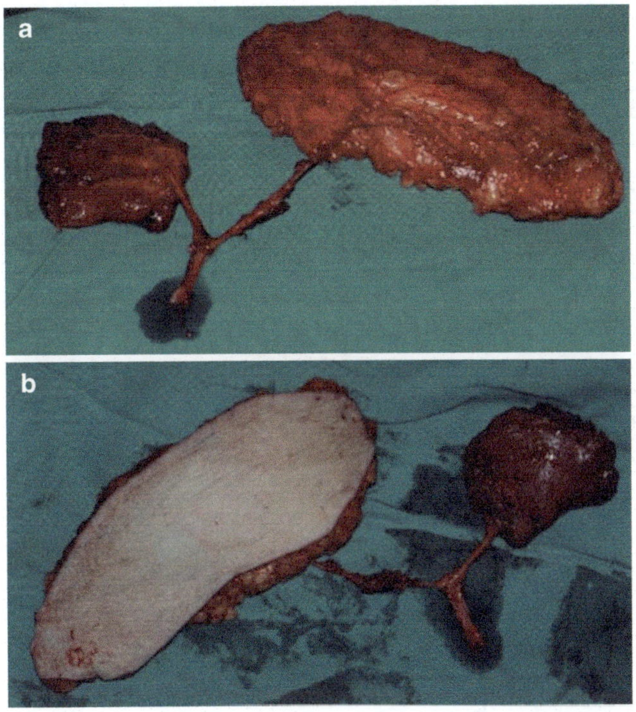

Fig. 20.22 The preparation of the profunda femoral artery pedicled adductor longus perforator chimeric gracilis myocutaneous flap is completed

20.7 Typical Case 5: An Example of Excision of the Gracilis Muscle Perforator Chimeric Myocutaneous Flap

The profunda femoral artery usually sends out three main perforating branches, the first perforating branch supplies the adductor and gracilis, and the second and third perforating branches supply the rest of the hamstring muscle groups [15]. When the required vascular pedicle is not long and there is a large amount of tissue, the gracilis perforator myocutaneous flap can be dissected directly if there is no obvious large perforator vessel on the surface of the gracilis muscle (Figs. 20.23, 20.24, 20.25, 20.26, 20.27, 20.28, and 20.29).

When the width of the flap is >6 cm with longitudinal design, it can easily incorporate most perforating branches of appropriate size along the profunda femoral artery. Therefore, in this case, accurate perforator localization by preoperative imaging may be less important [6]. The posteromedial femoral perforator flap designed vertically and longitudinally can be used for autologous breast reconstruction in women with medium breast size. The vertical posterior medial femoral perforator flap avoids some problems compared with other transverse flaps. The vertically designed free posteromedial femoral perforator flap can be a valuable choice in specific patients with breast reconstruction [21].

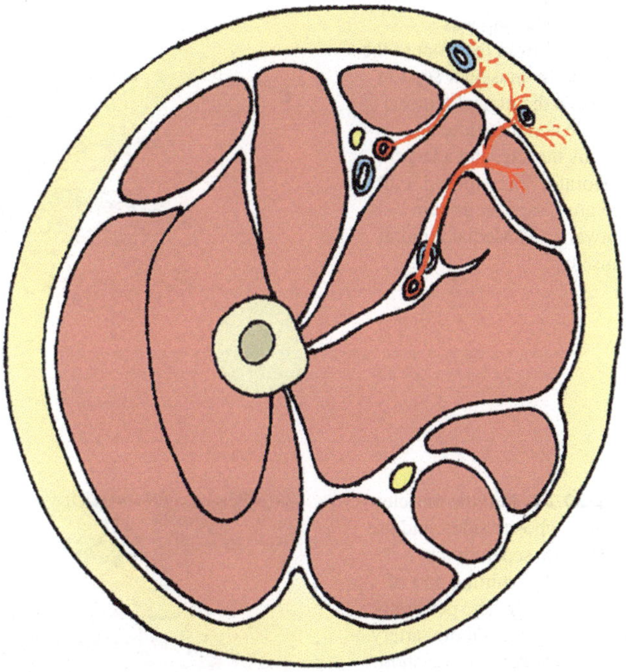

Fig. 20.23 Schematic diagram of anatomical types of perforating branches into the skin from both femoral artery and gracilis muscle branches

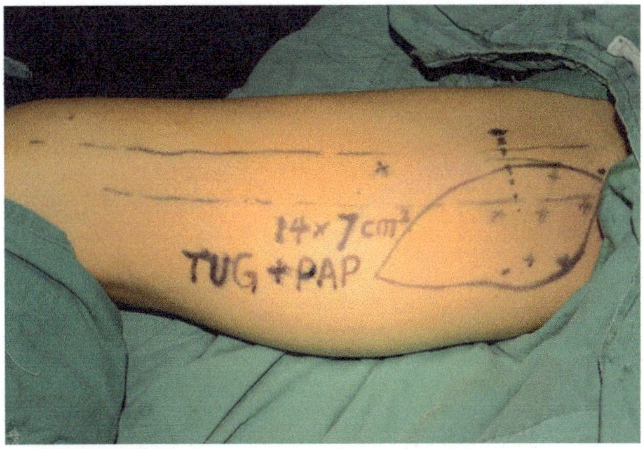

Fig. 20.24 The design of the medial femoral perforator flap. Try to carefully dissect the fascia flap and gracilis muscle pedicle

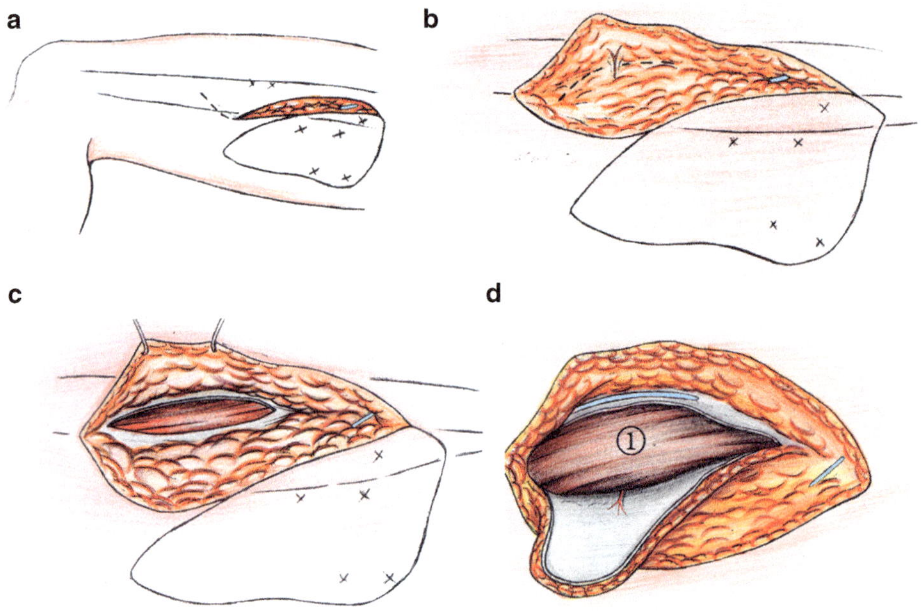

Fig. 20.25 Separating the fascial flap forward at the subdermal vascular network plane to the predetermined range. Dissecting the subcutaneous deep fascia to the surface of the medial femoral muscle and sartorius muscle. The flap was separated from the front to the back at the muscular septum between the medial femoral muscle and the adductor longus muscle, and a large perforator was exposed. Pull the great saphenous vein outward. (1) Medial femoral muscle

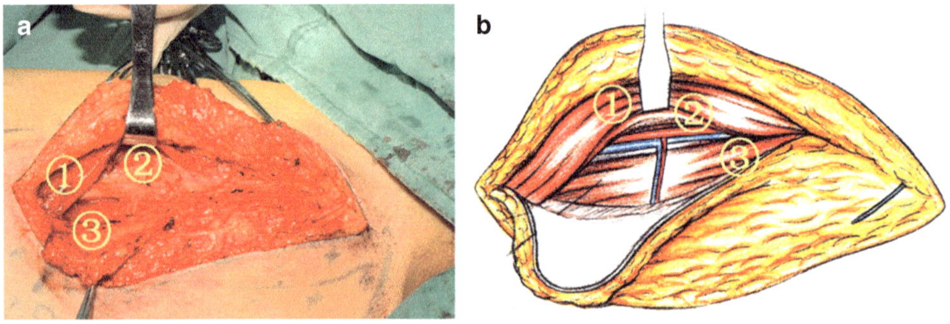

Fig. 20.26 Pull the muscles on the opposite sides, and use retrograde separation to explore the emitting part of the perforator. The perforator came from the femoral artery. The perforator was too short. It should be ligated and disconnected at the emitting plane for standby. (1) Medial femoral muscle. (2) Femoral vessels. (3) Adductor longus

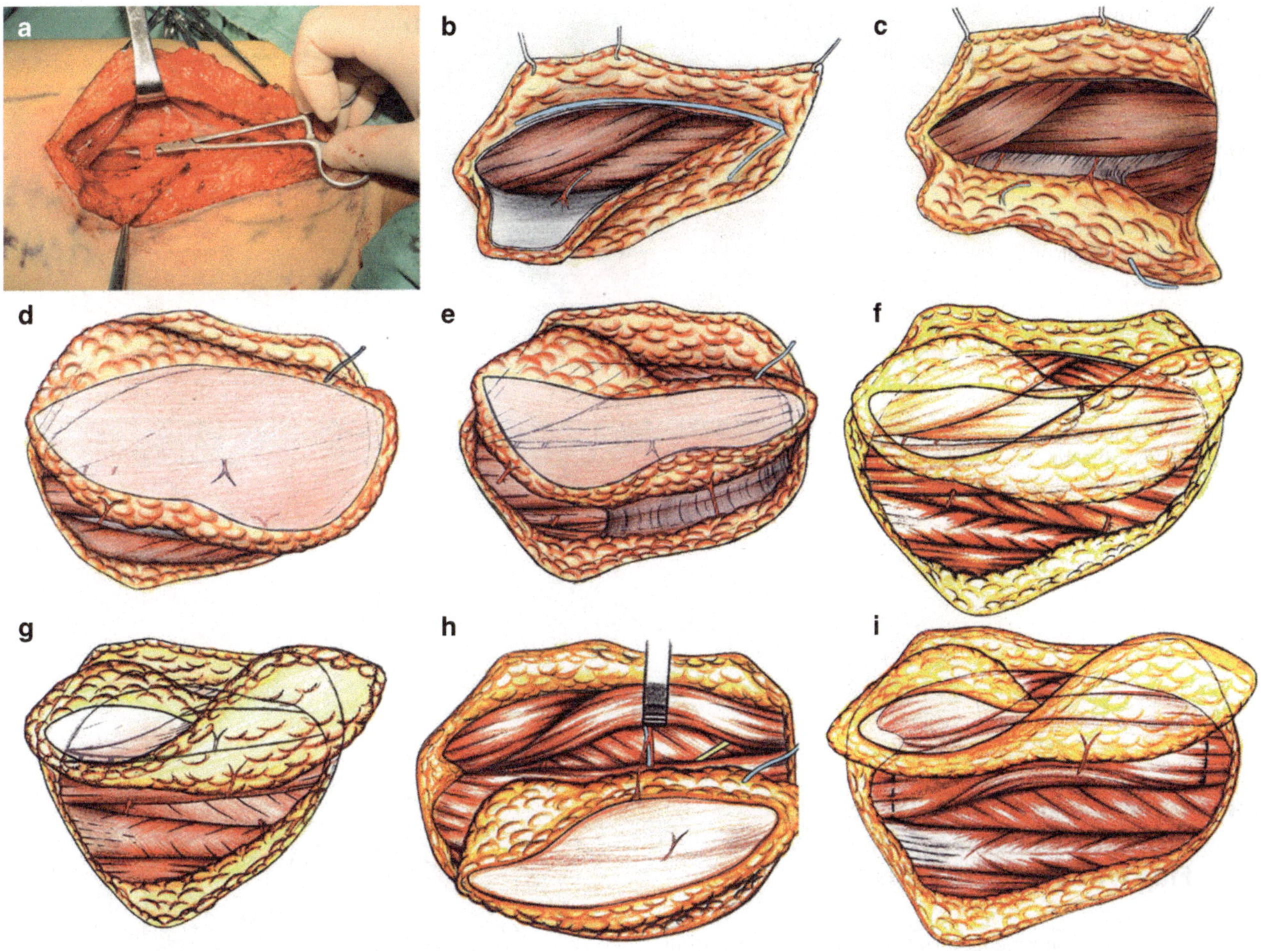

Fig. 20.27 Separate the flap posteriorly and medially, and expose the thick generic branch of the great saphenous vein along the surgical path. Dissect the long segment to its interval plane and ligate and disconnect the branches. The continuity and integrity of the main trunk of the great saphenous vein were preserved. The flap was further separated to the plane of the muscular septum between the adductor longus and the gracilis femoris. Through the muscular septum, the main blood vessels, nerve bundles, and a small perforating blood vessel were observed entering the skin on the surface of the gracilis femoris. Then, we switched to cut the proximal and distal edges of the flap to reveal a thin perforator between the adductor major and semimembranosus muscle at the distal and proximal ends of the flap, which drained into the flap. After judgment, it was ligated and disconnected. The flap was separated from proximal to distal and from deep to superficial layers. The layer was between the deep fascia and myomembrane. A relatively small perforator at the proximal end was exposed and ligated to facilitate further separation of the flap forward and outward. A perforator at the distal end of the flap was exposed between the adductor major and the semimembranosus muscle. Considering that its position was too far away, it was ligated and disconnected. Another perforator was exposed between the semitendinosus and semimembranosus muscles at the proximal end of the flap, which was too small and ligated. Lift the flap to the posterior edge of the gracilis muscle, and a thin perforating branch can be seen crossing the posterior edge of the gracilis muscle and incorporated into the skin, and this perforating branch was retained. The vascular pedicle of the gracilis muscle and the anterior and posterior perforating vessels were completely separated, and the subcutaneous tissue of the gracilis muscle and its surface skin were completely separated. Dissect the long segment of the gracilis muscle, and reserve the anterior branch of the long segment of the obturator nerve which crossed into the muscle for standby. After pulling the adductor longus upward, three larger branches can be seen entering the muscle medially, but only the first branch enters the gracilis muscle and the second and third branches entered the adductor magnus. Be careful not to choose the wrong vascular pedicle of the myocutaneous flap

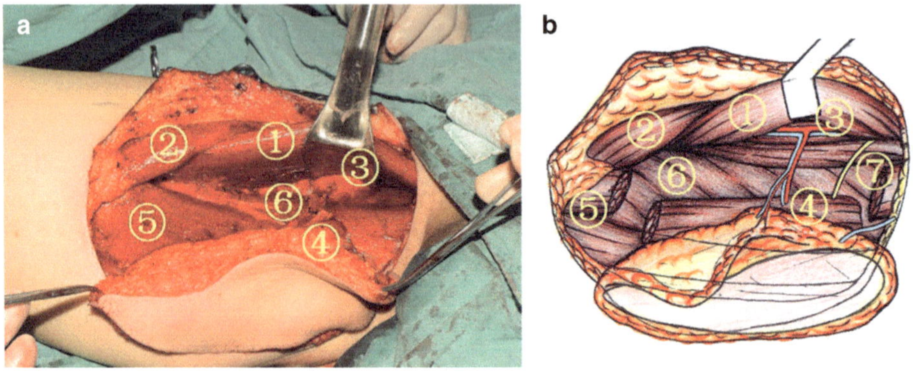

Fig. 20.28 Retrograde separation of the vascular pedicle to the plane of profunda femoral vessels. (1) Adductor longus. (2) Sartorius muscle. (3) Profunda femoral vessels. (4) Perforating vessels. (5) Gracilis muscle. (6) Adductor major. (7) Anterior branch of the obturator nerve

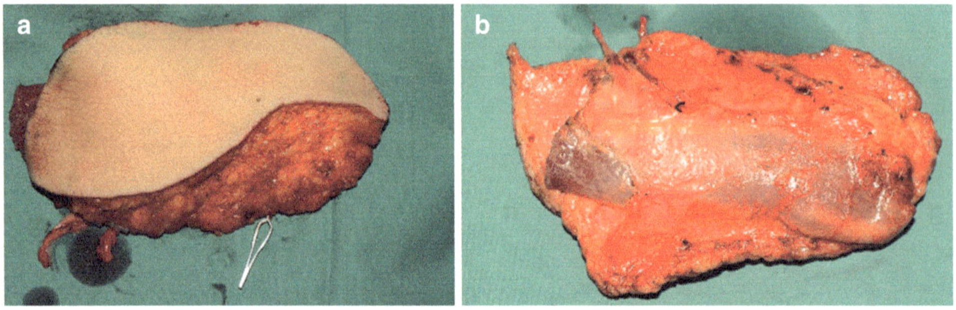

Fig. 20.29 The gracilis muscle perforator chimeric myocutaneous flap was cut

20.8 Typical Case 6: Multi-Perforator Profunda Femoral Artery Perforator Flap with Partial Gracilis Muscle

There are certain anatomical variations where perforating vessels arise from the profunda femoral artery and enter the gracilis muscle. In addition, the number of these perforating vessels is generally limited and the diameter is small. It is safe and reliable to use gracilis myocutaneous flap when small perforating vessels are found during operation (Figs. 20.30, 20.31, 20.32, 20.33, 20.34, 20.35, and 20.36) [22, 23].

The vascular pedicle length of the gracilis myocutaneous flap is significantly shorter than that of conventional perforator flap and is less flexible to be adjusted. However, it is suitable for cases with unsatisfactory vascular anatomical conditions and tissue filling [15, 24, 25]. At present, it is considered that there are a number of small perforating vessels on the surface of gracilis muscle, which results in obvious overlap of body area among perforating vessels, so the diameter of perforating vessels becomes smaller accordingly [26, 27]. When encountering multiple small perforators, the gracilis myocutaneous flap with partial gracilis muscle can be dissected, which not only ensures the blood supply but also minimizes the injury of the donor site.

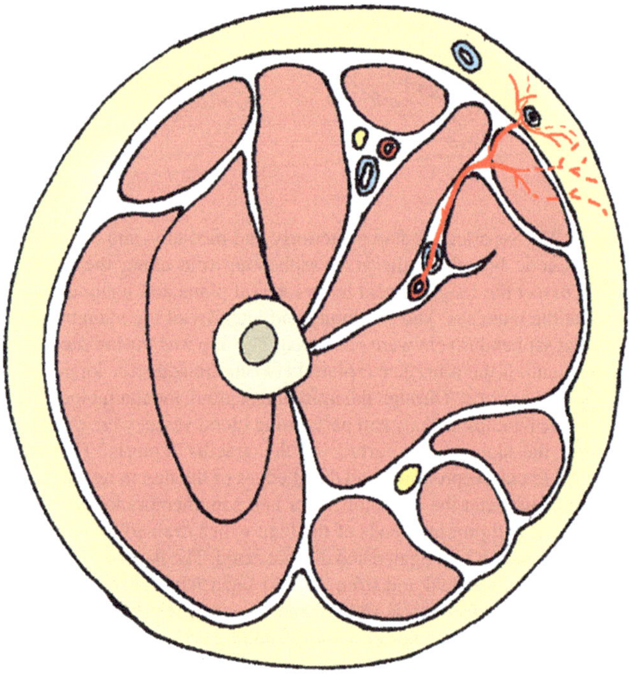

Fig. 20.30 Schematic diagram of anatomical types with small and large number of perforating vessels on the surface of the gracilis muscle

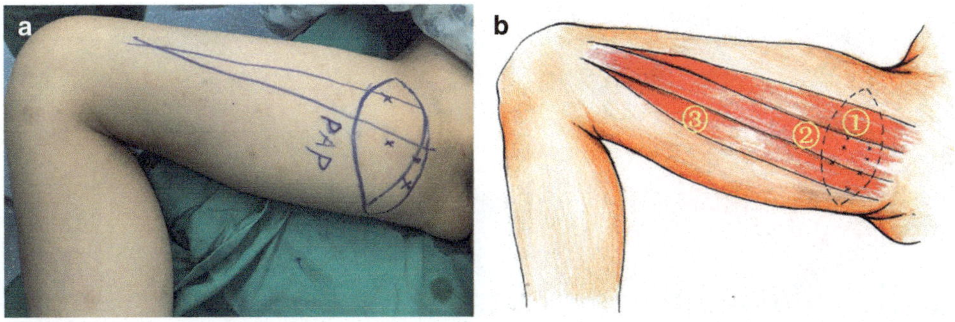

Fig. 20.31 Based on the preoperative Doppler detection, the perforator flap of the profunda femoral artery was designed accordingly. First, the great saphenous vein is separated and exposed to the proximal end after the distal incision, and the great saphenous vein was retained and carried the branch entering the flap

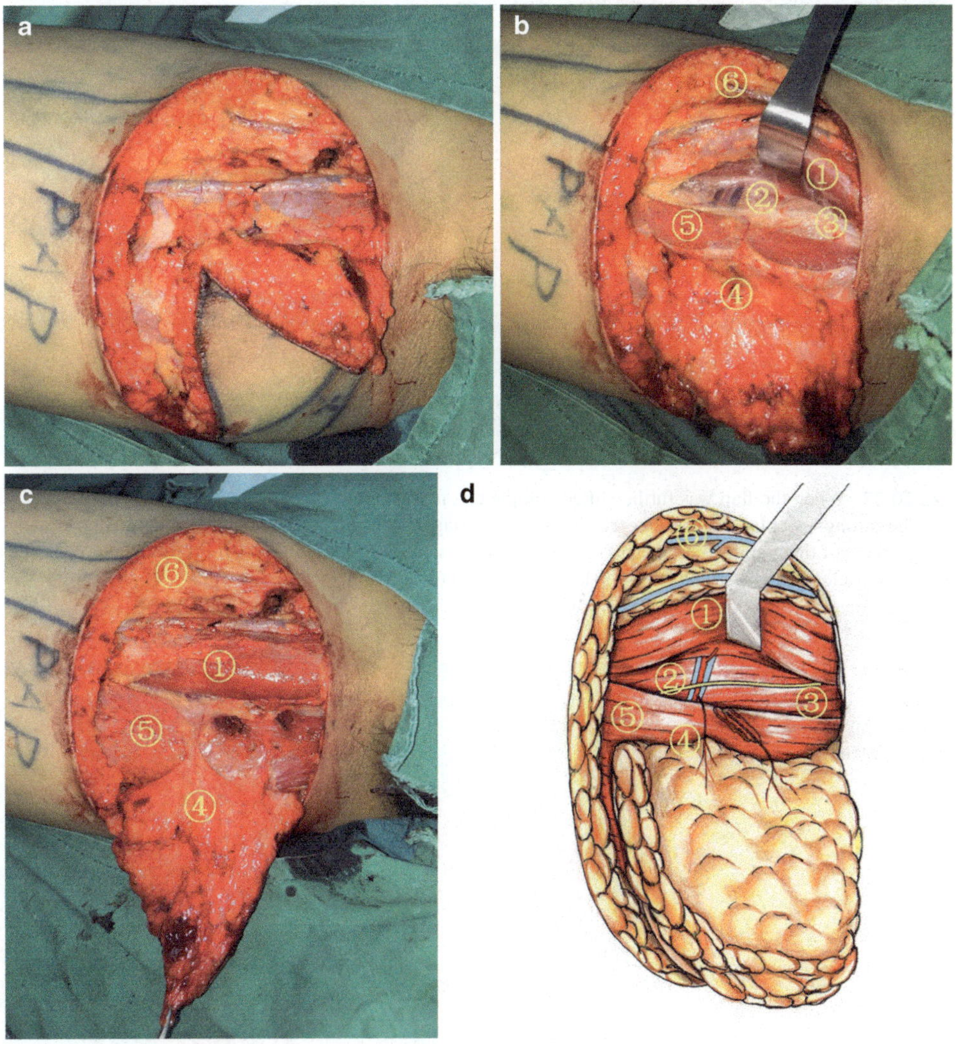

Fig. 20.32 Lift the flap from front to back to expose the two small perforating branches on the surface of gracilis muscle and the strong vascular pedicle entering gracilis muscle, and expose the anterior branch of obturator nerve. (1) Adductor longus. (2) Anterior branch of the obturator nerve. (3) Adductor major. (4) Perforating vessels of the gracilis muscle. (5) Gracilis muscle. (6) Great saphenous vein

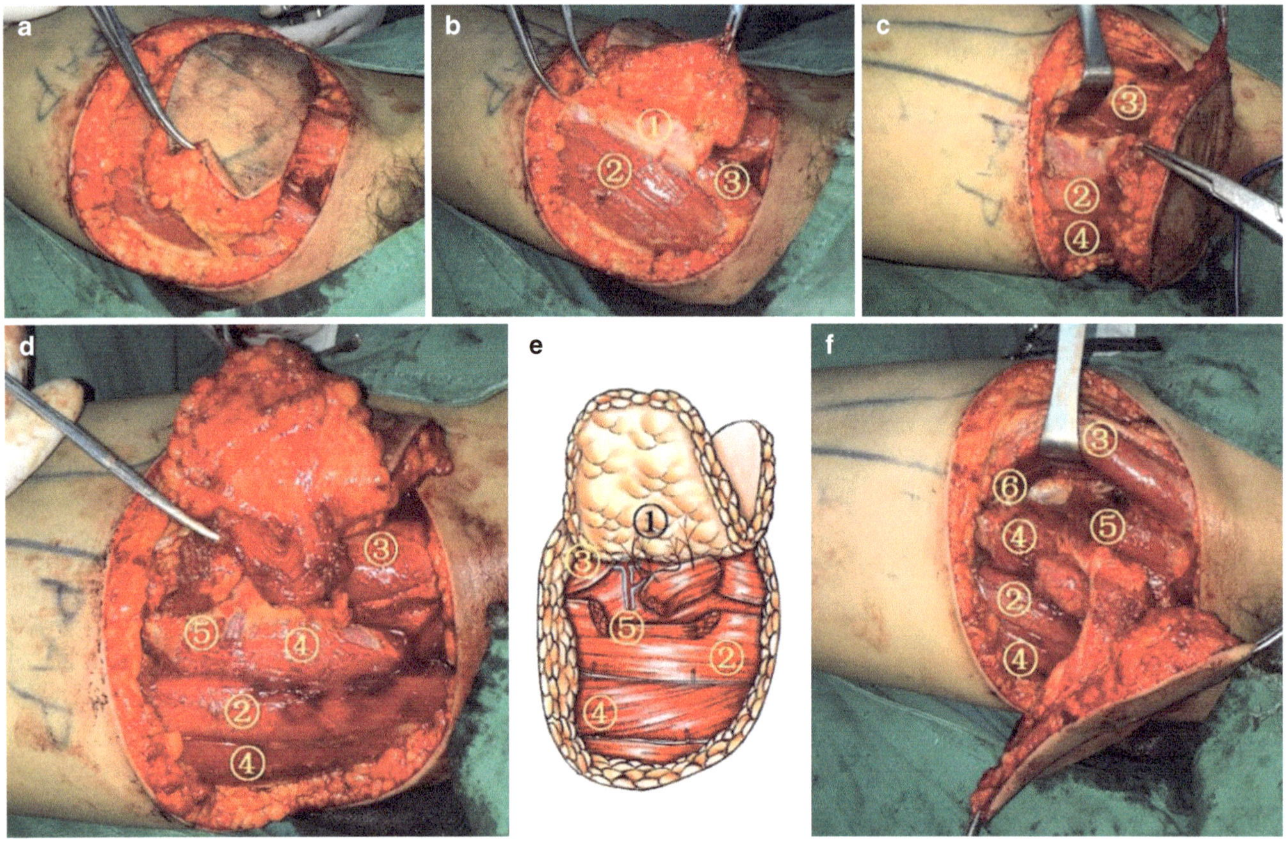

Fig. 20.33 When the flap was further lifted completely, it was found that the strong vascular pedicle entered the adductor magnus on the deep surface of the gracilis muscle, and one of its branches entered the gracilis muscle and further divided into skin branches. (1) Perforating vessels of the gracilis muscle. (2) Gracilis muscle. (3) Adductor longus. (4) Adductor major. (5) Vascular pedicle of the musculus adductor major. (6) Profunda femoral vessels

Fig. 20.34 The excision of the gracilis perforator chimeric myocutaneous flap was completed

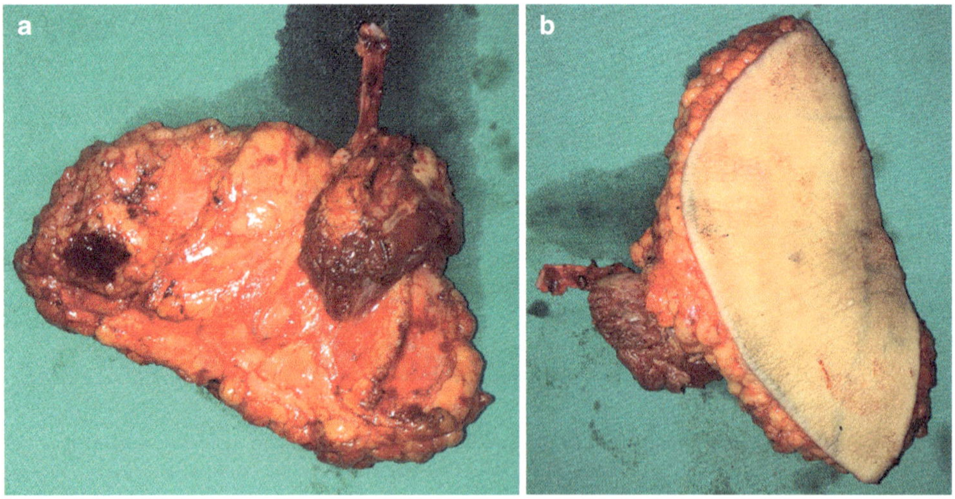

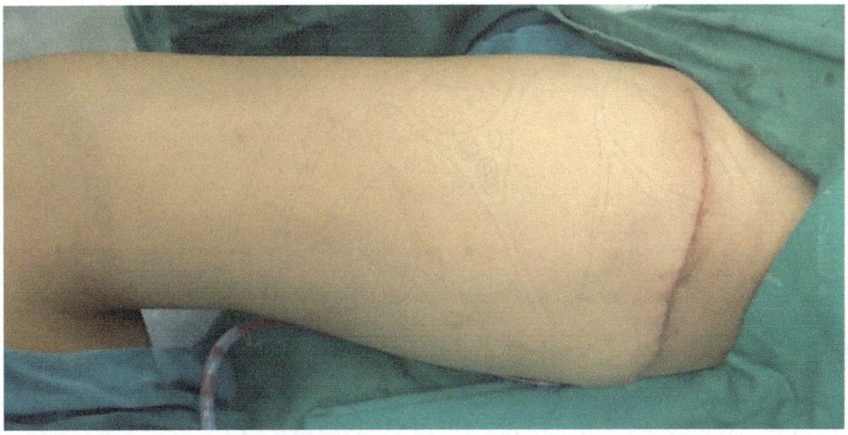

Fig. 20.35 Primary closure of the flap donor area

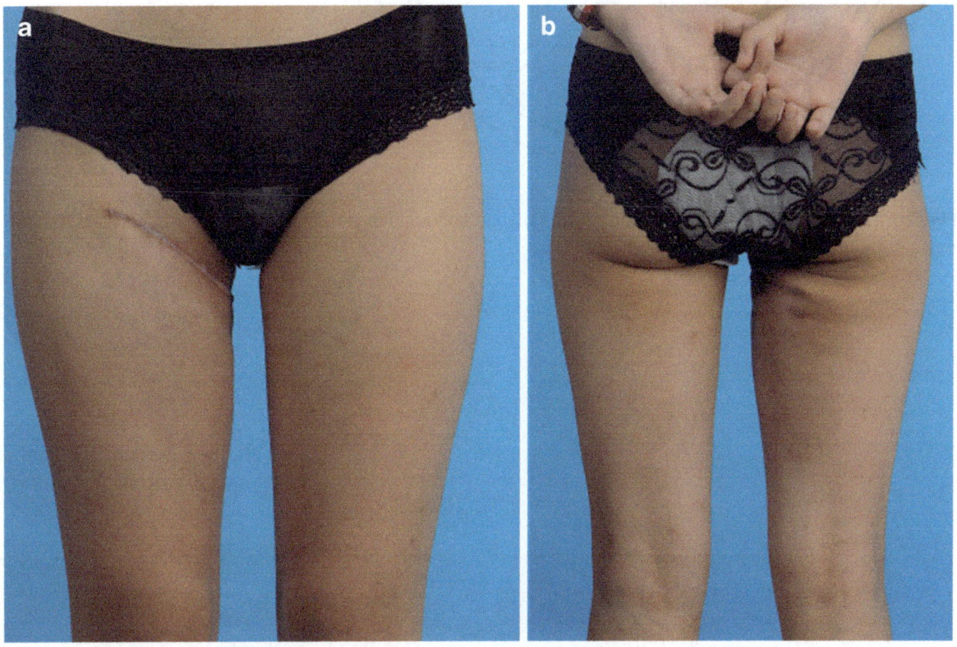

Fig. 20.36 Follow-up of the flap donor site 3 months after operation

20.9 Typical Case 7: Gracilis Myocutaneous Flap for Muscle Functional Reconstruction

The use of the gracilis myocutaneous flap to reconstruct facial muscle function was first reported by Chuang [28] in 2004 (Fig. 20.37). The gracilis myocutaneous flap with the anterior branch of the obturator nerve is the most preferred surgical method to treat facial paralysis (Figs. 20.38, 20.39, and 20.40).

As for breast reconstruction, an alternative is the transverse crescent-shaped gracilis myocutaneous flap (TUG) composed of tissues above the thigh (Fig. 20.41) [29, 30]. However, TUG flap for breast reconstruction is considered to have some disadvantages. The amount of tissue available in the thigh is scarce, and the length of vascular pedicle is short, generally 6–7 cm, and the donor area is prone to infection, wound dehiscence, and lymphatic leakage [31].

PAP flap is based on the musculocutaneous or septal perforator from the second or third perforator of the profunda femoral artery. They converge in the posterior gracilis and supply blood to the skin and subcutaneous fat under the gluteal sulcus. According to clinical observation and preoperative imaging studies, about 97% of the thighs have at least one suitable perforating branch with an average diameter of 1.9 mm in this area. The medial perforator was adjacent to the adductor magnus, with an average distance of 3.8 cm from the midline and 5 cm below the gluteal sulcus, and the lateral perforator was close to the biceps femoris and lateral femoral muscle, with an average distance of 1.2 cm from the midline and 5 cm below the gluteal sulcus. Even if the abdominal tissue is not enough, the flap still provides rela-

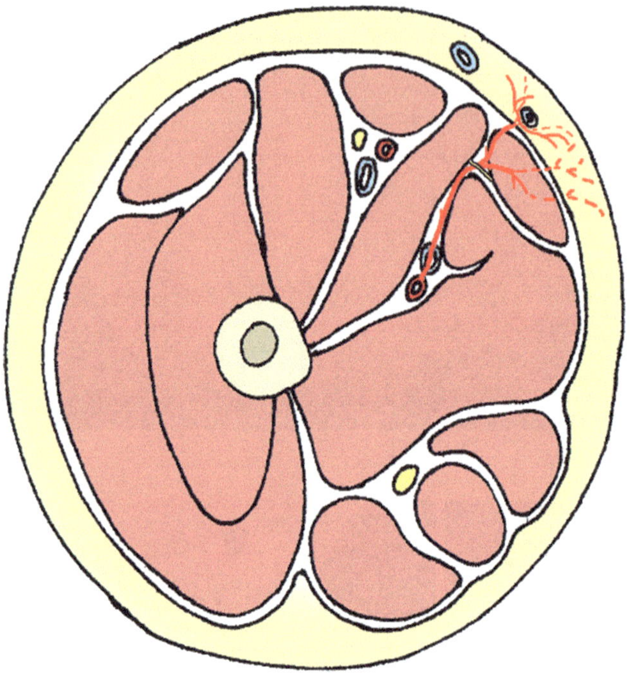

Fig. 20.37 Anatomical diagram of the gracilis myocutaneous flap for muscle functional reconstruction

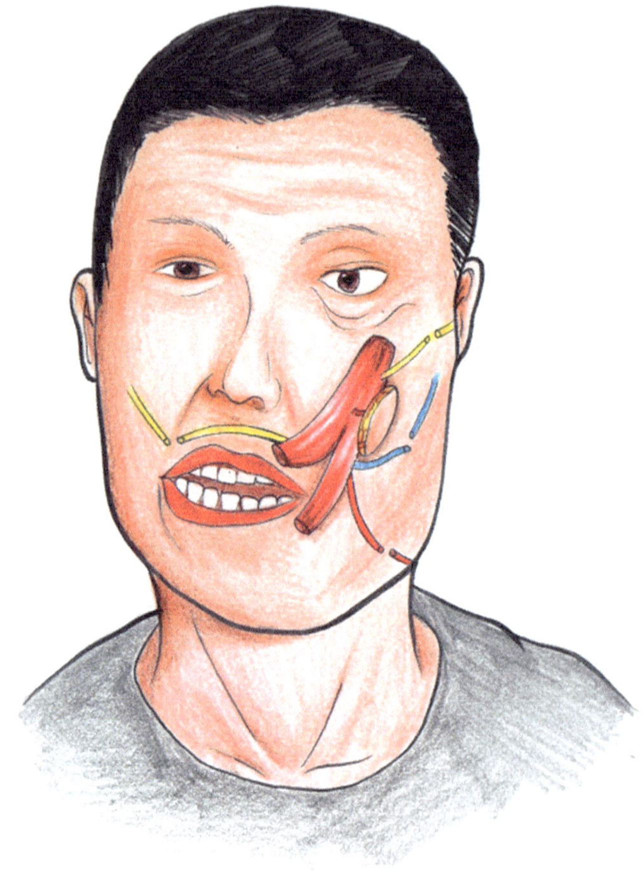

Fig. 20.38 Schematic diagram of the gracilis myocutaneous flap for facial muscle dynamic reconstruction

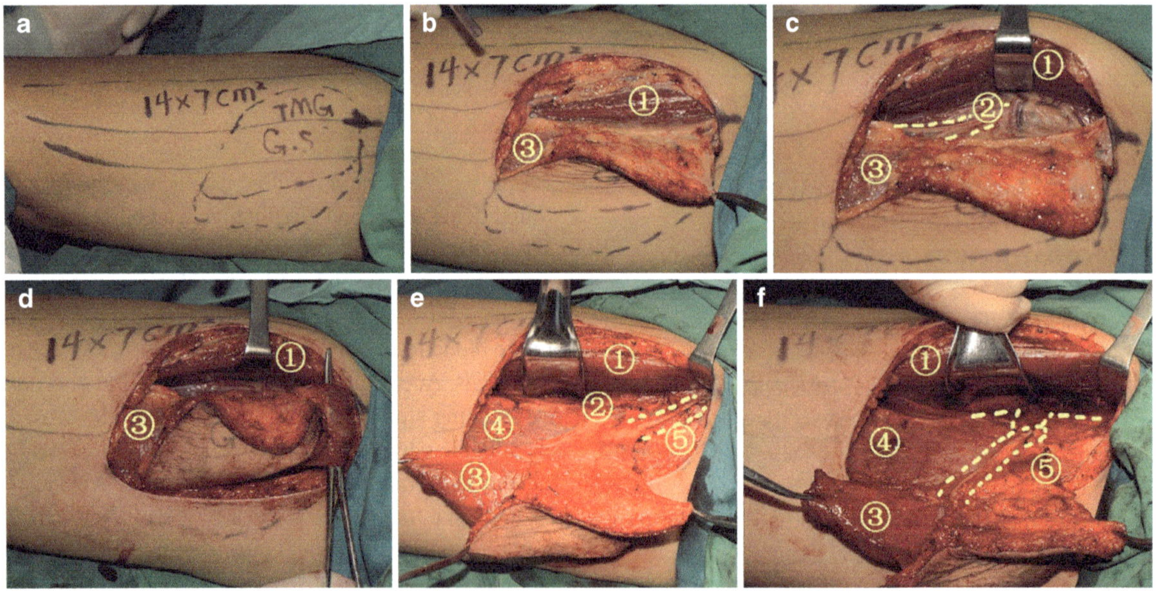

Fig. 20.39 (**a**) Gracilis myocutaneous flap design for muscle power reconstruction. (**b**) Lift the flap from front to back to expose the adductor longus and gracilis and the space between them. (**c**) Pull the gracilis muscle backward to expose the gracilis muscle branch and the anterior branch of the obturator nerve. (**d**) Turn to the posterior edge of the flap. (**e**) The gracilis muscle was cut off and the gracilis muscle flap was cut off. (**f**) The vascular pedicle was separated retrogradely to the level of profunda femoral vessels. (1) Adductor longus. (2) Gracilis muscle branch. (3) Gracilis muscle. (4) Adductor major. (5) Anterior branch of the obturator nerve

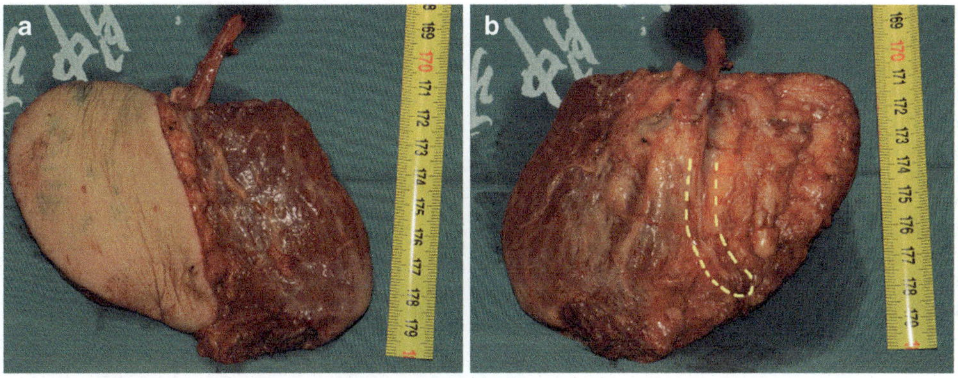

Fig. 20.40 The gracilis myocutaneous flap that can be used to reconstruct muscle function and tissue shape has been modified

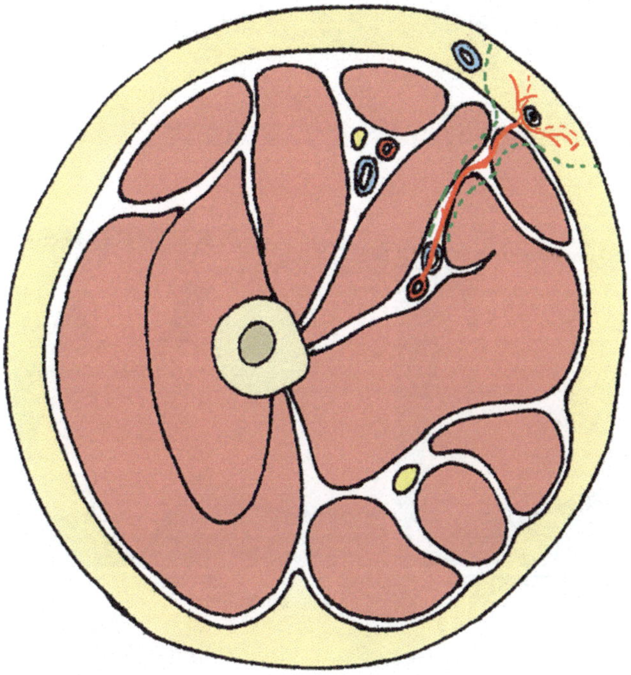

Fig. 20.41 Anatomical cross-sectional diagram of the anterior perforating branch of gracilis muscle

tively abundant soft tissue from the donor area. Similarly, it can be regarded as an evolved and improved technique of TUG flap, which further expands the indications and reduces donor site injury. Also, it offers longer vascular pedicle and more flexible dissection methods [16]. In terms of the effect of reconstructed breast and donor area, PAP flap should have more advantages than TUG flap in theory [25]. However, due to the variation of anatomical vessels in PAP flap. The gracilis perforator flap should be the most fitting one as the improved technique for TUG flap.

20.10 Typical Case 8: Pure Gracilis Perforator Flap

When a small area of the skin flap is needed, the design of the skin island position can be moved forward appropriately, and the best perforator vessel can be selected through sufficient exploration incision. In clinical practice, an obvious perforator vessel at the front edge of the gracilis muscle can always be found, and the gracilis muscle is preserved. The surgical position is convenient and the operation is relatively simplified. However, the perforator vessel is often not bulky, so it cannot be used as a vascular pedicle of a larger tissue flap (Figs. 20.42, 20.43, 20.44, and 20.45) [32–35].

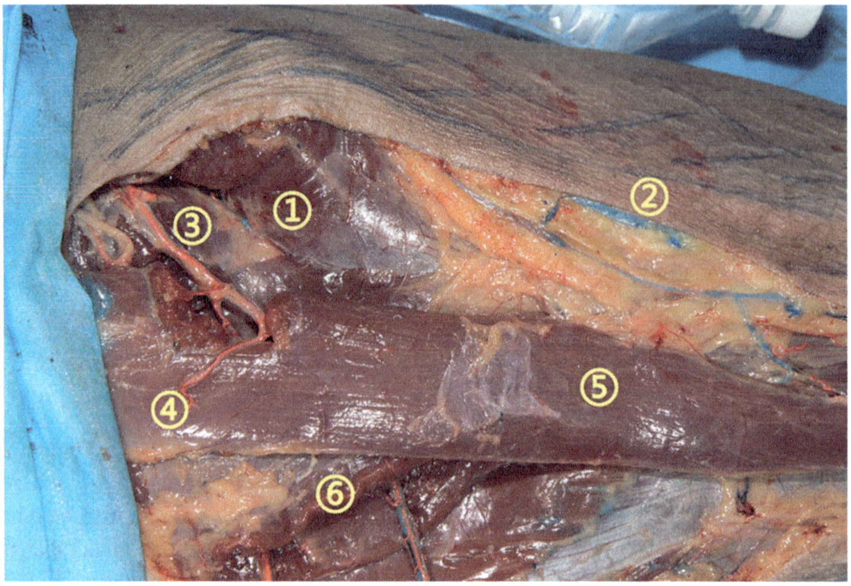

Fig. 20.42 In clinical practice, it is common to send a perforator of the profunda femoral artery into the skin near the front edge of the gracilis muscle. (1) Adductor longus. (2) Great saphenous vein. (3) Gracilis muscle branch. (4) Perforating branch of the gracilis muscle. (5) Gracilis muscle. (6) Adductor major

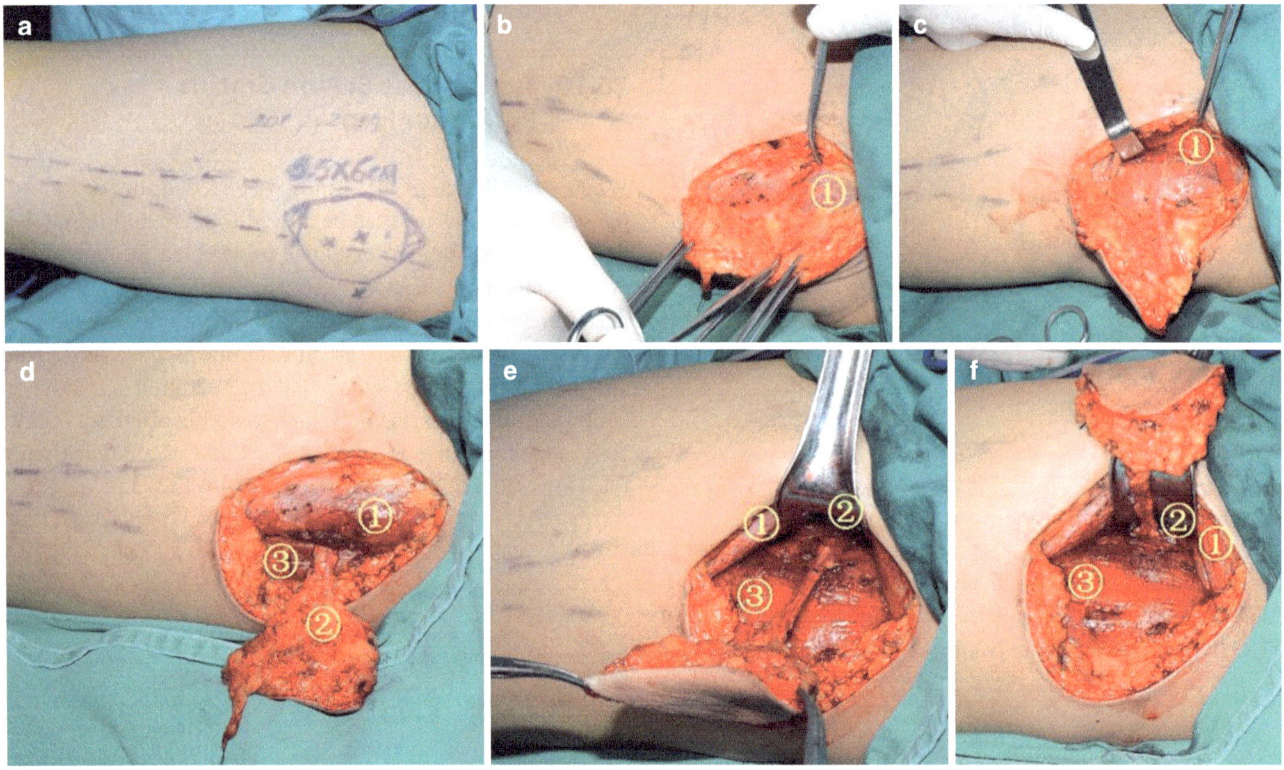

Fig. 20.43 Design and dissection of a pure gracilis perforator flap. (1) Adductor longus. (2) Perforating vessels of the gracilis muscle. (3) Gracilis muscle. (**a**) Flap design. (**b**) Lift the flap and expose the adductor longus. (**c**) Further lift the flap backward. (**d**) A perforator vessel was exposed on the surface of the gracilis muscle. (**e**) The main branches of the gracilis muscle were ligated on the surface of the gracilis muscle, and the vascular pedicle was separated retrogradely. (**f**) The vascular pedicle was separated retrogradely to the plane of the profunda femoral artery

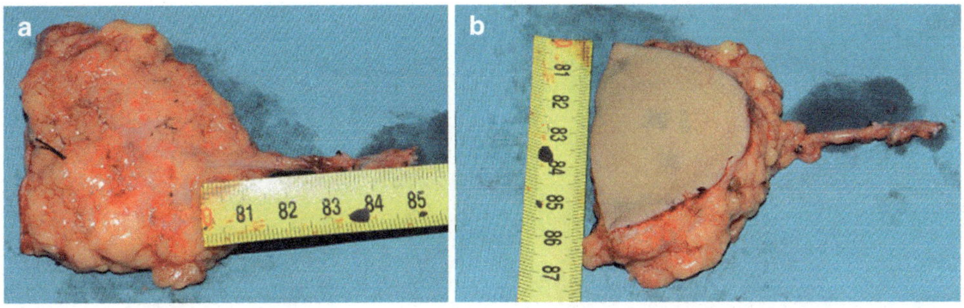

Fig. 20.44 The pure gracilis perforator flap was dissected

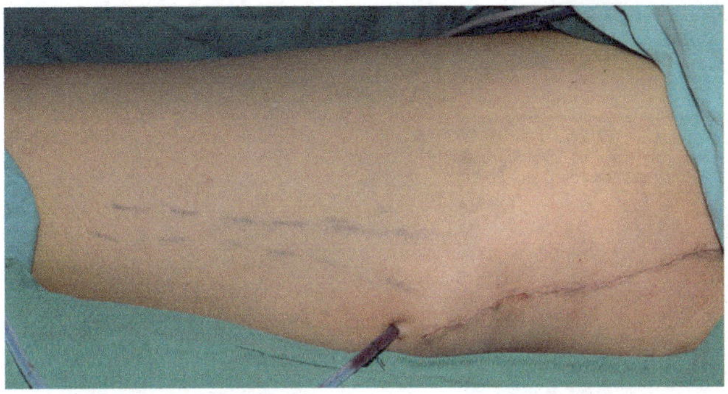

Fig. 20.45 Direct closure of the flap donor area

20.11 Typical Case 9: Profunda Femoral Artery Pedicled Gracilis Perforator Chimeric Myocutaneous Flap

When the presence of the gracilis musculocutaneous perforator is revealed and confirmed, it is relatively simple to cut the profunda femoral artery pedicled gracilis perforator chimeric myocutaneous flap, and the design is flexible. It can carry the whole segment of the gracilis musculocutaneous perforator or only a part of the gracilis musculocutaneous perforator according to clinical needs (Fig. 20.46). Another common clinical perforator of the gracilis muscle is from the middle segment of the muscle. In this case, although it is necessary to dissect the muscle fiber between the perforator and the front edge of the gracilis muscle, the procedures are not complex, and the gracilis muscle flap can be dissected, while the complex defect is repaired (Figs. 20.47, 20.48, 20.49, and 20.50).

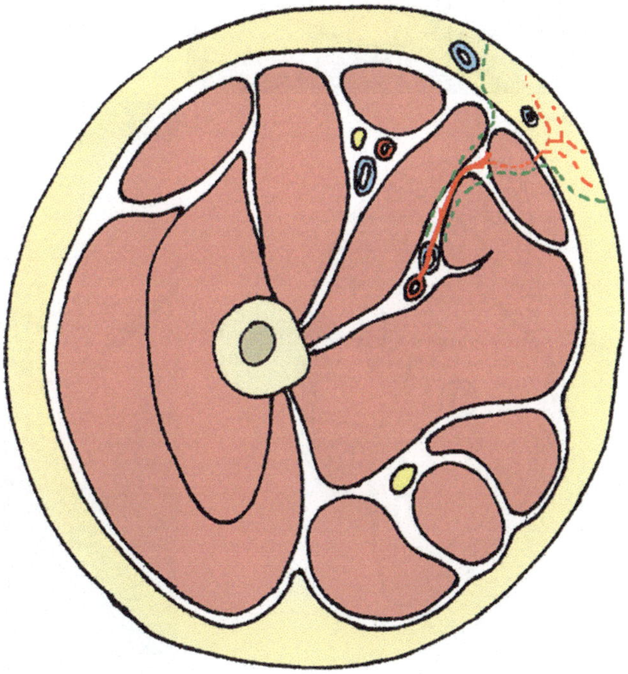

Fig. 20.46 Anatomical diagram of the middle perforator of the gracilis muscle

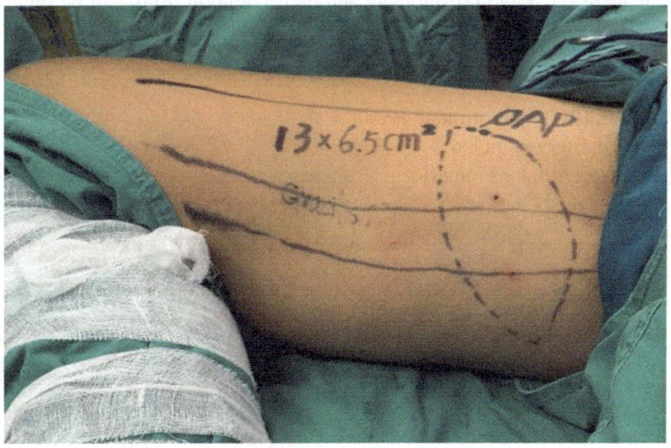

Fig. 20.47 Flap design

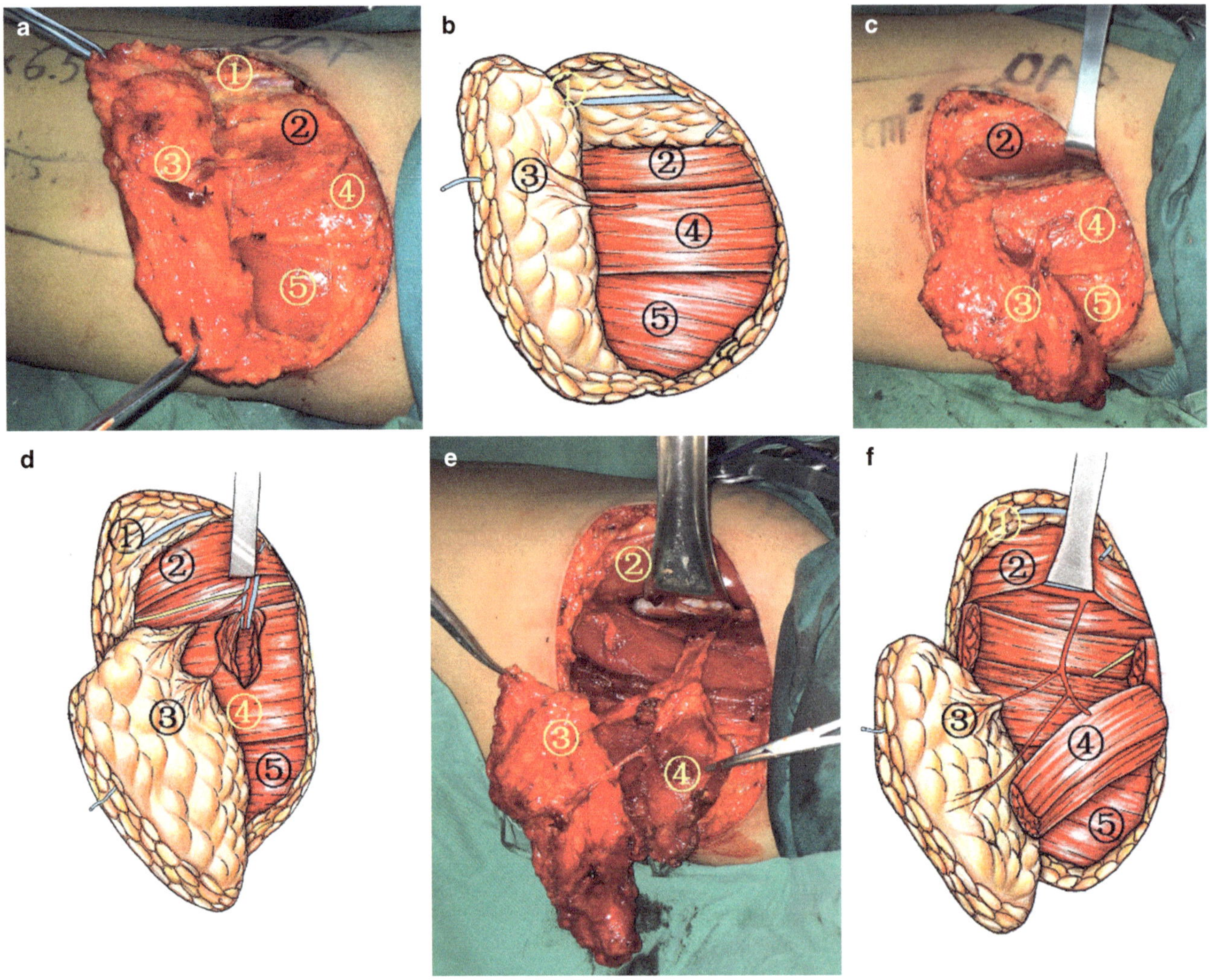

Fig. 20.48 Lift the flap from the proximal end to the distal end to explore the blood vessels. There were the two perforator vessels traveling from the surface of gracilis muscle and the muscle septum between adductor longus and gracilis muscle, respectively. The perforator vessels were separated retrogradely and their common trunk can be seen. The flap was dissected with the two perforator vessels as the pedicle and the gracilis muscle flap was incised with the gracilis muscle branch trunk as the pedicle. (1) Great saphenous vein. (2) Adductor longus. (3) Perforating vessels. (4) Gracilis muscle. (5) Adductor major

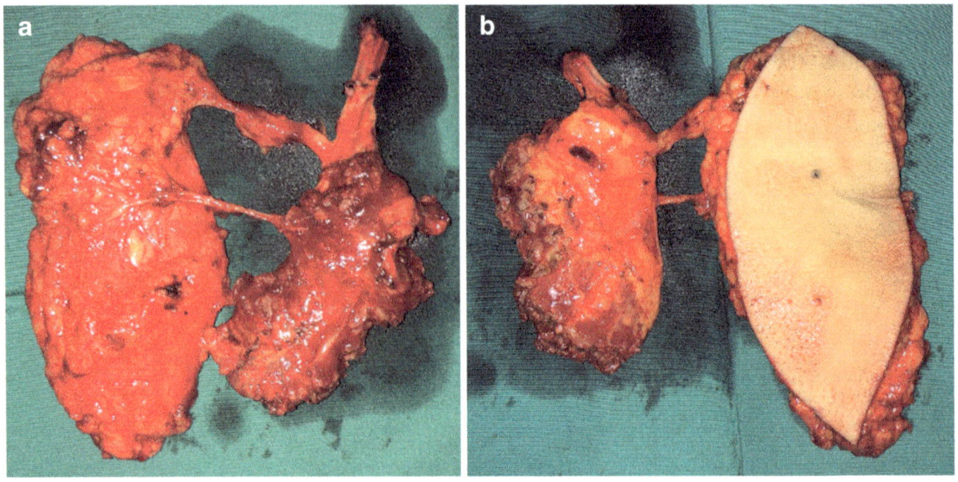

Fig. 20.49 The profunda femoral artery pedicled gracilis perforator chimeric myocutaneous flap was dissected

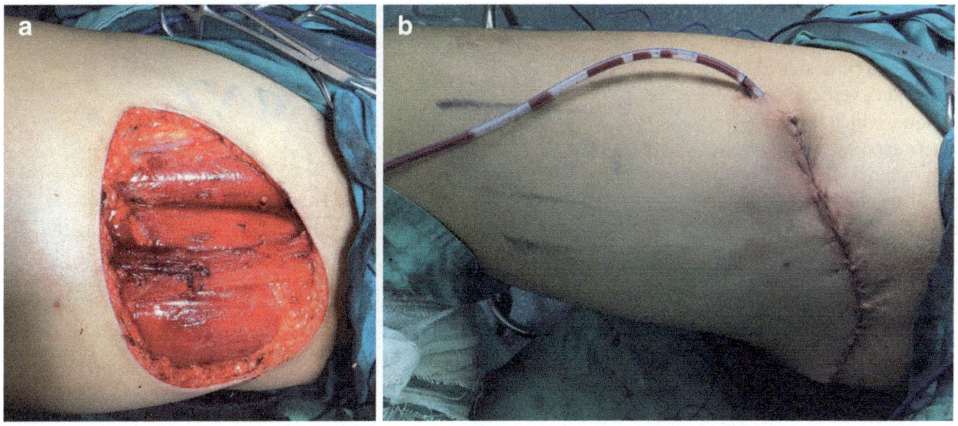

Fig. 20.50 Direct closure of the flap donor area

20.12 Typical Case 10: Gracilis Perforator Chimeric Myocutaneous Flap (Figs. 20.51, 20.52, 20.53, 20.54, 20.55, and 20.56)

Similar to the anterolateral femoral perforator flap, the posteromedial femoral deep artery perforator flap can be prepared for a chimeric flap composed of one skin island and one muscle or two skin islands to better fill the dead space or manage three-dimensional tissue flap placement. The most used posteromedial femoral myocutaneous flap is the chimeric gracilis myocutaneous flap (Fig. 20.51) [6].

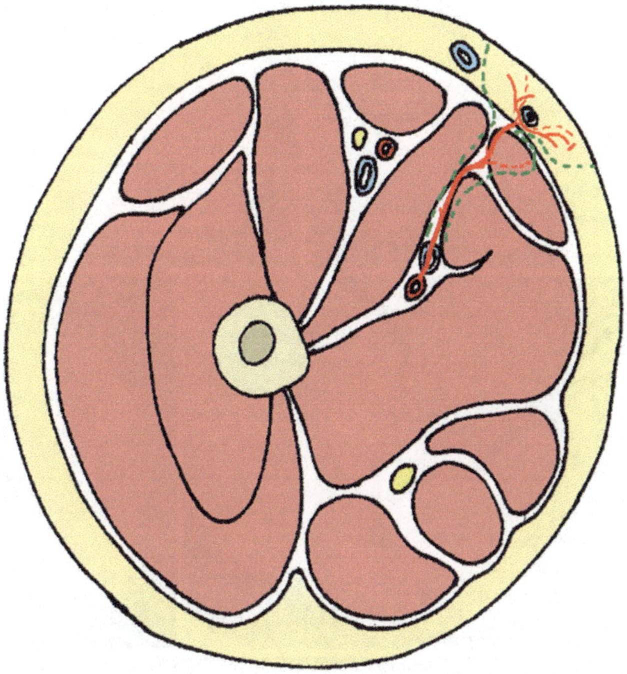

Fig. 20.51 Anatomical diagram of the cutting range of the chimeric myocutaneous flap with the anterior perforator of the gracilis muscle

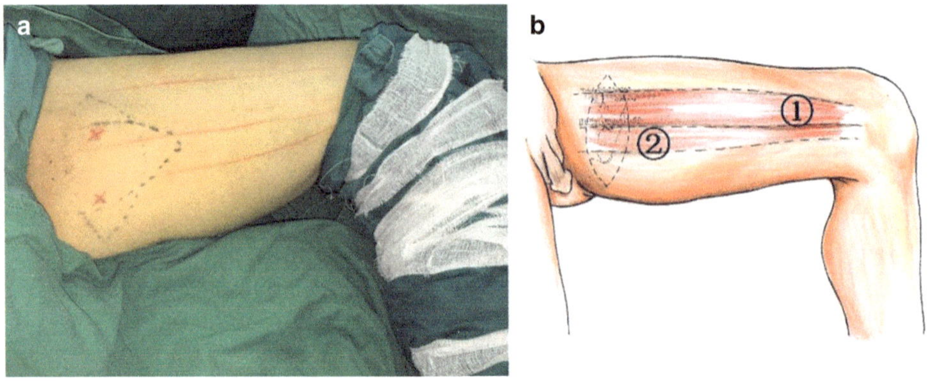

Fig. 20.52 Design of the medial femoral perforator flap. It can be designed as horizontal, vertical, or oblique, which is mainly determined by the shape and size of the flap. In addition, the distribution of perforators detected before perforator surgery is also an important reference

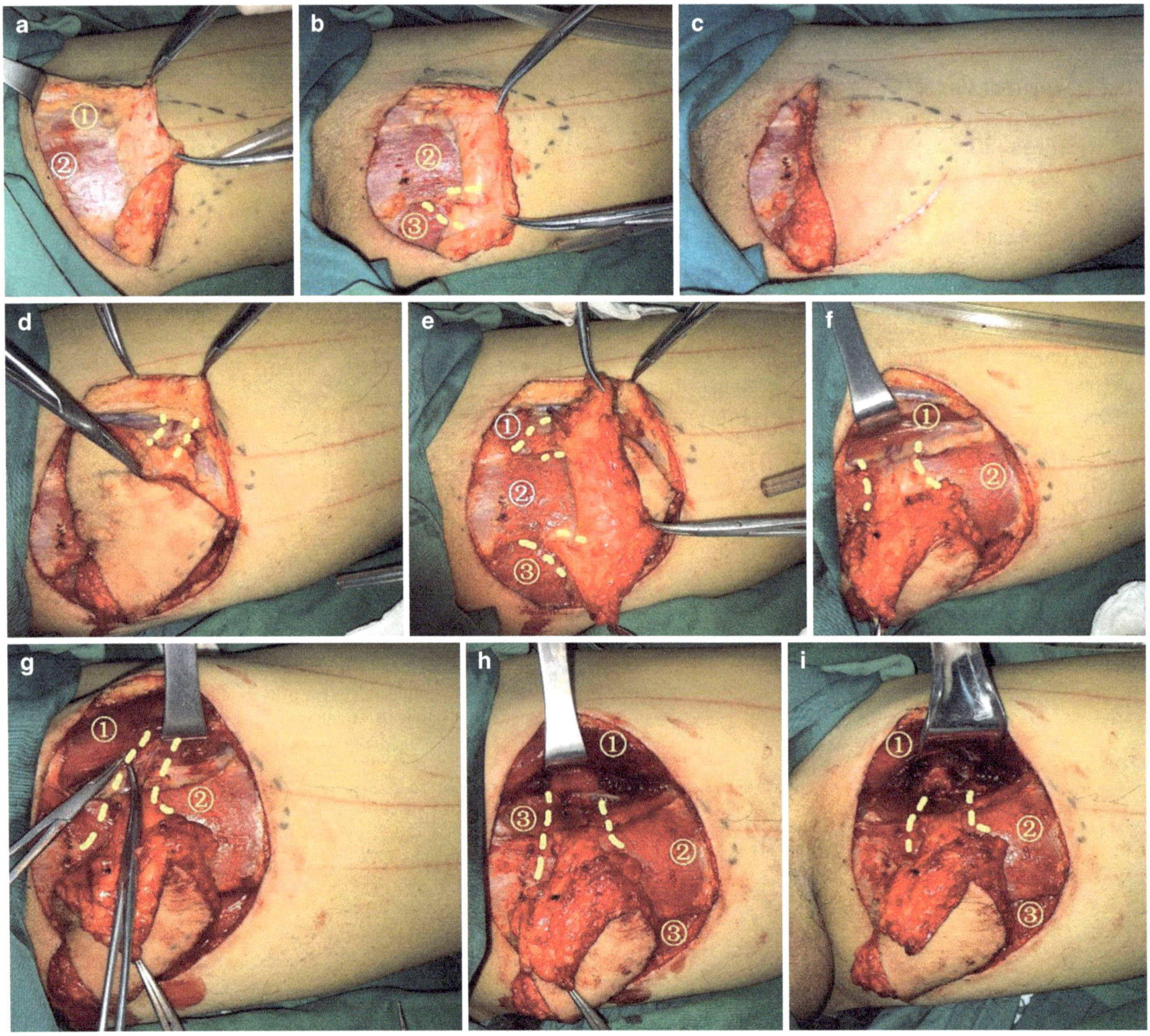

Fig. 20.53 Separate and expose the anterior and posterior perforating vessels of the gracilis muscle. First, retrograde separate the pedicle of the anterior perforating vessel to the plane of the profunda femoral vessel. (1) Adductor longus. (2) Gracilis muscle. (3) Adductor major

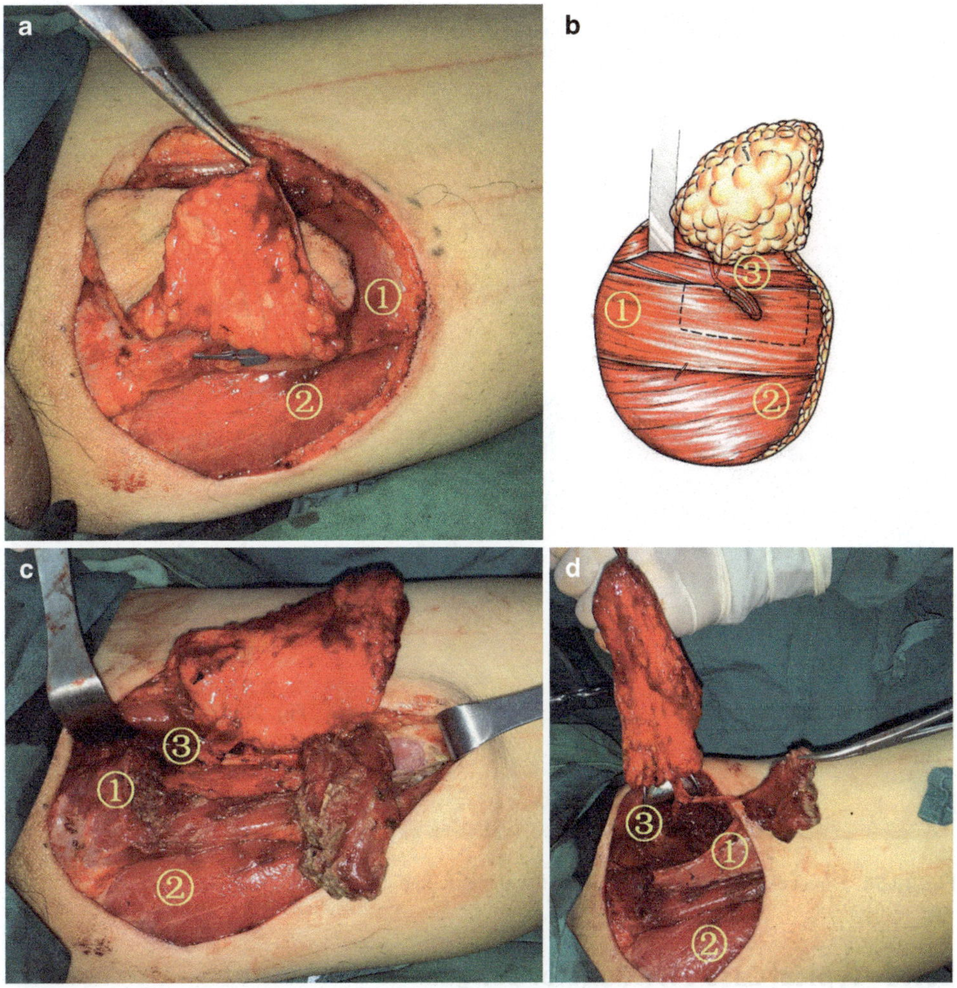

Fig. 20.54 Clamping experiment shows that the posterior perforator can be ligated and disconnected without carrying it. The flap and gracilis muscle flap are cut only with the anterior perforator vessel as the pedicle. (1) Gracilis muscle. (2) Adductor major. (3) Vascular pedicle

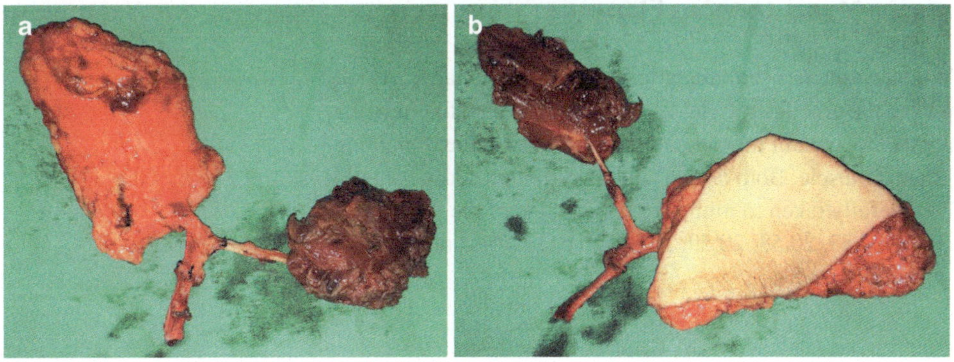

Fig. 20.55 The gracilis myocutaneous flap pedicled with profunda femoral artery was dissected

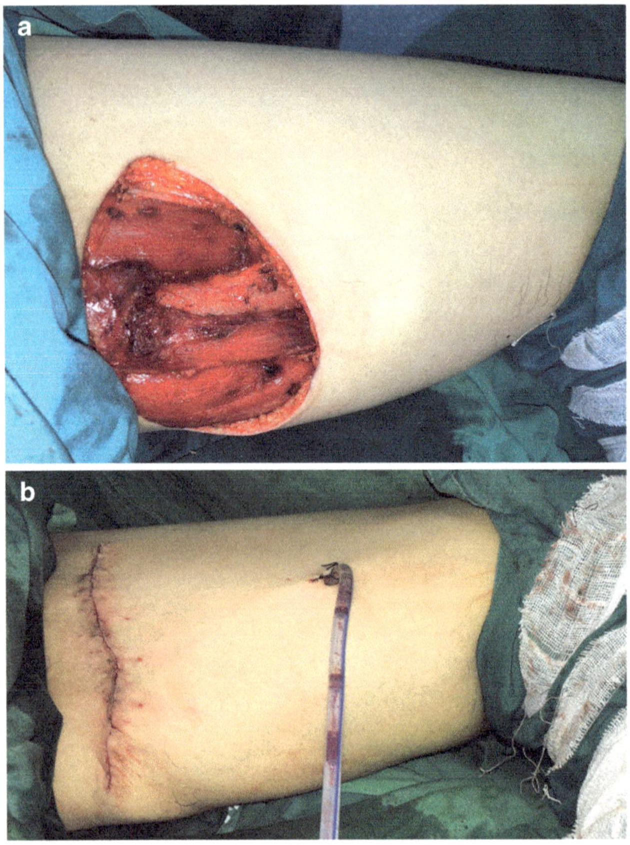

Fig. 20.56 Direct closure of the donor site of the chimeric flap

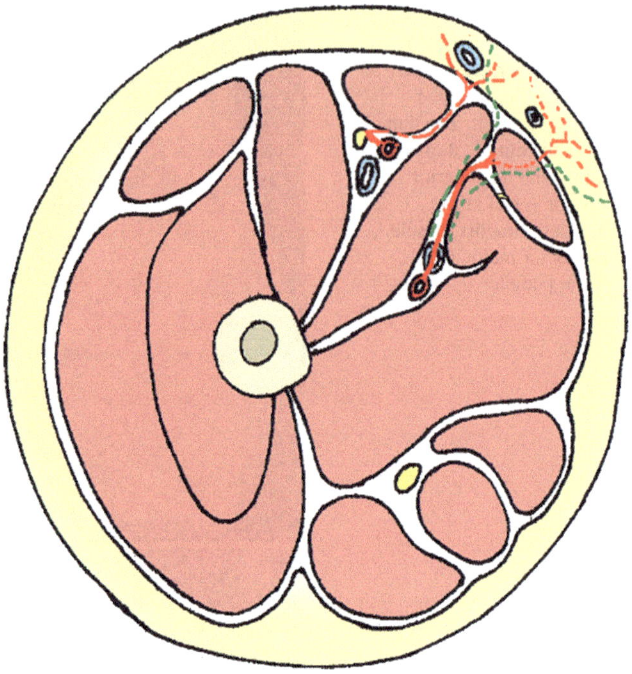

Fig. 20.57 The anterior branch of the obturator nerve entering the remaining gracilis muscle is preserved when the chimeric gracilis muscle myocutaneous flap is dissected

20.13 Typical Case 11: Adductor Longus Perforator Chimeric Gracilis Myocutaneous Flap

When dissecting the chimeric myocutaneous flap carrying part of the gracilis muscle, attention is to be paid to retain the anterior branch of the obturator nerve entering the remaining gracilis muscle. Both design and operation procedure should be carefully taken to minimize the damage of the donor area (Figs. 20.57, 20.58, 20.59, 20.60, 20.61, 20.62, and 20.63).

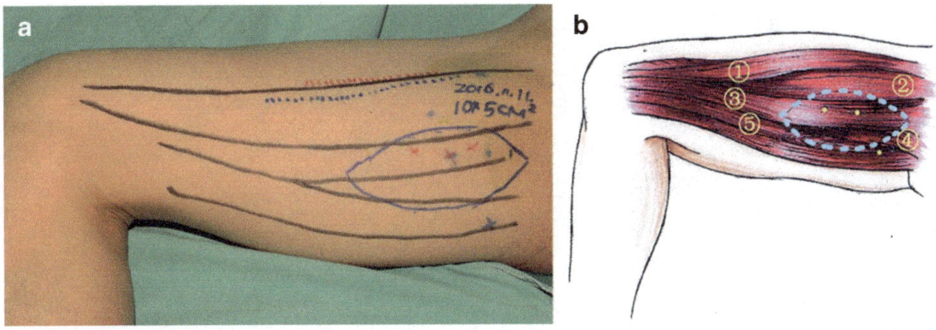

Fig. 20.58 Longitudinal profunda femoral artery pedicle embedded with gracilis perforator myocutaneous flap was designed on the surface of gracilis according to the preoperative Doppler detection sites. (1) Sartorius muscle. (2) Adductor longus. (3) Gracilis muscle. (4) Adductor major. (5) Semimembranosus muscle

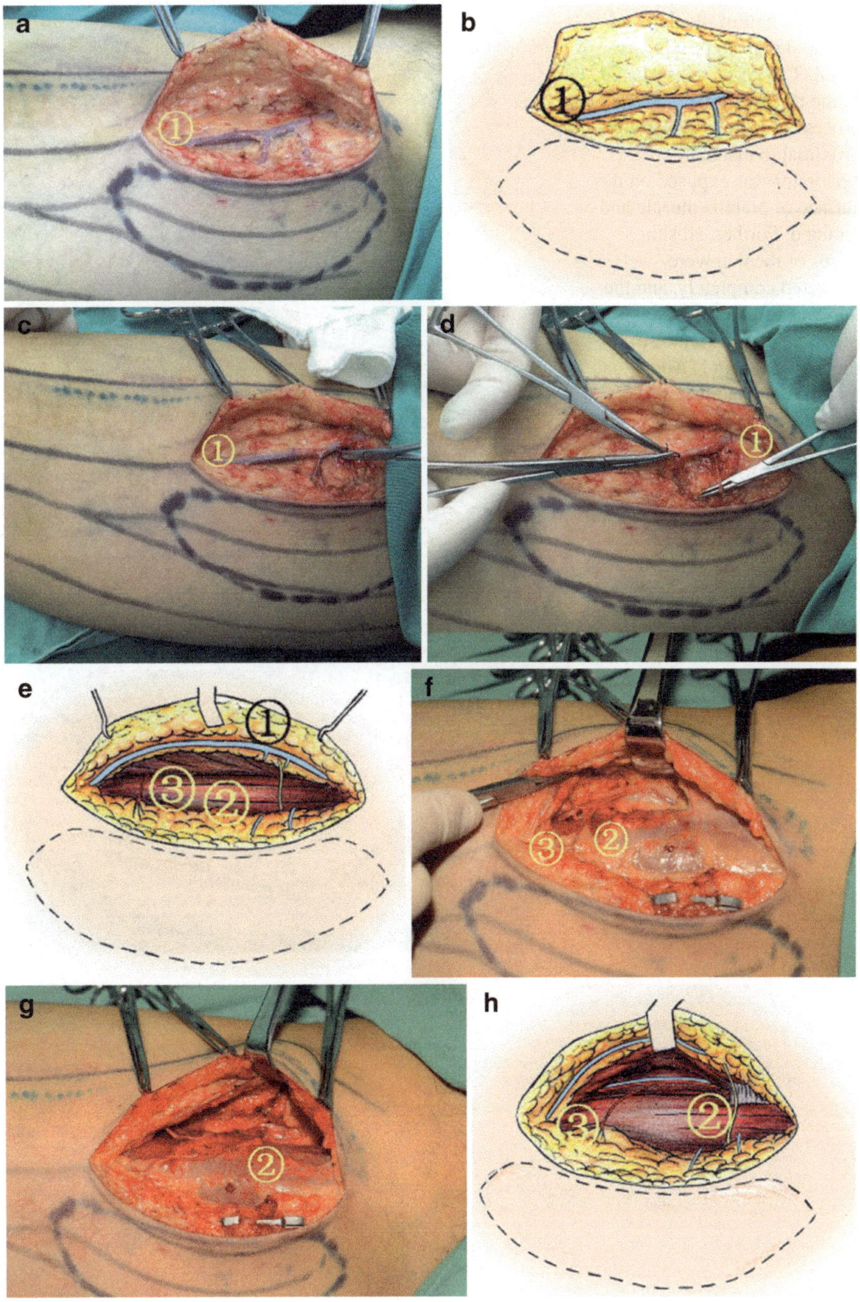

Fig. 20.59 Separate the skin subcutaneous tissue along the frontal edge of the flap, lift the anterior flap, expose the subcutaneous superficial great saphenous vein and its two thick vein branches entering the flap, ligate and disconnect the branches from the issuing plane, and leave them in the flap for standby. Pull the great saphenous vein forward, dissect the fascia to the surface of the deep fascia within the predetermined range, lift the fascia flap backward, and expose a slightly thin perforating branch of the middle and upper thigh between the medial femoral muscle and the adductor longus muscle. Dissect the deep fascia along the perforating branch and pull the muscles to the opposite sides. A perforating branch originating from the nourished vessel of the saphenous nerve was observed. After long segment division, the perforator is ligated and disconnected, and left in the flap for standby to preserve the integrity of the saphenous nerve. (1) Great saphenous vein. (2) Adductor longus. (3) Perforating vessels

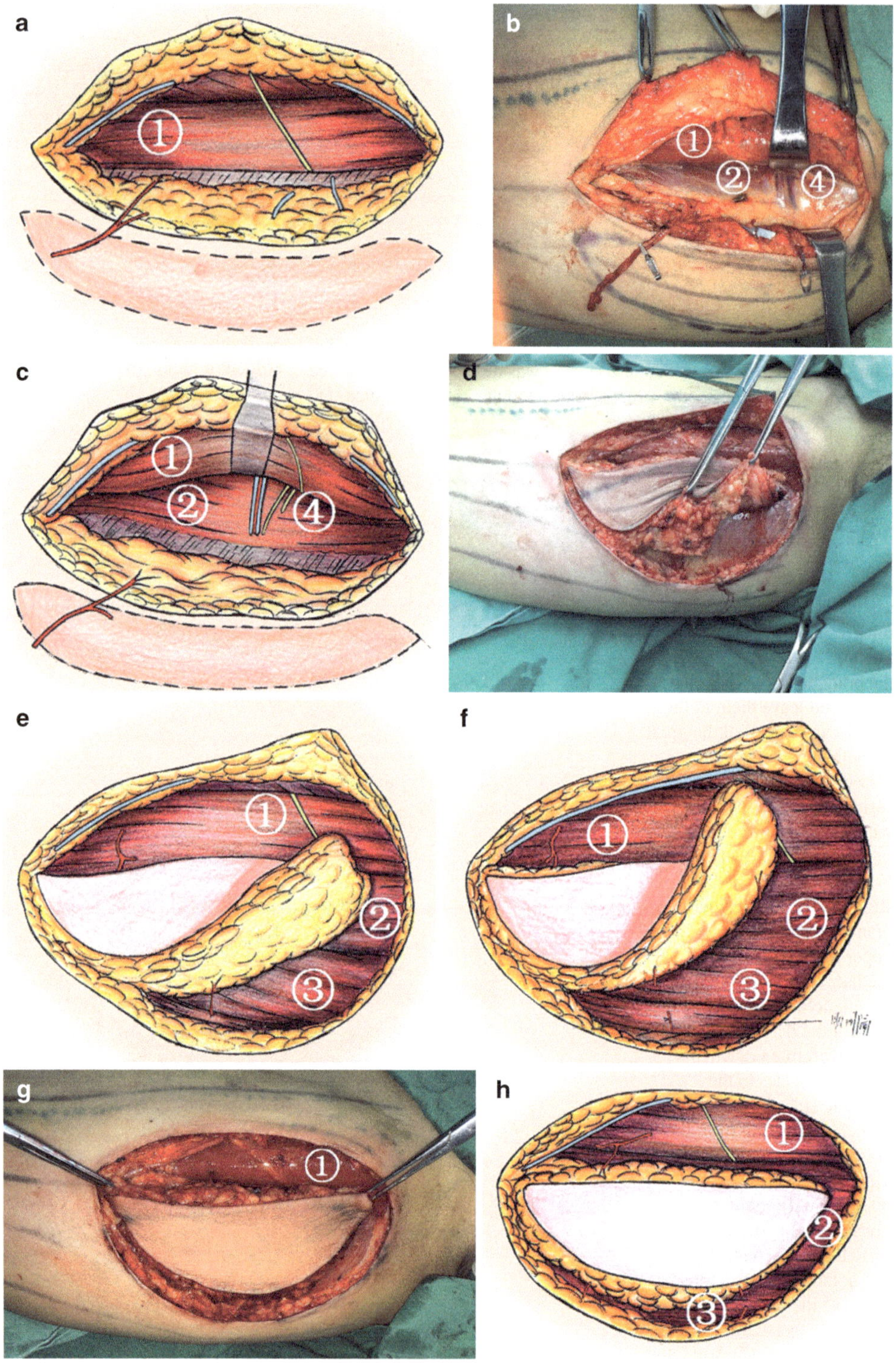

Fig. 20.60 Further separate the flap to the muscular septum between adductor longus and gracilis femoris, separate the muscular septum tissue, and no obvious perforating vessels were found. Moreover, no obvious perforating vessels were found on the surface of musculus septum and adductor longus. Further separate the muscle septum, lift the adductor longus and gracilis to the opposite sides, and expose the thick branch of the profunda femoral artery entering the gracilis. Then switch to cut the medial proximal half of the flap and lift the flap from proximal to distal. The layer: the surface of the myomembrane. In the process of lifting the flap from proximal to distal, a perforator was exposed on the surface of gracilis muscle and retained. Further, all skin edges of the flap were dissected completely, and the flap was lifted from distal to proximal on the surface of the myomembrane. (1) Adductor longus. (2) Gracilis muscle. (3) Adductor major

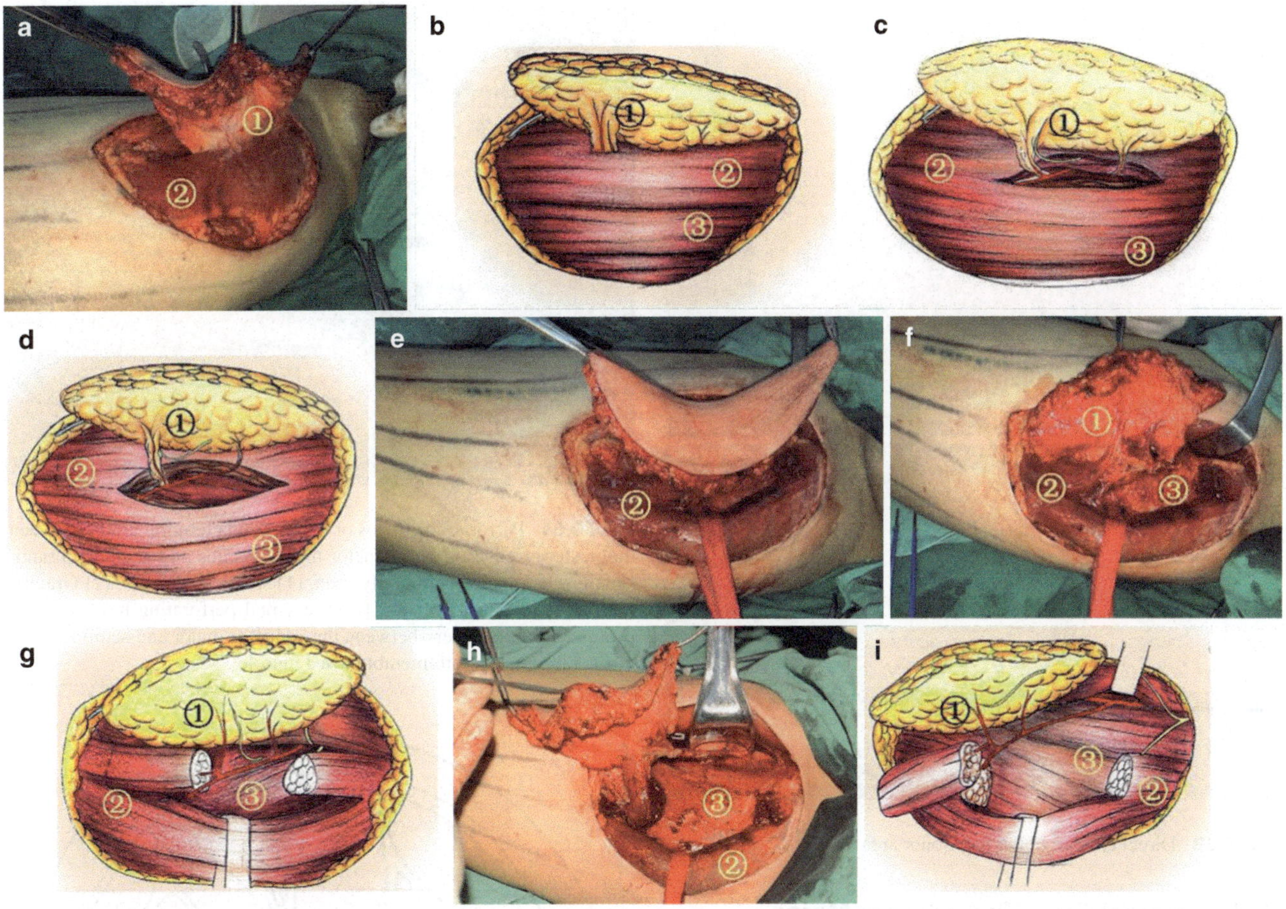

Fig. 20.61 Another perforator vessel entering the flap was exposed on the surface of the gracilis muscle. The skin branch of the anterior branch of the obturator nerve entered the flap. Lift the flap from the posterior to the anterior on the surface of the muscle membrane, ligate and disconnect several small perforating branches between the adductor major and the semimembranosus muscle, completely separate the flap, and the flap was connected to the donor area only through two perforating branches. The gracilis muscle was separated along the medial side of the two perforating branches and retrogradely dissociated to the plane of main branch entering the muscle. The main branch continued to course medial far away from the perforating branch and was ligated and disconnected at an appropriate plane. (There are viewpoints that the muscle flap can be dissected with the distal end of the trunk as the pedicle, but in this case, we prefer to cut it off as soon as possible for three reasons: (1) The trunk has obviously traveled inward, and we only need a small muscle bundle on the external in this case. (2) The chimeric flap has two perforating branches. According to the needs of the recipient area, the second perforating branch and the muscle flap need no complete separation, and the blood supply is reliable. (3) Leave as much muscle trunk as possible in the gracilis muscle, which is conducive to muscle blood perfusion.) The gracilis muscle was dissected along the surface of the first perforating branch, and the anterior branch of the obturator nerve was retained in the remaining gracilis muscle, and the vascular pedicle was separated. Completely dissected the vascular pedicle at the plane of the profunda femoral vessel, cut the pedicle and transfer, and properly revise it. Remember to use a suture to mark on the skin at the position where the branch enter the skin. (1) Perforating vessels. (2) Gracilis muscle. (3) Adductor major

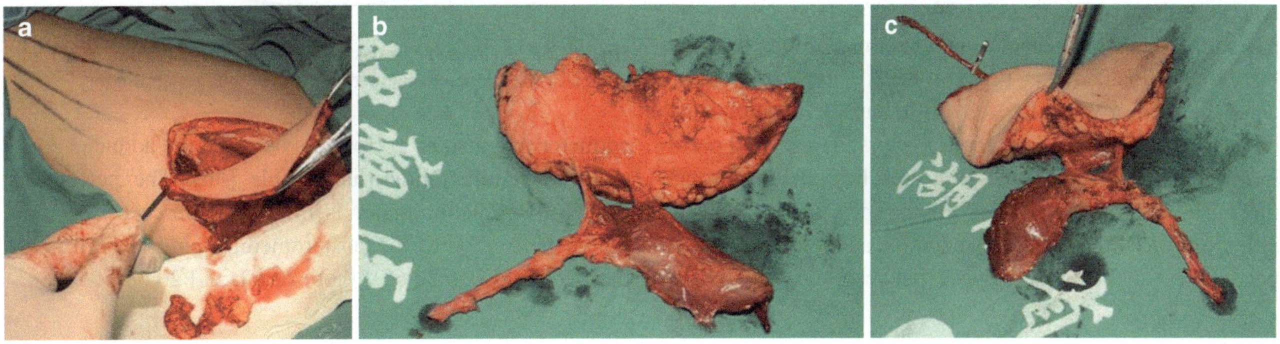

Fig. 20.62 The profunda femoral artery pedicled perforator gracilis myocutaneous flap was dissected

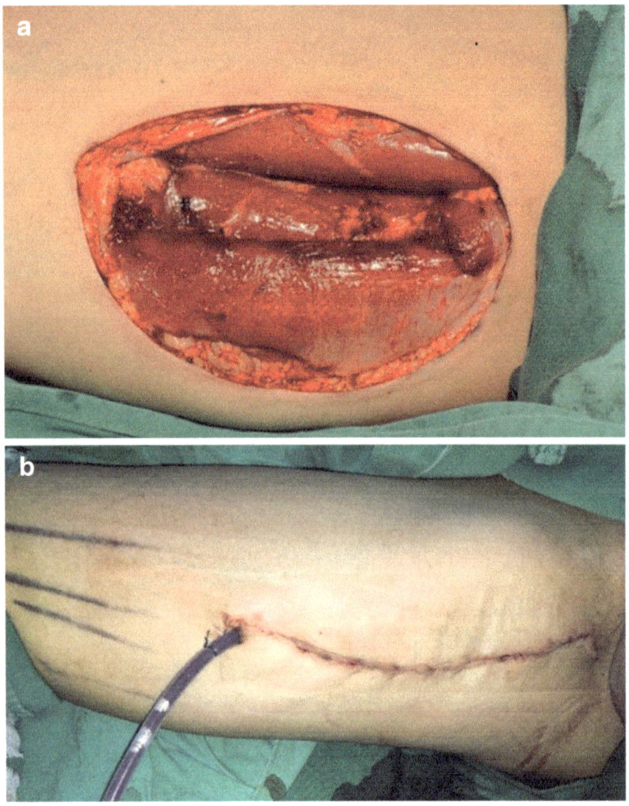

Fig. 20.63 Direct closure of the flap donor area

20.14 Typical Case 12: Adductor Major Perforator Flap Pedicled with Profunda Femoral Artery

The profunda femoral artery has four perforators behind the branches of the medial and lateral femoral circumflex arteries. The first perforator is sent out above the adductor brevis or between it and the pubic muscle, arising branches to the adductor magnus and gracilis. The second perforator crosses in front of the adductor brevis; the third branch travels under it. The second and third perforators supply the semimembranosus muscle, biceps femoris muscle, and lateral femoral muscle (Fig. 20.64). The fourth perforator is reported to have the most unstable anatomy in its donor area and is considered to be the terminal branch of the profunda femoral artery, passing through the muscular septum or resembling the other three musculocutaneous perforators. All these perforators enter the skin or muscular septum to supply the subcutaneous tissue and skin. Among them, the first and second perforating branches usually have skin branches passing through the posterolateral side of the thigh. These perforators are either muscle skin perforators from the adductor magnus, or perforators in the muscle space between the gracilis and adductor magnus, or perforators between the adductor magnus and semimembranosus muscle [36]. The perforating branch of adductor major is often the source of the most potent perforator of the posteromedial femoral perforating branch flap (Figs. 20.65, 20.66, 20.67, and 20.68).

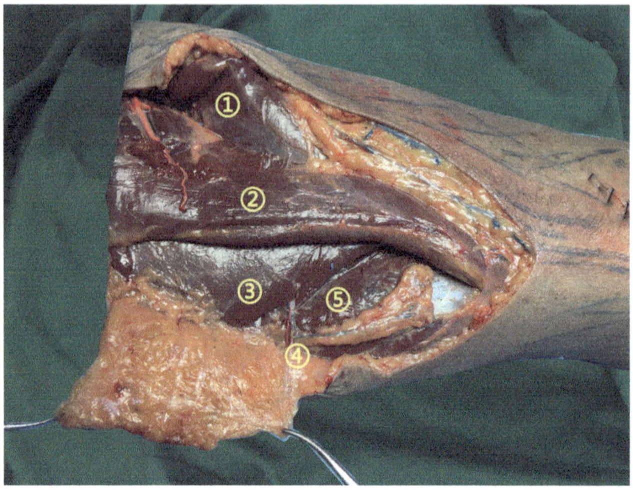

Fig. 20.64 Perforating vessels of the profunda femoral artery between the posterior edge of the adductor megacephalus and semimembranosus muscle are also commonly seen. (1) Adductor longus. (2) Gracilis muscle. (3) Adductor major. (4) The septal perforating branch of the profunda femoral artery between the adductor major and semimembranosus muscle. (5) Semimembranosus muscle

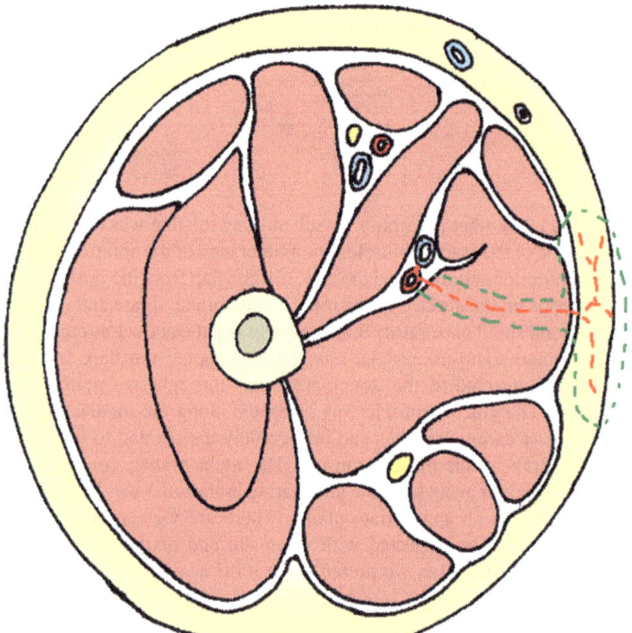

Fig. 20.65 Anatomical cross-sectional diagram of the perforating branch of the adductor major from the profunda femoral artery

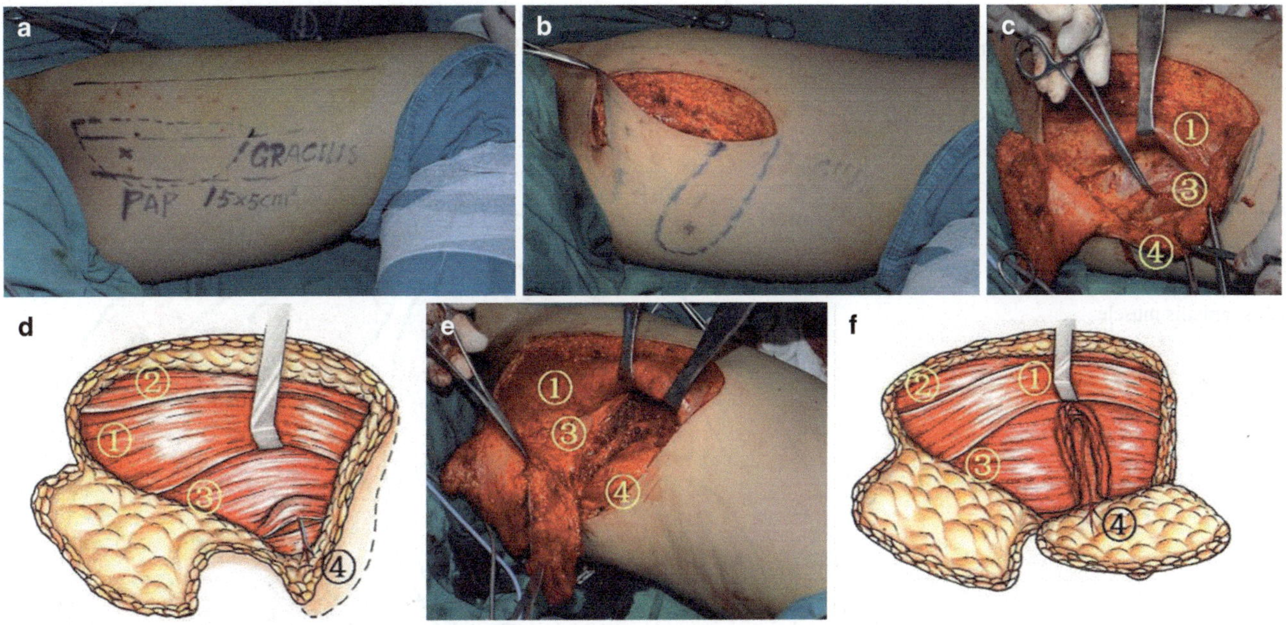

Fig. 20.66 (**a**) Design of the medial femoral perforator flap. (**b**) No suitable perforator vessel was found in the anterior exploration incision. A perforator vessel was found on the surface of the adductor major behind the gracilis muscle, and the medial femoral flap was re-designed. (**c**) Lift the flap and separate the perforating vessels of the adductor major muscle. (**d**) The origin of the perforator vessel was located behind the adductor magnus. (**e**) Retrograde separation of perforating vessels into the adductor major muscle. (**f**) The vessel pedicle was separated to the profunda femoral vessel plane to obtain sufficient length and diameter of the vessel pedicle. (1) Gracilis muscle. (2) Adductor longus. (3) Adductor major. (4) Perforating vessels

Fig. 20.67 The perforator flap of the adductor major was cut off

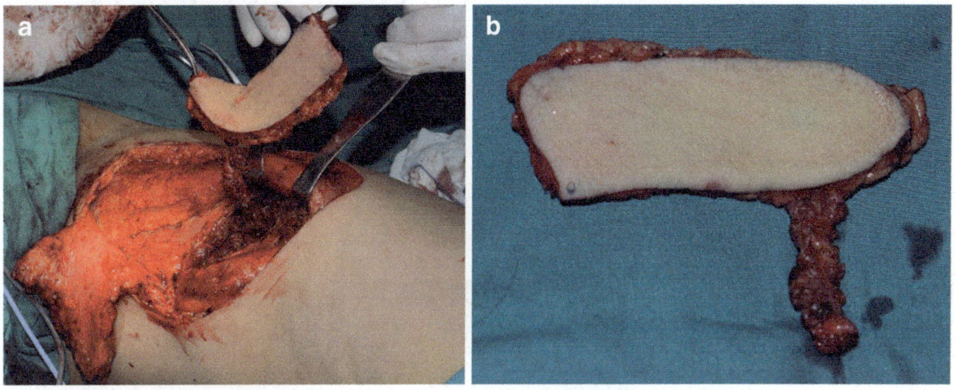

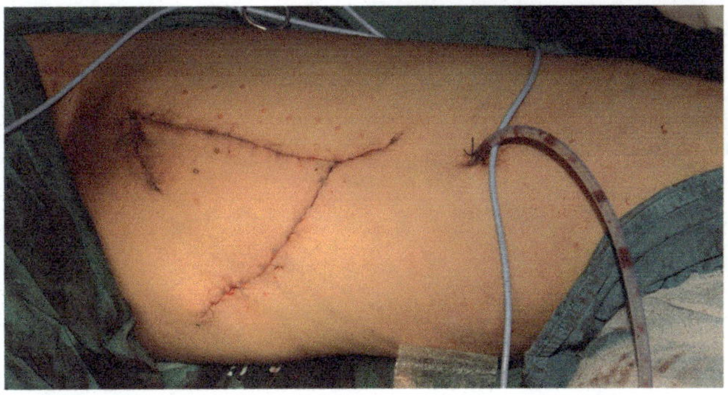

Fig. 20.68 Direct closure of the flap donor area

20.15 Typical Case 13: Chimeric Gracilis Myocutaneous Flap Pedicled with Perforating Branch of the Adductor Major

Most of the important perforating vessels of the profunda femoral artery in the posterior femoral area are the perforating vessels from the adductor major, which arise from the front of the gracilis based on the variable distribution to the skin. In most cases, the perforating vessels of the adductor major are located behind the gracilis. When the perforating vessels of the adductor major originate from the frontal area of the gracilis, the adductor major muscle flap and gracilis muscle flap can be dissected, respectively, to prepare the posterior medial femoral chimeric myocutaneous flap according to the perforating branch and branch of the adductor major (Figs. 20.69, 20.70, 20.71, 20.72, 20.73, 20.74, and 20.75) [23, 29].

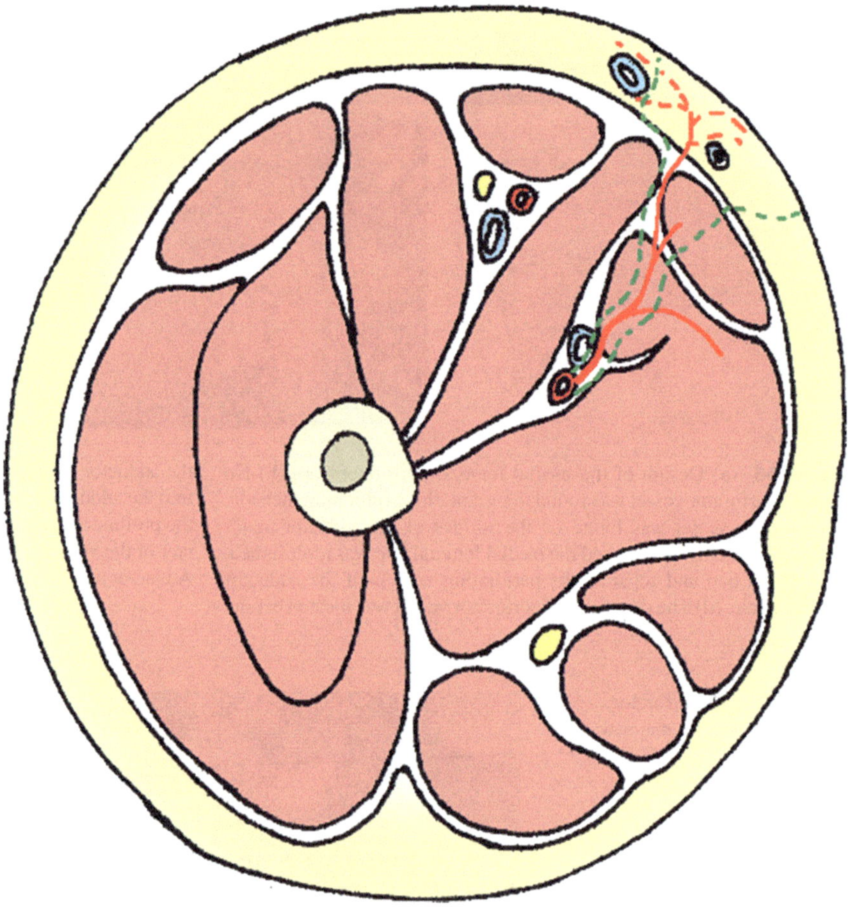

Fig. 20.69 Anatomical cross-sectional diagram of the perforating branch of the adductor major from the front of the gracilis muscle

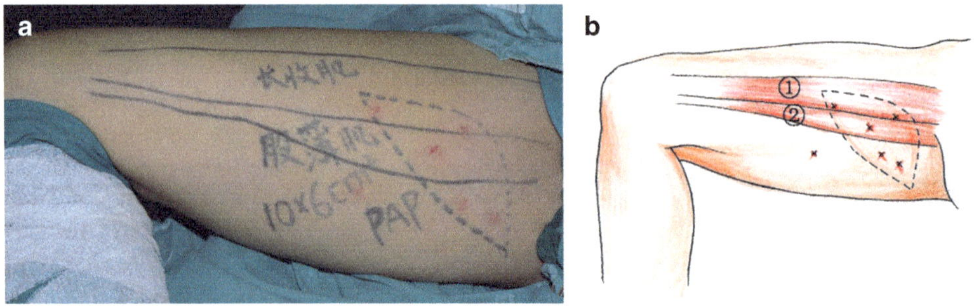

Fig. 20.70 Design of the chimeric gracilis myocutaneous flap. (1) Adductor longus. (2) Gracilis muscle

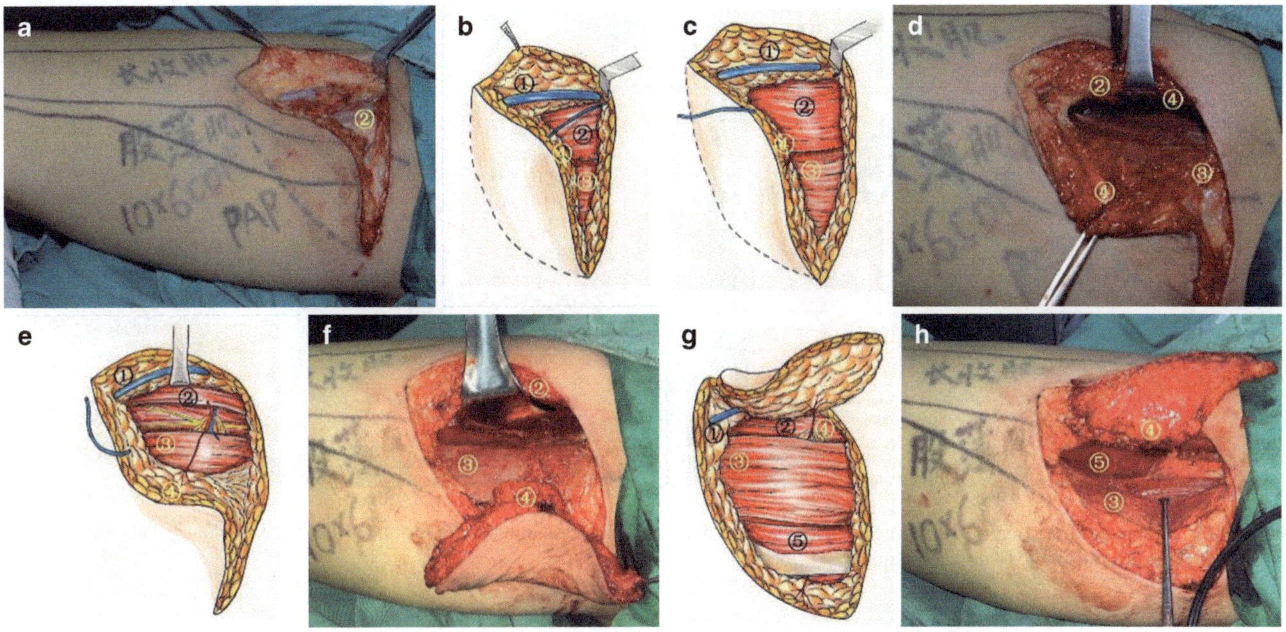

Fig. 20.71 It is important to design the exploration incision. The first incision is determined according to the shape of the flap and the number of perforations. The main saphenous vein and a long branch were exposed and carried in the flap after long segmental separation, but it was difficult to apply as a normal practice. Lift the flap from anterior to posterior and from proximal to distal to expose a perforator vessel between the gracilis and adductor longus, which was not thick. The perforator trunk of profunda femoral vessels was separated from the muscle space along the perforator branch. It was found that the perforator branch sent out two fascial branches after entering the skin, and the trunk entered the muscle. The retrograde separation of the trunk showed that multiple muscle branches were sent out into the adductor longus and adductor magnus. It was difficult to further separate the vascular pedicle. We then switch to dissect the remaining skin edge of the flap, and no large perforator was found. The only one was that a large perforator coursing between the adductor megacephalus and semimembranosus muscle after the posterior edge of the flap, which was temporarily retained. (1) Great saphenous vein. (2) Adductor longus. (3) Gracilis muscle. (4) Perforator vessel pedicle. (5) Adductor major

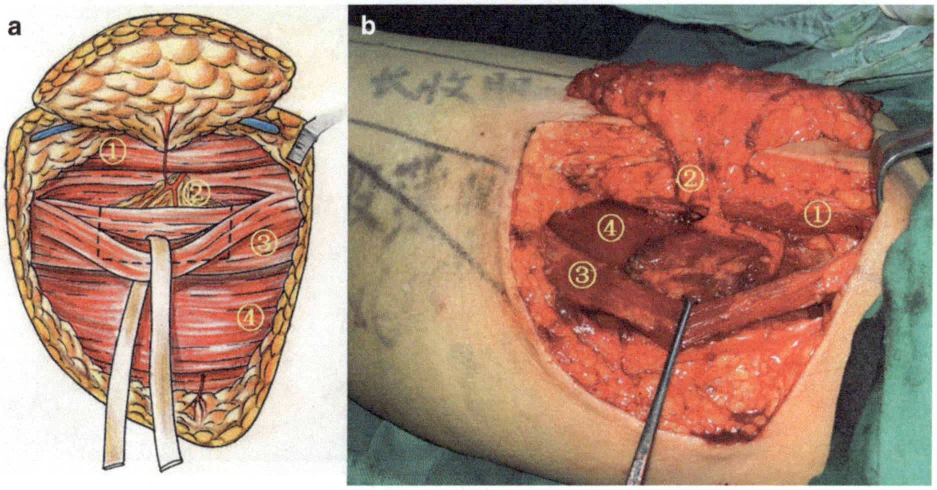

Fig. 20.72 Retain the muscle bundle in front of the gracilis muscle and pull it away. Cut the perforator of the profunda femoral blood vessel into the fascia muscle flap near the muscle hilus. (1) Adductor longus. (2) Vascular pedicle. (3) Gracilis muscle. (4) Adductor major. The dotted line indicates the range of the gracilis muscle flap to be cut

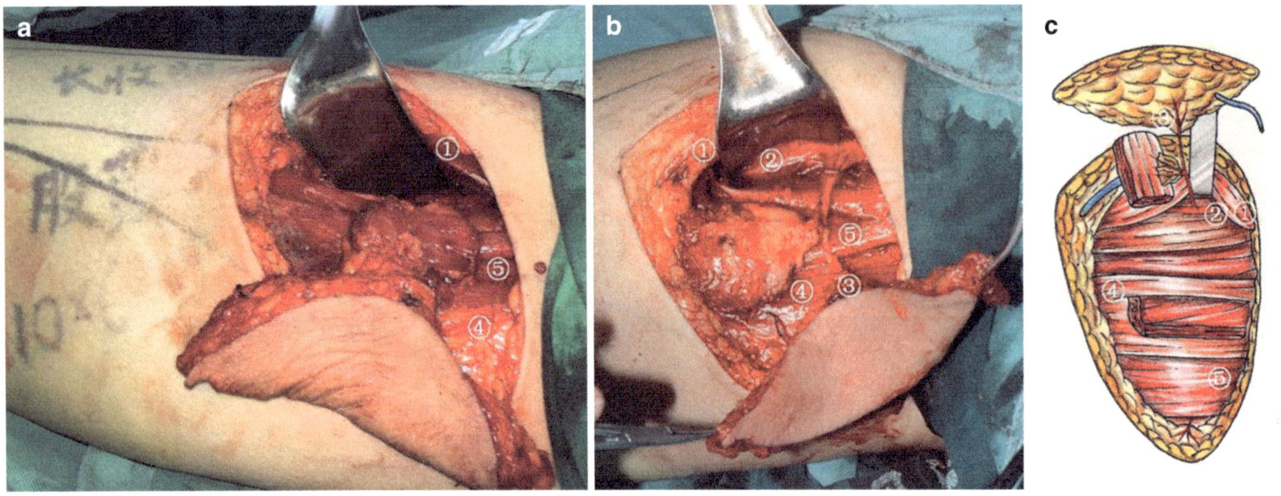

Fig. 20.73 Complete dissection of the chimeric myocutaneous flap. (1) Adductor longus. (2) Profunda femoral vessels. (3) Perforator vessel pedicle. (4) Gracilis muscle. (5) Adductor major

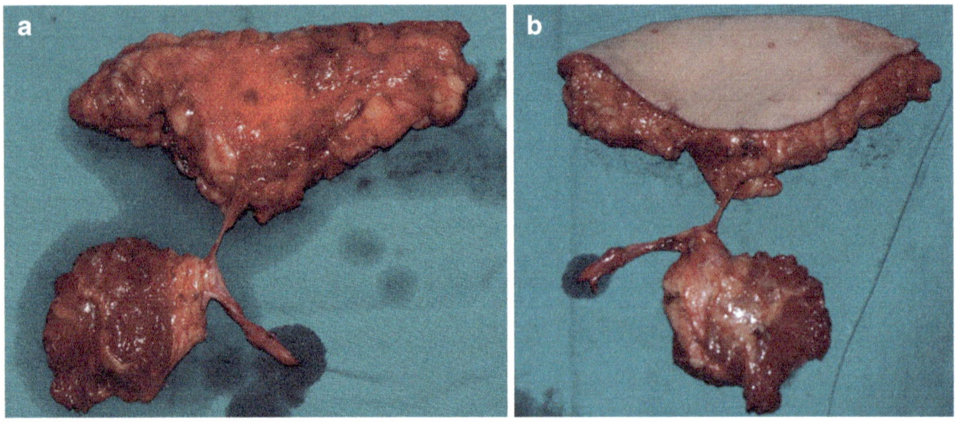

Fig. 20.74 The profunda femoral artery pedicled perforator gracilis myocutaneous flap was dissected

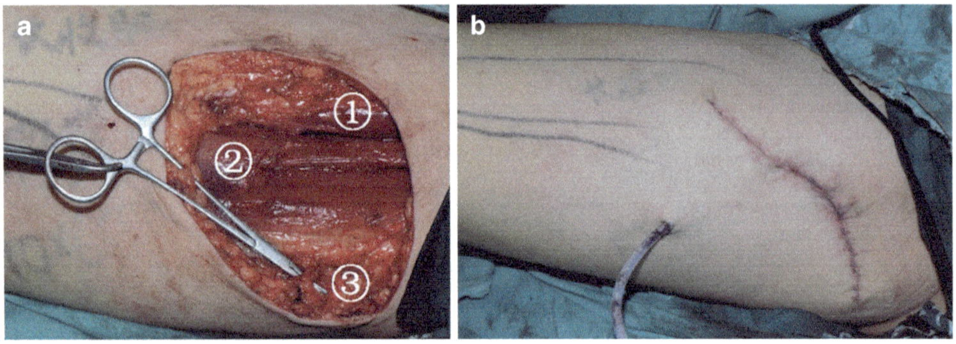

Fig. 20.75 Direct closure of the flap donor area. (1) Adductor longus. (2) Gracilis muscle. (3) Adductor major

20.16 Typical Case 14: Chimeric Gracilis Myocutaneous Flap Pedicled with the Perforating Branch of the Adductor Major While Preserving the Anterior Branch of the Obturator Nerve

When the musculocutaneous perforating branch and musculocutaneous branch of the gracilis major adductor muscle branch are sent out in front of the gracilis muscle, the flap and gracilis muscle flap can be dissected according to the actual clinical needs. If the required muscle flap is small, the nerve supplying the remaining gracilis muscle can be retained to minimize the damage of the donor area (Figs. 20.76, 20.77, and 20.78).

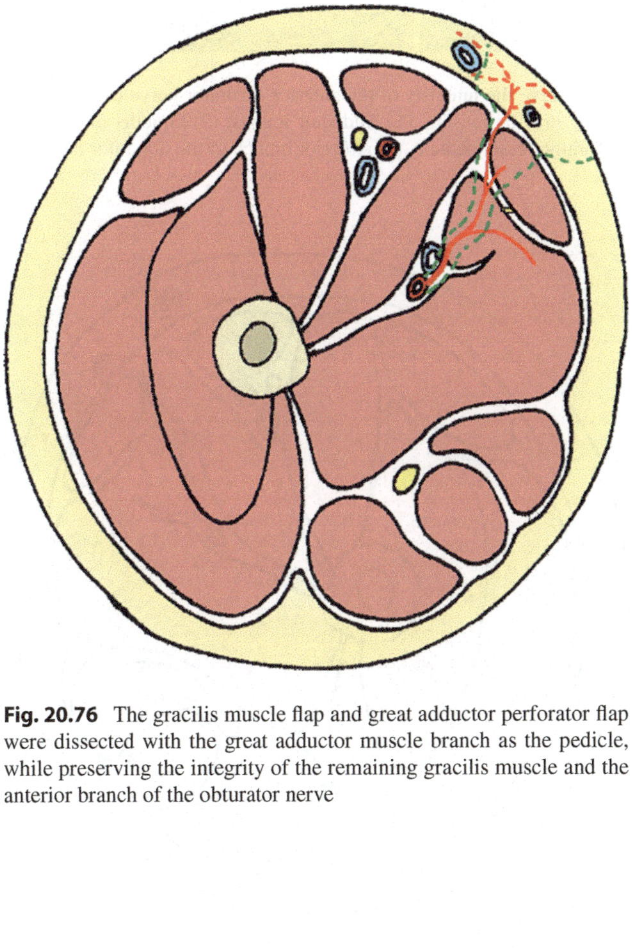

Fig. 20.76 The gracilis muscle flap and great adductor perforator flap were dissected with the great adductor muscle branch as the pedicle, while preserving the integrity of the remaining gracilis muscle and the anterior branch of the obturator nerve

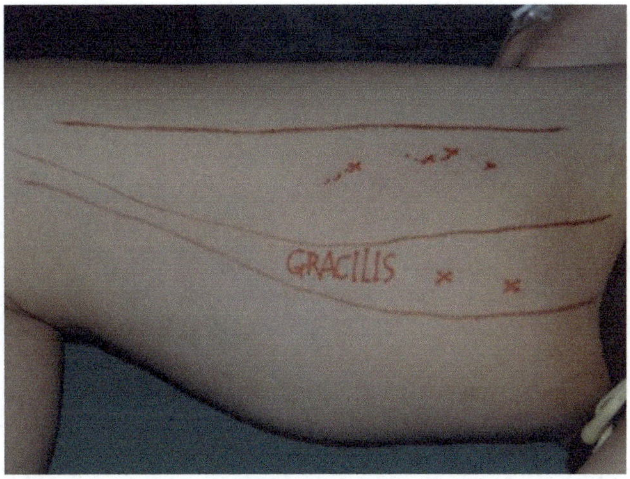

Fig. 20.77 Design of the chimeric gracilis myocutaneous flap

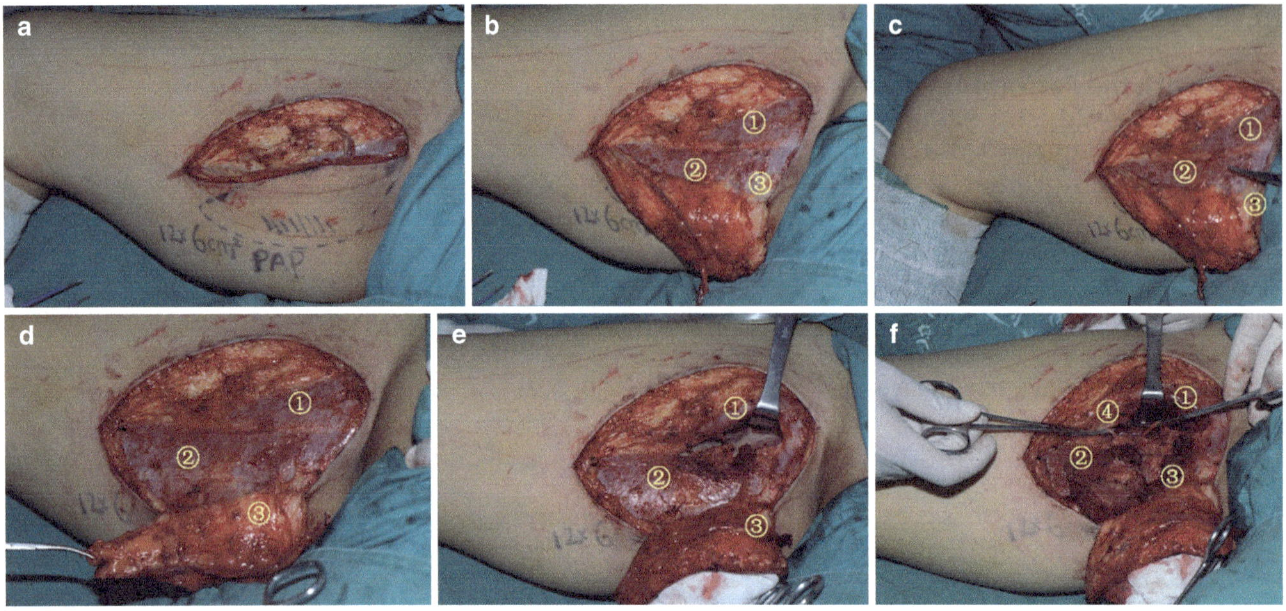

Fig. 20.78 Lift the flap from anterior to posterior to expose the adductor longus and gracilis muscle and the perforating vessels between them, retrograde separate the perforating vessels to the emitting plane, and preserve the integrity of the anterior obturator nerve branch entering the gracilis muscle. (1) Adductor longus. (2) Gracilis muscle. (3) Perforator vessel pedicle. (4) Anterior branch of the obturator nerve

20.17 Typical Case 15: Great Adductor Perforator-Embedded Gracilis Myocutaneous Flap

The posteromedial thigh regional flap was first reported by Conway and Griffith, conwa and kraissl in 1947. Later, Angrigiani et al. [17] conducted a cadaver study to evaluate the posteromedial thigh flap based on the perforator of the proximal adductor major muscle. The flap, in which the donor artery is the first medial branch of the profunda femoral artery, is named the "adductor flap." Although the profunda femoral artery is the main source artery of the posteromedial region of the thigh, the following arteries also supply this region: the medial circumflex femoral artery, the pudendal artery, the perforator of the semimembranosus and semitendinosus muscles, and the inferior gluteal artery [7].

The most important perforator vessel of the posteromedial thigh is the great adductor musculocutaneous perforator vessel from the profunda femoral artery. It has the advantages of large diameter, long vascular pedicle, and multiple branches. The separation process is relatively simple and does not damage the structures of important tissue. The great adductor perforator flap is also the most commonly used posteromedial femoral perforator flap for breast reconstruction (Fig. 20.79).

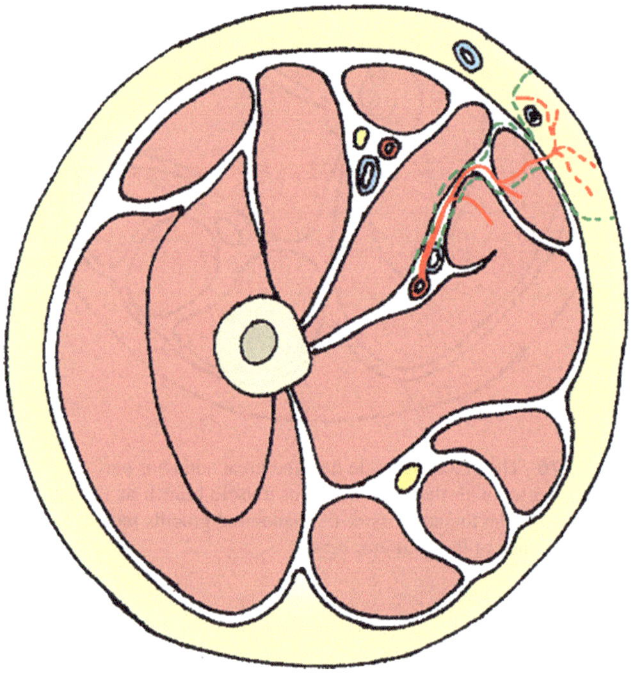

Fig. 20.79 Gracilis muscle flap and gracilis perforator flap were dissected and pedicled with the adductor major branch, while preserving the integrity of the remaining gracilis muscle and the anterior branch of obturator nerve

In this typical case, the perforating branch of the muscular septum between the great adductor muscle and the gracilis muscle is exposed behind the gracilis muscle. The perforating branch is from the great adductor muscle branch. The great adductor muscle branch sends out a large gracilis muscle branch at the same time. The great adductor muscle branch can be ligated far away from the perforating branch vessel, and the flap can be dissected and transferred from the deep surface of the gracilis muscle to the frontal area of the gracilis muscle. The gracilis muscle flap was then dissected to prepare a chimeric gracilis muscle flap pedicled with the great adductor muscle branch. You can also dissect the great adductor muscle flap with the great adductor muscle branch as the pedicle and transfer the muscle flap to the front of the gracilis muscle. After further dissecting the flap, the vascular pedicle is separated in retrograde fashion to the plane of the profunda femoral artery, and the preparation of the myocutaneous flap is completed (Figs. 20.80, 20.81, 20.82, 20.83, and 20.84).

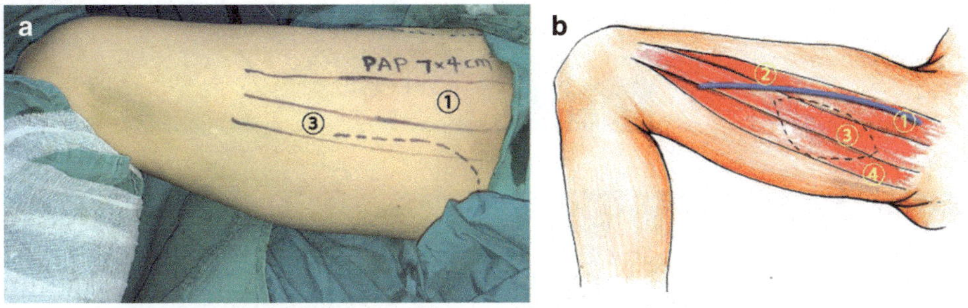

Fig. 20.80 Design and dissection of the medial femoral chimeric myocutaneous flap. (1) Adductor longus. (20 Great saphenous vein. (3) Gracilis muscle. (4) Adductor major

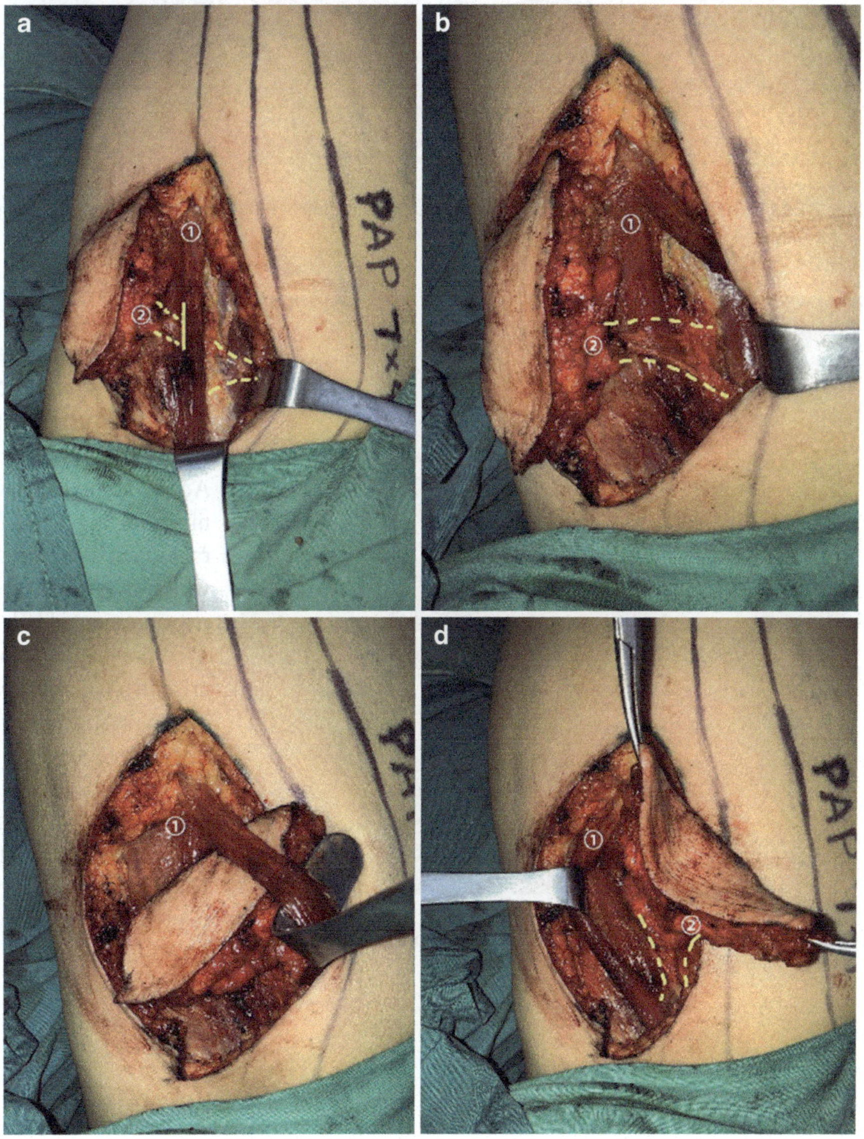

Fig. 20.81 Lift the flap from anterior to posterior to expose the perforator vessels from the center of the gracilis muscle, retrograde, separate the perforator vessel pedicle in the gracilis muscle in reverse direction, completely dissociate the flap, and transfer it from the intramuscular tunnel of the gracilis muscle to the same side of the vascular pedicle. (1) Gracilis muscle. (2) Perforator vessel pedicle

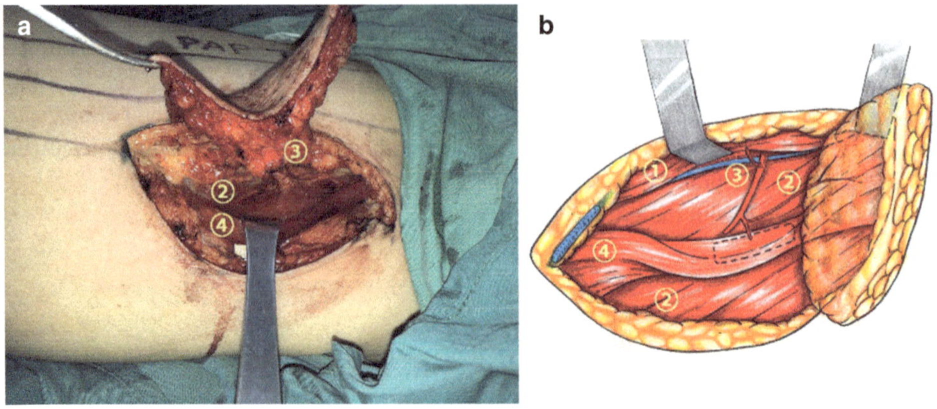

Fig. 20.82 The flap was cut off. (1) Adductor longus. (2) Adductor major. (3) Vascular pedicle of the musculus adductor major. (4) Gracilis muscle

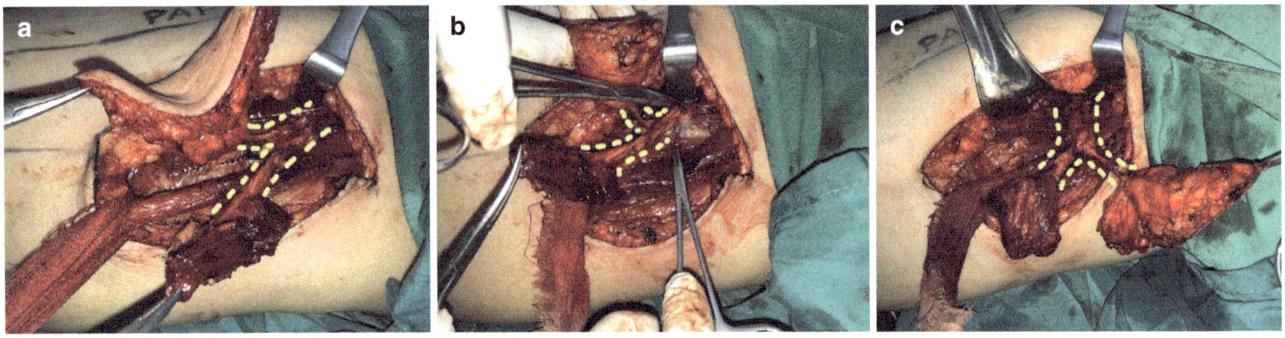

Fig. 20.83 After dissecting the adductor major muscle flap, retrograde separation of the vascular pedicle to the level of profunda femoral vessels was conducted

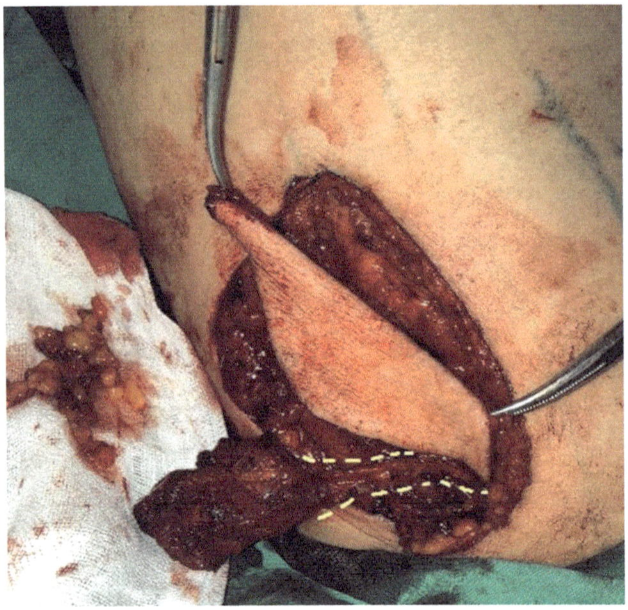

Fig. 20.84 The flap can be trimmed according to the actual needs of the receiving area

20.18 Typical Case 16: Profunda Femoral Artery Pedicled Adductor Major Perforator Chimeric Adductor Major Myocutaneous Flap

According to anatomical and imaging reports, the most common and largest perforator vessel in the posteromedial femoral region is located on the surface of the adductor major, which is basically consistent with the results of our clinical measurements [18].

When the perforating branch of the great adductor muscle arise from gap between the gracilis muscle and the long adductor muscle, the difficulty of preparing the chimeric myocutaneous flap is significantly reduced. First, the main branch of the great adductor muscle is separated retrogradely along the perforating branch vessel, and then the main branch of the great adductor muscle is separated in anterograde fashion and the great adductor muscle flap is dissected (Figs. 20.85, 20.86, 20.87, 20.88, 20.89, 20.90, 20.91, 20.92, 20.93, and 20.94).

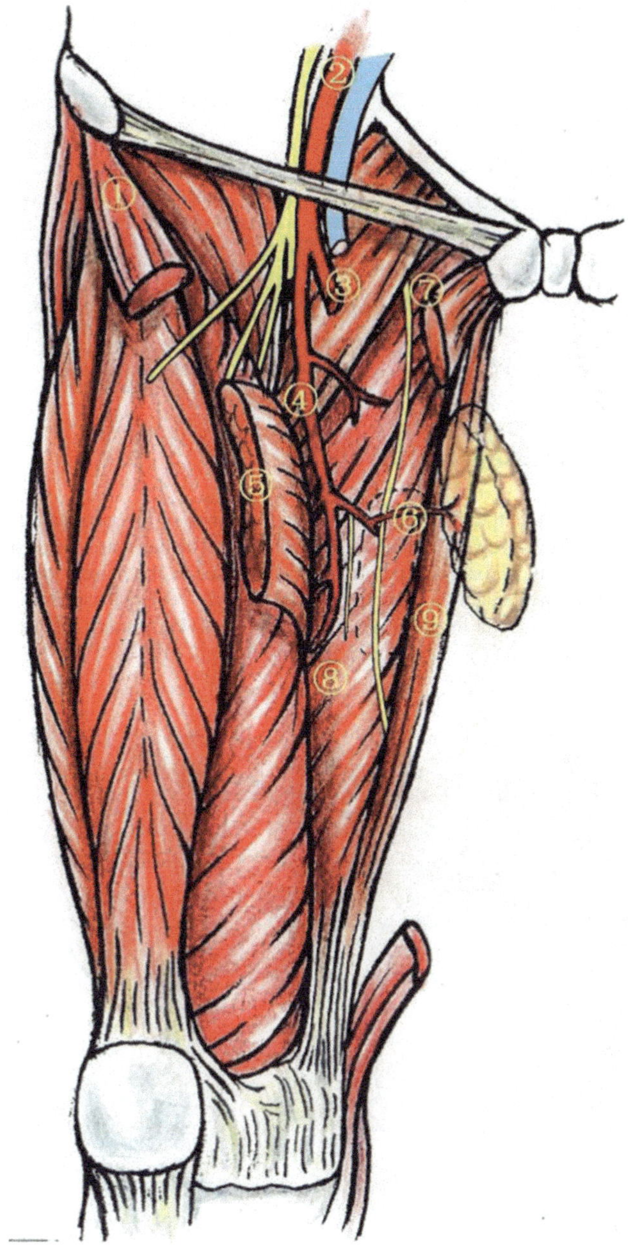

Fig. 20.85 Anatomical features of the profunda femoral artery pedicled adductor major perforator chimeric adductor major myocutaneous flap: the profunda femoral artery sends out a thick branch at the proximal thigh and enters the adductor major. Before entering the adductor major, it sends out a skin perforator (coursing between the adductor longus, gracilis and adductor major) into the flap. (1) Sartorius muscle. (2) Femoral artery. (3) Superficial femoral artery. (4) Profunda femoral artery. (5) Adductor longus. (6) Cutaneous perforator of the adductor major. (7) Anterior branch of the obturator nerve. (8) Adductor major. (9) Gracilis muscle. Key points of operation: for the safe blood supply of both muscle flap and skin flap, the vascular pedicle should be extended as long as possible

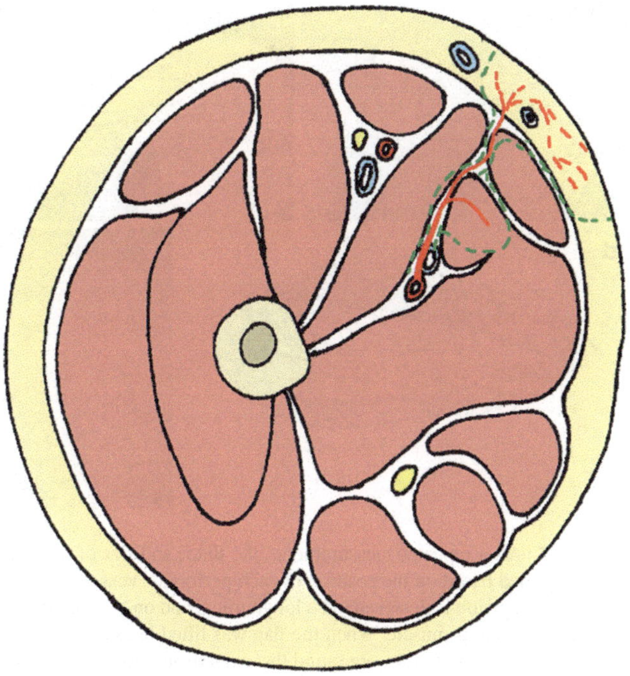

Fig. 20.86 Schematic diagram of chimeric cutting of the adductor major perforator flap and adductor major flap in front of the gracilis muscle

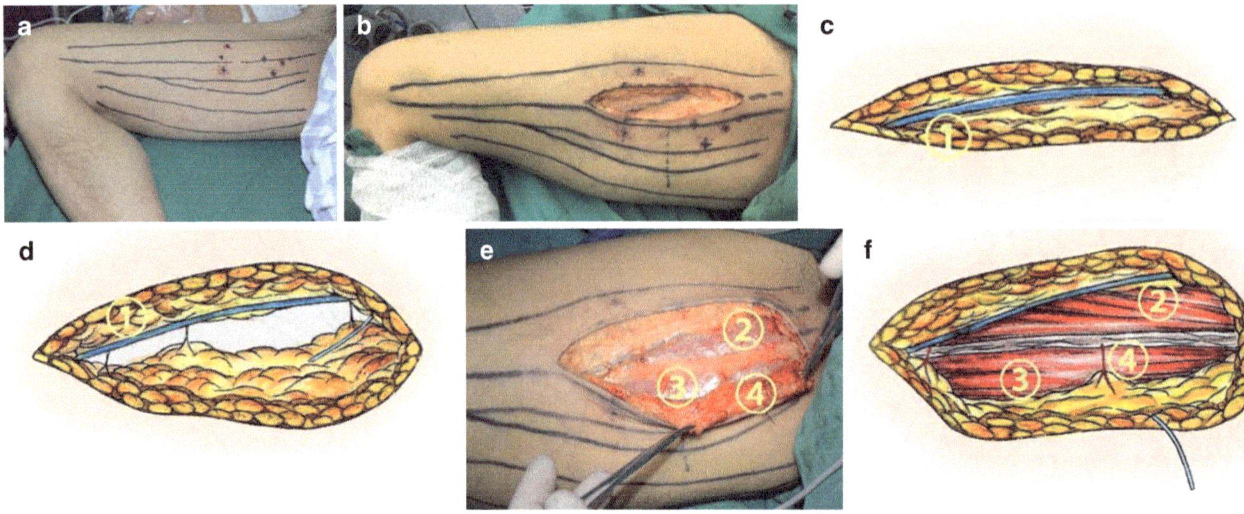

Fig. 20.87 After repeated measurements, the shape and size of the flap are determined based on the position of each perforator vessel, and the exploration incision is designed to be longitudinal and on the surface of the adductor longus muscle. When the flap was lifted backward, many small perforating branches were found that came from the nutrient vessels alongside the great saphenous vein. A branch of the great saphenous vein was separated and carried by the flap. The flap was separated retrogradely, and a small perforator was exposed in the muscle space between the adductor longus and gracilis femoris. (1) Great saphenous vein. (2) Adductor longus. (3) Gracilis muscle. (4) Perforating vessels

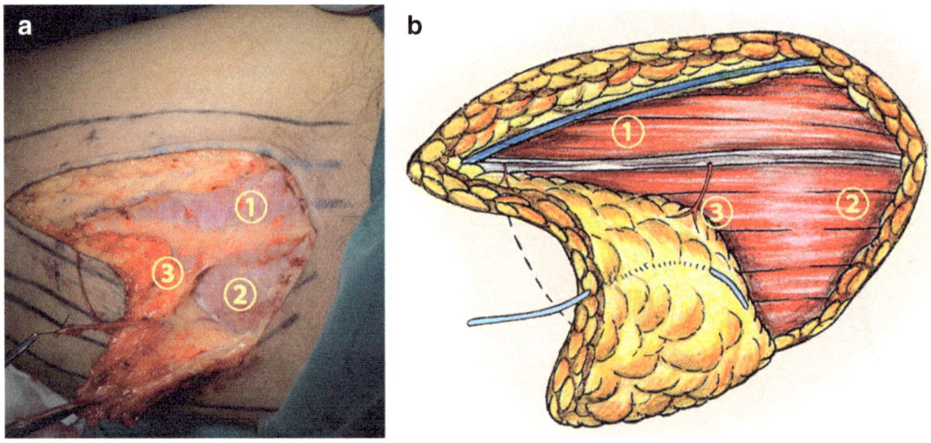

Fig. 20.88 Lift the flap from proximal to distal away from the surface of gracilis muscle, and no other obvious perforators were found. (1) Adductor longus. (2) Gracilis muscle. (3) Perforating vessels

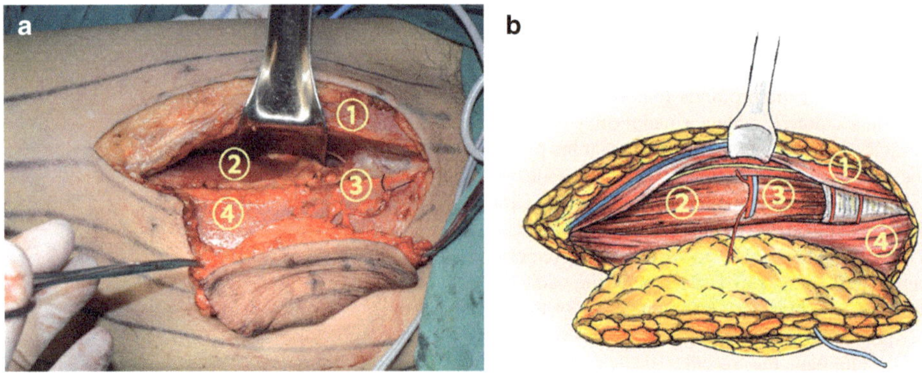

Fig. 20.89 Separate the tissue in the space between the adductor longus and gracilis femoris, and expose the main stem and nerve of the perforator vessel pedicle. The perforator vessel came from the thick adductor magnus muscle branch of the profunda femoral vessel. There were two muscle branches of the profunda femoral vessel entering the gracilis muscle, both of which had a high emitting plane, and there was no cutaneous perforator. (1) Adductor longus. (2) Adductor major. (3) Perforating branch of the adductor major. (4) Gracilis muscle

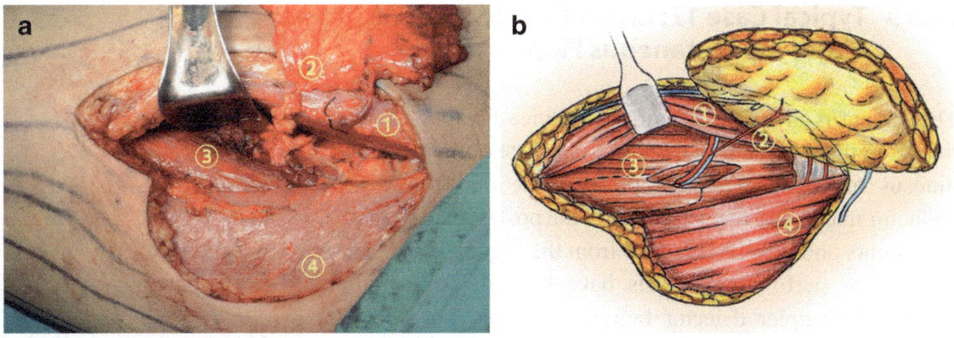

Fig. 20.90 Anterograde separation along the vascular pedicle of adductor major to determine the cutting edge of the myocutaneous flap (take the muscular branch of the adductor major as the trunk and the distal end as the pedicle). (1) Adductor longus. (2) Perforating vessels of the adductor major. (3) Adductor major. (4) Gracilis muscle

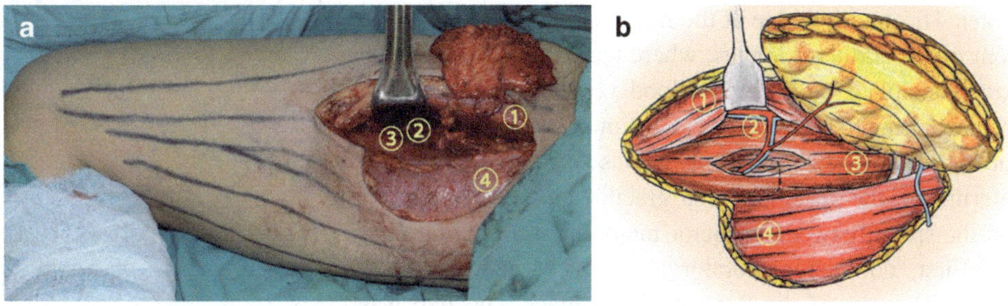

Fig. 20.91 Retrograde separation of the vascular pedicle to the profunda femoral artery trunk. (1) Adductor longus. (2) Profunda femoral vessels. (3) Adductor major. (4) Gracilis muscle

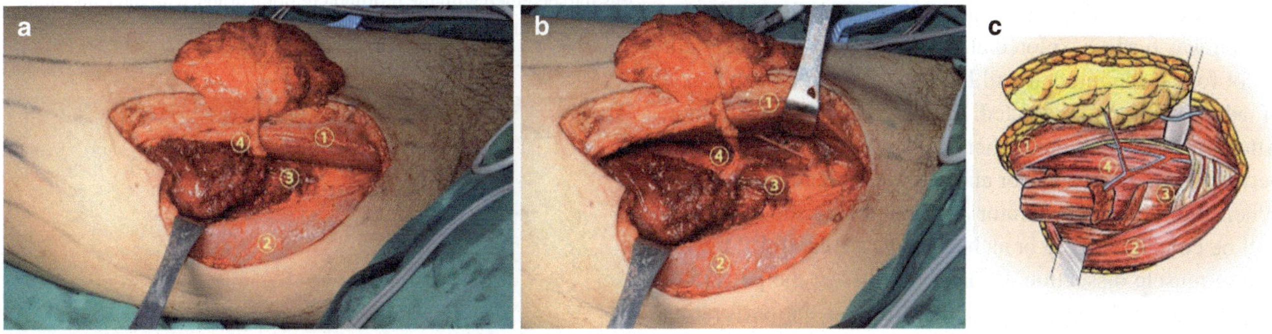

Fig. 20.92 The preparation of the chimeric myocutaneous flap was completed. (1) Adductor longus. (2) Gracilis muscle. (3) Adductor major. (4) Vascular pedicle

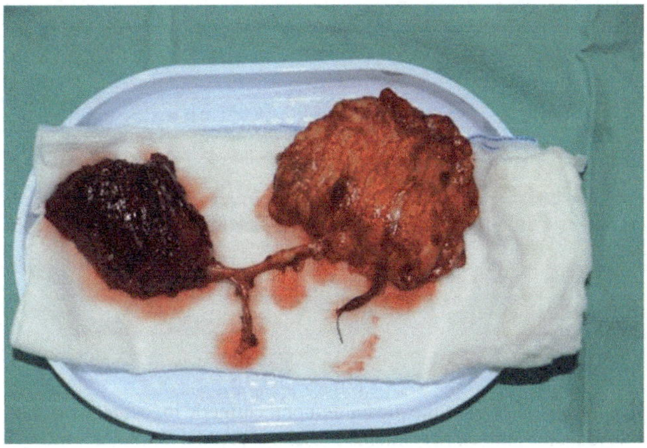

Fig. 20.93 The preparation of the profunda femoral artery pedicled chimeric adductor magnus perforator myocutaneous flap was completed

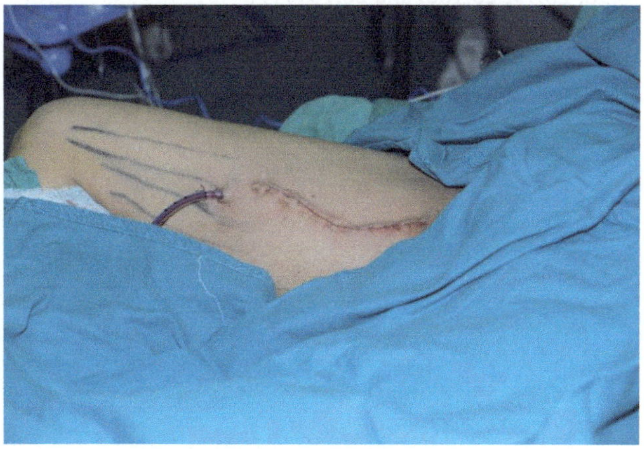

Fig. 20.94 Direct closure of the flap donor area

20.19 Typical Case 17: Chimeric Adductor Major Myocutaneous Flap

The patient is in supine position with knee flexion. Draw a line from the perineum to the distal interface of the semitendinosus muscle. This line represents the midline of the adductor major, and the perforator of the posteromedial thigh flap occurs about 8–10 cm away from the inguinal fold. The position of perforating vessels have been determined by hand-held Doppler detector before operation. For defects with width $\leq$ 7 cm and length $\leq$ 15 cm, the posteromedial flap can be designed laterally with the perforator set at the center. The anterior edge of the flap should not extend to the front of the adductor longus, where the anterior edge of the skin is supplied by different blood vessels. After reaching and separating to the deep fascia, the inferior skin edge of the flap was cut. The following two muscle intervals must be determined: the space between gracilis and adductor major and the space between adductor major and semimembranosus. First, conduct exploratory surgery at anterosuperior region. The rest of the flap remained intact. The flap was dissected at the fascia layer until it reached the muscular septum between gracilis and adductor major, and the perforator branch was further explored at this interval. If the perforator is not found, the interval will be opened and the deep fascia of adductor major dissected to search for the perforator. Attention should be paid when finding the septal perforator between the adductor major and semimembranosus muscles. When a fairly large perforator is found, retrograde dissection will be conducted. The branches should be carefully ligated during muscle dissection. Continue to dissect the perforator until the desired length is reached. Most of the perforating vessels of the adductor major in the clinic penetrate from behind the gracilis muscle, so the gracilis muscle can be simply pulled forward to prepare the chimeric adductor major myocutaneous flap behind it (Figs. 20.95, 20.96, 20.97, 20.98, 20.99, 20.100, and 20.101) [7].

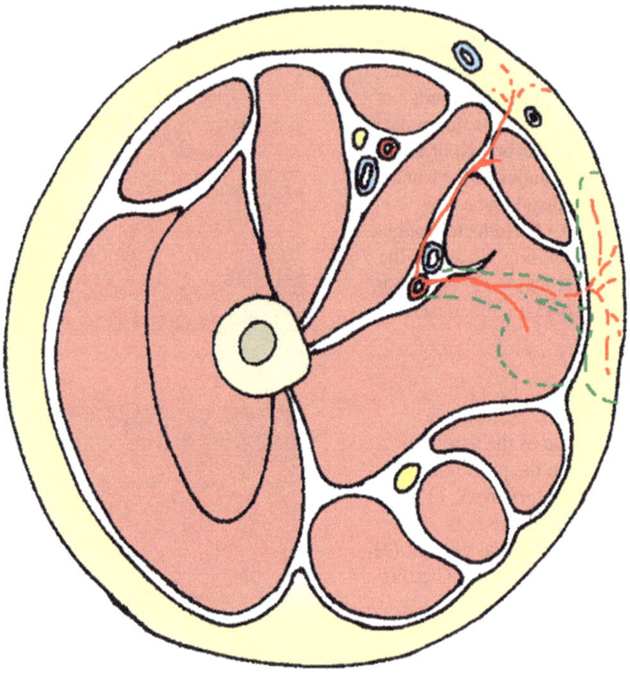

Fig. 20.95 Schematic diagram of the resection of the musculocutaneous flap pedicled with the profunda femoral artery with musculocutaneous branch of the adductor major

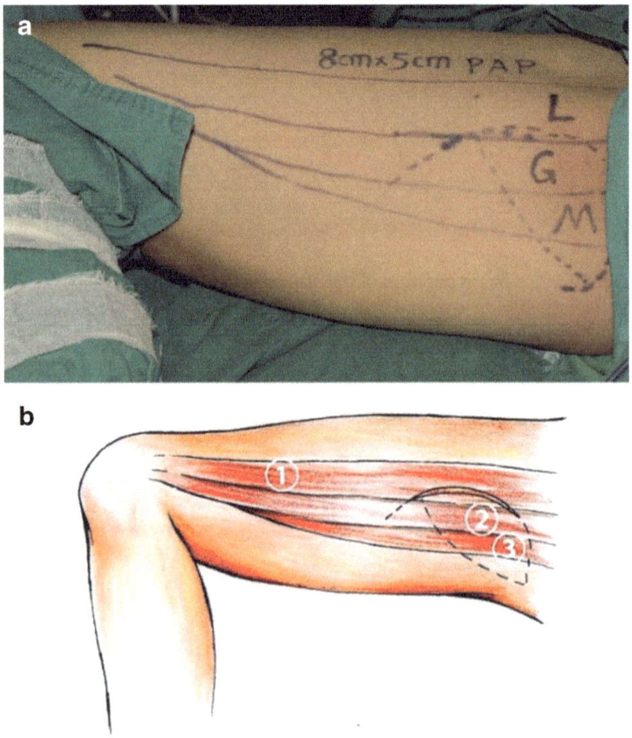

Fig. 20.96 Design of the medial femoral chimeric myocutaneous flap. (1) Adductor longus. (2) Gracilis muscle. (3) Adductor major

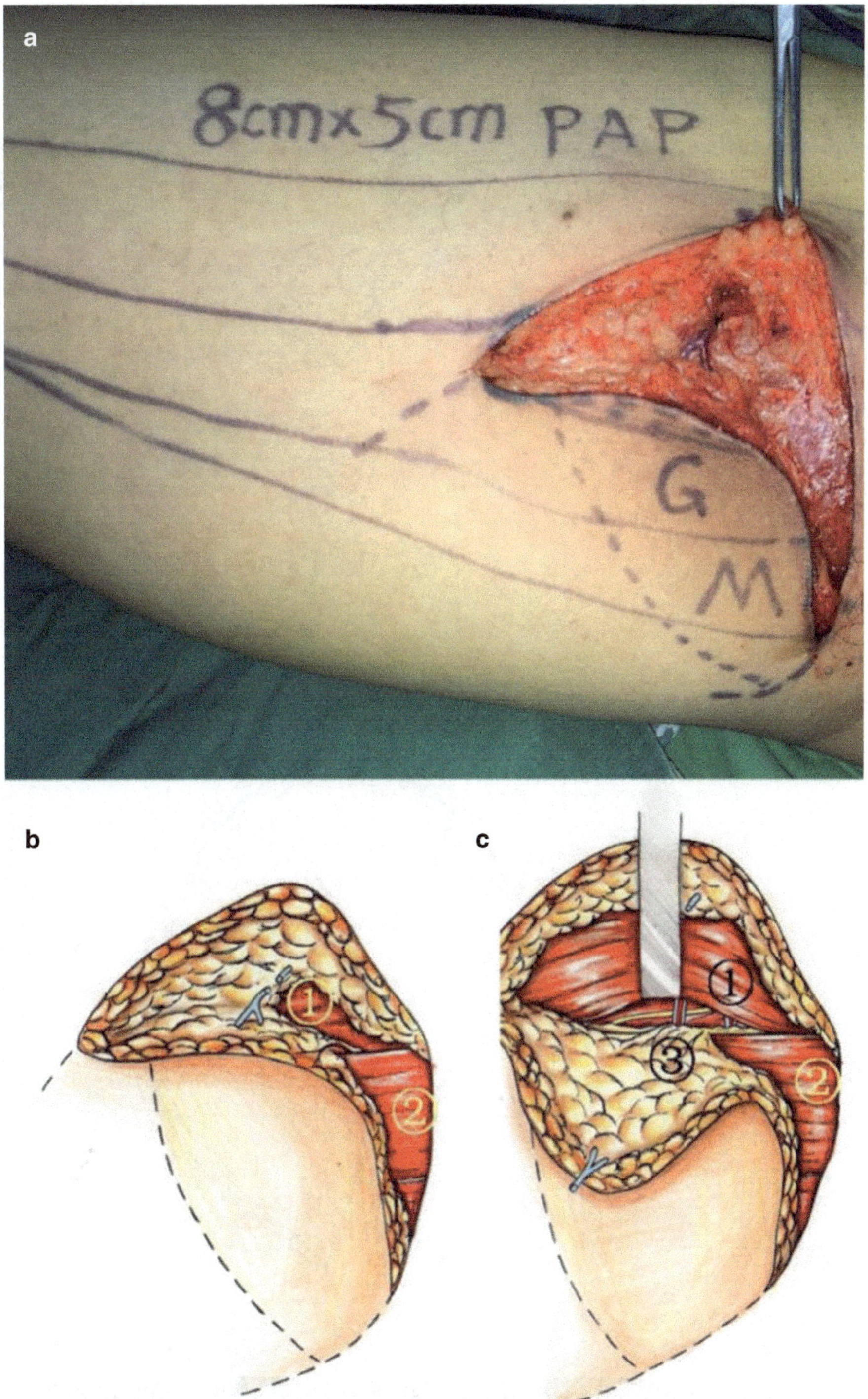

Fig. 20.97 Showing two small perforating vessels between the adductor longus and gracilis. (1) Adductor longus. (2) Gracilis muscle. (3) Perforating vessels

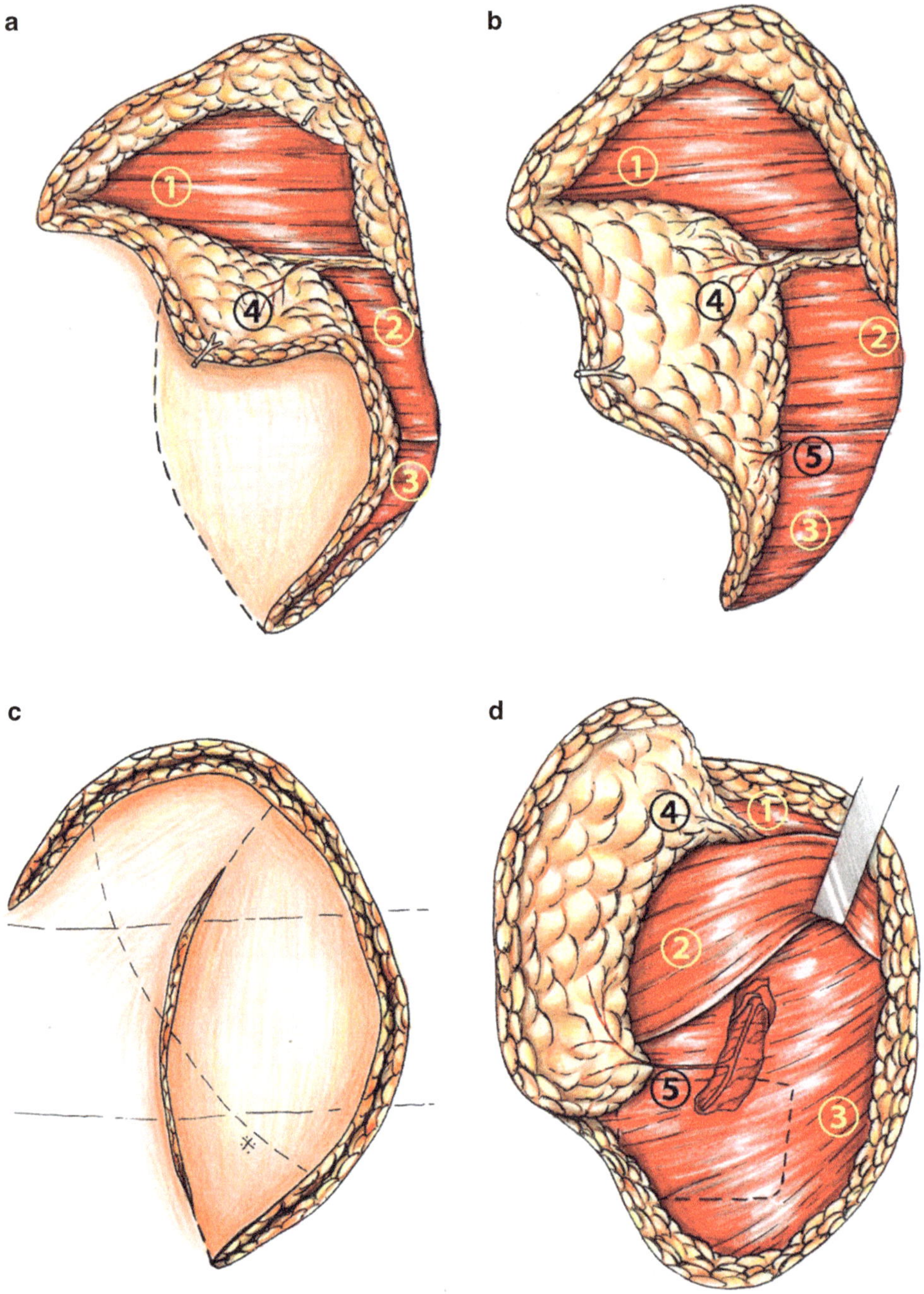

Fig. 20.98 Further separate and expose two thick vascular pedicles, extend the exploration incision, and further expose a thicker perforator on the surface of the adductor major. The flap was re-designed and the whole edge of the flap was cut. The adductor major myocutaneous flap was dissected. The perforating branch of adductor magnus was separated retrogradely to the plane of profunda femoral vessels. (1) Adductor longus. (2) Gracilis muscle. (3) Adductor major. (4) Perforating vessels of the gracilis muscle. (5) Adductor major perforator vessel

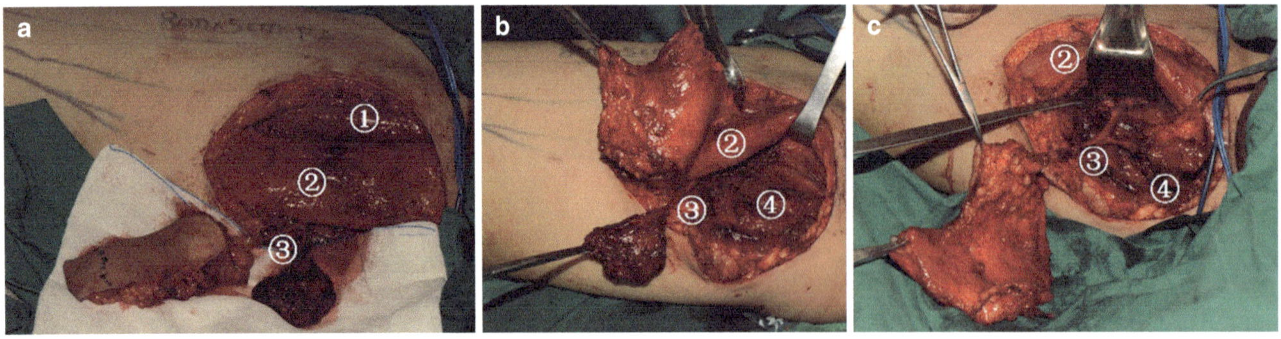

Fig. 20.99 Retrograde separation of the vascular pedicle of the chimeric myocutaneous flap. (1) Adductor longus. (2) Gracilis muscle. (3) Vascular pedicle. (4) Adductor major

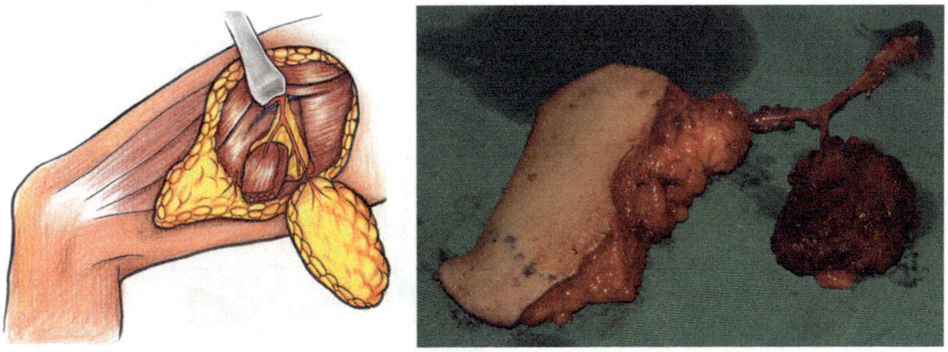

Fig. 20.100 The profunda femoral artery pedicled chimeric adductor magnus myocutaneous flap was separated

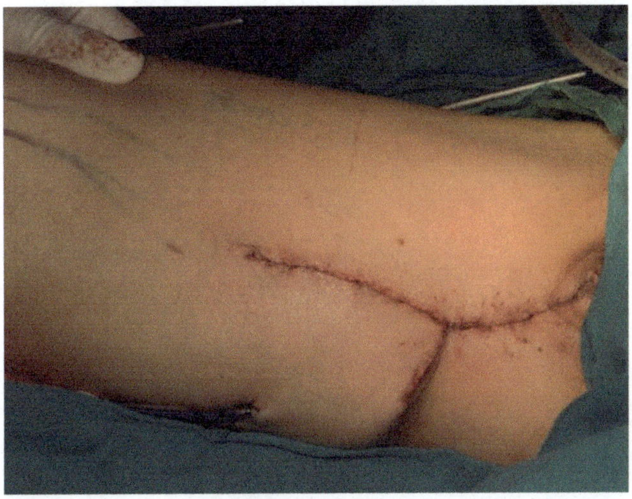

Fig. 20.101 Direct closure of the donor area of the posteromedial femoral flap by advancing the local flap

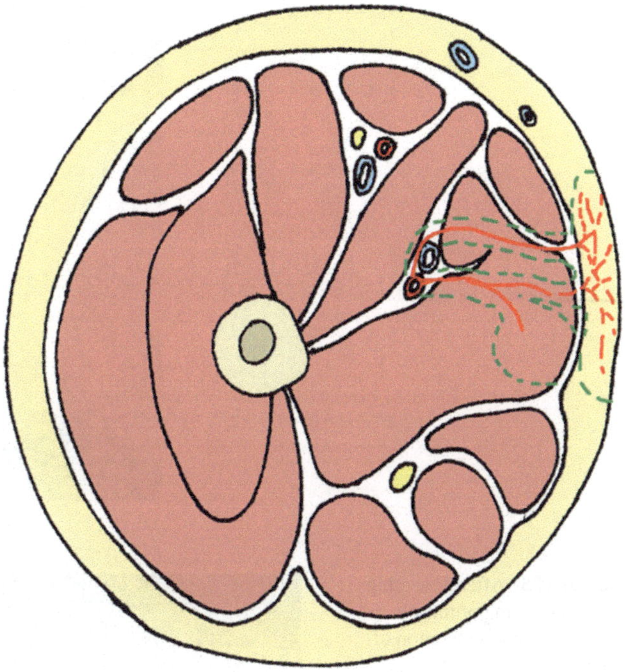

Fig. 20.102 A multi-vessel pedicled chimeric adductor major perforator flap is dissected according to different adductor major perforators. Supercharging can be used to ensure the blood supply of the flap for different vascular pedicles

20.20 Typical Case 18: Supercharged Adductor Major Perforator Myocutaneous Flap

The concept of supercharging has been introduced in detail in the chapter of the perforator flap of the inferior abdominal artery. This technology is also applicable to the flap in the posteromedial region of thigh. According to anatomical research, the number of perforator vessels in the posteromedial region of thigh is more than that in the anterolateral region of thigh. Different perforator vessels can be freely combined to provide better blood supply for the flap (Figs. 20.102, 20.103, 20.104, 20.105, 20.106, and 20.107) [29].

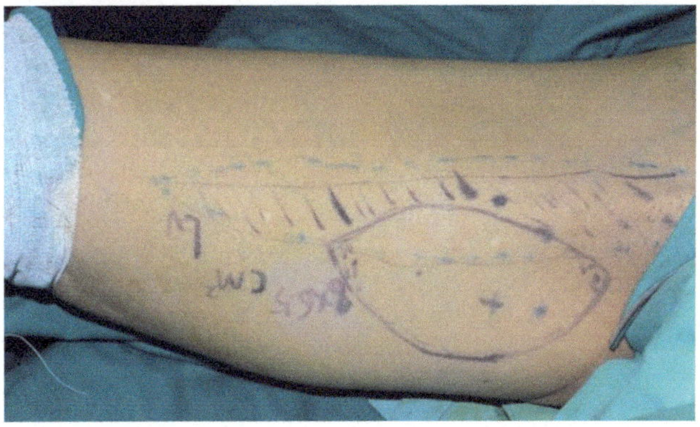

Fig. 20.103 Design of the medial femoral perforator myocutaneous flap

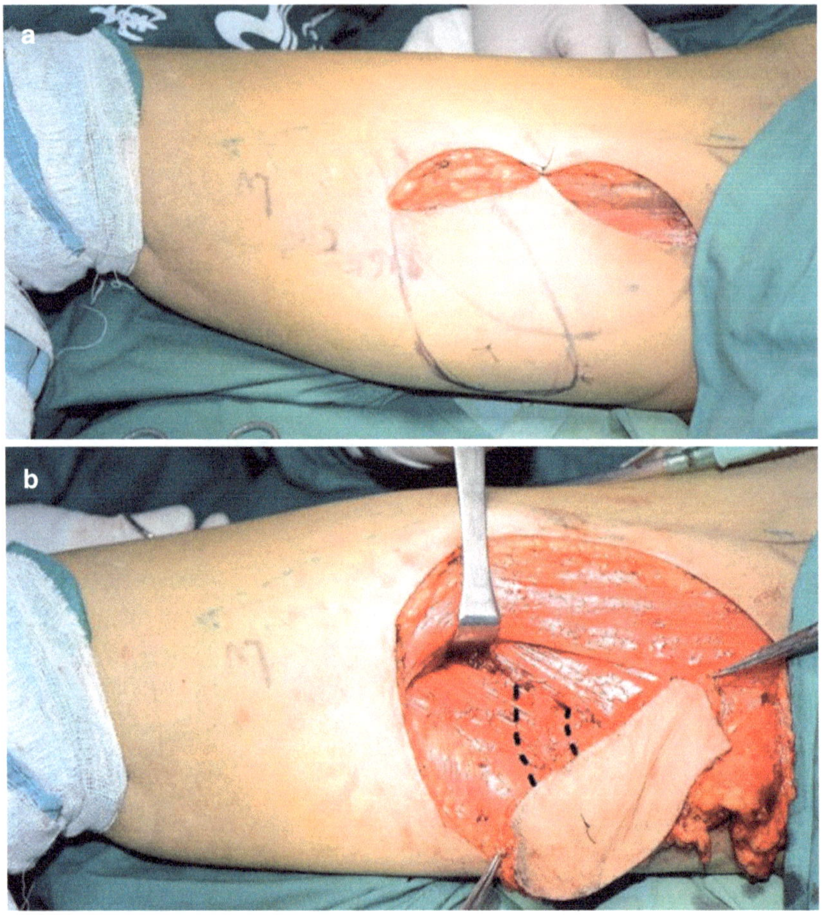

Fig. 20.104 It was found that the perforating vessels came from the posterior edge of the gracilis and the surface of the adductor major. The flap design was modified, the flap was dissected, and the vascular pedicle was separated retrogradely

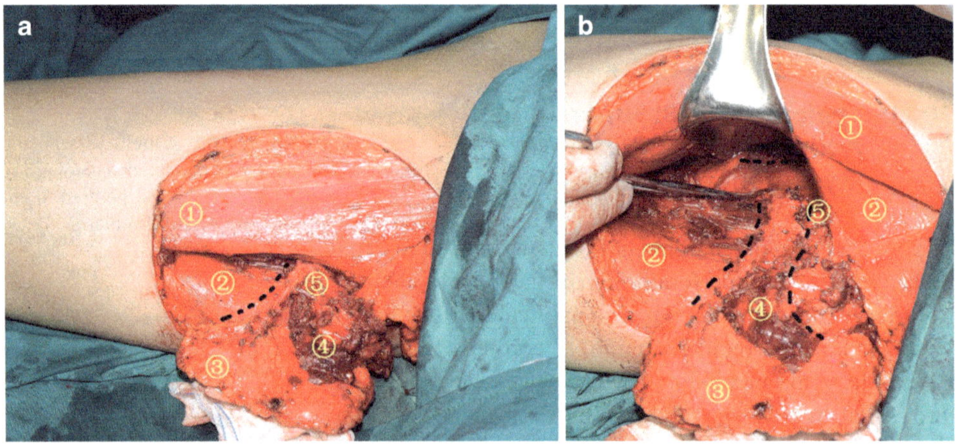

Fig. 20.105 After dissecting the adductor major muscle flap, retrograde separation of the vascular pedicle to the level of profunda femoral vessels was conducted. (1) Gracilis muscle. (2) Adductor major. (3) Flap. (4) Adductor major flap. (5) Vascular pedicle of the muscular branch of the adductor major

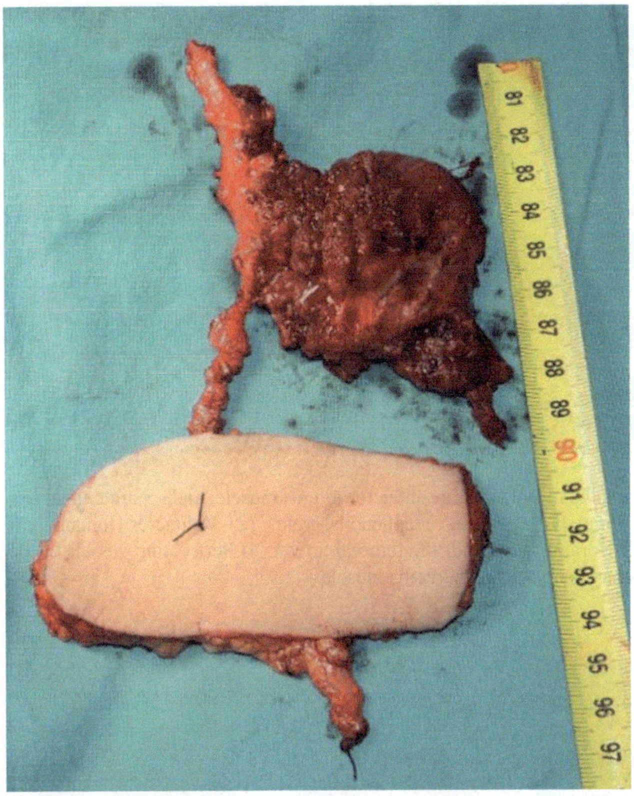

Fig. 20.106 The profunda femoral artery pedicled adductor major chimeric myocutaneous flap was dissected, carrying two perforating vessels of the adductor major at the same time which supercharging the vascularization of the flap

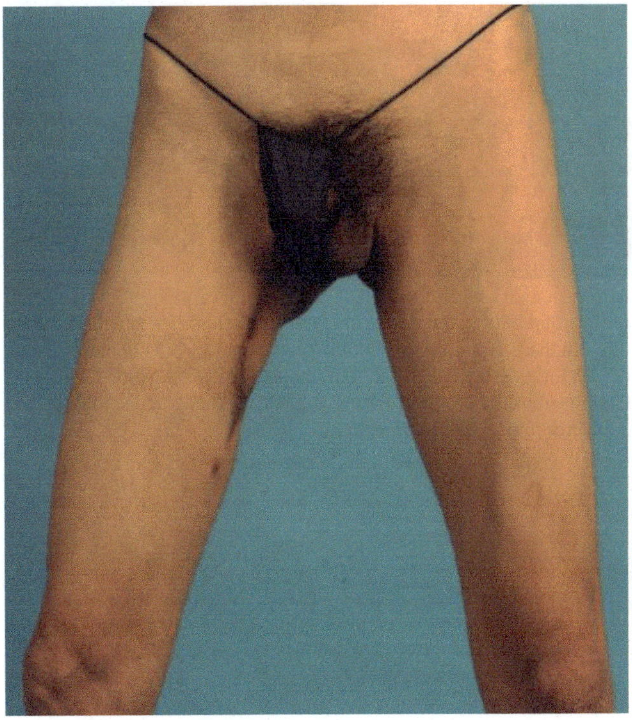

Fig. 20.107 The donor area of the flap was closed directly, and the appearance was presented 1 year after operation

20.21 Typical Case 19: Supercharged Chimeric Adductor Major Myocutaneous Flap

The most common perforating branch of the great adductor muscle arises from behind the gracilis muscle and passes over the surface of the great adductor muscle. However, the perforating branch vessels on the surface of the gracilis muscle can also be exposed in front of the flap during the exploration and separation, which can be carried together for the supercharging of the flap. With an increased number of vessels carried by vascular pedicles, the dissection methods and the design of chimeric myocutaneous flap can be extend further (Figs. 20.108, 20.109, 20.110, 20.111, 20.112, and 20.113) [32–35].

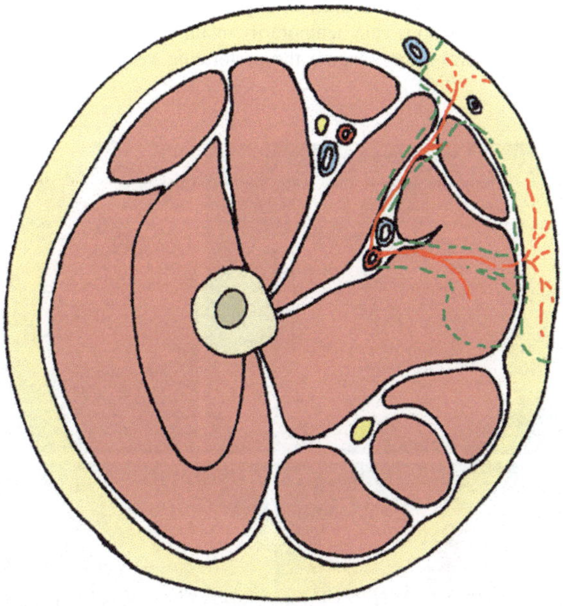

Fig. 20.108 Dissect the conjoined posterior medial femoral perforator flap with the perforator of the gracilis and adductor major from the profunda femoral artery to ensure the blood supply of the flap by supercharging

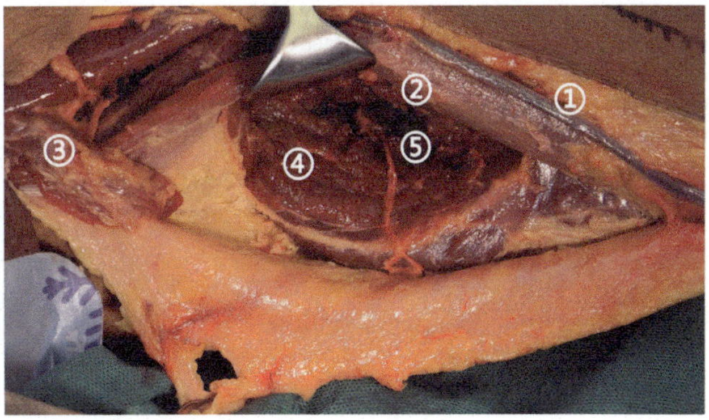

Fig. 20.109 The coarsest perforator from the profunda femoral artery often crosses through the adductor magnus into the skin. (1) Great saphenous vein. (2, 3) Gracilis muscle. (4) Adductor major. (5) Perforating branch of the profunda femoral artery

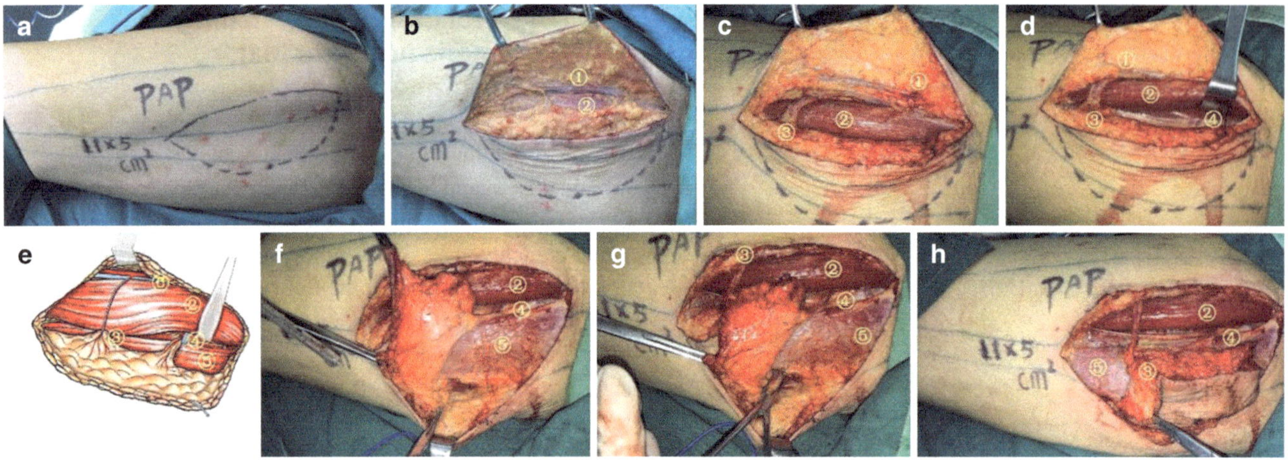

Fig. 20.110 A medial femoral chimeric myocutaneous flap was designed. Lift the flap from anterior to posterior, preserve the integrity of the great saphenous vein, temporarily retain the perforating vessels from the femoral artery, expose the perforating vessels between the gracilis muscle and the adductor longus muscle, and separate them retrogradely. (1) Great saphenous vein. (2) Adductor longus. (3) Perforating branch of the femoral artery. (4) Perforating vessels of the gracilis muscle. (5) Gracilis muscle

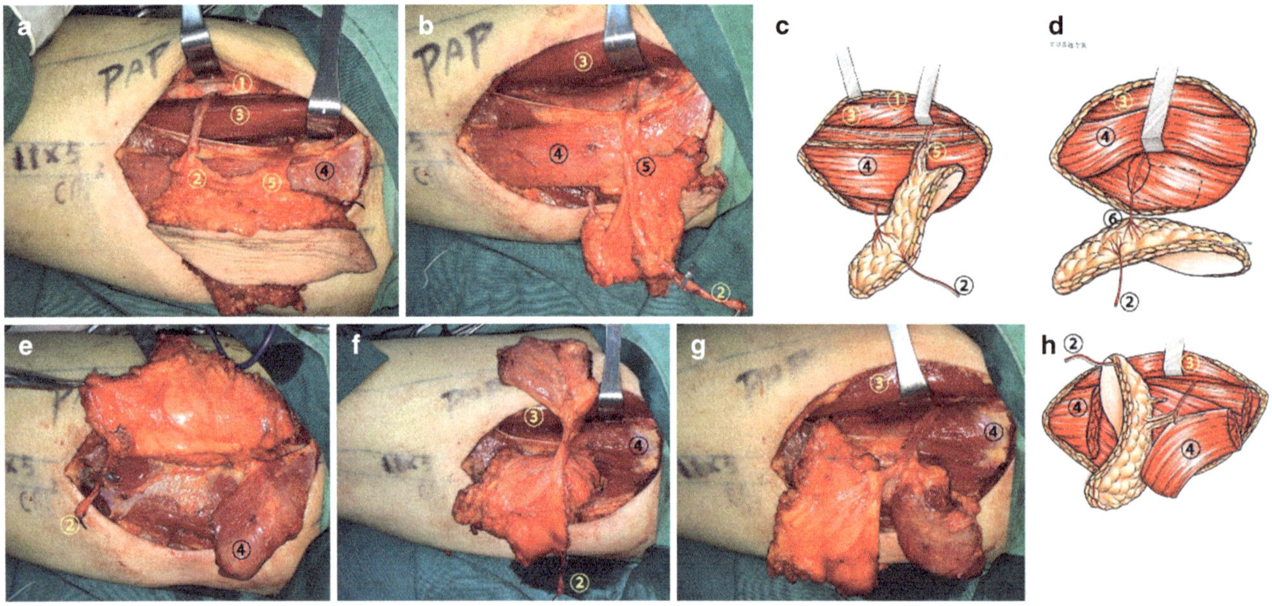

Fig. 20.111 Further separate the flap to its posterior edge to expose a perforator vessel arising from the surface of the great adductor muscle. After the confirming that the blood supply of the flap was safe by clamping experiment, ligate the perforator of the femoral artery and the perforator vessel of the great adductor muscle, and cut off the gracilis muscle flap. So far, the chimeric gracilis muscle flap was pedicled only through the perforator vessel of the gracilis muscle. (1) Femoral artery. (2) Perforating branch of the femoral artery. (3) Adductor longus. (4) Gracilis muscle. (5) Perforating branch of the gracilis muscle. (6) Adductor major perforator vessel

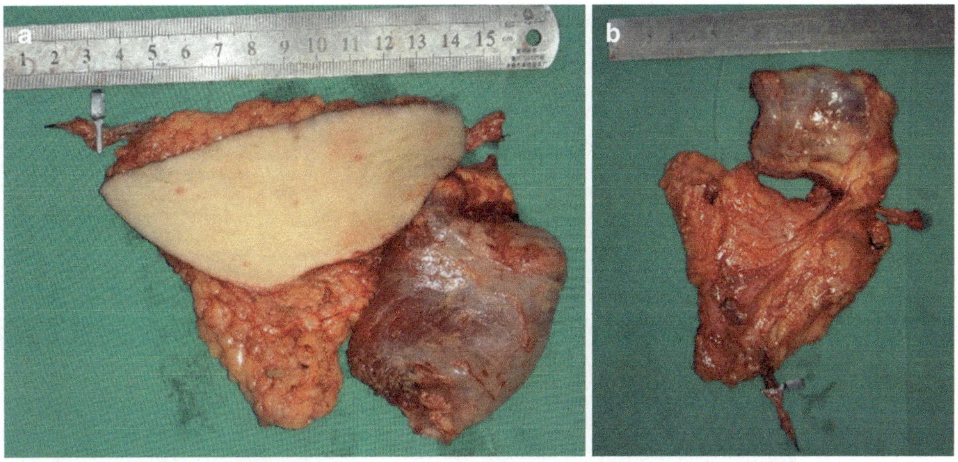

Fig. 20.112 The profunda femoral artery pedicled gracilis perforator myocutaneous flap was dissected

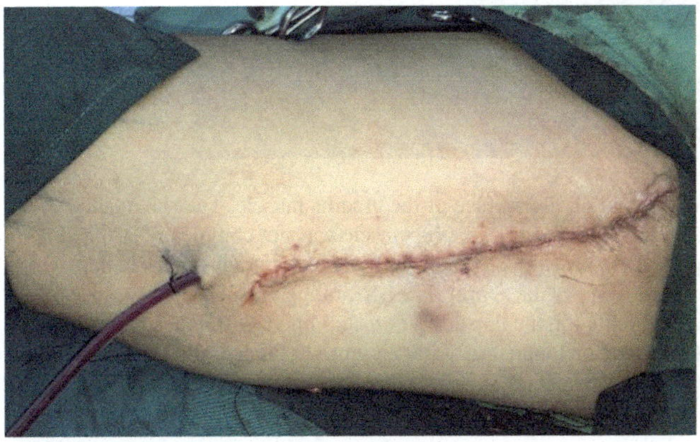

Fig. 20.113 Direct closure of the flap donor area

20.22 Typical Case 20: Supercharged Dual-Perforator Pedicled Adductor Major Perforator Flap and Donor Area Reconstructed by the Gracilis Myocutaneous Flap in Relay

The posterior thigh tissue is horizontally connected with iliotibial tract and adductor group, and is adjacent to gluteal sulcus and popliteal fossa in vertical direction. The profunda femoral artery usually sends out three main perforating branches after entering the inter-tissue space of the posterior thigh. The first perforating branch supplies the adductor magnus and gracilis, and the second and third perforating branches supply the semimembranosus muscle, biceps femoris, and lateral femoral muscle [15].

According to our previous experience and literature reports, the exploration of the posterior medial femoral perforator vessels often follows the direction from the anterosuperior to the posteroinferior. When the position of the perforator vessels is relatively low, the exploration flap should be further lifted. After dissecting the perforator flap, the exploration flap can be transferred and repaired in the form of muscle flap, rotary flap, or island flap.

In this typical case, no thick perforating vessels were found on the surface of gracilis muscle. Further retrograde exploration found that multiple perforating branches of adductor major could be used to prepare supercharged medial femoral perforating flap, and the donor area was repaired by pedicled gracilis muscle advancement flap (Figs. 20.114, 20.115, 20.116, 20.117, 20.118, and 20.119).

The design of exploratory incision in either horizontal or vertical direction cannot solve the problem of exploring perforators. It is necessary to constantly adjust the exploratory incision to expose and select perforating vessels during operation.

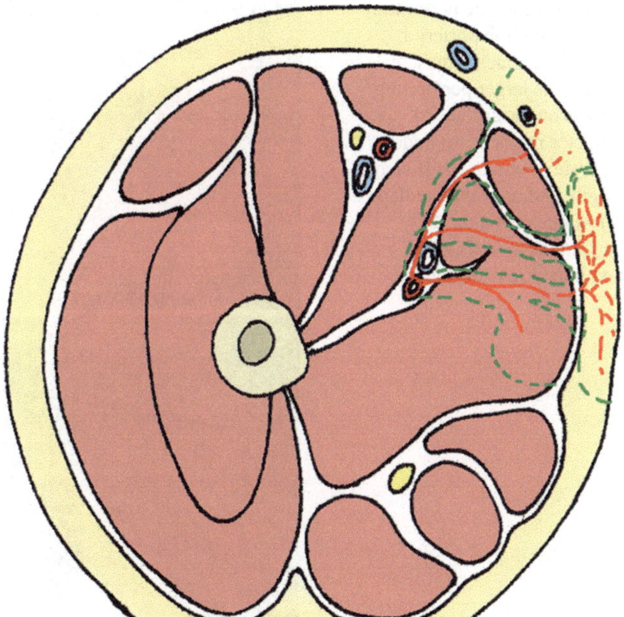

Fig. 20.114 There are many small perforating branches on the surface of gracilis muscle, and there are many perforating branches of the adductor major, which is a common anatomical form in clinic

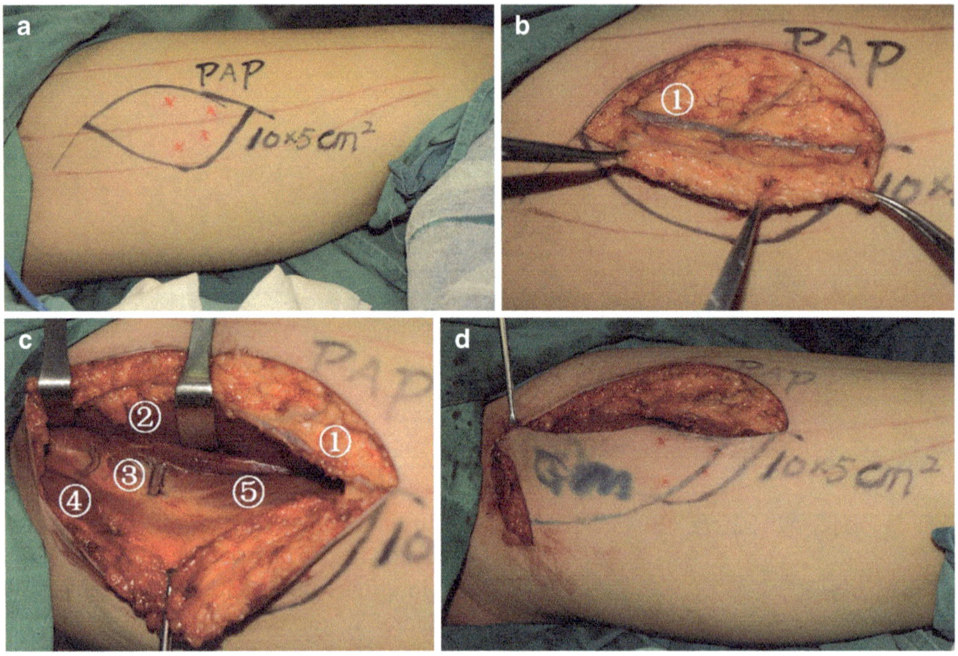

Fig. 20.115 (**a**) Flap design. (**b**) The markings were made by multiple puncture points using Doppler during preoperative exploration, in which the nutrient vessel of the great saphenous vein with thin diameter and short length was confirmed. Therefore, the vessel cannot be used for free flap transplantation. (**c**) No suitable perforator vessel was found at the proximal end of gracilis muscle. Further exploring for the perforator vessel on the deep surface of deep fascia, and no good perforator was found on the surface of the gracilis muscle. The subcutaneous tissue on the surface of gracilis muscle was not completely stripped temporarily to prepare the possibility of making gracilis muscle flap. (**d**) In order to expose the appropriate perforating vessels on the surface of the adductor major, the flap design was modified. (1) Great saphenous vein. (2) Adductor longus. (3) Gracilis muscle branch. (4) Gracilis muscle. (5) Adductor major

Fig. 20.116 Preserve the integrity of the skin island on the surface of gracilis muscle, further explore the perforating vessels from the posterior edge of the gracilis muscle, expose the larger perforating vessels on the surface of adductor major, retrograde separate to obtain a sufficient length, and redesign the flap. (1) Adductor major. (2) Perforating vessels. (3) Semimembranosus muscle

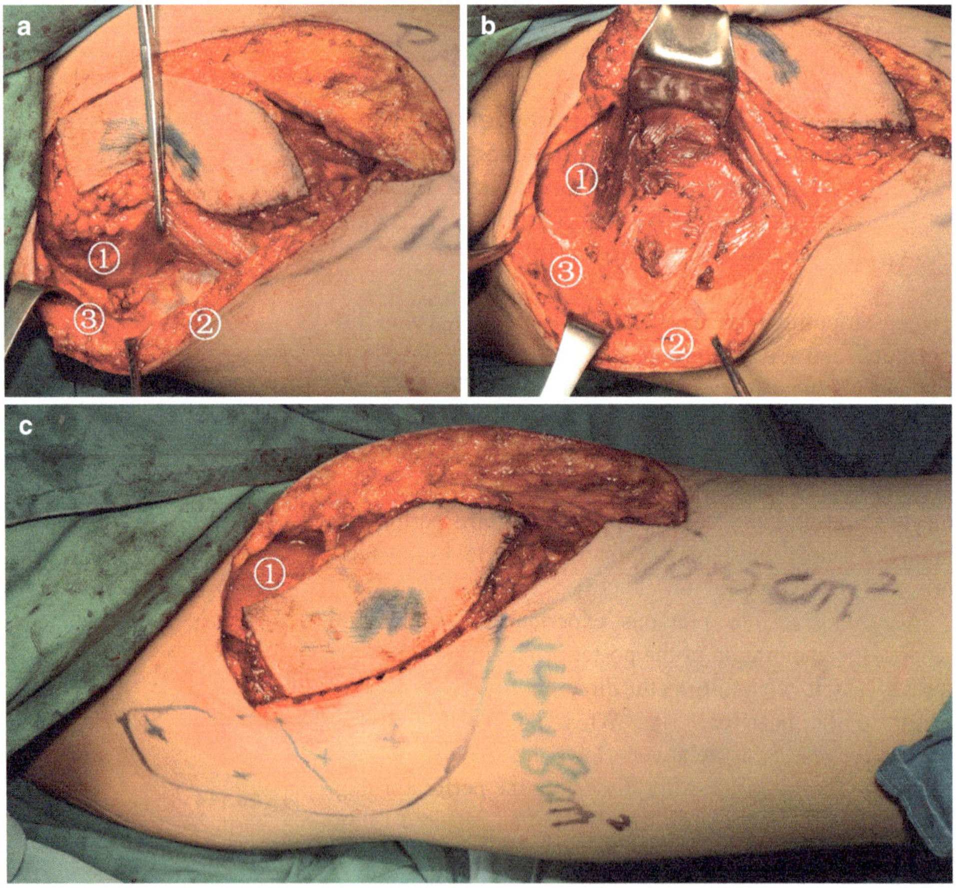

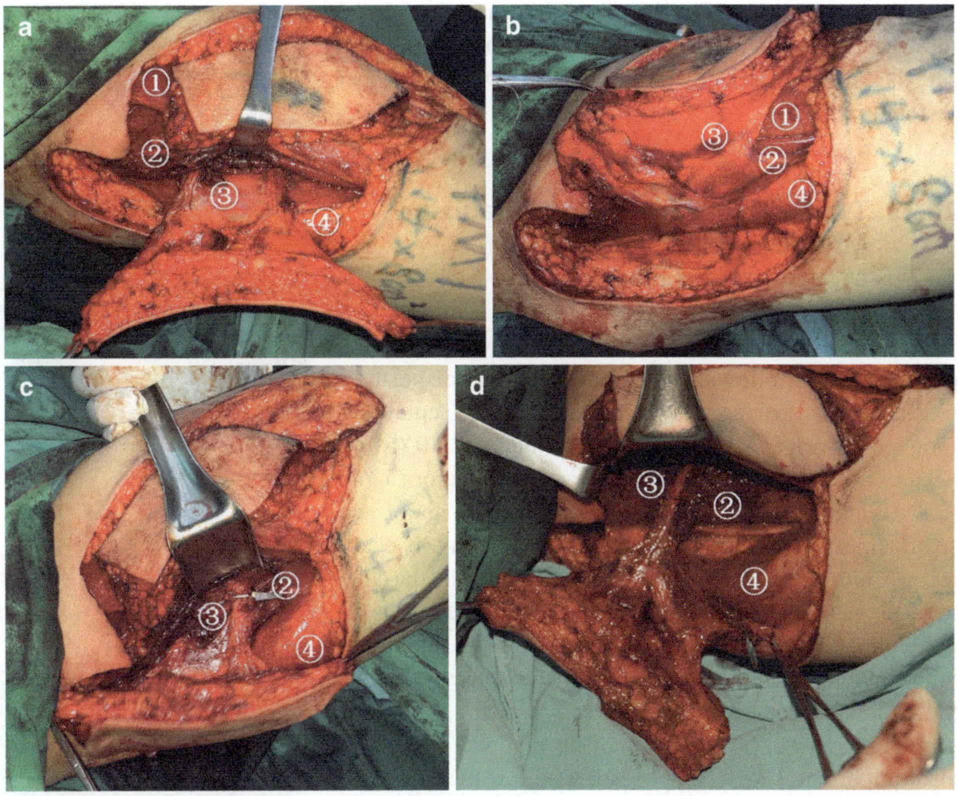

Fig. 20.117 Complete the dissection and preparation of the adductor major perforator flap, and separate the vascular pedicle to the plane of the profunda femoral vessel. (1) Gracilis muscle. (2) Adductor major. (3) Perforating vessels. (4) Semimembranosus muscle

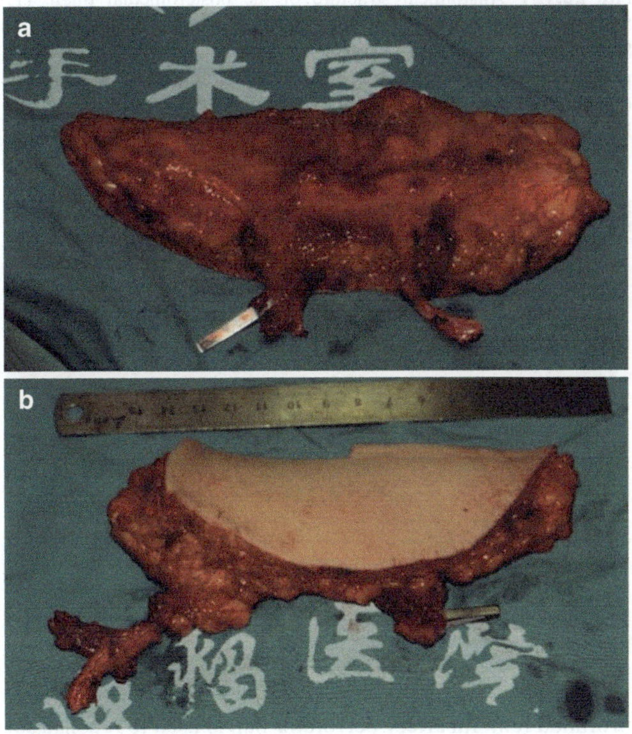

Fig. 20.118 The perforator flap of the adductor major pedicled with bilateral blood vessels was cut off

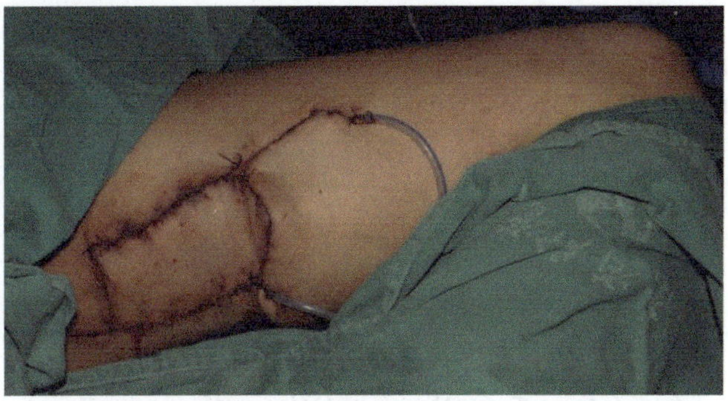

Fig. 20.119 Local advancement and transferring of the gracilis myocutaneous flap to directly close the donor area defect of the adductor major perforator flap

20.22.1 Clinical Thinking

As an alternative, the TUG flap is lifted from the anterior to the proximal without finding a suitable perforator near the frontal edge of the gracilis muscle. Do not rashly separate and explore the perforators on the surface of the gracilis muscle. Dissect the TUG skin island first, and strictly design the rear edge of the skin island to coincide with the rear edge of the gracilis muscle. Pull the skin island forward together with the gracilis muscle, and explore the perforator on the surface of the adductor major. If there is a suitable perforator, cut the PMT. Free tug was removed without proper perforator.

20.23 Typical Case 21: Semimembranosus Muscle Chimeric Perforator Myocutaneous Flap

According to clinical anatomy reports based on foreign population, the following three large patterns of posteromedial femoral perforators were found: (1) the septal perforator between gracilis and adductor major (2/40 (5%)); (2) musculocutaneous perforator of adductor major (32/40 (80%)); and (3) septal perforators of adductor major and semimembranosus muscles (6/40 (15%)) [7]. In this chapter, we introduce the clinical findings in which the anatomical patterns are far more than these three types. In particular, the septal perforator arising from the semimembranosus muscle and the adductor major muscle and the musculocutaneous perforator directly arising from the semimembranosus muscle cannot be ignored, which are also important blood supply sources for the posterior medial perforator flap of the thigh (Figs. 20.120, 20.121, 20.122, 20.123, and 20.124).

In our case, the thickness of the perforator flap of the posterior medial femoral artery of the thigh varied significantly, ranging from 15 to 35 mm [6]. When a thick posteromedial

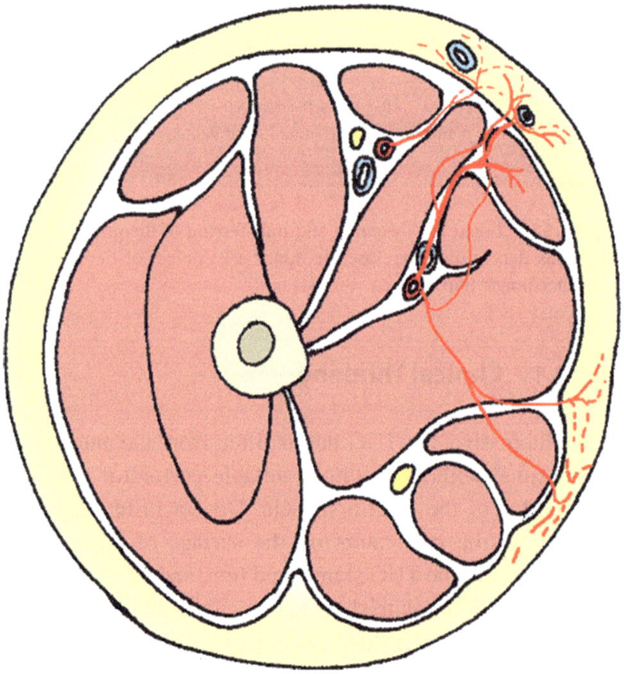

Fig. 20.120 Schematic cross-sectional anatomy of the medial femoral perforator vessel pattern

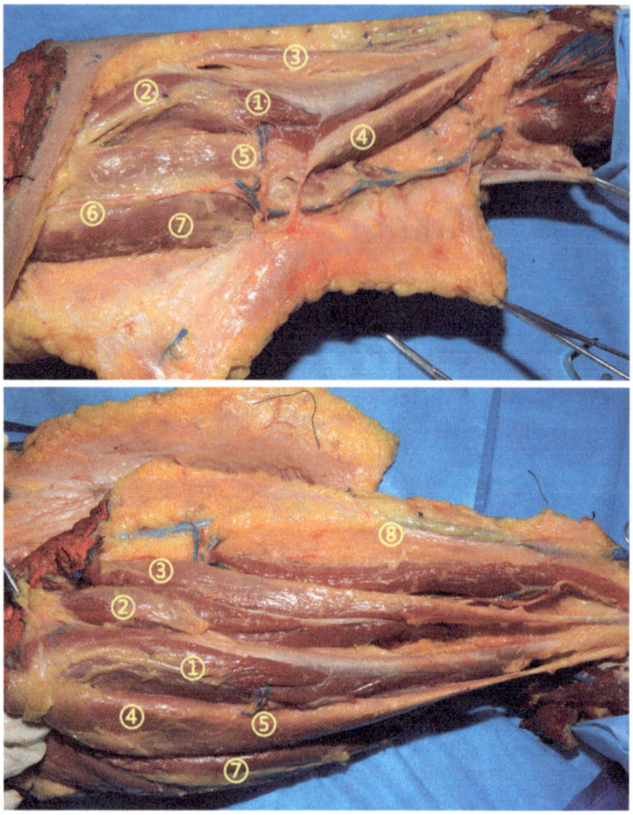

Fig. 20.121 Anatomical structure of the posteromedial thigh. (1) Semimembranosus muscle. (2) Adductor major. (3) Gracilis muscle. (4) Semitendinosus muscle. (5) The musculocutaneous perforator from the profunda femoral artery passing through the semimembranosus muscle. (6) Posterior femoral cutaneous nerve and its nutrient vessels. (7) Biceps femoris. (8) Great saphenous vein

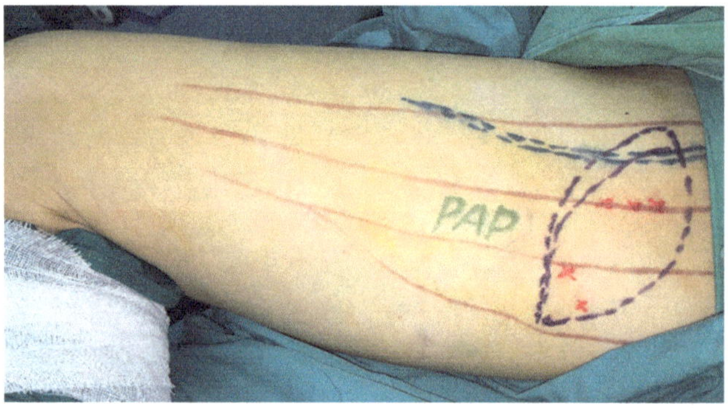

Fig. 20.122 Design of the oblique medial femoral chimeric myocutaneous flap according to the position of perforating vessels detected by preoperative Doppler

profunda femoral artery perforator flap is used to reconstruct the superficial defect, the flap can be trimmed and become thinner, just as we usually perform in the anterolateral femoral perforator flap [37].

Although the donor area of anterolateral femoral flap is rarely grafted, the lateral thigh often has a looser skin mobil-

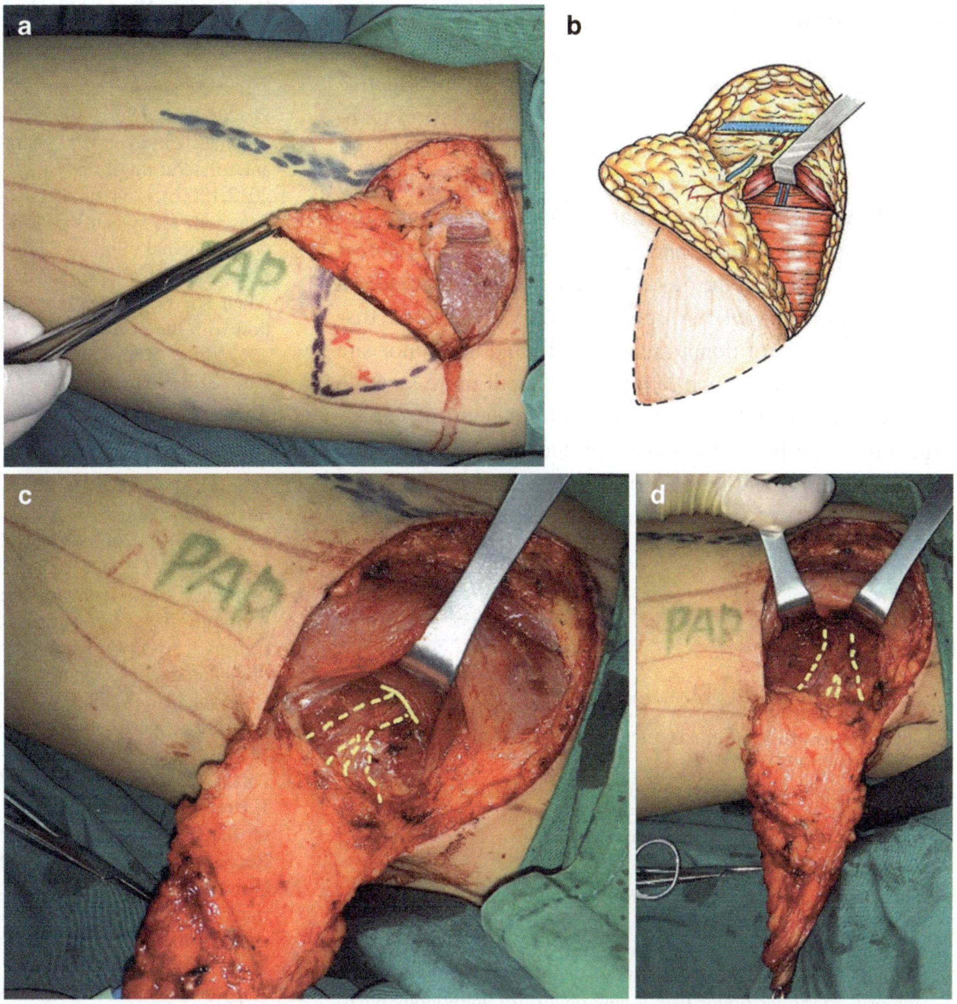

Fig. 20.123 Lift the flap from the anterior to the posterior to separate the great saphenous vein. Only perforating vessel in front of the flap was sent from the nutrient vessel of the great saphenous vein which cannot be used. We then switched to continue to separate to the posterior region. Two thicker perforating vessels were sent out behind the adductor megacephalus, and further retrograde separation was determined that the perforating vessels traveled in the long segment of the semimembranosus muscle

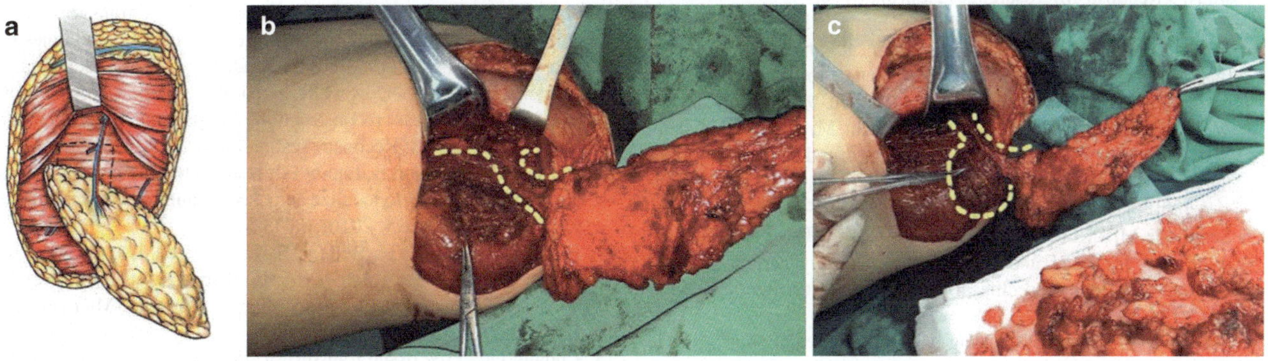

Fig. 20.124 Dissect the hemimembranous muscle chimeric myocutaneous flap pedicled with profunda femoral artery, and properly trim the flap according to the needs of the recipient area

ity, and a wider flap can be easily closed. So far, the largest flap we have cut is 9 cm in width. The donor site of this flap was primarily closed without dehiscence, which fully proved the excellent ductility of the skin and soft tissue of the posterior medial thigh. The flap boundary is not clearly defined. If the flap exceeds the perforator vessel body area, it may lead to partial necrosis of the flap. The size limit of flap is not defined at present. The largest flap we measured was 25 cm × 9 cm, while the donor site injury did not increase significantly.

20.24 Conclusion

In general, the posteromedial femoral flap is an effective supplement to our choice of free flap transplantation techniques. It cannot replace the major roles played by anterolateral thigh flap and perforator flap of inferior abdominal artery. However, we believe that for the soft tissue reconstruction of limbs, head, and neck, and even trunk defect breast reconstruction, the posteromedial thigh flap provides a favorable choice based on vascular anatomy. It is easy to dissect. The damage of donor area is small, and the donor site scar is hidden. Its soft and rich tissue make it more suitable for breast reconstruction than anterolateral femoral flap. A large number of literatures have introduced the anatomy and skin blood supply of these perforating branches in detail. We should be aware of the significance of expanding their further clinical application.

References

1. Mayo JL, Canizares O, Torabi R, Allen RJ, St HH. Expanding the applications of the profunda artery perforator flap. Plast Reconstr Surg. 2016;137(2):663–9.
2. Ahmadzadeh R, Bergeron L, Tang M, Geddes CR, Morris SF. The posterior thigh perforator flap or profunda femoris artery perforator flap. Plast Reconstr Surg. 2007;119(1):194–200; discussion 201–2.
3. Hurwitz ZM, Montilla R, Dunn RM, Patel NV, Akyurek M. Adductor magnus perforator flap revisited: an anatomical review and clinical applications. Ann Plast Surg. 2011;66(5):438–43.
4. Saad A, Sadeghi A, Allen RJ. The anatomic basis of the profunda femoris artery perforator flap: a new option for autologous breast reconstruction—a cadaveric and computer tomography angiogram study. J Reconstr Microsurg. 2012;28(6):381–6.
5. DeLong MR, Hughes DB, Bond JE, Thomas SM, Boll DT, Zenn MR. A detailed evaluation of the anatomical variations of the profunda artery perforator flap using computed tomographic angiograms. Plast Reconstr Surg. 2014;134(2):186e–92e.
6. Wu JC, Huang JJ, Tsao CK, Abdelrahman M, Kolios G, Cheng MH. Comparison of posteromedial thigh profunda artery perforator flap and anterolateral thigh perforator flap for head and neck reconstruction. Plast Reconstr Surg. 2016;137(1):257–66.
7. Scaglioni MF, Kuo YR, Yang JC, Chen YC. The posteromedial thigh flap for head and neck reconstruction: anatomical basis, surgical technique, and clinical applications. Plast Reconstr Surg. 2015;136(2):363–75.
8. Scaglioni MF, Chen YC, Yang JC. Posteromedial thigh (PMT) propeller flap for perineoscrotal reconstruction: a case report. Microsurgery. 2015;35(7):569–72.
9. Scaglioni MF, Enrique CJL, Kuo YR, Chen YC. Pedicled posteromedial thigh (PMT) flap: a new alternative for groin defect reconstruction. Microsurgery. 2017;37(4):339–43.
10. Wei FC, Jain V, Celik N, Chen HC, Chuang DC, Lin CH. Have we found an ideal soft-tissue flap? An experience with 672 anterolateral thigh flaps. Plast Reconstr Surg. 2002;109(7):2219–26; discussion 2227–30.
11. Song YG, Chen GZ, Song YL. The free thigh flap: a new free flap concept based on the septocutaneous artery. Br J Plast Surg. 1984;37(2):149–59.
12. Koshima I, Yamamoto H, Hosoda M, Moriguchi T, Orita Y, Nagayama H. Free combined composite flaps using the lateral circumflex femoral system for repair of massive defects of the head and neck regions: an introduction to the chimeric flap principle. Plast Reconstr Surg. 1993;92(3):411–20.
13. Lakhiani C, Lee MR, Saint-Cyr M. Vascular anatomy of the anterolateral thigh flap: a systematic review. Plast Reconstr Surg. 2012;130(6):1254–68.
14. Scaglioni MF, Chen YC, Lindenblatt N, Giovanoli P. The vertical posteromedial thigh (vPMT) flap for autologous breast reconstruction: a novel flap design. Microsurgery. 2017;37(5):371–6.
15. Allen RJ, Haddock NT, Ahn CY, Sadeghi A. Breast reconstruction with the profunda artery perforator flap. Plast Reconstr Surg. 2012;129(1):16e–23e.
16. Park JE, Alkureishi LW, Song DH. TUGs into VUGs and friendly BUGs: transforming the Gracilis territory into the best secondary breast reconstructive option. Plast Reconstr Surg. 2015;136(3):447–54.
17. Angrigiani C, Grilli D, Thorne CH. The adductor flap: a new method for transferring posterior and medial thigh skin. Plast Reconstr Surg. 2001;107(7):1725–31.
18. Haddock NT, Greaney P, Otterburn D, Levine S, Allen RJ. Predicting perforator location on preoperative imaging for the profunda artery perforator flap. Microsurgery. 2012;32(7):507–11.
19. Collins J, Ayeni O, Thoma A. A systematic review of anterolateral thigh flap donor site morbidity. Can J Plast Surg. 2012;20(1):17–23.
20. Ratanshi I, McInnes CW, Islur A. The proximal superficial femoral artery perforator flap: anatomic study and clinical cases. Microsurgery. 2017;37(6):581–8.
21. Satake T, Muto M, Ko S, Yasumura K, Ishikawa T, Maegawa J. Breast reconstruction using free posterior medial thigh perforator flaps: intraoperative anatomical study and clinical results. Plast Reconstr Surg. 2014;134(5):880–91.
22. Fansa H, Schirmer S, Warnecke IC, Cervelli A, Frerichs O. The transverse myocutaneous gracilis muscle flap: a fast and reliable method for breast reconstruction. Plast Reconstr Surg. 2008;122(5):1326–33.
23. Kappler UA, Constantinescu MA, Büchler U, Vögelin E. Anatomy of the proximal cutaneous perforator vessels of the gracilis muscle. Br J Plast Surg. 2005;58(4):445–8.
24. Schoeller T, Huemer GM, Wechselberger G. The transverse musculocutaneous gracilis flap for breast reconstruction: guidelines for flap and patient selection. Plast Reconstr Surg. 2008;122(1):29–38.
25. Hunter JE, Lardi AM, Dower DR, Farhadi J. Evolution from the TUG to PAP flap for breast reconstruction: comparison and refinements of technique. J Plast Reconstr Aesthet Surg. 2015;68(7):960–5.
26. Hupkens P, Van Loon B, Lauret GJ, et al. Anteromedial thigh flaps: an anatomical study to localize and classify anteromedial thigh perforators. Microsurgery. 2010;30(1):43–9.
27. Hupkens P, Ozturk E, Wittens S, Hoevenaren IA, Kooloos JG, Ulrich DJ. Posterior thigh perforator flaps: an anatomical study to localize and classify posterior thigh perforators. Microsurgery. 2013;33(5):376–82.
28. Chuang DC. Free tissue transfer for the treatment of facial paralysis. Facial Plast Surg. 2008;24(2):194–203.
29. Hunter JE, Mackey SP, Boca R, Harris PA. Microvascular modifications to optimize the transverse upper gracilis flap for breast reconstruction. Plast Reconstr Surg. 2014;133(6):1315–25.
30. Hupkens P, Westland PB, Ulrich DJO. The combined transverse upper gracilis and profunda artery perforator flap for breast reconstruction-letter to the editor. Ann Plast Surg. 2017;79(1):124–5.
31. Lakhiani C, DeFazio MV, Han K, Falola R, Evans K. Donor-site morbidity following free tissue harvest from the thigh: a systematic review and pooled analysis of complications. J Reconstr Microsurg. 2016;32(5):342–57.

32. Dajiang Song, Zan Li, Xiao Zhou. Clinical application of free medial femoral chimeric perforator myocutaneous flap in the repair of postoperative defect of tongue cancer in the repair of defects after tongue cancer surgery. Chin J Otorhinolaryngol Head Neck Surg2017. 52(4): 278–282.
33. Song D, Li Z, Zhou X. Observation of curative effect of different forms of free profunda femoral artery pedicle chimeric perforator myocutaneous flap in the repair of defects after tongue cancer surgery. Chin J Reparat Reconstr Surg. 2017;31(06):696–701.
34. Song D, Li Z, Zhou X. Free profunda femoral artery pedicled gracilis chimeric musculocutaneous perforator flap for repair of defects after oral and buccal cancer surgery. Chin J Plast Surg. 2017;33(4):242–7.
35. Dajiang Song, Zan Li, Xiao Zhou. Application of profunda femoral artery perforator flap in breast reconstruction. Chin J Plast Surg 2017. (6): 412–416.
36. Ito R, Huang JJ, Wu JC, Lin MC, Cheng MH. The versatility of profunda femoral artery perforator flap for oncological reconstruction after cancer resection—clinical cases and review of literature. J Surg Oncol. 2016;114(2):193–201.
37. Kimura N, Satoh K, Hasumi T, Ostuka T. Clinical application of the free thin anterolateral thigh flap in 31 consecutive patients. Plast Reconstr Surg. 2001;108(5):1197–208; discussion 1209–10.

21 Transverse Gracilis Musculocutaneous Flap for Breast Reconstruction

Dajiang Song and Narushima Mitsunaga

At present, there are many options for breast reconstruction. Autologous tissue transfer includes transverse rectus abdominis myocutaneous flap, latissimus dorsi myocutaneous flap, inferior abdominal artery perforator flap, superior gluteal artery perforator flap, inferior gluteal artery perforator flap, and lumbar artery perforator flap.

Transverse gracilis myocutaneous flap (TMG) has been widely used in Europe and America because of many advantages, but it has not been universally adopted in China [1, 2].

The advantages of TMG include reliable vascular anatomy, shorter operation times due to simpler anatomy compared with other flaps, no reposition of the patient during operation, and less function loss. Also, the donor tissue of TMG is generally loose and therefore easy for skin suture [3].

However, the disadvantage of TMG for autologous breast reconstruction is its small volume. Therefore, it is only applicable to small-to-moderate breast reconstruction or partial breast reconstruction.

It has also been reported that there were some surgical refinements to increase the volume of TMG. The methods are mainly to obtain the flap from a more posterior position, that is, to design and cut the flap from the thicker posterior thigh tissue [1, 4, 5].

In addition, Fattah et al. [5] described a method of immediately dissociating the subcutaneous tissue of the skin and carried as much subcutaneous tissue in the posterior thigh and periphery as possible in the flap.

Peek et al. [6] reported that the vertical expansion of the gracilis perforator flap (the expansion border does not include the gracilis), which is achieved by incorporating the connecting branches between the primary and secondary blood vessels of muscles together, because it can maintain the small perforators of the adjacent blood vessels and expand the cutaneous angiosome of the tissue flap.

Vega et al. added that transverse partial tissue transformed into an L-shaped flap can expand the gracilis myocutaneous flap [7, 8].

According to Schoeller et al., the volume of the gracilis myocutaneous flap ranges from 180 to 550 mL, and the maximum skin island is about 30 cm × 10 cm [4].

Despite the above methods, surgeons still need to expand bilateral gracilis myocutaneous flaps in certain cases for the sufficient volume of tissue required for one-side breast reconstruction [4, 5].

21.1 Applied Anatomy

The posterior thigh tissue is horizontally connected with iliotibial tract and adductors, and vertically adjacent to gluteal sulcus and popliteal fossa.

The size and distribution of all perforating branches on the posterior medial thigh must be fully understood preoperatively.

The internal mammary artery were commonly divided into three main perforating branches after entering the thigh space.

The first perforating branch supplies the adductor major and gracilis, and the second and third perforating branches supply the semimembranosus, biceps femoris, and lateral femoral muscles. The medial perforator of the internal mammary artery usually sends out two branches: medial and lateral. The medial perforator was often chose by the authors.

The medial perforator normally enters the gracilis muscle backward. In some cases, posterior and lateral perforating branches can also be used if these branches are more developed (Fig. 21.1).

The average length and diameter of the vascular pedicle of the main branch from the internal mammary artery entering the gracilis muscle is 6.7 cm and 2.2 mm, and the distance to the pubis is 8.6 cm [9].

D. Song (✉)
Department of Oncology Plastic Surgery, Hunan Cancer Hospital, Changsha, Hunan, China

N. Mitsunaga
Mie University Graduate School of Medicine Plastic and Reconstructive Surgery, Tsu, Mie, Japan
e-mail: sancho-ps@umin.ac.jp

Z. Li, D. Song (eds.), *Oncoplastic Flap Surgery*, https://doi.org/10.1007/978-981-19-8926-1_21

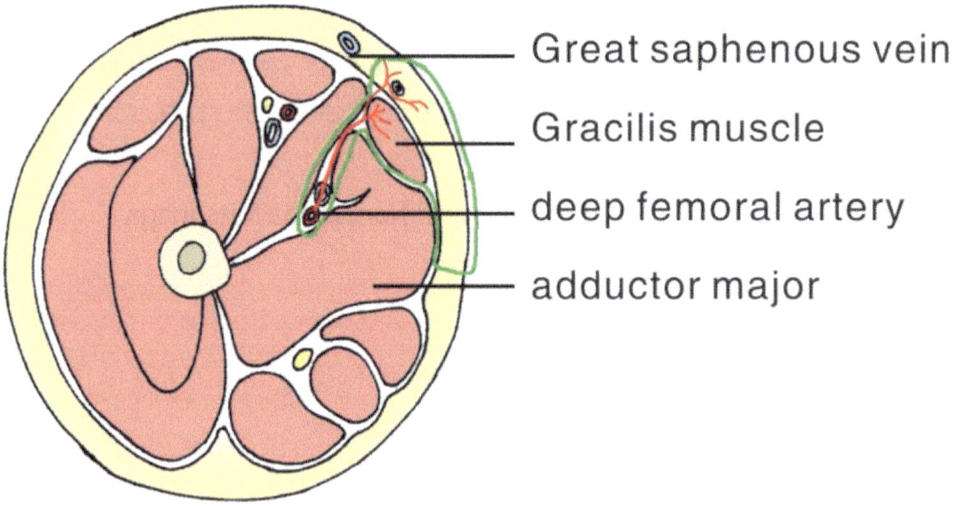

Fig. 21.1 Schematic diagram of anatomical cross section of tug flap. The green marking line indicates the cutting range of myocutaneous flap

21.2 Flap Design

Preoperative imaging examination, especially CTA, can locate the posterior thigh perforator from the perforator of internal mammary artery.

The midline of the adductor longus is a line from the pubic tubercle to the medial femoral condyle. The surface where the perforating branches of the internal mammary artery appear is normally 8–10 cm below the iliac inguinal fold behind this line.

The location and number of perforating vessels are further verified and marked by audible Doppler 1 day before operation. The mark at the upper end of the designed flap was 1 cm below the gluteal sulcus.

The lower mark is about 7 cm below the upper mark. The flap is usually designed transversely, with a maximum length of 27 cm (Fig. 21.2).

The gracilis myocutaneous flap can be expanded horizontally or vertically. The vertical design can obtain more tissue from the inner thigh by reducing the lower transverse incision of the skin or performing a trefoil flap.

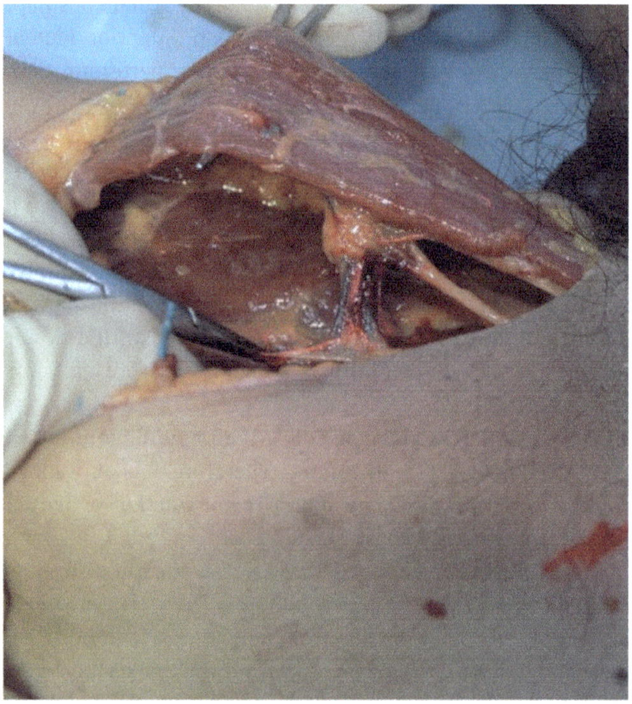

Fig. 21.2 Vascular pedicle and anterior obturator nerve branch of the main branches of the internal mammary artery entering the gracilis muscle

21.3 Tumor Resection and Recipient Site Preparation

The patient is treated in supine position, with the lower limb of donor site abducted and the hip and the knee in flexion (Fig. 21.3). After general anesthesia, the two teams of surgeons will operate simultaneously. The lesion resection team undergo radical excision of the breast cancer in order to completely remove the tumor and its surrounding tissue with safe resection.

The volume of tumor should be estimated according to intraoperative observation. If the affected side will be treated with radiotherapy, the contralateral vessels should be considered as the recipient vessels.

When selecting the internal thoracic artery as the recipient vessel, the intercostal space between the third and fourth costal cartilage is marked, and then the third or fourth costal cartilage is partially removed for about 2–3 cm during operation so that the internal thoracic artery can be fully exposed.

Lateral thoracic vessels or thoracodorsal vessels can also be chosen as the vascular pedicle of the receiving area according to the intraoperative assessment (refer to the chapter on vascular selection of the receiving area for details).

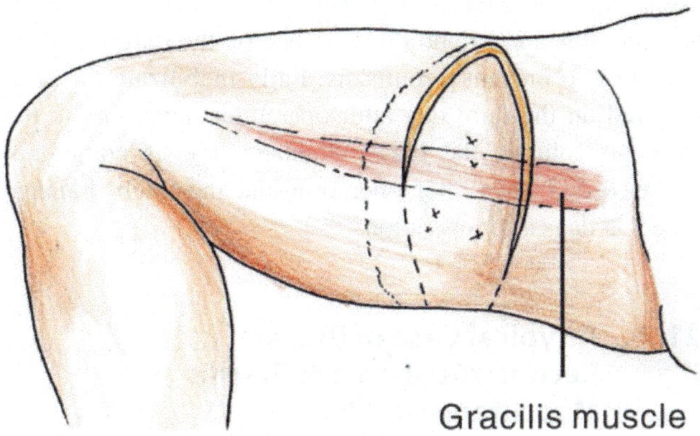

Fig. 21.3 Schematic diagram of design and predetermined cutting range of free transverse gracilis myocutaneous flap. The modified supine position with hip abduction and knee flexion was used to obtain the myocutaneous flap

21.4 Flap Cutting

As for the surgeons in the flap-obtaining team, free transverse gracilis myocutaneous flap is prepared.

According to the range and shape of the secondary breast defects, the free transverse gracilis myocutaneous flap is designed, the skin is incised along the designed markings of the flap to the superficial layer of the subcutaneous tissue, and the subcutaneous tissue is dissected around in order to harvest as much tissue volume in the flap as possible. Next, the flap is elevated from the proximal end to the distal end from the deep fascia plane to expose the perforating vessels, and the adductor longus and gracilis myocutaneous are further dissociated anatomically. After the dissection proceeding to the deeper part, the adductor longus muscle is then stretched to expose the internal mammary vessel which enters the vascular pedicle of the gracilis muscle (Fig. 21.4). Then, the distal end of the flap is dissected, and the flap is completely lifted from the distal end to the proximal end when reaching perforator vessels by separation. A retrograde dissection into the gracilis muscle along the perforator vessel to the main vascular pedicle is followed, and the retrograde separation continues along the vascular pedicle to the plane where the internal mammary vessel arises. After ligation and disconnection of the vascular pedicle, the myocutaneous flap was wrapped with heparin-saline gauze and transferred to the breast defect area. After adequate hemostasis in the flap supply area, a vacuum drainage tube is placed, and the subcutaneous tissue and skin are closed by layers and covered with sterile dressing.

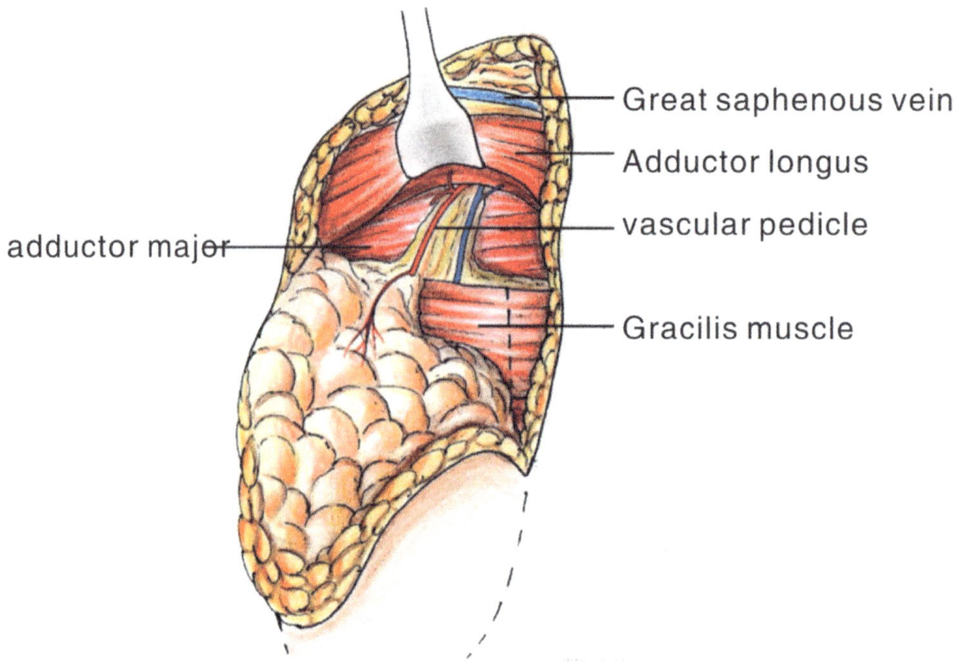

Fig. 21.4 Schematic diagram exposing the vascular pedicle of the myocutaneous flap

21.5 Breast Reconstruction and Vascular Anastomosis

The skin flap is placed in the breast defect area, and the skin flap is de-epithelialized according to the skin defect range of the recipient area. The skin flap is fixed in the recipient area with 4-0 absorbable sutures in an interrupted fashion. The blood vessels are anastomosed under the microscope. The perforating arteries of internal mammary vessels are anastomosed with the internal thoracic artery from the recipient area, and the accompanied veins were anastomosed to the internal thoracic artery. After confirming that the blood supply of the skin flap is reliable, the skin flap is transferred to the defect. After assessing that there is no tortuous torsion of the vascular pedicle, the flap is further fixed with 4-0 absorbable interrupted sutures. Additional re-check is performed to ensure that there is no active bleeding on the wound surface, and several vacuum drainage tubes are placed, followed by skin closure by layers.

21.6 Postoperative Treatment

The patient is kept warm in the operation area and rested in bed. The patient is treated with low-molecular-weight dextran for blood volume expansion, celecoxib analgesia, aspirin and heparin anticoagulation, papaverine antispasmodic, broad-spectrum antibiotics, and anti-inflammatory. The blood supply of the flap should be monitored every hour for the first 3 days after the operation, and every 4 h since the fourth day after operation. In the case of vascular congestion and swelling of the flap, the ischemic complication should be assessed and treated in time. The patient encouraged to lift legs and flex and extend knees in bed on the third day after operation to prevent thrombosis. Early mobilization is also required on the third day after operation. According to the drainage volume, the breast drainage tube is commonly removed 5–7 days after operation and the thigh drainage tube 3–5 days after operation.

21.7 A Typical Case of Breast Reconstruction with Gracilis Myocutaneous Flap

The patient, a 40-year-old female, found a left breast tumor for more than 8 months. A hard tumor measuring about 3 cm × 3 cm can be palpated on the outer upper quadrant of the left breast with unclear boundary, poor activity, and no obvious tenderness. There was no obvious abnormality in the right breast and no palpable axillary lymph nodes. Left breast coarse needle aspiration: histological grade II–III of left breast invasive ductal carcinoma. After admission, simple left breast resection with nipple areola preservation + sentinel lymph node biopsy + free gracilis myocutaneous flap resection and breast reconstruction were performed.

Five sentinel lymph nodes were resected during the operation and sent for rapid frozen section examination: no cancer was found in the left sentinel lymph nodes, and no cancer was found in the nipple, skin, and basal margin. The left breast gland and pectoralis major fascia were removed from inside to outside. The cartilage of the left third rib was about 4 cm long, and the internal thoracic arteries and veins were dissected for standby.

According to the preoperative evaluation of the perforating branches of the internal mammary artery, the medial femoral flap from the inner side of the right thigh to the posterior gluteal sulcus was designed, with an area of about 21 cm × 7 cm. The subcutaneous fat layer of the skin around the flap was cut and separated backward along the surface of the medial muscle. A perforator vessel of the gracilis muscle was raised from the surface of the gracilis muscle. This perforator vessel was retrogradely dissected to the internal mammary artery, and the vascular pedicle was cut off at the bifurcation of the internal mammary artery. The gracilis myocutaneous flap was completely transferred to the defect after left mastectomy. The vascular pedicle of the myocutaneous flap was sutured with the proximal end of the internal thoracic artery and vein, respectively, using end-to-end anastomosis. The blood supply of the flap was abundant after anastomosis. The flap was folded and shaped, making it symmetrical with the right breast in shape, and the epidermis was partially removed for further shaping. The wound was closed using sutures by layers, and three negative pressure drainage tubes were placed in the wound cavity.

Postoperative pathological examination showed that (1) the histology of left breast-invasive ductal carcinoma was grade II–III, and the size of the mass was 1 cm × 1 cm × 1 cm; (2) no cancer involvement was found in the nipple, skin, and basal margin; and (3) no cancer was found in five left sentinel lymph nodes and six left axillary lymph nodes. Immunohistochemistry showed Er (−), PR (−), CerbB-2 (3+), and Ki-67 about 20%. The patient was transferred to internal medicine for chemotherapy. The appearance of breast reconstruction was satisfactory during follow-up, and there was no tumor recurrence (Figs. 21.5, 21.6, 21.7, 21.8, 21.9, 21.10, 21.11, and 21.12).

One of the flap options for breast reconstruction is the transverse gracilis myocutaneous flap (TUG) on the upper inner thigh. The volume of tissue in the medial thigh donor area is relatively adequate. The advantages of TUG flap for breast reconstruction include the following: (1) The flap is soft and resembles breast tissue. Generally, 300–400 g of flap can be obtained, and the volume is enough to meet the needs of breast reconstruction in most female breast cancer patients in China. (2) The vascular body area of the skin on the inner thigh is large, and the skin island can be long and wide, which has advantages for secondary breast reconstruction and remedial reconstruction. (3) TUG is less difficult to obtain, and the vascular pedicle is thicker, with a more matched diameter to internal thoracic vessels.

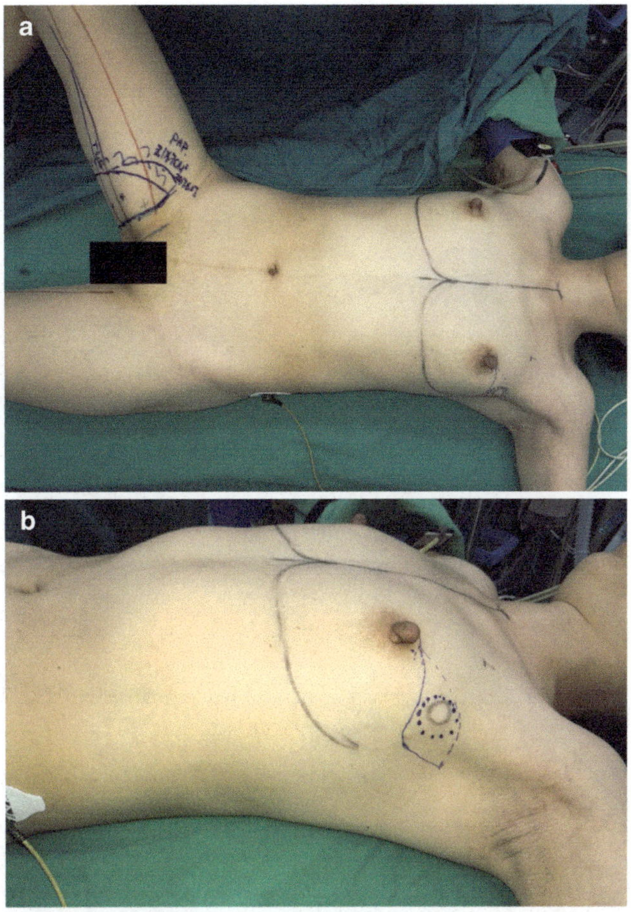

Fig. 21.5 Preoperative design and patient position

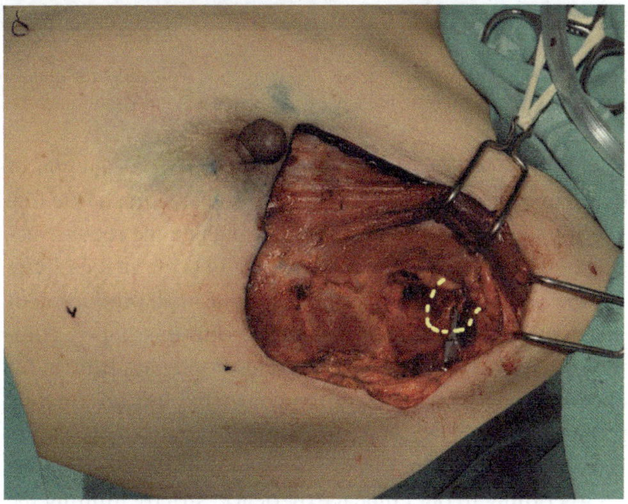

Fig. 21.6 Preparation of recipient vessels after modified radical mastectomy for left breast cancer

The disadvantages of TUG flap include the following: (1) The length of vascular pedicle is short and the placement of myocutaneous flap is restricted. (2) The donor site has the

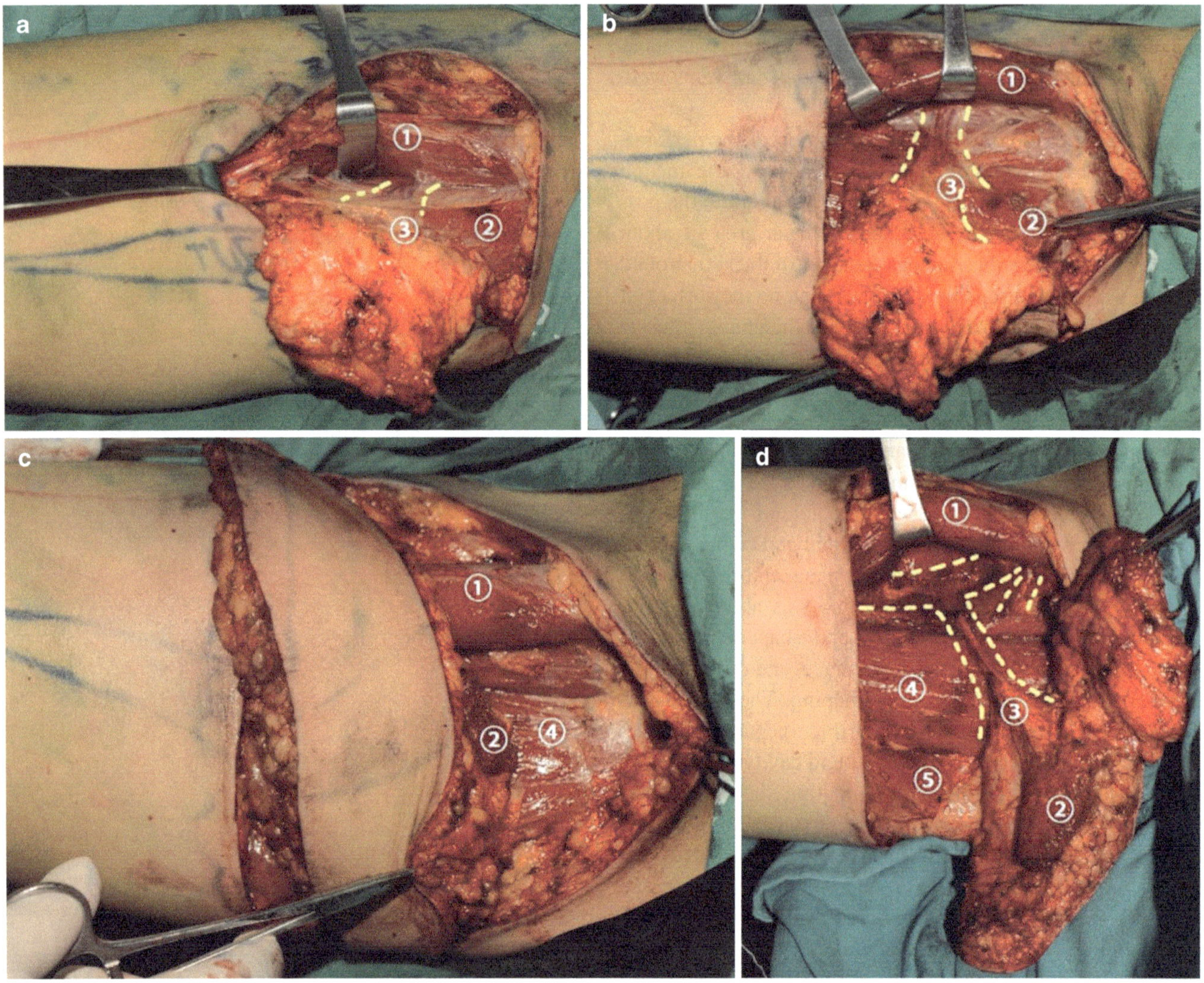

Fig. 21.7 Gracilis myocutaneous flap combined with adductor major perforator flap. (1) Adductor longus. (2) Gracilis muscle. (3) Vascular pedicle of the gracilis muscle branch. (4) Adductor major. (5) Semimembranosus muscle

possibility of dehiscence and infection. (3) The function of donor muscle is sacrificed. (4) The transplantation of the free gracilis myocutaneous flap does not include the reconstruction of the muscle nerve, and atrophy will occur in the future. Yet the gracilis muscle constitutes only a small proportion of the flap, and the breast recontructed with this flap is commonly small-sized, therefore, muscle atrophy has little influence on long-term aesthetic outcome. Reports of surgical refinements in TUG flap have further promoted its use in breast reconstruction.

According to our clinical experience, strictly limiting the size of the flap can reduce the complications of the donor site. The precautions include the following: (1) The width of TUG flap should be kept within 8–10 cm and may be extended to 12 cm in patients with loose skin. The primary closure of the donor site can avoid the adverse effects of skin graft repair on function and appearance. (2) During the separation of the front edge of the flap, be careful not to damage the great saphenous vein. The median line at the back side of the thigh is regarded as the boundary for posterior end of the incisal edge. Once beyond this boundary, the risks of complications such as flap necrosis and nerve injury will increase. (3) The proximal end of the flap should be incised. The tissue volume of TUG flap is based on the skin relaxation and the volume of fat in the inner thigh of the patient, which can basically meet the requirements for small-to-medium volume breast reconstruction. If available, bilateral TUG flap or the flap carrying total gracilis muscle can also be harvested for larger breast reconstruction. In addition, if the breast is not in full-shape after operation, fat transplantation can be performed to improve the breast appearance.

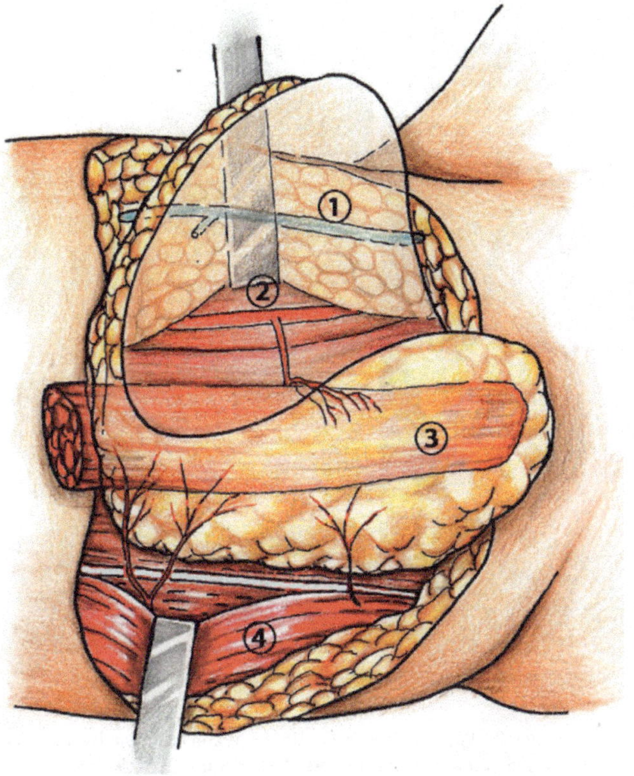

Fig. 21.8 Schematic diagram of the operating process for the gracilis perforator myocutaneous flap. The perforator vessels from the posterior semimembranosus muscle can be used after clamping experiment. (1) Great saphenous vein. (2) Internal mammary vessels. (3) Gracilis muscle. (4) Semimembranosus muscle

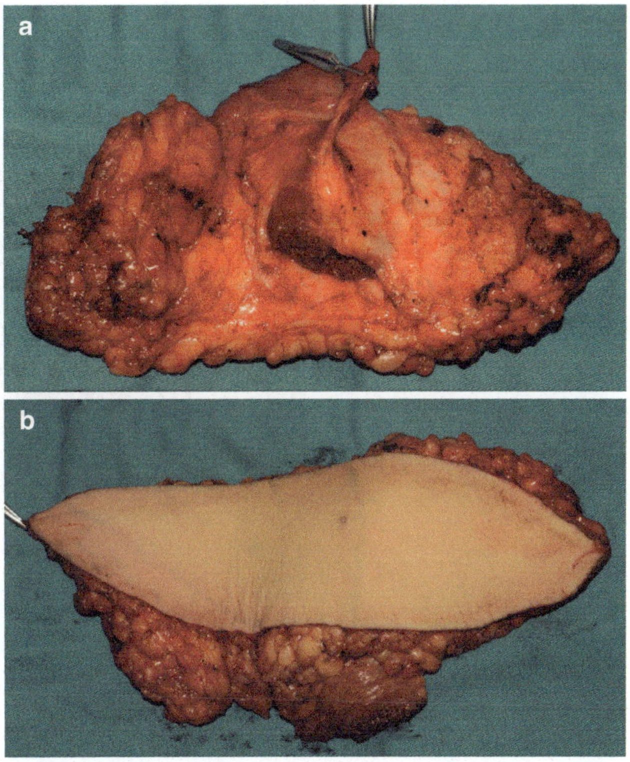

Fig. 21.9 The free gracilis myocutaneous flap was cut

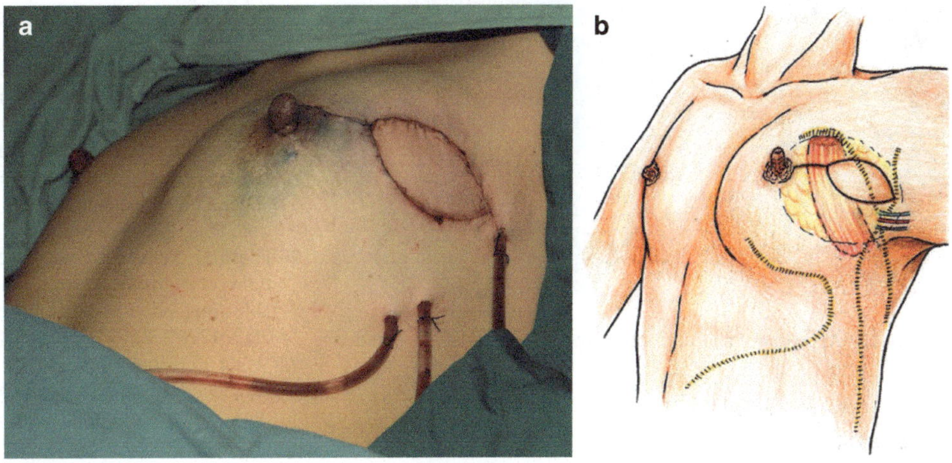

Fig. 21.10 (a) Immediate view after skin flap shaping. (b) Revascularization pattern. The vascular pedicle of the gracilis muscle branch was anastomosed with the lateral thoracic vessel (1a2v)

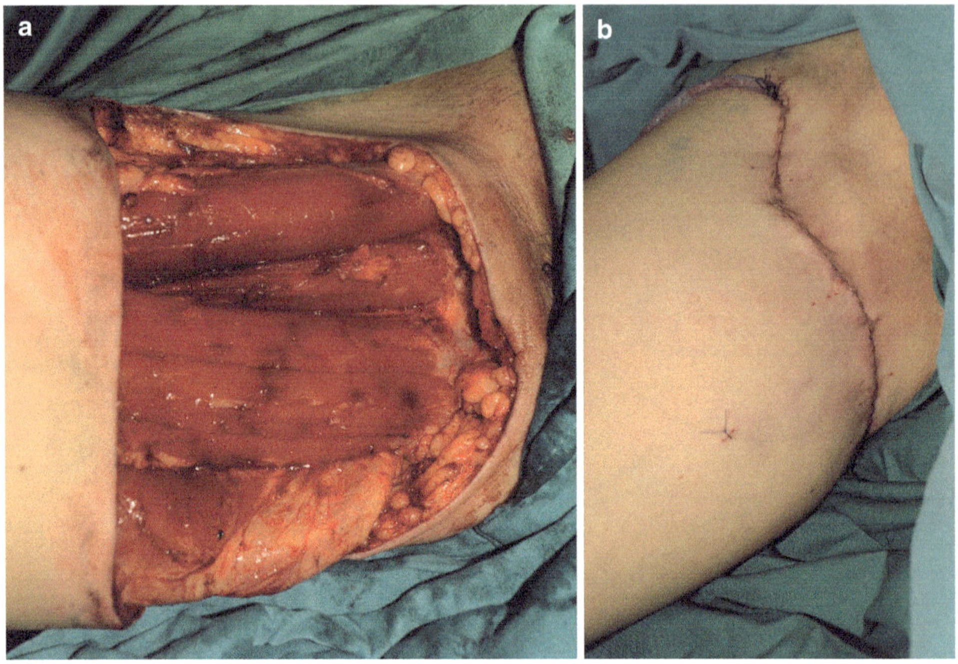

Fig. 21.11 Direct closure of the flap donor area

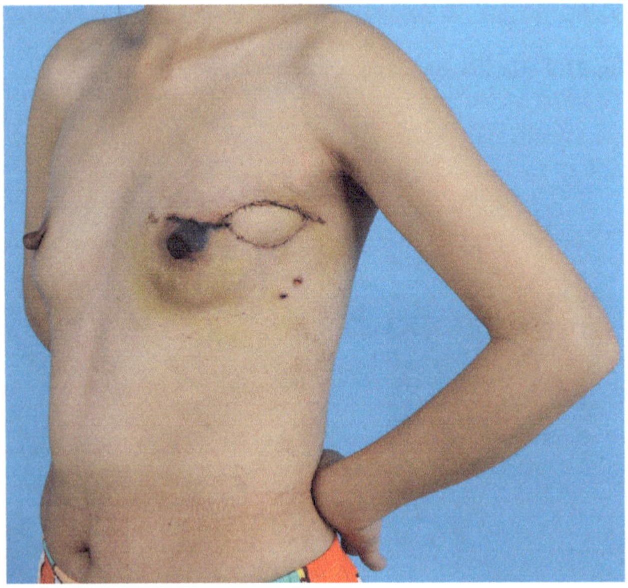

Fig. 21.12 Appearance and function recovery 2 weeks after operation

References

1. Schoeller T, Wechselberger G. Breast reconstruction by the free transverse gracilis (TUG) flap. Br J Plast Surg. 2004;57(5):481–2.
2. Wechselberger G, Schoeller T. The transverse myocutaneous gracilis free flap: a valuable tissue source in autologous breast reconstruction. Plast Reconstr Surg. 2004;114(1):69–73.
3. Yousif NJ, Matloub HS, Kolachalam R, Grunert BK, Sanger JR. The transverse gracilis musculocutaneous flap. Ann Plast Surg. 1992;29(6):482–90.
4. Schoeller T, Huemer GM, Wechselberger G. The transverse musculocutaneous gracilis flap for breast reconstruction: guidelines for flap and patient selection. Plast Reconstr Surg. 2008;122(1):29–38.
5. Fattah A, Figus A, Mathur B, Ramakrishnan VV. The transverse myocutaneous gracilis flap: technical refinements. J Plast Reconstr Aesthet Surg. 2010;63(2):305–13.
6. Peek A, Müller M, Ackermann G, Exner K, Baumeister S. The free gracilis perforator flap: anatomical study and clinical refinements of a new perforator flap. Plast Reconstr Surg. 2009;123(2):578–88.
7. Vega SJ, Sandeen SN, Bossert RP, Perrone A, Ortiz L, Herrera H. Gracilis myocutaneous free flap in autologous breast reconstruction. Plast Reconstr Surg. 2009;124(5):1400–9.
8. Fansa H, Schirmer S, Warnecke IC, Cervelli A, Frerichs O. The transverse myocutaneous gracilis muscle flap: a fast and reliable method for breast reconstruction. Plast Reconstr Surg. 2008;122(5):1326–33.
9. Wong C, Mojallal A, Bailey SH, Trussler A, Saint-Cyr M. The extended transverse musculocutaneous gracilis flap: vascular anatomy and clinical implications. Ann Plast Surg. 2011;67(2):170–7.

Single Pedicled Profunda Femoral Artery Perforator Flap for Breast Reconstruction

22

Dajiang Song and Narushima Mitsunaga

For patients who need autologous breast reconstruction after mastectomy, it is a common choice to use the perforator flap of inferior abdominal artery based on abdominal free flap. However, not all patients have sufficient abdominal tissue, either because of low body mass index, scars, inappropriate perforations, or because they have had DIEP or abdominal wall plastic surgery before [1]. An alternative is the transverse crescent-shaped upper gracilis myocutaneous flap (TUG) composed of upper tissue above the thigh [2–4]. However, TUG flap is considered to have some disadvantages. The amount of tissue available in the thigh is scarce, the vascular pedicle is short (6–7 cm in length), and the donor area is prone to wound dehiscence and infection [5–7]. As reported in the successful cases, a number of solutions against these constraints have been described from many aspects, among which the profunda artery perforator flap (PAP) reported by Allen is the most interesting refinement [8]. PAP flap is based on the musculocutaneous or septal perforator of the second or third perforator of profunda femoral artery. They converge behind the gracilis muscle and supply blood to the skin and subcutaneous fat under the gluteal sulcus. According to clinical observation and preoperative imaging studies, about 97% of the thighs have at least one suitable perforating branch with an average diameter of 1.9 mm in this area. The medial perforator is close to the adductor magnus, with an average distance of 3.8 cm from the midline and 5 cm below the gluteal sulcus, and the lateral perforator is close to the biceps femoris and lateral femoral muscle, with an average distance of 1.2 cm from the midline and 5 cm below the gluteal sulcus [9, 10]. When the abdominal tissue is insufficient, the flap can also be used as an alternative to provide soft tissue from the medial thigh donor area with relatively abundant tissue to complete breast reconstruction. It can be regarded as an evolutionary form of TUG flap. According to the evaluation of reconstructed breast and donor area, PAP flap should have more advantages than TUG flap in theory [8].

As for the flap design, placing the perforator vessel in the center of the flap can optimize the blood supply of the flap to the greatest extent. Generally, it can carry 300–400 g tissue, which is equal to the weight of resected tissue after most mastectomies, so it is suitable for most patients. The skin island that can be dissected is long, and the general safety range is about 27 cm × 7 cm, which has prominent advantages for secondary breast reconstruction and remedial breast chest wall reconstruction. The vascular pedicle is longer, with an average length of 9.9 cm, which makes the tissue flap implantation more flexible. Also, the vessels are well matched with those in the receiving area. As for the donor area, the scar is well hidden in the hip sulcus. There is no need to sacrifice the muscle like dissection TUG flap, and the anatomical range is farther away from lymphatic vessels, which can reduce the potential risk of subcutaneous seroma. The operation is more complicated than gracilis myocutaneous flap, but you can master it quickly after understanding the anatomical basis. The anatomy and surgical methods have been previously elaborated.

22.1 A Typical Case of Breast Reconstruction with Single Vessel Pedicled Profunda Femoral Artery Perforator Flap

The patient was a 60-year-old female with right breast mass found in physical examination for 1 week. The pathological diagnosis is invasive ductal carcinoma, histological grade I–II. After admission, she underwent modified radical mastectomy for right breast cancer and breast reconstruction with left profunda femoral artery perforator flap. The operation

D. Song (✉)
Department of Oncology Plastic Surgery, Hunan Cancer Hospital, Changsha, Hunan, China

N. Mitsunaga
Mie University Graduate School of Medicine Plastic and Reconstructive Surgery, Tsu, Mie, Japan
e-mail: sancho-ps@umin.ac.jp

Z. Li, D. Song (eds.), *Oncoplastic Flap Surgery*, https://doi.org/10.1007/978-981-19-8926-1_22

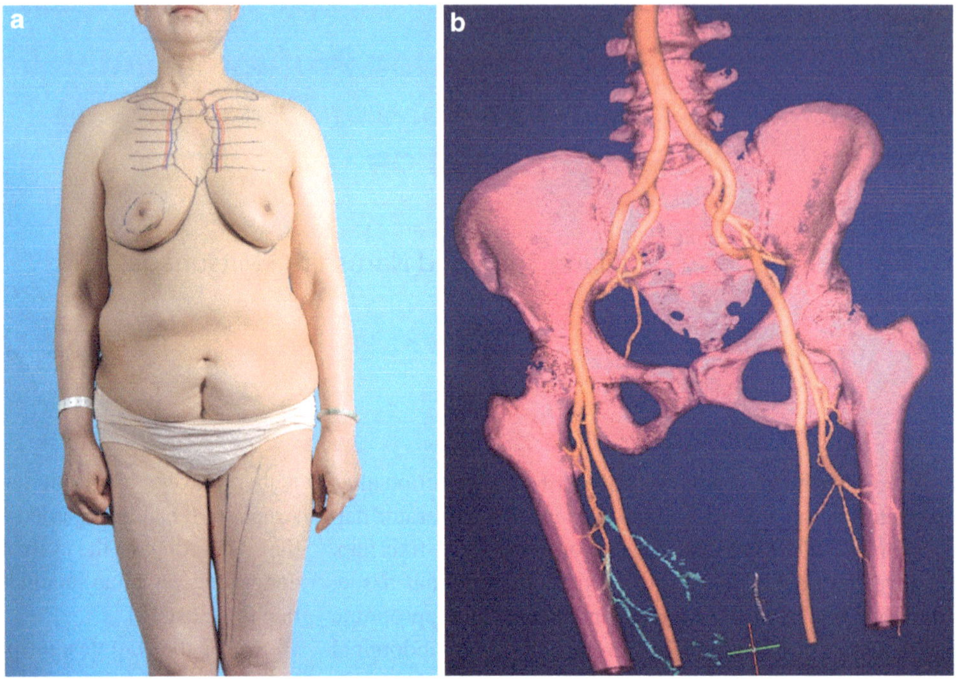

Fig. 22.1 Preoperative patient condition (**a**) and CTA angiography showing bilateral medial thigh perforator vessels (**b**)

was successful and the flap survived well. The patients was transferred to internal medicine department for chemotherapy. The appearance of reconstructed breast was satisfactory during follow-up, and no tumor recurrence was found (Figs. 22.1, 22.2, 22.3, 22.4, 22.5, 22.6, 22.7, 22.8, 22.9, 22.10, and 22.11).

The single vessel pedicled profunda femoral artery perforator flap for breast reconstruction has its characteristics and precautions: (1) There is the largest and most consistent profunda femoral artery perforator on the surface of adductor major, so the design center point of the flap should be properly moved backward when dissecting the profunda femoral artery perforator flap. (2) As long as the site of the perforator is reasonably designed near the central area of the flap, the reliable blood supply of the larger flap can be ensured, because the blood supply of the medial femoral is abundant, which is different from the vascular distribution of the lower abdomen. Also, there is no obvious restriction on the vascular perforating body area. (3) Preoperative Doppler detection of the location of perforating vessels is often not highly accurate, especially in female patients with thick fat on the inner thigh. If possible, CTA of the inner thigh should be used to determine the size, quantity, location, and source of perforating vessels.

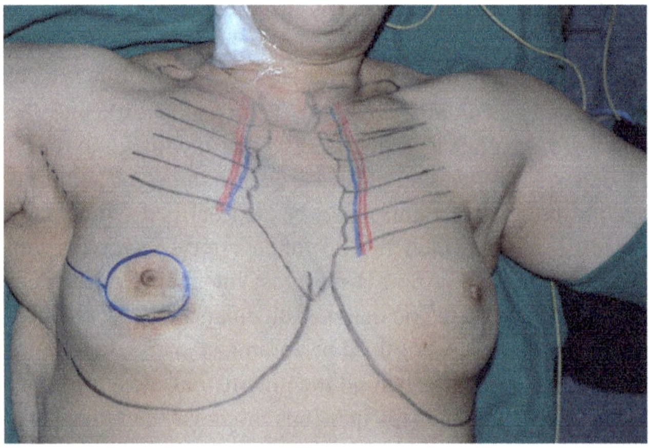

Fig. 22.2 Design mark of intraoperative receiving area

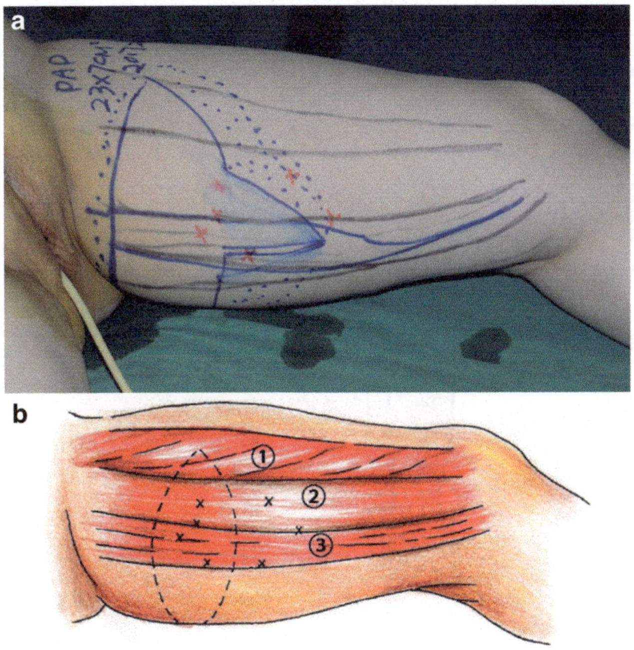

Fig. 22.3 Design of medial femoral perforator flap. The multi-leaf shape design can carry the inner thigh tissue to the greatest extent, but it will expand the scar. Finally, A transverse incision in shuttle shape was chosen. (1) Medial femoral muscle. (2) Adductor longus. (3) Gracilis muscle

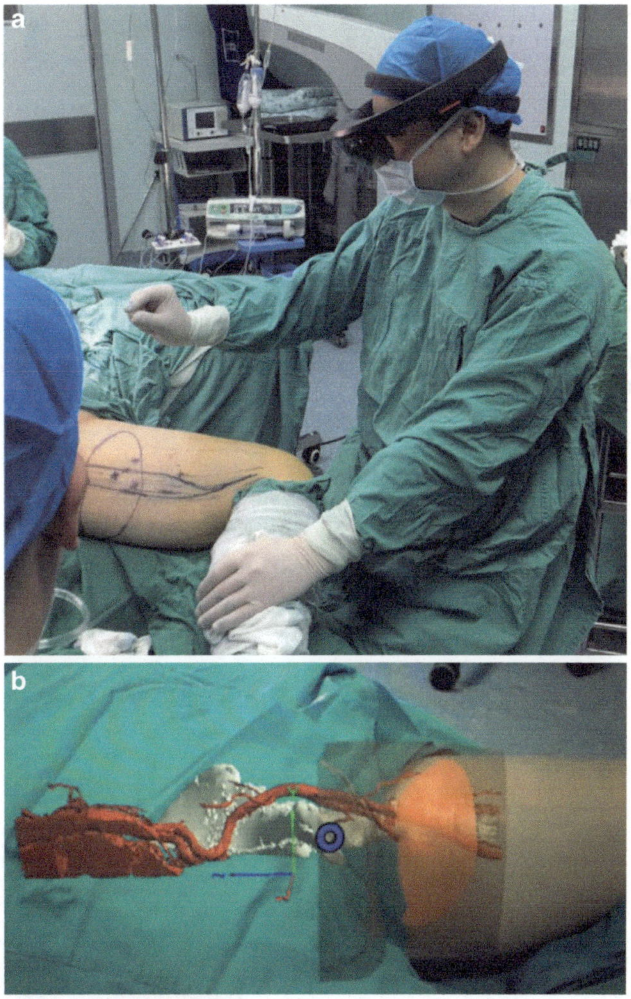

Fig. 22.4 Intraoperative use of VR hybrid reality technology to assist in guiding the design of flap dissection

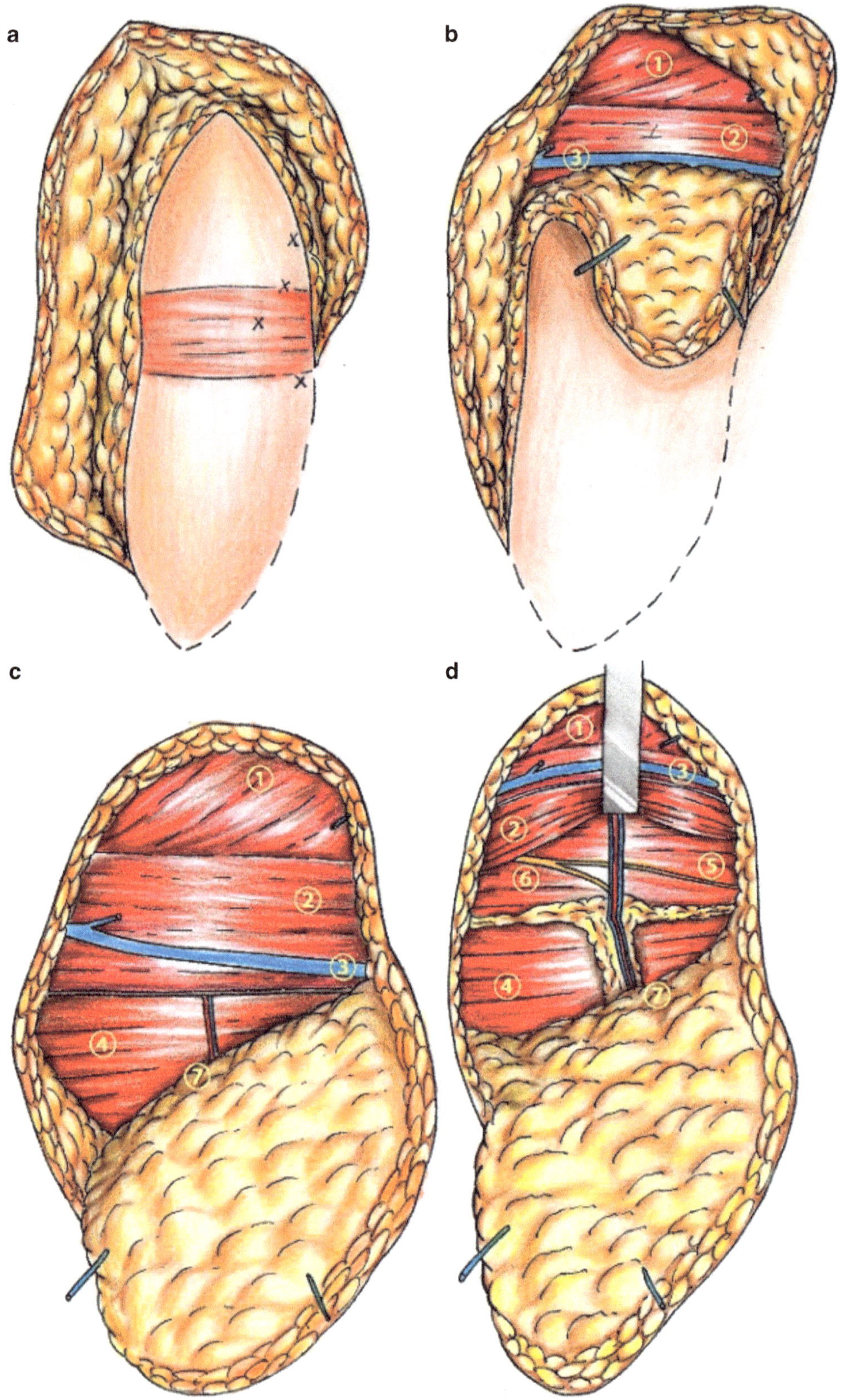

Fig. 22.5 Lift the flap from the anterior to the posterior, reserve as much subcutaneous adipose tissue as possible in the flap, then expose the large perforating vessels between the gracilis and adductor longus, and separate them retrogradely. (1) Medial femoral muscle. (2) Adductor longus. (3) Great saphenous vein. (4) Gracilis muscle. (5) Adductor major. (6) Anterior branch of obturator nerve. (7) Perforating vessels

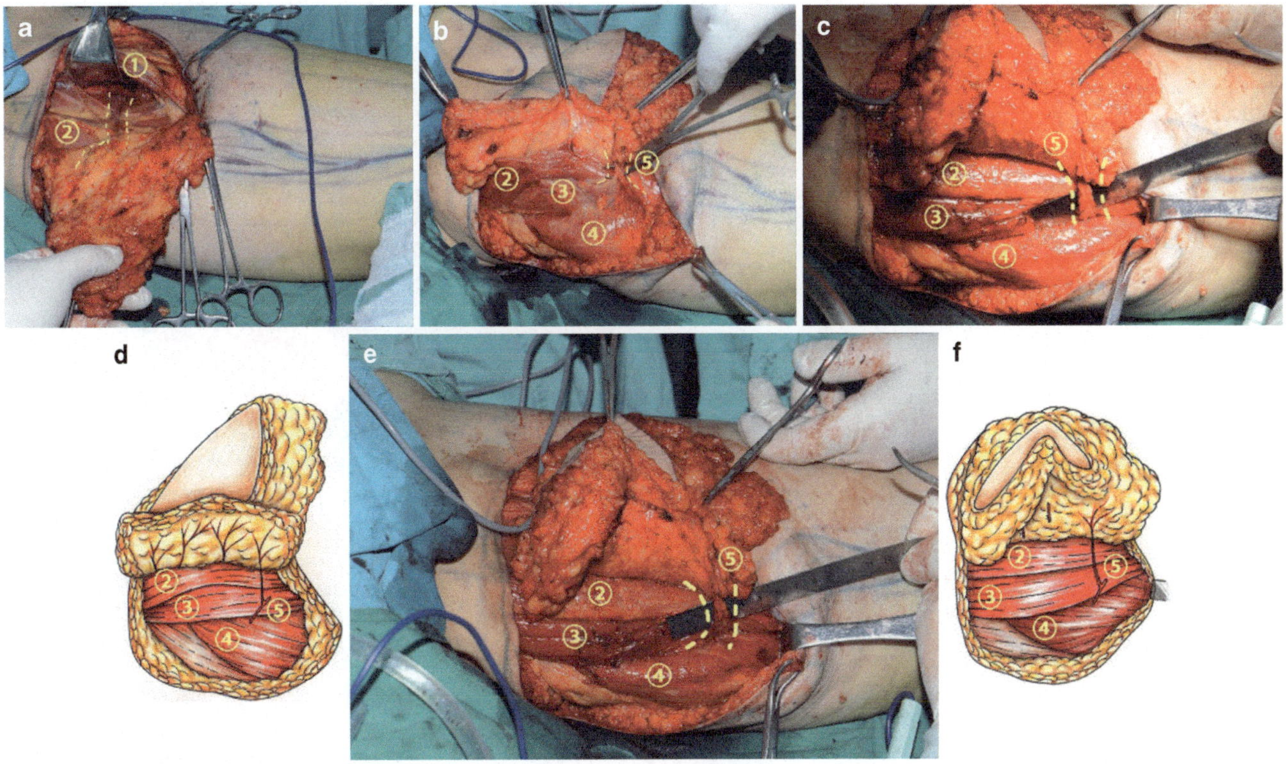

Fig. 22.6 After the retrograde separation of the vascular pedicle of the gracilis muscle branch to the plane of the profunda femoral vessel, we switch to lift the posterior edge of the flap to expose a perforator vessel between the great adductor muscle and the semimembranosus muscle. (1) Adductor longus. (2) Gracilis muscle. (3) Adductor major. (4) Semimembranosus muscle. (5) Adductor major perforator vessel

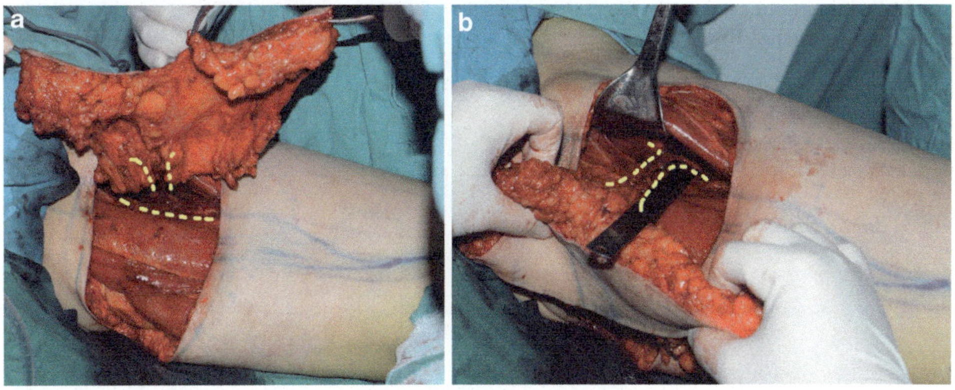

Fig. 22.7 After confirming the blood supply of the flap by the vascular clamping experiment, the perforating vessels of the adductor major were ligated and disconnected, and the perforating vessels of the gracilis muscle were separated retrogradely to the plane of the profunda femoral vessels

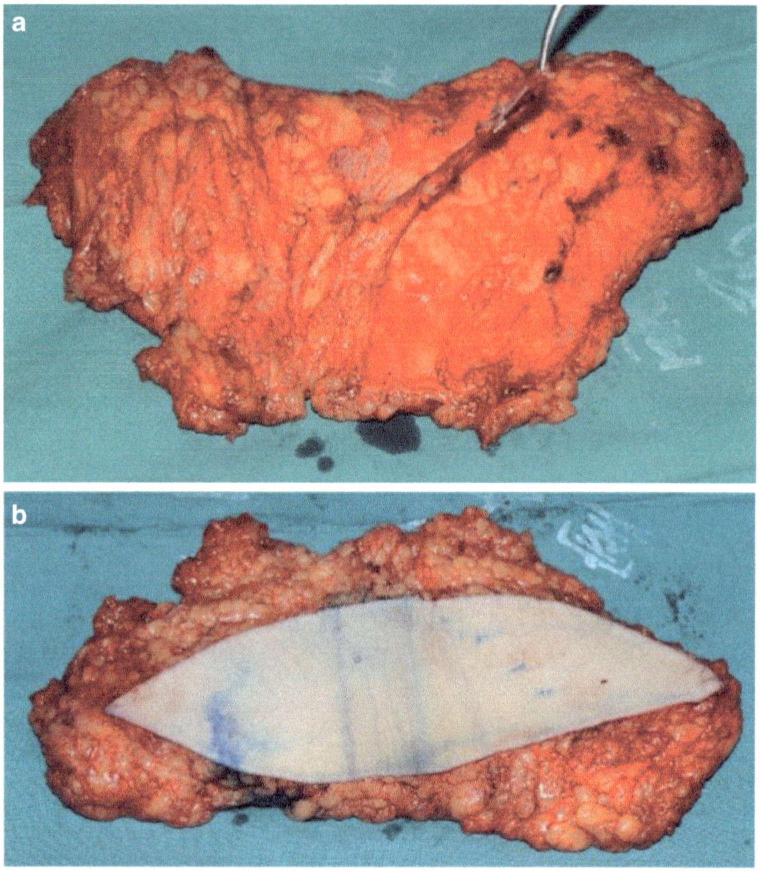

Fig. 22.8 The gracilis perforator flap was dissected

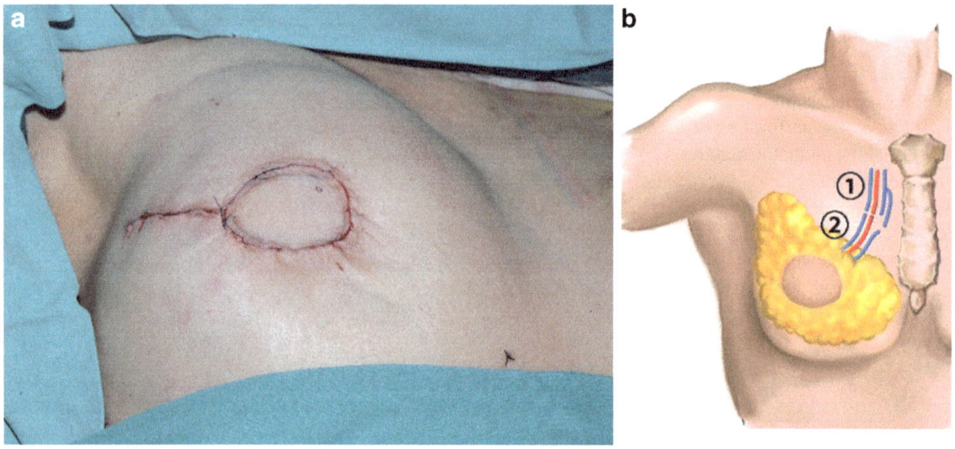

Fig. 22.9 (**a**) Immediate view of breast reconstruction after skin flap shaping. (**b**) The pattern of flap revascularization. (1) Internal mammary vessels. (2) Vascular pedicle of gracilis muscle branch

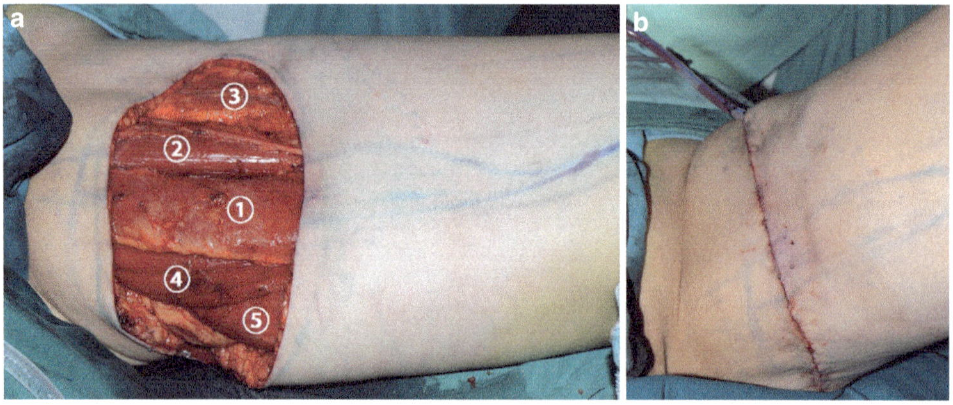

Fig. 22.10 Direct closure of the flap donor area. (1) Gracilis muscle. (2) Adductor longus. (3) Medial femoral muscle. (4) Adductor major. (5) Semimembranosus muscle

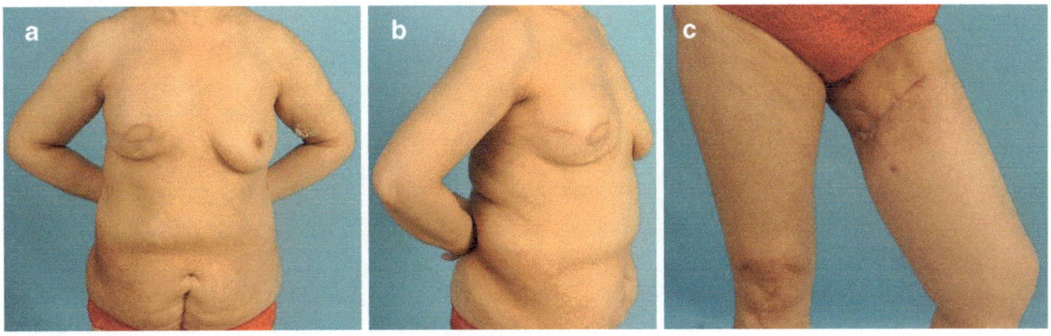

Fig. 22.11 The appearance and function 6 months after operation

References

1. Hunter JE, Lardi AM, Dower DR, Farhadi J. Evolution from the TUG to PAP flap for breast reconstruction: comparison and refinements of technique. J Plast Reconstr Aesthet Surg. 2015;68(7):960–5.
2. Yousif NJ, Matloub HS, Kolachalam R, Grunert BK, Sanger JR. The transverse gracilis musculocutaneous flap. Ann Plast Surg. 1992;29(6):482–90.
3. Schoeller T, Huemer GM, Wechselberger G. The transverse musculocutaneous gracilis flap for breast reconstruction: guidelines for flap and patient selection. Plast Reconstr Surg. 2008;122(1):29–38.
4. Fattah A, Figus A, Mathur B, Ramakrishnan VV. The transverse myocutaneous gracilis flap: technical refinements. J Plast Reconstr Aesthet Surg. 2010;63(2):305–13.
5. Wong C, Mojallal A, Bailey SH, Trussler A, Saint-Cyr M. The extended transverse musculocutaneous gracilis flap: vascular anatomy and clinical implications. Ann Plast Surg. 2011;67(2):170–7.
6. Schoeller T, Wechselberger G. Breast reconstruction by the free transverse gracilis (TUG) flap. Br J Plast Surg. 2004;57(5):481–2.
7. Locke MB, Zhong T, Mureau MA, Hofer SO. Tug 'O' war: challenges of transverse upper gracilis (TUG) myocutaneous free flap breast reconstruction. J Plast Reconstr Aesthet Surg. 2012;65(8):1041–50.
8. Allen RJ, Haddock NT, Ahn CY, Sadeghi A. Breast reconstruction with the profunda artery perforator flap. Plast Reconstr Surg. 2012;129(1):16e–23e.
9. Haddock NT, Greaney P, Otterburn D, Levine S, Allen RJ. Predicting perforator location on preoperative imaging for the profunda artery perforator flap. Microsurgery. 2012;32(7):507–11.
10. Ahmadzadeh R, Bergeron L, Tang M, Geddes CR, Morris SF. The posterior thigh perforator flap or profunda femoris artery perforator flap. Plast Reconstr Surg. 2007;119(1):194–200; discussion 201–2.

23 Free Gracilis Myocutaneous Flap Combined with Profunda Femoral Artery Perforator Flap for Breast Reconstruction

Dajiang Song and Narushima Mitsunaga

Compared with prosthetic breast reconstruction, autologous tissue breast reconstruction is more recommended. Autologous tissue transfer includes the pedicled latissimus dorsi and rectus abdominis. There are also free flaps, such as the perforator flap of the inferior abdominal artery, gracilis free flap [1], and gluteus maximus flap [2, 3]. The perforator flap of inferior abdominal artery is the gold standard for breast reconstruction. Its most fitting indication is female patients with sufficient abdominal fat and without serious comorbidities and history of abdominal surgery. However, emaciated women with thin abdominal fat layer cannot provide the amount of fat required for breast reconstruction. Non-pregnant young female patients often reject the selection of abdominal donor area. Because Asian women tend to be thin and the group of breast cancer patients is younger, there is an increasing number of patients who are not suitable for breast reconstruction with the inferior abdominal artery perforator flap but have strong desire to breast reconstruction. This is why breast cancer plastic surgeons are looking for other donor sites for breast tissue reconstruction by autologous tissue [4].

The medial thigh is a potential flap donor area. As a flap donor area for breast reconstruction, it is easy to hide the scars which is more aesthetically acceptable. The vascular perforators supplying the medial thigh region originate from the profunda femoral artery. Thigh-based flaps such as transverse upper gracilis (TUG) [1, 5–8], transverse gracilis perforator flap [9], longitudinal gracilis flap (VUG) [10], and profunda artery perforator flap (PAP) [11–13] are the second most commonly used options for autologous breast reconstruction. Detailed techniques for dissecting TUG and PAP flaps have been reported, respectively, before. Skin flaps based on these perforating branches have been widely used in pressure ulcer and breast reconstruction. Although both flaps are supplied by the profunda femoral artery system, their respective vascular body areas are different and have their own advantages and disadvantages. The anatomy of the gracilis myocutaneous flap is relatively simple, and there is no need to dissect the perforating branches in the muscle. Also, the damage of the donor area is small, and the scar is hidden. It is especially suitable for small- to medium-sized breast reconstruction in patients with less inferior abdominal tissue and thin body. The disadvantages of the gracilis myocutaneous flap mainly include short vascular pedicle and limited amount of tissue, so it only applied for small-sized breast reconstruction. Some reports have also introduced the improved dissecting method of gracilis myocutaneous flap, but the limitation due to anatomical basis is still difficult to be completely solved [5]. In 1992, Yousif et al. studied the vascular anatomy of TUG flap [1], and the results showed that the vascular pedicle entered the gracilis muscle 8–12 cm below the pubic tubercle. The length of vascular pedicle is 6–8 cm [14, 15]. The average volume of the flap was 350 mL [6]. The anatomy of TUG flap is relatively simple, usually untapped, need not to dissect perforator within muscle, along with minimal functional defects and hidden scar in donor area. It is suitable for small- to medium-sized breast reconstruction in patients with thin body and less lower abdominal tissue [8]. The disadvantages of TUG flap include short vascular pedicle, possible complications in donor area, wound dehiscence, ugly scar, sensory disturbance, volume loss due to denervation atrophy, and small-to-medium amount of flap tissue [16].

Recently, Bodin et al. [17] reported that when dissecting the gracilis myocutaneous flap, an additional vascular pedicle of the profunda femoral artery was carried in order to increase the reliability of the blood supply of the gracilis myocutaneous flap.

In the report, the gracilis myocutaneous flap was further extended and dissected posteriorly. They used this method in four patients and further extended the cutting range of the

D. Song (✉)
Department of Oncology Plastic Surgery, Hunan Cancer Hospital, Changsha, Hunan, China

N. Mitsunaga
Mie University Graduate School of Medicine Plastic and Reconstructive Surgery, Tsu, Mie, Japan
e-mail: sancho-ps@umin.ac.jp

Z. Li, D. Song (eds.), *Oncoplastic Flap Surgery*, https://doi.org/10.1007/978-981-19-8926-1_23

flap. The authors believed that anastomosing additional perforator pedicle of profunda femoral artery could prevent partial necrosis of the flap. However, despite the inclusion of a second vascular pedicle, the volume of the gracilis myocutaneous flap dissected in this report did not significantly increase compared with traditional applications [18, 19]. The profunda femoral artery perforator flap reported by Allen et al. is a new progress of concern, which overcomes many shortcomings compared with the conventional gracilis myocutaneous flap [20, 21]. A series of reports confirmed that the profunda femoral artery perforator flap was supplied by the musculocutaneous or septal perforator of the second or third perforator of the profunda femoral artery. They converged behind the gracilis and supply blood to the skin and subcutaneous fat under the gluteal sulcus. According to clinical observations and preoperative imaging studies [22, 23], about 97% of the thighs have at least one perforating branch with an average diameter of 1.9 mm over the surface of the adductor megacephalus in this area, with an average distance of 3.8 cm from the midline and 5 cm below the gluteal sulcus. Up to about 27.0 cm × 7.0 cm of the adductor major perforator pedicled long skin island can be dissected, which has advantages for secondary breast reconstruction and remedial reconstruction. Moreover, the vascular pedicle of the perforating branch of the adductor major is longer, with an average length of 9.9 cm, which makes the implantation more flexible. The vascular diameter can be well matched with that of the vessels in the recipient area. The scar of the flap donor area is hidden in the gluteal sulcus, which is more concealed than the scar of the gracilis flap donor area. There is no need to sacrifice muscles, and the dissecting area is far away from lymphatic vessels, which can reduce the risk of potential donor lymphatic leakage. However, the long segment of separation of perforator vessel pedicle in adductor major increases the difficulty of operation and prolongs the operation time. In this context, gracilis myocutaneous flap has more advantages, and there is no need to deliberately separate perforator in muscle, which significantly reduces the difficulty of operation [24]. In previous reports, the average length of the vascular pedicle of the PAP flap in cadaveric study was 10.6 cm and 9.9 cm in clinical study [20, 21]. In our current study, the average perforator length was 11 cm on anatomical specimens and 9.6 cm in clinical studies. The mean arterial diameter was 1.9 mm and the mean venous diameter was 2.4 mm, while previously reported clinical studies showed that they were 2.4 mm and 2.8 mm, respectively [20]. Delong et al. evaluated computed tomography of the perforating branch of the profunda femoral artery and found a larger average vessel diameter of 2.7 mm [25]. Scaglioni et al. [26] used PAP flaps in head and neck reconstruction, and they found similar anatomical results in this group of patients mainly consisting of male. The factors associated to the diameter of the profunda femoral artery perforator were age, gender, perforator location, and body mass index.

TUG + PAP flap is a combination of two commonly recognized flaps: transverse upper gracilis myocutaneous flap (TUG) and profunda artery perforator flap (PAP). According to anatomical and clinical studies [5–9, 11, 14, 15, 20, 24, 27–29], although both TUG flap and PAP flap originate from profunda femoral artery system, they supply blood to different skin areas. We used the combined TUG and PAP flap as the second flap donor for autologous breast reconstruction, and several significant advantages were developed. TUG + PAP flap can provide softer tissue without affecting the shape of hip. The operation procedures of vascular pedicle were simpler, and the flap can be bent freely during implantation. Also, there is no need to change body position during operation. We examined the possibility of combining these flaps and tried to increase the tissue volume of unilateral breast reconstruction to overcome the shortage due to medium tissue volume of the flap. Although refined methods to increase the volume of TUG flap have been reported previously, such as extending the flap downward or vertically, it is impossible to significantly increase its tissue volume due to the restriction by vascular body area [30]. PAP flap is based on the perforating branch of deep artery. The length of the vascular pedicle was 9 cm, and the pedicle is located 3 cm behind the gracilis muscle. Preoperative imaging is helpful to identify the dominant perforator in order to design the flap centered on the perforator. The upper boundary of the flap is 1 cm below the gluteal sulcus, and the incision area can reach 7 cm × 27 cm. Allen et al. believed that compared with TUG flap, PAP flap has the advantages of increasing the length of vascular pedicle and avoiding injury to inguinal lymph nodes [15, 20]. The average volume of PAP flap was 385 ML, which was equivalent to that of TUG flap. Another advantage of PAP is the hidden scars on the thighs and lower hips. Its oval design makes the reconstructed breast ideal and natural in shape. More importantly, the PAP flap is a perforator flap, thus the muscle is retained and the complication rate in donor site is reduced. In some cases, bilateral thigh flaps can be used for unilateral large breast reconstruction. The shapes of TUG and PAP flap are almost identical, and breast reconstruction with either TUG or PAP flap shares the same problem of limited size. If the amount of tissue is too large, not only the donor area of the flap cannot be closed primarily but also the blood perfusion of the whole flap will become unreliable. Moreover, dissecting wide skin islands and fat to increase the amount of tissue may result in more complications in donor site. In order to avoid these complications, the cutting range of each flap should be limited to ensure the reliability of the flap. The largest area of TUG + PAP flap in the report was 30 cm × 9 cm. Using dual sets of the vascular pedicle for the elliptical flap, the area and the volume of the flap are increased safely and reliably through combined vascular perfusion. As for bilateral large-sized breast reconstruction, both sides can be reconstructed with TUG + PAP flap without looking for other flap donor areas, and the donor areas are also symmetrical. The fascial flap can be dissected beyond the skin boundary of the flap to obtain more soft tissue without affecting the closure of the donor wound and additional shaping of the thigh as needed. The anatomical location of PAP perforator is the key to dissect TUG + PAP flap. The perforator should be located in the center of the PAP flap. When dissecting the TUG + PAP flap, it is not necessary to identify the TUG perforator or expose it, because TUG is not a perforator flap.

TUP + PAP flap is a new surgical scheme, which shortens the operation time of large-volume breast reconstruction. It requires only one flap donor area. Also, the anatomy for dissecting the flap is simple and there is no need to change the body position during operation. The two groups of surgeons can operate on the donor area and recipient area of breast reconstruction simultaneously. Although the second vascular pedicle needs to be dissected, the time of dissection only prolonged for 15 min in our cases, which is acceptable. Of course, it takes time to anastomose the second set of vessels. A possible complication of TUG + PAP flap is the potential damage of thigh lymphatic reflux. As mentioned in some reports of TUG flap, it is necessary to design the flap as posterior as possible, away from the area of lateral thigh lymphatic tissue system, and be away from this area during anatomical separation [30, 31]. After the flap was dissected, the vascular pedicle of the perforating branch of gracilis muscle was blocked with a microvascular clamp, and the distal and proximal blood perfusion of the flap were evaluated for a few minutes. We then changed to block the blood flow of the perforating branch of the adductor major by turns. It was determined that choosing only one perforating branch would reduce the blood flow in the corresponding part of the flap. Therefore, we believe that it is the safest choice for the flap to carry two vascular pedicles at the same time. Because the adductor group has five muscles, sacrificing the gracilis muscle and cutting part of the adductor major at the same time did not significantly affect the thigh function. Moreover, because the medial thigh donor area is far from the knee joint and no important muscle, ligament, or fascia structures that affect the movement of the knee joint were dissected, the postoperative patients did not complain about the adverse impact on thigh function.

In all cases, the area of the gracilis myocutaneous flap combined with adductor major perforator flap was determined by the volume of specimens after mastectomy. The gracilis myocutaneous flap combined with the great adductor perforator flap can be used for ipsilateral or contralateral breast reconstruction, as well as the internal thoracic artery or thoracodorsal artery. In our cases, only the proximal and distal ends of internal mammary vessel of one side were used, and the arterial and venous diameters were matched.

23.1 Gracilis Myocutaneous Flap Combined with Profunda Femoral Artery Perforator Flap for Breast Reconstruction: A Typical Case

The patient, a 33-year-old female, found a left breast mass for more than 8 months and received mass resection in other hospital in 1 month. Physical examination: the breasts were symmetrical. A scar with a length of about 3 cm can be seen below the left areola. Scar hyperplasia can be touched below it, and no obvious mass is touched and no obvious dimple sign or lemon peel sign; and no obvious redness, swelling or rash. Nipples were symmetrical, without depression and obvious overflow. Consultation and pathological examination revealed left breast-invasive ductal carcinoma, histological grade II. After her admission, modified radical mastectomy plus free TUG + PAP skin flap transplantation plus breast reconstruction was performed.

Five sentinel lymph nodes were resected during operation and sent to rapid frozen section for pathological examination: no obvious cancer metastasis was found in sentinel lymph nodes 0/5. The oval incision sizing 5 cm × 4 cm including nipple areola was designed and the incision was extend outward. The left breast gland, nipple areola specimens, and pectoralis major fascia were removed from the internal to external. The wound received complete hemostasis and was washed twice with 1000 mL of distilled water. The cartilage of the left third rib was about 2.5 cm long, and the internal thoracic arteries and veins were dissected for standby.

According to the preoperative detection of the location of the profunda artery perforator (PAP), the PAP flap from the lateral right thigh to the posterior gluteal sulcus was designed, with an area of about 20 cm × 7 cm in size. The subcutaneous fat layer of the skin around the flap was dissected and separated backward along the surface of the medial muscle. A perforator vessel of the gracilis muscle was found on the surface of the gracilis muscle. The perforator vessel was retrogradely dissected to the profunda femoral artery, and the vascular pedicle was cut off at the bifurcation of the profunda femoral artery. Continue to separate backward from the surface of gracilis, and two perforator vessels were found on the surface of posterior adductor major of gracilis. The perforator vessels were retrogradely dissected to the bifurcation of profunda femoral artery, where the vascular pedicle was cut off and double ligated near the distal end. The PAP flap was completely transferred to the defects after left mastectomy, and the transverse upper gracilis (TUG) perforator artery and vein and PAP perforator artery were sutured end-to-end with the proximal and distal ends to the internal thoracic artery and vein, respectively. The blood supply of the flap was satisfactory after anastomosis. The flap was folded and assembled. Two triangular flaps were designed at the overlap of the flap to form a new nipple by crossing the flap. A piece of costal cartilage was placed under the new nipple, fixed with silk thread, and the position was adjusted to be consistent with the opposite side. The flap was shape to make it consistent with the right breast defect, then a part of the skin was removed, followed by the wound closure in layers. Three negative-pressure drainage tubes were placed in the operation cavity. The donor area of the right thigh was directly closed and sutured, and a negative pressure drainage tube was placed in the operation cavity. The results of routine pathological examination showed (Part1) left breast intraductal carcinoma; (Part2) ductal carcinoma, histological grade II; and (Part3) intraductal papilloma with moderate to severe atypical hyperplasia. No cancer metastasis was found in six left sentinel lymph nodes and three left axillary deep lymph nodes. No cancer invasion was found in the skin, nipple, base, and lower cutting edge. Immunohistochemistry showed Er (strongly positive, 80%), pr (strongly positive, 80%), CerbB-2 (2 +), and Ki-67 about 20% +. The patient recovered well after operation and was further transferred to comprehensive treatment. The function and appearance of the reconstructed breast were satisfactory during follow-up, and only linear scars were left in the thigh donor area (Figs. 23.1, 23.2, 23.3, 23.4, 23.5, 23.6, 23.7, 23.8, 23.9, 23.10, 23.11, 23.12, and 23.13).

When there is more than one perforator, the selected perforator is based on the following standards: the perforator is located at the center of the flap. The diameter is large and located in the muscular septum. In the process of dissecting the perforator, the outermost part of the flap is retained to protect the spare perforator from the profunda femoral artery and the inferior abdominal artery.

Pay attention to avoid the posterior femoral cutaneous nerve running under the deep fascia.

When the flap is separated to only the vascular pedicle bifurcation, indocyanine green fluoroscopy can be used to ensure sufficient tissue perfusion of the flap.

Once the flap is separated, the vascular pedicle is anastomosed with the recipient vessels, and then the shaping and implantation of the flap are completed.

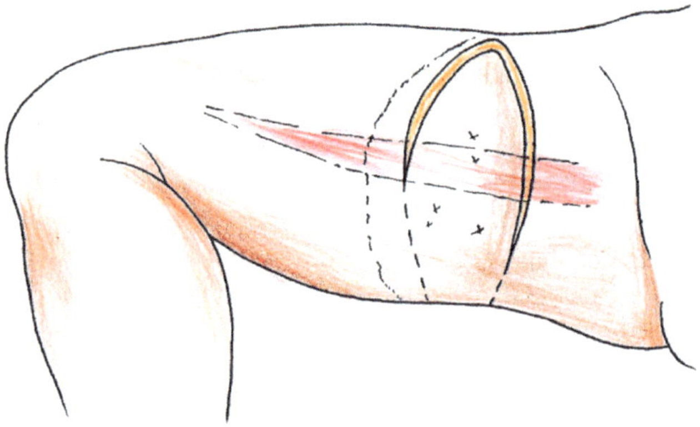

Fig. 23.2 First incision of the subcutaneous tissue of the skin at the frontal edge of the flap

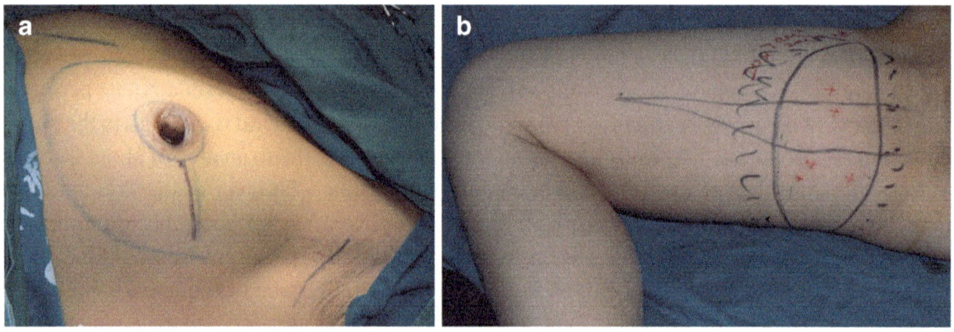

Fig. 23.1 Preoperative design of the transverse medial femoral perforator flap: the proximal end shall be as far away from the groin area as possible to avoid lymphedema. The proximal skin edge shall be incised vertically rather than expanding by dissociation. The flap size was 20 cm × 7 cm. (**a**) markings on the affected breast; (**b**) flap design

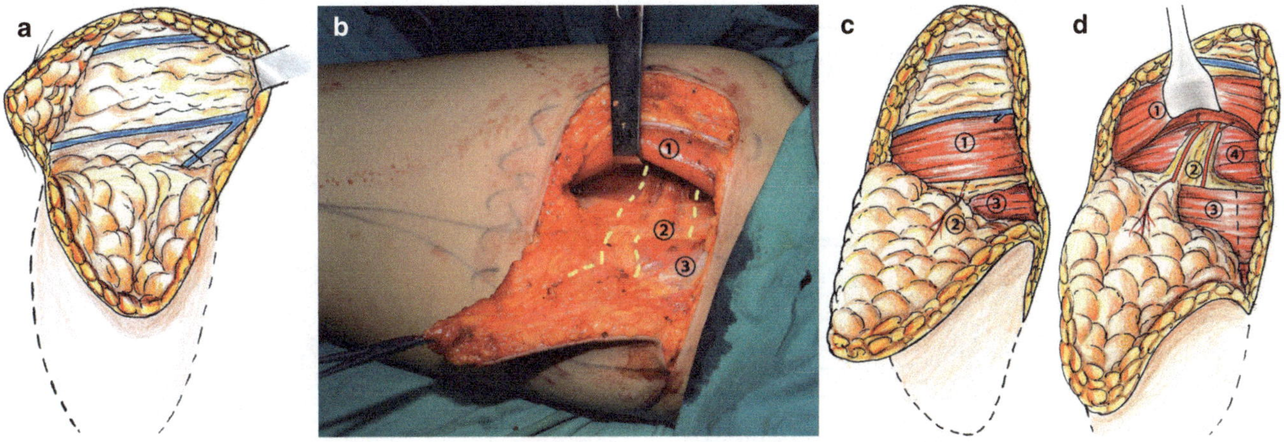

Fig. 23.3 Lift the flap from the anterior to the posterior. First dissect the proximal skin edge. Do not cut deep in order to protect the great saphenous vein. Then lift the flap from the anterior to the posterior, exposing the main trunk of the great saphenous vein. After careful dissociation, pull off the large venous branches for protection and ligate the branches entering the flap and carry them in the flap. After the vein was preserved, the dissecting layer of the flap became deeper. Directly cut to the surface of the long adductor muscle membrane, and lift the flap from the anterior to the posterior to the septum between the long adductor muscle and the gracilis muscle. Through the muscle septum, it was vaguely visible that the profunda femoral vessel entered the gracilis muscle branch and sent a thin perforator into the skin. (1) Adductor longus. (2) Vascular pedicle of the gracilis muscle branch. (3) Gracilis muscle. (4) Adductor major

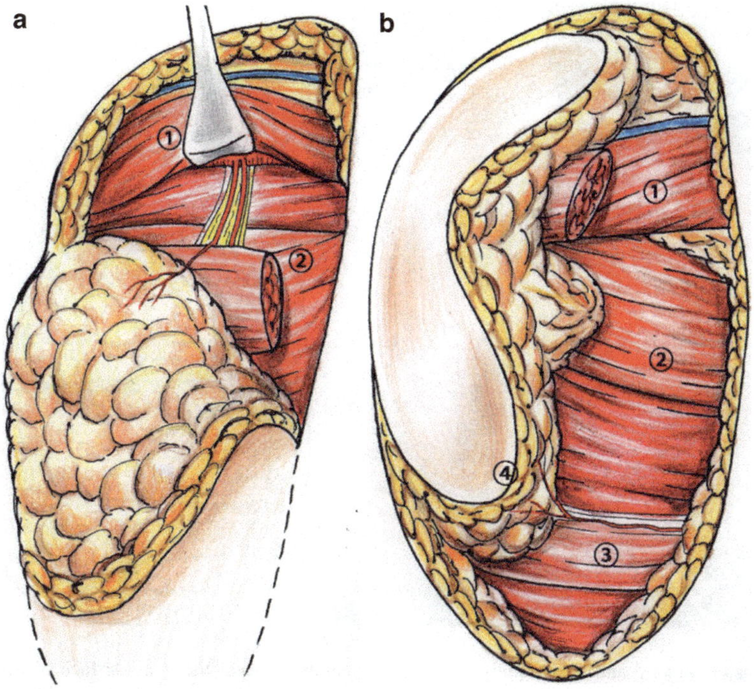

Fig. 23.4 Dissect the muscle septum and expose two larger muscle branches entering the gracilis muscle. The distal muscle branch sends a thinner skin branch into the flap before entering the muscle. The two muscle branches were separated deep along the muscle gap, and more branches that entering the adductor longus and adductor magnus were observed. Considering that no desired perforator was found on the surface of the gracilis muscle by preoperative CTA, we decided to dissect the gracilis muscle flap. Retrogradely separate the two vascular pedicles to the plane from the profunda femoral vessel, and carefully ligate and disconnect the branches along their courses. Do not separate the tissue between the two muscle branches so as to retain enough fascia tissue around the vascular pedicle. Cut off the gracilis muscle at the proximal end. Because the pedicle cannot be dissected, it is difficult to further separate the flap from the anterior to the posterior. We then switched to cut the whole layer of the flap and lifted the flap from the posterior to the anterior. During this process, expose the branches of the posterior femoral cutaneous nerve and nutrient vessels between the semitendinosus and semimembranosus muscles, and retain them, but do not carry them in the flap. The flap was further separated from the posterior to the anterior to expose a thick perforator between the semimembranosus muscle and the adductor magnus muscle, and the posterior edge of the adductor magnus muscle passed through the muscle into the flap. At this stage, the flap separation was not suitable in the superficial layer of deep fascia, because it was difficult to separate subcutaneous fat from deep fascia. Therefore, we chose to separate the flap in the deep surface of deep fascia. (1) Adductor longus. (2) Adductor major. (3) Semimembranosus muscle. (4) Adductor major perforator vessel

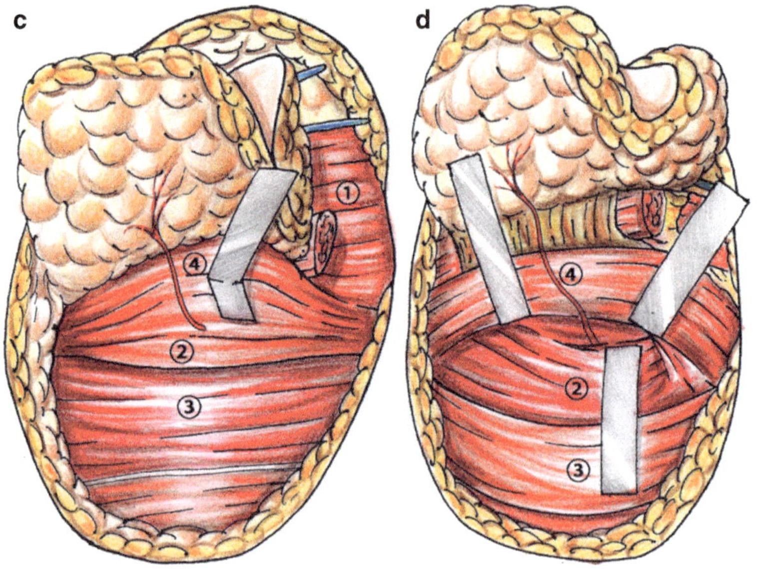

Fig. 23.4 (continued)

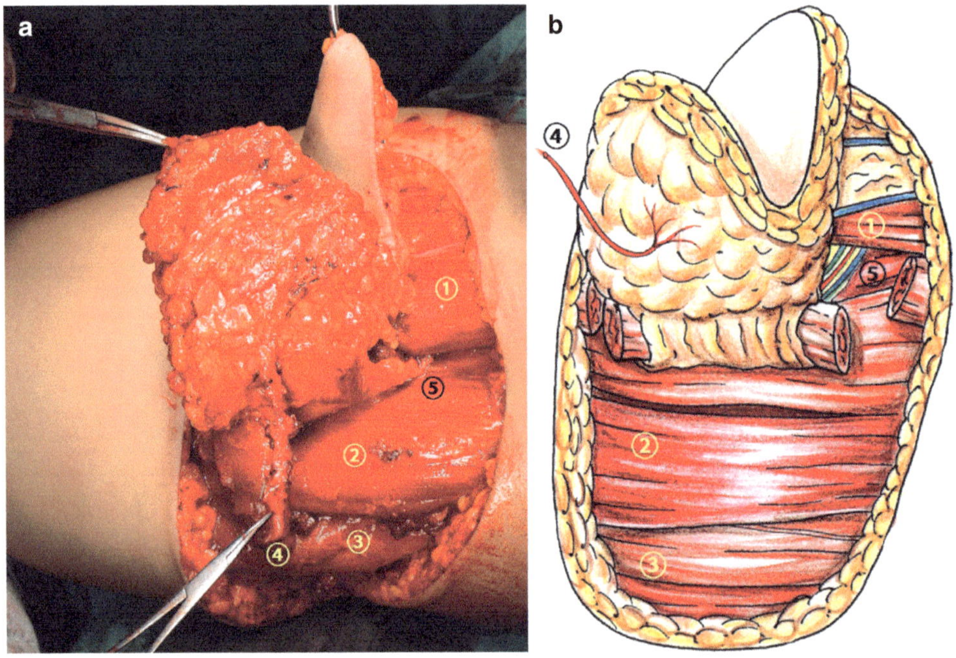

Fig. 23.5 Pull the adductor major forward and retrogradely separate the long segment of perforating vessels in the muscle. It can be seen that it commonly coursed horizontally in the adductor major muscle. It was difficult to separate the vascular pedicle to the length of 7 cm. It was rather circuitous and difficult to separate further. It was fairly close to the plane from the profunda femoral vessel. It was very difficult to separate the vascular pedicle here and the blood vessels were too tight to separate. Dissect the deep surface of the blood vessel on the deeper plane. The perforating branch of adductor major was ligated and disconnected, and the flap was further separated from the back to the back edge of gracilis muscle. The distal end of the gracilis muscle was dissected. (1) Adductor longus. (2) Adductor major. (3) Semimembranosus muscle. (4) Adductor magnus perforator vascular pedicle. (5) Vascular pedicle of the gracilis muscle branch

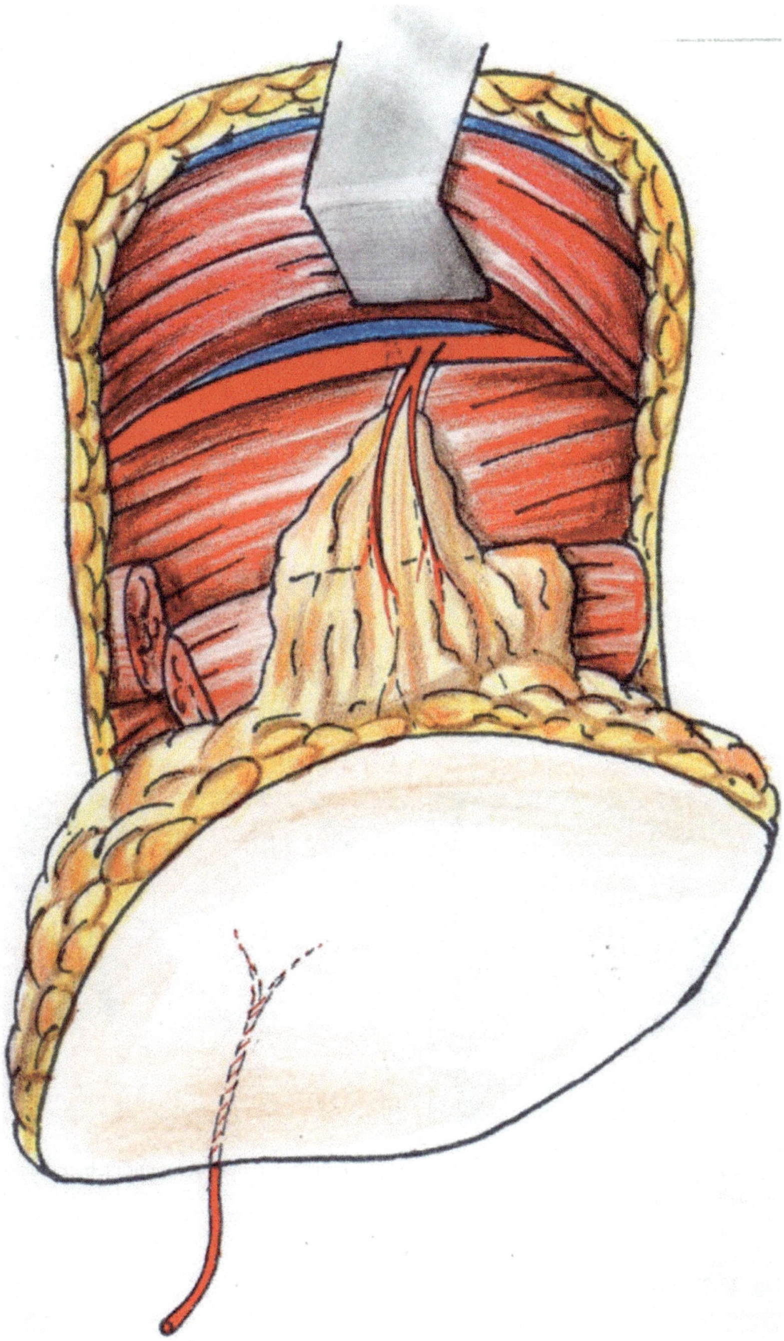

Fig. 23.6 Showing the complete separation of the skin flap and the muscle flap

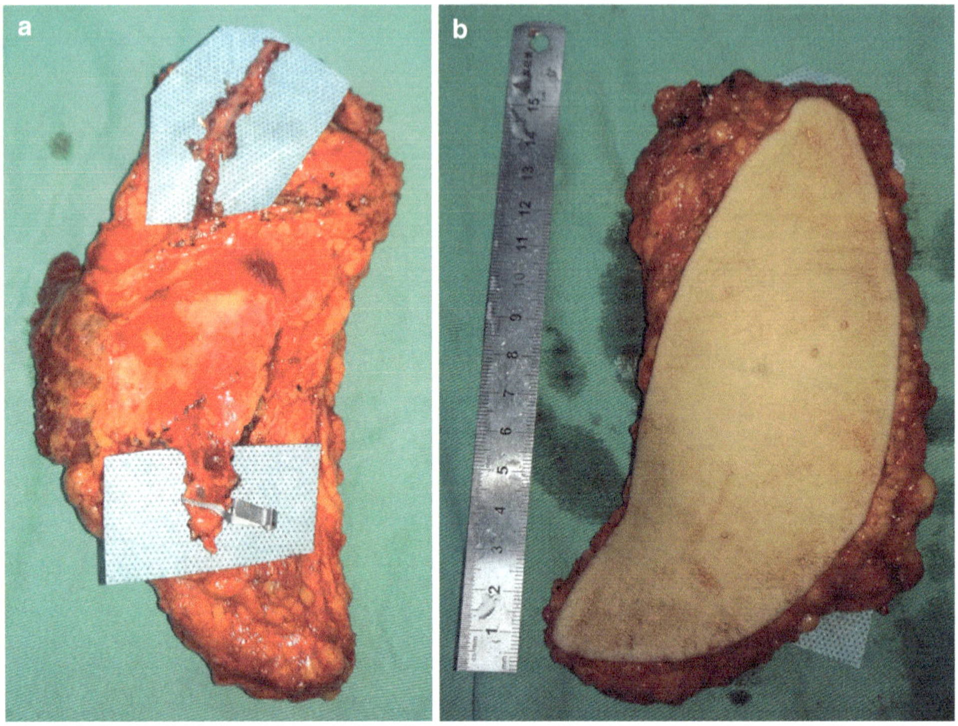

Fig. 23.7 The gracilis myocutaneous flap combined with the perforator flap of the adductor major was dissected

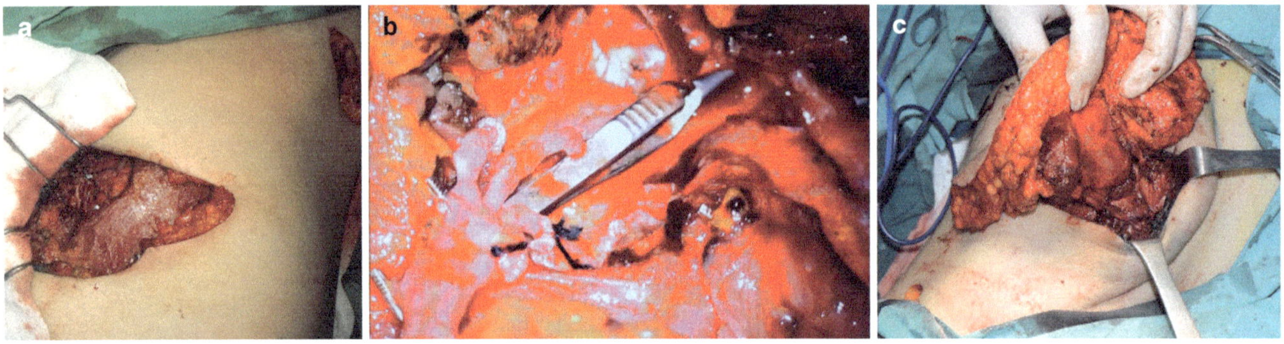

Fig. 23.8 Vascular pedicle of the gracilis muscle branch and perforating branch of the adductor major were anastomosed with proximal and distal thoracic vessels, respectively

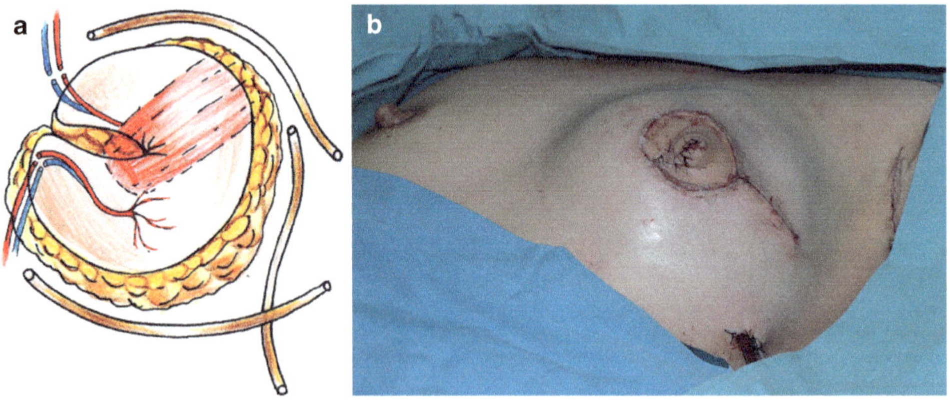

Fig. 23.9 (**a**) Schematic illustration of flap revascularization, flap shaping, and drainage tube placement. (**b**) The skin flap shaping and nipple reconstruction must be performed, while the patient is in sitting position, and the fullness of the lower quadrant should be paid attention to

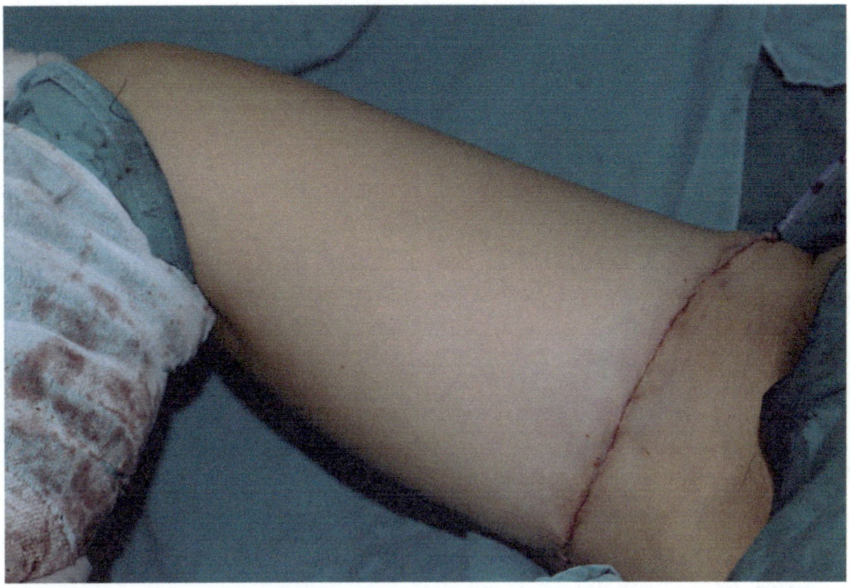

Fig. 23.10 Direct closure of the flap donor area

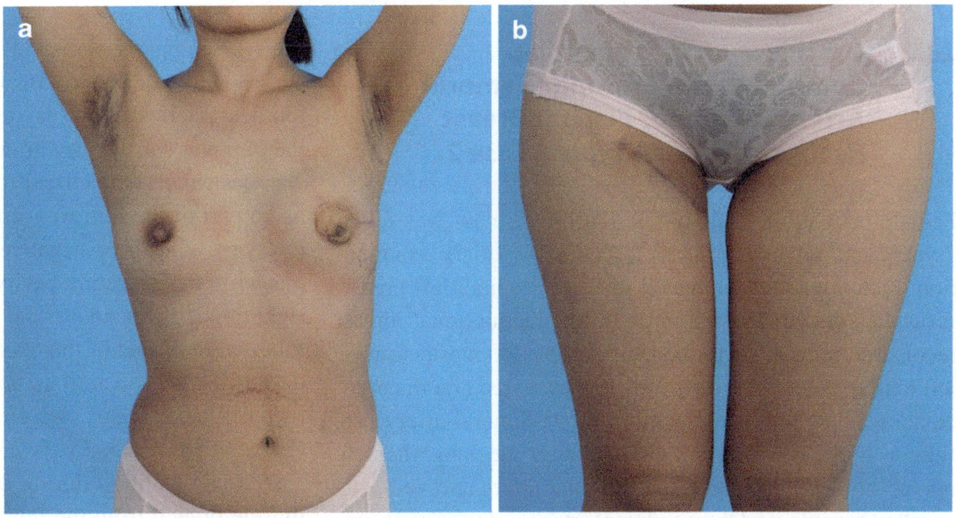

Fig. 23.11 Four-month follow-up after operation

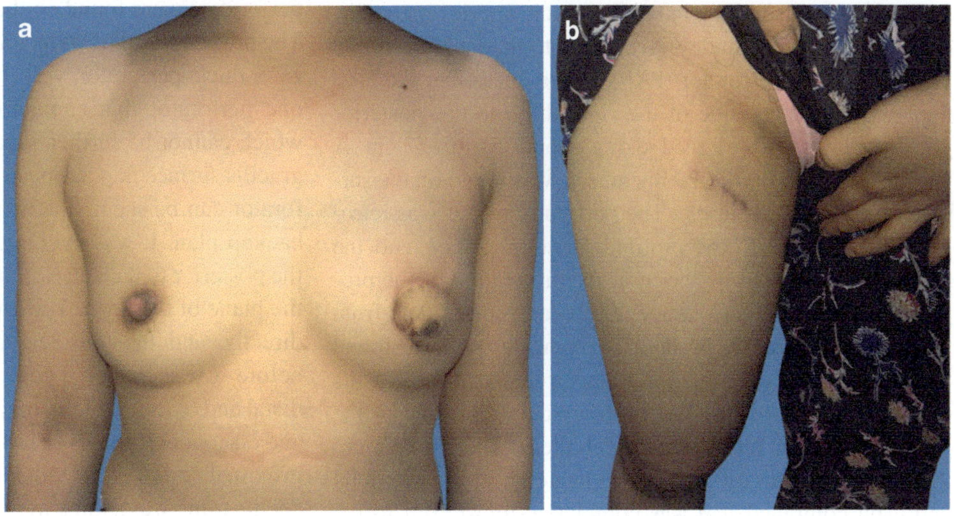

Fig. 23.12 Fourteen-month follow-up

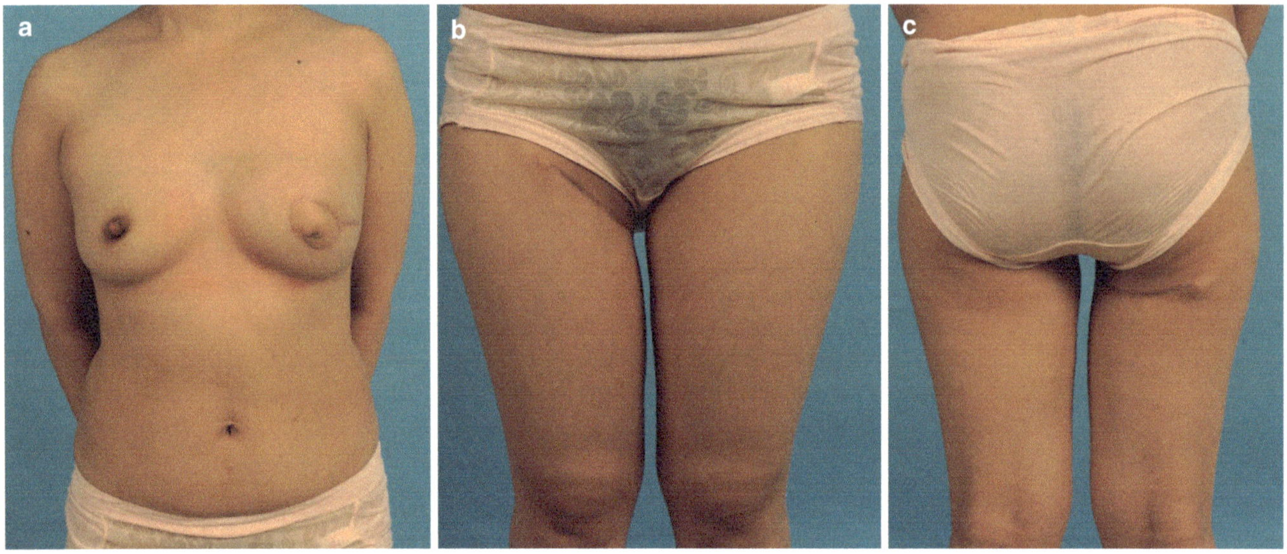

Fig. 23.13 Re-examination 24 months after operation

23.2 Gracilis Myocutaneous Flap Combined with Profunda Femoral Artery Perforator Flap for Breast Reconstruction: A Typical Case 2

Female patient, 48 years old. A left breast mass was found 2 years and 4 days after mass resection. Auxiliary examination: pathological examination of local hospital: left breast-invasive ductal carcinoma. After admission, breast reconstruction was performed with simple left mastectomy + left axillary sentinel lymph node biopsy + free gracilis myocutaneous flap combined with profunda femoral artery perforator flap. After the left mastectomy, the long thoracic nerve, thoracodorsal nerve, subscapular artery and vein, circumflex scapula, and thoracodorsal artery and vein were preserved. The 4-cm-long cartilage of the left third rib was further removed, and the internal thoracic arteries and veins were dissected for standby. According to the location of the profunda artery perforator (PAP) before operation, the PAP flap from the inner side of the right thigh to the posterior gluteal sulcus was designed sizing about 25 cm × 7 cm. A perforator vessel of the gracilis muscle was found on the surface of the gracilis muscle. The perforator vessel was retrogradely dissected to the profunda femoral artery, and the vascular pedicle was dissected at the bifurcation of the profunda femoral artery. Continue to separate retrogradely from the surface of gracilis muscle. Two perforators were found on the surface of the posterior adductor major of the gracilis muscle. The perforators were retrogradely dissected to the bifurcation of the profunda femoral artery, where the vascular pedicle was cut off and double ligated near the proximal end. The combined flap was completely transferred to the left breast defect, and the perforating arteries and veins of the transverse upper gracilis (TUG) and PAP were anastomosed end-to-end with the proximal and distal ends of the internal thoracic arteries and veins, respectively. The blood supply of the flap was satisfactory after anastomosis. After shaping, it was basically symmetrical to the defect of the right breast and a part of the skin was removed. The wound was sutured in layers, and three negative-pressure drainage tubes were placed in the operation cavity. Hemostasis at the root of the right thigh, direct suture, and two negative-pressure drainage tubes were placed in the operation cavity. The flap survived decently after operation, and the shape and function of reconstructed breast were satisfactory during follow-up (Figs. 23.14, 23.15, 23.16, 23.17, 23.18, and 23.19).

Actual condition during operation: The adductor longus muscle branch from the femoral artery was injured by mistake, and it can't be used even if it is preserved. No obvious perforators were found on the surface of the gracilis muscle. The proximal end of adductor major near the upper thigh had zero thick perforator vessel. Retrograde separation found one perforator that came from the inferior gluteal artery, which cannot be further separated and utilized. Half of the gracilis surface flap has been stripped, and only one fine perforator can be seen, which cannot be further separated as a backup plan. It was extremely difficult to lift the flap from the posterior to the anterior. It is important to pay attention to the plane of the layer. The gluteal fascia should be dissected directly, and the muscle septum tissue should be cut off before it was loosened completely. A thin perforator at the distal end of the adductor major was exposed and then ligated and disconnected so as to further expose a perforator near the proximal end of the gracilis major. The course was complex, and its trunk was a thick muscular branch entering the adductor major.

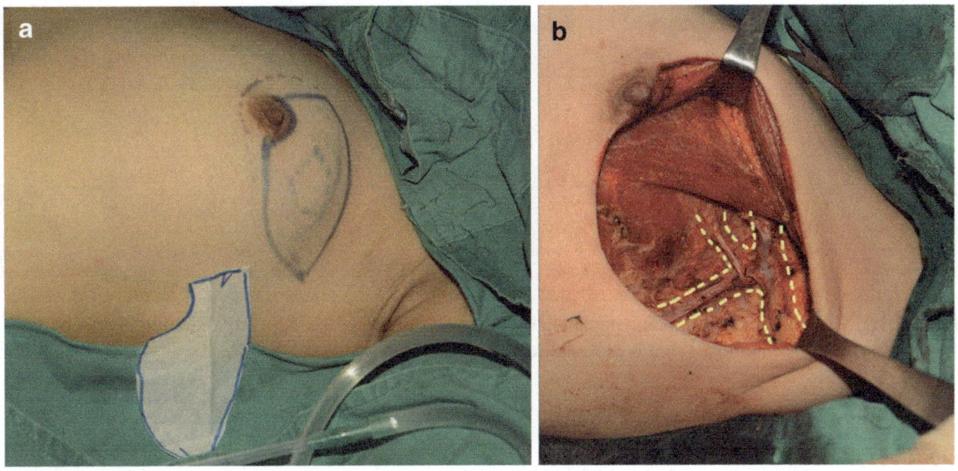

Fig. 23.14 (**a**) Preoperative design. (**b**) Finish modifying the radical mastectomy and prepare the blood vessels in breast cancer area

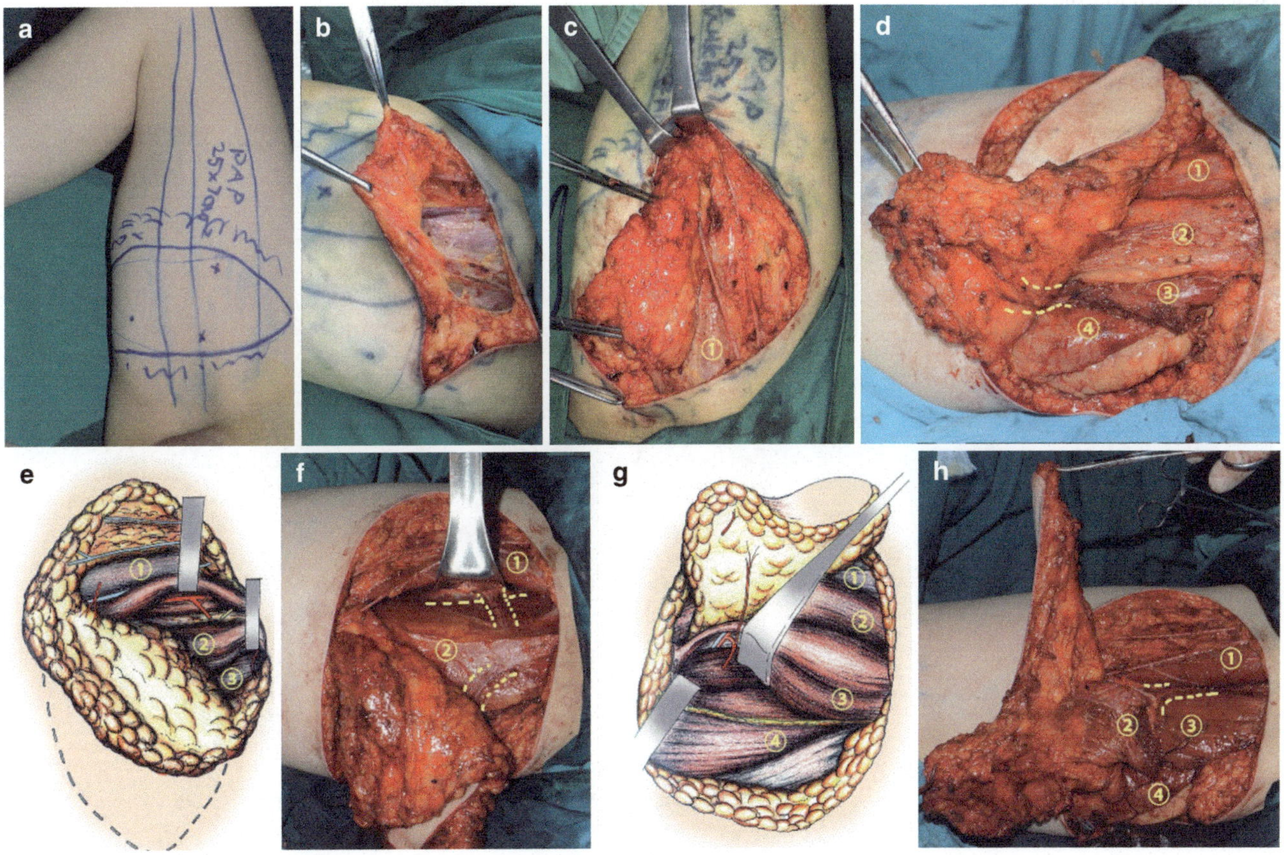

Fig. 23.15 The medial femoral perforator flap was designed and dissected. Depending on the specific condition during the operation, the gracilis myocutaneous flap combined with the adductor major perforator flap was applied. (1) Adductor longus. (2) Gracilis muscle. (3) Adductor major. (4) Semimembranosus muscle

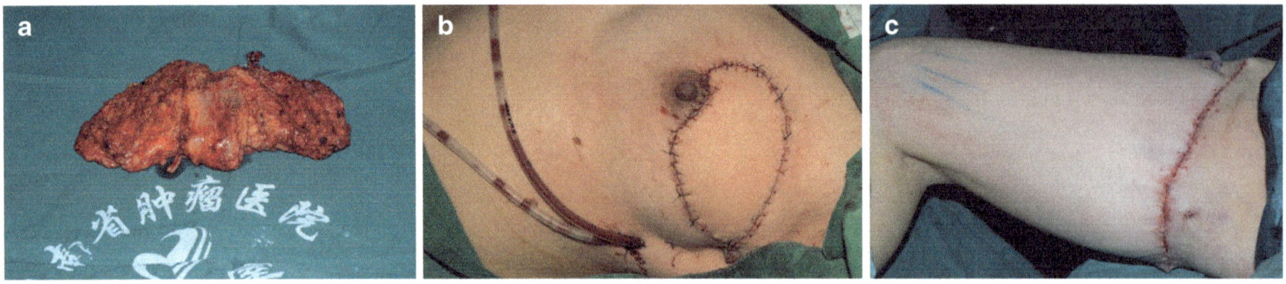

Fig. 23.16 Breast reconstruction is completed after the preparation of the flap. After shaping, it can be seen that the appearance and function are satisfactory, and the flap donor area is closed directly

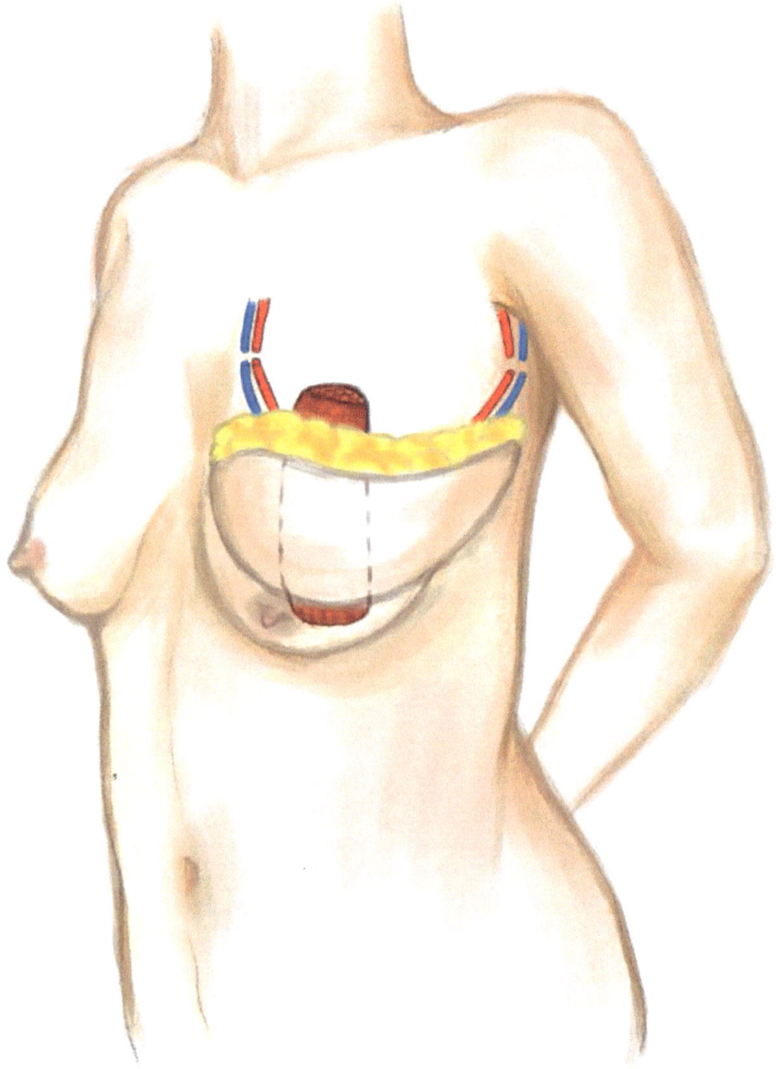

Fig. 23.17 Revascularization mode. The vascular pedicle of the gracilis muscle branch was anastomosed with the internal thoracic vessel (1A1V), and the vascular pedicle of the adductor major perforator was anastomosed with the lateral thoracic vessel (1A1V)

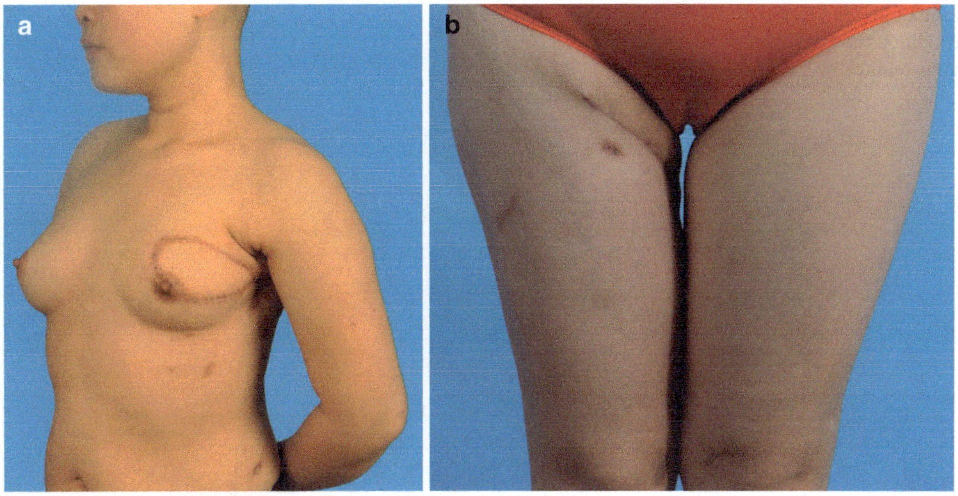

Fig. 23.18 The appearance and function after 1-year follow-up

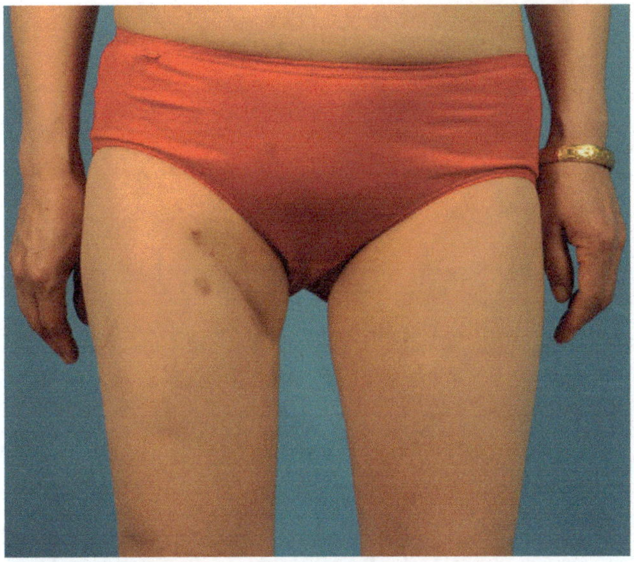

Fig. 23.19 The appearance and function after 18 months of follow-up

23.3 Gracilis Myocutaneous Flap Combined with Profunda Femoral Artery Perforator Flap for Breast Reconstruction: Typical Case 3

The patient was a female, 47 years old. Twenty days after four rounds of neoadjuvant chemotherapy for right breast cancer, pathological diagnosis showed (right breast) invasive ductal carcinoma, histological grade II; immunohistochemistry revealed Er (−), PR (−), C-erbB-2 (−), p53 (+), Ki-67 (+ 70%), CK5/6 (−), p63 (−), p120catenin (membrane +), top2 (+), E-cadherin (+), AR (−), GATA-3 (+), GCDFP-15 (−), EGFR (+), CD34 (vascular +), and special staining: pas (−).

After admission, breast cancer was reconstructed by modified radical mastectomy plus free profunda artery perforator (PAP) flap and thin flap transplantation.

During the operation, the medial femoral flap sizing 33 cm × 7 cm from the inner side of the right thigh to the posterior gluteal sulcus was designed to dissected, the perforating vessels of the transvers upper gracilis (TUG) and PAP were anastomosed end-to-end with the proximal and distal ends of the internal thoracic arteries and veins, respectively. The blood supply of the flap was satisfactory after anastomosis. The flap was folded and assembled. Two triangular flaps were designed at the overlap of the flap to cross to form a new nipple. A piece of costal cartilage was placed under the new nipple, fixed with silk thread, and the position was adjusted to be consistent with the opposite side. After shaping, the appearance of the right breast was consistent with the left breast. The unnecessary part of the skin was removed, and the wound was sutured in layers. Three negative-pressure drainage tubes were placed in the operation cavity. Hemostasis at the root of the right thigh, direct suture, and two negative-pressure drainage tubes were placed in the operation cavity.

Postoperative pathological examination report: (1) (Right breast) the residual breast showed proliferative changes, chronic inflammatory cell infiltration was seen in the area, and cancer thrombus formation in the vessel was seen. There was no clear residual cancer nest, which was consistent with the postoperative changes. (2) Cancer metastasis was found in 1/16 of the lymph nodes (right axillary), and no cancer metastasis was found in 2 lymph nodes in group 3. (3) No cancer invasion was found in the skin, basal margin, nipple area, and intermuscular tubercle. Further comprehensive treatment progressed smoothly. The function and appearance of the reconstructed breast of patients were satisfactory during follow-up, and only one linear scar was left in the donor area (Figs. 23.20, 23.21, 23.22, 23.23, 23.24, 23.25, 23.26, and 23.27).

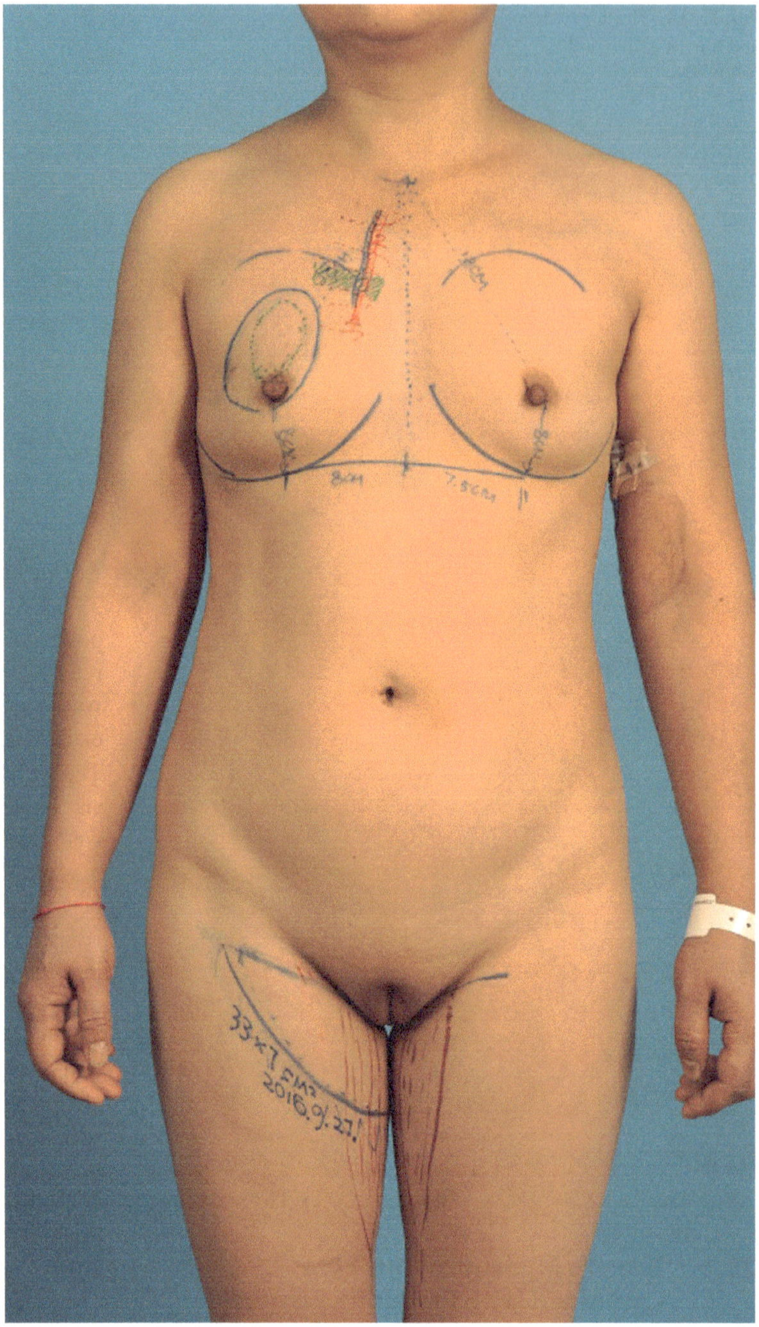

Fig. 23.20 Preoperative conditions and design preparation

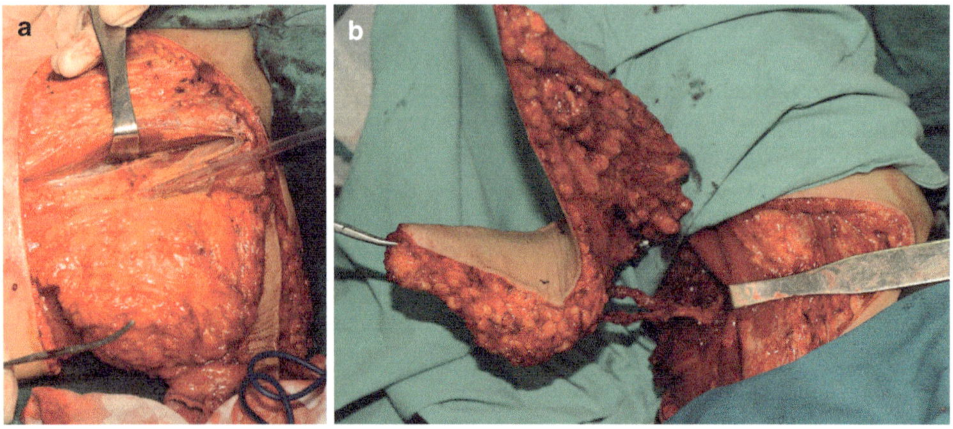

Fig. 23.21 Design of the gracilis myocutaneous flap combined with adductor major perforator flap

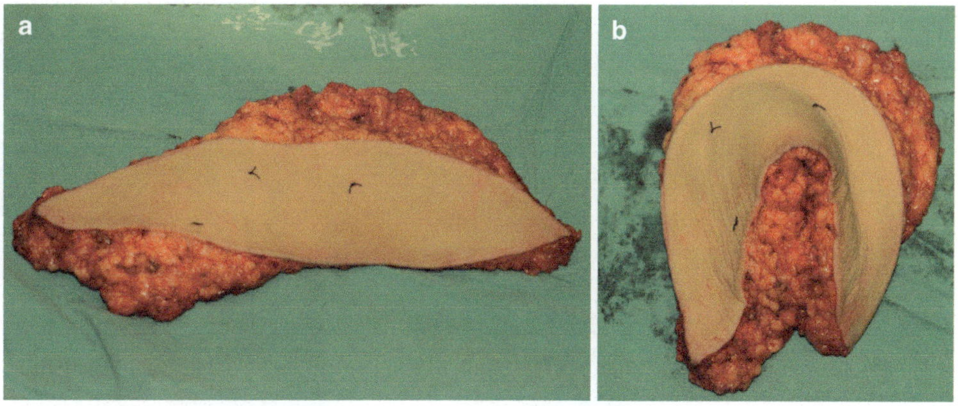

Fig. 23.22 The flap was dissected and further shaped

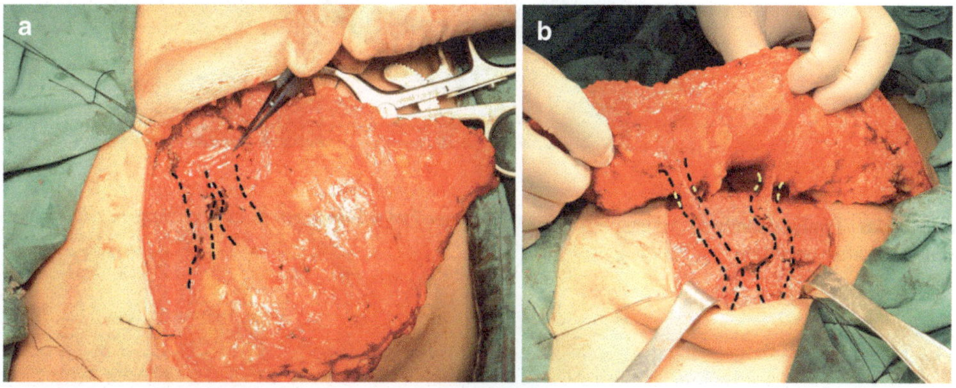

Fig. 23.23 Bilateral vascular pedicle anastomosed with proximal and distal thoracic vessels, respectively

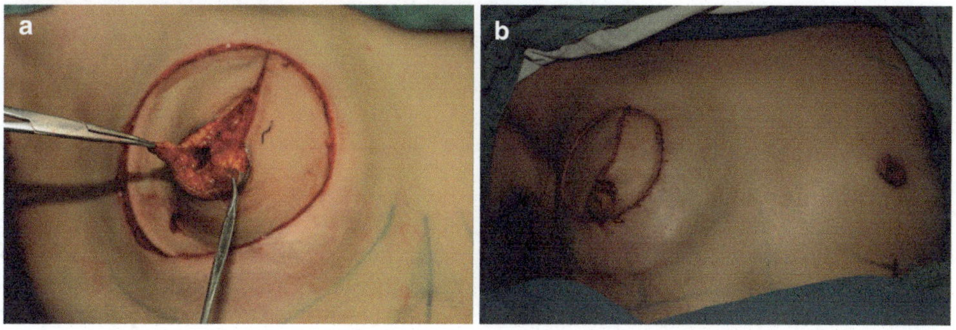

Fig. 23.24 Skin flap shaping and nipple reconstruction in one stage

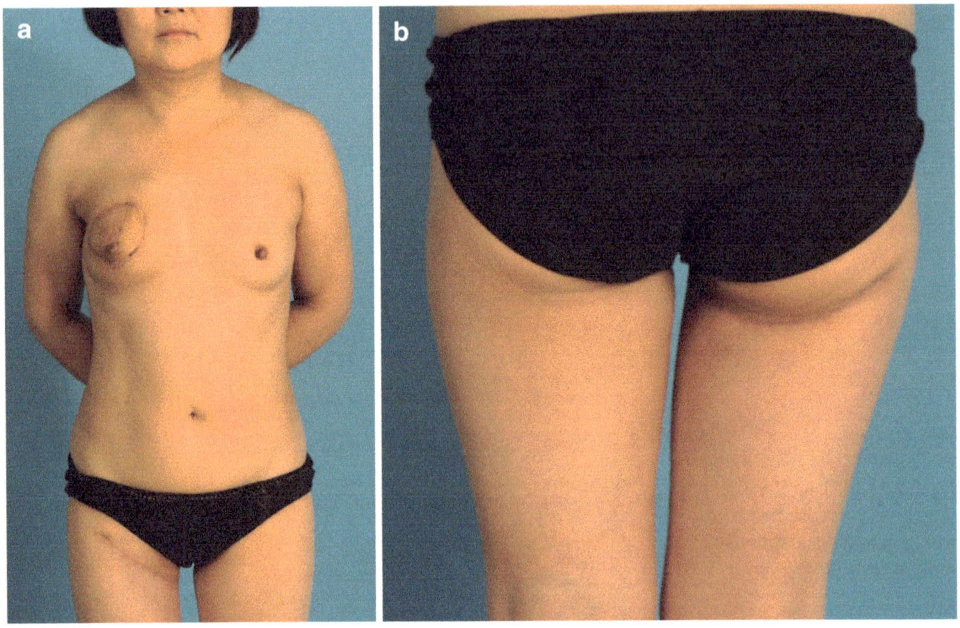

Fig. 23.25 Six-month follow-up after operation

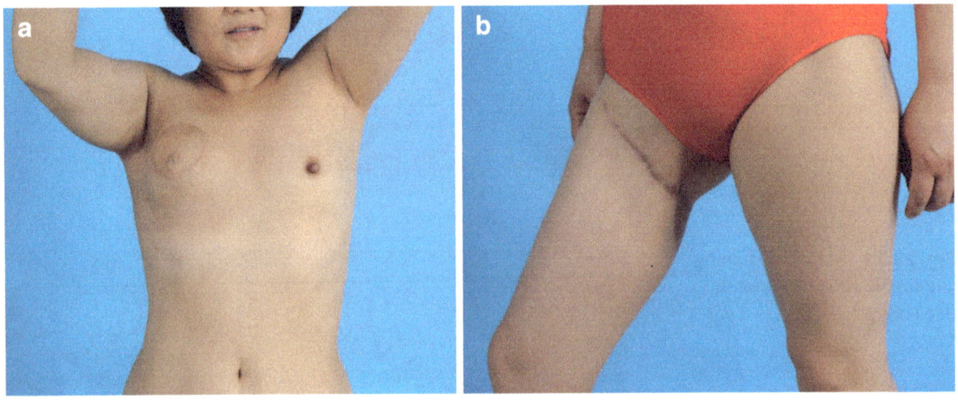

Fig. 23.26 Twelve-month follow-up after operation

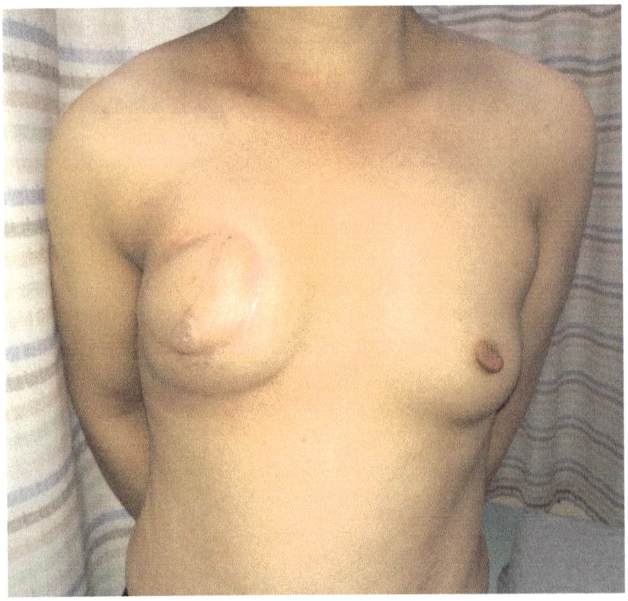

Fig. 23.27 Eighteen-month follow-up

23.4 Gracilis Myocutaneous Flap Combined with Profunda Femoral Artery Perforator Flap for Breast Reconstruction

The patient was a female, 37 years old. Left breast mass was found in 6 months. Physical examination: The upper quadrant of the left breast was palpated and a mass sizing 4.5 cm × 3.0 cm was found. The mass was about 0.5 cm from the nipple, hard, uneven surface, clear boundary, tenderness, and with palpable enlarged lymph nodes under the left armpit. No mass was palpated in the right breast, and the enlarged lymph nodes were not palpable in the right armpit and on the double clavicle. Auxiliary examination: color Doppler ultrasound in our hospital: The malignant possibility of the left breast tumor was high. After admission, breast reconstruction with modified radical mastectomy of left breast cancer + free profunda artery perforator flap (PAP) combined with gracilis myocutaneous flap was performed.

The operation was divided into two groups: donor area and primary defect area. Both operation groups were performed at the same time. One group completed the modified radical mastectomy and preservation of the long thoracic nerves, the thoracodorsal nerve, and the inferior scapular artery and vein. The left third costal cartilage was further removed for about 3 cm long, and the left internal thoracic artery and vein were dissected for standby.

In the other group, the flap in shuttle shape about 26 cm × 7 cm in size was designed at the root of the right thigh according to the preoperative location of the profunda femoral artery perforator. The vascular pedicle of the flap was separated to the plane from the profunda femoral artery to form a double vascular pedicle flap pedicled with two perforator vessels (the pedicle length was 7.0 cm). The flap was completely dissociated and transferred to the left breast defect. The two perforator vessels and arteriovenous vessels carried by the flap were anastomosed end to end with the proximal and distal ends of the reserved internal thoracic artery and vein. The blood supply of the flap was good after vascular anastomosis. In the sitting position, the skin flap was used for shaping to make the reconstructed breast basically symmetrical with the right breast. A part of the skin was removed. Three negative pressure drainage tubes were placed in the chest wall wound, and the wound was sutured in layers. The leg was abducted, and the proximal and distal edges of the donor flap area at the root of the thigh were closed and sutured in layers. Two negative pressure drainage tubes were placed in the operation cavity. After operation, breast specimens and axillary lymphoid adipose tissue were sent to pathological examination. The results showed that (1) (left breast) invasive ductal carcinoma was histologically grade III, tumor thrombus was seen in the vessel, and the size of the mass was 5 cm × 2.5 cm × 1.8 cm; (2) cancer metastasis can be seen in 1/1 of the lymph nodes: (between the pectoral muscles) and 5/14 of the left armpit, and no cancer metastasis can be seen in 1 of the lymph nodes (between the armpits); and (3) skin, basal margin, and nipple: no cancer invasion. Immunohistochemistry: Er (weak, medium and strong, about 80%), PR (weak, medium and strong, about 60%), CerbB-2 (+), and Ki-67 (about 60%). The postoperative recovery was smooth, and the further chemotherapy process went well. The appearance and function of the reconstructed breast were satisfactory. There was no tumor recurrence. Only linear scars were left in the donor area (Figs. 23.28, 23.29, 23.30, 23.31, 23.32, 23.33, 23.34, 23.35, 23.36, and 23.37).

Intraoperative conditions: There were three to four perforating branches of different sizes arising from the profunda femoral artery between the adductor longus and gracilis femoris. There were two main branches entering the gracilis muscle and crossing each other (the vascular pedicle must be completely separated under the microscope. The blood vessels in the thorax should be completely separated in long sections for standby, so as to avoid tortuous traction or kinking compression. The blood vessels were thin and cannot be excessively extended. Washing with water was required during anastomosis. The thread can be left first, and finally tied uniformly to avoid avulsion. The whole procedures were very difficult to operate.) There were two potent perforating branches in the muscle interval between gracilis and adductor major. Unfortunately, both vessels were not used. The size and length of the vascular pedicle should be measured in the first place. The posterior femoral cutaneous nerve and its nutrient vessels between semitendinosus and semimembranosus muscle and biceps femoris muscle entered the skin as the second vascular pedicle. The saphenous nerve was located in the deep fascia at the proximal end of the thigh.

For the preparation techniques of internal mammary vessels, refer to the chapter of rectus abdominis flap and the chapter of the recipient vessel selection.

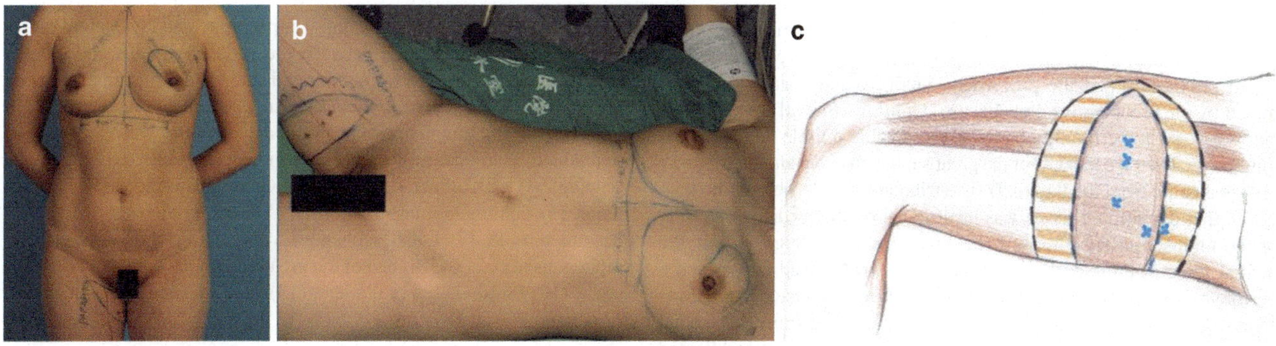

Fig. 23.28 Preoperative design. The inferior fold of the breasts of both affected and contralateral sides and the amount of skin and tissue missing from the affected breast were determined from the patient's standing position before operation so as to evaluate the potential volume of resected tissue after operation

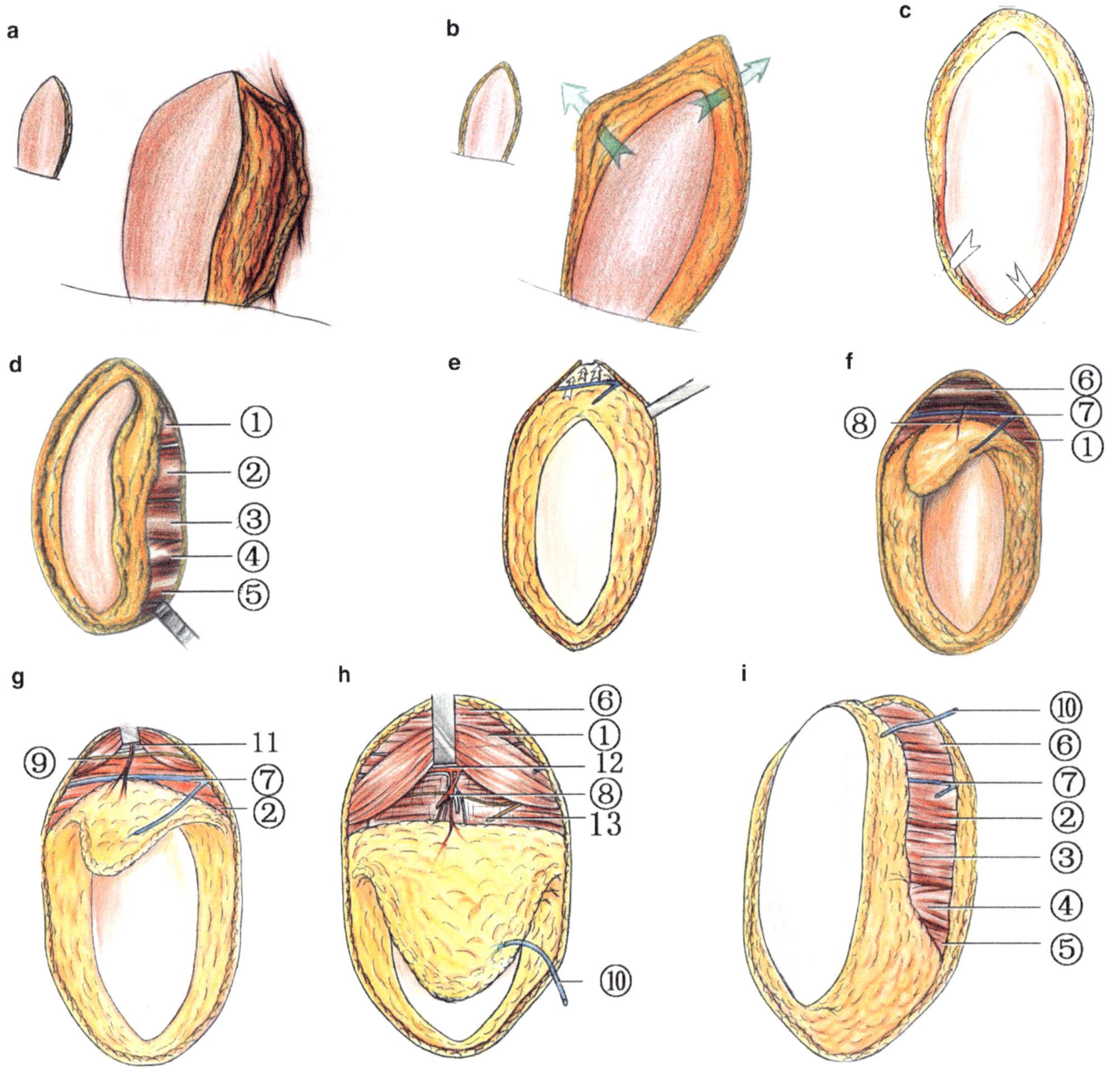

Fig. 23.29 Flap raising started with opening the medial margin (**a**), followed by wide undermining of the flap off the skin (**b**). The undermining began proximally and the proceeded anteriorly and distally as determined by the preoperative drawings (**c**). Uplift the flap off the deep fascia to reveal the perforators between the gracilis muscle and adductor longus (**d**). Then we looked for the great saphenous vein and its tributary (10) that came from the flap (**e**, **f**). The tributary was carried on the flap. Given that the adipose tissue was insufficient on the medial thigh, flap undermining continued toward the anterior lateral thigh. Upon the medial femoral muscle, the flap was raised off the deep fascia, and a perforator between the medial femoral muscle and adductor longus was found (**g**). Later, we found that this perforator came from the medial femoral circumflex artery, however, the perforator was short and ligated (**h**). Further undermining of the flap was performed and two small perforators were observed to run between the adductor longus and gracilis muscle. These perforators were separated. Next, we turned to lift the flap off the deep fascia at the proximal margin, two small perforators travelling between the gracilis muscle and adductor major were viewed and maintained. Flap undermining was continued according to preoperative drawings (**i**). 1: Adductor longus. (2) Gracilis muscle. (3) Adductor major. (4) Semimembranosus muscle. (5) Semitendinosus. (6) Medial femoral muscle. (7) Great saphenous vein. (8) Perforator vessel. (9) Saphenous nerve. (10) Branch of the great saphenous vein. (11) Femoral artery. (12) Profunda femoral artery. (13) Anterior branch of the obturator nerve

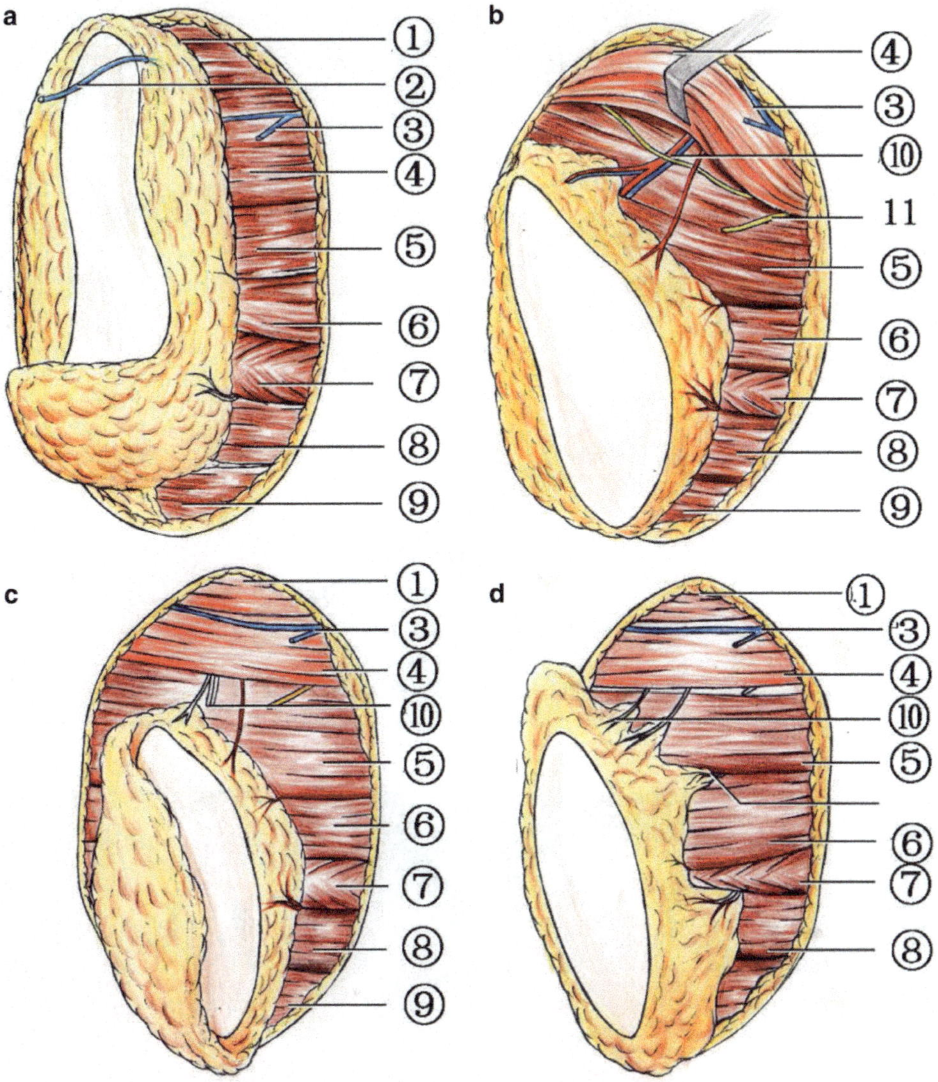

Fig. 23.30 Flap undermining continued inferiorly and medially, a large perforator concomitant with nerves between the semitendinosus and semimembranosus muscles were spotted (**a**). Then, we pulled the adductor longus aside and found two intermuscular perforators and a large branch of the deep femoral vessel that penetrated the gracilis muscle (**b**). We separated these perforators off the anterior branch of the obturator nerve. Finally, we the intermuscular perforator between the semitendinosus and semimembranosus muscles were preserved and used as the flap pedicle (**c**, **d**). The second perforating artery of the profunda femoral artery traveled closely with the branch of the posterior femoral cutaneous nerve running in the space between the semimembranosus muscle and semitendinosus muscle. (1) Medial femoral muscle. (2) Branch of the great saphenous vein. (3) Great saphenous vein. (4) Adductor longus. (5) Gracilis muscle. (6) Adductor major. (7) Semimembranosus muscle. (8) Semitendinosus. (9) Biceps femoris. (10) Perforator vessel. (11) Anterior branch of the obturator nerve

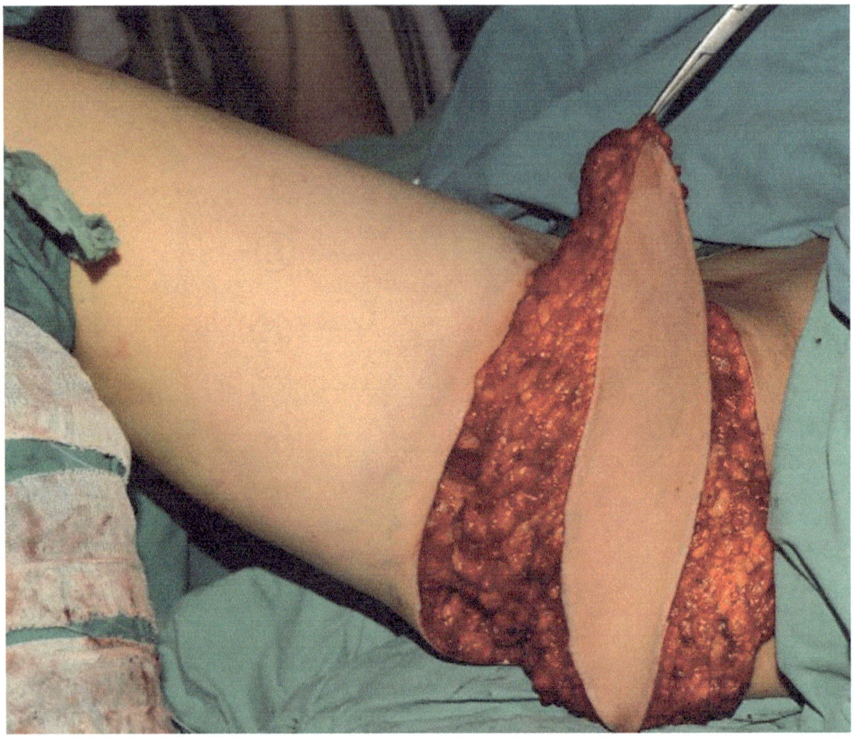

Fig. 23.31 The dissection of the flap was completed

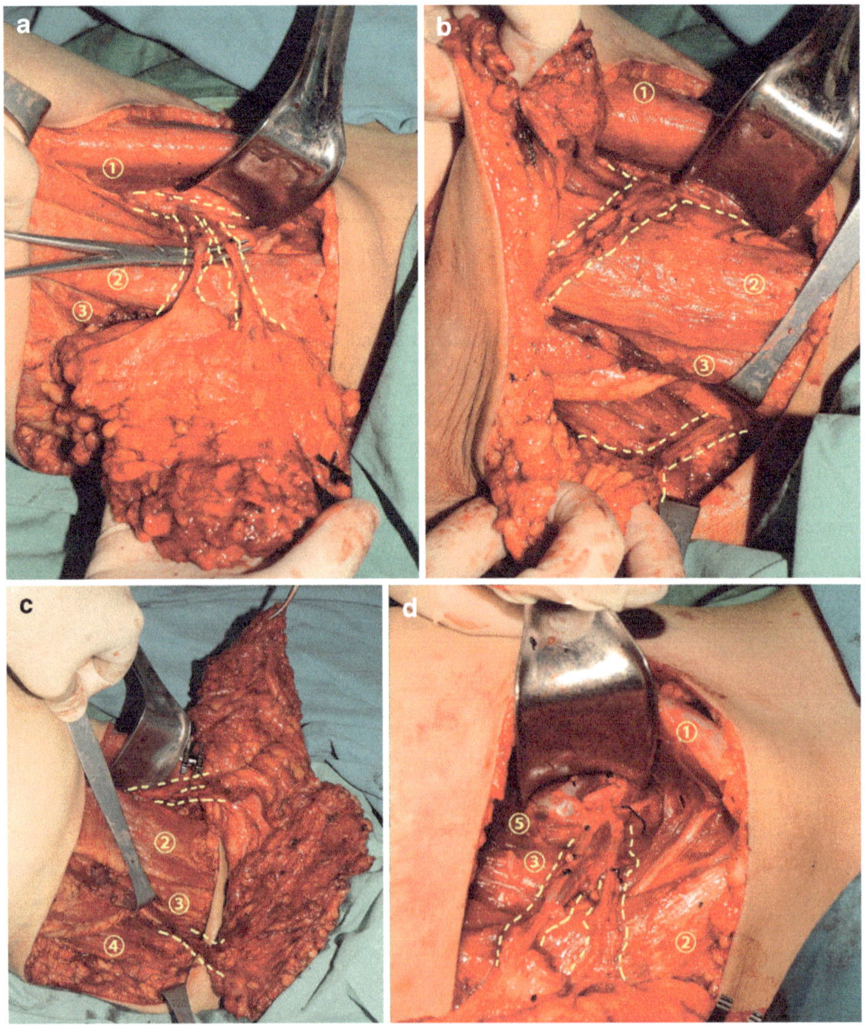

Fig. 23.32 Retrograde separation of the bilateral vascular pedicle to the plane from profunda femoral vessels. (1) Adductor longus. (2) Gracilis muscle. (3) Adductor major. (4) Semimembranosus muscle. (5) Profunda femoral vessels

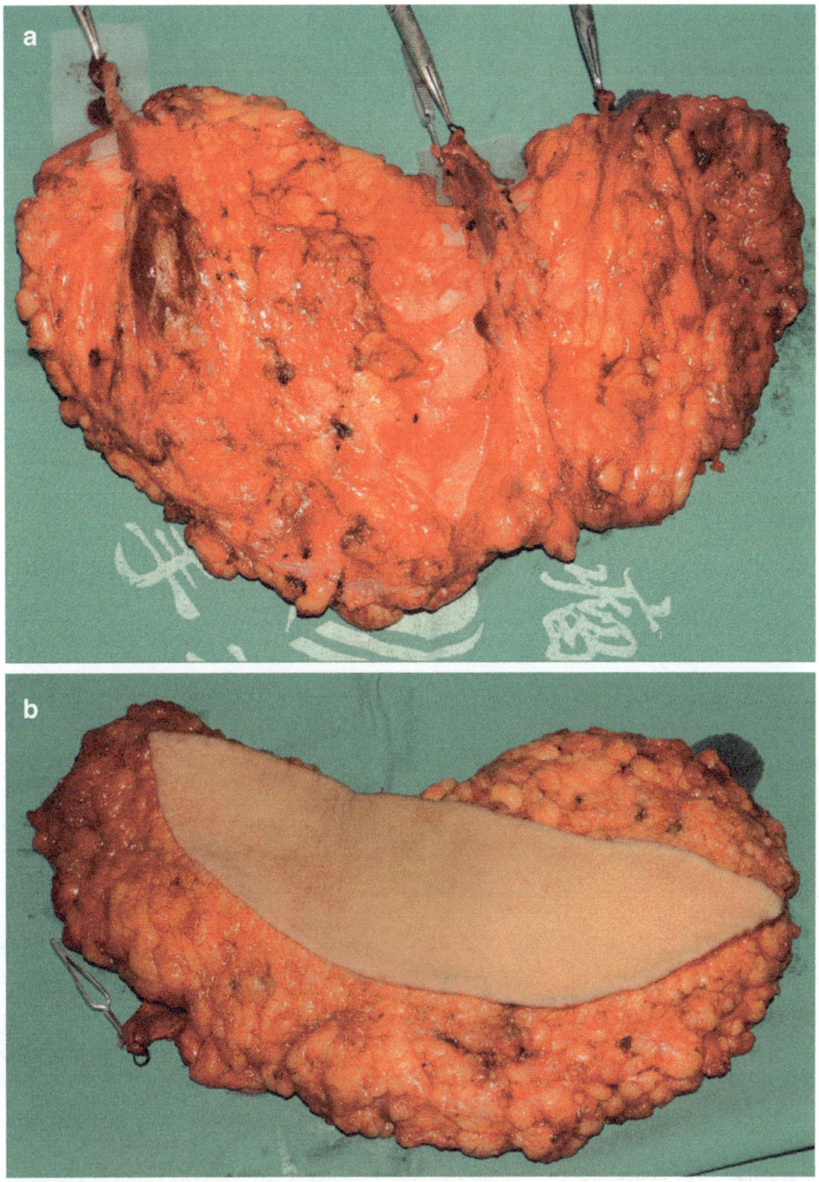

Fig. 23.33 The perforator flap of profunda femoral artery pedicled with bilateral vessels has been cut off

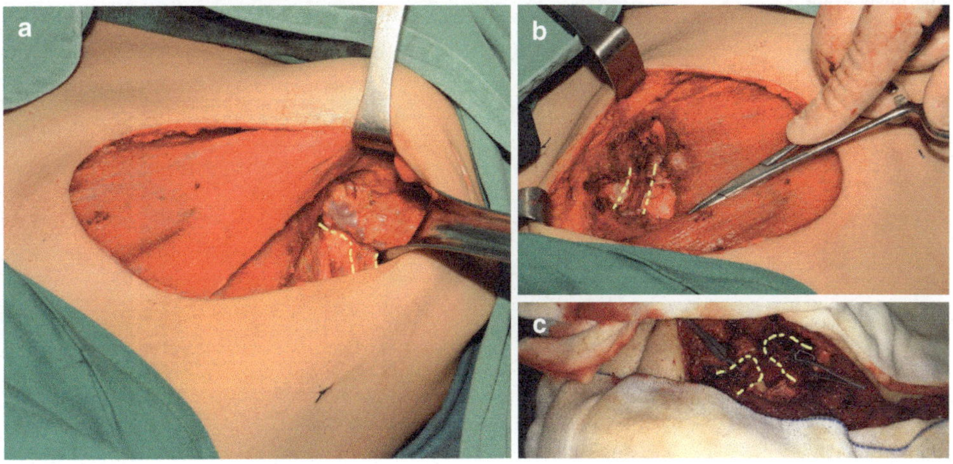

Fig. 23.34 After modified radical mastectomy for left breast cancer, the further recipient blood vessels were prepared

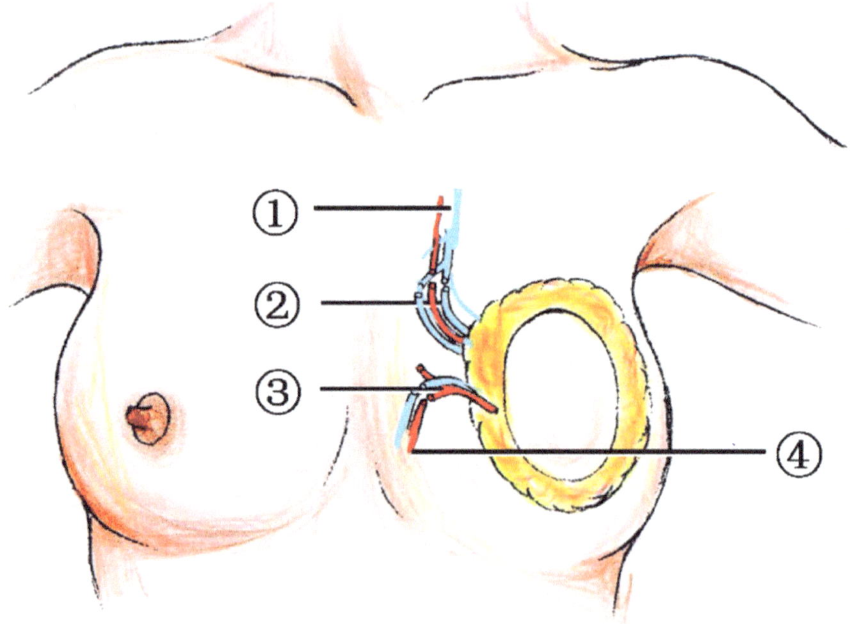

Fig. 23.35 Pattern of flap revascularization. (1) Proximal end of the internal mammary vessels. (2) Perforator of the profunda femoral artery. (3) Perforator of the second perforator artery of the profunda femoral artery. (4) Distal end of internal mammary vessels

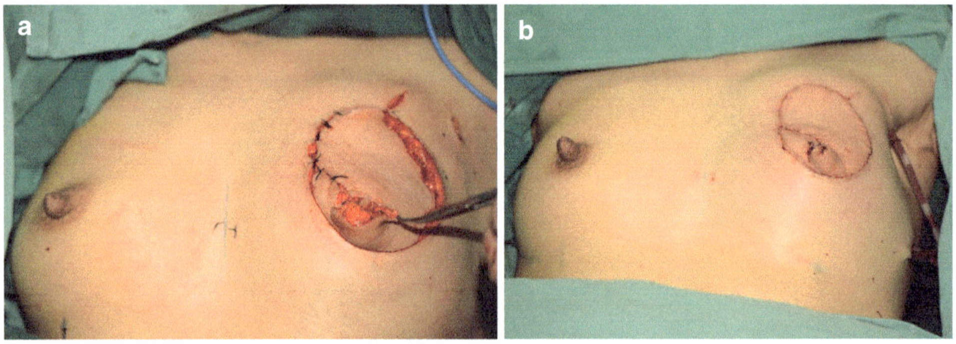

Fig. 23.36 Flap shaping and nipple reconstruction in one stage during operation

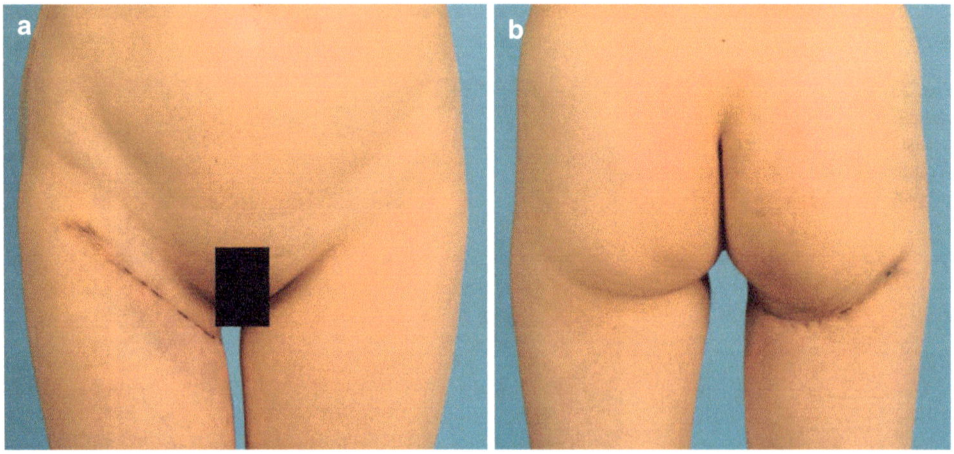

Fig. 23.37 The donor site was directly closed, leaving only linear scars

23.5 Discussion

The combination of transverse upper gracilis muscle and profunda artery perforator flap (TUG + PAP) is mainly used for unilateral donor area for ipsilateral medium or large volume breast reconstruction. The gracilis combined with profunda femoral artery flap consists of two kinds of flaps, including transverse crescent gracilis myocutaneous flap (TUG) and PAP. All gracilis combined with profunda femoral artery perforator flaps are composed of two vascular pedicles: the gracilis muscle branch of the profunda femoral artery supplying the gracilis muscle flap and the adductor major perforator of profunda femoral artery supplying the profunda femoral artery perforator flap. According to international reports and statistics, the average dissecting area of the skin island is 28.6 cm × 8 cm (range from 27 cm × 7 cm to 30 cm × 9 cm). The average length of the vascular pedicle of the gracilis myocutaneous flap was 7 cm (range 6–8 cm), and the length of vascular pedicle of perforator flap of profunda femoral artery was 9 cm (range 8.5–10 cm). Our clinical data are consistent with it. The independent technique of dissecting TUG and PAP flaps has been described in detail in the previous chapters.

23.6 Conclusion

The gracilis combined with profunda femoral artery perforator flap is a valuable alternative for autologous breast reconstruction.

References

1. Yousif NJ. The transverse gracilis musculocutaneous flap. Ann Plast Surg. 1993;31(4):382.
2. Healy C, Allen RJ. The evolution of perforator flap breast reconstruction: twenty years after the first DIEP flap. J Reconstr Microsurg. 2014;30(2):121–5.
3. LoTempio MM, Allen RJ. Breast reconstruction with SGAP and IGAP flaps. Plast Reconstr Surg. 2010;126(2):393–401.
4. Allen RJ, Treece P. Deep inferior epigastric perforator flap for breast reconstruction. Ann Plast Surg. 1994;32(1):32–8.
5. Schoeller T, Huemer GM, Wechselberger G. The transverse musculocutaneous gracilis flap for breast reconstruction: guidelines for flap and patient selection. Plast Reconstr Surg. 2008;122(1):29–38.
6. Fansa H, Schirmer S, Warnecke IC, Cervelli A, Frerichs O. The transverse myocutaneous gracilis muscle flap: a fast and reliable method for breast reconstruction. Plast Reconstr Surg. 2008;122(5):1326–33.
7. Vega SJ, Sandeen SN, Bossert RP, Perrone A, Ortiz L, Herrera H. Gracilis myocutaneous free flap in autologous breast reconstruction. Plast Reconstr Surg. 2009;124(5):1400–9.
8. Buntic RF, Horton KM, Brooks D, Althubaiti GA. Transverse upper gracilis flap as an alternative to abdominal tissue breast reconstruction: technique and modifications. Plast Reconstr Surg. 2011;128(6):607e–13e.
9. Peek A, Müller M, Ackermann G, Exner K, Baumeister S. The free gracilis perforator flap: anatomical study and clinical refinements of a new perforator flap. Plast Reconstr Surg. 2009;123(2):578–88.
10. Scaglioni MF, Chen YC, Lindenblatt N, Giovanoli P. The vertical posteromedial thigh (vPMT) flap for autologous breast reconstruction: a novel flap design. Microsurgery. 2017;37(5):371–6.
11. Ahmadzadeh R, Bergeron L, Tang M, Geddes CR, Morris SF. The posterior thigh perforator flap or profunda femoris artery perforator flap. Plast Reconstr Surg. 2007;119(1):194–200; discussion 201–2.
12. Fosseprez P, Gerdom A, Servaes M, Deconinck C, Pirson G, Berners A. [Profunda artery perforator flap: reliable secondary option for breast reconstruction?]. Ann Chir Plast Esthet. 2017;62(6):637–45.
13. Haddock N, Nagarkar P, Teotia SS. Versatility of the profunda artery perforator flap: creative uses in breast reconstruction. Plast Reconstr Surg. 2017;139(3):606e–12e.
14. Wong C, Mojallal A, Bailey SH, Trussler A, Saint-Cyr M. The extended transverse musculocutaneous gracilis flap: vascular anatomy and clinical implications. Ann Plast Surg. 2011;67(2):170–7.
15. Fattah A, Figus A, Mathur B, Ramakrishnan VV. The transverse myocutaneous gracilis flap: technical refinements. J Plast Reconstr Aesthet Surg. 2010;63(2):305–13.
16. Pülzl P, Schoeller T, Kleewein K, Wechselberger G. Donor-site morbidity of the transverse musculocutaneous gracilis flap in autologous breast reconstruction: short-term and long-term results. Plast Reconstr Surg. 2011;128(4):233e–42e.
17. Bodin F, Dissaux C, Dupret-Bories A, Schohn T, Fiquet C, Bruant-Rodier C. The transverse musculo-cutaneous gracilis flap for breast reconstruction: how to avoid complications. Microsurgery. 2016;36(1):42–8.
18. Hupkens P, Hameeteman M, Westland PB, Slater NJ, Vasilic D, Ulrich DJ. Breast reconstruction using the geometrically modified profunda artery perforator flap from the posteromedial thigh region: combining the benefits of its predecessors. Ann Plast Surg. 2016;77(4):438–44.
19. Date S, Ciudad P, Maruccia M, Chen HC. Breast reconstruction using the geometrically modified profunda artery perforator flap from the posteromedial thigh region: combining the benefits of its predecessors. Ann Plast Surg. 2017;79(1):124.
20. Allen RJ, Haddock NT, Ahn CY, Sadeghi A. Breast reconstruction with the profunda artery perforator flap. Plast Reconstr Surg. 2012;129(1):16e–23e.
21. Saad A, Sadeghi A, Allen RJ. The anatomic basis of the profunda femoris artery perforator flap: a new option for autologous breast reconstruction—a cadaveric and computer tomography angiogram study. J Reconstr Microsurg. 2012;28(6):381–6.
22. Hupkens P, Van Loon B, Lauret GJ, et al. Anteromedial thigh flaps: an anatomical study to localize and classify anteromedial thigh perforators. Microsurgery. 2010;30(1):43–9.
23. Hupkens P, Ozturk E, Wittens S, Hoevenaren IA, Kooloos JG, Ulrich DJ. Posterior thigh perforator flaps: an anatomical study to localize and classify posterior thigh perforators. Microsurgery. 2013;33(5):376–82.
24. Haddock NT, Greaney P, Otterburn D, Levine S, Allen RJ. Predicting perforator location on preoperative imaging for the profunda artery perforator flap. Microsurgery. 2012;32(7):507–11.
25. DeLong MR, Hughes DB, Bond JE, Thomas SM, Boll DT, Zenn MR. A detailed evaluation of the anatomical variations of the profunda artery perforator flap using computed tomographic angiograms. Plast Reconstr Surg. 2014;134(2):186e–92e.
26. Scaglioni MF, Kuo YR, Yang JC, Chen YC. The posteromedial thigh flap for head and neck reconstruction: anatomical basis, surgical technique, and clinical applications. Plast Reconstr Surg. 2015;136(2):363–75.
27. Satake T, Muto M, Ko S, Yasumura K, Ishikawa T, Maegawa J. Breast reconstruction using free posterior medial thigh perfora-

tor flaps: intraoperative anatomical study and clinical results. Plast Reconstr Surg. 2014;134(5):880–91.
28. Trignano E, Fallico N, Dessy LA, et al. Transverse upper gracilis flap with implant in postmastectomy breast reconstruction: a case report. Microsurgery. 2014;34(2):149–52.
29. Hurwitz ZM, Montilla R, Dunn RM, Patel NV, Akyurek M. Adductor magnus perforator flap revisited: an anatomical review and clinical applications. Ann Plast Surg. 2011;66(5):438–43.
30. Saint-Cyr M, Wong C, Oni G, et al. Modifications to extend the transverse upper gracilis flap in breast reconstruction: clinical series and results. Plast Reconstr Surg. 2012;129(1):24e–36e.
31. Ciudad P, Maruccia M, Orfaniotis G, et al. The combined transverse upper gracilis and profunda artery perforator (TUG+PAP) flap for breast reconstruction. Microsurgery. 2015;36:359.

Double-Pedicled Profunda Femoral Artery Perforator Flap for Breast Reconstruction

24

Dajiang Song and Narushima Mitsunaga

Since the first description of breast reconstruction with deep inferior epigastric artery perforator (DIEP) flap in 1992, the choice of autologous breast reconstruction has been developed [1]. DIEP flap has been the first choice for autologous breast reconstruction for a long time, and its advantages are obvious [2]. However, not all patients can be treated with DIEP flap [3, 4]. With the ongoing progress of microsurgical technology, the continuous development of tumor plastic surgery, and the emergence of novel flaps, it is important to analyze the results and compare them with the previous methods when new flaps are created. Different forms of various flaps have distinct indications and have their own subtle variations and characteristics. Hurwitz and Walton first described the profunda artery perforator flap in 1980 [5]. Later, Angrigiani et al. improved and applied it in clinic as a free flap for burn and bedsore reconstruction [6]. It was not until 2010 that the profunda femoral artery perforator flap was first reported for breast reconstruction. The landmark event was that the profunda artery perforator flap was first demonstrated for breast reconstruction at the International Conference of Perforator Flap in Mexico City in 2010 [7, 8]. The perforator flap of profunda femoral artery has been popularized, and there is an increasing number of reports in the literature. Since 2010, we have performed a series of profunda artery branch flap transplantation, and a lot of knowledge, details, and experience have been gained and understood about its advantages, disadvantages, and surgical techniques in the process of leveraging this flap [9–11]. In order to overcome the restrictions of small tissue volume and insufficient blood supply of the profunda artery perforator flap, we prepared external pressurized profunda femoral artery perforator flap with larger tissue volume and more reliable blood supply by dissecting double-vascular pedicle at the same time according to the anatomical basis of large number of perforator vessels in the posterior medial femoral region, and the clinical effects are satisfactory.

D. Song (✉)
Department of Oncology Plastic Surgery, Hunan Cancer Hospital, Changsha, Hunan, China

N. Mitsunaga
Mie University Graduate School of Medicine Plastic and Reconstructive Surgery, Tsu, Mie, Japan
e-mail: sancho-ps@umin.ac.jp

24.1 Surgical Technique

All patients underwent preoperative thigh magnetic resonance or computed tomography angiography to determine the key perforating branches and assist in determining the volume of tissue available for reconstruction. The preoperative markings were made in the patient's standing position the day before the operation. The upper edge of the flap is located at the gluteal sulcus, and the inferior edge of the flap is about 6–7 cm below the upper edge, depending on the required flap size and tissue volume. The key perforations were explored with a handheld Doppler probe in the patients supine position. Try to detect as many perforating branches on the lateral and posterior of the thigh as possible, the perforating branches should be designed near the center of the flap as much as possible. On the day of operation, the patient was in the lithotomy position under general anesthesia. We have two methods to dissect the double vessel pedicled profunda femoral artery perforator flap, which are different from the previous international reports [12].

First, incise the skin subcutaneous tissue at the front edge and proximal end of the flap along the designed markings. Dissect the deep fascia from the surface of the adductor longus, and lift the flap from the deep surface of the deep fascia from the anterior to the posterior, from the proximal end to the distal end. Explore whether there is a suitable perforator on the surface of the gracilis. If a suitable perforator is found, separate it as long as possible, and then carry it in the flap after ligation. Further separate to the surface of the adductor magnus to expose the perforating vessels of the adductor magnus. Generally, the main perforating vessels in the posterior of the thigh are the perforating vessels of the adductor magnus, but pay attention to the location and type of the

Z. Li, D. Song (eds.), *Oncoplastic Flap Surgery*, https://doi.org/10.1007/978-981-19-8926-1_24

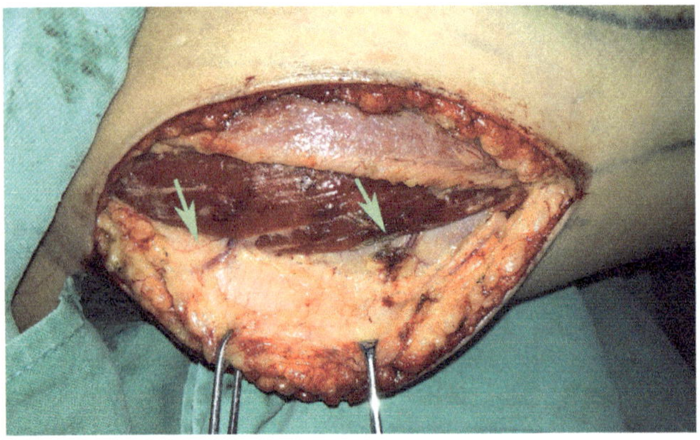

Fig. 24.1 Lift the flap to expose the two perforators of the profunda femoral artery from the surface of the great adductor muscle

perforating vessels of the adductor magnus. The perforating vessels of the muscular septum are rare. In most cases, they are the perforating vessels of the musculocutaneous adductor magnus. Sufficient length can be obtained by retrograde intramuscular separation to the plane of the profunda artery perforator pedicle of profunda femoral artery with sufficient diameter (Figs. 24.1, 24.2, and 24.3) (details are presented in pictures of typical cases for the description of operation process).

Conventionally, the vascular pedicle of the recipient area is prepared as the proximal and distal end of the internal thoracic vessels. But in the clinical practice, the lateral thoracic vessels, thoracodorsal vessels, intercostal vessels, anterior thoracic shoulder vessels, transverse carotid arteries, and veins, etc. can be selected flexibly according to the specific situation of the donor recipient area. The double-vessel pedicled profunda artery perforator flap with larger tissue volume can be shaped into a cone and embedded into the chest to reshape the ideal shape and contour of the breast.

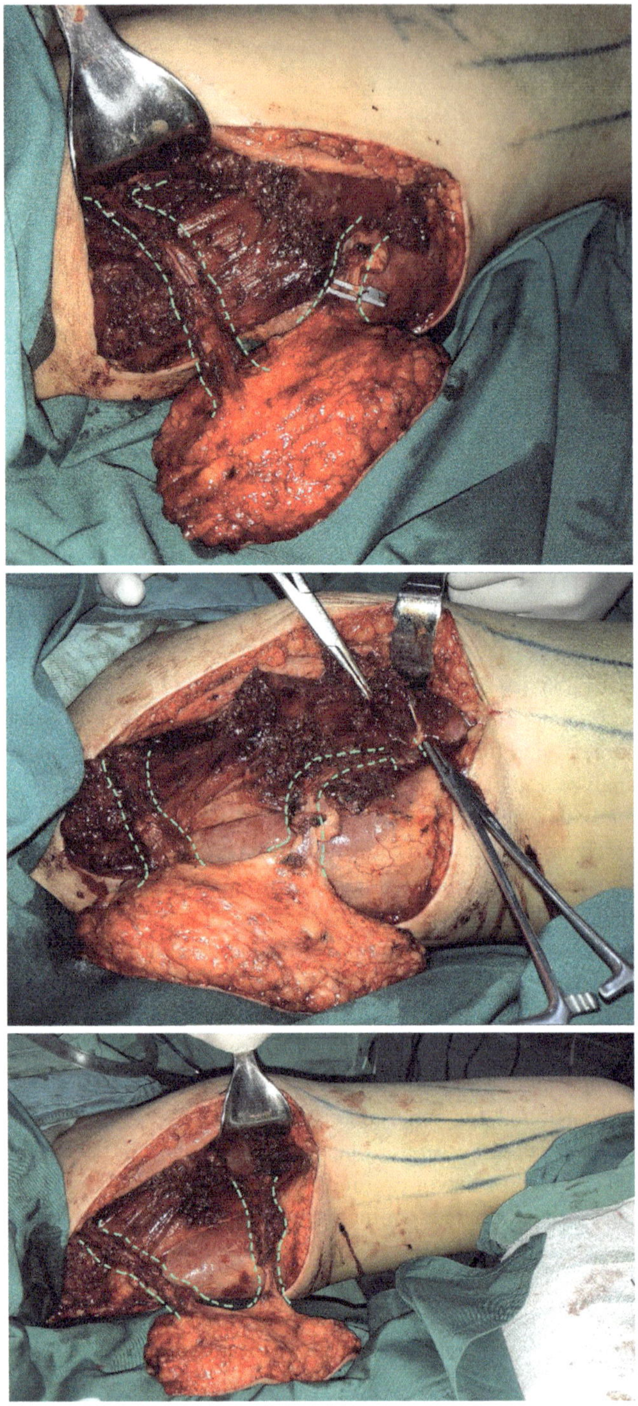

Fig. 24.2 Retrograde separation of two perforating vessels in adductor major to the plane from profunda femoral vessels

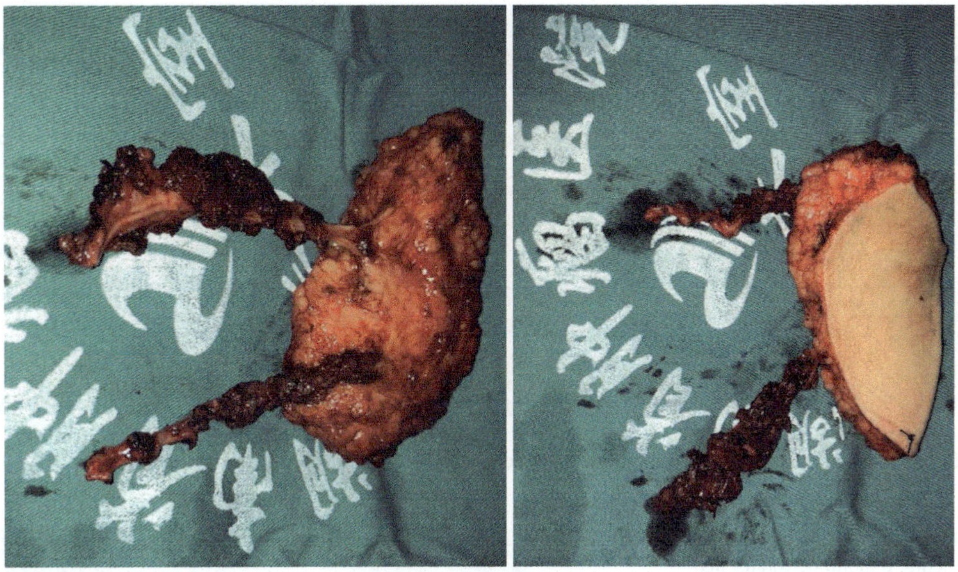

Fig. 24.3 Preparation of double-vessel pedicled profunda femoral artery perforator flap is dissected

24.2 Double-Vessel Pedicled Profunda Femoral Artery Perforator Flap for Breast Reconstruction: A Typical Case

A 41-year-old female patient found a right breast mass for 7 days. The lower quadrant of the right breast can be palpable at 4 o'clock, with a size of about 1 cm × 1 cm, medium mass, clear boundary, poor activity, and no tenderness. Enlarged lymph nodes were not palpable in bilateral axilla and supraclavicle, and other superficial lymph nodes were not palpable. Mass biopsy showed invasive ductal carcinoma and the immunohistochemistry results were E-cadherin (+) er (+), PR (+), c-erb-2 (+), Ki-67 (10–20%) +, p53 cells +, bcl-2 +, and ck-l +. The patient refused to preserve the breast and underwent modified radical mastectomy of right breast cancer and breast reconstruction with right profunda femoral artery perforator flap. After the modified radical mastectomy for right breast cancer, the right profunda artery perforator flap was designed with a size of about 27 cm × 7 cm (as shown in Fig. 24.6). The right perforator located by CTA before operation was marked on the body surface. The vascular pedicle of the flap was end-to-end anastomosed with the internal thoracic artery and vein (1A2V). After successful vascular anastomosis, the blood supply of the flap was good [13]. The flap edge and defect edge were sutured intermittently for breast shaping. Three negative pressure drainage tubes were placed in the operation cavity. The donor area was closed directly. The patient recovered well after operation. Pathological results showed that (1) the histology of invasive ductal carcinoma (right breast) was grade II, and the size of the mass was about 2.0 cm × 0.9 cm × 1.3 cm; (2) no cancer metastasis was found in three right axillary lymph nodes and sentinel lymph nodes; and (3) no cancer was found at the skin margin, nipple, and basal margin. Immunohistochemistry showed Er (2 +, about 60%), PR (2 +, about 40%), CerbB-2 (2 +) Ki67 about 20%, and p63-CK5/6-EGFR-syn-. The function and appearance of the reconstructed breast were satisfactory, and only linear scars were left in the donor area (Figs. 24.4, 24.5, 24.6, 24.7, 24.8, 24.9, 24.10, and 24.11).

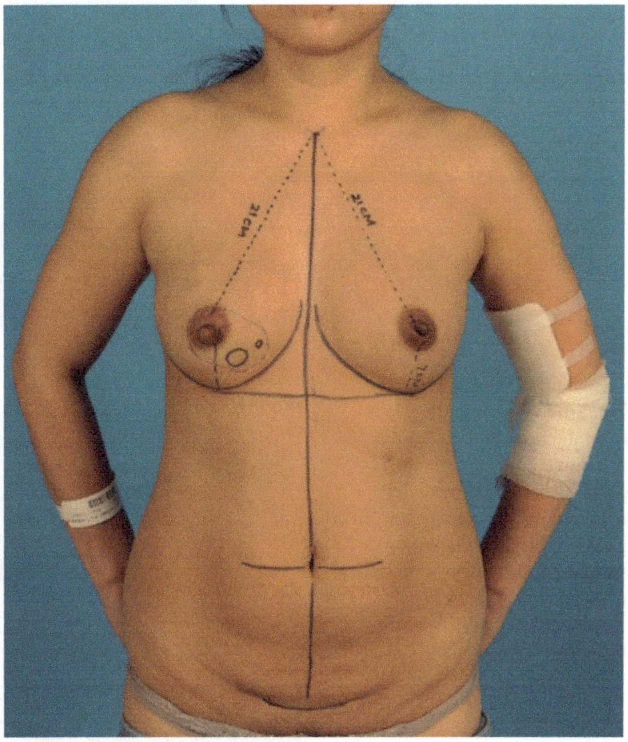

Fig. 24.4 Preoperative design. (The inferior fold of both the affected and contralateral breast and the amount of the skin and tissue to be resected from the affected breast were determined from the patient in standing position before operation, and the volume of missing tissue after operation was evaluated)

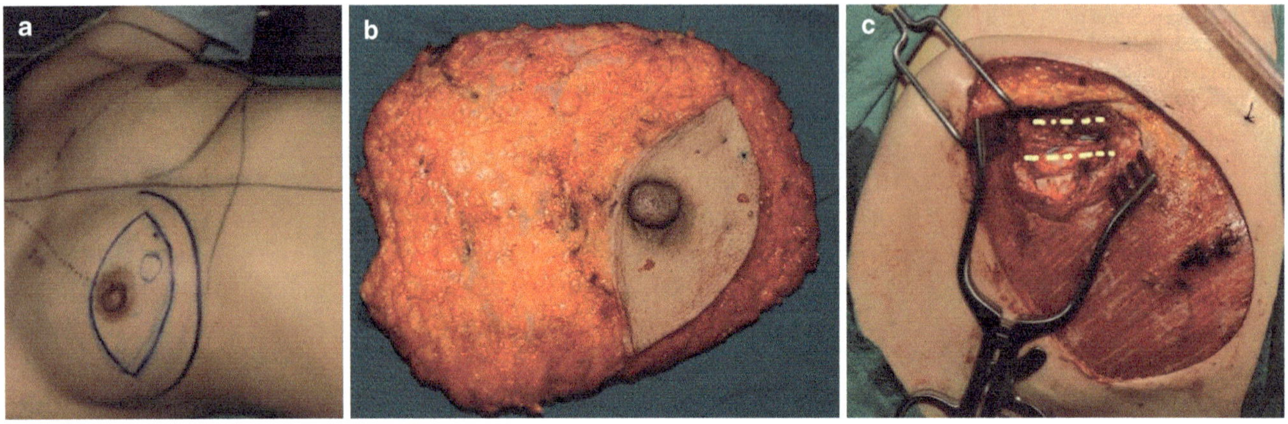

Fig. 24.5 Modified radical mastectomy and recipient vessel preparation during operation

Fig. 24.6 Design of the right medial femoral perforator flap

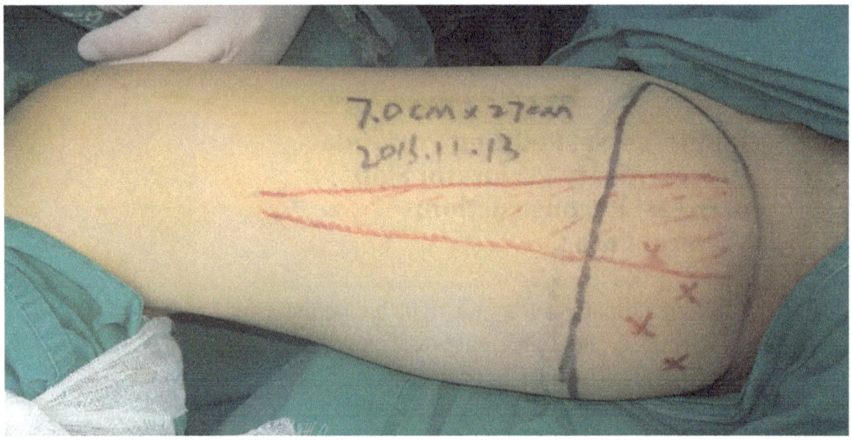

Fig. 24.7 Separate the flap from the proximal end to the distal end, and expose two perforator vascular pedicles from the frontal edge of the gracilis muscle and the surface of the adductor major muscle, respectively. (1) Adductor longus. (2) Gracilis muscle

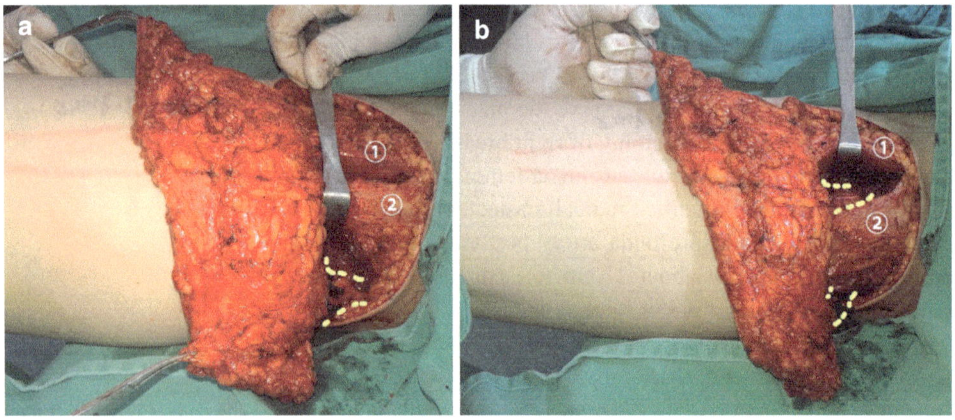

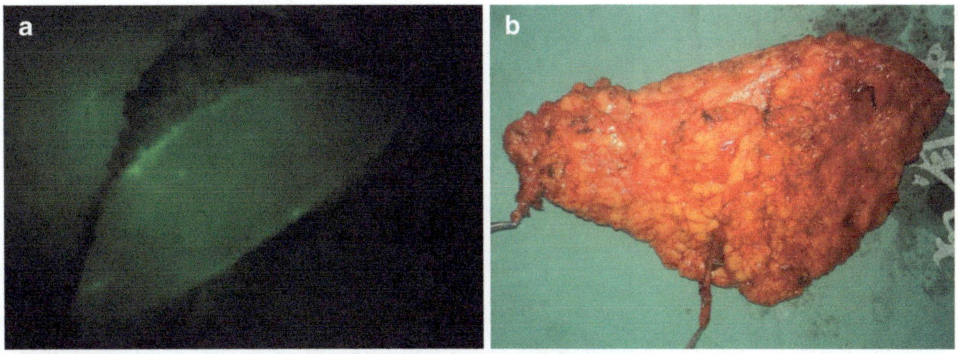

Fig. 24.8 During the operation, ICG determined that the blood supply of the flap was reliable only when both perforator vascular pedicles were supplied. It was decided to use the bilateral vascular pedicled medial femoral perforator flap. Then, the vascular pedicles were ligate and disconnect

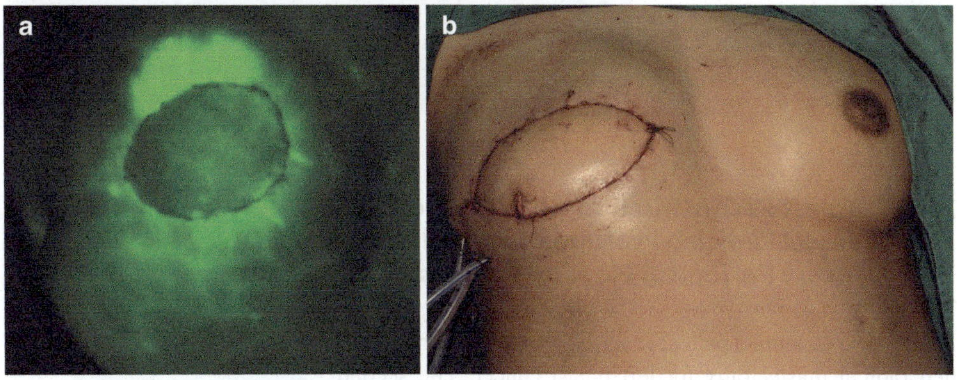

Fig. 24.9 After revascularization, ICG determined that the blood supply of the flap was acceptable, and the appearance of the reconstructed breast was satisfactory after intraoperative shaping

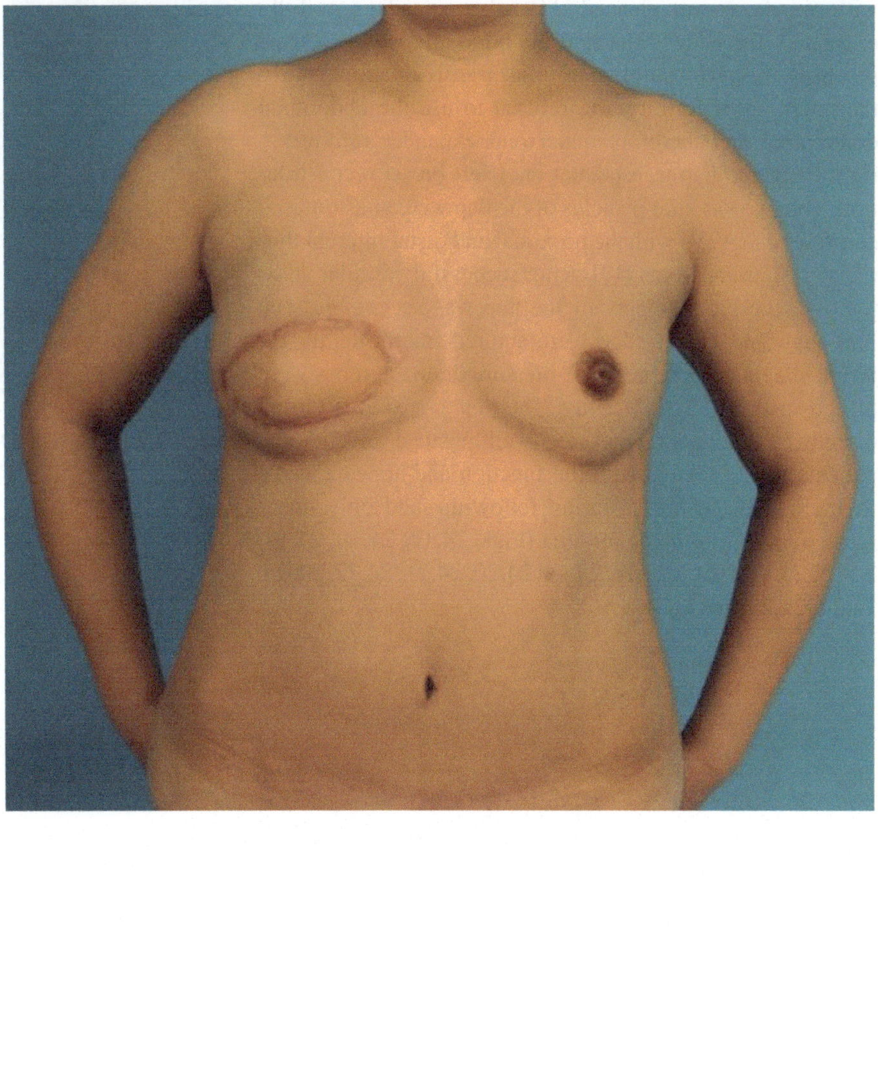

Fig. 24.10 The appearance of reconstructed breast was satisfactory after 12-month follow-up

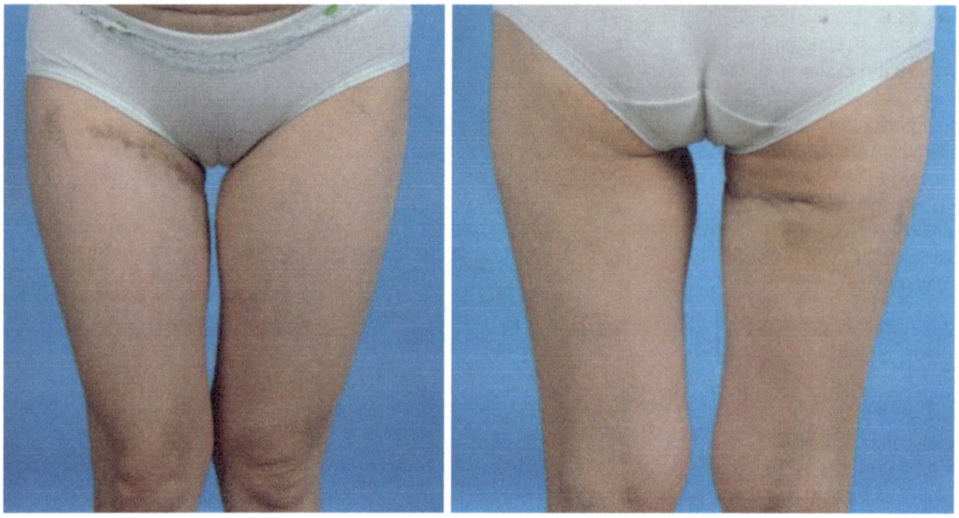

Fig. 24.11 Only a linear scar was left in the flap donor area

24.3 Breast Reconstruction with Double-Vessel Pedicled Profunda Femoral Artery Perforator Flap: Typical Case 2

A 30-year-old female patient received 1 year after the modified radical mastectomy for left breast cancer. The second stage expander had been implanted and breast reconstruction with prosthesis was planned. After the expander was fully expanded, the patient changed his mind and wanted breast reconstruction with autologous tissue transplantation. Due to the intention of fertility, she refused to use the abdominal donor area and therefore underwent expander removal + right PAP free flap transplantation + left breast reconstruction. The two vascular pedicles of the flap were anastomosed end-to-end (2A2V) with the proximal and distal internal thoracic arteries and veins [13]. After successful vascular anastomosis, the blood supply of the flap was acceptable. The flap edge and defect edge were sutured intermittently for breast shaping. Three negative-pressure drainage tubes were placed in the operation cavity. The donor area was closed directly. The patient recovered well postoperatively. The patients were satisfied with the function and appearance of the reconstructed breast during follow-up, and only linear scars were left in the donor area (Figs. 24.12, 24.13, 24.14, 24.15, 24.16, 24.17, 24.18, 24.19, 24.20, 24.21, 24.22, 24.23, 24.24, 24.25, and 24.26).

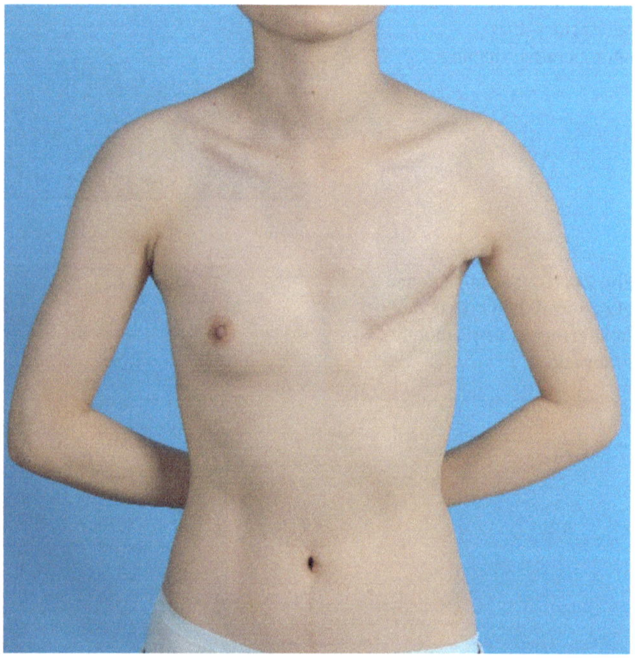

Fig. 24.12 The appearance after modified radical mastectomy for breast cancer and before secondary expander implantation

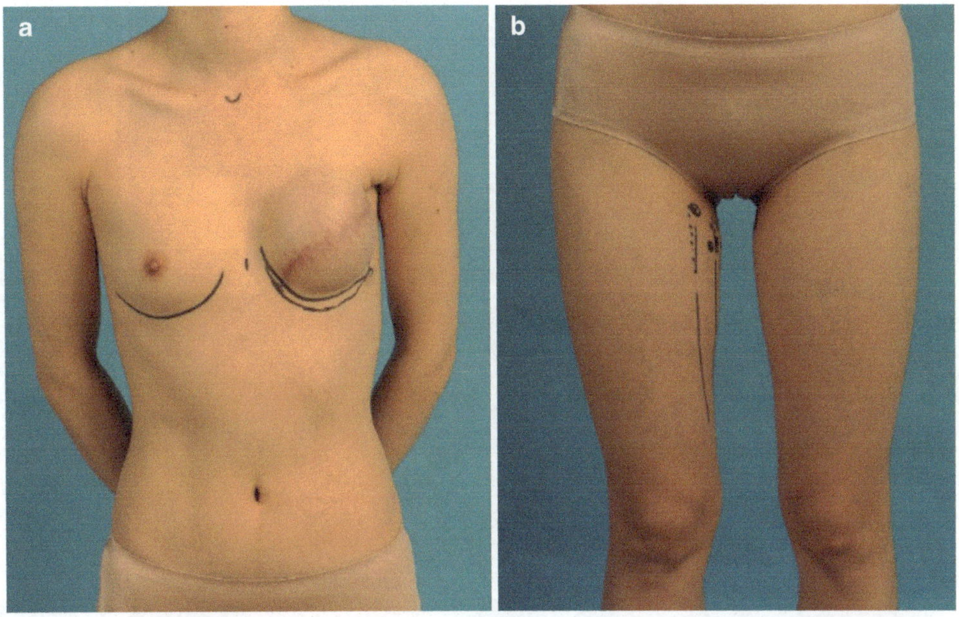

Fig. 24.13 Preoperative findings and incision design

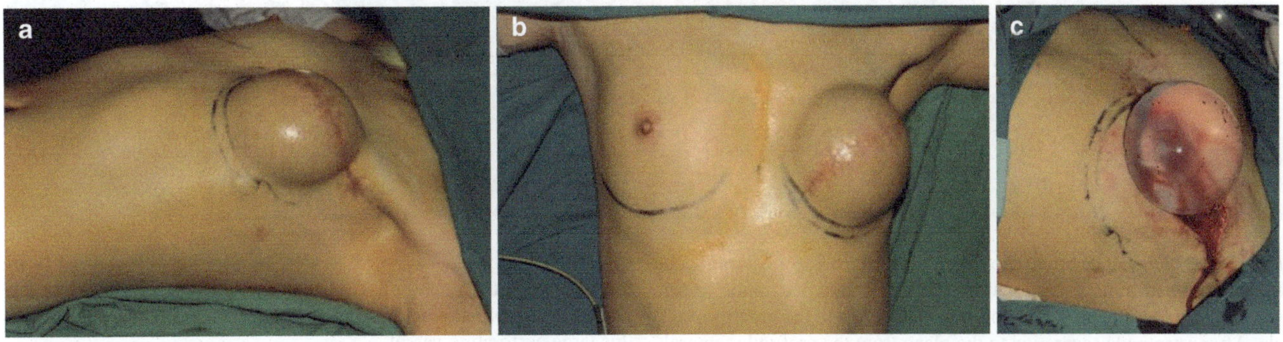

Fig. 24.14 Removal of the left chest expander during operation

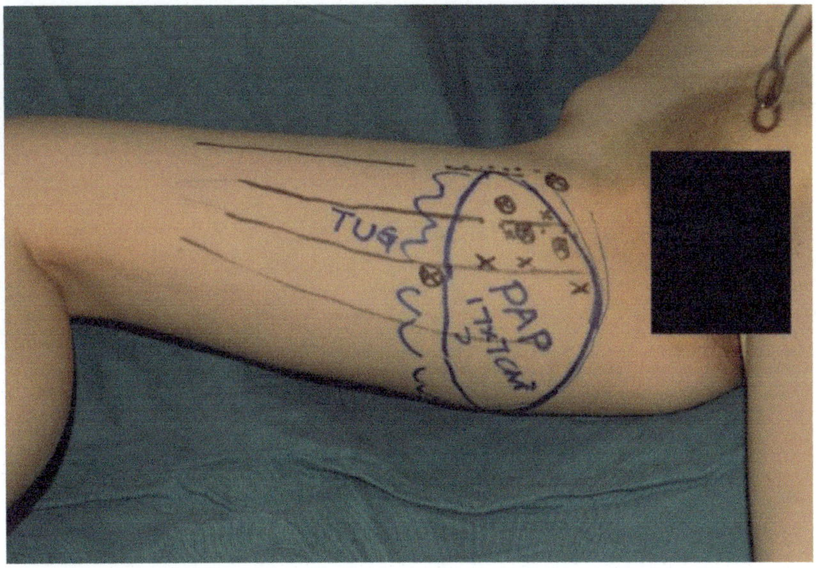

Fig. 24.15 Design of the right thigh medial perforator flap

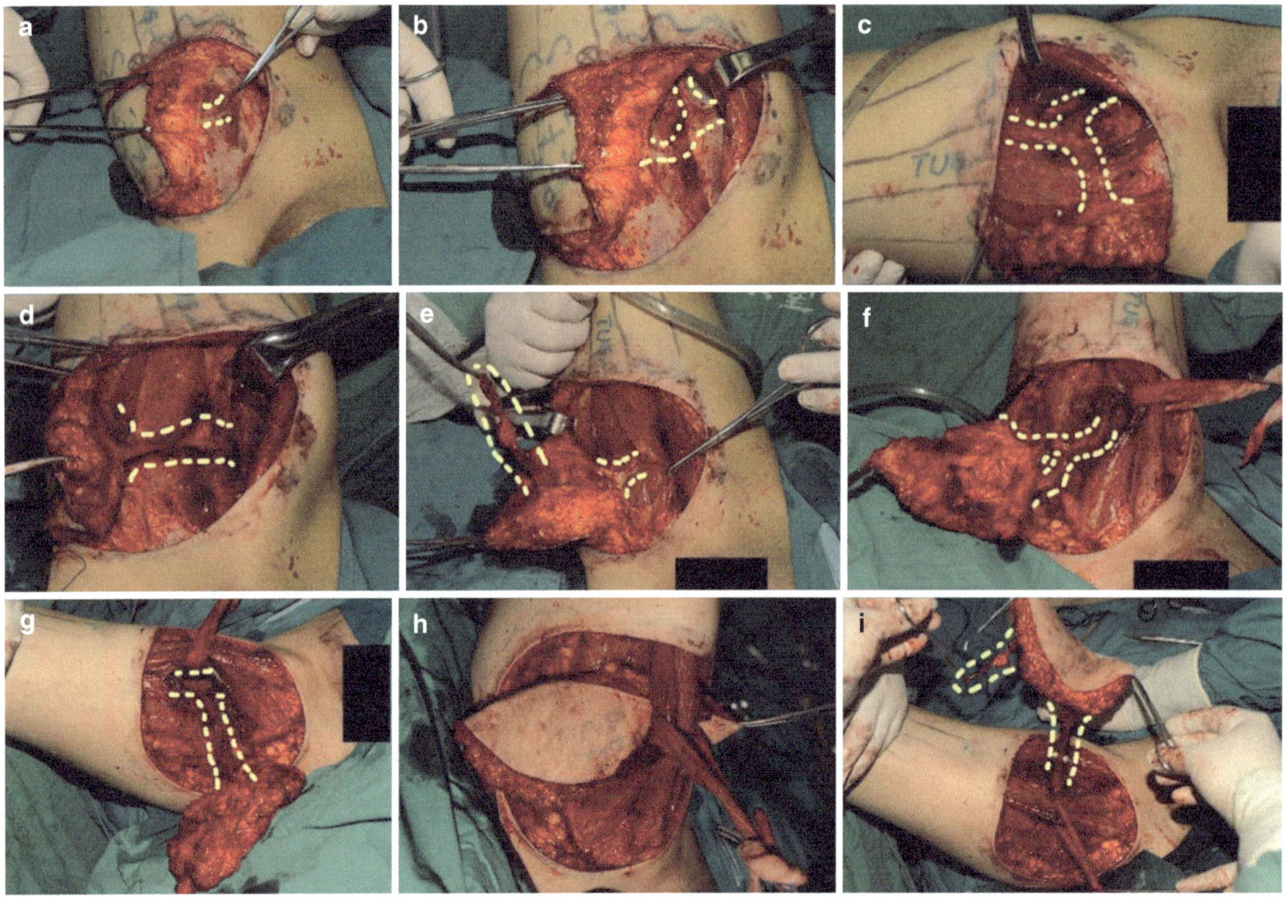

Fig. 24.16 Dissect the flap from the anterior to the posterior and explore the perforating vessels. It can be seen that a perforator vessel was sent out between the adductor longus muscle and the gracilis muscle. After retrograde separation to the plane from the profunda femoral vessel, the perforators were then ligated and disconnected. Further separate and explore backward. A large perforating vessel came from the surface of the great adductor muscle. Retrograde separate to the plane of the profunda femoral vessel and then ligated and disconnected this large perforating vessel

Fig. 24.17 Preparation of the bilateral vascular pedicled profunda femoral artery perforator flap

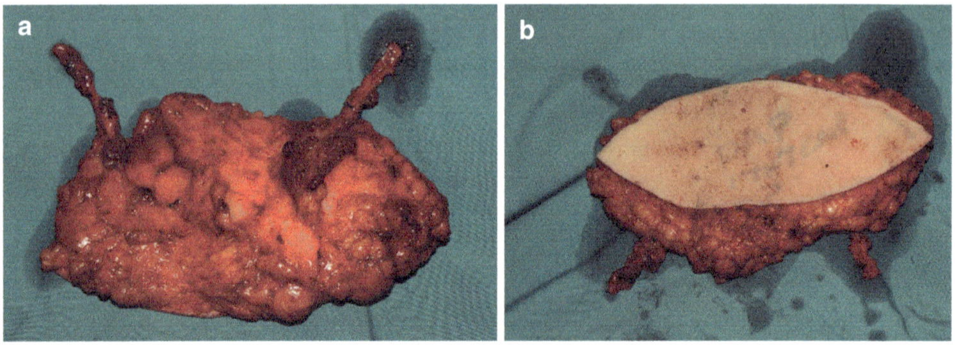

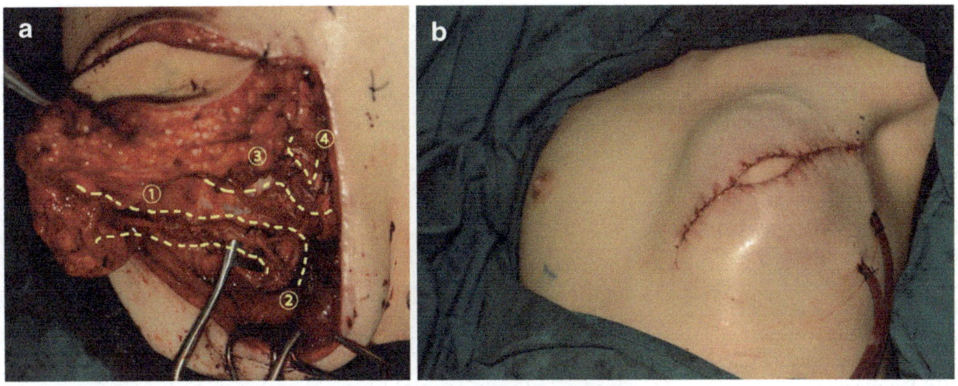

Fig. 24.18 The bilateral vascular pedicles of the flap were anastomosed with the proximal and distal ends of the internal thoracic vessels, respectively. After shaping, a small skin island is reserved for flap blood supply monitoring. (1) Perforating vessels of the adductor major. (2) Proximal thoracic vessels. (3) Perforating vessels of the gracilis muscle. (4) Distal thoracic vessels

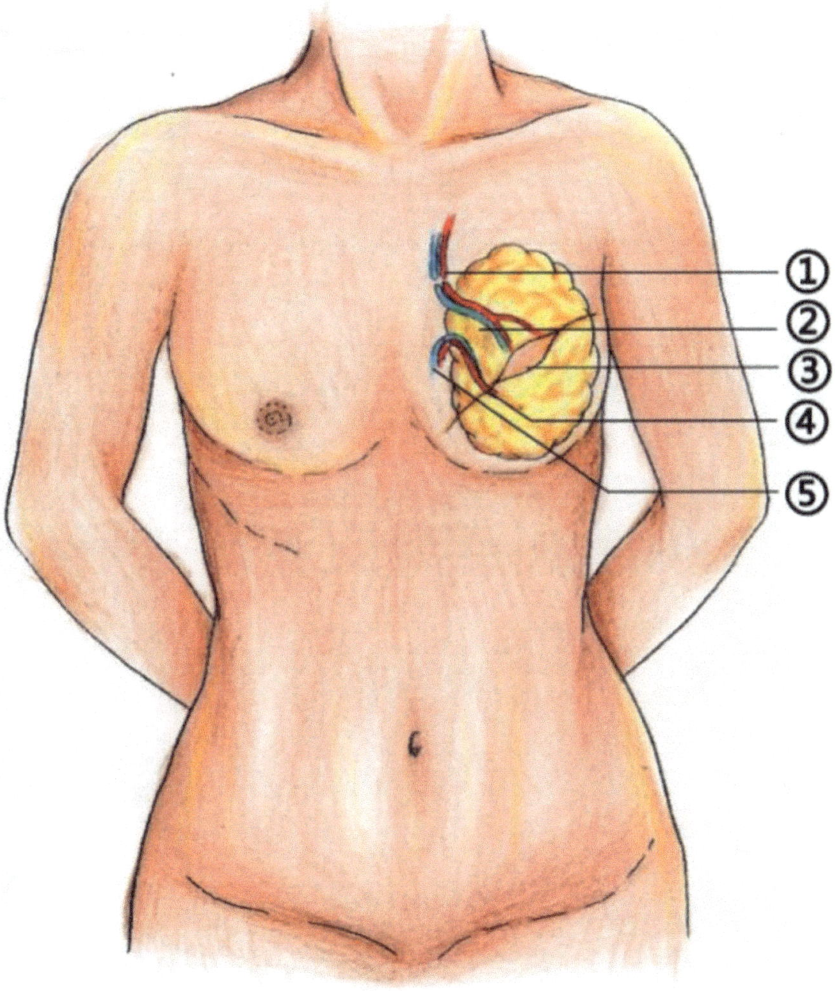

Fig. 24.19 Illustration of flap revascularization. (1) Proximal thoracic vessels. (2) Perforating vessels of the adductor major. (3) Monitoring PI island. (4) Perforating vessels of the gracilis muscle. (5) Distal thoracic vessels

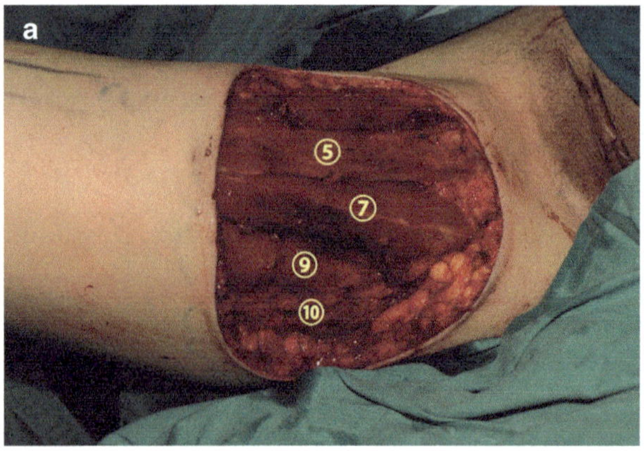

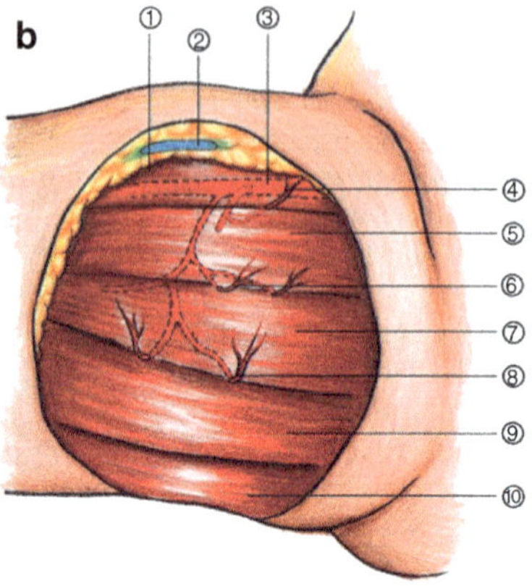

Fig. 24.20 The muscle damage in the flap donor area was mild. (1) Adductor longus. (2) Great saphenous vein. (3) Profunda femoral artery. (4) Anterior perforator vessel of the gracilis muscle. (5) Gracilis muscle. (6) Posterior perforator vessel of the gracilis muscle. (7) Adductor major. (8) Perforating vessels of the adductor major. (9) Semimembranosus muscle. (10) Semitendinosus

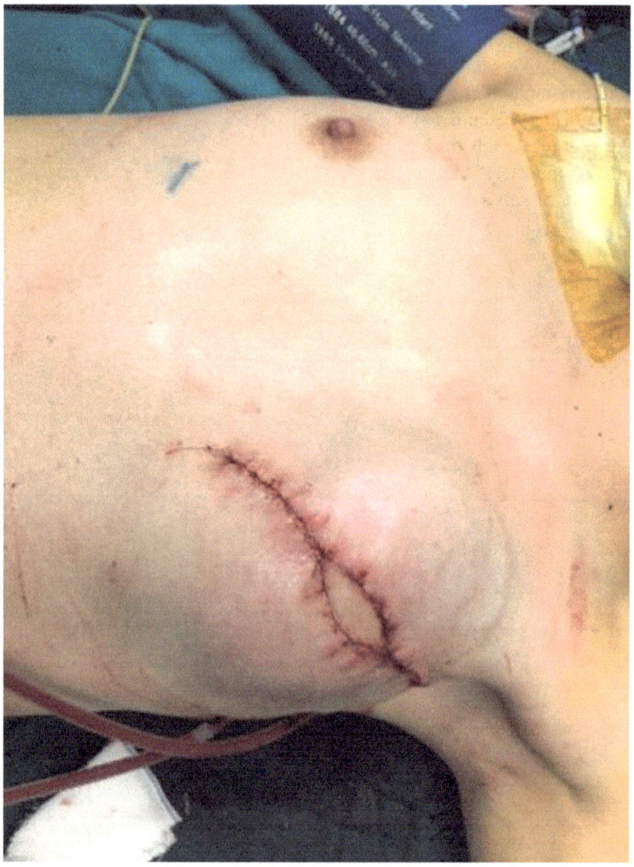

Fig. 24.21 The postoperative course was consistent and the blood supply of the flap was satisfactory

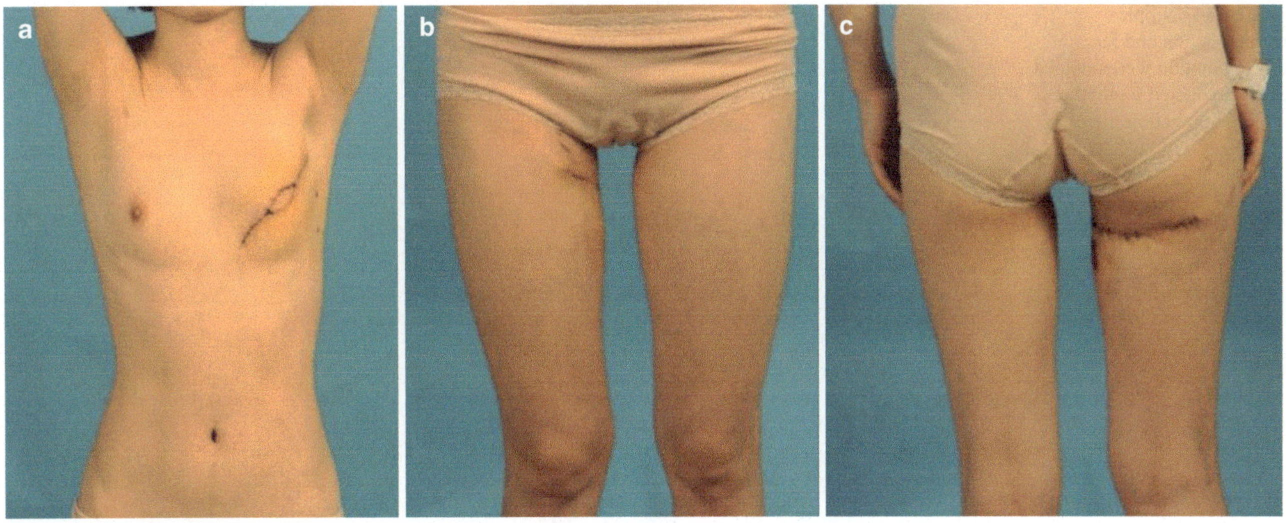

Fig. 24.22 One-month follow-up after operation

Fig. 24.23 (**a**, **b**) Two-month follow-up after operation. (**c**, **d**) Six-month follow-up after operation

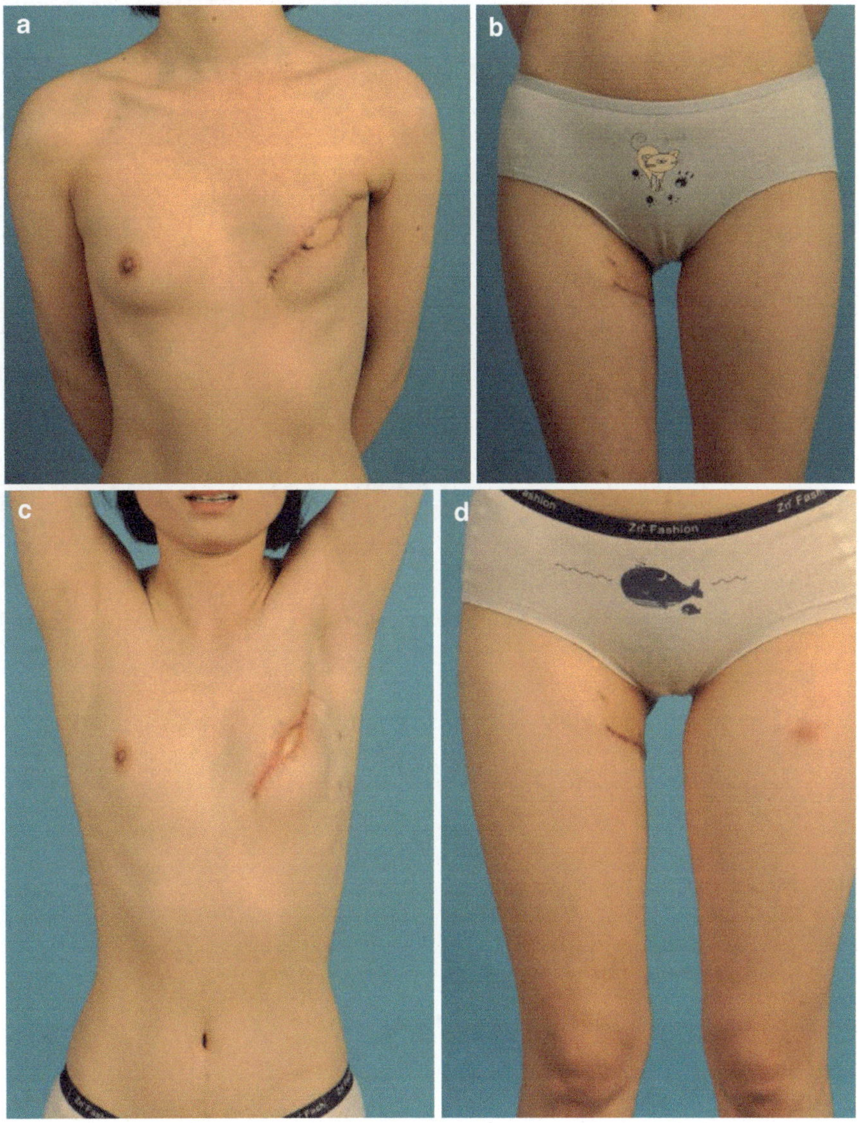

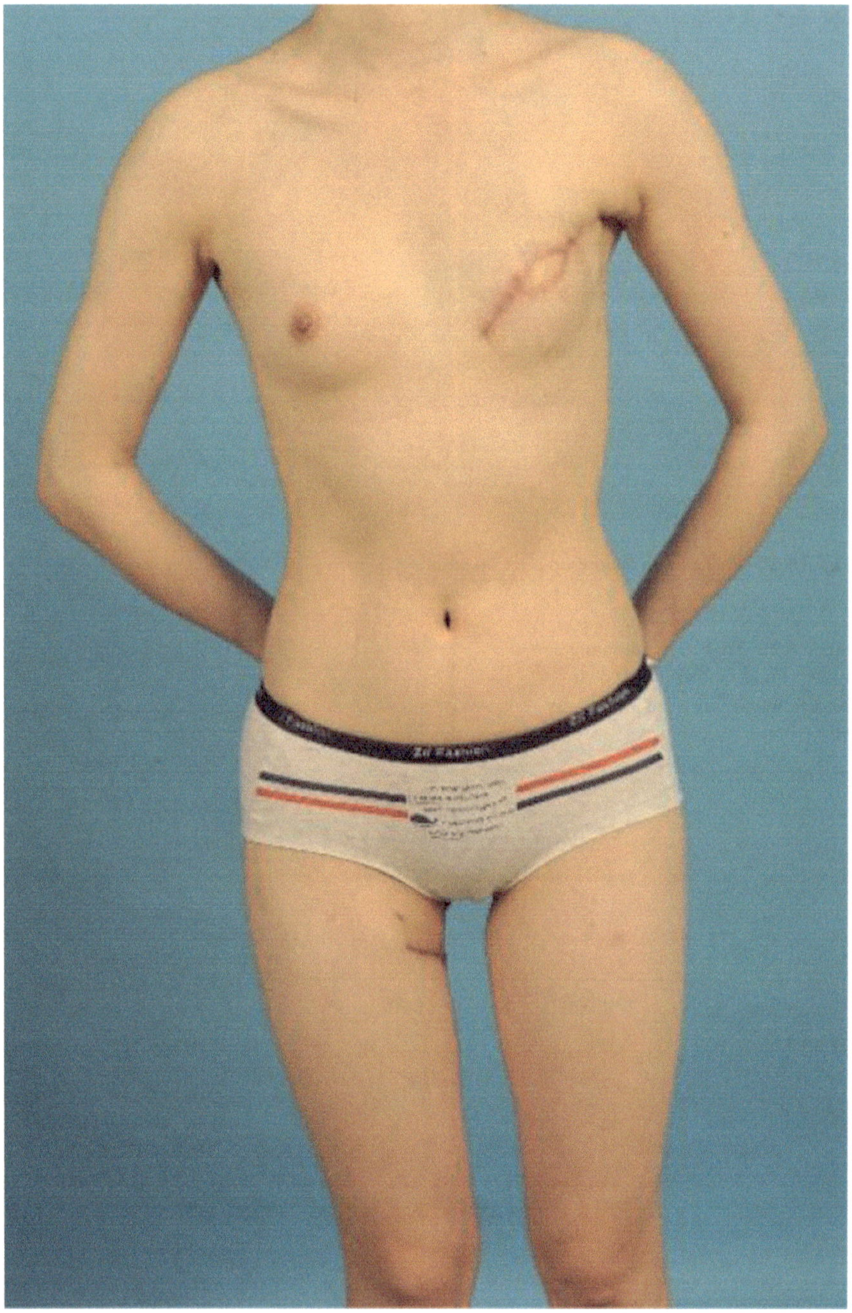

Fig. 24.24 Nipple reconstruction and fat transplantation were planned to be conducted 9 months after the operation

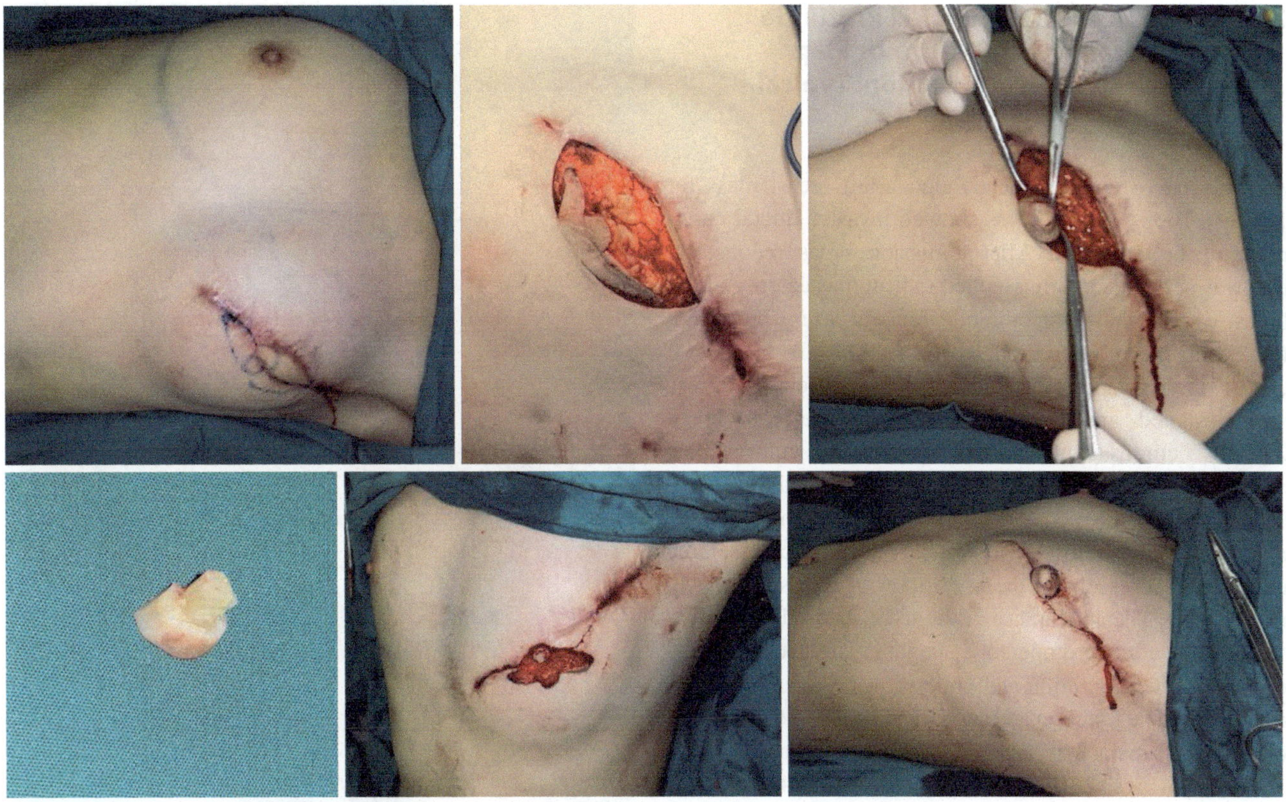

Fig. 24.25 Reconstruction of nipple with trilobal flap combined with reserved costal cartilage as preoperative design

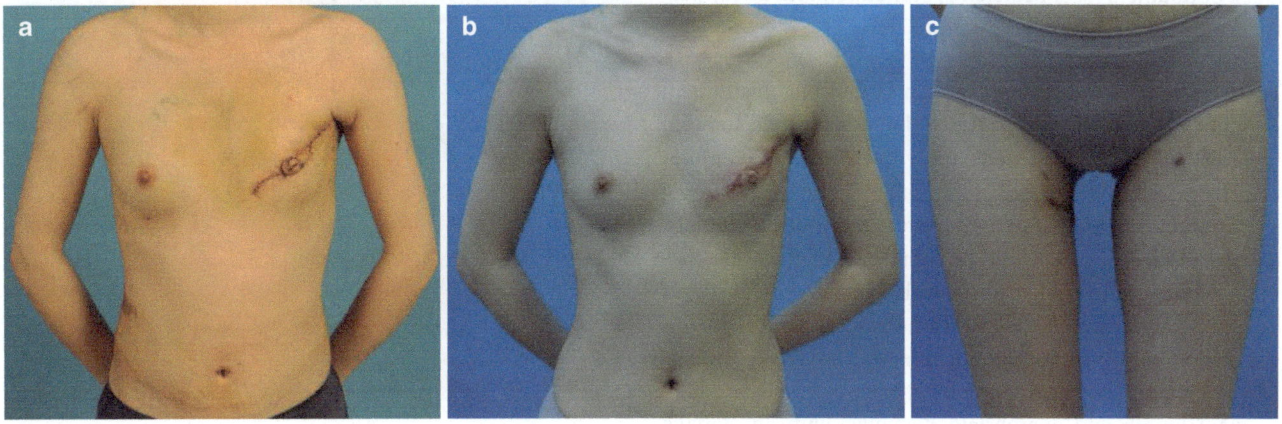

Fig. 24.26 (**a**) The appearance 3 days after operation. (**b**) Breast and nipple reconstruction 3 months after stage two operation. (**c**) The appearance of donor site 12 months after operation

24.4 Double-Vessel Pedicled Profunda Femoral Artery Perforator Flap for Breast Reconstruction: Typical Case 3

A 60-year-old female patient found a left breast mass for 14 days. Biopsy of the mass showed invasive ductal carcinoma of the left breast. After admission, breast reconstruction was performed with modified radical mastectomy of left breast cancer and right profunda femoral artery perforator flap. After the modified radical mastectomy for left breast cancer, the right perforator flap of profunda femoral artery was designed and dissected, and the size was about 27 cm × 7 cm (as shown in Fig. 24.28). The vascular pedicle of the perforating branches of gracilis muscle and the vascular pedicle of the perforating branches of two adductors major were anastomosed with the lateral thoracic vessel, the thoracodorsal vessel, and the anterior serratus muscle branch, respectively. The appearance of the reconstructed breast was satisfactory after intraoperative shaping. The patient recovered well after operation and underwent postoperative chemotherapy. The function and appearance of the reconstructed breast were satisfactory, and only linear scars were left in the donor area (Figs. 24.27, 24.28, 24.29, 24.30, 24.31, 24.32, 24.33, 24.34, and 24.35).

Based on our experience, we found several key advantages of double-vessel pedicled profunda femoral artery perforator flap in breast reconstruction.

1. According to the anatomical report and our anatomical clinical findings, the perforator flap of profunda femoral artery has a reliable blood supply from profunda femoral artery. Using computed tomography or magnetic resonance angiography before operation, the key perforator of perforator flap can always be found, with an average distance of 4.5 cm (range, 1–6 cm) below the gluteal sulcus and 3.4 cm (range, 2–9 cm) from the midline [15, 16].

   Our research and anatomical reports are basically consistent with previous studies. These vessels have sufficient length and appropriate diameter, with an average length of 10.2 cm, an average diameter of 1.4 cm in arteries, and an average diameter of 2.1 cm in veins. Compared with the data reported in the international literatures, these vessels are relatively small. Taking into considerations the differences of ethnic groups, these variations have clinical guiding significance. In breast reconstruction, vascular pedicle and recipient vessels can be well matched. Other anatomical studies have also confirmed the anatomical consistency of the perforator flap of the profunda femoral artery. Delong et al. confirmed that there are at least two perforators of profunda femoral artery on each thigh, of which 85% of patients have more than three perforators. The average diameter measured by computed tomography is slightly larger than the average diameter of 2.7 mm. In addition, Hunter et al. also found similar favorable results, especially compared with gracilis myocutaneous flap, cutting flap can obtain sufficient vascular pedicle length [17].

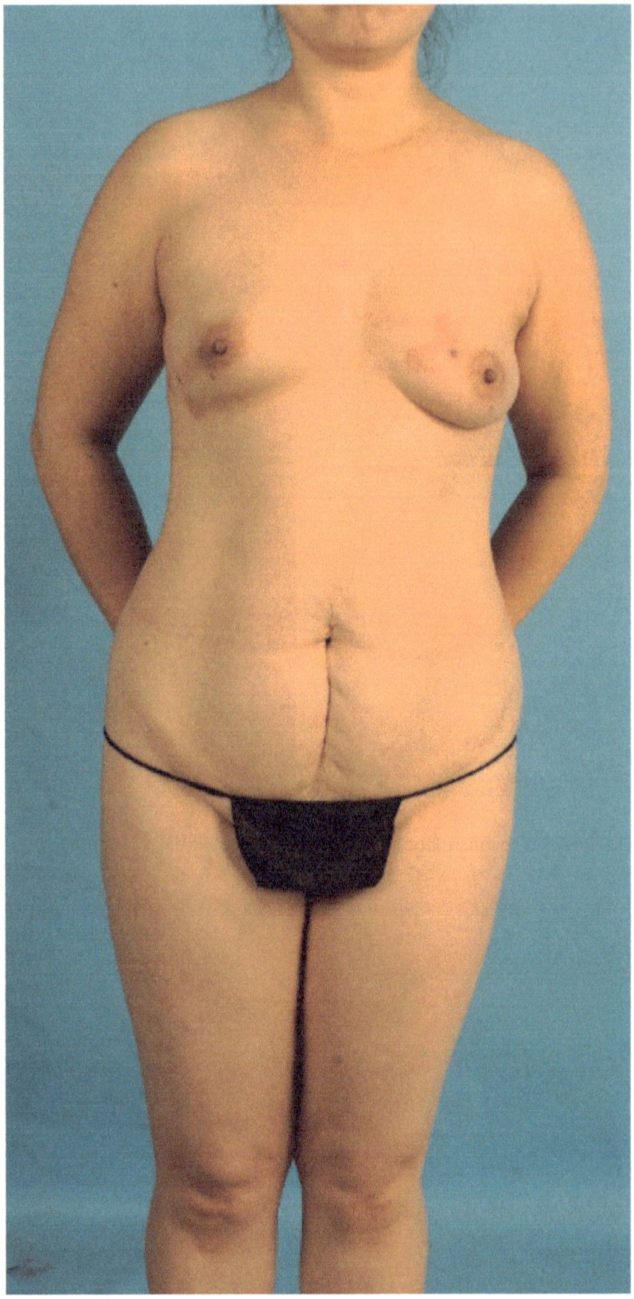

Fig. 24.27 Preoperative conditions

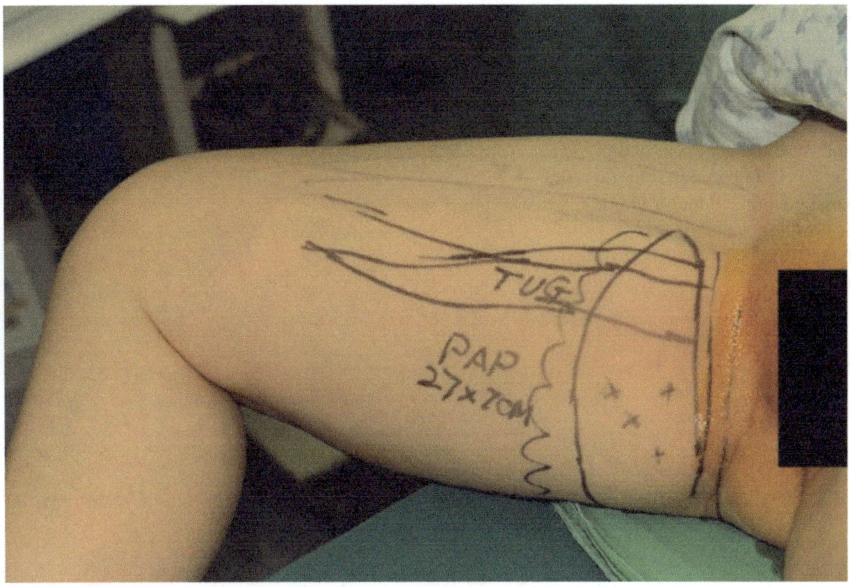

Fig. 24.28 Design of the posterior medial femoral perforator flap

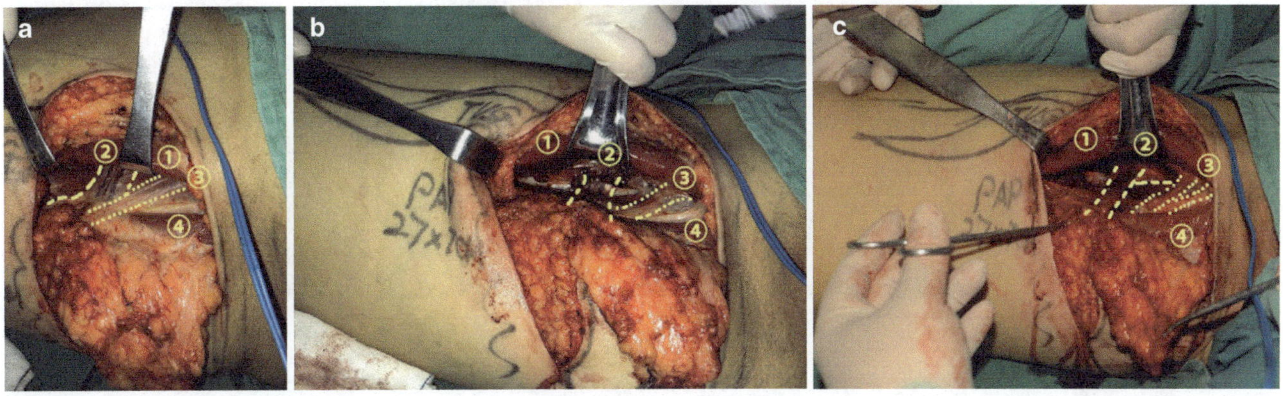

Fig. 24.29 Lift the flap from the anterior to the posterior to expose the perforating vessels of gracilis muscle, and retrograde separate it to the plane from the profunda femoral vessels. (1) Adductor longus. (2) Vascular pedicle of the perforating branch of gracilis muscle. (3) Anterior branch of the obturator nerve. (4) Gracilis muscle

2. This flap allows two surgical teams to operate at the same time. Mastectomy and regional blood vessels preparation can be done at the same time. In addition, bilateral profunda femoral artery perforator flaps can be dissected in the same position simultaneously.
3. We found that the profunda artery perforator flap provided softer tissue than the gluteal artery perforator flap. These tissues can be easily shaped to reconstruct the breast with better elasticity and more natural shape.

We believe that the flap size is the only comparative disadvantage. Although the average flap size is merely about 350 g, Asian women usually have smaller breasts, and the smaller flap size has no significant impact on the reconstruction effects. Patients may have leg discomfort within 2–6 weeks after surgery, but it can usually be tolerated by patients.

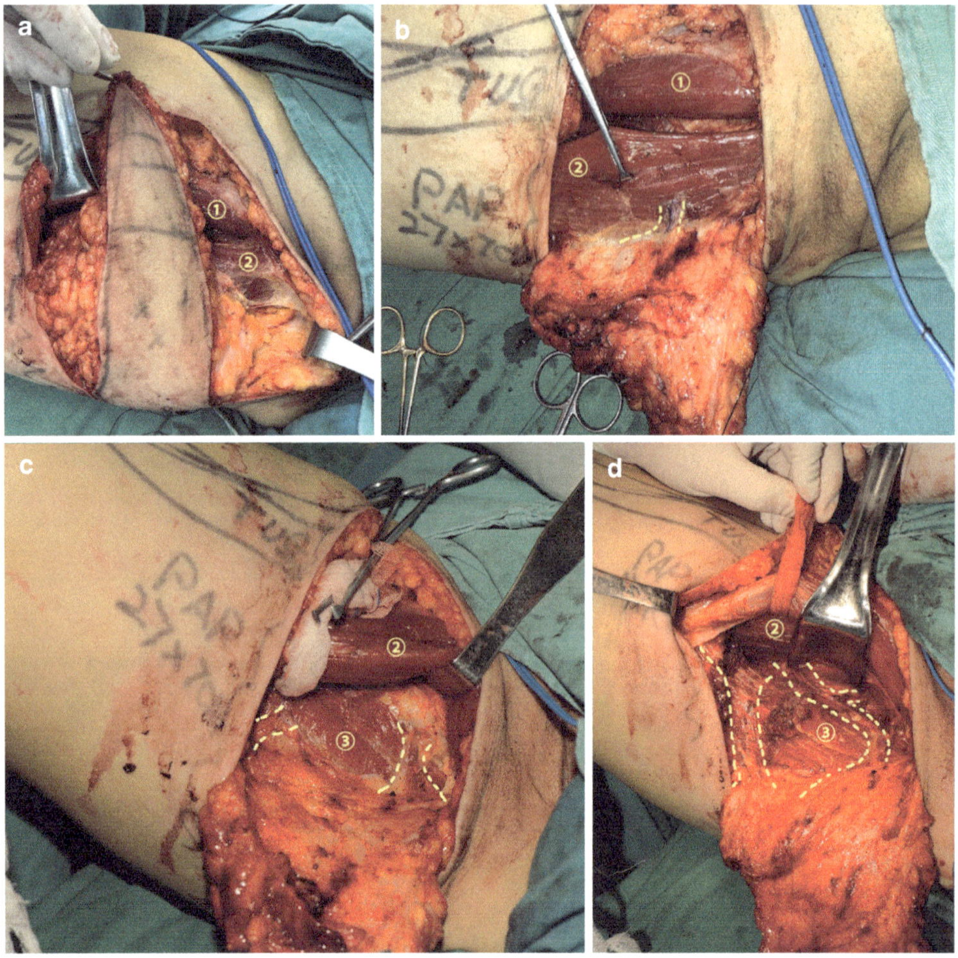

Fig. 24.30 The flap was further separated backward. Two other large perforating vessels were found on the surface of the adductor major and retrogradely separated to the level of profunda femoral vessels in the adductor major. (1) Adductor longus. (2) Gracilis muscle. (3) Adductor major

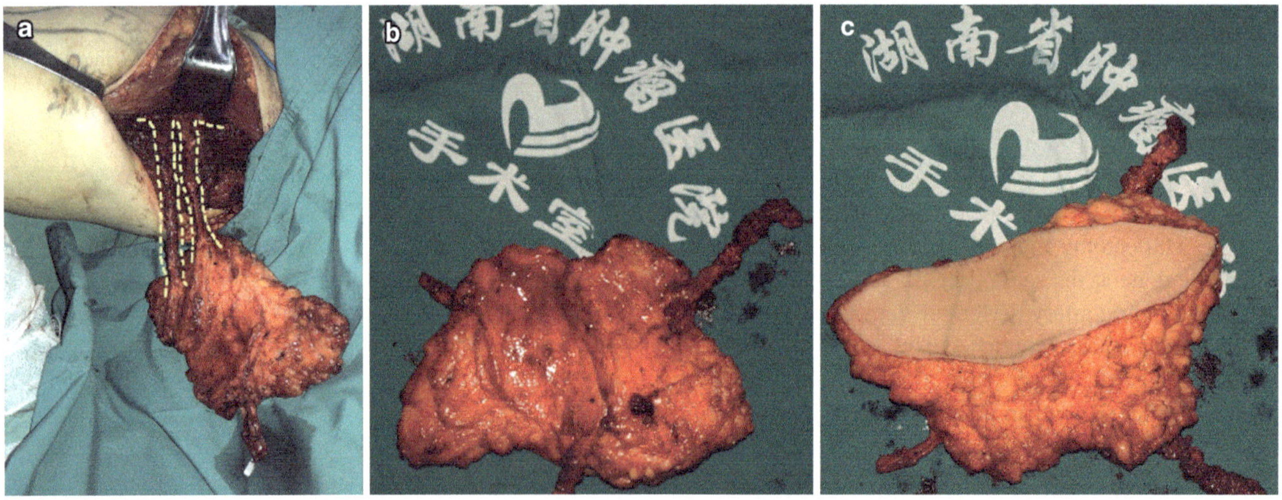

Fig. 24.31 The perforator flap of profunda femoral artery pedicled with bilateral vessels has been dissected

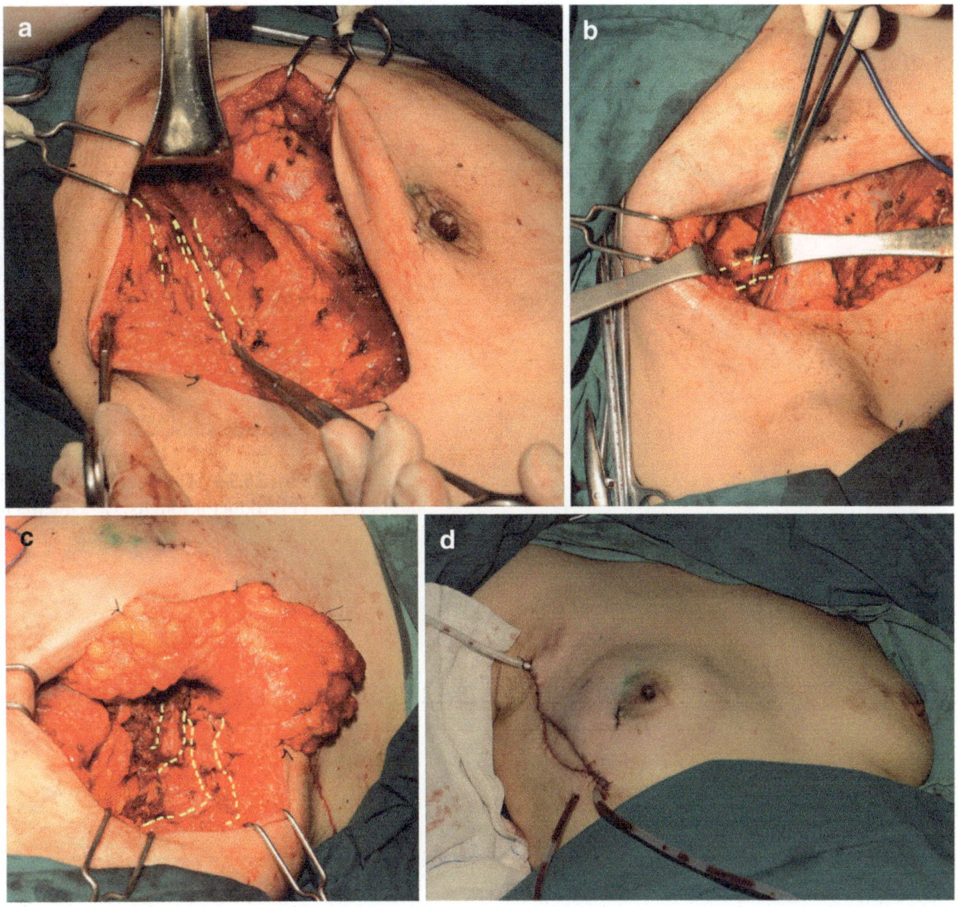

Fig. 24.32 Vascular pedicle of the gracilis perforator and two adductor major perforator was anastomosed with lateral thoracic vessels, thoracodorsal vessels, and anterior serratus branches, respectively. The appearance of reconstructed breast was satisfactory after intraoperative shaping

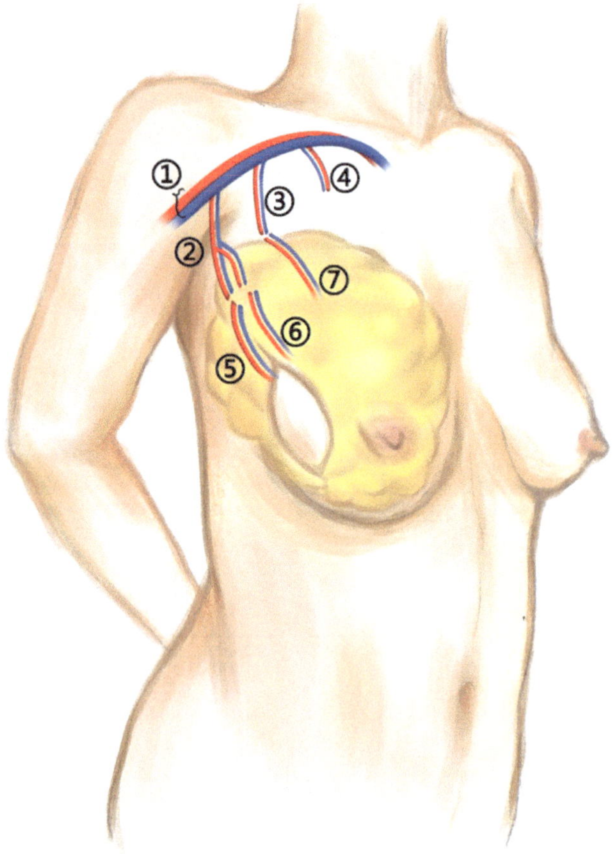

Fig. 24.33 Schematic diagram of revascularization: bilateral vascular pedicles were anastomosed with lateral thoracic vessels, thoracodorsal vessels and anterior serratus muscle branches (3A3V). (1) Axillary artery and vein. (2) Thoracodorsal vessels and their branches of the anterior serratus muscle. (3) Lateral thoracic vessels. (4) Thoracic acromial vessels. (5) Perforating branch of the adductor major 1. (6) Perforating branch of the adductor major 2. (7) Perforating branch of the gracilis muscle

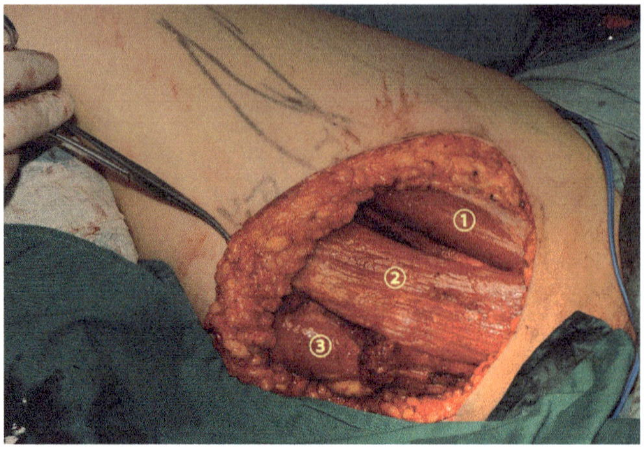

Fig. 24.34 The degree of muscle injury in the donor area is small [14]. (1) Adductor longus. (2) Gracilis muscle. (3) Adductor major

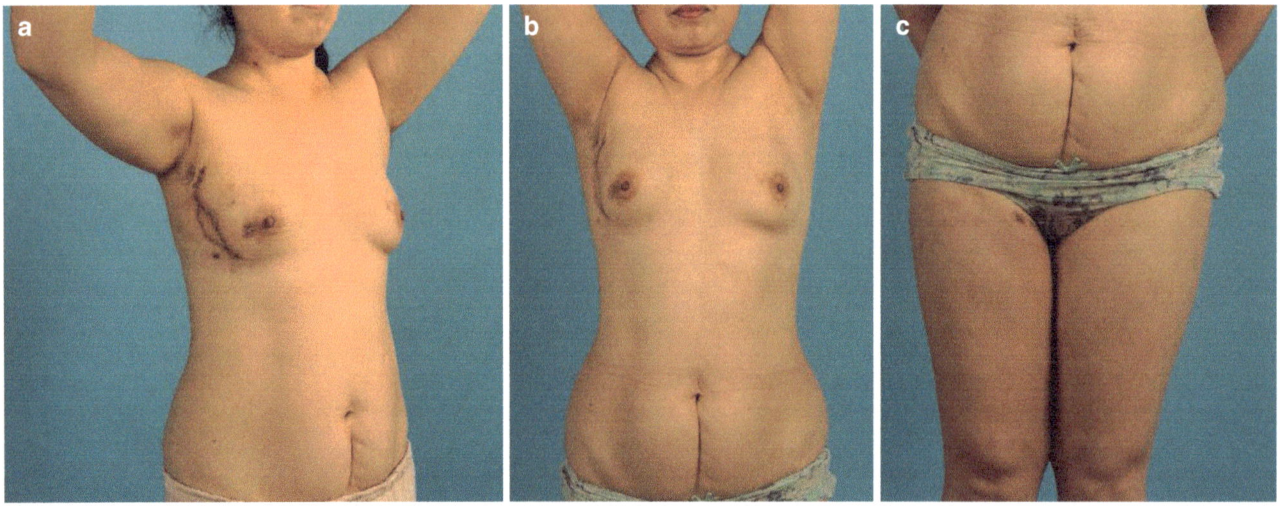

Fig. 24.35 (a) After 1-month follow-up, the appearance and function were satisfactory. (b) The shape and function of reconstructed breast were satisfactory 6 months after operation. (c) The scar location of the medial thigh donor area was hidden 6 months after operation

24.5 Conclusion

Profunda artery perforator flap is a good choice for breast reconstruction. Its advantages include reliable blood supply, long vascular pedicle, more optional vascular pedicle, and flexible dissecting forms, thick and soft tissue in the donor area, and hidden donor area. At present, the profunda femoral artery perforator flap is second only to the inferior abdominal artery perforator flap in the application for breast reconstruction by the authors [12].

References

1. Allen RJ, Treece P. Deep inferior epigastric perforator flap for breast reconstruction. Ann Plast Surg. 1994;32(1):32–8.
2. Healy C, Allen RJ. The evolution of perforator flap breast reconstruction: twenty years after the first DIEP flap. J Reconstr Microsurg. 2014;30(2):121–5.
3. Gill PS, Hunt JP, Guerra AB, et al. A 10-year retrospective review of 758 DIEP flaps for breast reconstruction. Plast Reconstr Surg. 2004;113(4):1153–60.
4. Healy C, Ramakrishnan V. Autologous microvascular breast reconstruction. Arch Plast Surg. 2013;40(1):3–10.
5. Hurwitz DJ, Walton RL. Closure of chronic wounds of the perineal and sacral regions using the gluteal thigh flap. Ann Plast Surg. 1982;8(5):375–86.
6. Angrigiani C, Grilli D, Thorne CH. The adductor flap: a new method for transferring posterior and medial thigh skin. Plast Reconstr Surg. 2001;107(7):1725–31.
7. Haddock NT, Greaney P, Otterburn D, Levine S, Allen RJ. Predicting perforator location on preoperative imaging for the profunda artery perforator flap. Microsurgery. 2012;32(7):507–11.
8. Allen RJ, Haddock NT, Ahn CY, Sadeghi A. Breast reconstruction with the profunda artery perforator flap. Plast Reconstr Surg. 2012;129(1):16e–23e.
9. Song D, Li Z, Zhou X. Application of profunda femoral artery perforator flap in breast reconstruction. Chin J Plast Surg. 2017;6:412–6.
10. Song D, Li Z, Zhou X. Free profunda femoral artery pedicled gracilis chimeric musculocutaneous perforator flap for repair of defects after oral and buccal cancer surgery. Chin J Plast Surg. 2017;33(4):242–7.
11. Song D, Li Z, Zhou X. Clinical application of free medial femoral chimeric perforator myocutaneous flap in the repair of defects after tongue cancer surgery. Chin J Otorhinolaryngol Head Neck Surg. 2017;52(4):278–82.
12. Allen RJ, Lee ZH, Mayo JL, Levine J, Ahn C, Allen RJ. The profunda artery perforator flap experience for breast reconstruction. Plast Reconstr Surg. 2016;138(5):968–75.
13. Stalder MW, Lam J, Allen RJ, Sadeghi A. Using the retrograde internal mammary system for stacked perforator flap breast reconstruction: 71 breast reconstructions in 53 consecutive patients. Plast Reconstr Surg. 2016;137(2):265e–77e.
14. Momoh AO, Colakoglu S, Westvik TS, et al. Analysis of complications and patient satisfaction in pedicled transverse rectus abdominis myocutaneous and deep inferior epigastric perforator flap breast reconstruction. Ann Plast Surg. 2012;69(1):19–23.
15. Saad A, Sadeghi A, Allen RJ. The anatomic basis of the profunda femoris artery perforator flap: a new option for autologous breast reconstruction—a cadaveric and computer tomography angiogram study. J Reconstr Microsurg. 2012;28(6):381–6.
16. Ahmadzadeh R, Bergeron L, Tang M, Geddes CR, Morris SF. The posterior thigh perforator flap or profunda femoris artery perforator flap. Plast Reconstr Surg. 2007;119(1):194–200; discussion 201–2.
17. Hunter JE, Lardi AM, Dower DR, Farhadi J. Evolution from the TUG to PAP flap for breast reconstruction: comparison and refinements of technique. J Plast Reconstr Aesthet Surg. 2015;68(7):960–5.

25 Greater Omental Flap for Breast Reconstruction

Nengbing Wan and Shihong Ma

25.1 Background

Greater omental flap is one of the earliest-applied free tissue flaps, and it was also the first used for repair and reconstruction inside and outside the abdominal cavity [1]. In 1963, Romania surgeon Kiricuta used pedicled omental flap to perform breast reconstruction for ten patients with breast cancer. Among them, four cases did not use prosthesis implantation, and the effect was satisfactory. Since then, it has been reported that the free greater omentum flap was used to conduct the reconstruction of facial deformity for Romberg's patients. Since then, the application field of the greater omental flap has become more and more extensive [2, 3].

Advances in surgical anatomy and technology allow reconstruction in the chest wall more thorough and less restricted than that in other domains to remove tumors, infection foci, and radiation necrosis [4, 5]. The applications of local muscle flap, omental transposition, and free tissue transplantation have eliminated many taboos in chest wall surgery [6–9]. Pedicled omentum flap has been proved to be a reliable method for repairing complex chest wall defects. It can provide blood-rich tissue with less complications [10–15]. However, the cost of greater omentum removal is rather high. It is only considered when other flaps or myocutaneous flaps are not available, and the amount of tissue is insufficient. Especially when cutting with pedicle, a considerable amount of omentum tissue is left in the abdominal cavity and tunnel [16]. Therefore, although the application of the greater omental flap is becoming increasingly popular, most of the improvement of cutting technology is committed to reduce donor site damage [17–20].

N. Wan (✉)
Department of Oncoplastic Surgery, Hunan Province Cancer Hospital, Changsha, Hunan, China
e-mail: wannengbing@hnca.org.cn

S. Ma
Department of Thyroid and Breast Surgery, Center Hospital of Xuhui District, Shanghai, China

25.2 Indications

Because of its shape and unique blood supply, omentum has become an ideal donor area for breast reconstruction. The chest skin is often damaged by biopsy, and the omentum has rich blood supply, which can protect the surface of the skin. The omentum also protects the deep prosthesis and reduce the risks of prosthesis exposure. The breast tissue removed in most patients is much larger than the prosthesis. If you want the skin to fit the prosthesis after contraction, it will eventually lead to a disaster in appearance. Omentum has many advantages: skin grafting on omentum is easy to survive; wide cutting range; and donor site defect is less. The omentum can provide blood-rich tissue to cover necrotic, radioactive, malignant, or infected wounds, and the effect is reliable. It has abundant lymphatic reflux and theoretically has the advantages of anti-infection and antitumor. It is reported that the omentum was used to cover the wound after tumor resection, and the recurrence, if occurred, was usually located at the edge of omentum flaps [14]. Another method of breast reconstruction using omentum is to fill the breast with omentum and using skin graft by taking advantages of the special properties of the omentum. The omentum was transferred to the chest wall for reshaping and covered with skin graft.

The omentum can not only provide an effective reconstruction method for curative surgery but also improve the quality of life of patients with advanced ulcerative and complex wounds. For example, it can be used for various wounds after chest wall resection: primary tumor, recurrent breast cancer, and progressive radiation-induced necrosis. For breast reconstruction or repair of infectious chest wall dehiscence, it can provide a reliable method if the latissimus dorsi or pectoralis major are not available or the covers are insufficient.

Specific indications include (1) immediate one-stage reconstruction of unilateral or bilateral subcutaneous mastectomy, with or without prosthesis according to the size of the breast. (2) After mastectomy or delayed reconstruction

Z. Li, D. Song (eds.), *Oncoplastic Flap Surgery*, https://doi.org/10.1007/978-981-19-8926-1_25

after radical mastectomy, there is no other good method. For example, the chest skin has extensive burns or extensive radioactive skin necrosis and/or radiodermatitis [11].

25.3 Anatomy

The greater omentum originates from the dorsal mesentery of the stomach. There are two main blood vessels (left and right gastroepiploic arteries) for nutrition. They are sent out by gastroduodenal and splenic arteries, respectively, and courses along the great curvature of the stomach to form the gastroepiploic arch. The right, middle, and left omental arteries and many small omental vessels are sent out from the arch. Each omental artery joins in the formation of another vascular arch, so the omental flap can be divided into two parts. Mastering the five main variants of vascular arch can selectively retain and utilize the contralateral blood flow, so as to transfer with pedicle to remoter parts [21, 22].

Main blood supply: right omental artery. Length: 20 cm (range 10–30 cm). Vessel diameter: 2.2 mm (range 1.5–3 mm). The right gastroepiploic artery comes from gastroduodenal artery. It passes through the greater curvature of the stomach and sends four main branches to the omentum and sends several short branches of the gastric artery to the stomach and finally joins the left omental artery [2].

Secondary blood supply: left omental artery. Length: 20 cm (range 10–30 cm). Vessel diameter: 2 mm (range 1.2–2.9 mm). The left omental artery originates from the splenic artery, passes through the greater curvature of the stomach and anastomoses with the right omental artery.

Main venous reflux of omental flap: right omental vein. Length: 20 cm (range 10–30 cm). Vessel diameter: 2.7 mm (range 2–3.4 mm). The right omental vein flows back into the superior mesenteric vein and courses along the great curvature of the stomach from left to right, parallel to the right omental artery. The diameters of arteries and veins are similar, but the wall of the vein is thinner, which increases the difficulty of vascular anastomosis [20]. Second venous reflux: left omental vein. Length: 20 cm (range 10–30 cm). Vessel diameter: 2.7 mm (range 2–3.4 mm). The left omental vein courses along the great curvature of the stomach from right to left, parallel to the left omental artery, and flows into the splenic vein.

The omental flap had no motor and sensory innervation.

The volume of the omentum is only suitable for unilateral breast reconstruction, and the volume problem can be overcome by using prosthesis. Therefore, the omentum is mainly used as a protective membrane with blood supply and sometimes provides filling with partial volume. The average length of female omentum is 33 cm and the width is 32.5 cm. At least a size of 16 cm × 16 cm of the omentum can be obtained on each side to cover the breast [23]. It is reported that even the smallest omentum can reach 19 cm × 20.4 cm which is also enough to cover both breasts [24], but our clinical measurements based on Asian women were inconsistent.

The size of the omentum can be estimated according to the patient's height and weight before operation. However, if the patient has a history of abdominal surgery and may have omental adhesion, it is difficult to predict the size of the omentum. Even if the patient has omental adhesion, the omental flap can still be prepared by careful dissection.

The omentum in 75% of patients can reach the level of the nipple, and that of 40% of patients can reach the sternal angle level. Only about 10% of patients reach the inguinal ligament level after partial dissociation of the omentum and colon. The omentum can be used to cover the wounds in the dorsum and waist through the retroperitoneal tunnel. The omentum can be separated and extended to the head, the middle of the thigh, and forearm. However, for wounds in remote area, it is more practical to use free tissue transplantation than to sacrifice the distal area for the excessive length of the pedicle [23].

According to our clinical findings, the greater omentum flaps are divided into four types according to its tissue characteristics (Fig. 25.1):

1. Thin type: fat is sparse and transparent, showing a network.
2. Intermediate type: slightly more fat, translucent.
3. Hypertrophic type: rich in fat which is in plate shape.
4. Absent type: the amount of the omentum is rare.

Key points in anatomy:

1. The diameter of the right gastroepiploic artery is usually larger than that of the left, so the right side is usually used as the vascular pedicle. Extensive separation of the left gastroepiploic vessels increases the risk of spleen injury.
2. The gastroomental arch has four main branches: accessory omental artery, right omental artery, middle omental artery, and left omental artery.
3. The middle omental artery coincides with the left and right omental arteries. This anatomical basis is very important when the omental flap requires to be extended or the multi-leaf omental flap is to be made [2].

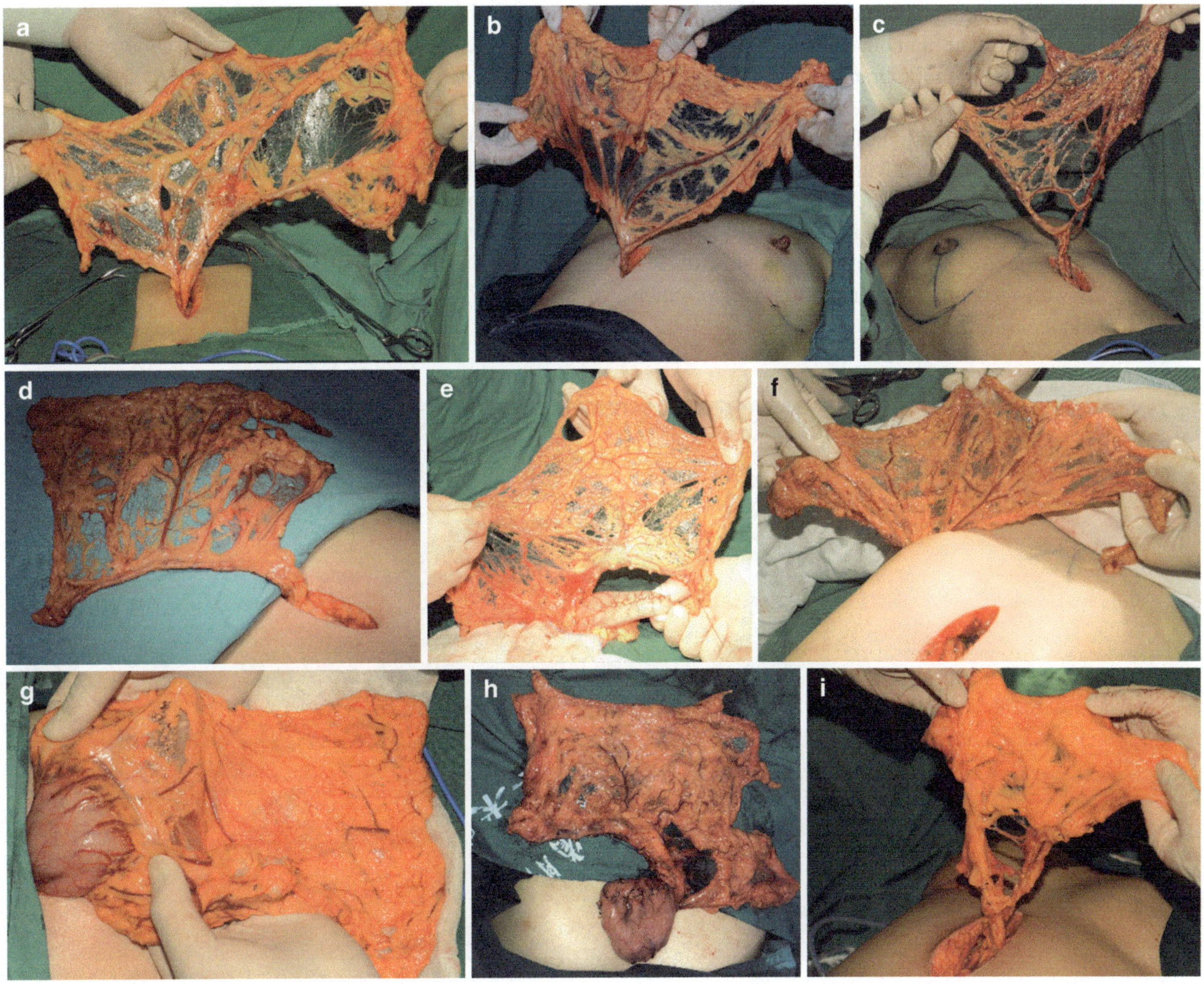

Fig. 25.1 Characteristics and types of omentum tissue: (**a**–**c**) thin type; (**d**–**f**) intermediate type: slightly more fat, translucent; (**g**–**i**) hypertrophic type: rich in fat, in plate shape

25.4 Advantages and Disadvantages of the Greater Omental Flap and Preoperative Preparation

Advantages of omental flap include the following [3, 18]:

1. It can be used as free transplantation or dissected with pedicle.
2. The tissue is thin and soft with good plasticity.
3. Large surface area, which can cover a larger area of defects.
4. Long vascular pedicle.
5. It has angiogenic and immune characteristics.
6. The operation is simple and fast, and the operation time is short.
7. Abundant blood supply.
8. Less damages in the donor site.
9. After abdominal flap transplantation, the greater omentum flap can still be designed and dissected.

Disadvantages include the following:

1. Laparotomy is required.
2. The size and tissue volume of the omental flap could not be evaluated before operation.

Preoperative preparation includes the following:

1. Omental flap design, anatomical markings of inferior costal margin and midline of the abdomen
2. Omental flap size: Length: average 35 cm. Width: average 25 cm. Thickness: average 1 cm
3. Omental flap design

The omental flap is designed according to the defect size of the recipient area. The amount of omental flap tissue required varies, and the vascular branches carried by the flap are also different.

When a large area of body surface defect needs to be repaired, omental flap combined with intermediate-thickness skin graft is the best choice (Fig. 25.2).

Free omental flap can be used to repair a wide range of craniofacial defects, lower limb, or head and neck defects. The currently well-recognized features of the greater omental flap include the following:

1. Easy to shape and repair irregular defects.
2. The tissue has good ductility and the vascular pedicle can be prolonged.
3. There are two sets of vascular pedicles for anastomosis.
4. It has unique advantages in the repair of wounds with poor blood circulation such as infection, pollution, and radioactivity.

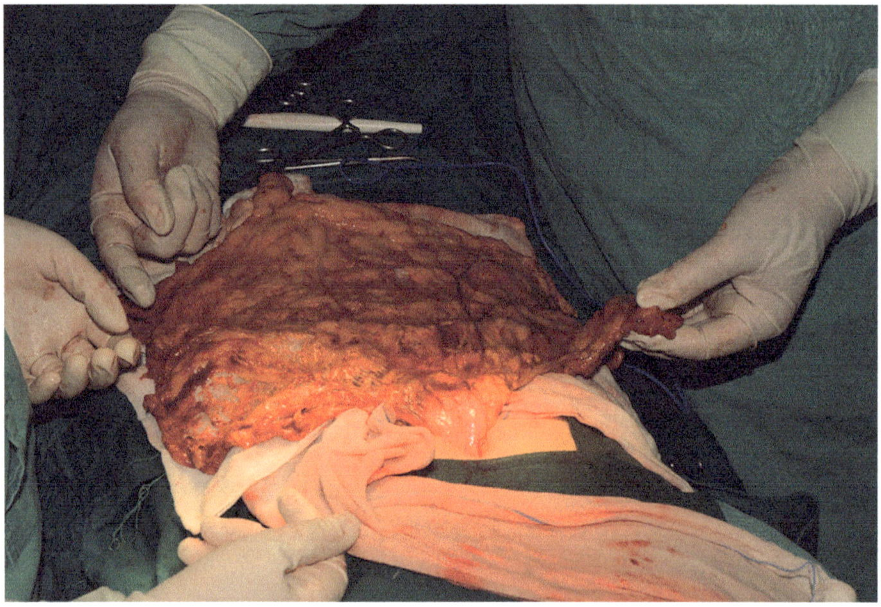

Fig. 25.2 Greater omental flap generally has a large area

25.5 Typical Cases of Free Greater Omental Flap

A 49-year-old male patient had a large area of ulceration around the right leg. The local hospital recommended amputation, and the measured ulcer area was 25 cm × 20 cm. The results of pathological examination was well differentiated squamous cell carcinoma. After anti-infection treatment, the cancerous ulcer of the right lower limb was fully resected under general anesthesia + free greater omentum flap transplantation, and moist dressing was used after operation. After the granulation tissue grew satisfactorily, the skin was grafted on the granulation tissue wound. The skin graft survived well. No tumor recurrence was found in the following 24 months after operation, and the appearance and function of the right lower limb were satisfactory (Figs. 25.3, 25.4, 25.5, 25.6, and 25.7) [25].

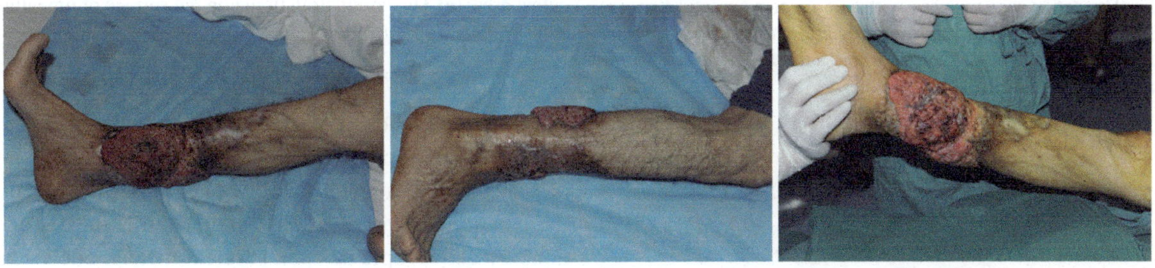

Fig. 25.3 Large area cancerous ulcer of the right leg can be seen before operation

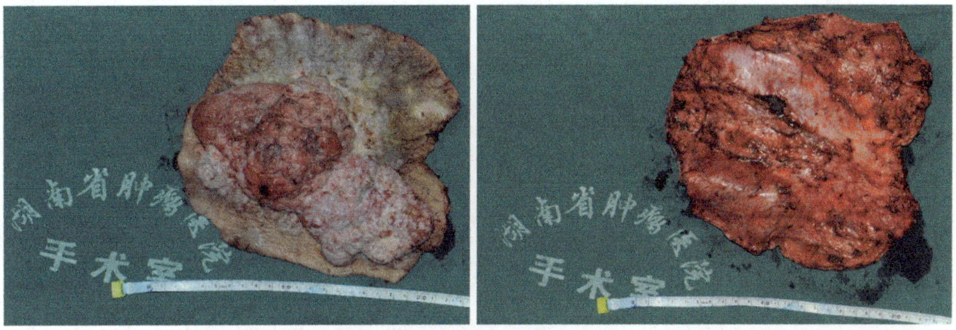

Fig. 25.4 Full-thickness extended and radical resection of cancerous ulcer tissue and its surrounding normal tissue

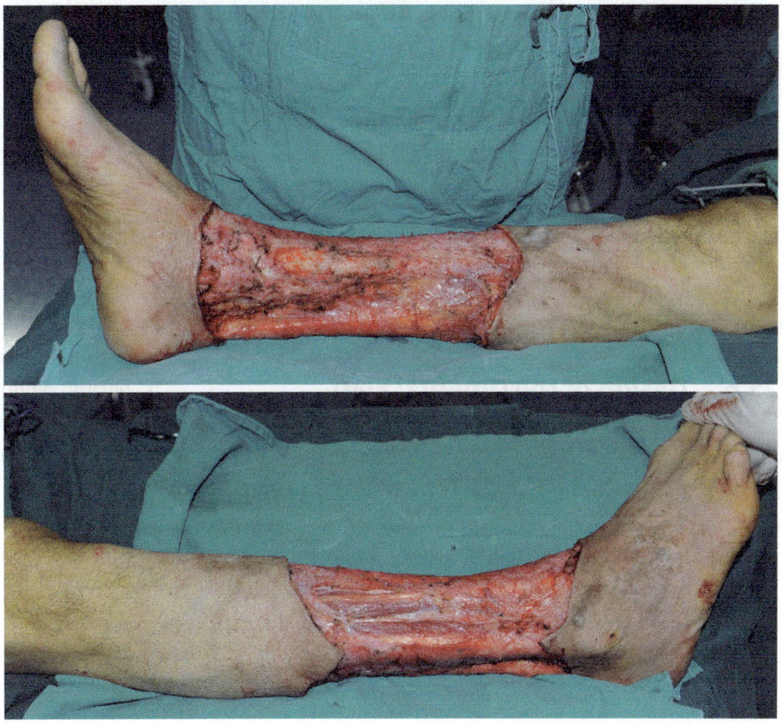

Fig. 25.5 Large skin and soft tissue defects around the right leg

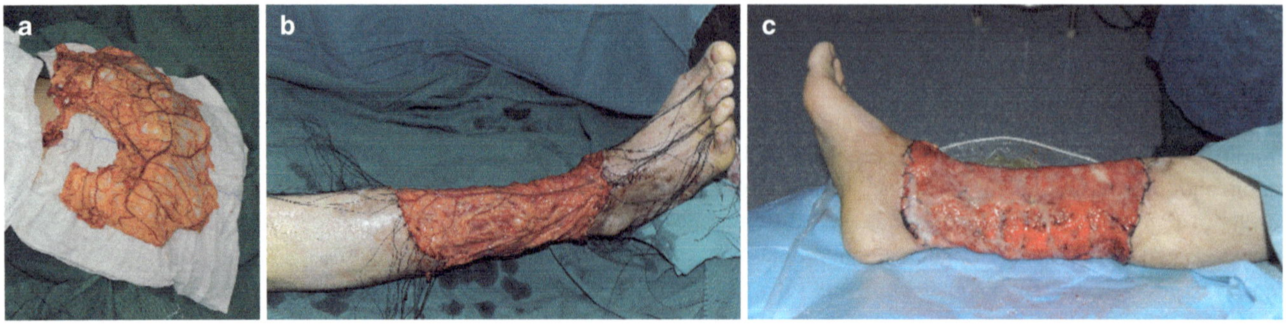

Fig. 25.6 The defect was repaired with free greater omental flap. (**a**) Free greater omental flap was cut during operation. (**b**) After vascular anastomosis, the greater omental flap was sutured and fixed in the defect area. (**c**) The granulation tissue on the surface of omentum grew well 10 days after operation

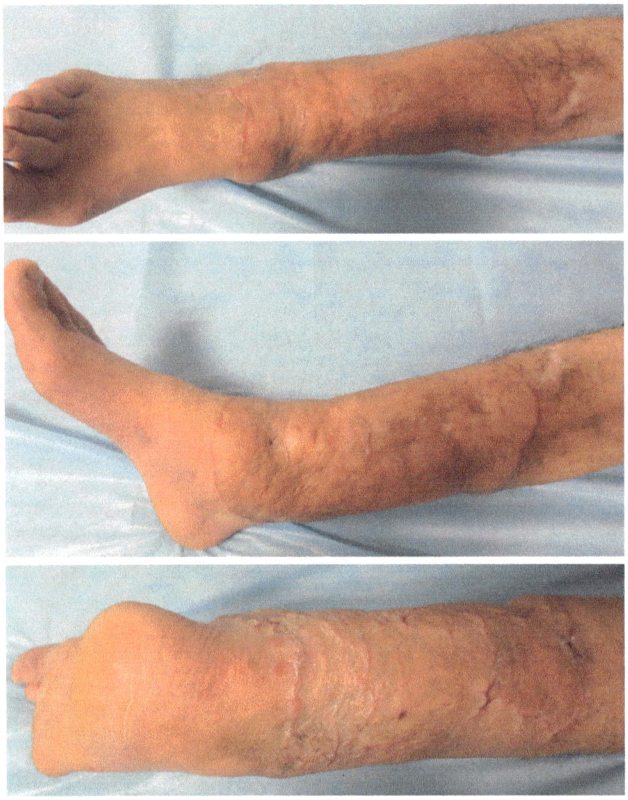

Fig. 25.7 The skin graft survived well after two-stage operation. No tumor recurrence was found during the follow-up of 24 months after operation, and the function and appearance of the right lower limb were satisfactory

25.6 Design of the Omental Flap for Special Requirements

Free greater omentum flap can be used to repair intraoral or oropharyngeal defects [20, 26].

Pedicled omental flap can be used for chest wall, abdominal wall reconstruction, and breast reconstruction—the omental flap is dissected through a small surgical incision of the diaphragm and transferred through subcutaneous tunnel. Whether in free form or pedicled form, the dissecting method of transplanted omental flap does not vary dramatically, but there is influence on the donor area whether the dissection is done by endoscopic or open surgical means. The size of the greater omental flap will change significantly according to the patient's body shape. A history of abdominal surgery or abdominal infection before operation will have a great impact on the omental properties and tissue volume. Due to its flexible ductility, the omental flap can be further folded to increase its thickness. Therefore, it is particularly suitable for breast reconstruction.

25.7 Omental Flap Markings

A complete piece of greater omentum is usually dissected for transplantation, but its size can only be determined after intraoperative exposure. Patients usually take the supine position, and the omental flap often needs to be rearranged and reshaped after transfer.

25.8 Surgical Methods

After separating the omentum to a sufficient length, carefully form a subcutaneous tunnel through the laparotomy incision and another separate incision in the anterior sheath of the rectus abdominis, or an incision between ribs adjacent to the recipient area. The latter two incisions can avoid the risks of hernia. Many doctors have penetrated the pedicle on the left side of the sickle ligament, which can also prevent hernia formation. In the process of omental transposition, pay attention to avoid damaging and twisting the pedicle, duodenum, and gastric antrum. Pull out the omentum to the edge of the wound guided by wire to avoid omental protrusion and hyperactivity.

When the scope and position of the omentum are appropriate, fix the omentum near the tunnel in the recipient area.

Expose the omentum and cover it with moist gauze. After closing the abdominal wound, turn your attention to the chest wall. Carefully remove all necrotic, infected, radioactive, or tumor tissue. In particular, the involved costal cartilage should also be widely removed.

After the defect of chest wall is covered by flap, one or two layers of Prolene mesh can be sutured on the inner surface of the costal arch to reconstruct the strength of the chest wall. This material is relatively more resistant to contamination. For large full-thickness defects, the ribs can be transplanted for bone support to prevent "reverse movement" and abnormal appearance of chest wall.

After the omentum is sutured to the edge of the wound, the surface of the omentum can be directly covered with Prolene mesh, rib graft, chest drainage tube, and reticular full-thickness skin to drain the postoperative exudation. The postoperative wound was packed with moist dressing without additional pressure.

Subcutaneous mastectomy was performed through a lower external incision. Separate the skin and a thin layer of fat from the breast surface to the clavicle. Pay extra attention when reaching the lateral axillary extension and the thinned medial quadrant. The whole breast was removed from the surface of the pectoral muscle for complete hemostasis.

The surgical strategy of chest wall reconstruction with omentum includes evaluating and transferring the omentum before removing infectious chest wall wounds or extensive resection. Through the incision of the abdominal wall and thorough exploration the peritoneum, the non-vascularized tissue that connects the omentum and the colon is dissociated with the assistance of pulling the omentum. Because the left side of the omentum usually has less adhesion with the body and tail of the pancreas, most doctors recommend moving the omentum from the left. During the operation, try to avoid the damages of the colonic diverticulum and the wrapping of appendix, transverse colon, and middle colon vessels by the omentum. Ligate the blood vessels in time and avoid electrocoagulation, so as to prevent the injury of these thin blood vessels and the secondary injury of gastrocolonic arch caused by thrombosis.

If the mobilization of omentum is not enough, the following methods can be used. Separating the omentum from the migrating part of the stomach and some gastrocolonic vessels is the simplest and most commonly used method to prolong the omentum. Be careful not to distort the gastrocolonic vessels when separating and ligating the omentum and gastric migrating segment. Short blood vessels between stomach and gastrocolonic vessels should be ligated one by one as far away from the duodenum and gastric antrum as possible. More importantly, the left and right blood vessels of the stomach and colon need to be blocked by turn to assess the blood supply capacity of the arterial arch. The right gastrocolonic artery is usually thicker with stronger pulsation. Therefore, the left gastrocolonic artery is usually sacrificed during operation. Finally, the method of expanding the omentum includes the selective separation of omentum (according to the course of blood vessels) as being discussed in the anatomical part.

The omentum was taken out from the median incision of the upper abdomen and pay attention to the distribution of blood vessels. Previous abdominal diseases may cause omental adhesion. At this time, enough amount of the omentum needs to be carefully separated. Then dissociate the omentum from the transverse colon along the avascular area, so as to protect the blood vessels of the colon from damage [24].

If only one side of the breast needs reconstruction, the omentum and greater curvature of the stomach can be separated with the right gastroepiploic vessel as the pedicle. If you need to reconstruct bilateral breasts, separate the omentum and stomach from the middle of the great curvature of the stomach to both sides, so that the vascular pedicle on both sides can be preserved.

The separation plane is close to the greater curvature of the stomach to ensure that the gastroepiploic vessels are connected to the omentum [26]. At this time, the omentum is enough to reach the breast level through the subcutaneous tunnel. Unfold the omentum to form a fan-like shape and embed it on the inner surface of the skin. Check the torsion of the pedicle. The fan-shaped omentum is fixed through the catgut sutures or subcutaneous fixations or through the skin and fixed with tension-reduced sutures cushioned by Vaseline gauze. After the prosthesis was placed in the deeper surface of the omentum, the breast incision was closed layer by layer. Dissect and close the posterior omentum and subcutaneous tissue. Drainage was placed accordingly. The abdominal incision was closed in layers, leaving a small crack above the incision through which the omental pedicle passed. The wound was covered with elastic bandage. Because the omental pedicle passes through the costal edge, a bra could not be worn so as to avoid the compression to the vascular pedicle.

Steps of Omental Flap for Breast Reconstruction:

1. Omental collection
2. Primary defect resection
3. Breast reconstruction
4. Axillary lymph node dissection through minor incision

The steps of omental flap for breast reconstruction are explained in detail in typical cases.

The patient, a 43-year-old female, found a right breast mass for 10 days. Breast color Doppler ultrasound showed (1) solid mass in the upper quadrant of the right outer breast, BI-RADS 4B. (2) No obvious enlarged lymph nodes were found in bilateral axillary areas. Under general anesthesia, breast-conserving radical mastectomy + one-stage reconstruction of pedicled omental breast for right breast cancer was reported as invasive cancer of the right breast. No obvious cancer tissue was found around the conserving margin of the affected breast. The patient was then transfer to internal medicine for comprehensive treatment. The appearance and function of the reconstructed breast were satisfactory during follow-up (Figs. 25.8, 25.9, 25.10, 25.11, 25.12, 25.13, 25.14, 25.15, 25.16, 25.17, 25.18, 25.19, 25.20, and 25.21).

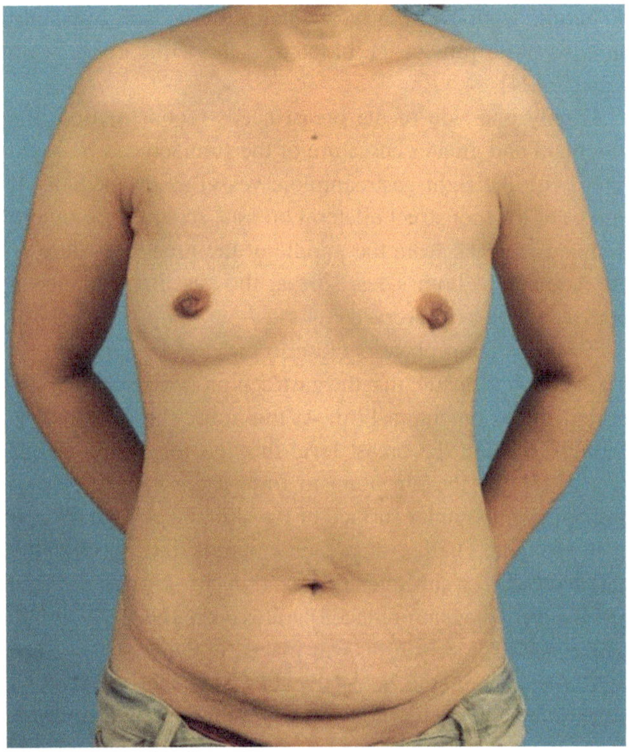

Fig. 25.8 Preoperative conditions

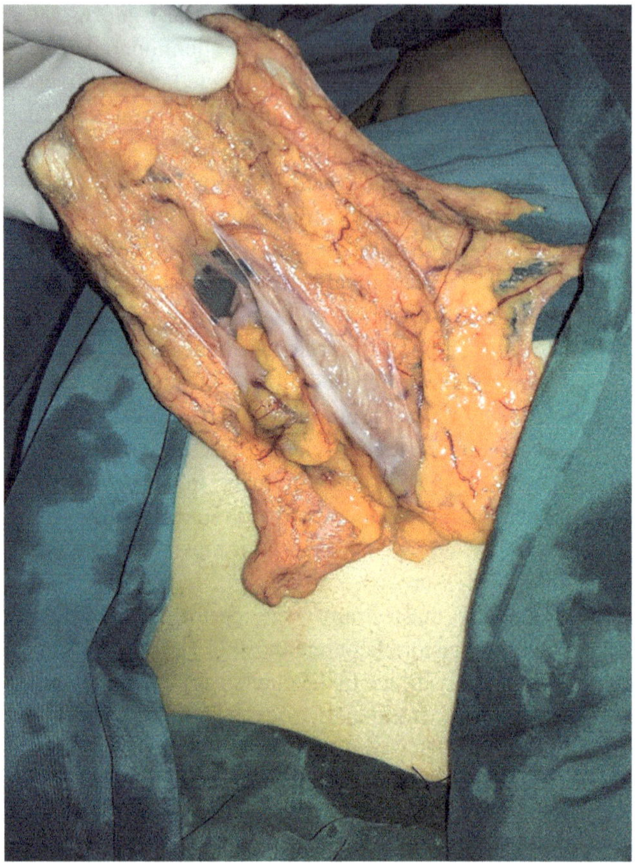

Fig. 25.9 Expose the greater omentum and pull it out

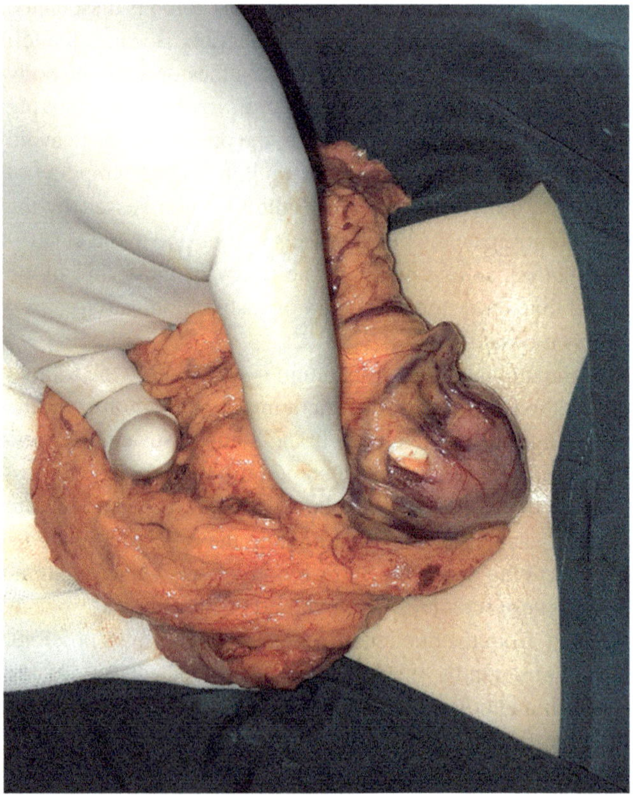

Fig. 25.10 Ligate the short gastric artery branch along the way

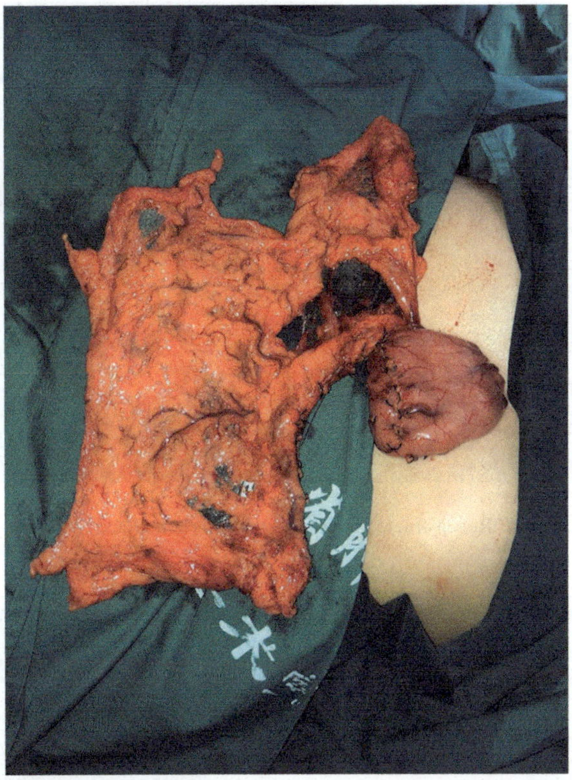

Fig. 25.11 The greater omentum was only connected to the donor area with the vascular pedicle of the left and right gastroepiploic arteries

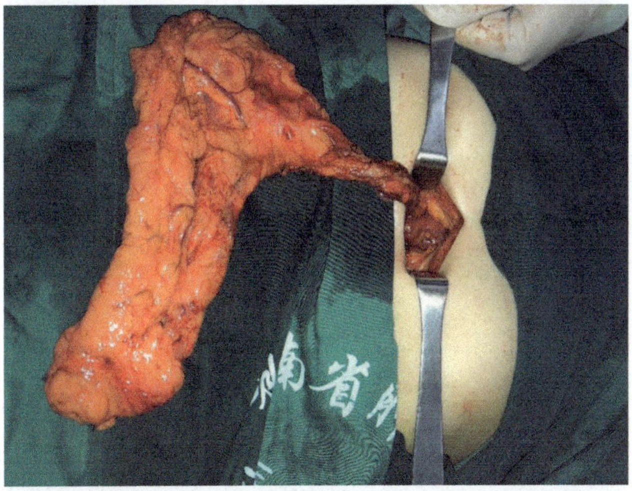

Fig. 25.12 In order to prolong the length of vascular pedicle of the omental flap, the left gastroepiploic artery was ligated and disconnected, and the omental flap pedicled the right gastroepiploic artery was prepared

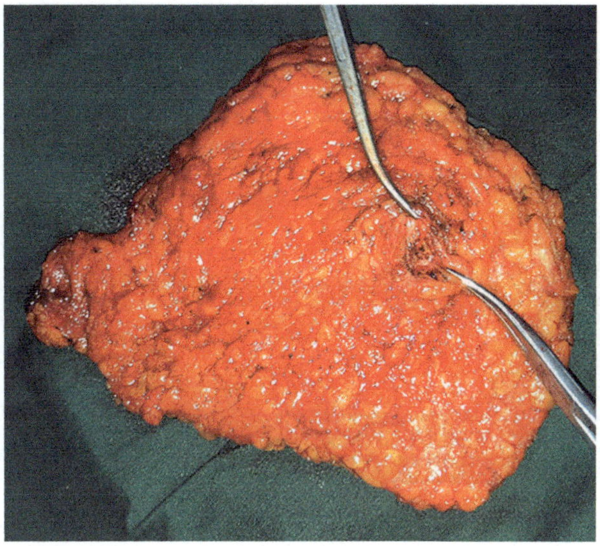

Fig. 25.13 Modified radical mastectomy for breast cancer with the nipple and areola preserved

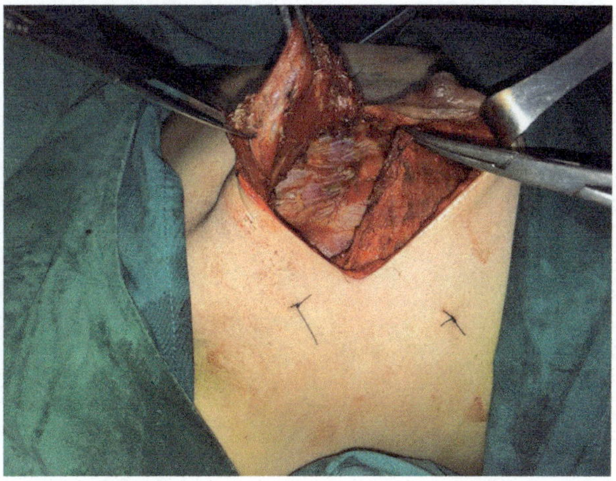

Fig. 25.14 Lift the pectoralis major and part of the anterior serratus muscle to prepare the cavity to accommodate the prosthesis

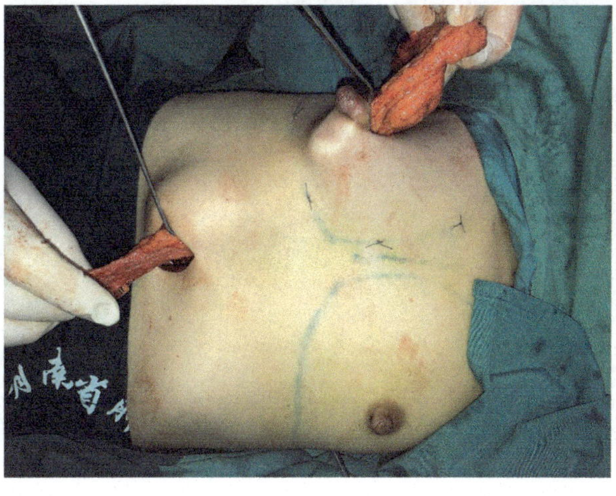

Fig. 25.15 Transfer of the omental flap to the right chest wall through a narrow subcutaneous tunnel

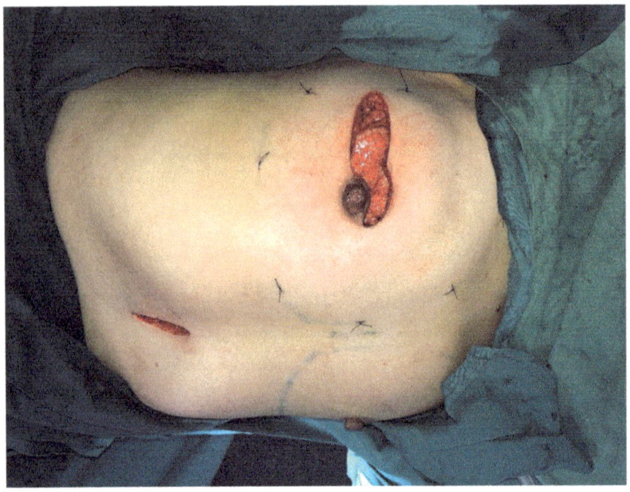

Fig. 25.16 After confirming that the vascular pedicle is tension-free, place the omental flap in the receiving area to determine its coverage

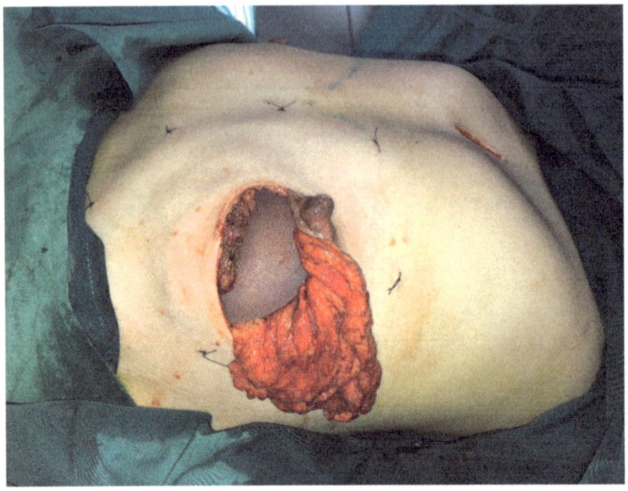

Fig. 25.17 Implant prosthesis in the deep surface of the pectoralis major and omental flap

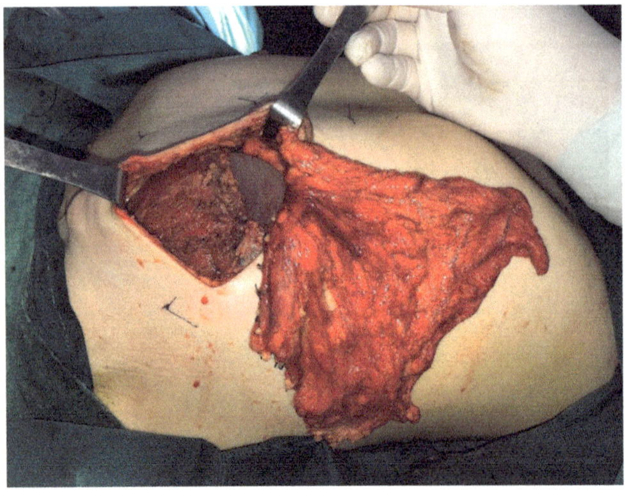

Fig. 25.18 Breast shaping with the pectoralis major and omental flap covering the prosthesis

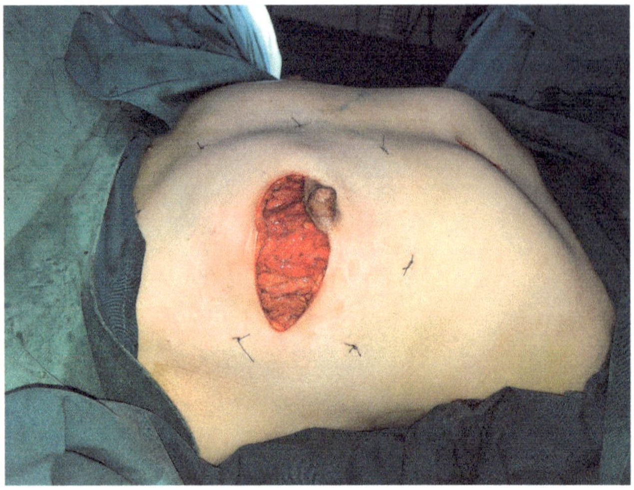

Fig. 25.19 Reconstructed breast shaping was completed

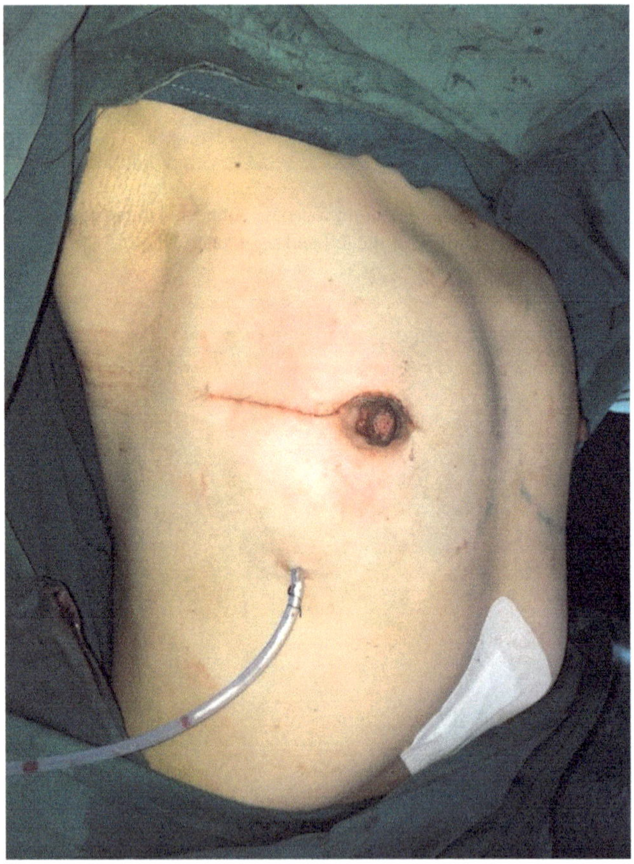

Fig. 25.20 Lymph node dissection through a small axillary incision after cosmetic suture of the wound

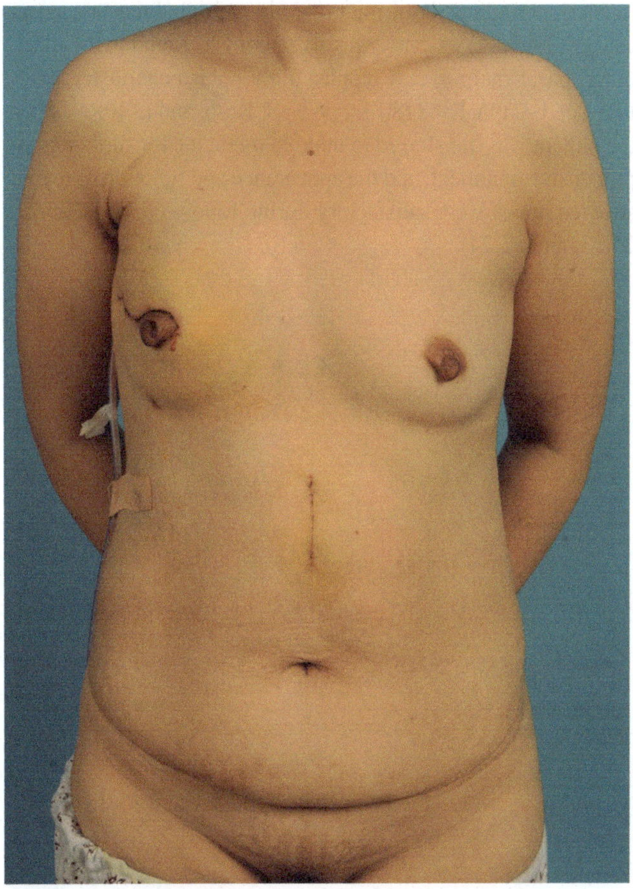

Fig. 25.21 Discharge 4 days after operation

25.9 Precautions for Omental Flap Dissection Technique [27]

1. The abdominal cavity is explored through the median incision of the upper abdomen. The area, tissue volume, and vascular pedicle length of the greater omentum should be evaluated. The flap is dissected from the transverse colon, and the transfer and shaping are adjusted above the gastric omental arch.
2. Blunt separation and bipolar hemostasis are used. The larger branches must be ligated with titanium clips or sutures.
3. The short gastric artery branches are ligated throughout the procedures, and the lateral splenic septal tissue should be carefully separated. Finally, the left or right omental vessels are used as the pedicle.
4. Special care should be given to avoid clamping and kinking the vascular pedicle when transferring the omental flap.

25.10 Endoscopic Harvest of the Omental Flap

The standard omental endoscopic resection uses four trocars that are placed on the umbilicus, pubis, and bilateral external iliac depression. During the operation, the pressure of CO_2 for pneumoperitoneum is maintained at 10–12 mmHg. The stomach was lifted and the right omental artery was separated. Ligate and disconnect the short gastric artery along the greater curvature of the stomach until the left omental artery is exposed. Carefully separate the greater omentum from the transverse colon while preserving the mesenteric blood supply. The left gastroepiploic artery is ligated and disconnected at the edge of the left colonic curvature, and the omental flap is pulled out through one of the four incisions of trocar [17].

25.11 Omental Flap Monitoring

Based on the fact that the gastroepiploic artery sends out several short branches into the greater curvature of the stomach, the gastric mucosal flap can be taken from one of the branches for intraoral or oropharyngeal reconstruction [20, 26].

25.12 Special Instruments

Endoscopic dissection of the omental flap can significantly reduce donor site injury [17, 28].

25.13 Donor Closure and Postoperative Management

The intestinal volvulus should be avoided after the dissection of the free omental flap. Standard endoscopic closure technique was used to repair abdominal incision of the donor area. Generally, there is no need for placing drainage in the donor area. When dissecting the pedicled omental flap, the abdominal fascia layer requires a small gap for the vascular pedicle to pass through. This can lead to abdominal wall hernia, but surgical intervention in particular is generally not required.

25.14 Postoperative Treatment

Avoid heavy physical work 6–8 weeks after operation. Abdominal bandage is recommended to be retained for 4 weeks. Most of the complications of the omentum flap are rather small and easy to deal with. They include temporary gastrointestinal obstruction, partial omental, or skin graft separation or necrosis, and occasional recurrence of infection. Although granulation tissue growth and epithelization occur quickly at most wound margin, repeated flap debridement and repositioning may still be required.

Possible complications of pedicled omental reconstruction include hernia formation and omental movement at the peritoneal exit. As with any transabdominal procedure, a certain risk is the presence of adhesive intestinal obstruction, although this is not a major problem. It was reported that a patient had died due to the cecal torsion by omental adhesion after thoracic wall reconstruction with pedicled omentum flap [15].

There are many [16, 24–34] techniques for breast plastic surgery after partial breast reconstruction after breast cancer. Since 2010, we have performed more than 200 cases of omental flap transplantation and immediate breast reconstruction with satisfactory results.

25.15 Simple Transposition of Pedicled Omental Flap for Breast Reconstruction: Typical Case 1

A 29-year-old female patient found a right breast mass for half a month and received mass resection for 14 days. Under general anesthesia, breast-conserving surgery for right breast cancer + one-stage breast reconstruction of greater omentum were performed. The postoperative pathological examination showed (1) right breast mass combined with immunohistochemistry accorded with histological grade III of invasive ductal carcinoma, and the size of the mass was about 1.3 cm × 1.7 cm × 1.4 cm; (2) (axillary lymph nodes) 2/13 showed cancer metastasis; (3) (posterior quadrant tissue after resection of right breast mass) no cancer tissue; (4) no cancer involvement was found in the inner, outer, basal margin, and nipple. Immunohistochemistry: Er−, PR−, cerb-2 (+), Ki67 (80%), p63 +, CK5/6, and EGFR−. Then the patient was transferred to internal medicine for further comprehensive treatment, and the appearance and function of reconstructed breast were satisfactory during follow-up (Figs. 25.22, 25.23, and 25.24).

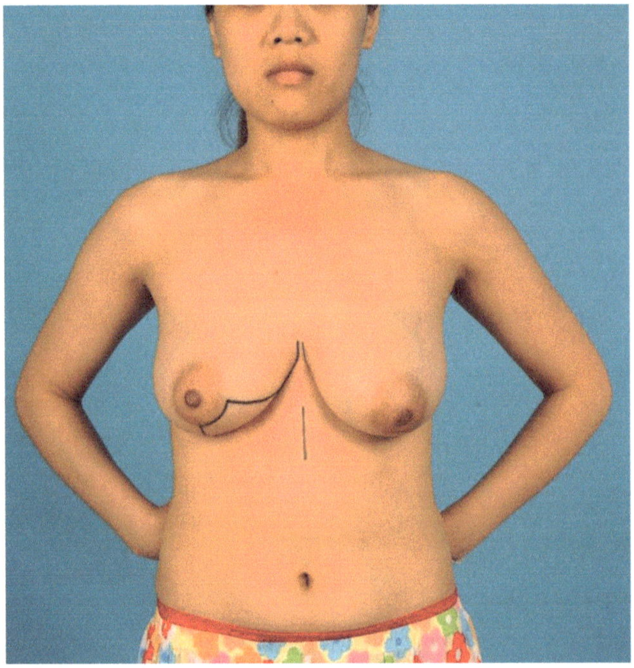

Fig. 25.22 Preoperative conditions

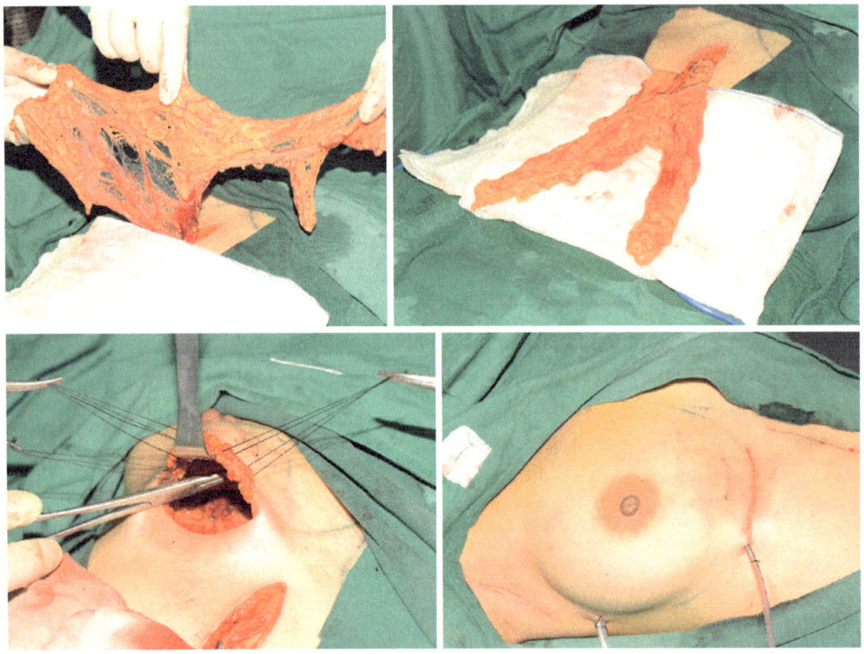

Fig. 25.23 The dissection and shaping of the greater omental flap were completed, and the modified radical mastectomy for breast cancer was conducted. Transfer the greater omental flap and reconstruct the breast shape and volume

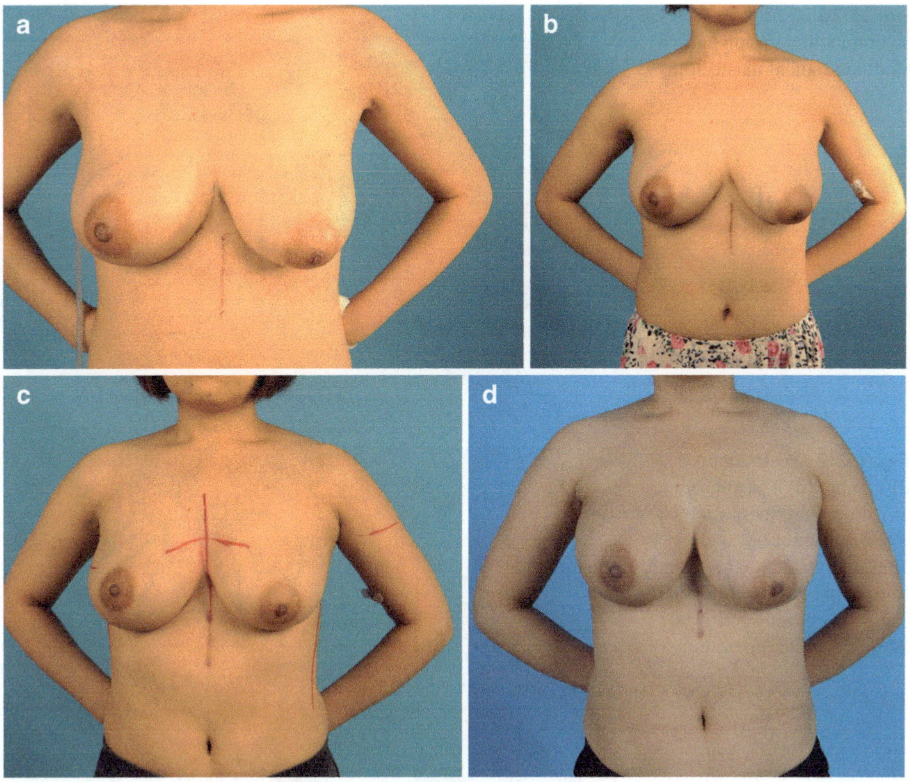

Fig. 25.24 Postoperative follow-up. (**a**) Appearance 5 days after operation. (**b**) Appearance 15 days after operation. (**c**) Three-month follow-up after operation. (**d**) The patients were followed up 18 months after operation

25.16 Simple Transposition of Pedicled Omental Flap for Breast Reconstruction: Typical Case 2

The patient, a 41-year-old female, found a right breast mass for 1 month. Breast color Doppler ultrasound showed (1) solid mass in the lower quadrant of the right outer breast, BI-RADS 4B; (2) bimodal lobular hyperplasia; and (3) no obvious enlarged lymph nodes were found in bilateral axillary areas. Under general anesthesia, breast-conserving radical mastectomy plus one-stage breast reconstruction with pedicled omentum were performed. The pathological reports showed right breast ductal cancer. No obvious cancer tissue was found at the breast-conserving margin. The patient was transferred to internal medicine for further comprehensive treatment. The appearance and function of the reconstructed breast were satisfactory during follow-up (Figs. 25.25, 25.26, and 25.27).

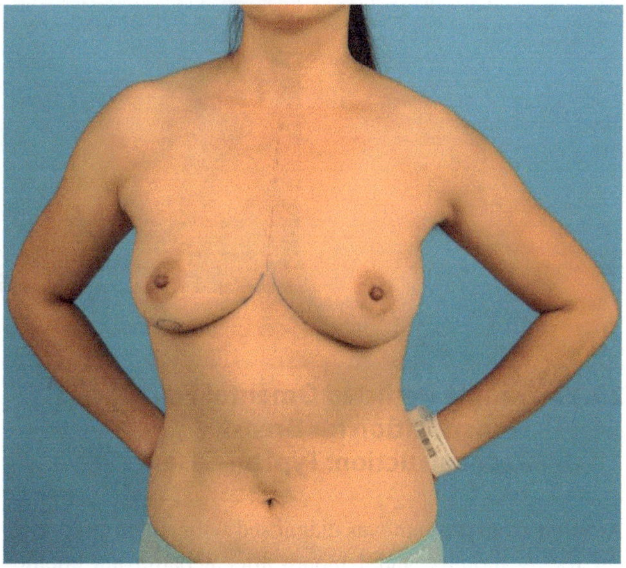

Fig. 25.25 Preoperative conditions

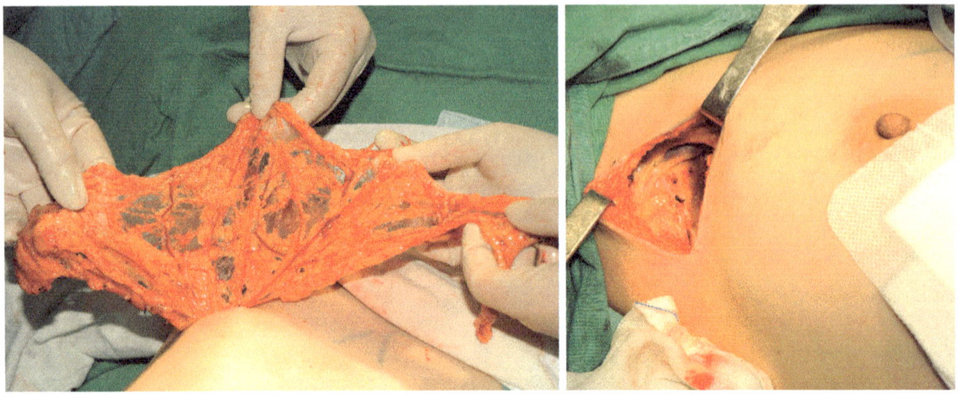

Fig. 25.26 Complete omentum preparation and modified radical mastectomy

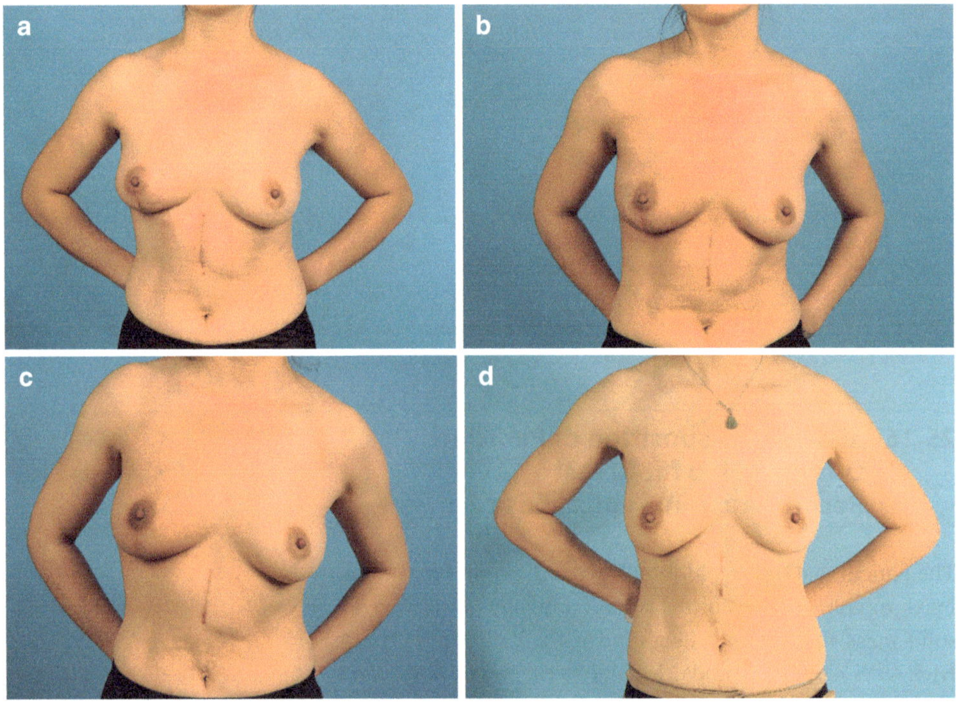

Fig. 25.27 Postoperative follow-up. (**a**) The appearance at 7 days after operation. (**b**) The appearance at 20 days after operation, (**c**) Six-month follow-up after operation. (**d**) The patients were followed up 24 months after operation

25.17 Simple Pedicled Omental Flap Transposition for Breast Reconstruction: Typical Case 3

A 34-year-old woman was diagnosed with right breast cancer for 6+ months, and 1 month after neoadjuvant chemotherapy for six rounds. Under general anesthesia, modified radical mastectomy for right breast cancer + breast reconstruction with pedicled greater omental flap were performed. The results of pathological examination (right breast puncture biopsy) showed invasive cancer with poor differentiation. Immunohistochemical results showed Er (−), PR (−), CerbB-2 (3 +), EGFR (−), CK5/6 (−), p63 (−), and Ki-67 were about 60%. Cytological examination of right axillary lymph nodes showed that metastatic cancer cells were found in the smear. The patient was transferred to internal medicine for further comprehensive treatment, and the appearance and function of the breast were satisfactory during follow-up (Figs. 25.28, 25.29, and 25.30).

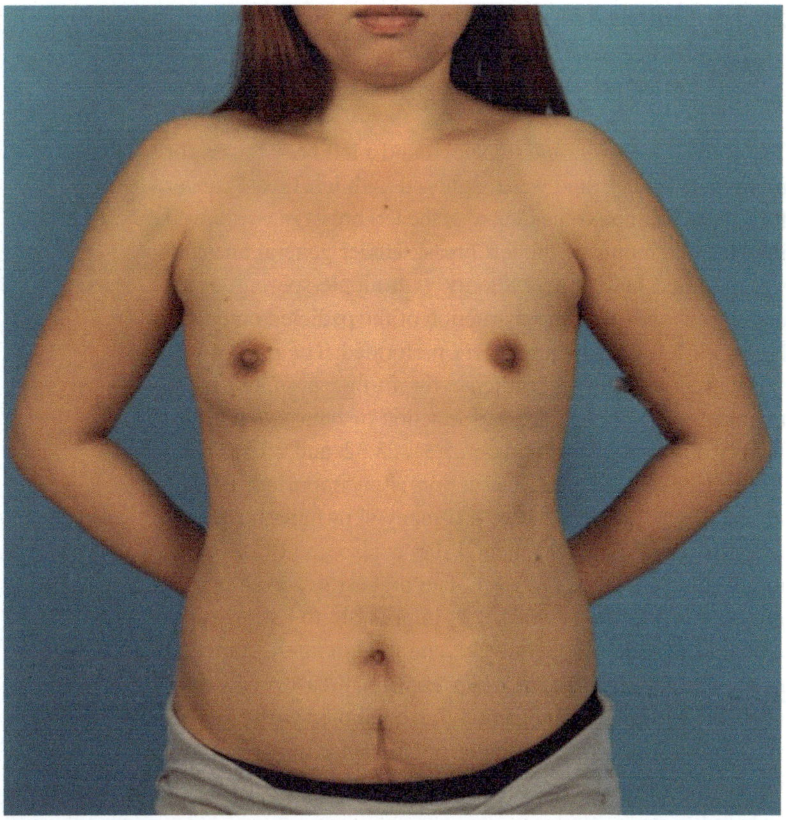

Fig. 25.28 Preoperative conditions

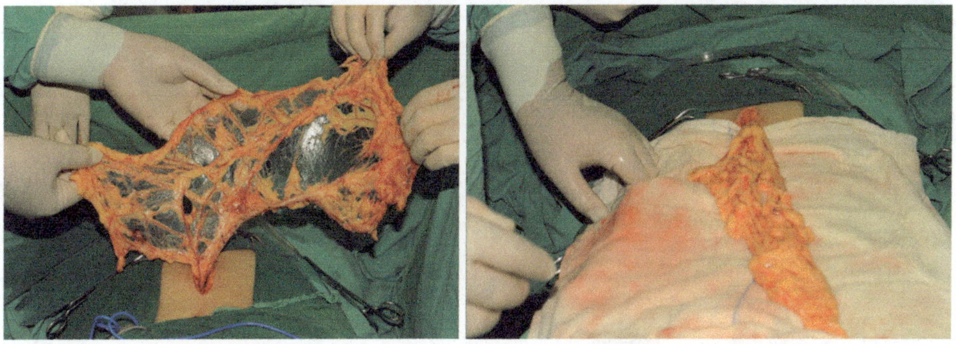

Fig. 25.29 Complete dissection and shaping of the greater omental flap

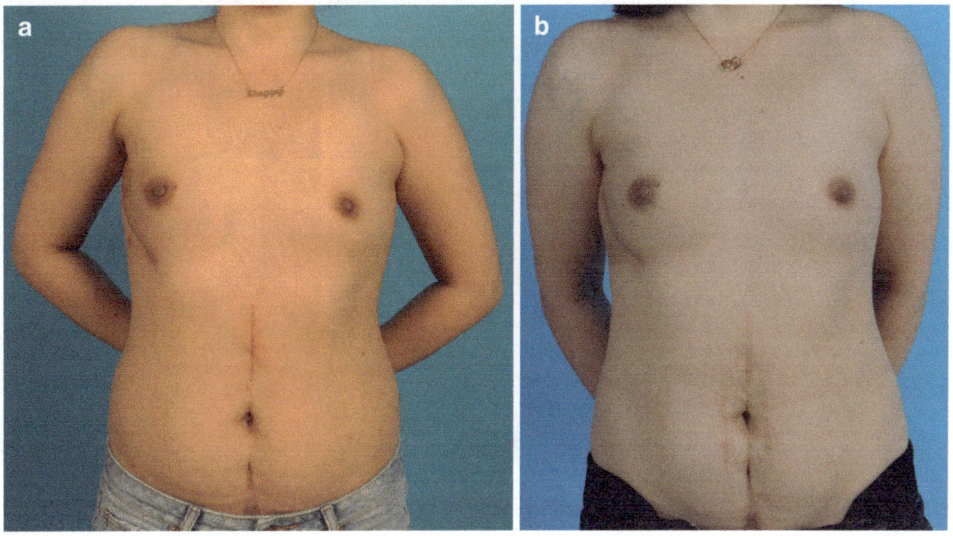

Fig. 25.30 Postoperative follow-up. (**a**) The appearance at 30 days after operation. (**b**) The appearance at 3 months followed up after operation

25.18 Simple Transposition of the Pedicled Omental Flap for Breast Reconstruction: Typical Case 4

The patient, a 42-year-old female, found a left breast mass for more than 10 days and was diagnosed with left breast cancer for 7 days. Mammotome biopsy of the left breast mass showed invasive carcinoma of the left breast. Under general anesthesia, modified radical mastectomy with nipple-sparing areola complex + one-stage reconstruction of the pedicled omentum breast for left breast cancer were performed. The patient was transferred to internal medicine for further comprehensive treatment. The appearance and function of breast were satisfactory during follow-up (Figs. 25.31, 25.32, and 25.33).

Immediate breast reconstruction is an important part of tumor plastic surgery. There are many skin flaps for breast reconstruction. Greater omental flap is also one of the commonly used methods [35, 36]. The biggest disadvantage of greater omental flap is that it is impossible to estimate the amount of tissue preoperatively, and the amount of omental tissue may be insufficient when used for breast reconstruction. Therefore, greater omental flap combined with prosthesis implantation is increasingly popular in clinical primary breast reconstruction [32–34].

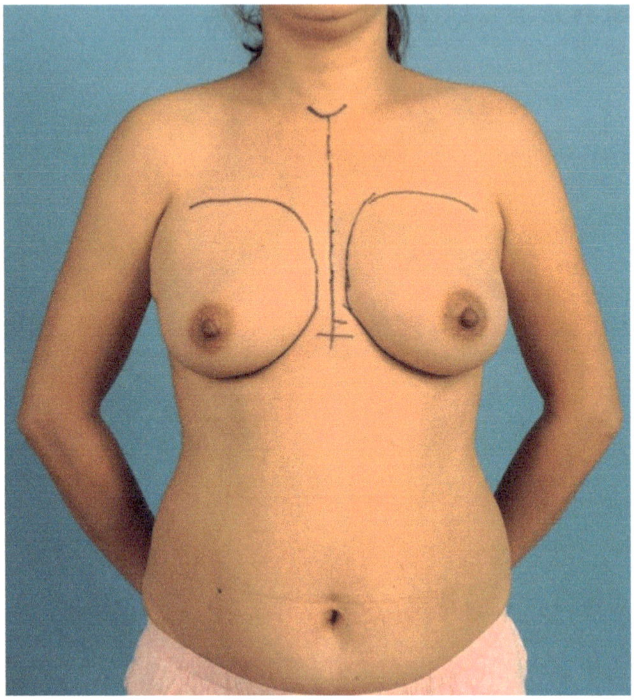

Fig. 25.31 Preoperative conditions

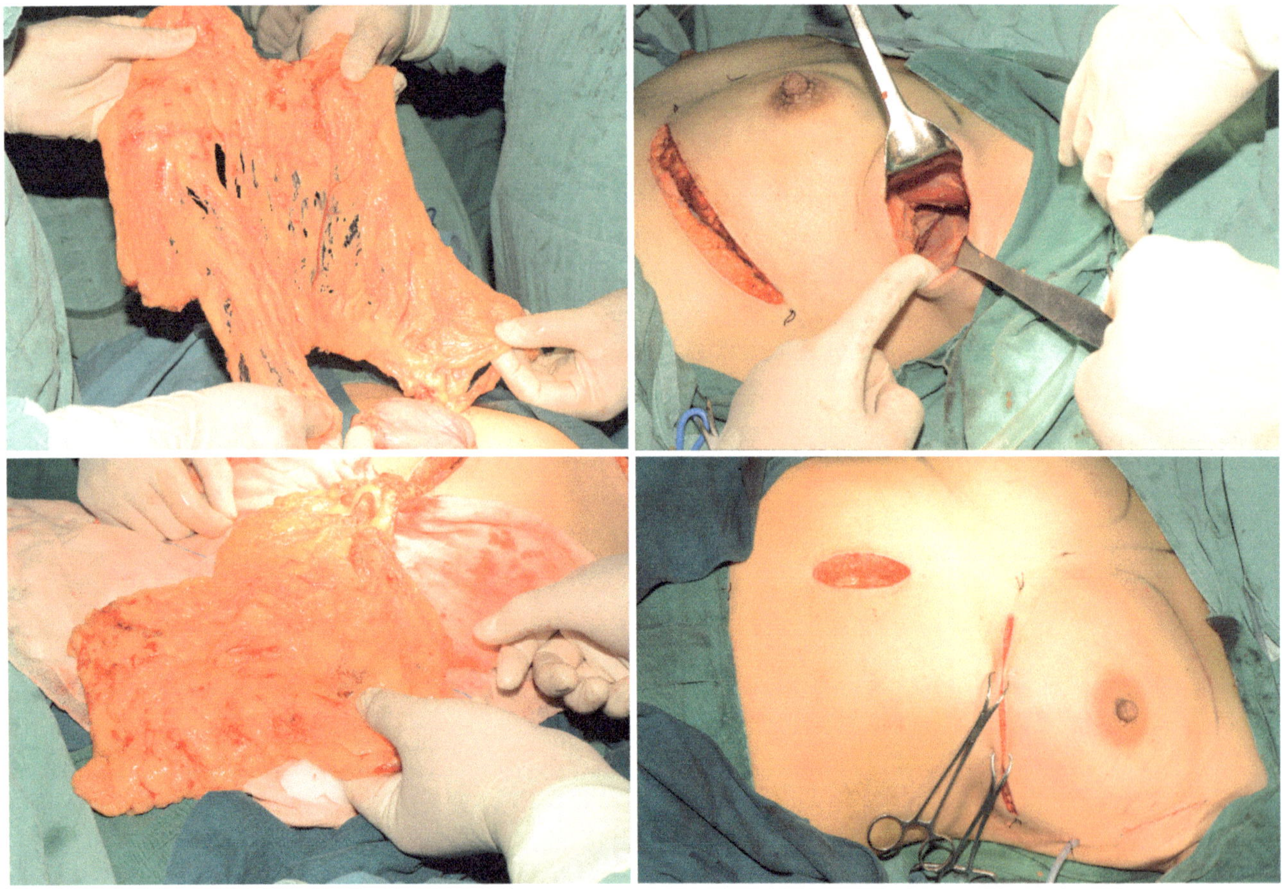

Fig. 25.32 The omentum flap and breast cancer-modified radical mastectomy were performed

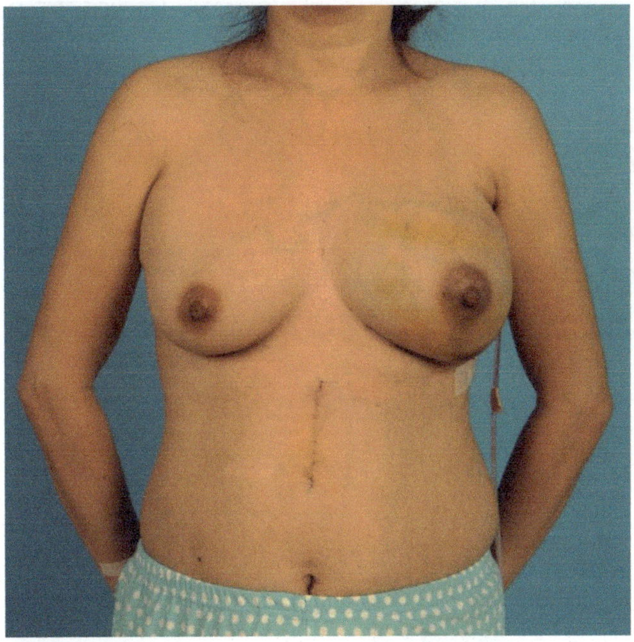

Fig. 25.33 Five-day follow-up after operation

25.19 Transposition of Pedicled Greater Omentum Flap Combined with Prosthesis Implantation for Breast Reconstruction: Typical Case 1

The patient was a 23-year-old female. The right breast mass was found for 2 months. The biopsy report showed that the right breast mass was grade II invasive ductal carcinoma, and some areas were high-grade ductal carcinoma in situ. No clear intravascular tumor thrombus was found. Three rounds of neoadjuvant chemotherapy were performed according to AC-T regimens. Under general anesthesia, modified radical mastectomy + prosthesis combined with omental primary reconstruction of right breast cancer with the nipple-areola preservation were performed. Postoperative pathological examination showed (1) grade II–III invasive ductal carcinoma (right breast), mass size 2 cm × 1.5 cm × 1.5 cm. (2) Cancer metastasis was seen in 2/11 of the right axilla. (3) The nipple and basal margin: no cancer invasion was found. The pathological stage was pt2n1m0 IIB.

Special inspection results revealed Er (+ ~ 2 + about 80%), pr (2 + ~ 3 + about 80%), CerbB-2 (2 +), and Ki-67 about 20% p63-CK5/6-E-cad +. The appearance and function of the breast were satisfactory during follow-up (Figs. 25.34, 25.35, and 25.36).

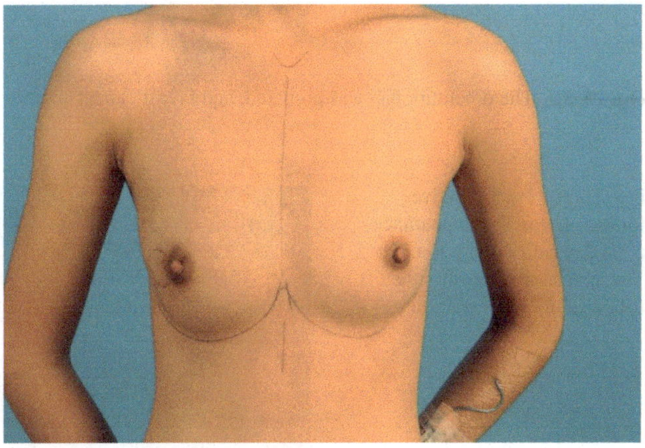

Fig. 25.34 Preoperative conditions

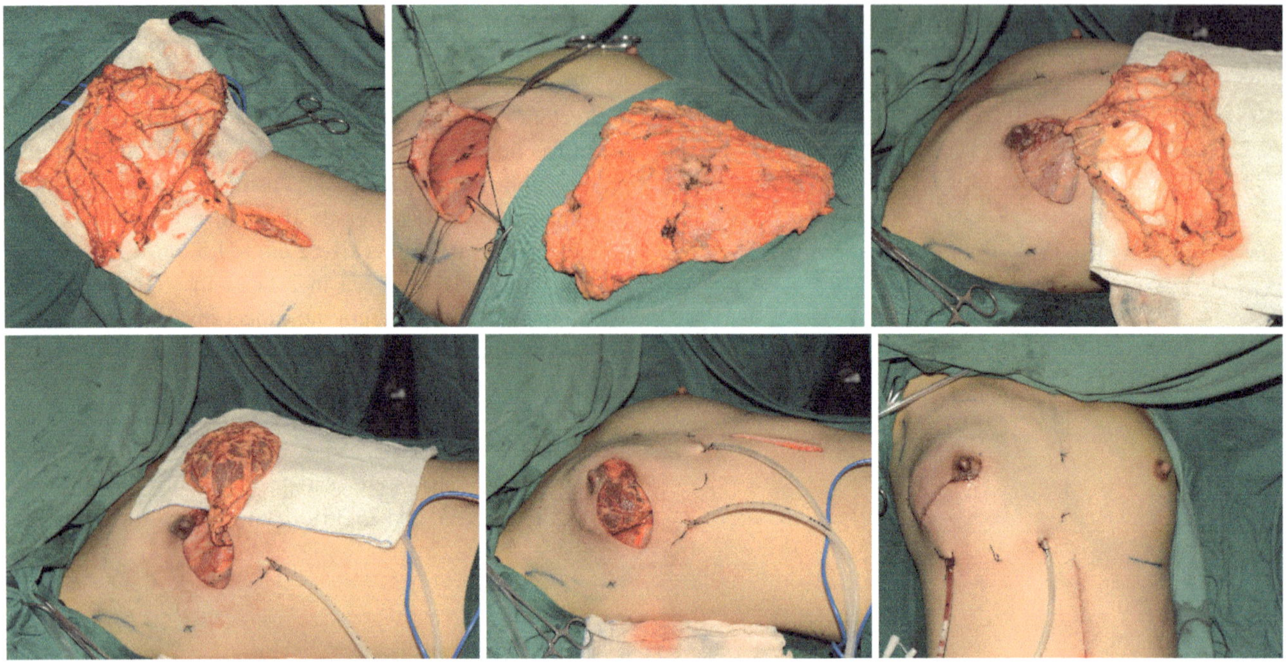

Fig. 25.35 The omentum flap was prepared, and breast cancer-modified radical mastectomy was completed

Fig. 25.36 Postoperative follow-up. (**a**) The appearance at 10 days after operation. (**b**) The appearance at 9 months followed up after operation

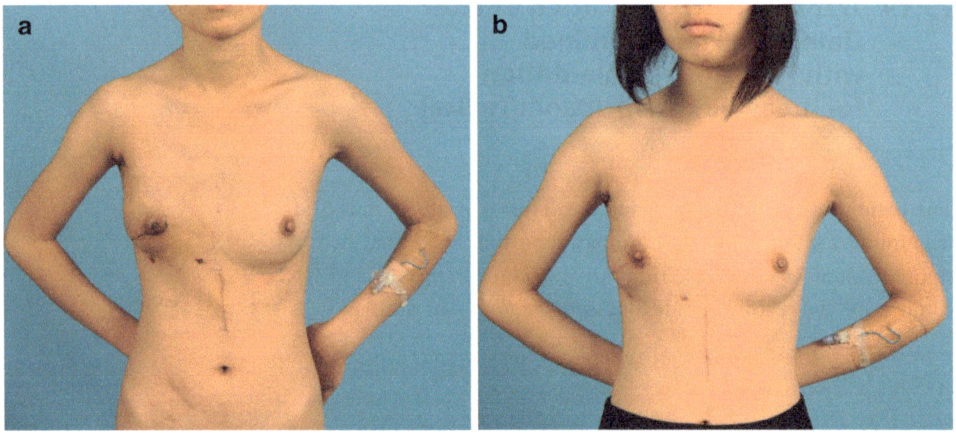

25.20 Transposition of the Pedicled Omental Flap Combined with Prosthesis Implantation for Breast Reconstruction: Typical Case 2

The patient, a 41-year-old female, found a right breast mass for more than 1 month. The right breast mass was resected under general anesthesia. Rapid intraoperative examination showed invasive carcinoma. Therefore, we switched to perform modified radical mastectomy with nipple-areola sparing and right breast cancer + prosthesis implantation combined with greater omentum breast phase I reconstruction. Postoperative pathological examination showed that the invasive ductal carcinoma of the right breast was grade II–III, and the size of the mass was about 1.3 cm × 1.2 cm × 1 cm, lymph node 0/9. Immunohistochemistry showed ER + + 30%, PR + 10%, CerbB-2 +, Ki-67 25%, and pathological grade pT1N0M0 I. The patient recovered well and was discharged from the hospital. The appearance of the reconstructed breast was satisfactory during follow-up (Figs. 25.37, 25.38, and 25.39).

The self-shaping ability of omentum is strong, and surprisingly satisfactory results will be achieved after operation.

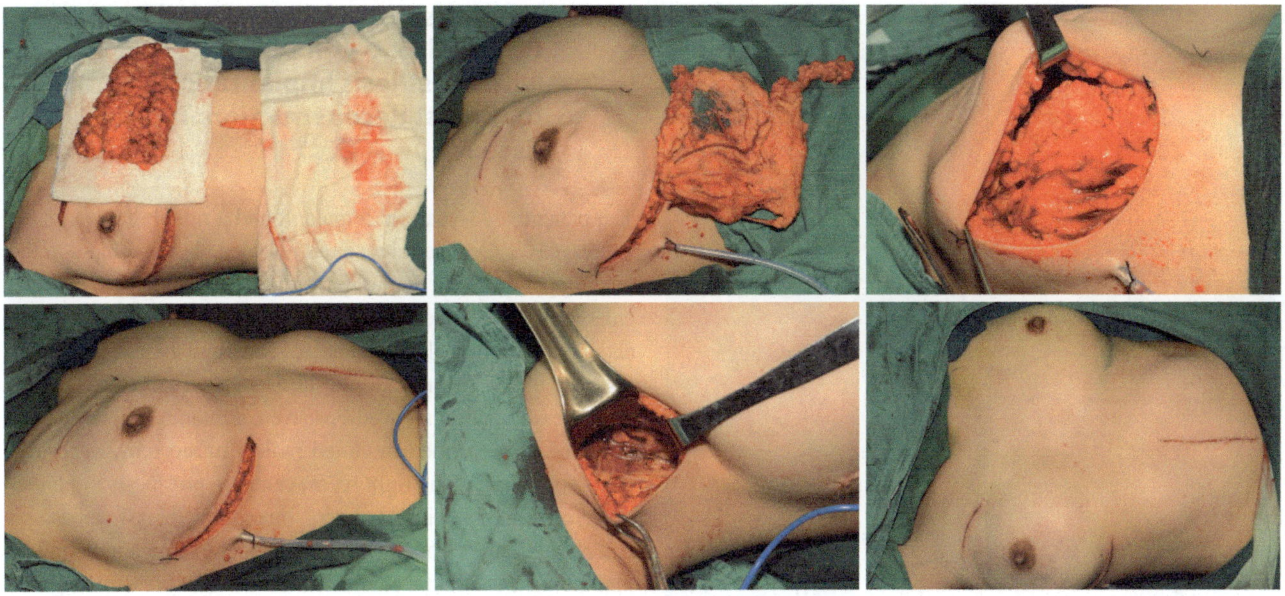

Fig. 25.37 The omentum flap was prepared, and breast cancer-modified radical mastectomy was completed

Fig. 25.38 Postoperative follow-up. (**a**) The appearance at 7 days after operation. (**b**) The appearance at 20 days after operation. (**c**) Six-month follow-up after operation. (**d**) Twenty-four-month follow-up after operation

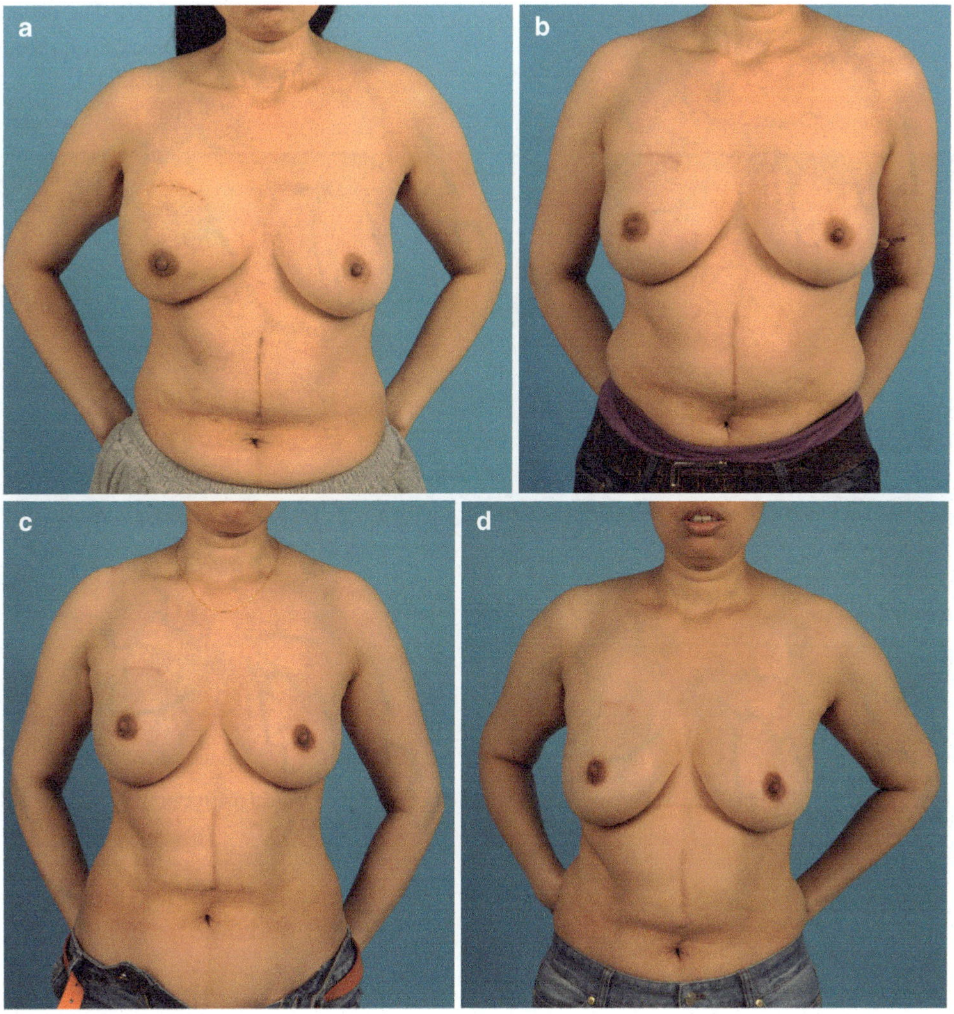

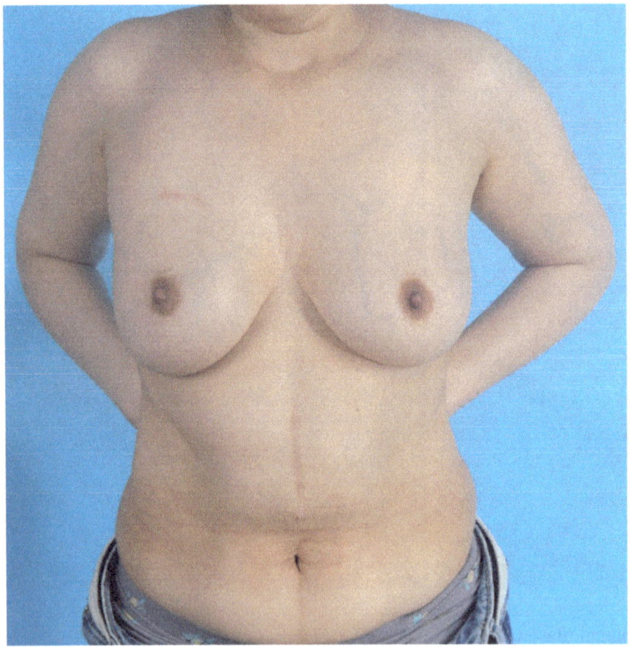

Fig. 25.39 45-month follow-up

25.21 Transposition of the Pedicled Omental Flap Combined with Prosthesis Implantation for Breast Reconstruction: Typical Case 3

The patient, a 43-year-old female, found a right breast mass for 7 days. Color Doppler ultrasound revealed (1) Solid mass in the outer upper quadrant of the right breast, bi-rads5. (2) No obvious enlarged lymph nodes were found in the bilateral axillary area and bilateral supraclavicular area. The right breast mass was resected under general anesthesia. Rapid intraoperative pathological examination showed invasive carcinoma. Therefore, we switched to performed modified radical mastectomy with nipple-areola sparing and right breast cancer + prosthesis implantation combined with greater omentum breast phase I reconstruction. Postoperative pathological examination showed that the invasive ductal carcinoma of the right breast was grade II–III, and the size of the mass was about 2.5 cm × 2.0 cm × 2.0 cm, lymph node 2/15. Immunohistochemistry showed ER + + + 70%, PR + + + 90%, CerbB-2 + +, Ki-67 10%, and pathological stage pt2n1m0 IIB. The patient recovered well postoperatively, and the appearance of reconstructed breast was satisfactory (Figs. 25.40 and 25.41).

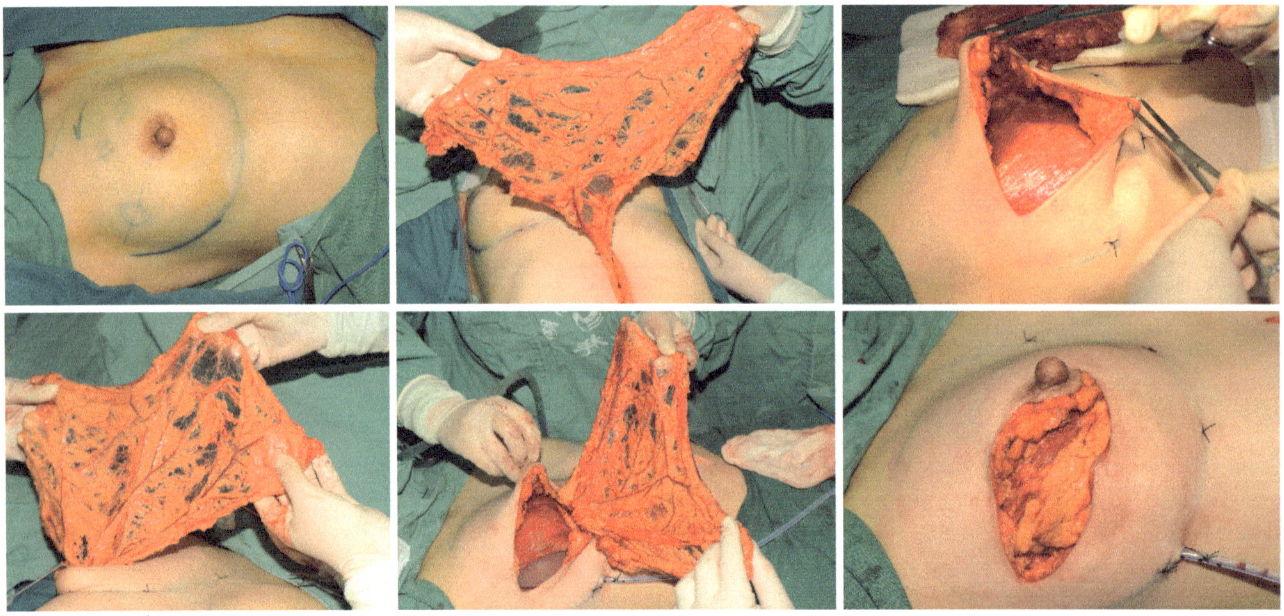

Fig. 25.40 The omentum flap was prepared, and breast cancer modified radical mastectomy was completed

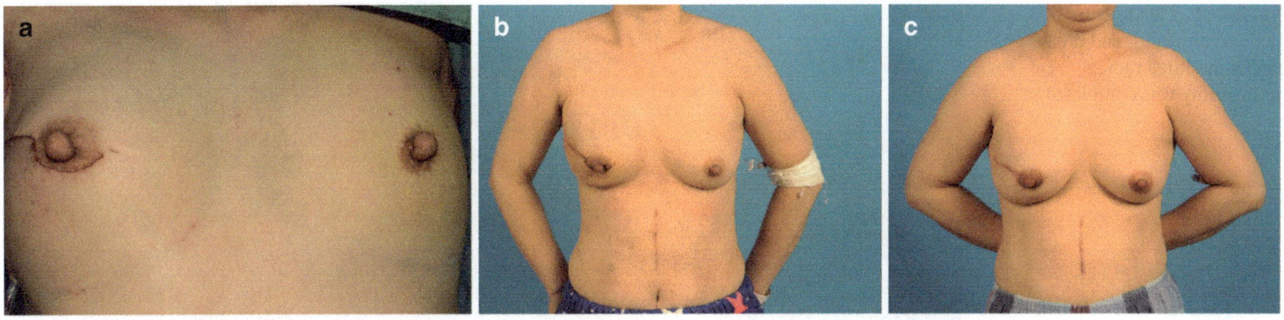

Fig. 25.41 Postoperative follow-up. (**a**) The appearance of immediate breast reconstruction during operation. (**b**) The appearance at 12 days after operation. (**c**) The patients were followed up 5 months after operation

25.22 Transposition of Pedicled Greater Omentum Flap Combined with Prosthesis Implantation for Breast Reconstruction: Typical Case 4

A 40-year-old woman found a left breast mass for 9 days without obvious inducement. The mass was about the size of a broad bean, without redness, pain, and nipple discharge. The MRI of the breast suggested that the left breast lump was considered to be BI-RADS 4C. Biopsy pathology showed left breast invasive ductal carcinoma. Under general anesthesia, the left breast subcutaneous gland total resection with nipple and areola sparing + prosthesis combined with omentum one-stage breast reconstruction were performed. Supportive treatments were given after operation, and the recovery was smooth. The breast function and appearance were satisfactory during the follow-up (Figs. 25.42, 25.43, and 25.44).

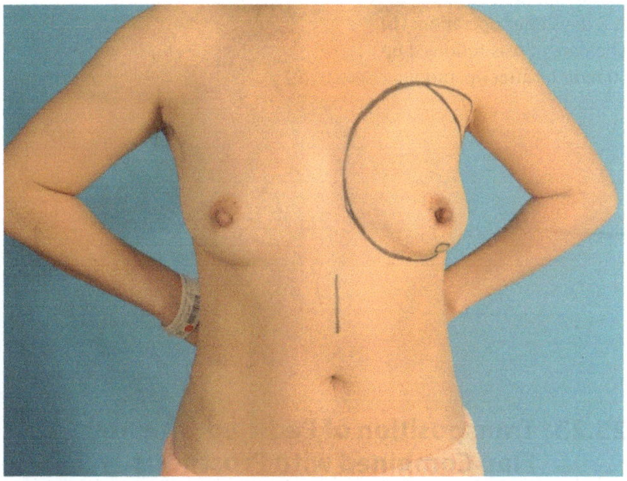

Fig. 25.42 Preoperative conditions

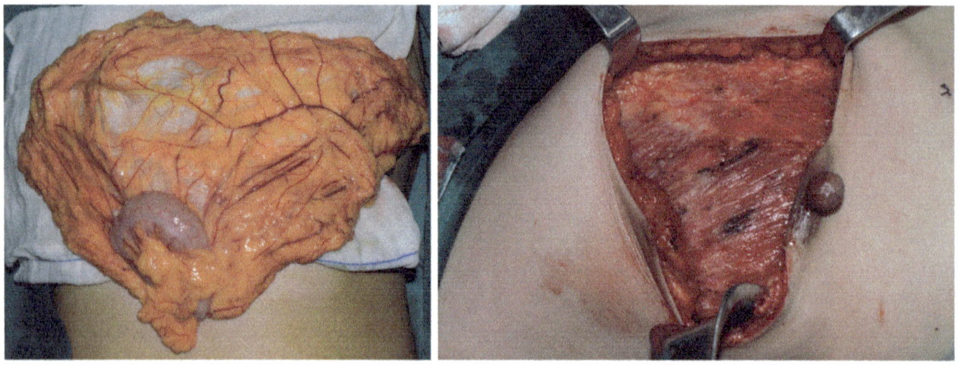

Fig. 25.43 The omentum flap was prepared, and breast cancer modified radical mastectomy was completed

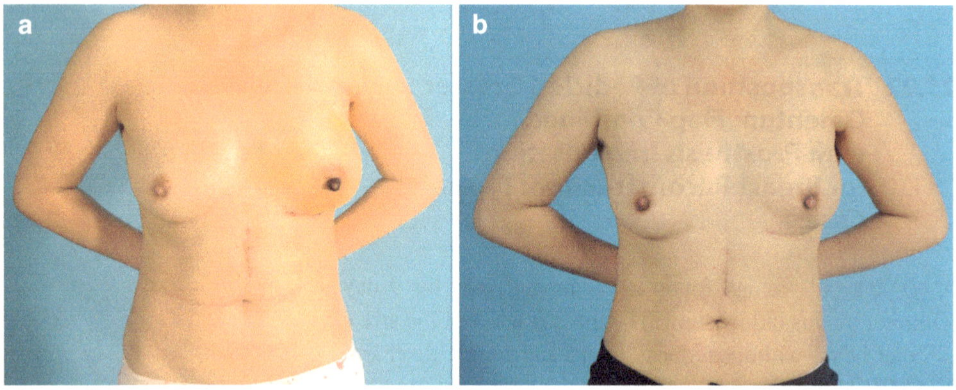

Fig. 25.44 Postoperative follow-up. (**a**) The appearance at 8 days after operation. (**b**) The patient was followed up 10 months after operation

25.23 Transposition of Pedicled Omental Flap Combined with Prosthesis Implantation for Breast Reconstruction: Typical Case 5

The patient, a 49-year-old female, found a left breast mass for 2 months. Biopsy showed that (left breast) invasive ductal carcinoma was histologically grade III. Under general anesthesia, modified radical mastectomy for left breast cancer (preserving nipple and areola) and one-stage breast reconstruction with pedicled greater omentum combined with prosthesis were performed. The postoperative pathological examination results showed that the invasive ductal carcinoma was grade II–III and the mass size was 2.5 cm × 2.0 cm × 1.5 cm; axillary lymph node 1/15 metastasis. Immunohistochemical results showed Er (−), PR (20% +), cerb2 (2 +), Ki67 (80% +), and pathological stage pt2n1m0 IIB. The recovery was smooth. The breast function and appearance were satisfactory during follow-up (Figs. 25.45, 25.46, and 25.47).

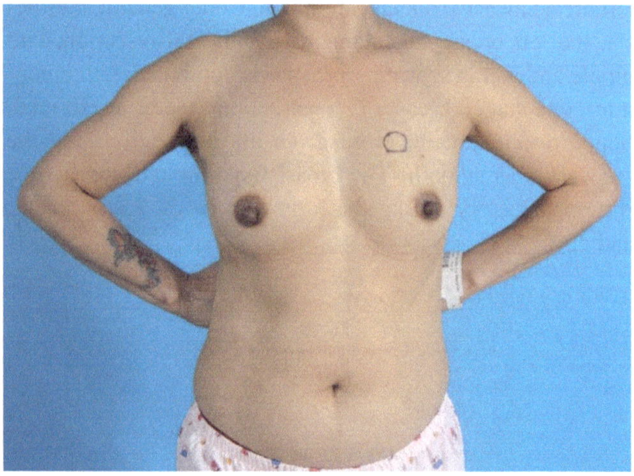

Fig. 25.45 Preoperative conditions

The greater omental flap can provide tissue with rich blood supply and is easy to shape. It can be used for the repair of various defects, especially for the repair of large-area defects, chronic wounds with poor blood supply, or radioactive ulcer wounds [18, 37, 38]. Possible complications, including abdominal wall hernia and abdominal adhesion, should be prevented [17, 20].

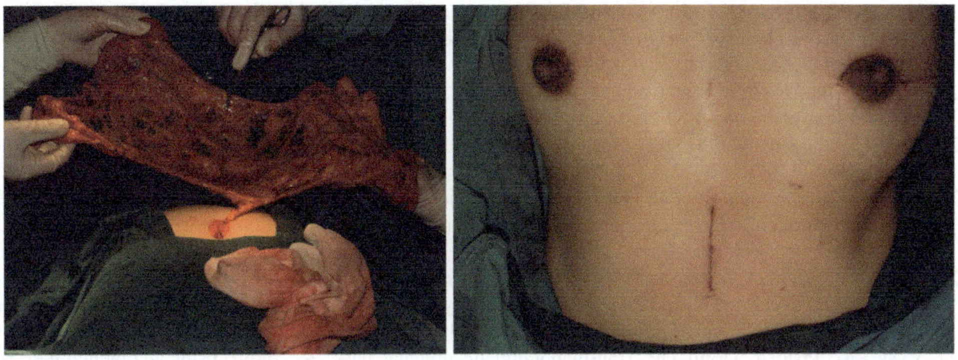

Fig. 25.46 The omentum flap was prepared, and breast cancer modified radical mastectomy was completed

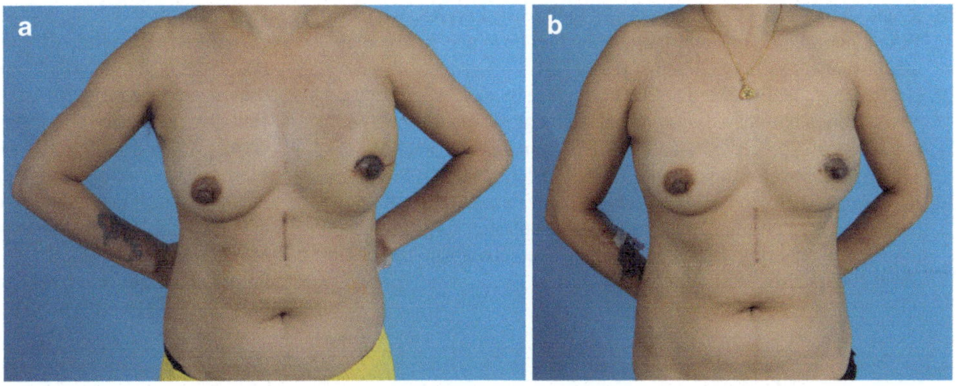

Fig. 25.47 Postoperative follow-up. (**a**) The appearance at 7 days after operation; (**b**) The patient was followed up 4 months after operation

References

1. McLean DH, Buncke HJ. Autotransplant of omentum to a large scalp defect, with microsurgical revascularization. Plast Reconstr Surg. 1972;49(3):268–74.
2. Upton J, Mulliken JB, Hicks PD, Murray JE. Restoration of facial contour using free vascularized omental transfer. Plast Reconstr Surg. 1980;66(4):560–9.
3. Jurkiewicz MJ, Nahai F. The omentum: its use as a free vascularized graft for reconstruction of the head and neck. Ann Surg. 1982;195(6):756–65.
4. Lopez R, Didolkar MS, Karakousis C, Baffi R, Bakamjian V. Problems in resection of chest wall sarcomas. Am Surg. 1979;45(7):471–7.
5. Woods JE, Arnold PG, Masson JK, Irons GB, Payne WS. Management of radiation necrosis and advanced cancer of the chest wall in patients with breast malignancy. Plast Reconstr Surg. 1979;63(2):235–41.
6. Starzynski TE, Snyderman RK, Beattie EJ. Problems of major chest wall reconstruction. Plast Reconstr Surg. 1969;44(6):525–35.
7. Leonard AG. Reconstruction of the chest wall using a de-epithelialised "turn over" deltopectoral flap. Br J Plast Surg. 1980;33(2):187–9.
8. Arnold PG. Reconstruction of the sternum and anterior chest wall: aesthetic considerations. Clin Plast Surg. 1981;8(2):384–97.
9. Salo JTK, Tukiainen EJ. Oncologic resection and reconstruction of the chest wall: a 14-year experience in a single center. Plast Reconstr Surg. 2018;142(2):536–47.
10. Dupont C, Menard Y. Transposition of the greater omentum for reconstruction of the chest wall. Plast Reconstr Surg. 1972;49(3):263–7.
11. Arnold PG, Hartrampf CR, Jurkiewicz MJ. One-stage reconstruction of the breast, using the transposed greater omentum. Case report. Plast Reconstr Surg. 1976;57(4):520–2.
12. Jurkiewicz MJ, Arnold PG. The omentum: an account of its use in the reconstruction of the chest wall. Ann Surg. 1977;185(5):548–54.
13. Arnold PG, Irons GB. The greater omentum: extensions in transposition and free transfer. Plast Reconstr Surg. 1981;67(2):164–76.
14. Newing RK, Pribaz JJ, Bennett RC, Buls J. Omental transposition and skin graft in the management of chest wall recurrence of carcinoma of the breast. Aust N Z J Surg. 1979;49(5):546–51.
15. Hakelius L. Fatal complication after use of the greater omentum for reconstruction of the chest wall: case report. Plast Reconstr Surg. 1978;62(5):796–7.
16. Jimenez AG, Germain PS, Sirois M, Hatheway M, Lethbridge R. Free omental flap for skin-sparing breast reconstruction harvested laparoscopically. Plast Reconstr Surg. 2002;110(2):545–51.
17. dos Santos Costa S, Blotta RM, Mariano MB, Meurer L, Edelweiss MI. Aesthetic improvements in Poland's syndrome treatment with omentum flap. Aesthet Plast Surg. 2010;34(5):634–9.
18. Horch RE, Horbach T, Lang W. The nutrient omentum free flap: revascularization with vein bypasses and greater omentum flap in severe arterial ulcers. J Vasc Surg. 2007;45(4):837–40.
19. Boyd JB, Taylor GI, Corlett R. The vascular territories of the superior epigastric and the deep inferior epigastric systems. Plast Reconstr Surg. 1984;73(1):1–16.
20. Bayles SW, Hayden RE. Gastro-omental free flap reconstruction of the head and neck. Arch Facial Plast Surg. 2008;10(4):255–9.
21. Alday ES, Goldsmith HS. Surgical technique for omental lengthening based on arterial anatomy. Surg Gynecol Obstet. 1972;135(1):103–7.

22. Powers JC, Fitzgerald JF, McAlvanah MJ. The anatomic basis for the surgical detachment of the greater omentum from the transverse colon. Surg Gynecol Obstet. 1976;143(1):105–6.
23. Das SK. The size of the human omentum and methods of lengthening it for transplantation. Br J Plast Surg. 1976;29(2):170–44.
24. Das SK. Assessment of the size of the human omentum. Acta Anat (Basel). 1981;110(2):108–12.
25. Li X, Ouyang Z, Yang S, et al. Omental transplantation improves surgical outcome of large squamous cell carcinoma: a case report. Oncol Lett. 2015;9(6):2805–8.
26. Gallagher J, Webb A, Ilankovan V. Gastro-omental free flaps in oral and oropharyngeal reconstruction: surgical anatomy, complications, outcomes. Br J Oral Maxillofac Surg. 2002;40(1):32–6.
27. Vyas RM, Prsic A, Orgill DP. Transdiaphragmatic omental harvest: a simple, efficient method for sternal wound coverage. Plast Reconstr Surg. 2013;131(3):544–52.
28. Reade CC, Meadows WM, Bower CE, Lalikos JF, Zeri RS, Wooden WA. Laparoscopic omental harvest for flap coverage in complex mediastinitis. Am Surg. 2003;69(12):1072–6.
29. Hoffmann J, Wallwiener D. Classifying breast cancer surgery: a novel, complexity-based system for oncological, oncoplastic and reconstructive procedures, and proof of principle by analysis of 1225 operations in 1166 patients. BMC Cancer. 2009;9:108.
30. Kronowitz SJ, Kuerer HM, Buchholz TA, Valero V, Hunt KK. A management algorithm and practical oncoplastic surgical techniques for repairing partial mastectomy defects. Plast Reconstr Surg. 2008;122(6):1631–47.
31. Munhoz AM, Montag E, Arruda E, et al. Assessment of immediate conservative breast surgery reconstruction: a classification system of defects revisited and an algorithm for selecting the appropriate technique. Plast Reconstr Surg. 2008;121(3):716–27.
32. Zaha H, Inamine S, Naito T, Nomura H. Laparoscopically harvested omental flap for immediate breast reconstruction. Am J Surg. 2006;192(4):556–8.
33. Song XY, Guan DD, Lin H, et al. [Immediate breast reconstruction using laparoscopically harvested omental flap after breast-conserving surgery]. Zhonghua Zheng Xing Wai Ke Za Zhi. 2011;27(6):401–5.
34. Zaha H, Sunagawa H, Kawakami K, Touyama T, Yonaha T, Ohshiro N. Partial breast reconstruction for an inferomedial breast carcinoma using an omental flap. World J Surg. 2010;34(8):1782–7.
35. Arnold PG, Witzke DJ, Irons GB, Woods JE. Use of omental transposition flaps for soft-tissue reconstruction. Ann Plast Surg. 1983;11(6):508–12.
36. Cartier R, Brunette I, Hashimoto K, Bourne WM, Schaff HV. Angiogenic factor: a possible mechanism for neovascularization produced by omental pedicles. J Thorac Cardiovasc Surg. 1990;99(2):264–8.
37. López-Monjardin H, de-la-Peña-Salcedo A, Mendoza-Muñoz M, López-Yáñez-de-la-Peña A, Palacio-López E, López-García A. Omentum flap versus pectoralis major flap in the treatment of mediastinitis. Plast Reconstr Surg. 1998;101(6):1481–5.
38. Maloney CT, Wages D, Upton J, Lee WP. Free omental tissue transfer for extremity coverage and revascularization. Plast Reconstr Surg. 2003;111(6):1894–904.

Application of ICG in Flap Surgery for Oncoplasty

26

Juanjuan Li, Huawei Yang, and Youmao Zheng

Breast reconstructions after mastectomy can be divided into prosthesis, tissue expander, and/or autologous free tissue transfer reconstruction. Regardless of the type of reconstruction, the major cause of early complications is insufficient perfusion of flap tissue [1–3]. Ischemia due to insufficient tissue perfusion in breast reconstruction may cause flap necrosis, higher risks of infection, poor wound healing, anastomotic thrombosis, and fat liquefaction [4, 5].

There are many methods to evaluate tissue perfusion and predict necrosis. Evaluation by clinical experience is the most used method to assess tissue perfusion [6]. However, it is not reliable to evaluate tissue perfusion only based on clinical experience [7]. Other intraoperative methods that can be used to evaluate perfusion include handheld Doppler, laser Doppler flowmeter, and fluorescence contrast agents [8, 9]. However, these methods have their own defects, which limit their application in intraoperative evaluation of perfusion [10]. It is necessary to find other more reliable technical means to evaluate perforator and tissue perfusion in breast reconstruction.

In the recent 10 years, indocyanine green (ICG) angiography and fluorescence perfusion evaluation system have been applied in breast reconstruction surgery [1, 3, 5–14]. Indocyanine green (ICG) is a fluorescent substance used in medical diagnosis and various surgical fields. Its characteristics are as follows: (1) It is negatively charged and can tightly bind to plasma proteins, making it only exist in blood vessels. (2) The spectral absorption peak of ICG is 800 nm, which is in infrared spectrum. It can be detected and imaged by scanning diode infrared laser. (3) The pharmacokinetics of ICG showed that its half-life was 150–180 s, it could be quickly removed from the tissue, and it was only metabolized by the liver and excreted with bile without entering hepatointestinal circulation. Therefore, it can repeatedly evaluate perfusion in the one particular operation. The above features show that it is particularly suitable for intraoperative angiography. Recent studies have shown that in breast reconstruction surgery, ICG angiography and fluorography system significantly increase the accuracy in predicting the necrosis of breast flap than clinical judgment [15]. This chapter reviews the application and evidence of ICG angiography in evaluating tissue perfusion in breast reconstruction.

26.1 History of Clinical Application of ICG Angiography

26.1.1 Initial: 1950s, 1960s, and 1970s

ICG technology was originally used as a tricarbocyanine dye in color printing and optical filters. In the 1950s, coincidentally, a Kodak employee recommended ICG to his cardiologist Irwin Fox for research. This is the first time to introduce ICG into medicine and diagnostic physiology. It is found that ICG has an absorption peak at near-infrared light, which endows it with strong penetration and the ability to detect different tissues. The emission wavelength of this dye is the same in oxygenated and deoxygenated blood, which avoids the interference of plasma protein on ICG spectral analysis, and ICG concentration can be directly measured in blood despite the oxygen saturation [16]. The pharmaceutical companies of Hynson Wescott and Dunning have further modified ICG into a stable lyophilized state, which has been used since then [17]. The Food and Drug Apartment approved the use of ICG in cardiac and hepatic angiography in 1956. In the following year, ICG was used to measure cardiac output as its first medical application. Because ICG is only metabolized through the liver and excreted by bile, there is no hepatointestinal circulation involved. This makes ICG a reliable

J. Li (✉)
Department of Breast and Thyroid Surgery, Renmin Hospital of Wuhan University, Wuhan, Hubei Province, China

H. Yang
Department of Breast Surgery, Affiliated Cancer Hospital of Guangxi Medical University, Nanning, China

Y. Zheng
Hand and Foot Surgery, Taizhou Hospital, Taizhou, Zhejiang, China

Z. Li, D. Song (eds.), *Oncoplastic Flap Surgery*, https://doi.org/10.1007/978-981-19-8926-1_26

tracer to detect liver blood flow and its function [17–20]. Kogure and choromokos used ICG for animal angiography for the first time [21, 22]. David et al. first applied ICG in human angiography to analyze carotid blood flow [23].

26.1.2 Development: Application in Ophthalmology in the 1970s and 1980s

The application of ICG image has greatly promoted the development in ophthalmology. In 1972, Flower and Hochheimer first used ICG angiography for human choroidal imaging [24]. In the mid-1980s, Hayashi et al. improved the infrared filter to improve the resolution of ICG, which marked a significant transformation of the application of ICG from film and television to angiography [25–27]. In 1989, ICG angiography was applied to scanning laser ophthalmoscopy [28]. Instant high-resolution images were first applied by Yannuzzi et al. in 1992, which laid a solid foundation for the development of ICG perfusion imaging [29].

26.1.3 Wide Application: After the 1990s

Since its refinement in the 1990s, ICG has been widely used in various fields, including cardiovascular (evaluation of aortic and coronary artery bypass), colorectal (evaluation of gastrointestinal anastomosis), transplantation surgery (prediction of the prognosis of living donor liver transplantation), urinary system (perfusion of allograft kidney, ureterography, urinary calculi and obstruction), tumor surgery (sentinel lymph node biopsy, tumor markers), gynecology (identification of endometriosis), and general surgery (cholangiography) [30–35]. In addition, surgeons from other fields, including plastic and reconstructive surgery, begin to realize the practicability of this image technology. Newman and Samson first used ICG angiography in breast reconstruction microsurgery in the United States in 2006 [11]. Since then, many reports on the application of ICG in evaluating tissue perfusion and reconstruction of free flap perfusion have been published [1, 11, 13–15].

At present, the commonly used imaging systems in plastic reconstruction surgery include ICG image capture and analysis system [36]. The system was first used to evaluate the patency of coronary artery bypass grafting (CABG) and began to be used in plastic, reconstruction, and microsurgery in 2007 [37].

26.1.4 Clinical Application of ICG in China

It is reported that in the 1990s, China began to use ICG clinically, mainly for hepatobiliary surgery and ophthalmology [38, 39]. In the early twenty-first century, ICG was used for intracranial vascular imaging in brain surgery and gradually applied in other departments. In the recent 5 years, ICG has been used for sentinel lymph node tracing in cancer, especially in sentinel lymph nodes of breast cancer as mentioned in many literatures [40, 41]. In the recent 3 years, relevant literatures have successively reported the applications of ICG in vascular perfusion evaluation of flap surgery, including the uses in free and pedicled flaps in breast reconstruction [41]. Due to the late start of breast reconstruction in China, the current reconstruction rate is less than 4.5%, so the reports on the use of ICG in breast reconstruction are less in China than in foreign countries. However, with the improvement of people's living standards, the proportion of breast reconstruction also increases. According to the advantages of ICG reported abroad, it is promising that ICG will be more popularized in breast reconstruction in China with broad prospects in its applications [42].

26.2 Characteristics of ICG

Indocyanine green is a negatively charged amphiphilic tricarbocyanine dye [43], which is characterized as follows (as shown in Fig. 26.1):

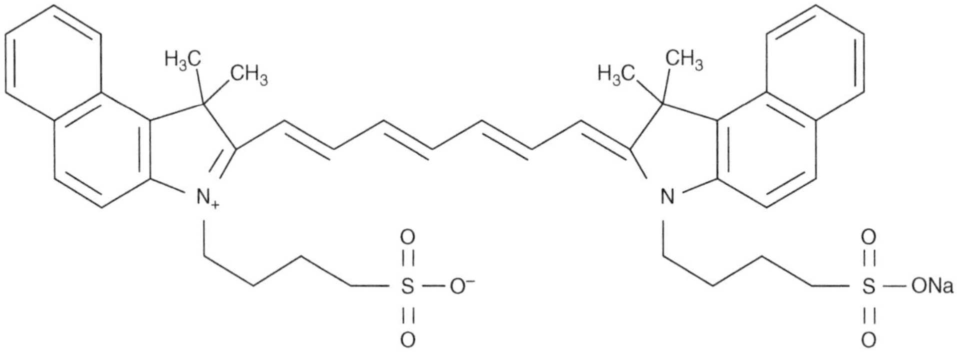

Fig. 26.1 Molecular formula of ICG

1. After injection into the blood vessel, ICG is rapidly and completely associated with α-lipoprotein-based plasma protein binding and rarely penetrates into the vascular space, making it only exist in the blood vessels. Therefore, it is an ideal dye for evaluating tissue perfusion.
2. ICG is only ingested by liver cells and secreted into bile for excretion. There is no hepatointestinal circulation involved and is not excreted through the kidney. Therefore, it can also be safely used in patients with renal insufficiency.
3. The half-life of ICG in human body is short, about 3–5 min. Therefore, it can repeatedly evaluate perfusion in the same operation.
4. The safety of ICG is promising, and adverse reactions such as allergy are rare, with an incidence of only 1/42,000. However, because ICG contains iodine, patient's allergic to iodine should avoid using ICG. In fact, most of the complications after clinical application of ICG are rather mild, and only some patients may encounter fever or throat pain.
5. The spectral absorption peak of ICG is 800 nm, which is infrared spectrum. It can be detected and imaged by scanning diode infrared laser.

26.3 Application of ICG Imaging in Breast Reconstruction

26.3.1 Prediction Models and Comparison of Tissue Perfusion During Reconstruction

Breast reconstruction after mastectomy in breast cancer patients can reduce the psychological trauma caused by losing the breast and significantly improve the quality of life of patients. Breast reconstructions after mastectomy can be divided into immediate reconstruction and delayed reconstruction by time order. Based on the surgical techniques, breast reconstructions can be divided into prosthesis, tissue expander, and/or autologous-free tissue (latissimus dorsi flap, rectus abdominis flap, perforator flap of inferior abdominal artery, etc.) [1–3, 44]. Regardless of the types of reconstruction, the primary cause of early complications is insufficient tissue perfusion of the flap, resulting in partial or total necrosis of the flap, increased risks of infection, poor wound healing, anastomotic thrombosis, and fat liquefaction [45–48]. In brief, the accurate prediction of flap perfusion greatly affect clinical decision-making and reduce postoperative complications, which will considerably improve the life quality of patients and reduce overall costs.

The most used prediction method is the clinical observation by surgeons. The position of perforating branch can be assessed according to anatomical knowledge. For the flap perfusion area, the objective indexes including tissue color, vascular filling, temperature, and bleeding in skin margin are used to evaluate the tissue perfusion and changes. However, the position of perforator may be affected by anatomical variation. The measurement of perfusion area is still dependent on the surgeon influenced by subjective views. For this reason, the auxiliary method of evaluating tissue perfusion has been studied and applied in clinic. CTA can accurately locate the position of perforating branches and decide whether there is anatomical variation. However, it cannot be used intraoperatively to evaluate the perfusion area, but is only considered as a preoperative examination.

The commonly used intraoperative auxiliary examinations are Doppler, tissue oxygen measurement, sodium fluorescein angiography, and ICG angiography. Handheld ultrasound Doppler is a safe, simple, and widely used method to evaluate the location of vascular perforations during operation, but it is dependent on the operator, and its application in judging the perfusion body area and accurately designing the size of flap is limited [9, 49, 50]. The laser Doppler flowmeter can estimate the survival of the flap, but the perforator cannot be detected during the operation [49, 50], and it is easy to be affected by small movements. Postoperative use of percutaneous oxygen measurement can successfully monitor flap survival, but its intraoperative use is time-consuming and overworked [51, 52]. Fluorescein sodium has been widely used to evaluate tissue perfusion. However, this technique is limited by its pharmacokinetics. Its half-life is 12–18 h, so it cannot be used repeatedly in the one operation. Fluorescein sodium also has a certain false positive rate [53]. A recent prospective study reported that the accuracy of fluorescein sodium in predicting flap necrosis after mastectomy was lower than that of ICG [15]. The limitations of these techniques show the need for a safe, accurate, and intraoperative method to evaluate perfusion volume. The emergence of ICG makes a new breakthrough in intraoperative monitoring of tissue perfusion. At present, the following literature has reported the comparison of various methods (see Table 26.1):

In conclusion, the prediction of flap necrosis merely by clinical judgment is inaccurate, which is not enough to prevent flap necrosis. Sodium fluorescein may be over predicted [15]. Underprediction leads to an increased risks of necrosis, and overprediction results in the removal of potentially viable tissues. Other methods have certain limitations. In contrast (see Table 26.2), ICG can effectively overcome most limitations, with good sensitivity and specificity, and therefore plays an important role in evaluating flap perfusion in breast reconstruction.

Table 26.1 Related references on comparison of prediction methods of tissue perfusion

Researchers (Year)	Content	Findings
Philip (2012) [15]	In 51 cases of breast reconstruction with expander implantation (32 patients), clinical judgment, ICG angiography, and fluorescein were used to judge the intraoperative flap perfusion. Compare the differences between the three methods	1. Twenty-one cases of necrosis in total, including 9 cases of flap removal due to ischemia 2. ICG predicted necrosis: sensitivity 90%, specificity 50%, positive predictive value 55.9%, negative predictive value 88.2% 3. Fluorescein predicted necrosis: sensitivity 90%, specificity 30%, positive predictive value 47.5%, negative predictive value 81.8% 4. Clinical judgments: sensitivity 42.8%, specificity 100%
Ludolph (2016) [54]	A total of 35 cases of TRAM or DIEP. Comparing the effects of ICG angiography and laser Doppler spectroflowmeter in predicting flap necrosis	Clinical judgment and Doppler jointly predicted three cases of necrosis, but ICG angiography showed good perfusion so the flaps were not removed. All flaps survived without partial necrosis Specificity: ICG 100%, Doppler 91.3%

26.3.2 Application of ICG in Breast Reconstruction

In general, a series of cases and prospective studies reported that ICG angiography can reduce the probability of postoperative flap necrosis compared with clinical judgment in the reconstruction by free pedicled skin flap and implant. Conservatively, necrosis often occurs in areas where ICG angiography is rather negative but not corrected intraoperatively [55].

26.3.2.1 ICG Is Used for Breast Reconstruction with Expander and Prosthesis Implantation

In breast reconstruction with tissue expander and prosthesis implantation, it is particularly important to evaluate the flap of mastectomy. With the increasing proportion of skin and nipple-preserving mastectomy, the incidence of nipple and skin necrosis is also rising year by year, and the incidence is even as high as 40% in some studies [23, 29–32]. Generally, this is due to the disconnection of axial blood flow in the flap caused by excessive separation or traction of the flap, and ICG can distinguish this potential risks of necrosis. If there is no fluorescence in the breast skin and nipple, it indicates relative ischemia, so the corresponding incidence of necrosis will be higher. Software analysis can also further clarify such high-risk areas. When such ischemic area is found in clinical examination, the ischemic area needs to be removed and skin

Table 26.2 Prediction methods and comparison of tissue perfusion

	Sensitivity of predicting necrosis	Specificity of predicting necrosis	Positioning perforator	Cost	Used intraoperatively	Repeated use in operation	Notes
ICG	88–100% [49]	50–86% [15, 49]	√ Superficial positioning, within 1 cm subcutaneously [55]	Expensive	√	√	Renal insufficiency can be used with less adverse reactions
Fluorescein sodium	90%	30% [15]	√	Relatively expensive	√	×	
Clinical judgment	42.8% [15]	91.3–100% [15, 54]	×	–	√	√	Excessively high operator dependence
Handheld Doppler	×	×	√ Superficial location	Cheap	√	√	High operator dependence
Laser Doppler flowmeter	No data yet	91.3% [54]	√	Cheap	√	×	High operator dependence
Percutaneous oxygen measurement	No data yet	No data yet	×	Cheap	×	×	
CTA	×	×	√ Deep location	Medium	×	×	Preoperative examination

Table 26.3 Literatures on ICG for breast reconstruction with tissue expander and prosthesis implantation

Researchers (Year)	Research contents	Findings
Komorowska (2010) [1]	There were 24 cases in the ICG group (16 tissue expanders, 2 latissimus dorsi muscles, and 6 DIEP/SIEA), compared with 206 cases before the introduction of ICG technology	The incidence of complications was 15% in the unused group and 4% in the ICG-used group ($P < 0.01$)
Sood and Glat (2013) [56]	Breast reconstruction with one-stage prosthesis implantation in 91 cases There were 39 cases in ICG group and 52 cases in group without ICG application	1. The necrosis rate of skin flap after mastectomy was 36.5% in the unused group and 17.9% in the ICG-used group. $P = 0.0631$ 2. The number of re emergencies after operation: 1.21 ± 1.47 in the unused group and 0.41 ± 0.71 in the use group; $P = 0.0023$
Duggal (2014) [57]	There were 184 cases in ICG group and 184 cases in unused group A total of 368 cases (including 129 cases of expander implantation, 91 cases of latissimus dorsi + expander implantation, 19 cases of latissimus dorsi, 84 cases of TRAM, and 46 cases of free TRAM or DIEP, there was no significant difference between the two groups, $P = 0.202$)	1. The necrosis rate of skin flap after mastectomy was 23.4% in the unused group and 13.0% in the ICG-used group. $P = 0.010$ 2. The re-emergency rate after operation was 14.1% in the unused group and 5.9% in the ICG-use group, $P = 0.009$ 3. TRAM or DIEP: 71 cases in the unused group and 59 cases in the ICG-used group. The probability of partial flap necrosis: 22% in the unused group and 14% in the ICG-used group, $P = 0.237$
Gustave (2016) [58]	A total of 114 cases of breast reconstruction with one-stage prosthesis implantation ICG was used in 61 cases and not in 53 cases	1. The severe necrosis rate of skin flap after mastectomy was 18.9% in the unused group and 4.9% in the ICG-used group. $P = 0.02$ 2. There was no significant difference in the overall incidence of complications and the probability of returning to the operating room
Chattha (2017) [60]	Among 110,320 cases of breast reconstruction from multicenter database in the United States, 107,005 cases (97.0%) in the non ICG group and 3315 cases (3.0%) in the use group	1. The application rate of ICG has an increasing trend. (750 cases in 2012, accounting for 1.9%, 1257 cases in 2013, accounting for 3.7%, $P < 0.01$) 2. Smokers, hypertension, and obesity were more likely to undergo ICG 3. The rate of ICG angiography: autologous tissue reconstruction (4.5%) was higher than expander reconstruction (2.1%). $p < 0.001$

flap transplantation if necessary. Komorowska-Timek et al. [1], Sood and Glat et al. [56], Duggal et al. [57], Gustave [58], and Chatha [59] et al. showed that the application of ICG angiography can reduce the occurrence of flap necrosis and postoperative emergency after breast reconstruction with expander and prosthesis implantation (see Table 26.3).

26.3.2.2 ICG for Breast Reconstruction with Autologous Tissue Transfer

ICG used in autologous tissue transfer for reconstruction started relatively late compared with prosthesis or expander implantation. At the moment, ICG played a relatively minor role in evaluating the perfusion of mastectomy flap, because autologous tissue can make up for the resected breast flap. However, if the deepithelialization of autologous tissue is excessive, it is still necessary to evaluate the blood perfusion of mastectomy flap. The main functions of ICG angiography in autologous tissue reconstruction are as follows:

Locate the Vascular Perforator

Researchers often compare the results of indocyanine green angiography with those of CT angiography (CTA) and magnetic resonance angiography (MRA). The detective depth of ICG angiography is only a few millimeters, which is served as a surface detecting technique. Therefore, for thin perforator flap, the effect of ICG imaging is equivalent to that of CTA imaging. Because ICG angiography has the advantages of real-time imaging, it can provide more intuitive markings for the position of perforating branches on the flap tissue. However, for the flap with thickness >1 cm, the accuracy of ICG angiography perforator positioning is not satisfactory [55].

If CTA and MRA are used to search the "roots and stems of trees," ICG imaging is like looking for the "leaves of trees." Usually, we can design the flap based on the assessment of the location of the perforators by the imaging position, but with the increase in its depth of the layer, the position of the perforators in the subcutaneous fascia becomes increasingly uncertain. Although it is believed that the location with the earliest fluorescence is the tissue with best perfusion, it has not been confirmed by medical research. Similarly, there is no research to prove that the largest perforator located by CTA and MRA is considered to be the best perforator for perfusion and distribution. However, in CTA and MRA, the position of the perforator must be given by the radiologist with reference to the positioning point. The advantage of ICG angiography is that the surgeon can mark the perforator area independently during the operation.

The Perforator Perfusion Area Was Recorded in Real Time

This is the biggest advantage of ICG angiography, which enables surgeons to observe perfusion and ischemia in real time without empiricism by human eyes.

Vascular body area refers to the range and size of tissue flap supplied by a single blood vessel. When the blood supply vessel is a perforator vessel, the tissue mass is called the perforator area [61].

Also, independent blood vessels may supply adjacent or "secondary" blood vessels at the same time. The tissue separated by the two vascular bodies is called the tertiary vascular body, and its blood supply is often unreliable [10]. Through ICG angiography, these vascular bodies and perforator areas can be observed in real time. After ICG was injected into the tissue, the first imaging of fluorescence was the first-stage blood vessel. After the darkening of the first vascular body, the second vascular body starts to become visible, but the brightness is slightly dark. The third-stage vascular body is only weakly lighted or not imaged. At this moment, the slight changes in brightness that are difficult to observe by the human eyes but are quite obvious under the detection of the infrared camera. The fluorescence brightness is affected by vasospasm in the dissected perforator vessels, but the position and range of the vascular body remain unchanged unless the surgical intervention is delayed for more than 1 week. By locating all the main perforating branches and testing the perfusion of the tissue by selectively clamping the blood vessels, the dominant perforating branches can be selected. If the tissue perfusion is insufficient, the number of reserved perforators can be employed to ensure blood supply. The real-time recorded image data can also be saved as medical documents, which is not only the scientific research data but also can served as insurance and court evidence. Also, the images with fluorescent contrast can be used to help the patients and their families understand the operation procedures.

Komorowska et al. [1], Duggal et al. [57], Munabi et al. [62], and ludolph [54] used ICG in autologous breast reconstruction to evaluate the perfusion of perforator area (mainly latissimus dorsi, TRAM and DIEP flaps) with ideal results (see Tables 26.1 and 26.3). Quilchini et al. [62] also used ICG angiography to improve the reliability of breast reconstruction with superficial deep inferior epigastric artery perforator (SIEA) flap. The pedicle of SIEA flap and its vascular body area have considerable variability, which makes its application less popular than other flaps. However, SIEA flap without abdominal fascia is a desired donor area for autologous breast reconstruction. In conclusion, in various forms of autologous breast reconstruction, ICG can record the perforator perfusion area in real time to improve the reliability of the flap. Even the rate of ICG angiography in autologous tissue reconstruction (4.5%) was higher than that in expander reconstruction (2.1%) ($P < 0.001$) [59].

To Evaluate the Effect of Microsurgical Anastomosis

ICG angiography was first used to evaluate arteriovenous blood flow in plastic surgery. ICG angiography can directly observe the flow of blood in the flap. In some cases, due to the slow blood flow after vasospasm, the venous outflow is not obvious, and the Doppler probe cannot detect the blood flow signal despite the good condition of the flap. These temporary changes can be improved with the attenuation of spasm or the reorganization and recanalization of blood vessels. ICG angiography can evaluate the inflow and outflow of blood immediately after vascular anastomosis and avoid the opening of the anastomosis for evaluation. Therefore, it saves time and avoids unnecessary procedures and tissue damage. The sensitivity and specificity of ICG in detecting anastomotic thrombus were 100% and 86%. The published literature has well proved the important role of ICG in evaluating the microscopic anastomosis (see Table 26.4).

Postoperative Observation

Although ICG angiography is conducive to the observation of postoperative flap, it is limited by the use of ICG contrast and fluorescence imaging machine in the ward [65]. For some cases, the results of implantable Doppler probe are not reliable because the subcutaneous perforators are too small. For other cases, it is difficult to use the surface probe to detect blood oxygenation. In these cases, ICG angiography has obvious advantages. At present, some clinical centers have begun to use ICG angiography as routine observation after operation [49]. With the popularization of ICG angiography and infrared photography in clinical application, it will undoubtedly be increasingly popularized in postoperative observation. It can also be used to predict the postoperative flap ischemia and reduce the risks of secondary exploration. This technique has a direct impact on the monitoring of postoperative flap. With the wider application, ICG postoperative

Table 26.4 Literature related to ICG evaluation of microsurgical anastomosis effect

Researchers (Year)	Research content	Findings
Holm (2010) [63]	The secondary exploration cases after free flap operation (20 cases in total) were selected Evaluation of anastomotic vascular thrombosis by ICG angiography	Anastomotic thrombus occurred in 11 of 20 cases (55%) The sensitivity and specificity of ICG in detecting anastomotic thrombus were 100% and 86%
Yan Liu (2016) [64]	In 17 cases of breast reconstruction with autologous tissue, 22 anastomotic arteries and 30 veins were anastomosed. The anastomotic conditions of blood vessels were monitored by ICG detection for 38 times	ICG showed that the blood circulation at the anastomosis of one artery and one vein was impaired. After re-anastomosis, the fluorescence and perfusion were good. All flaps survived without partial necrosis

monitoring can be used in ICU ward. When the patient is suspected of flap ischemia or venous congestion after operation, the application of this technique is of great guiding significance to judge whether it is necessary to conduct a second operation.

26.4 ICG Was Applied to Lower Abdominal Flap with Vertical Incision of Cesarean Section: A Typical Case

The patient was a 44-year-old female with right breast cancer. After admission, right NSM + sentinel lymph node biopsy + free DIEP flap transplantation + breast reconstruction were performed. The arteriovenous vessels under the left abdominal wall of the flap were anastomosed end-to-end with the internal thoracic arteriovenous vessels (1A1V). During ICG, it was confirmed that the unilateral vascular pedicle could not provide sufficient blood supply for the bilateral flaps. The tissues in area IV and part of area III were removed, and the flaps survived well. The results of pathological examination showed that the invasive ductal carcinoma of the right breast was graded with a maximum diameter of 2 cm, the right side of the subpapillary areola, and no cancer was found at the basal margin. There were four sentinel lymph nodes without cancer metastasis, ER < 1%, PR < 1%, HER-2 (−), Ki67 50% +, and pathological stage pT2N0M0 IIA. Adjuvant chemotherapy was followed. The flap survived well without obvious complications. The quality and appearance of the reconstructed breast were satisfactory, and the patient recovered well (Figs. 26.2, 26.3, 26.4, 26.5, 26.6, 26.7, 26.8, 26.9, 26.10, 26.11, 26.12, 26.13, 26.14, 26.15, 26.16, and 26.17).

The upper abdominal scar will affect the dissection of free abdominal flap and the closure of donor site.

The vertical surgical scar of the lower abdominal midline will damage the blood supply of the lower abdominal flap and restrict the size of the flap. If more than one side of the abdomen is required, the flap needs to be pedicled with bilateral subabdominal vessels for safety.

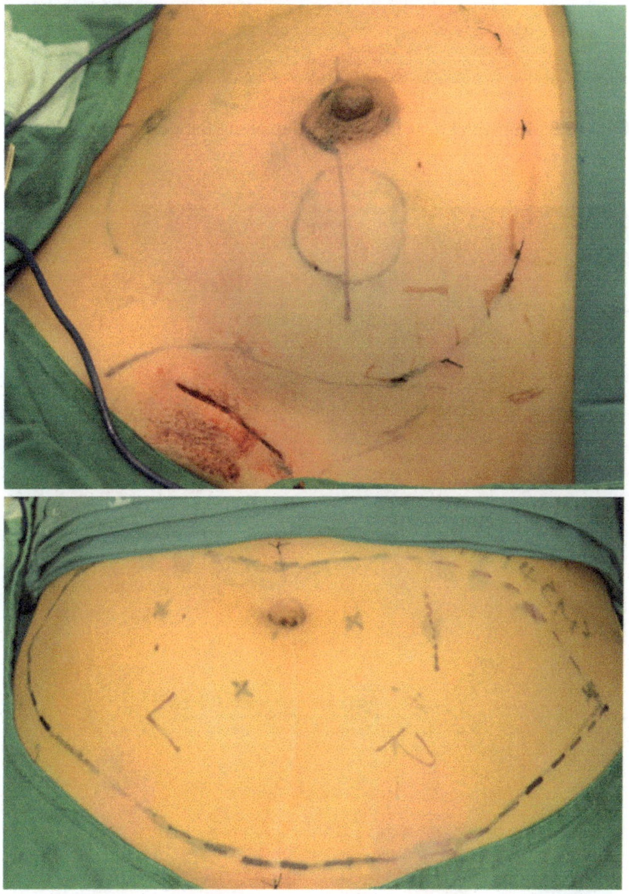

Fig. 26.2 Preoperative design. CTA identified vascular perforators

The lateral branches of perforator vessels can provide sufficient blood supply for the half lower abdominal flap, while the medial row of perforators are more capable of supplying blood to the contralateral area III tissue. Therefore, it should be determined which area of excess tissue should be removed according to the actual supply by perforator vessel.

In addition, whether it is the medial or lateral row perforator, the thickest one with the most potent pulsation should be preferred as the blood supply perforator.

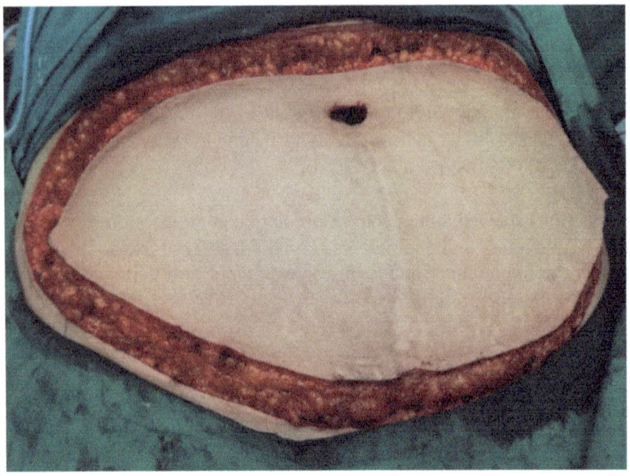

Fig. 26.3 Full-thickness incision of flap along the designed markings

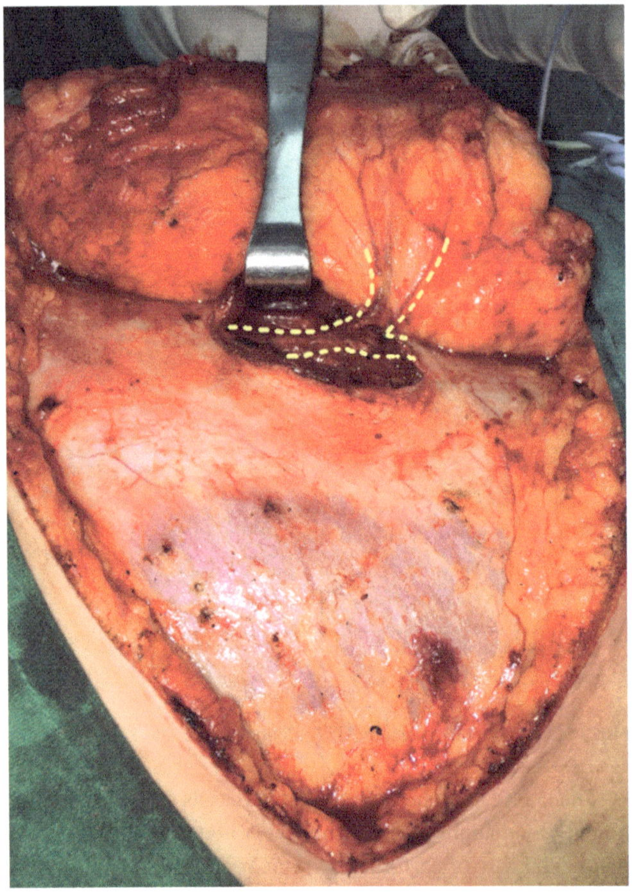

Fig. 26.4 The left lower abdominal perforator vessel was presented, and the long segment of rectus abdominis was separated as the vascular pedicle trunk

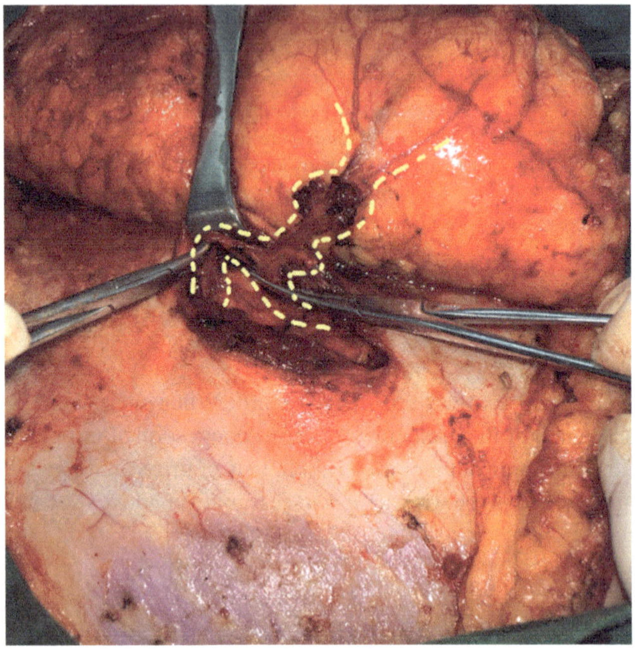

Fig. 26.5 The branch perforated the tendinous intersection. Carrying an appropriate part of the surrounding tissue of tendinous intersection to avoid excessive exposure of perforating vessels

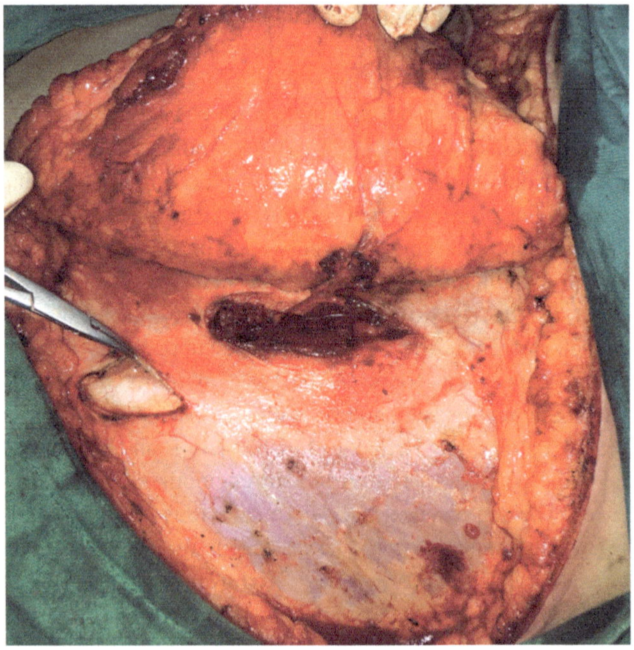

Fig. 26.6 Longitudinal auxiliary incision of the anterior sheath at the lateral edge of the rectus abdominis muscle

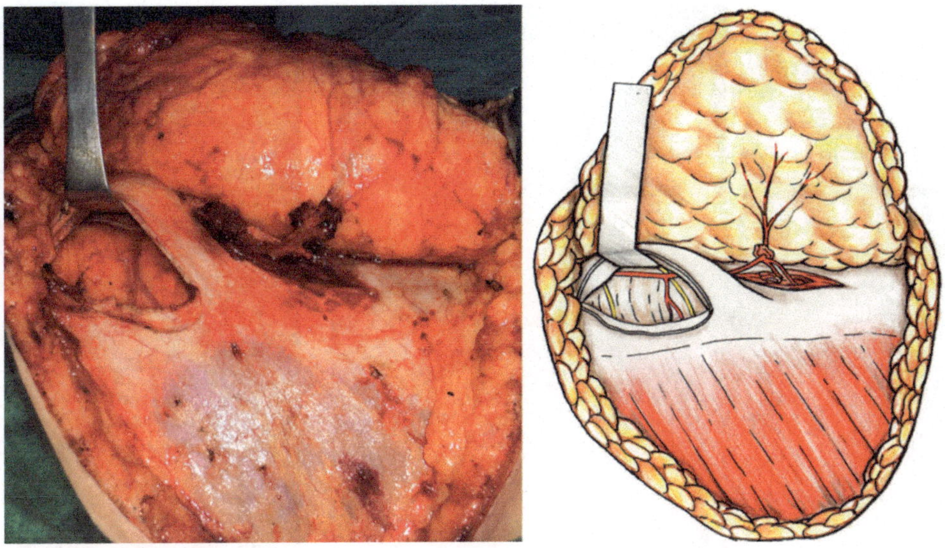

Fig. 26.7 Lift the rectus abdominis muscle from the external to expose the vascular pedicle during the whole process

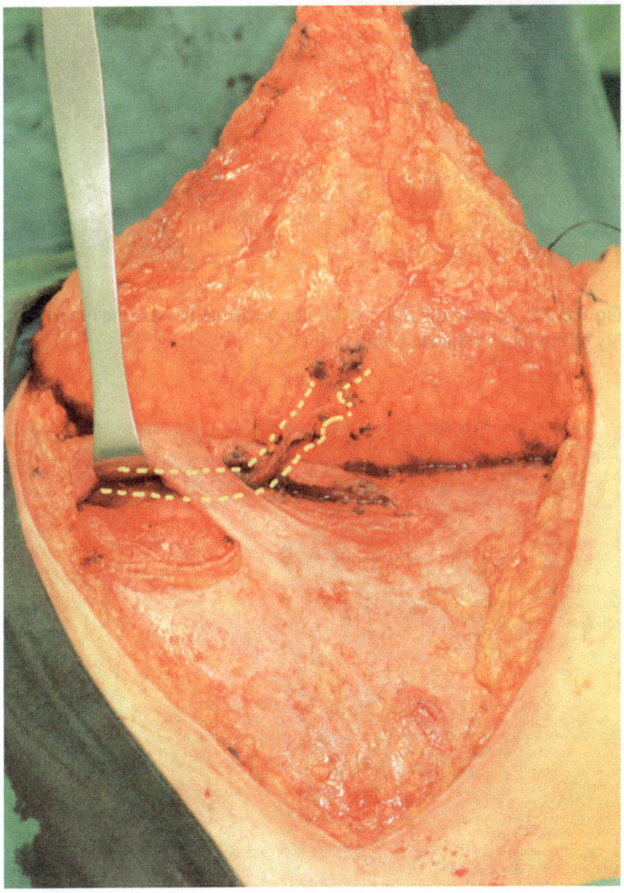

Fig. 26.8 Carefully separate and protect the intercostal nerve

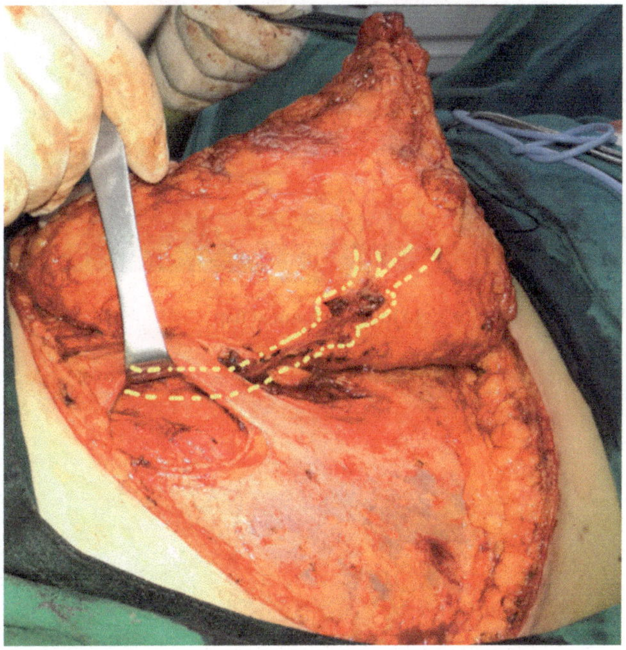

Fig. 26.9 Completely dissect vascular pedicle through tunnel

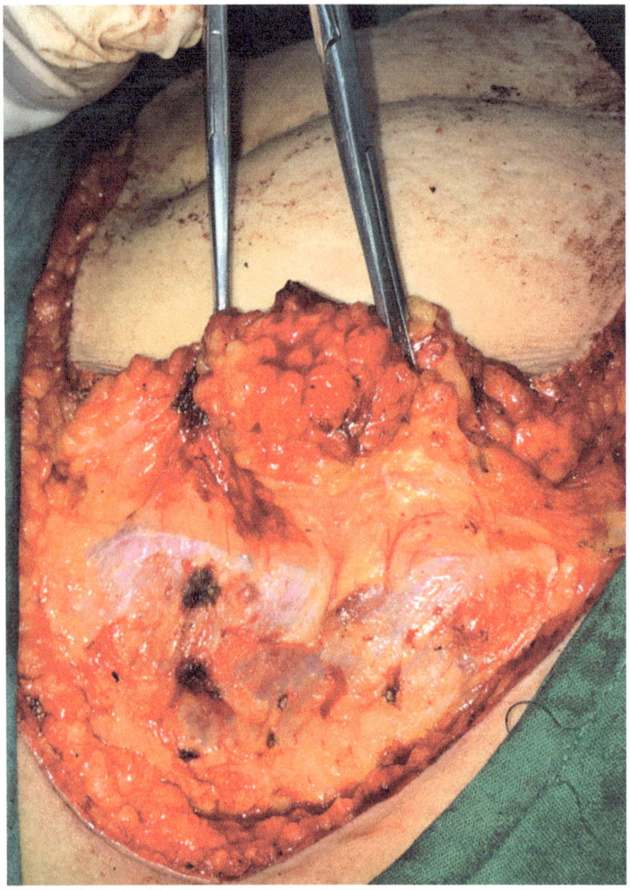

Fig. 26.10 Lift the right lower abdominal flap

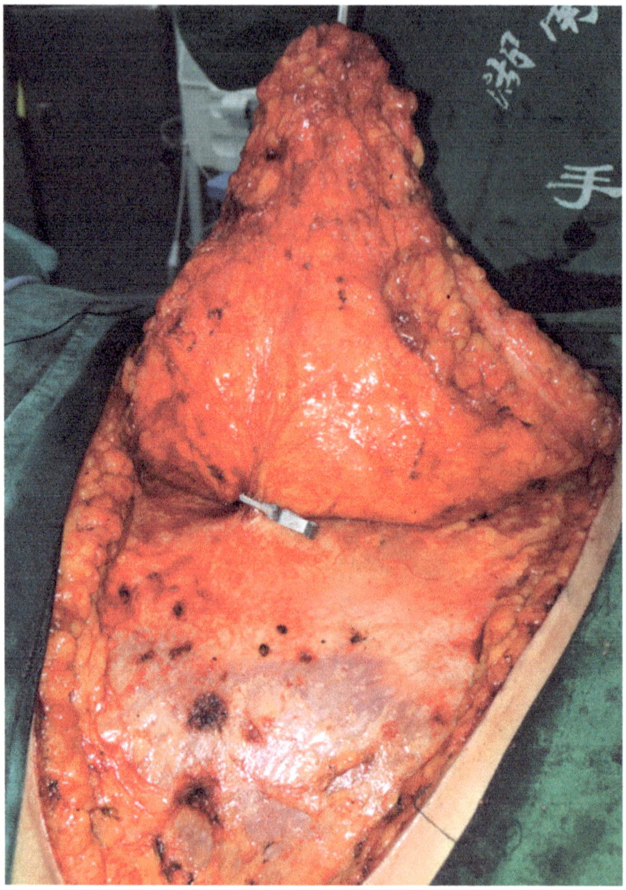

Fig. 26.11 Expose the right perforator vessel and assess the blood supply of the flap by the clamping test

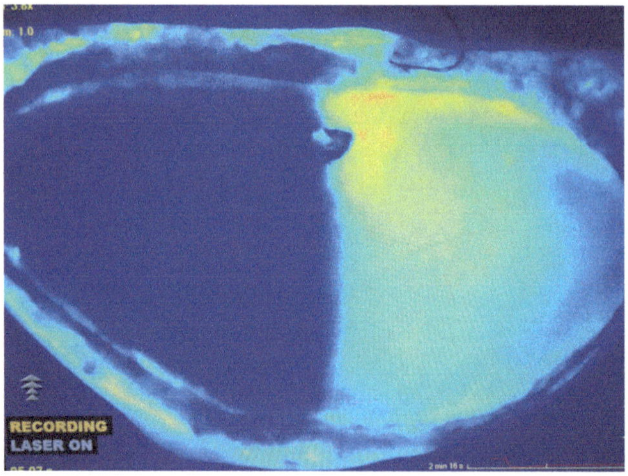

Fig. 26.12 The ICG imaging shows poor blood circulation in the right half of the flap

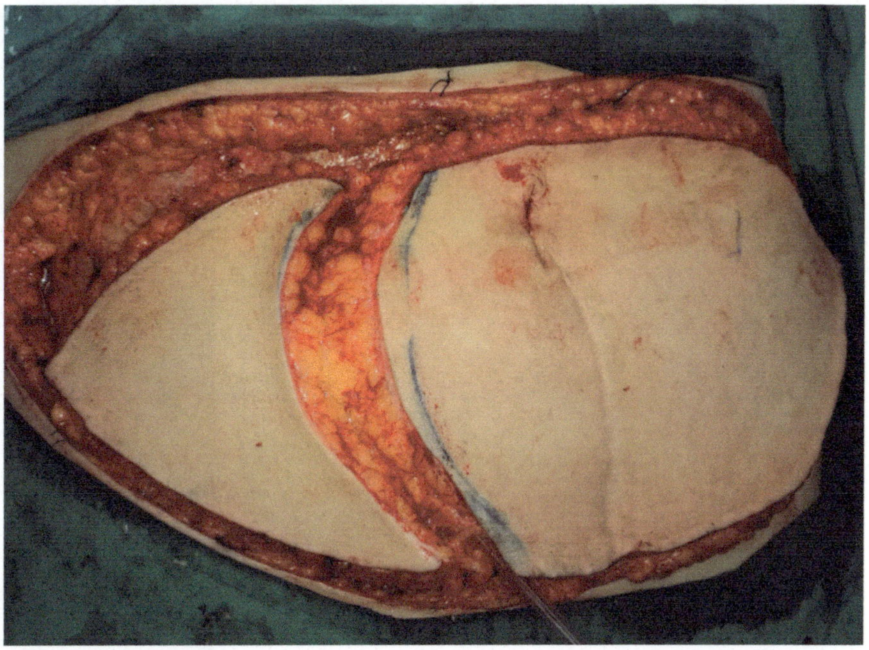

Fig. 26.13 Dissect most of the right side of the flap. The selection strategy of removing excessive part is very important. Since the left perforator in this case came from the lateral branches of inferior abdominal vessels, the excess tissue in contralateral area IV should be completely removed first, which was further confirmed by ICG intraoperative monitoring

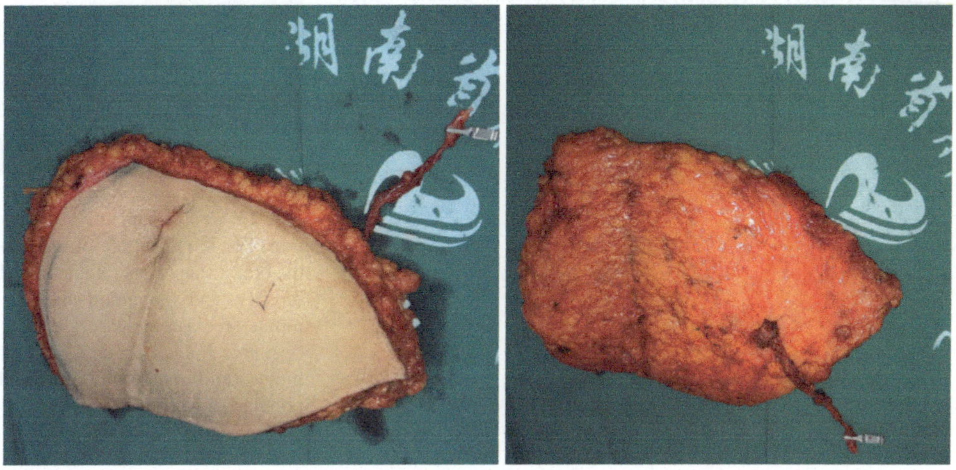

Fig. 26.14 The flap pedicled with the left deep inferior epigastric artery has been dissected

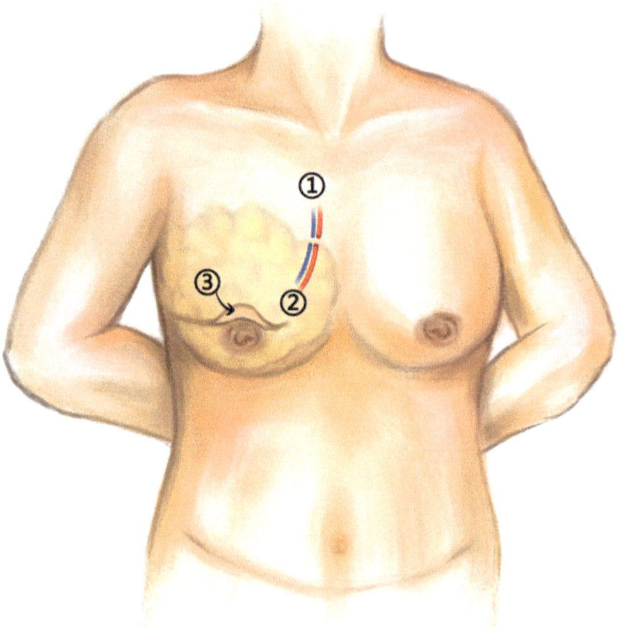

Fig. 26.15 Schematic diagram of revascularization: DIEAV + internal mammary AV (1A1V). (1) internal mammary vessels. (2) deep inferior epigastric vessels. (3) Observe skin island

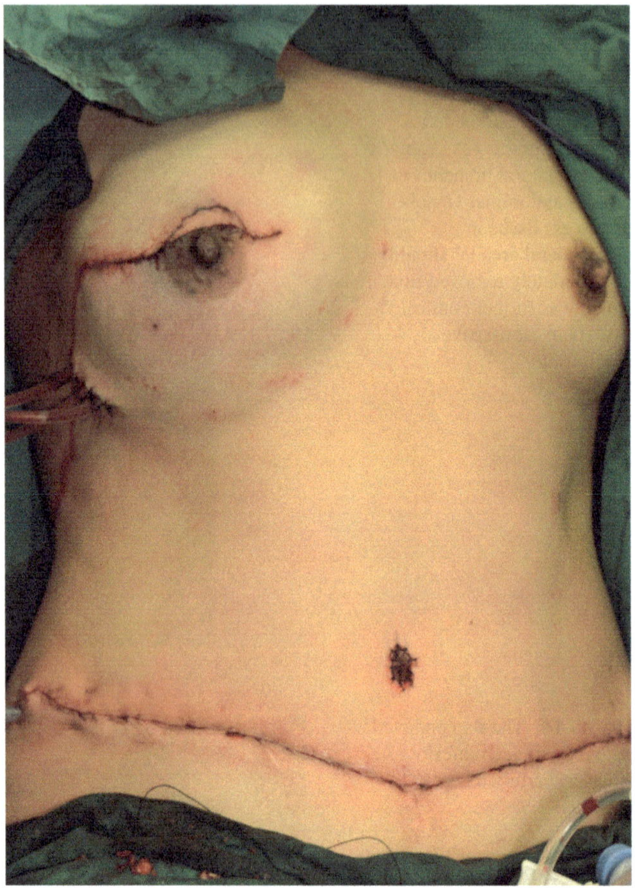

Fig. 26.16 Intraoperative observation immediately after reconstruction. The blood supply of the flap observation window was good, and the breast shape was satisfactory. The abdominal donor area was closed directly, and the umbilicus was repositioned and reconstructed. In nipple-areola complex-preserving mastectomy, the application of intraoperative fluorescence angiography to ensure the blood perfusion of nipple can improve the safety and effect of operation, which deserves popularizing

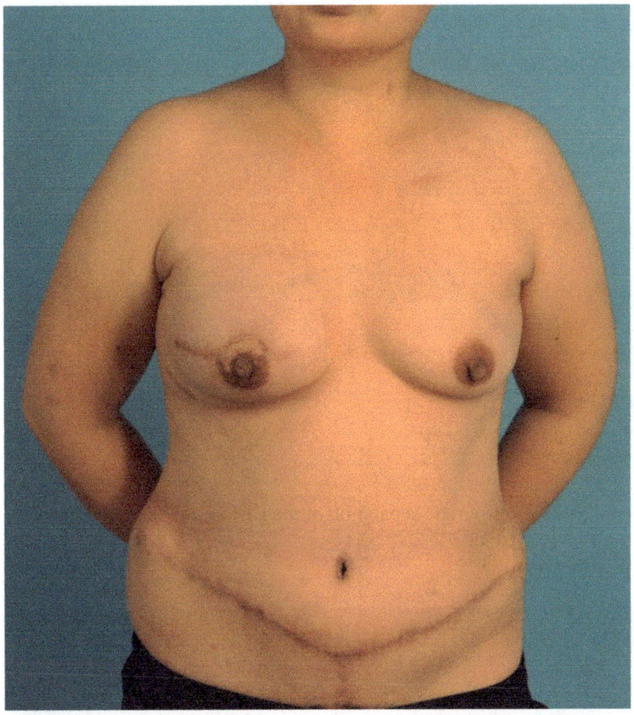

Fig. 26.17 The appearance and function were satisfactory after 12 months of follow-up

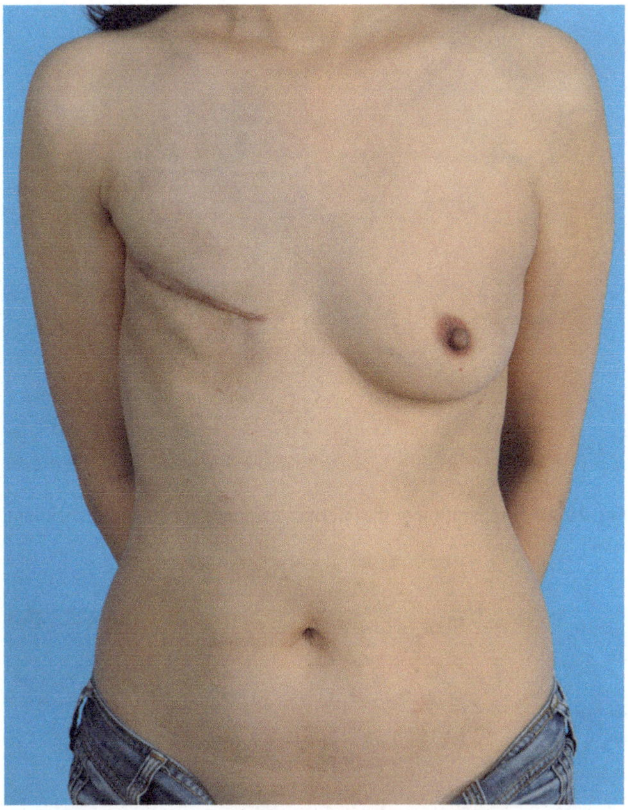

Fig. 26.18 Preoperative conditions

26.5 ICG Determined the Number of Vascular Pedicles Required for the Flap: A Typical Case

A 41-year-old female patient underwent two-stage breast reconstruction with bilateral vascular pedicle inferior abdominal artery perforator flap. Past history of right breast cancer was performed after modified radical mastectomy and 2 years after comprehensive treatment. Two-stage breast reconstruction was performed. After admission, the two-stage breast reconstruction was performed by free transplantation of inferior abdominal artery perforator flap. The right internal thoracic artery and its accompanying vein were exposed during the operation. The size of the designed flap was about 26 cm × 12 cm, and two sets of blood vessels were anastomosed: proximal end-to-end anastomosis (1A1V) between one side of inferior abdominal wall artery and vein and internal thoracic artery and vein carried by the flap, and distal end-to-end anastomosis (1A1V) between the other side of inferior abdominal wall artery and vein and internal thoracic artery and vein. The pathological report of rapid intraoperative examination suggested that (right chest wall nodule) the tested objects are fibers and lymphoid tissue, and there is no cancer. The flap survived well after operation, and the appearance and feeling of reconstructed breast recovered satisfactorily (Figs. 26.18, 26.19, 26.20, 26.21, 26.22, 26.23, 26.24, 26.25, 26.26, 26.27, 26.28, 26.29, 26.30, 26.31, and 26.32).

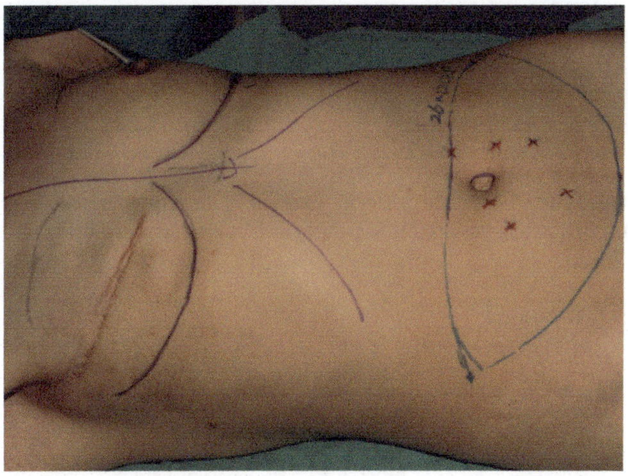

Fig. 26.19 Intraoperative design

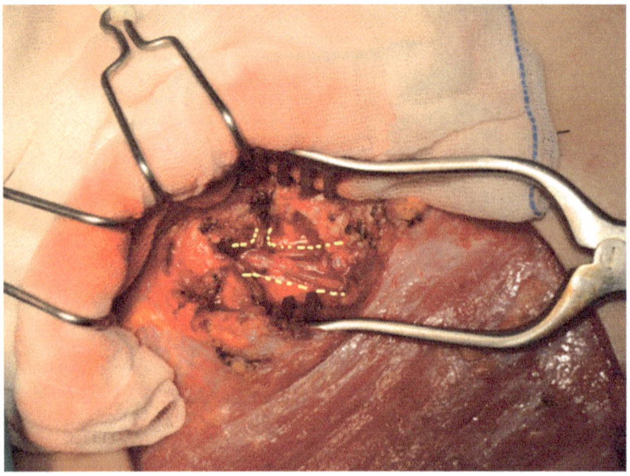

Fig. 26.20 Preparation of the internal mammary vessel in the recipient area

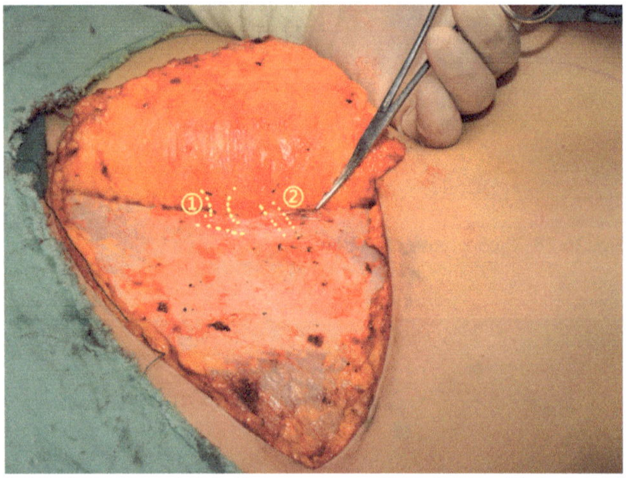

Fig. 26.21 Expose the perforating vessels of the left lower abdomen. (1) Perforating vessels. (2) Sensory branch of the intercostal nerve

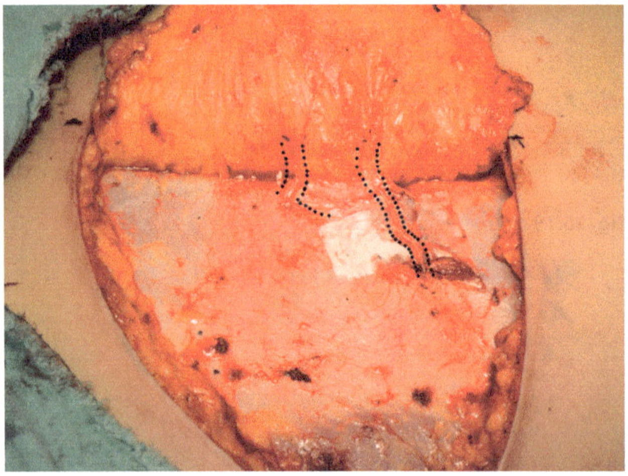

Fig. 26.22 Incise of the anterior sheath and separate intramuscularly for perforating branches. The superficial intercostal nerve branches were exposed along with the procedures. Separate the nerve near the deep surface of the anterior sheath, and protect it carefully

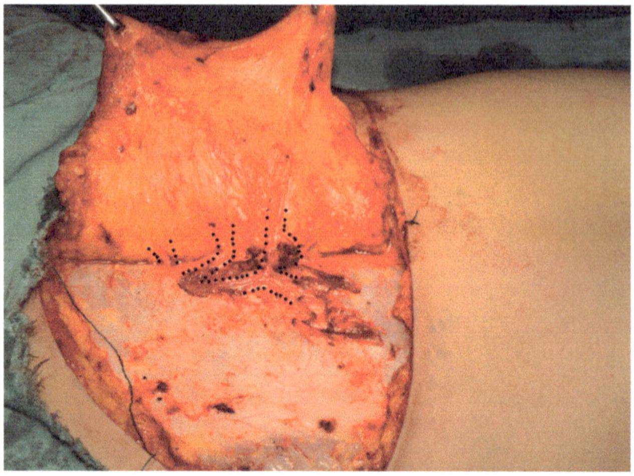

Fig. 26.23 Retrograde separation of the perforating branch to the vascular pedicle trunk

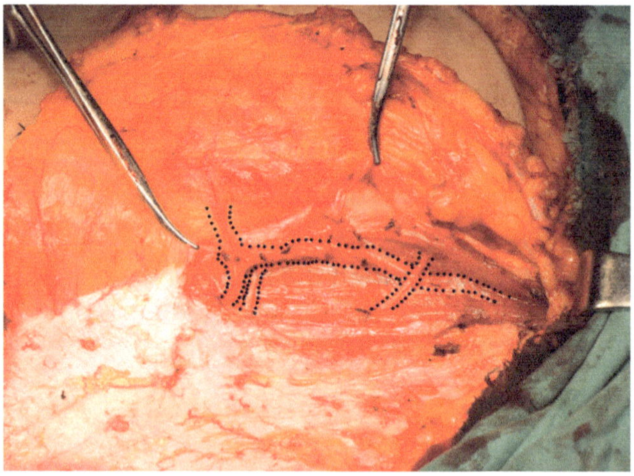

Fig. 26.24 Intercostal nerve was protected along with the procedures

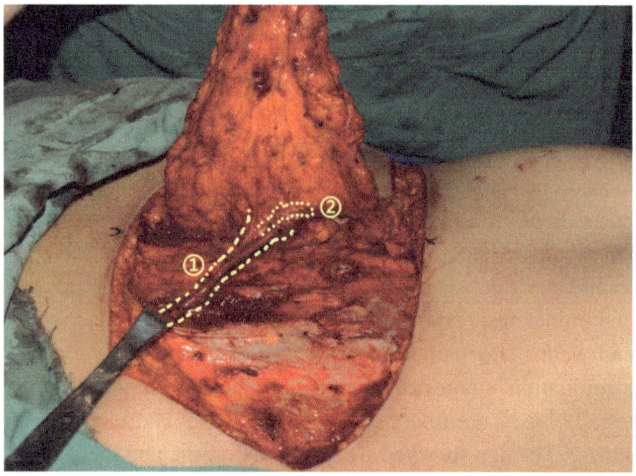

Fig. 26.25 Dissect the left inferior abdominal artery perforator flap. (1) Deep inferior epigastric vessels. (2) Sensory branch of the intercostal nerve

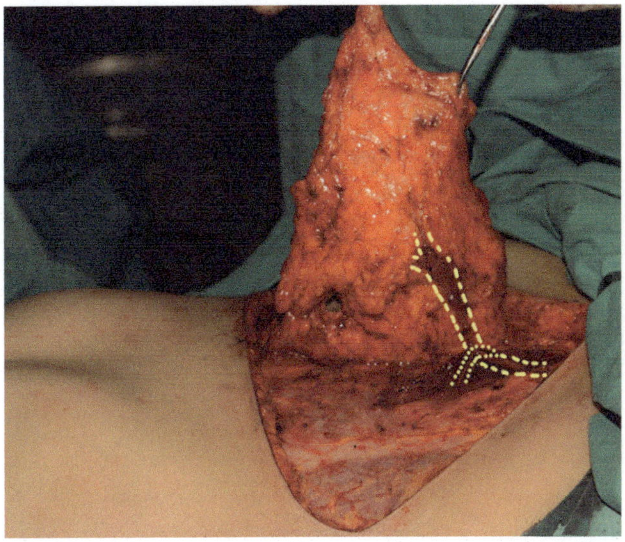

Fig. 26.26 The right inferior abdominal artery perforator flap was dissected with the complete preserving of the integrity of the intercostal nerve

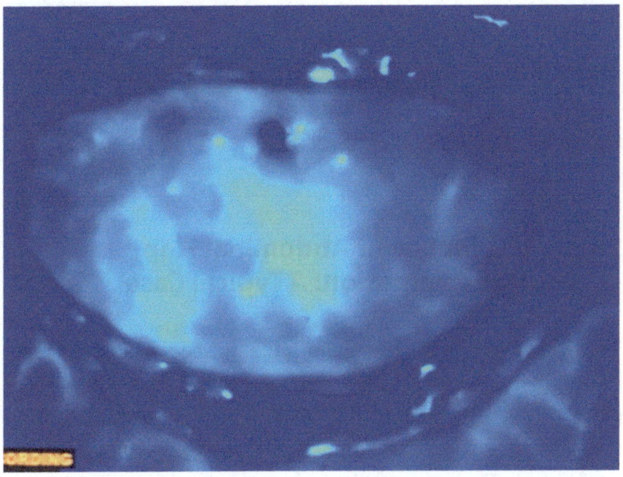

Fig. 26.27 ICG imaging showed that the left side of the flap has insufficient blood supply, whereas the reliable blood supply of the flap can only be obtained by the bilateral vascular pedicle

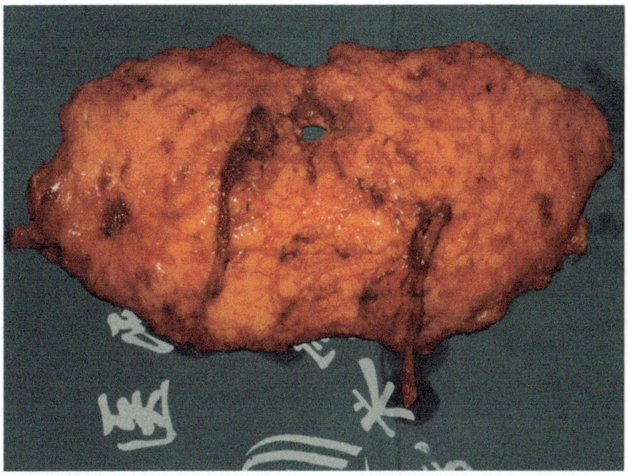

Fig. 26.28 Bilateral pedicled perforator flap of inferior abdominal artery was dissected

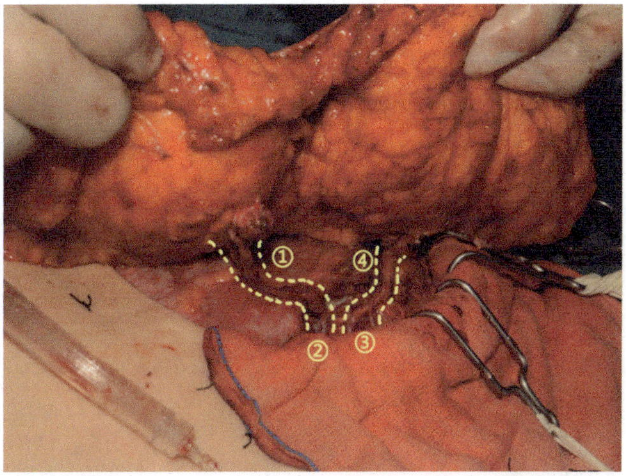

Fig. 26.29 Bilateral deep inferior epigastric artery perforators were anastomosed with proximal and distal thoracic vessels, respectively (1A1V). (1) Right deep inferior epigastric vessels. (2) Distal thoracic vessels. (3) Proximal thoracic vessels. (4) Left deep inferior epigastric vessel

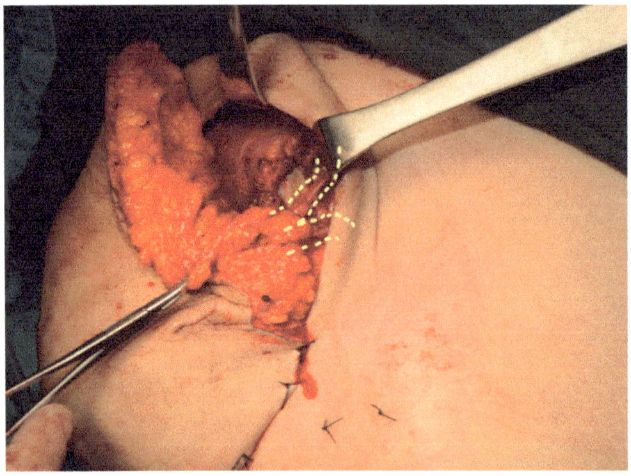

Fig. 26.30 After vascular anastomosis, attention should be given to further protect the flap and avoid tortuous tension and kinking. Then the flap was shaped

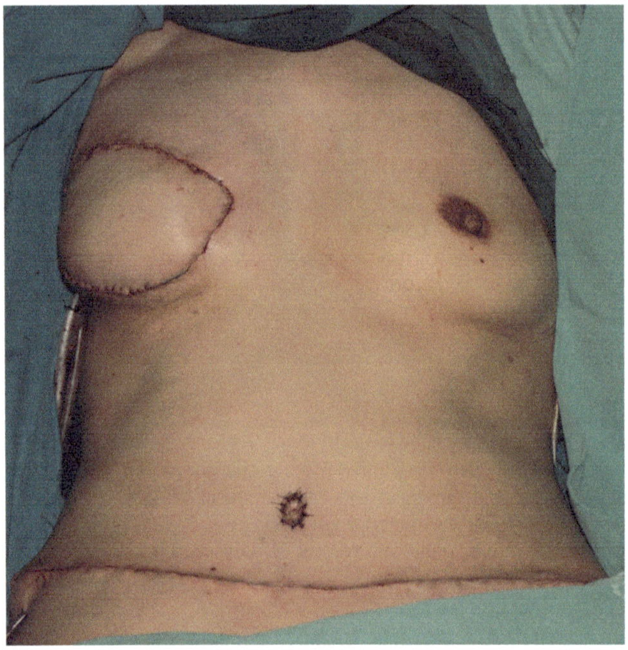

Fig. 26.31 Immediate view of intraoperative reconstruction

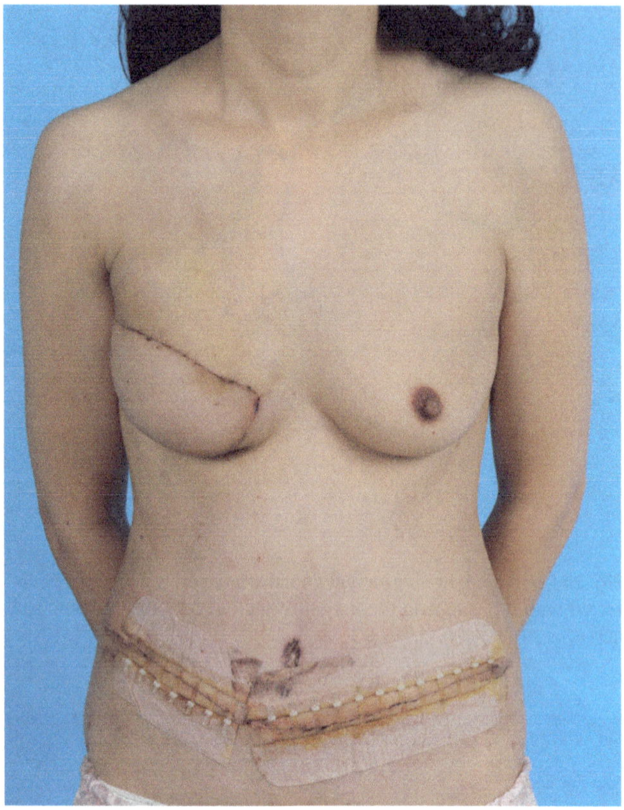

Fig. 26.32 Two weeks after operation

26.6 ICG for Lower Abdominal Flap Transplantation: A Typical Case

The patient was a 40-years-old female. She was hospitalized more than 3 years after modified radical mastectomy for right breast cancer. After admission, breast reconstruction with free deep inferior epigastric artery perforator flap was performed. The internal thoracic artery and its accompanying veins were exposed during the operation. The size of the designed flap was about 26 cm × 13 cm. The right inferior abdominal wall artery and vein were anastomosed with the distal end of the left inferior abdominal wall artery and vein (1A2V) to form internal pressurization. End-to-end anastomosis (1A2V) was performed between inferior abdominal wall artery and vein and internal thoracic artery and vein. Intraoperative ICG confirmed that the blood supply of the flap was good, and the flap survived well after operation. Results of pathological examination: (right chest wall mass) fibrous tissue hyperplasia and inflammatory cell infiltration were found in the specimens, and no definite malignancy was found. The flap survived well, and the breast function and appearance recovered satisfactorily (Figs. 26.33, 26.34, 26.35, 26.36, 26.37, and 26.38).

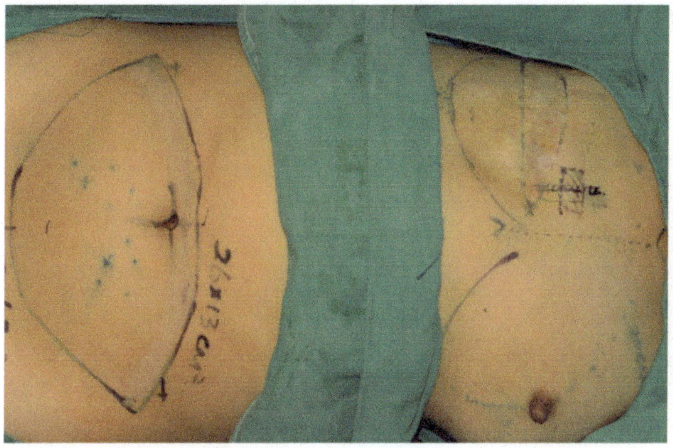

Fig. 26.33 Preoperative conditions

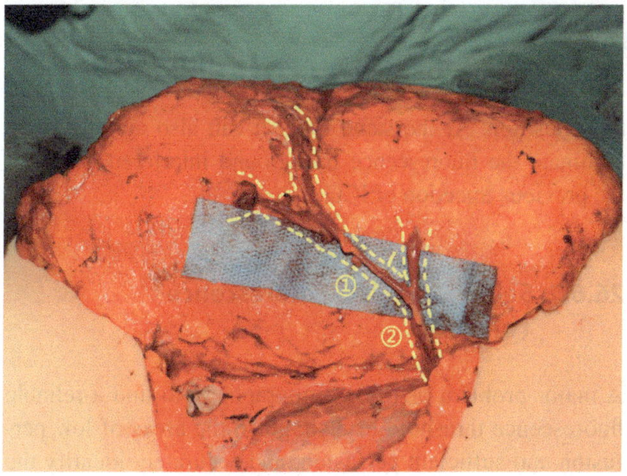

Fig. 26.34 After the separation of bilateral subabdominal vascular pedicle and perforating vessels, the left subabdominal vascular anastomosis with the distal end of the right subabdominal vascular trunk to form internal pressurization. (1) Left deep inferior epigastric vessel. (2) Right deep inferior epigastric vessel

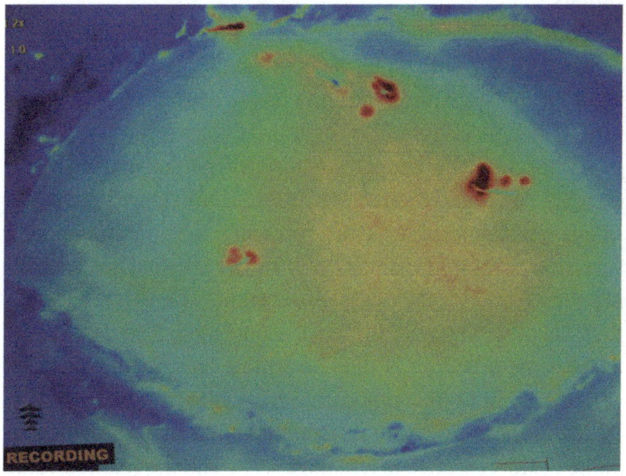

Fig. 26.35 ICG imaging showed that the blood supply of the flap was satisfactory

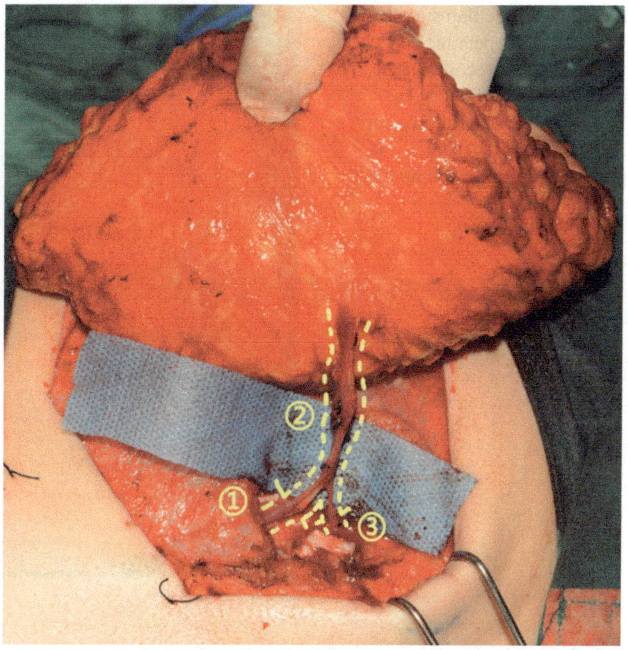

Fig. 26.36 The right deep inferior epigastric artery was anastomosed with the internal thoracic vein (1A2V), and the two accompanying veins of the deep inferior epigastric artery were anastomosed with the proximal and distal internal thoracic veins, respectively. (1) Proximal thoracic vessels. (2) deep inferior epigastric vessels. (3) Distal thoracic vessels

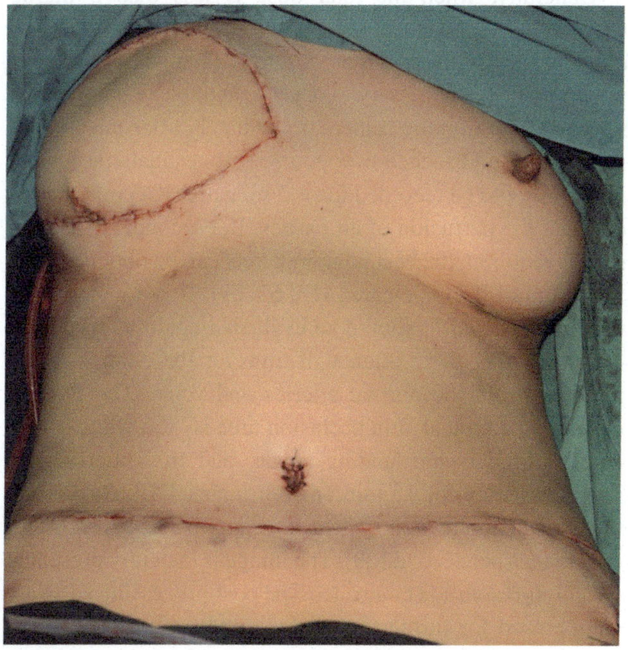

Fig. 26.37 Immediate intraoperative observation

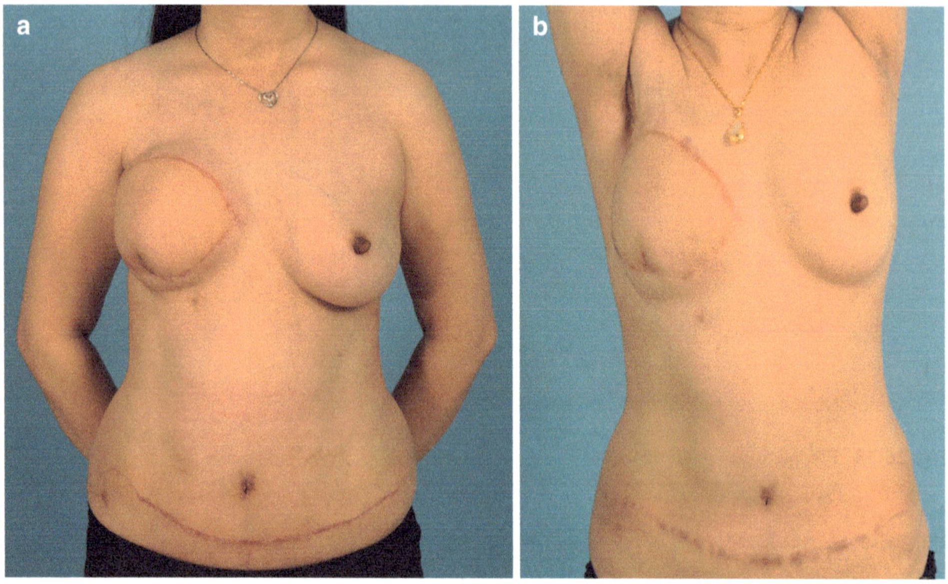

Fig. 26.38 The flap survived well and the appearance and function of the reconstructed breast were satisfactory. (**a**) The patients were followed up for 12 months. (**b**) The patients were followed up for 18 months

26.6.1 Application of ICG During Operation

During the operation, when the surgeon needs imaging, first place the probe perpendicular to the detection plane with a working distance of 30 cm [66], and a single injection of 25 mg of ICG and 10 mL of normal saline intravenously into the patient is given.

Generally, when the total dose is less than 5 mg/kg (400 mg/80 kg/person), patients will not have obvious side effects. The common acquisition time is about 1 min after injection. If it is necessary to observe and locate the perforator vessel, turn on the camera immediately after injection to record the fluorescence flow courses. To evaluate perfusion, images should be recorded for 1–3 min after ICG injection to evaluate the perfusion of all tissues. If a secondary imaging scan is required, the best imaging effect can be obtained after 10 min until ICG is cleared [13, 67–69]. If venous obstruction is suspected, it should be evaluated again after at least 4 min, so that there is enough time for the contrast to be removed from the normal arteries and veins. The fluorescence in the typical vein occlusion area is "too white" compared with the surrounding tissue, and this fluorescence signal will stay for 15 min or even longer [70]. At present, the clinical application system can capture 3.75–30 continuous images per second [28]. The image is instantly presented on a high-resolution controller. The post-processing software can be used for further comparison and analysis of images and numerical quantitative calculation of fluorescence intensity [70]. There are two ways of fluorescence value: relative and absolute. The relative value is calculated based on other regions of interest on the image. The absolute value only reflects the fluorescence signal intensity [70]. The software can automatically analyze the data and mark the strong fluorescence area representing the best perfusion area or perforator's position. At the same time, it can also automatically eliminate the fluorescence background interference left by the previous injection of ICG.

26.6.2 Selection of ICG Fluorescence Threshold

A major problem of ICG angiography is to find a reliable fluorescence threshold to distinguish the areas of low perfusion and sufficient perfusion, and accurately identify the tissues at risk of necrosis. Clinically, most surgeons will consider combining ICG imaging with clinical measuring instrument, and evaluate tissue perfusion based on these findings and their own clinical experience. The latest version of the spy system (spy-q)™ Analytical tools) can quantify the absolute and relative values of fluorescence signals.

Both absolute and relative values have clinical significance. The absolute value reflects the absolute fluorescence value of the study area, but it is easily affected by temperature, ICG concentration, plasma protein concentration, oxygen saturation, individual situation of patients, tissue, and equipment. Relative values offset these effects with the maximum perfusion area as the reference area. However, the selection of reference area is very subjective, and the selected reference area of each case is different. Therefore, in practice, absolute value and relative value should be considered at the same time, rather than determined lopsidedly.

According to the comprehensive analysis of related studies (see Table 26.5), it is recommended that the absolute value of fluorescence is less than 3.7–7 and the relative value is less than 30–33%, which means that there is a high risk of necrosis and relevant measures need to be taken.

Table 26.5 Literature on ICG fluorescence threshold

Researchers (Year)	Research content	Findings
Moyer and Losken (2012) [67]	Skin sparing mastectomy flap in 118 cases The objective was to explore the ICG fluorescence threshold of flap necrosis	1. Necrosis occurred in 17 cases (13%) 2. The mean relative fluorescence value of necrotic area was 24.6% (mean absolute value 6.3) 3. The average relative value of fluorescence in the active region was 46.1% (average absolute value 12.3) 4. Ninety percent of tissues with relative value ≤25% will not have vitality. Ninety-eight percent of tissues with relative value ≥45% were active 5. Under the threshold of 33% relative fluorescence value, the sensitivity was 84.6%, the specificity was 87.5%, the positive predictive value was 88% (i.e., the proportion of real necrosis in predicted necrotic tissue), and the negative predictive value was 16% (i.e., the proportion of real vitality in predicted viable tissue)
Philip (2012) [15]	In 51 cases of breast reconstruction with expander implantation (32 patients), ICG was used to assess the intraoperative flap perfusion. To investigate the fluorescence value related to necrosis	1. Necrosis occurred in 21 cases 2. Fluorescence absolute value <3.7, sensitivity 90%, and specificity 100% 3. The absolute value of fluorescence was <8.0, the sensitivity was 100%, and the specificity was 70% 4. According to the absolute value, there are three categories: dynamic organizations (absolute value >8.0); tissues that should be evaluated in combination with clinical presentation (3.7–8.0); high risk of necrosis (<3.7)
Munabi(2014) [68]	A total of 62 cases (including 48 expander implantation, 6 TRAM, 6 DIEP, and 2 prosthesis implantation) The objective was to explore the ICG fluorescence threshold of flap necrosis	1. One necrosis occurred in eight cases (13%) 2. The false positive rate was more likely to occur in smokers and intraoperative adrenaline users 3. When the threshold of absolute fluorescence value was 7, the sensitivity was 88%, the specificity was 83%, the positive predictive value was 44%, and the negative predictive value was 98% When the smokers and intraoperative adrenaline users were excluded, the sensitivity was 83%, the specificity was 98%, the positive predictive value was 83%, and the negative predictive value was 98%

26.6.3 Precautions for ICG Application

Some factors may affect the use of ICG fluorescence system [70, 71]: (1) factors related to ischemia (e.g., post-radiotherapy, recent smoking, peripheral vascular disease, obesity, diabetes, vascular disease, long-term use of glucocorticoid, breast flap after mastectomy) and factors affecting blood flow such as vasoconstriction (epinephrine). Guidelines for the use of spy show that vasoconstrictors [70], such as adrenaline, can affect methods that estimate tissue perfusion of all kinds, including ICG angiography. Wait at least 2 h after epinephrine when ICG is to be applied. Some commonly used dyes, such as methylene blue, can also affect angiography.

26.7 Economic Factors of ICG in Breast Reconstruction

The cost of dealing with postoperative complications is expensive. The cost of infection after breast reconstruction is estimated to exceed $4000 [72]. The use of ICG can significantly reduce postoperative complications, especially those related to flap necrosis, but the cost of ICG angiography is expensive. Does it have sufficient economic benefits?

In a retrospective study of 710 cases of prothesis reconstruction by Kanuri et al. [69], if all patients used ICG angiography, each patient received an average 1.4 times of ICG during operation, and the average increased cost was $1537.3. However, if ICG was used only in patients at high risk of necrosis, the average cost for smokers was $2098.80, $5162.30 (BMI > 30 kg/m^2) for obese patients, and $1892.70 for patients with breast volume more than 800 g. The data show that if all patients use ICG, there is no obvious benefit. However, for high-risk groups (smokers, obese people, large breasts), the economic benefits are obvious.

In breast reconstruction with free autologous tissue flap, Chatterjee [59] et al. showed that the incidence of postoperative complications without ICG was 26.5%. Only 5% of patients used ICG. In this analysis, the difference between the cost baseline is $773.66. Compared with ICG, the increased cost-effectiveness ratio is $3516.64/quality adjusted life year. The research of Chatha et al. [60] also showed that the rate of using ICG in autologous tissue reconstruction is higher than that of expander or prosthesis implantation reconstruction, and smokers and hypertensive and obese individuals are more likely to use ICG.

In conclusion, as a cost-effective method, ICG angiography significantly reduces postoperative flap necrosis, so as to reduce the cost to a large extent. In terms of economics, ICG is recommended for all high-risk people (smoking, obesity, BMI > 30, hypertension, large breast >800 g) and autologous tissue reconstruction. For those without high-risk factors, expanders or prosthesis implantation and reconstruction should be used according to the economic situation. In addition, the cost of ICG in China is much lower than that in foreign countries. Taking our hospital as an example, the average increased cost of each patient using ICG is about 500 RMB. This reinforces the economic benefits of ICG in breast reconstruction in China.

26.8 The Future of ICG in Breast Reconstruction

The progress of some new ICG technologies expand the visible field of the image, prolong the duration to capture the image, quantify the blood flow change, and provide colored coverage function. In particular, the color coverage function is one of the latest developments. It can use different colors in different spectrum on the perfusion map similar to contour topographic map to identify the value of bleeding flow and the intensity of fluorescence signal. This feature allows the surgeon to establish a translucent overlay layer on the patient's body surface tissue. Because the deep anatomical tissue was displayed by direct visualization, the surgeons can quickly evaluate the ischemic area and identify the boundary of dynamic tissue.

Although the flap transplantation needs to constantly pay attention to the inflow artery, the venous outflow is the key point to judge the flap necrosis and the success of the operation [5, 73]. Because ICG imaging can evaluate the venous outflow by the disappearance of ICG in tissue, its potential in this regard should not be underestimated. Usually, the venous area of the flap and the perforator area are not completely anastomosed, so the survival rate of the perforator flap can be improved by ensuring arterial perfusion and venous drainage [61]. Therefore, the clinical standard for evaluating the inflow and outflow of blood vessels is very important for intraoperative decision-making.

According to another characteristic of ICG clearance and excretion, the images of lymphatic system can also be obtained. Because breast reconstruction also includes lymphatic reconstruction, it is essential for breast reconstruction. Many researchers have reported successful cases in this field [74–77]. ICG can also outline and identify lymph nodes, so it can be used to evaluate patients with potential or existing lymphatic dysfunction.

26.9 Summary

The main cause of early complications after breast reconstruction is insufficient blood perfusion, including flap after mastectomy, which potentially leads to flap necrosis or other adverse consequences. Since ICG entered the medical field in the 1950s and the use of ICG in breast reconstruction in recent years, ICG has become an intraoperative image technology with its value and safety proven. Although clinical assessment is important, it is not enough to predict flap necrosis. Among many auxiliary methods for evaluating tissue perfusion, ICG has the following advantages: it can be evaluated repeatedly in one operation, high sensitivity and specificity, and less adverse reactions. ICG is widely used in various forms of breast reconstruction: in breast reconstruction with expander and prosthesis implantation, the blood perfusion of mastectomy flap can be evaluated. In breast reconstruction with autologous tissue, the perforator can be accurately located, and the perfusion area can be evaluated and recorded immediately. The tissue perfusion degree can be estimated by fluorescence signal, and the patency of vascular anastomosis can be evaluated. The blood supply of flap can be monitored after operation. Although the cost of ICG is relatively expensive, it has been proven to have high economic benefits in breast reconstruction, especially for high-risk people and autologous tissue reconstruction. In the future, new technologies of ICG imaging, such as color coverage function, will be widely used in breast reconstruction. In addition, the evaluation of venous perfusion and lymphatic reconstruction by ICG also facilitate the intraoperative decision-making of breast reconstruction.

References

1. Komorowska-Timek E, Gurtner GC. Intraoperative perfusion mapping with laser-assisted indocyanine green imaging can predict and prevent complications in immediate breast reconstruction. Plast Reconstr Surg. 2010;125(4):1065–73.
2. Garvey PB, Buchel EW, Pockaj BA, et al. DIEP and pedicled TRAM flaps: a comparison of outcomes. Plast Reconstr Surg. 2006;117(6):175–9; discussion 1720–1.
3. Pestana IA, Coan B, Erdmann D, Marcus J, Levin LS, Zenn MR. Early experience with fluorescent angiography in free-tissue transfer reconstruction. Plast Reconstr Surg. 2009;123(4):1239–44.
4. Kroll SS. Fat necrosis in free transverse rectus abdominis myocutaneous and deep inferior epigastric perforator flaps. Plast Reconstr Surg. 2000;106(3):576–83.
5. Blondeel PN, Arnstein M, Verstraete K, et al. Venous congestion and blood flow in free transverse rectus abdominis myocutaneous and deep inferior epigastric perforator flaps. Plast Reconstr Surg. 2000;106(6):1295–9.
6. Jallali N, Ridha H, Butler PE. Postoperative monitoring of free flaps in UK plastic surgery units. Microsurgery. 2005;25(6):469–72.
7. Olivier WA, Hazen A, Levine JP, Soltanian H, Chung S, Gurtner GC. Reliable assessment of skin flap viability using orthogonal polarization imaging. Plast Reconstr Surg. 2003;112(2):547–55.
8. Dorfman D, Pu LL. The value of color duplex imaging for planning and performing a free anterolateral thigh perforator flap. Ann Plast Surg. 2014;72(Suppl 1):S6–8.
9. Hallock GG. Doppler sonography and color duplex imaging for planning a perforator flap. Clin Plast Surg. 2003;30(3):347–57, v–vi.
10. Rozen WM, Phillips TJ, Ashton MW, Stella DL, Gibson RN, Taylor GI. Preoperative imaging for DIEA perforator flaps: a comparative

study of computed tomographic angiography and Doppler ultrasound. Plast Reconstr Surg. 2008;121(1):9–16.
11. Newman MI, Samson MC. The application of laser-assisted indocyanine green fluorescent dye angiography in microsurgical breast reconstruction. J Reconstr Microsurg. 2009;25(1):21–6.
12. Newman MI, Samson MC, Tamburrino JF, Swartz KA. Intraoperative laser-assisted indocyanine green angiography for the evaluation of mastectomy flaps in immediate breast reconstruction. J Reconstr Microsurg. 2010;26(7):487–92.
13. Murray JD, Jones GE, Elwood ET, Whitty LA, Garcia C. Fluorescent intraoperative tissue angiography with indocyanine green: evaluation of nipple-areola vascularity during breast reduction surgery. Plast Reconstr Surg. 2010;126(1):33e–4e.
14. Francisco BS, Kerr-Valentic MA, Agarwal JP. Laser-assisted indocyanine green angiography and DIEP breast reconstruction. Plast Reconstr Surg. 2010;125(3):116e–8e.
15. Phillips BT, Lanier ST, Conkling N, et al. Intraoperative perfusion techniques can accurately predict mastectomy skin flap necrosis in breast reconstruction: results of a prospective trial. Plast Reconstr Surg. 2012;129(5):778e–88e.
16. Fox IJ, Wood EH. Indocyanine green: physical and physiologic properties. Proc Staff Meet Mayo Clin. 1960;35:732–44.
17. Wheeler HO, Cranston WI, Meltzer JI. Hepatic uptake and biliary excretion of indocyanine green in the dog. Proc Soc Exp Biol Med. 1958;99(1):5–4.
18. Cherrick GR, Stein SW, Leevy CM, Davidson CS. Indocyanine green: observations on its physical properties, plasma decay, and hepatic extraction. J Clin Invest. 1960;39:592–600.
19. Villeneuve JP, Huot R, Marleau D, Huet PM. The estimation of hepatic blood flow with indocyanine green: comparison between the continuous infusion and single injection methods. Am J Gastroenterol. 1982;77(4):233–7.
20. Leevy CM, Smith F, Longueville J, Paumgartner G, Howard MM. Indocyanine green clearance as a test for hepatic function. Evaluation by dichromatic ear densitometry. JAMA. 1967;200(3):236–40.
21. Kogure K, Choromokos E. Infrared absorption angiography. J Appl Physiol. 1969;26(1):154–7.
22. Kogure K, David NJ, Yamanouchi U, Choromokos E. Infrared absorption angiography of the fundus circulation. Arch Ophthalmol. 1970;83(2):209–14.
23. Choromokos E, Kogure K, David NJ. Infrared absorption angiography. J Biol Photogr Assoc. 1969;37(2):100–4.
24. Flower RW, Hochheimer BF. Clinical infrared absorption angiography of the choroid. Am J Ophthalmol. 1972;73(3):458–9.
25. Hayashi K, Hasegawa Y, Tokoro T. Indocyanine green angiography of central serous chorioretinopathy. Int Ophthalmol. 1986;9(1):37–41.
26. Hasegawa Y, Hayashi K, Tokoro T, De Laey JJ. [Clinical use of indocyanine green angiography in the diagnosis of choroidal neovascular diseases]. Fortschr Ophthalmol. 1988;85(4):410–2.
27. Hayashi K, Hasegawa Y, Tazawa Y, de Laey JJ. Clinical application of indocyanine green angiography to choroidal neovascularization. Jpn J Ophthalmol. 1989;33(1):57–65.
28. Scheider A, Schroedel C. High resolution indocyanine green angiography with a scanning laser ophthalmoscope. Am J Ophthalmol. 1989;108(4):458–9.
29. Yannuzzi LA, Slakter JS, Sorenson JA, Guyer DR, Orlock DA. Digital indocyanine green videoangiography and choroidal neovascularization. 1992. Retina. 2012;32(Suppl 1):191.
30. Tanaka E, Chen FY, Flaumenhaft R, Graham GJ, Laurence RG, Frangioni JV. Real-time assessment of cardiac perfusion, coronary angiography, and acute intravascular thrombi using dual-channel near-infrared fluorescence imaging. J Thorac Cardiovasc Surg. 2009;138(1):133–40.
31. Hori T, Iida T, Yagi S, et al. K(ICG) value, a reliable real-time estimator of graft function, accurately predicts outcomes in adult living-donor liver transplantation. Liver Transpl. 2006;12(4):605–13.
32. Polom W, Markuszewski M, Rho YS, Matuszewski M. Use of invisible near infrared light fluorescence with indocyanine green and methylene blue in urology. Part 2. Cent European J Urol. 2014;67(3):310–3.
33. Ahmed M, Purushotham AD, Douek M. Novel techniques for sentinel lymph node biopsy in breast cancer: a systematic review. Lancet Oncol. 2014;15(8):e351–62.
34. Levey KA. Use of fluorescence imaging technology to identify peritoneal endometriosis: a case report of new technology. Surg Laparosc Endosc Percutan Tech. 2014;24(2):e63–5.
35. Dip F, Roy M, Lo ME, Simpfendorfer C, Szomstein S, Rosenthal RJ. Routine use of fluorescent incisionless cholangiography as a new imaging modality during laparoscopic cholecystectomy. Surg Endosc. 2015;29(6):1621–6.
36. Lee BT, Hutteman M, Gioux S, et al. The FLARE intraoperative near-infrared fluorescence imaging system: a first-in-human clinical trial in perforator flap breast reconstruction. Plast Reconstr Surg. 2010;126(5):1472–81.
37. Desai ND, Miwa S, Kodama D, et al. A randomized comparison of intraoperative indocyanine green angiography and transit-time flow measurement to detect technical errors in coronary bypass grafts. J Thorac Cardiovasc Surg. 2006;132(3):585–94.
38. Zhang HM. Indocyanine green fundus angiography operation and nursing cooperation. Chin J Nurs. 1999;4:220.
39. Liu Z, Liu Z. Evaluation of indocyanine green for diagnosis of liver diseases. J Clin Hepatol. 1994;2:92–3.
40. Ji Y, Jiang Y. Application of indocyanine green fluorescence navigation technology combined with methylene blue tracing in sentinel lymph node biopsy in breast cancer. Guangxi Med J. 2015;9:1275–7.
41. Yang K, Mu L. The value of indocyanine green angiography in skin flap surgery. Chin J Reparat Reconstr Surg. 2015;9:1113–6.
42. Chen Y, Chen J. Investigation report on the status of breast reconstruction after breast cancer surgery in China. Chin J Oncol. 2014;11:851–7.
43. Moody ED, Viskari PJ, Colyer CL. Non-covalent labeling of human serum albumin with indocyanine green: a study by capillary electrophoresis with diode laser-induced fluorescence detection. J Chromatogr B Biomed Sci Appl. 1999;729(1–2):55–64.
44. Newman MI, Samson MC, Tamburrino JF, Swartz KA, Brunworth L. An investigation of the application of laser-assisted indocyanine green fluorescent dye angiography in pedicle transverse rectus abdominus myocutaneous breast reconstruction. Can J Plast Surg. 2011;19(1):e1–5.
45. Kummer O, Widmer MK, Plüss S, et al. Does infection affect amputation rate in chronic critical leg ischemia. Vasa. 2003;32(1):18–21.
46. Jaccard Y, Walther S, Anderson S, et al. Influence of secondary infection on amputation in chronic critical limb ischemia. Eur J Vasc Endovasc Surg. 2007;33(5):605–9.
47. Baxter BT, Mesh CL, McGee GS, et al. Limb-threatening ischemia complicated by perigenicular infection. J Surg Res. 1993;54(2):163–7.
48. Olsen MA, Lefta M, Dietz JR, et al. Risk factors for surgical site infection after major breast operation. J Am Coll Surg. 2008;207(3):326–35.
49. Hedén P, Jurell G, Arnander C. Prediction of skin flap necrosis: a comparative study between laser Doppler flowmetry and fluorescein test in a rat model. Ann Plast Surg. 1986;17(6):485–8.
50. Schlosser S, Wirth R, Plock JA, Serov A, Banic A, Erni D. Application of a new laser Doppler imaging system in planning and monitoring of surgical flaps. J Biomed Opt. 2010;15(3):036023.

51. Keller A. A new diagnostic algorithm for early prediction of vascular compromise in 208 microsurgical flaps using tissue oxygen saturation measurements. Ann Plast Surg. 2009;62(5):538–43.
52. Keller A. Noninvasive tissue oximetry for flap monitoring: an initial study. J Reconstr Microsurg. 2007;23(4):189–97.
53. Rübben A, Eren S, Krein R, Younossi H, Böhler U, Wienert V. Infrared videoangiofluorography of the skin with indocyanine green—rat random cutaneous flap model and results in man. Microvasc Res. 1994;47(2):240–51.
54. Ludolph I, Arkudas A, Schmitz M, et al. Cracking the perfusion code?: laser-assisted Indocyanine Green angiography and combined laser Doppler spectrophotometry for intraoperative evaluation of tissue perfusion in autologous breast reconstruction with DIEP or ms-TRAM flaps. J Plast Reconstr Aesthet Surg. 2016;69(10):1382–8.
55. Azuma R, Morimoto Y, Masumoto K, et al. Detection of skin perforators by indocyanine green fluorescence nearly infrared angiography. Plast Reconstr Surg. 2008;122(4):1062–7.
56. Sood M, Glat P. Potential of the SPY intraoperative perfusion assessment system to reduce ischemic complications in immediate postmastectomy breast reconstruction. Ann Surg Innov Res. 2013;7(1):9.
57. Duggal CS, Madni T, Losken A. An outcome analysis of intraoperative angiography for postmastectomy breast reconstruction. Aesthet Surg J. 2014;34(1):61–5.
58. Newman MI, Jack MC, Samson MC. SPY-Q analysis toolkit values potentially predict mastectomy flap necrosis. Ann Plast Surg. 2013;70(5):595–8.
59. Chatterjee A, Krishnan NM, Rosen JM. Complex ventral hernia repair using components separation with or without biologic mesh: a cost-utility analysis. Ann Plast Surg. 2015;74(4):471–8.
60. Chattha A, Bucknor A, Chen AD, Lee BT, Lin SJ. Indocyanine green angiography use in breast reconstruction: a national analysis of outcomes and cost in 110,320 patients. Plast Reconstr Surg. 2018;141(4):825–32.
61. Saint-Cyr M, Schaverien M, Arbique G, Hatef D, Brown SA, Rohrich RJ. Three- and four-dimensional computed tomographic angiography and venography for the investigation of the vascular anatomy and perfusion of perforator flaps. Plast Reconstr Surg. 2008;121(3):772–80.
62. Quilichini J, Le MP, Guihard T. [Increasing the reliability of SIEA flap using peroperative fluorescent angiography with indocyanine green in breast reconstruction]. Ann Chir Plast Esthet. 2010;55(6):531–8.
63. Holm C, Mayr M, Höfter E, Dornseifer U, Ninkovic M. Assessment of the patency of microvascular anastomoses using microscope-integrated near-infrared angiography: a preliminary study. Microsurgery. 2009;29(7):509–14.
64. Liu Y, Mu L. The value of indocyanine green angiography during microsurgery vascular anastomosis to evaluate vascular patency. China Med. 2017;3:434–7.
65. Holm C, Tegeler J, Mayr M, Becker A, Pfeiffer UJ, Mühlbauer W. Monitoring free flaps using laser-induced fluorescence of indocyanine green: a preliminary experience. Microsurgery. 2002;22(7):278–87.
66. Chen Y, Gao W. The application of indocyanine green in medical imaging. Int J Biomed Eng. 2013;5:289–293, 316.
67. Moyer HR, Losken A. Predicting mastectomy skin flap necrosis with indocyanine green angiography: the gray area defined. Plast Reconstr Surg. 2012;129(5):1043–8.
68. Munabi NC, Olorunnipa OB, Goltsman D, Rohde CH, Ascherman JA. The ability of intra-operative perfusion mapping with laser-assisted indocyanine green angiography to predict mastectomy flap necrosis in breast reconstruction: a prospective trial. J Plast Reconstr Aesthet Surg. 2014;67(4):449–55.
69. Kanuri A, Liu AS, Guo L. Whom should we SPY? A cost analysis of laser-assisted indocyanine green angiography in prevention of mastectomy skin flap necrosis during prosthesis-based breast reconstruction. Plast Reconstr Surg. 2014;133(4):448e–54e.
70. Gurtner GC, Jones GE, Neligan PC, et al. Intraoperative laser angiography using the SPY system: review of the literature and recommendations for use. Ann Surg Innov Res. 2013;7(1):1.
71. Dashti R, Laakso A, Niemelä M, et al. Application of microscope integrated indocyanine green video-angiography during microneurosurgical treatment of intracranial aneurysms: a review. Acta Neurochir Suppl. 2010;107:107–9.
72. Olsen MA, Chu-Ongsakul S, Brandt KE, Dietz JR, Mayfield J, Fraser VJ. Hospital-associated costs due to surgical site infection after breast surgery. Arch Surg. 2008;143(1):53–60; discussion 61.
73. Krishnan KG, Schackert G, Steinmeier R. The role of near-infrared angiography in the assessment of post-operative venous congestion in random pattern, pedicled Island and free flaps. Br J Plast Surg. 2005;58(3):330–8.
74. Azuma S, Yamamoto T, Koshima I. Donor-site lymphatic function after microvascular lymph node transfer should be followed using indocyanine green lymphography. Plast Reconstr Surg. 2013;131(3):443e–4e.
75. Hara H, Mihara M, Seki Y, Todokoro T, Iida T, Koshima I. Comparison of indocyanine green lymphographic findings with the conditions of collecting lymphatic vessels of limbs in patients with lymphedema. Plast Reconstr Surg. 2013;132(6):165–8.
76. Becker C, Assouad J, Riquet M, Hidden G. Postmastectomy lymphedema: long-term results following microsurgical lymph node transplantation. Ann Surg. 2006;243(3):313–5.
77. Pons G, Masia J, Loschi P, Nardulli ML, Duch J. A case of donor-site lymphoedema after lymph node-superficial circumflex iliac artery perforator flap transfer. J Plast Reconstr Aesthet Surg. 2014;67(1):119–23.

Shaping for Breast Reconstruction with Autologous Tissue Transplantation

27

Tomoyuki Yano, Xiaoqing Lu, and Yanni Ding

Although a number of detailed reports have introduced autologous tissue and allogeneic transplantation in the domain of breast surgery, there are few reports on the aesthetic shaping of breast reconstruction. Similarly, despite abundant literatures regarding the technical points of anatomy related to breast plastic surgery, breast reconstruction of autologous tissue, and breast implants, there is hardly any monograph on the artistic techniques for shaping breasts in the process of breast plastic surgery and breast reconstruction. Most experienced breast surgeons would believe that the shape of a breast created or reconstructed during breast reconstruction and cosmetic surgery should be aesthetically satisfactory, such a view might seem self-evident. However, every surgeon has his or her own surgical techniques to achieve the great aesthetic results. Usually, techniques can be imparted to their students, whereas some specific surgical techniques cannot. In most cases, it needs a long process of trial and errors for the students to obtain "experience and mastership" [1].

As teachers, we often feel that it is sometimes difficult to teach this "artistry" to our surgical successors. The imparting of our own artistic insight and the artistic skills to the apprentices will be determined by the effectiveness of knowledge transfer and the ultimate surgical outcome. While artistic awareness is difficult to define and teach, we believe that analytical and methodological methods will help to overcome the problems of malformed breasts in a reliable and reproducible way. We present our own systematic approach to breast reconstruction and cosmetic surgery that can create a natural breast. The analytical methods described in different sections of this article enable the surgeon to break down, understand, and describe the different deformities that occur in problem breasts, regardless of their causes.

Before explaining the key points of breast shaping, it is important to understand the basics of normal breast anatomy. Everyone's breasts come in different shapes and sizes, so it's difficult to define exactly what constitutes the perfect breast shape. But we can still define what kinds of breasts will be considered beautiful by most people. We consider that there are several basic elements to define a beautiful breast: breast position, the ratio of the breast to trunk, beautiful contour, symmetry of shape, and volume between bilateral breasts [2]. Breasts positioned too high or too low will affect its beauty. Small-sized breasts may not be suitable for overweight women. Irregular breast shape is even more unsatisfactory. Whether the breast is beautiful varies from person to person, and affected by different races and national cultures [3]. Overall, the breast-to-trunk ratio should be appropriate, and the lateral margin of the breast should exceed the lateral contour of the trunk. The contour of the breast should naturally transition to the upper and inner side of the chest wall, while the aesthetic standard of the transition of the inframammary fold is well defined [4]. The angle of the inframammary fold should not be too sharp; otherwise, it will turn into breast ptosis. The tissue distribution of perfect breast should be mainly in the lower inner quadrant, while the distribution of tissue in the upper inner quadrant is the least [5].

Compared with breast shape, a more important cosmetic evaluation index is whether bilateral breasts are symmetrical [6]. In the process of writing all chapters of the book, we have been thinking about how to summarize and introduce the breast reconstruction and shaping methods that can be repeatedly applied in different reconstruction situations. Due to space constraints, we selected several examples and typical cases to explain the specific details of breast shaping during the operations.

T. Yano (✉)
Department of Plastic and Reconstructive Surgery, Cancer Institute Hospital, Tokyo, Japan

X. Lu
Center for Breast Cancer, Shanxi Provincial Cancer Hospital, Taiyuan, Shanxi Province, China

Y. Ding
Department of Breast Surgery, The Tumor Hospital of Shaanxi Province, Xi'an City, Shaanxi Province, China

Z. Li, D. Song (eds.), *Oncoplastic Flap Surgery*, https://doi.org/10.1007/978-981-19-8926-1_27

27.1 A Case Study of One-Stage Breast Reconstruction with DIEP Flap Transplantation

The patient, a 33-year-old female, found a right breast mass through physical examination and was diagnosed with right breast invasive ductal carcinoma by needle biopsy. She was admitted to hospital and underwent deep inferior epigastric artery perforator flap transplantation + right breast reconstruction + left breast lifting. The flap survived well after operation and was transferred to internal medicine for further comprehensive treatment. The appearance and function of the reconstructed breast were satisfactory during follow-up (Figs. 27.1, 27.2, 27.3, 27.4, 27.5, 27.6, 27.7, 27.8, 27.9, and 27.10).

Modified radical mastectomy with nipple-areola skin sparing is performed, followed by washing the wound, re-draping, and replacing the surgical instruments. The third costal cartilage of 3 cm in length is dissected, and the internal thoracic artery was fully exposed. Attention is required when exploring whether there were lymph nodes around the internal thoracic artery for pathological examination. Also surgeons need to determine whether the vascular condition is reliable, whether there is adhesion, whether the intima is sliced, and whether there are floating objects in the vascular cavity.

When the opening of the skin sack is small, the operation space for anastomosing blood vessels is accordingly small. At this time, the operative room is determined by the movable part of the skin sack. Full rotation of the flap can help to obtain the maximum operation space. Attention should be given to protect the edge of the skin sack by wrapping it with moist gauze.

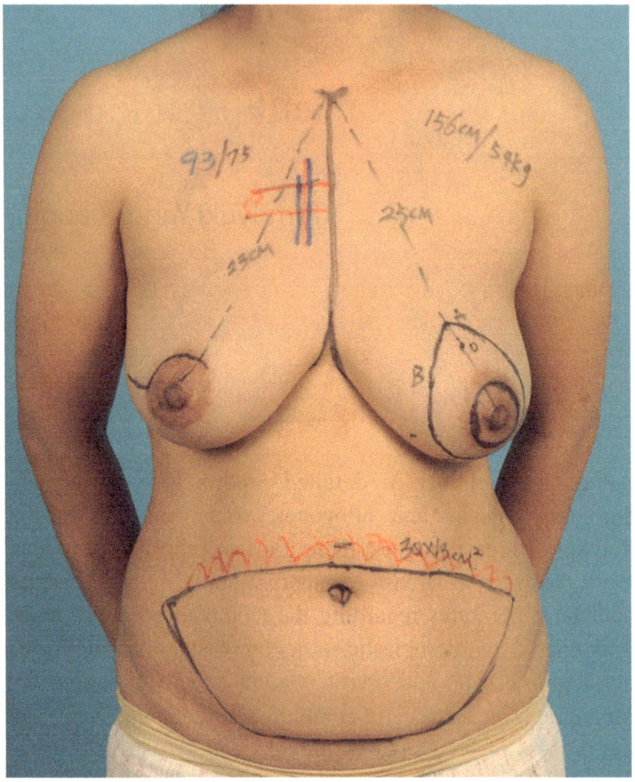

Fig. 27.1 Preoperative markings and scribing

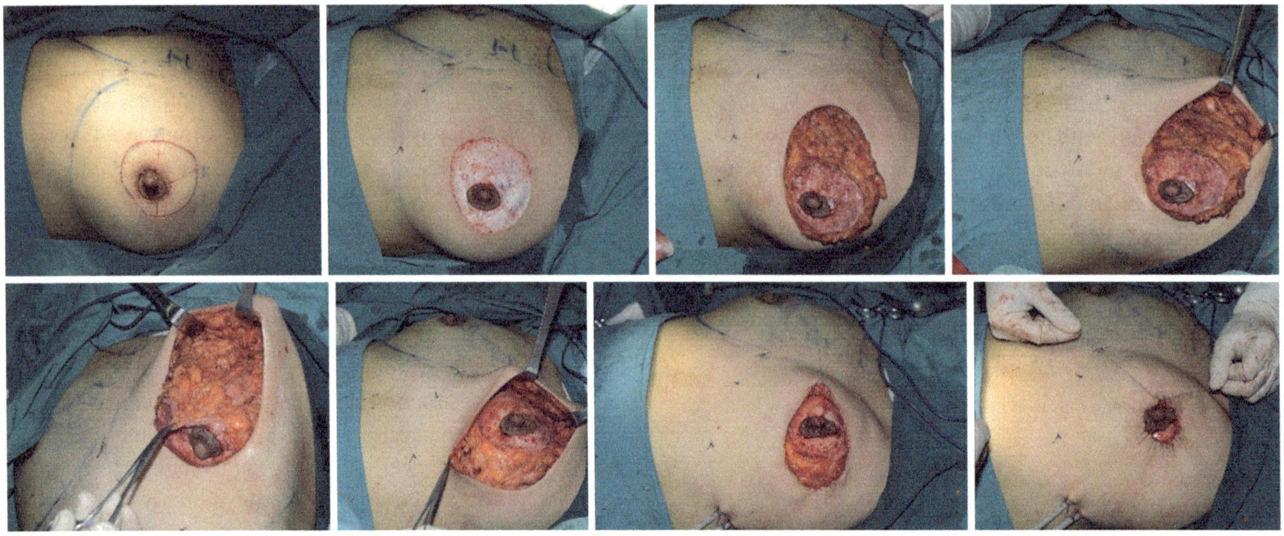

Fig. 27.2 Breast lifting on the healthy side first (we often use double-ring method)

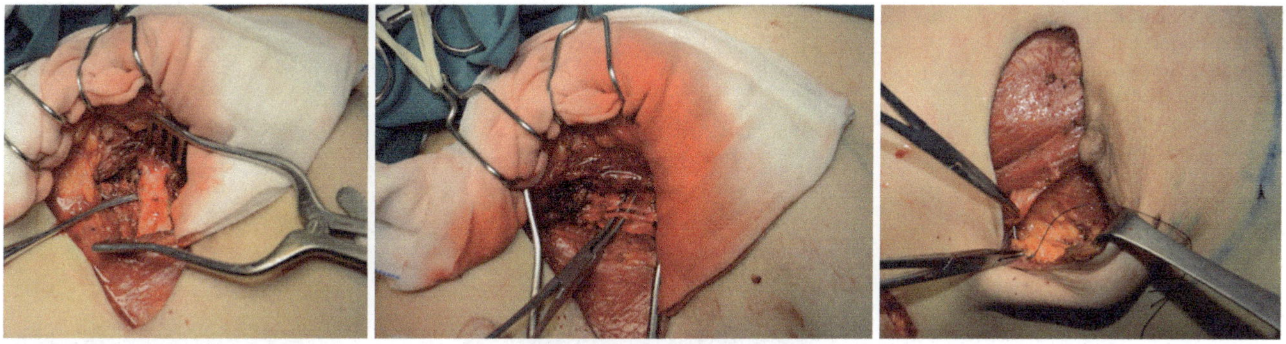

Fig. 27.3 Preparation of internal mammary vessels as recipient vessels after resection of right breast cancer lesions

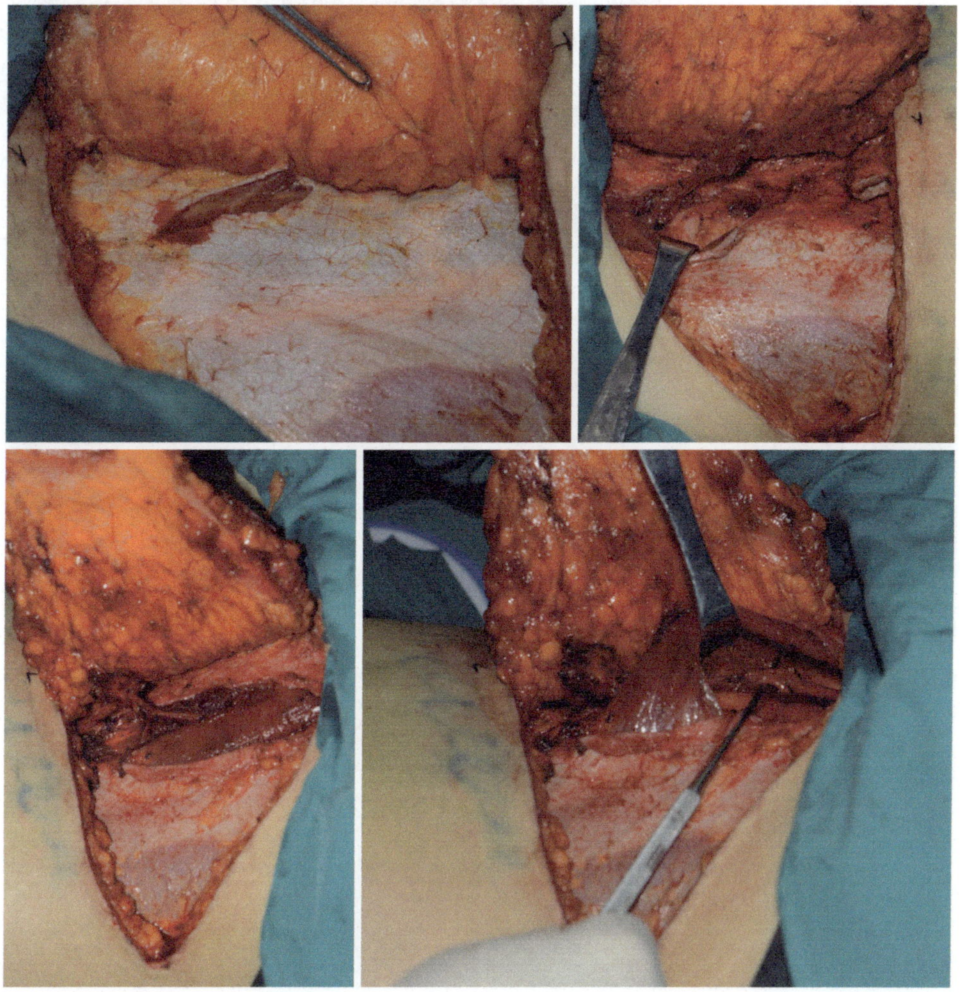

Fig. 27.4 Considering that a large breast was to be reconstructed, the deep inferior epigastric perforator flap with bilateral vascular pedicle was designed. The intramuscular courses of perforating branches of inferior abdominal vessels on both sides were different, which need to be treated in different ways. The long segment of the blood vessel under the left abdominal wall always courses in the medial area of the rectus abdominis muscle, and gradually reaches the superficial layer of the rectus abdominis muscle and sends out a thick perforator vessel. The perforator vessel does not vertically penetrate the anterior sheath into the subcutaneous tissue, but further runs for a long segment above the surface of the rectus abdominis muscle obliquely inward for a certain distance before penetrating the anterior sheath, which is very easy to be damaged. The perforating branch of the right inferior abdominal wall is a typical perforating branch of the tendinous intersection. After one side of the perforating branches and vascular pedicles are exposed in the tendinous intersection area, a part of the tendinous intersection tissue should be carried around the blood vessels to avoid injury

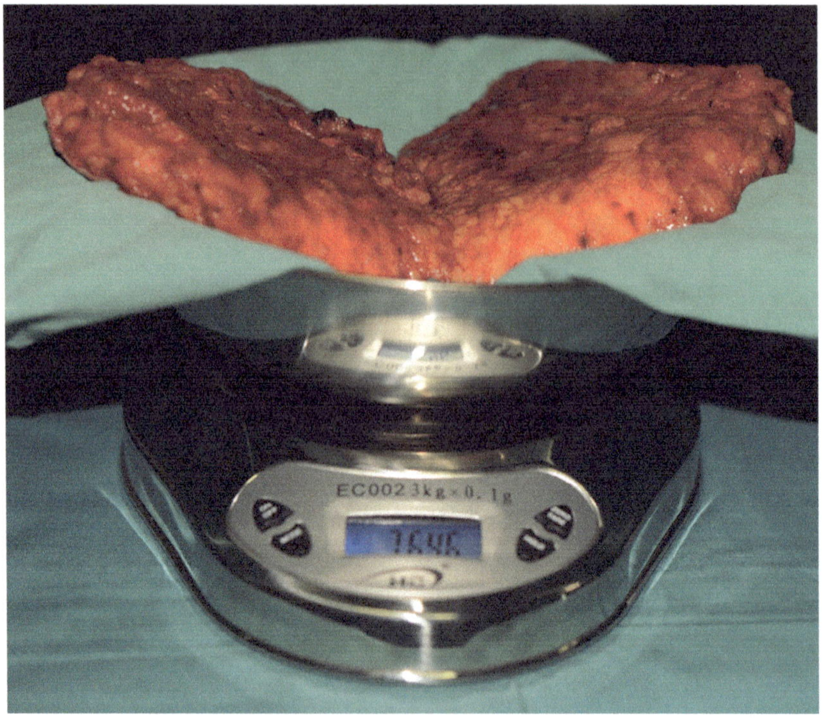

Fig. 27.5 The weighing after flap preparation and pedicle dissection. The proximal and distal part of the flap tissue was removed to make it slightly larger than the excised breast by about 10–50 g

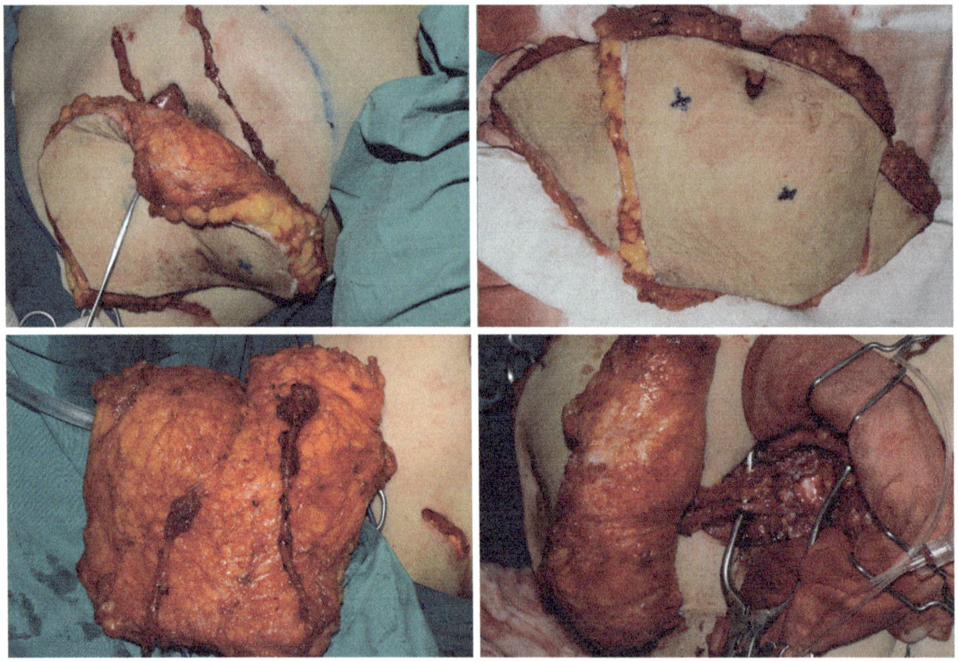

Fig. 27.6 Before transferring the perforator flap of the deep inferior epigastric artery with bilateral vascular pedicle to the recipient area, the inferior part of the skin sack of the chest must be dissociated the appropriate location of the inferior breast fold, and the position of the lateral breast fold on the outside of the skin sack shall be sutured and fixed intermittently. Also, a certain part of the flap should be resected according to the amount of tissue required by the recipient area. The position of the flap should be adjusted while considering whether the length of the vascular pedicle is sufficient. Place the vascular pedicle unaffectedly along the line to absolutely avoid torsion and compression. The vascular pedicle under the bilateral abdominal wall was anastomosed with the proximal and distal vessels in the right thorax, respectively

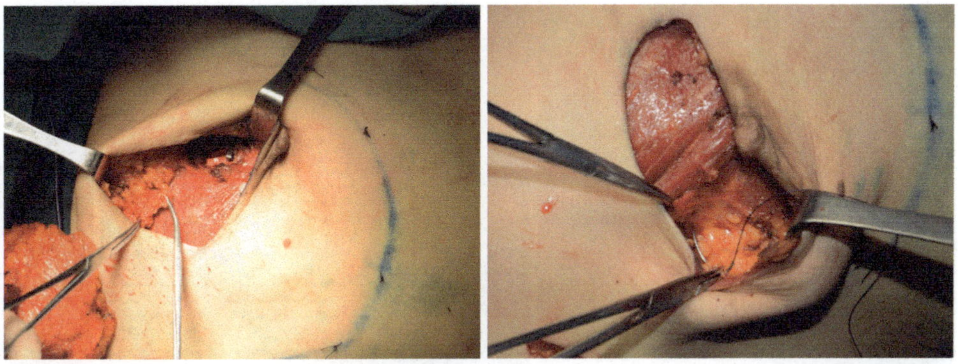

Fig. 27.7 First, dissociate the subclavian ligament for preparation, and then suture and fix the outer contour area of the breast skin sack with two sutures to avoid displacement to the lateral armpit after transferring of the skin flap

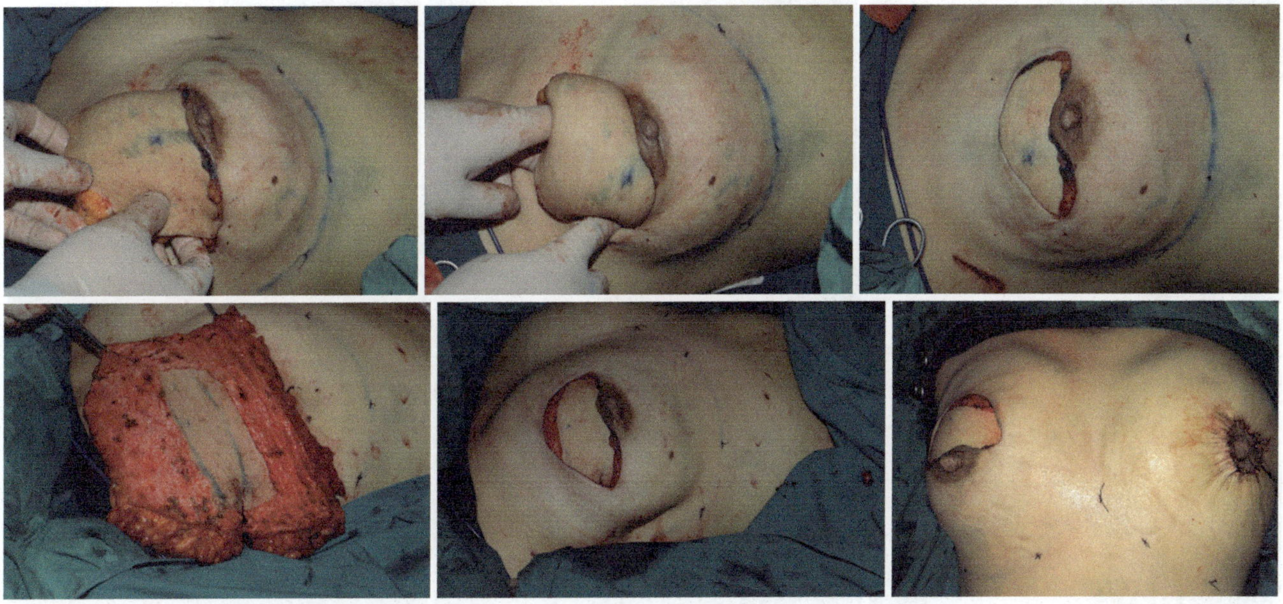

Fig. 27.8 After vascular anastomosis, monitor the blood supply of the flap, preliminarily determine the angle and placement position of the flap. Transfer the whole flap into the skin sack, and check the symmetry of bilateral breasts in seated position. Further shape the flap so as to adjust the placement position

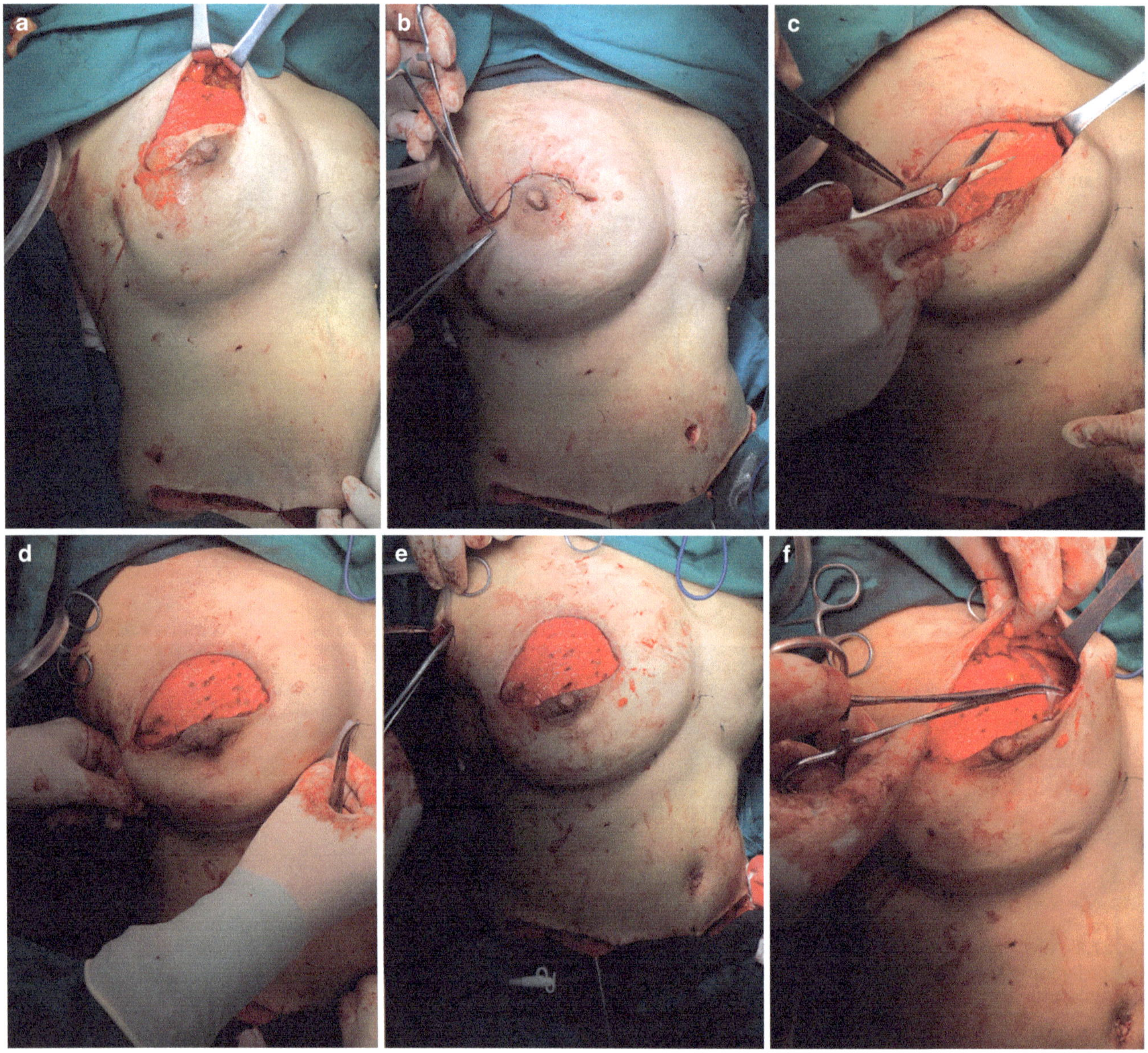

Fig. 27.9 First, the flap should be intermittently sutured and fixed with the prepared subclavian ligament, medial sternal ligament, and surrounding tissues. Otherwise, the flap will fall under the constant influence of gravity, and the subclavian ligament will naturally shrink upward, resulting in pits in the subclavian area, which would adversely affect the appearance. The subclavian area is an important detail for women's physical beauty, especially when wearing low chest or V-neck clothes. (**a**) The suture and fixation of the flap and the subclavian ligament need not be extremely tight. The subclavian ligament itself has a certain degree of movement with tough texture. Intermittent suture with one or two stitches can avoid obvious step-bunched appearance. (**b**) After observing the shape of the reconstructed flap and ensuring that the appearance and range of the lateral and inferior mammary folds are satisfactory, the skin edge of the sack is temporarily sutured and fixed to determine the shape, position, and area of the observed skin island to be retained. (**c**) Trim and remove the excess skin island, only keep the small skin island as the observation window, and use the de-epidermized lateral skin flap to fill the shape of the anterior axillary fold. (**d**) The shaping was basically completed, and the effect was satisfactory. The first drainage tube was placed at the lower edge of the flap. (**e**) The second drainage tube was placed in the axillary area. (**f**) The third drainage tube was placed on the upper space of the flap

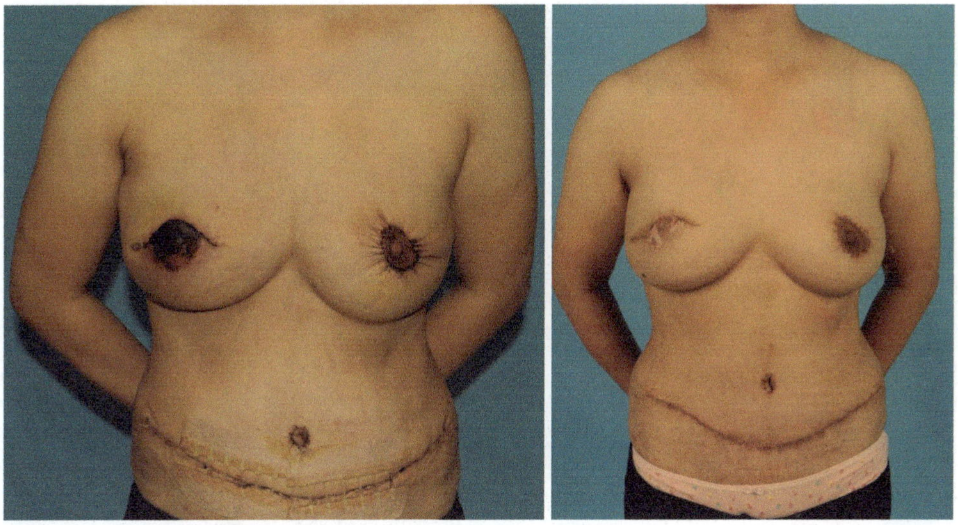

Fig. 27.10 One week after operation, the symmetry of bilateral breasts was satisfactory. The blood supply of the right nipple areola was poor, and the epidermis was necrotic. The wound healed after debridement. The appearance and function of bilateral breasts were satisfactory after 2 months of follow-up

27.2 DIEP Skin Flap Transplantation for Secondary Breast Reconstruction

The patient, a 37-year-old female, underwent modified radical mastectomy for left breast cancer in the local hospital 4 years ago. The pathological type was unknown. She was admitted to the hospital and underwent free deep inferior epigastric perforator flap transplantation + left breast reconstruction. The postoperative flap survived well, and the appearance and function of the reconstructed breast were satisfactory (Figs. 27.11 and 27.12).

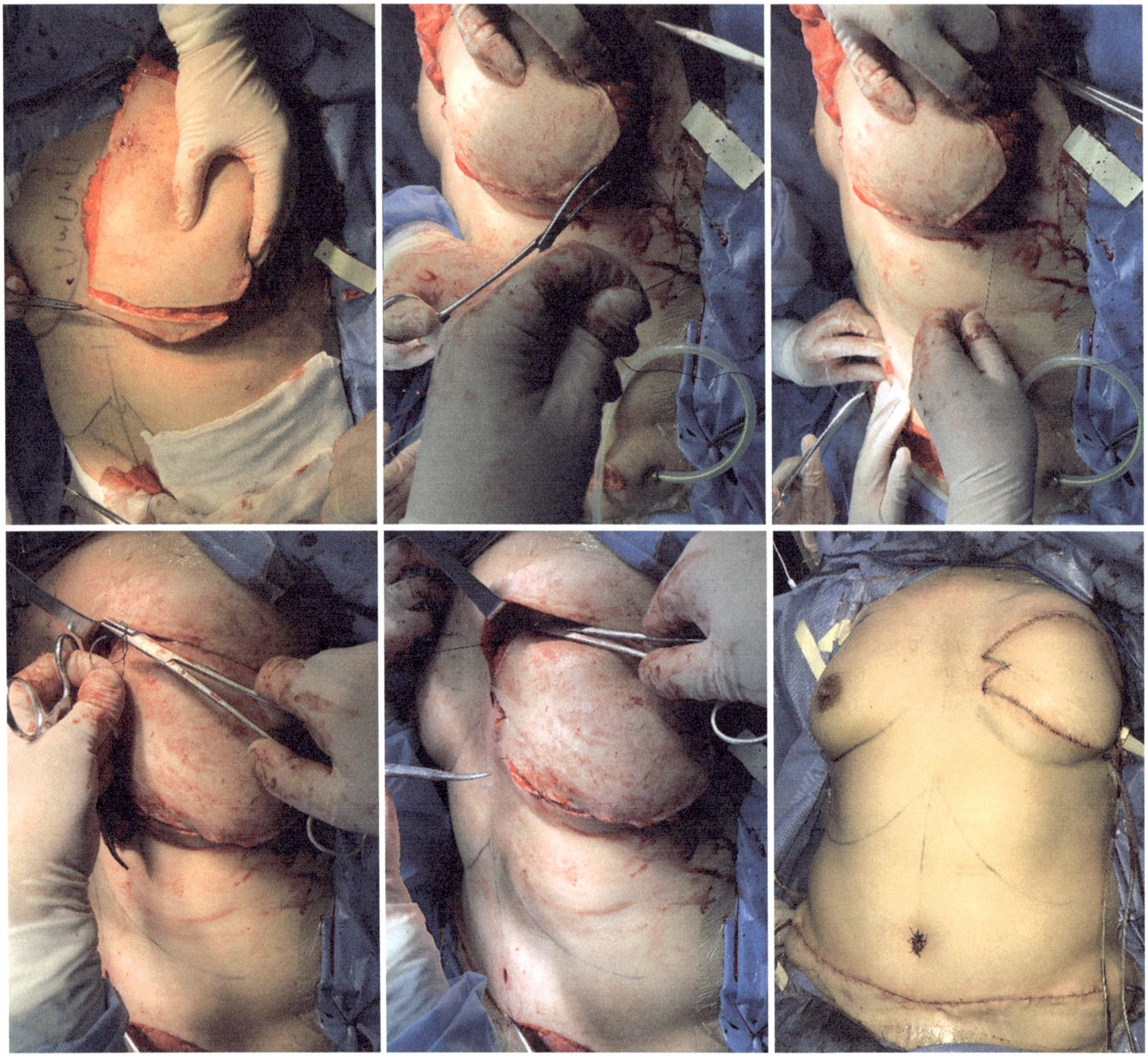

Fig. 27.11 The two-stage breast reconstruction with free skin flap transplantation is relatively difficult to shape, and the scar is more severe. Due to the large skin island required, the area for removing the skin of the flap was significantly reduced, and the shaping and fixation principle were basically the same as that of the one-stage reconstruction. However, in order to better shape the inferior mammary fold, the chest skin sack needed to be dissociated downward to the plane consistent with the contralateral inferior mammary fold. An increased amount of flap tissue was needed to reshape the sagging shape of the breast. In the medial and lateral corners of the chest, attention should be paid to applying the Z-shape modification method to avoid the occurrence of linear scar and webbed contracture

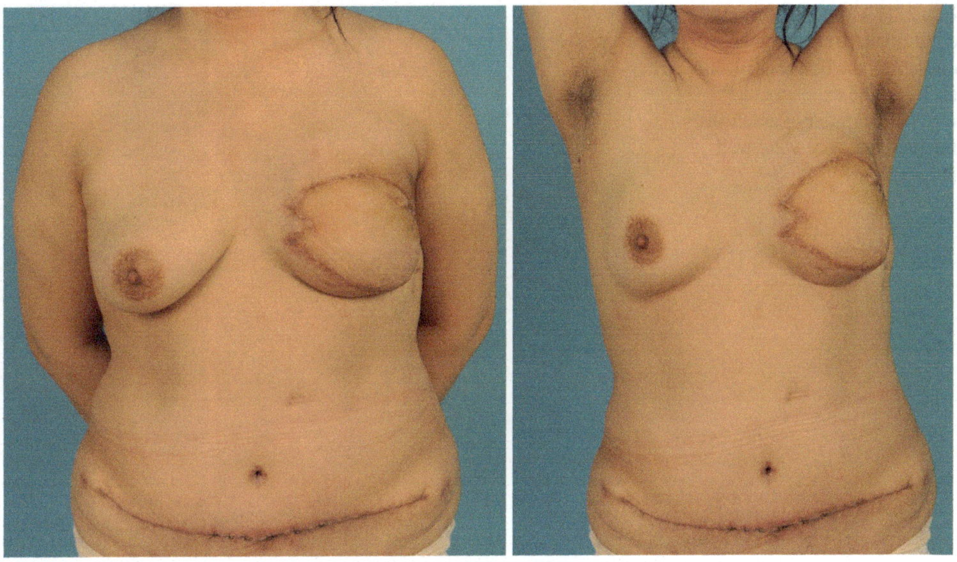

Fig. 27.12 One-month follow-up showed satisfactory appearance and function

27.3 DIEP Skin Flap Transplantation for Secondary Breast Reconstruction: A Complicated Case

The patient, a 41-year-old female, underwent modified radical mastectomy for left breast cancer in the local hospital 2 years ago. The pathological type was unknown. She was admitted to the hospital and underwent free deep inferior epigastric perforator flap transplantation + left breast reconstruction + right breast lifting. The postoperative flap survived well, and the appearance and function of the reconstructed breast were satisfactory (Figs. 27.13, 27.14, 27.15, 27.16, 27.17, and 27.18).

The skin sack cannot be formed if the longitudinal incision is taken. After the original incision, the inferior mammary fold is designed (1–2 cm higher than the contralateral side), and the skin is incised to form a triangular defect. The inferior part of the flap is trimmed into an arc-shape and sutured with the inferior skin edge of the chest wall to form a new inferior mammary fold.

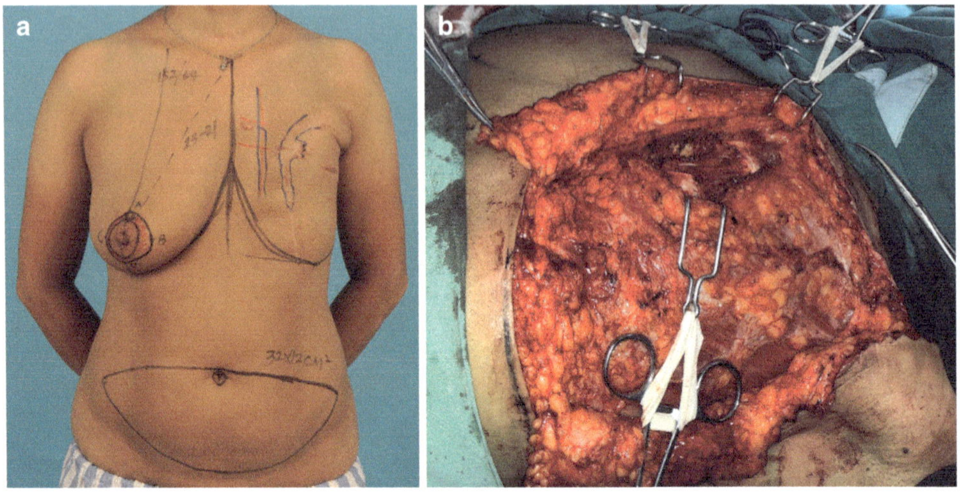

Fig. 27.13 (**a**) Preoperative conditions. (**b**) During the operation, the dissociated skin sack and the exposure of internal mammary vessels in the recipient area were well prepared

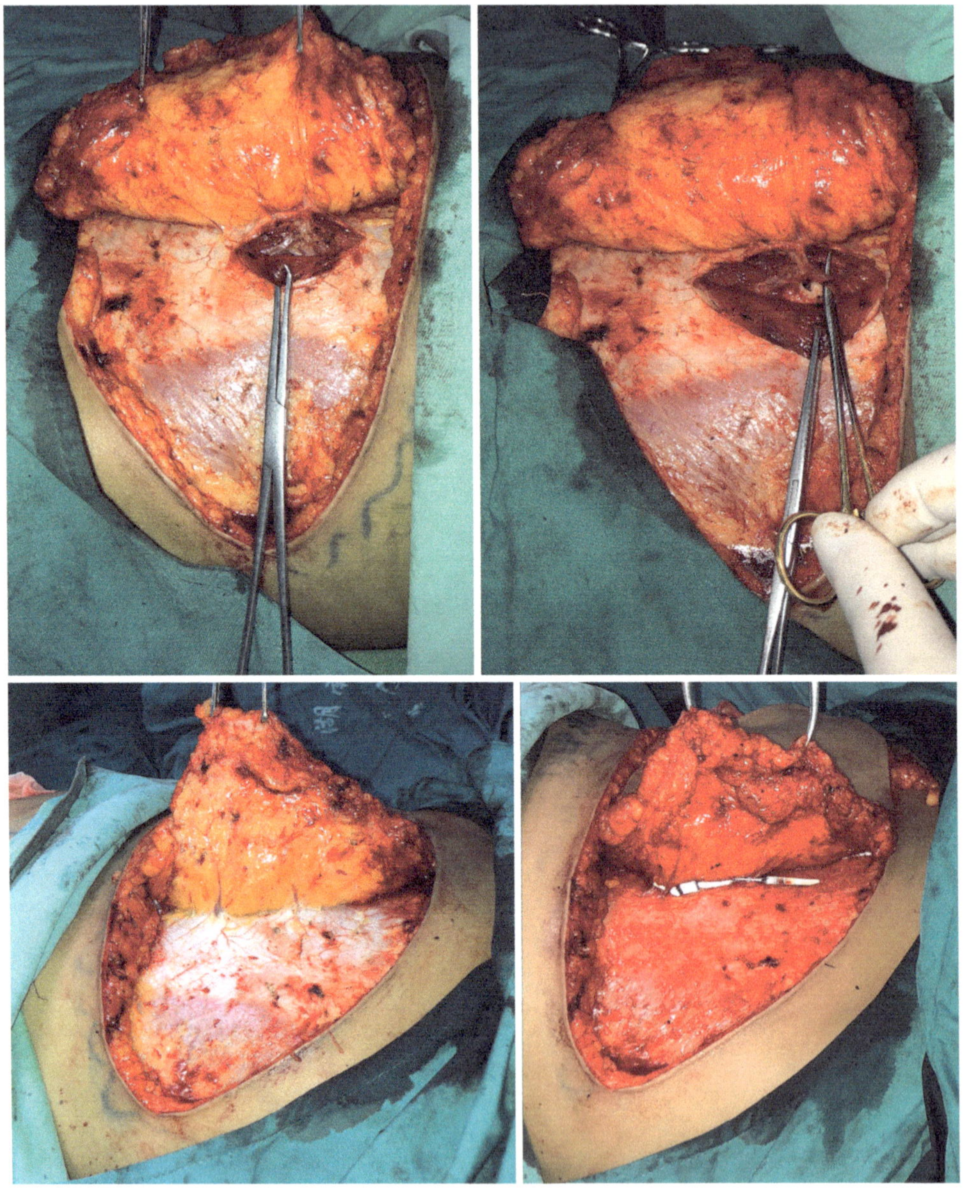

Fig. 27.14 Two perforating branches of the lateral row of the deep inferior epigastric artery were exposed in the left lower abdomen. After the separation of the perforating branches and vascular pedicle, the perforating branches of the right lower abdomen were further exposed. The clamping experiment confirmed that the blood supply of the flap was reliable and the perforating branch flap pedicled with the deep inferior epigastric artery on the left was prepared

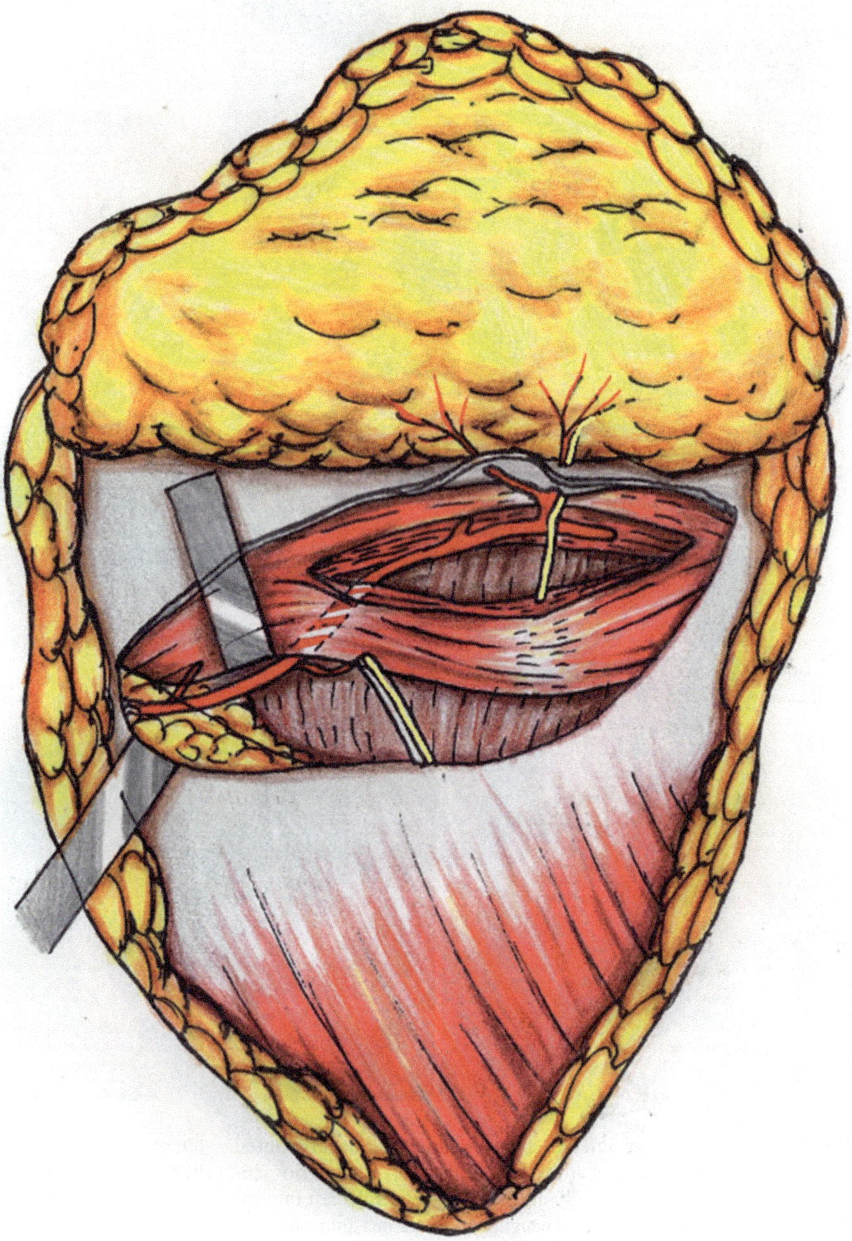

Fig. 27.15 The vascular and neural anatomy of this case provides a desired basis for the preparation of sensory deep inferior epigastric artery perforator flap

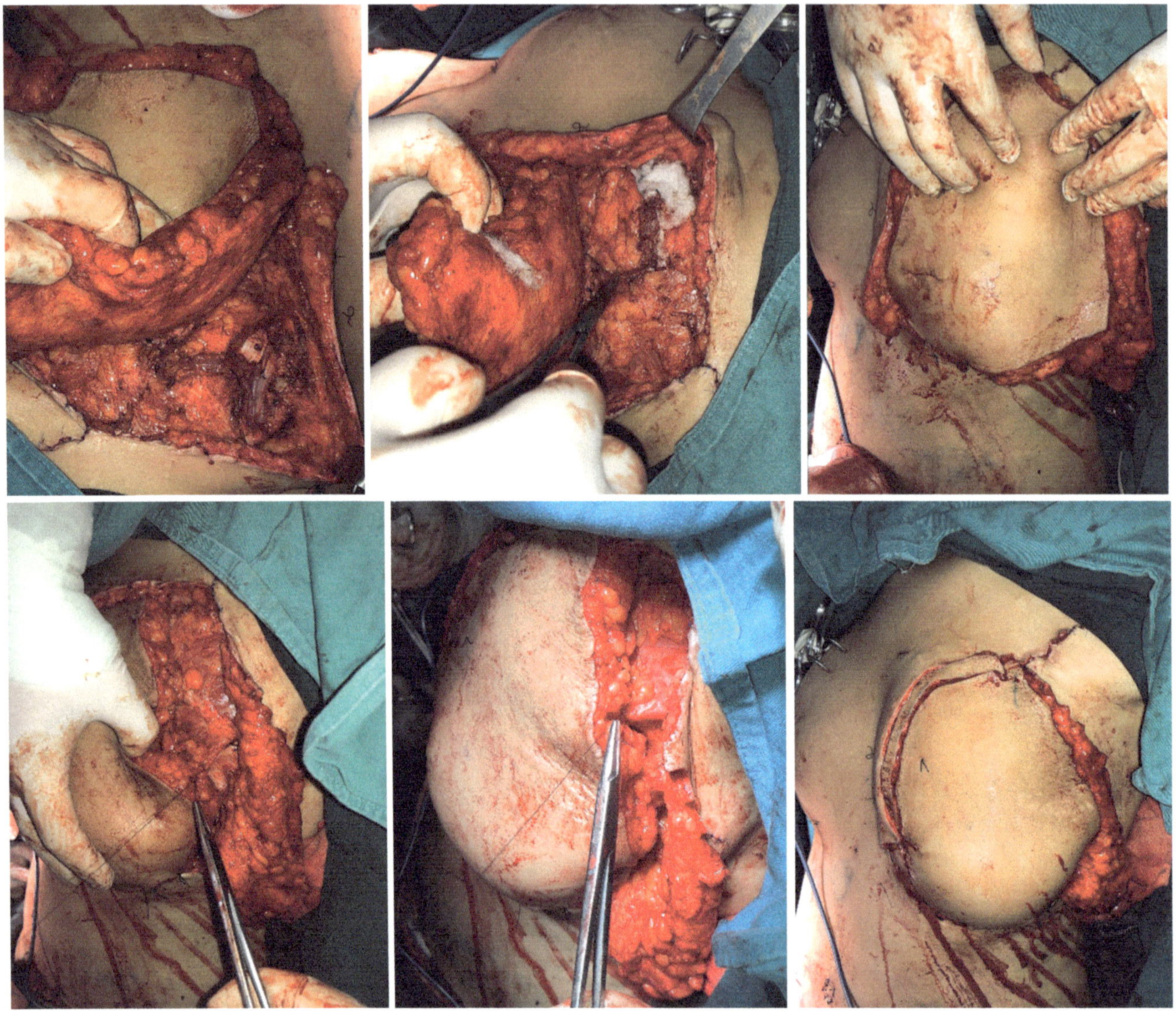

Fig. 27.16 The left deep inferior epigastric artery was anastomosed with the left internal thoracic artery (1A2V, the left deep inferior epigastric artery is anastomosed with the proximal end of the left internal thoracic artery, and the two accompanying veins are anastomosed with the proximal and distal ends of the left internal thoracic vein, respectively). After confirming that the blood supply of the flap was reliable, the flap was temporarily placed in the chest wall, and more tissue was reserved at the inferior pole of the flap to reconstruct the sagging of the breast. After determining the scope of the excess of the skin island, the flap was taken out and roughly trimmed, and then put the flap back into the skin sack. The posterior of the flap was intermittently sutured and fixed with the pectoralis major muscle and residual ligament of the breast according to the designed scope. The upper superior and inferior mammary folds were shaped, and the excessive tissue and skin were trimmed delicately

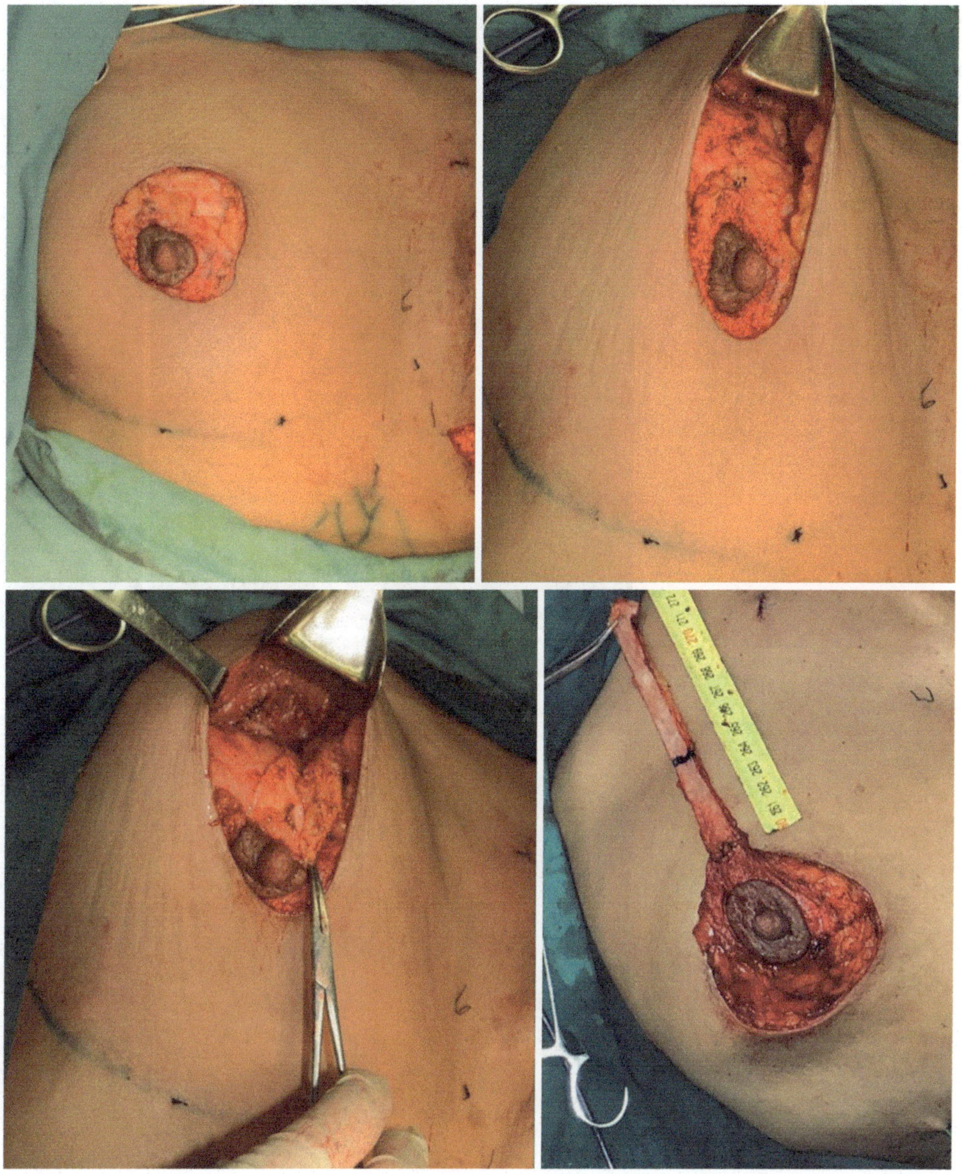

Fig. 27.17 Right breast was lifted according to the shape and size of the reconstructed left breast

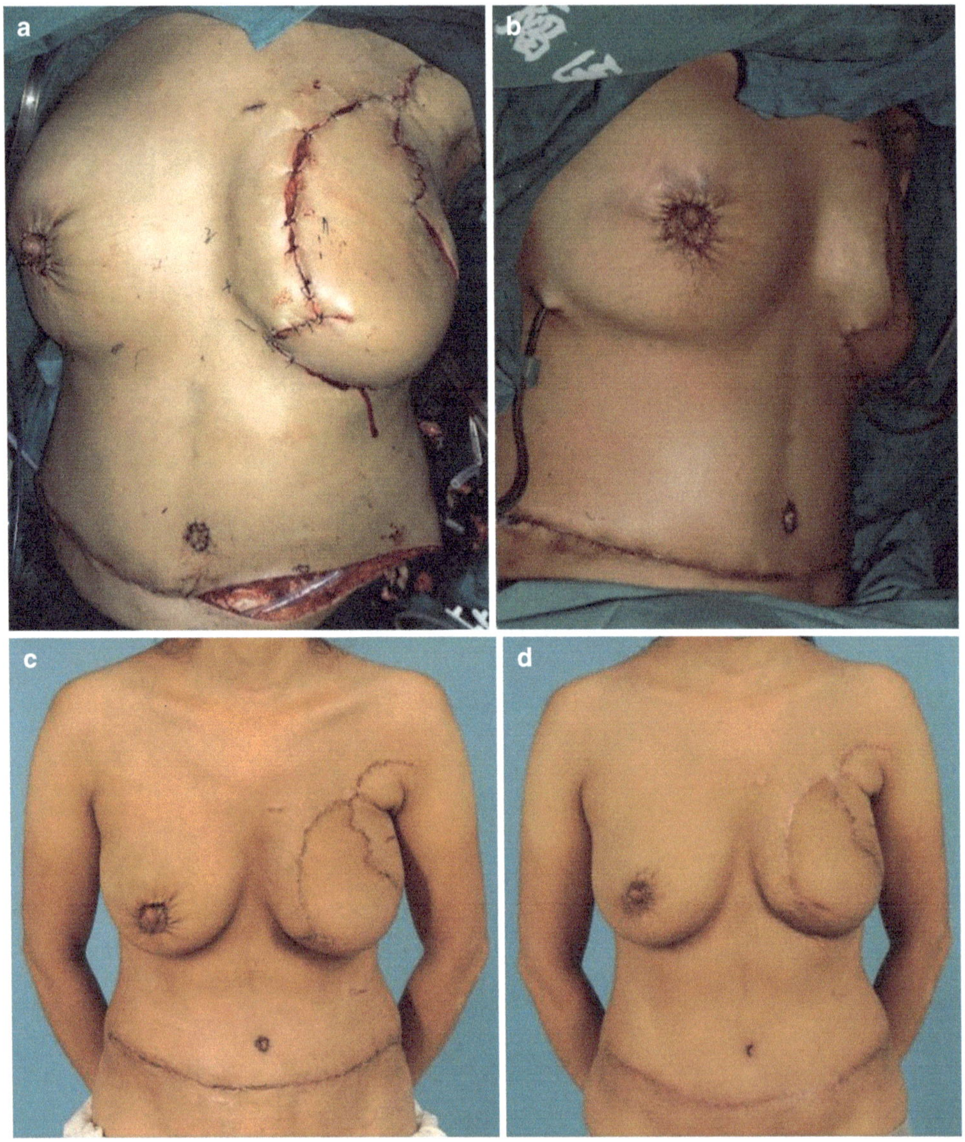

Fig. 27.18 (**a**, **b**) The intraoperative appearance of the breasts from a front and a side view. (**c**) Discharge 10 days after operation. (**d**) The appearance and function were followed up 2 months after operation

27.4 Extensive Scar Due to Chest Wall Radiotherapy Treated by Secondary Breast Reconstruction by Autologous Tissue Flap Transplantation

The patient, a 43-year-old female, underwent gland resection of right breast cancer with the nipple and areola preserved in the external hospital 8 years after radiotherapy and chemotherapy. Seven years ago, the expander was implanted subcutaneously in other hospital. Due to local infection, the expander was removed and skin necrosis occurred. After debridement and dressing change, the wound healed. After radiotherapy, the scar adhesion on the chest wall was severe, and the retained nipple was seriously displaced to the upper medial part. After the patient admitted to our hospital, the right chest wall scar was repaired under general anesthesia + breast reconstruction with free deep inferior epigastric perforator flap. After the operation, the blood supply of the flap was good, and the nipple was restored to the normal position. The appearance and function of the reconstructed breast were satisfactory, and the symmetry in terms of shape and volume was obtained between the left and right breasts. The position of the nipple-areola was satisfactory (Figs. 27.19, 27.20, 27.21, 27.22, 27.23, and 27.24).

27.4.1 Difficulties in Preoperative Evaluation

1. Extensive scar was attached to the right chest wall, and the amount of defect tissue was large.

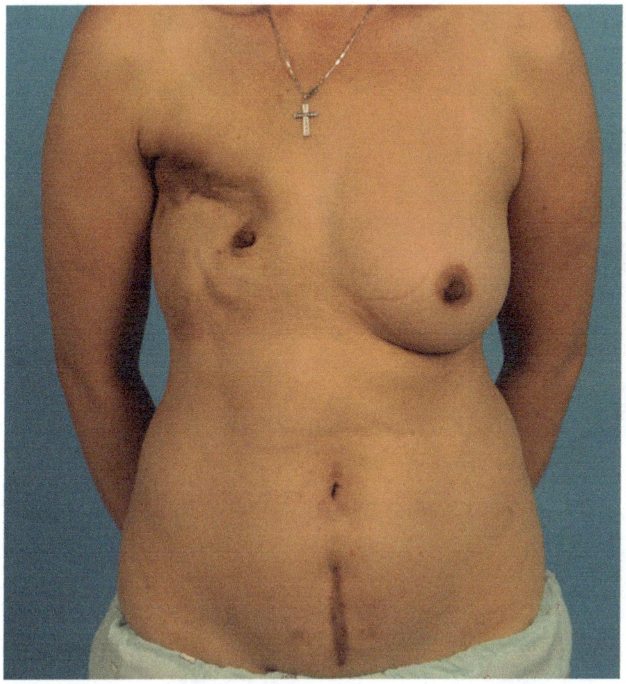

Fig. 27.19 Preoperative findings

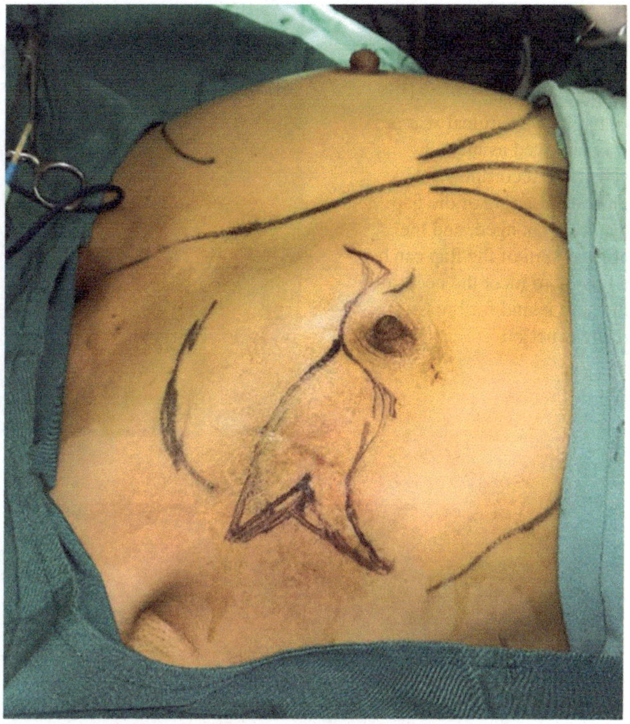

Fig. 27.20 Local flap design for removing chest wall scar before operation

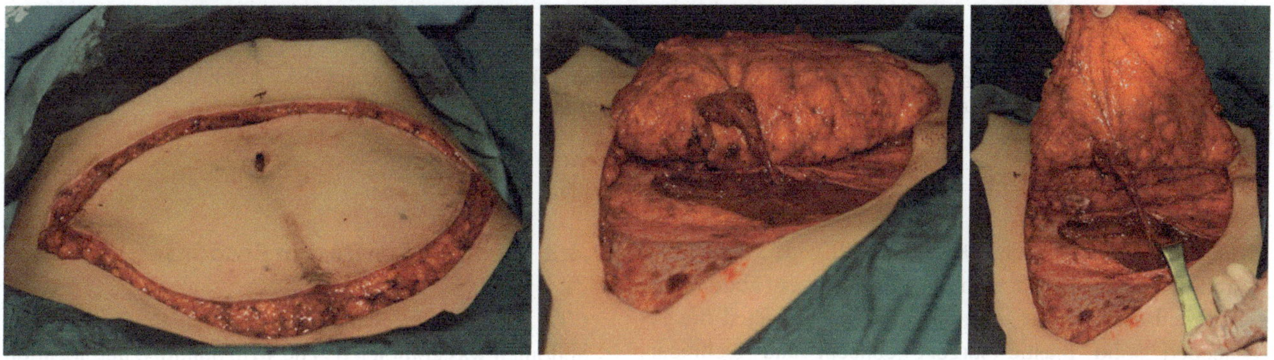

Fig. 27.21 The dissection of the deep inferior epigastric perforator flap with bilateral vascular pedicle was completed

2. After multiple radiotherapy on the right chest wall, the deep vascular injury may be extensive, and the risks for free tissue transplantation increases dramatically.
3. The patient liked sports and opposed to any method of breast reconstruction with myocutaneous flap transplantation.
4. The right chest wall had received expander implantation in the local hospital before, but postoperative infection resulted in further hyperplasia and adhesion of local tissue scars, which increased the difficulty of reoperation. The previously retained nipple-areola moves inward and upward, and patients want to retain her own nipple-areola. How to transfer the nipple-areola to the normal position while ensuring reliable blood supply was very challenging.
5. There were longitudinal cesarean section incision scars in the abdomen, which increased the difficulty and risks of operation. The patient had a strong request of transplanting the medial thigh flap to reconstruct the breast, but it belongs to two-stage breast reconstruction, which required a large amount of tissue and skin in which the medial thigh perforator flap was not suitable.
6. Patients do not want to use the lower abdominal flap carrying the existing surgical scar, but only the lower abdo-

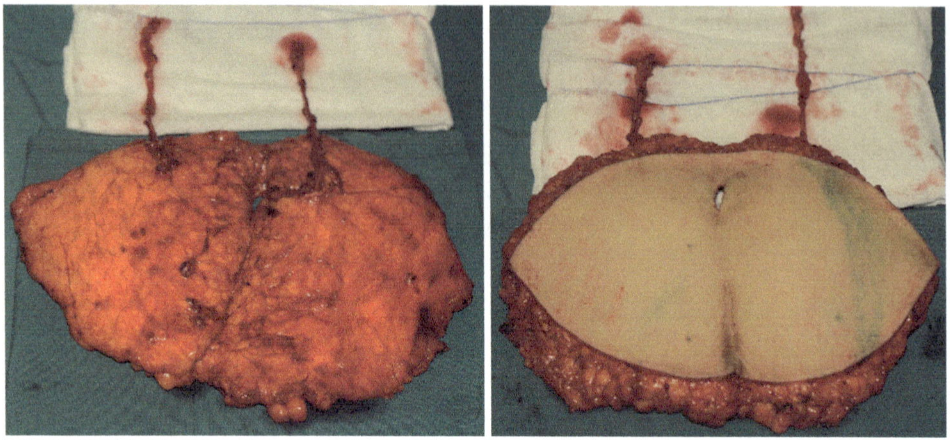

Fig. 27.22 After the dissection of the deep inferior epigastric perforator flap with bilateral pedicle, the skin island in the surgical scar area was removed as much as possible. Accordingly, the placement angle of the flap also was changed, and the normal skin of the flap can be adjusted to meet the needs of the skin island for breast reconstruction

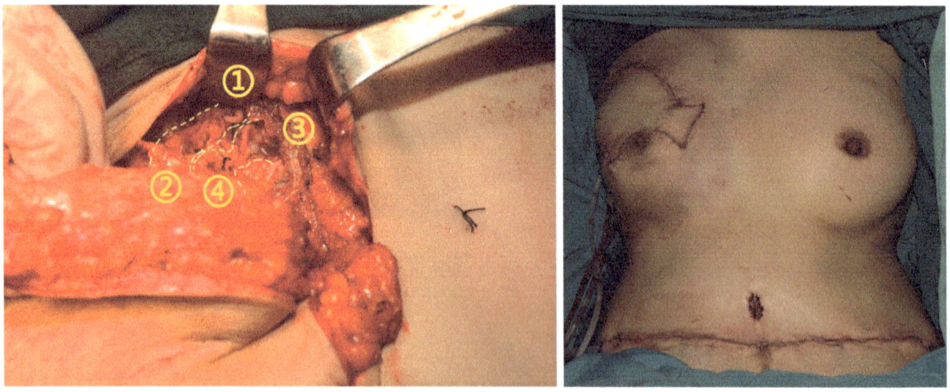

Fig. 27.23 The bilateral inferior abdominal wall arteries and veins were anastomosed with the proximal and distal parts of the right thoracic internal vessels, respectively (A: V = 1:1), and the wound margin was cosmetic sutured after placing the drainage tube. (1) Proximal end of the right internal mammary vessel. (2) Left deep inferior epigastric vessel. (3) Distal end of the right internal mammary vessel. (4) Right deep inferior epigastric vessel

men can offer the free tissue flap with wide skin island and rich tissue. How to eliminate the impact of abdominal surgical scar on the appearance of reconstructed breast needed solid plastic surgery concept and technical experience.

7. The patient hoped to retain the previously displaced nipple, which increased the difficulty of the operation. Because the local scar contracture was obvious, the blood supply disorder of the flap was likely to occur after lifting the skin sack, and the nipple areola may be necrotic. To possibly adjust and reset the position of nipple areola, an extremely precise design was required.

27.4.2 Preoperative Questions

How to ensure the blood supply of the flap when the patient has longitudinal surgical scar in the lower abdomen?

How to hide the abdominal wall scar to the greatest extent through reasonable design?

27.4.3 Preoperative Design Response

1. CTA angiography of the bilateral inner thigh and lower abdomen was completed. The size, quantity, and location of perforating vessels in the lower abdomen and bilateral inner thigh were accurately evaluated. The results showed that the perforators of multiple flap donor areas were satisfactory.
2. Patiently explain with the patient that if there was no suitable blood vessel in the recipient area, the contralateral pedicled rectus abdominis flap combined with ipsilateral free deep inferior epigastric perforator flap may be used for the right breast reconstruction;
3. After evaluating the amount of tissue and the size of skin island in the recipient area, if the medial thigh perforator flap was needed, both sides of the flap must be dissected simultaneously to meet the needs of tissue volume. The trauma was large, and the operation anesthesia time was long. The risks was also increased, so as the injury of donor area.

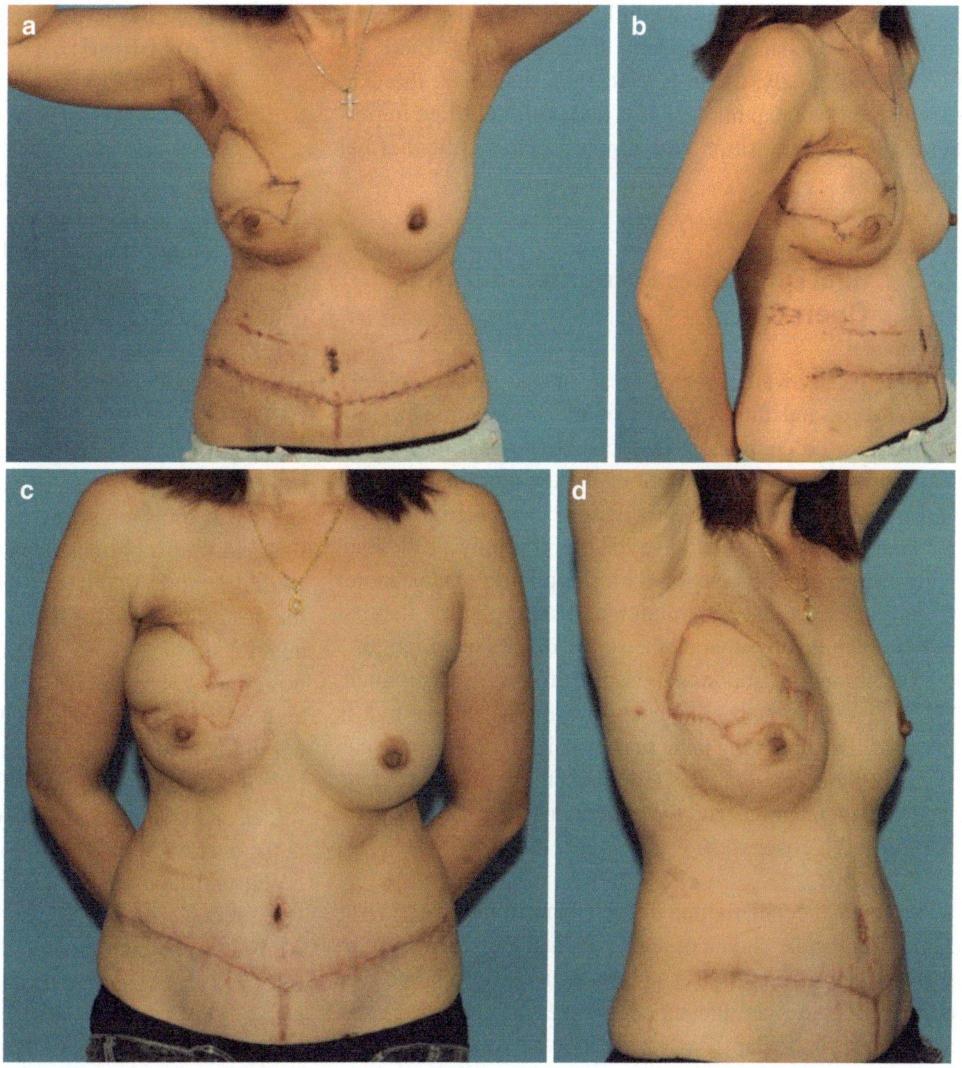

Fig. 27.24 (**a**, **b**) The patient was discharged 9 days after operation. (**c**, **d**) Three-month follow-up after operation

4. Scar excision and blood vessel preparation in the recipient area shall be carried out first, and free flap transplantation shall be carried out after confirming that the blood vessels in the receiving area were good. Even if the blood vessels in the recipient area were greatly affected by radiotherapy or infection, they shall not be abandoned easily. There were also thoracoacromial vessels and transverse cervical vessels to choose from (see the chapter on blood vessel selection in the recipient area for details).
5. The shape and design of the chest scar excision were the key point to ensure the postoperative aesthetics. After the chest wall adherent scar was completely excised by multiple Z-shaped incisions, the nipple-areola complex was located on the medial Z-shaped flap, which can not only transfer flexibly to the original position but also ensure the safety of blood supply to the greatest extent (see Fig. 27.20).
6. After determining the good condition of the blood vessels in the receiving area, the deep inferior epigastric perforator flap with the bilateral vascular pedicle was dissected and transplanted for breast reconstruction. There were two purposes: (1) The scar of the longitudinal operation of the lower abdomen may affect the blood supply of the crossing area between flaps, and a single vascular pedicle was difficult to ensure the blood supply safety of the whole lower abdominal flap. (2) After the deep inferior epigastric perforator flap with the maximum tissue volume cut from the bilateral vascular pedicle was transferred to the recipient area, the flap can be flexibly shaped to the greatest extent, and the scar skin island can be removed as much as possible. Only the subcutaneous tissue on the posterior surface of the scar skin island can be reserved for filling, and the breast appearance can be reconstructed with normal skin.

The designed incision can fully dissociate the scar and form multiple Z-shaped incisions simultaneously. There are two reasons: firstly, it can help to fully dissociate the skin sack to facilitate flap implantation and shaping. More importantly, it can reposition the nipple back to the normal location.

27.5 Real Difficulties Encountered During Operation

1. The chest wall-adherent scar must be completely removed, and the skin sack of the inframammary fold needs to be completely dissociated to reach the perfect shape of breast reconstruction, and the intraoperative use of electric knife should therefore be avoided. Thermal damage is likely to damage the blood supply of the flap. In fact, sharp dissociation with sharp knife blade can not only preserve the maximum blood supply of the flap but also completely separate the skin sack in a large range.
2. The amount of abdominal tissue of the patient is limited, and the tension by direct closure of the donor area is large. The operating table in the "knife-folding" state can reduce the tension of the donor area to the greatest extent. The patient can extend the abdomen 10 days after operation and recover well.

For breast reconstruction, the deep inferior epigastric perforator flap is the choice of most patients. However, in some patients, flaps from thighs and hips are the good choice. The common choices are the superior gluteal or inferior gluteal artery perforator flap [7, 8] and transverse gracilis muscle flap [9]. The posteromedial femoral perforator flap pedicled with profunda femoral artery is an evolutionary form of the gracilis myocutaneous flap, with less damage to the donor area, soft texture, and strong plasticity [10], but the size and distribution of all posteromedial femoral perforators must be fully understood before operation. The upper end is marked 1 cm below the gluteal sulcus. The lower mark is about 7 cm below the upper mark. The flap is designed to be oval, so the scar will not extend to the visible area outside the gluteal sulcus. The flap is usually designed horizontally, with a length of about 27 cm and a width of no more than 8 cm. The posteromedial femoral perforator flap is used to reconstruct the breast. In fact, it is not difficult to dissect the flap, but it is more difficult to shape. Firstly, it is necessary to strictly stick to the selection indications of the flap. It is only suitable for patients with small and medium breast size and those whose posteromedial femoral perforator flap is applicable. Secondly, the placement and shaping of the intraoperative skin flap are completely different from the DIEP flap.

27.6 Gracilis Myocutaneous Flap Combined with Profunda Femoral Artery Perforator Flap for Breast Reconstruction: A Typical Case

The patient was a 47-year-old female who experienced the fourth cycle of neoadjuvant chemotherapy for right breast cancer twenty days ago. Pathological diagnosis: (right breast) invasive ductal carcinoma, and histological grade II; immunohistochemistry: Er (−), PR (−), C-erbB-2 (−), p53 (+), Ki-67 (+ 70%), CK5/6 (−), p63 (−), p120catenin (membrane +), top2 (+), E-cadherin (+), AR (−), GATA-3 (+), GCDFP-15 (−), EGFR (+), CD34 (vascular +), and special staining: pas (−). After admission, breast cancer was resected, and the breast was reconstructed by modified radical mastectomy plus free profunda artery perforator (PAP) flap and thin flap transplantation. During the operation, the medial femoral flap from the inner side of the right thigh to the posterior gluteal sulcus was designed to be dissected for about 33 cm × 7 cm in size, and the perforating vessels from transverse upper gracilis (TUG) and PAP flaps were sutured end-to-end with the proximal and distal ends with the internal thoracic arteries and veins, respectively. The blood supply of the flap was good after anastomosis. The flap was folded and assembled, and two triangular flaps were designed at the overlap of the flap to form a new nipple. A piece of the costal cartilage was placed under the new nipple for two-stage reconstruction, which was fixed with silk thread and adjusted to be consistent with the opposite side. After shaping, a symmetrical outlook was reached between both breasts. The excess of the skin was removed, and the wound was sutured in layers. Three negative-pressure drainage tubes was placed in the operative cavity. Hemostasis at the root of the right thigh was complete, followed by direct closure and indwelling of two negative-pressure drainage tubes. Postoperative pathological examination report: (1) (right breast) the residual breast showed hyperplasia and pathological changes, with chronic inflammatory cell infiltration in the area and tumor thrombus formation in the vessel. There was no clear residual cancer nest, which was consistent with the postoperative changes. (2) Adenocarcinoma metastasis was found in 1/16 of the lymph nodes (right axillary), and no cancer metastasis was found in two lymph nodes in group 3. (3) No cancer invasion was found in the skin, basal margin, nipple area, and intermuscular tubercle. Further comprehensive treatment progressed smoothly. The function and appearance of the reconstructed breast were satisfactory, and only one linear scar was left in the donor area (Figs. 27.25, 27.26, 27.27, 27.28, 27.29, 27.30, 27.31, and 27.32).

The profunda artery perforator flap is characterized by constant anatomy, strong tissue plasticity, and soft texture. It

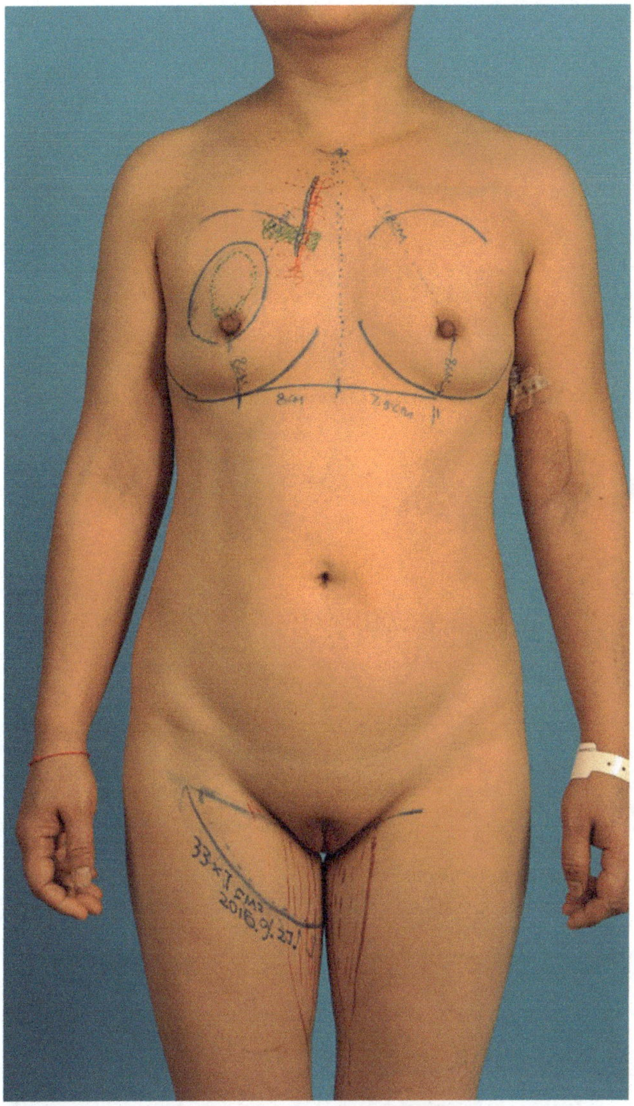

Fig. 27.25 Preoperative condition and design preparation

is especially suitable for patients who are unwilling or inappropriate to use abdominal flap. Moreover, the donor area is relatively hidden and easy for patients to accept. The main factor limiting its application is that the width of skin island cannot exceed 8 cm. Therefore, when using profunda artery perforator flap for breast reconstruction, a long skin island and U-shape design are needed to make up for its insufficient width. When dissecting the flap, carrying as much surrounding subcutaneous tissue as possible would facilitate the satisfactory shaping of the reconstructed breast.

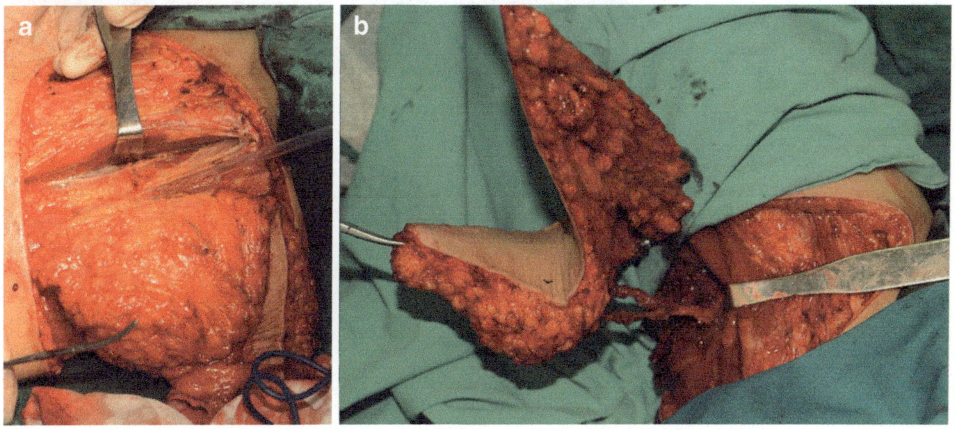

Fig. 27.26 Design of the gracilis myocutaneous flap combined with the adductor major perforator flap

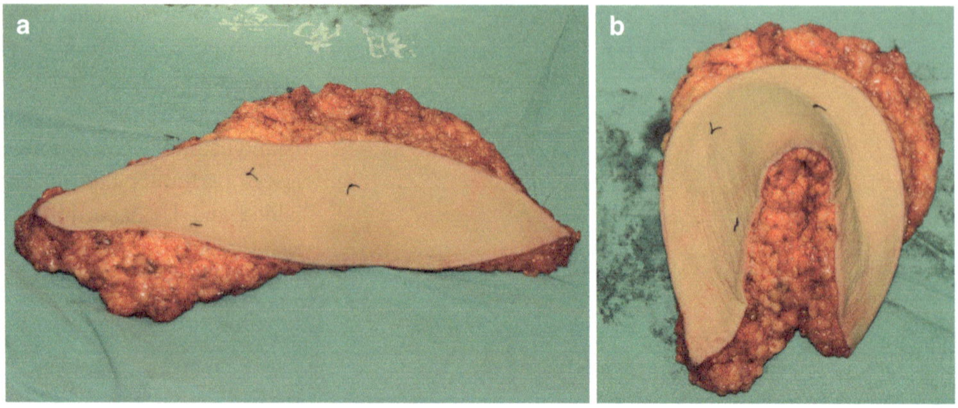

Fig. 27.27 The flap was dissected and further shaped

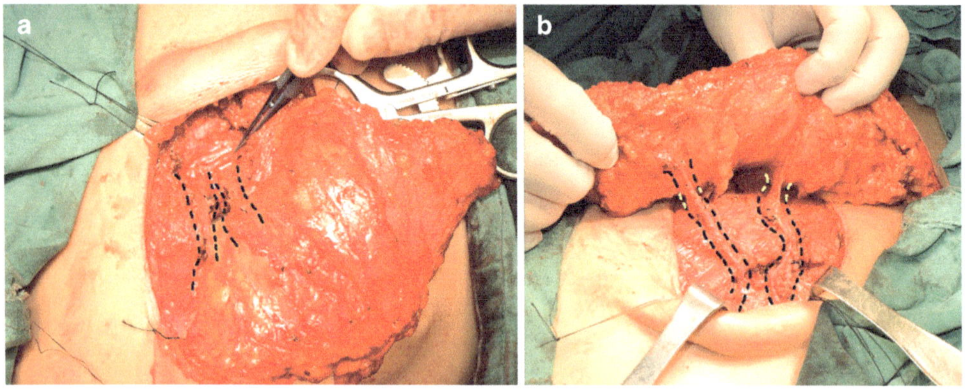

Fig. 27.28 Bilateral vascular pedicle anastomoses with proximal and distal thoracic vessels, respectively

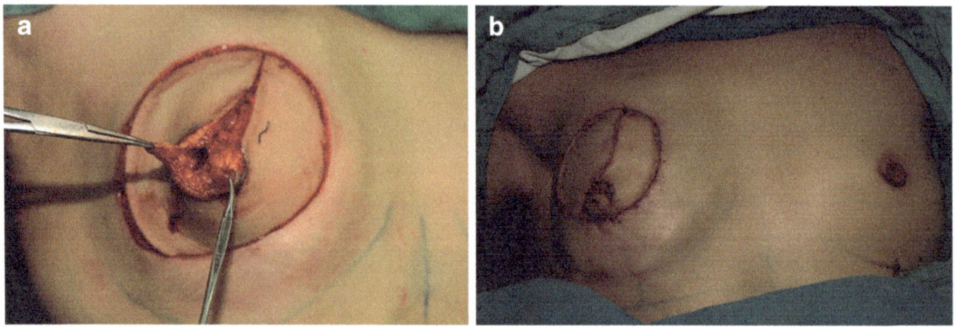

Fig. 27.29 One-stage skin flap shaping and nipple reconstruction

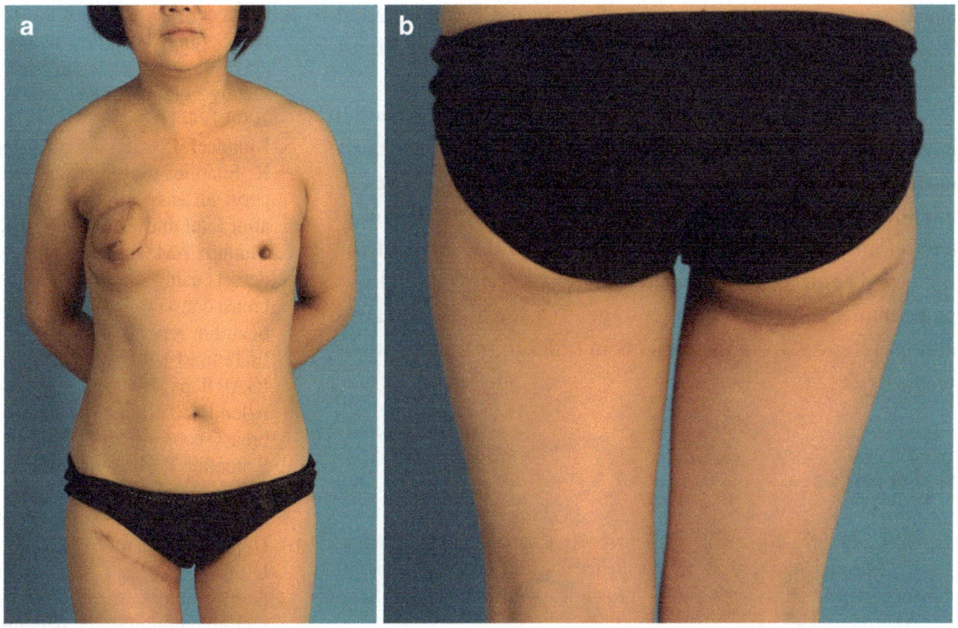

Fig. 27.30 Six-month follow-up after operation

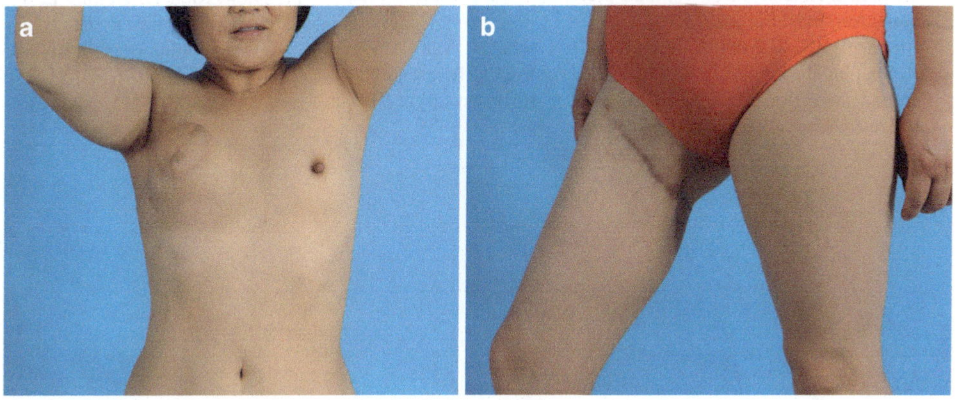

Fig. 27.31 Twelve-month follow-up after operation

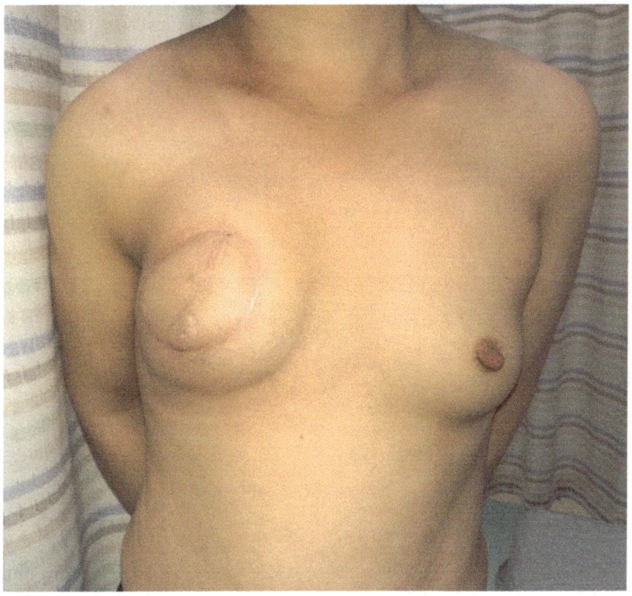

Fig. 27.32 Eighteen-month follow-up

27.7 Conclusion

The oval-shaped design can be made into a cone to provide an ideal shape for the breast. Unlike the hip flap, the posterior medial femoral perforator flap does not affect the hip contour. The plasticity of the posterior thigh tissue is better than that of the abdomen and hips, which affords the reconstructed breast a better three-dimensional shape. Although the ranges of height and weight of patients is less restricted, we routinely dissect flaps that are proportional to the tissue volume removed by mastectomy so as to match the defects. The shaping characteristics are different from those of DIEP flap transplantation. The vascular pedicle is relatively short compared with DIEP flap, but the crimp and conical design can compensate the lack of vascular pedicle length to the greatest extent. Through careful preoperative design, separation, carrying subcutaneous tissue exceeding the range of the skin island when dissecting the flap, and timely adjustment of the angle and position during shaping, the posteromedial femoral perforator flap can reconstruct a satisfactory breast shape.

At present, there are more advanced three-dimensional imaging with preoperative analysis in order to reconstruct a more beautiful and satisfactory breast [11]. However, whether the breast is beautiful always varies from person to person and affected by the changes due to the trend of the times and cultural habits and are different among nationalities and countries. We should never forget to listen to the demands and preferences from the patients in order to truly meet their wishes.

References

1. Blondeel PN, Hijjawi J, Depypere H, Roche N, Van Landuyt K. Shaping the breast in aesthetic and reconstructive breast surgery: an easy three-step principle. Plast Reconstr Surg. 2009;123(2):455–62.
2. Gill K, Mann R, Brunsworth L, Newman M. Aesthetic subunit of the breast: an analysis of women's preference and clinical implications. Ann Plast Surg. 2014;73(2):249.
3. Blondeel PN, Hijjawi J, Depypere H, Roche N, Van Landuyt K. Shaping the breast in aesthetic and reconstructive breast surgery: an easy three-step principle. Part IV—aesthetic breast surgery. Plast Reconstr Surg. 2009;124(2):372–82.
4. Blondeel PN, Hijjawi J, Depypere H, Roche N, Van Landuyt K. Shaping the breast in aesthetic and reconstructive breast surgery: an easy three-step principle. Part III—reconstruction following breast conservative treatment. Plast Reconstr Surg. 2009;124(1):28–38.
5. Blondeel PN, Hijjawi J, Depypere H, Roche N, Van Landuyt K. Shaping the breast in aesthetic and reconstructive breast surgery: an easy three-step principle. Part II—breast reconstruction after total mastectomy. Plast Reconstr Surg. 2009;123(3):794–805.
6. Munhoz AM. Practical guidelines for repair of partial mastectomy defects using the breast reduction technique in patients undergoing breast conservation therapy. Plast Reconstr Surg. 2008;122(2):675–6; author reply 676–7.
7. LoTempio MM, Allen RJ. Breast reconstruction with SGAP and IGAP flaps. Plast Reconstr Surg. 2010;126(2):393–401.
8. Allen RJ, Tucker C. Superior gluteal artery perforator free flap for breast reconstruction. Plast Reconstr Surg. 1995;95(7):1207–12.
9. Schoeller T, Huemer GM, Wechselberger G. The transverse musculocutaneous gracilis flap for breast reconstruction: guidelines for flap and patient selection. Plast Reconstr Surg. 2008;122(1):29–38.
10. Hupkens P, Hameeteman M, Westland PB, Slater NJ, Vasilic D, Ulrich DJ. Breast reconstruction using the geometrically modified profunda artery perforator flap from the posteromedial thigh region: combining the benefits of its predecessors. Ann Plast Surg. 2016;77(4):438–44.
11. Dionyssiou D, Demiri E, Tsimponis A, Boorman J. Predesigned breast shaping assisted by multidetector-row computed tomographic angiography in autologous breast reconstruction. Plast Reconstr Surg. 2014;133(2):100–8e.

GPSR Compliance

The European Union's (EU) General Product Safety Regulation (GPSR) is a set of rules that requires consumer products to be safe and our obligations to ensure this.

If you have any concerns about our products, you can contact us on ProductSafety@springernature.com

In case Publisher is established outside the EU, the EU authorized representative is:

Springer Nature Customer Service Center GmbH
Europaplatz 3
69115 Heidelberg, Germany

Batch number: 10808278

Printed by Printforce, the Netherlands